Clinical Electromyography

Second Edition

Clinical Electromyography

Second Edition

Edited by

WILLIAM F. BROWN, M.D., F.R.C.P.(C)

Professor of Neurology and Head of Neuromuscular
Unit, Department of Neurology, New England Medical
Center, Boston, Massachusetts; Professor, Faculty of
Kinesiology, University of Western Ontario, London,
Ontario

CHARLES F. BOLTON, M.D., C.M., F.R.C.P.(C)

Professor of Neurology, Department of Clinical
Neurological Sciences, University of Western Ontario;
Director, EMG Laboratory, and Consultant Neurologist,
Victoria Hospital, London

With 29 Contributing Authors

Butterworth-Heinemann
Boston   London   Oxford   Singapore   Sydney   Toronto   Wellington

Recognizing the importance of preserving what has been written, it is the policy of Butterworth-Heinemann to have the books it publishes printed on acid-free paper, and we exert our best efforts to that end.

Library of Congress Cataloging-in-Publication Data
Clinical electromyography / edited by William F. Brown, Charles F. Bolton; with 29 contributing authors.——2nd ed.
    p. cm.
   Includes bibliographical references and index.
   ISBN 0-7506-9204-9
   1. Electromyography. 2. Nervous system—Diseases—Diagnosis.
3. Nerves, Peripheral—Diseases—Diagnosis. I. Brown, William F.
(William Frederick), 1939- . II. Bolton, Charles Francis, 1932-.
[DNLM: 1. Electromyography. WE 500 C641]
RC77.5.C54 1993
616.8'047547—dc20
DNLM/DLC
for Library of Congress   92-49042
                                   CIP

British Library Cataloguing-in-Publication Data. A catalogue record for this book is available from the British Library.

Butterworth-Heinemann
313 Washington Street
Newton, MA 02158-1626

10 9 8 7 6 5 4 3

Printed in the United States of America

Contents

Contributing Authors

Michael J. Aminoff, M.D., F.R.C.P.
Professor of Neurology, University of California, Director, Clinical Neurophysiology Laboratories, University of California Medical Center, San Francisco, California

Henry Berry, M.D., D.Psych., M.R.C.P. (Lond.), F.R.C.P.(C)
Associate Professor, Faculty of Medicine (Neurology), University of Toronto; Director, Department of Neurophysiology, St. Michael's Hospital, Toronto, Ontario, Canada

Giorgio Cruccu, M.D.
Assistant Professor of Neurology, Department of Neurosciences, University of Rome, "La Sapienza," Rome, Italy

Andrew A. Eisen, M.D., F.R.C.P.(C)
Professor of Neurology, University of British Columbia; Head, Neuromuscular Disease Unit, Vancouver General Hospital, Vancouver, British Columbia, Canada

José M. Fernández, M.D.
Consultant, Department of Clinical Neurophysiology, University Hospital Vall D'Hebron, Barcelona, Spain

Morris A. Fisher, M.D.
Professor, Department of Neurology, Loyola University Stritch School of Medicine, Maywood, Illinois; Attending Physician, Hines Veterans Administration Hospital and Loyola University Medical Center, Hines and Maywood, Illinois

Charles K. Jablecki, M.D.
Associate Clinical Professor, Department of Neurosciences, University of California, San Diego, San Diego, California

H. Royden Jones, Jr., M.D.
Associate Clinical Professor, Department of Neurology, Harvard University; Director, EMG Lab, Neurology, Children's Hospital Medical Center, Boston, Massachusetts; Chairman, Neurology, Lahey Clinic Medical Center, Burlington, Massachusetts

John J. Kelly, Jr., M.D.
Professor and Chairman, Department of Neurology, George Washington University Medical Center, Washington, D.C.

Mikihiro Kihara, M.D.
Assistant Professor, Department of Neurology, MAYO Medical School; Assistant Professor, Department of Neurology, MAYO Clinic, Rochester, Minnesota

Jun Kimura, M.D.
Professor and Chairman, Department of Neurology, University of Kyoto School of Medicine; Director, Department of Neurology, Kyoto University Hospitals, Kyoto, Japan

Tetsuo Komori, M.D.
Professor of Neurology, Tokyo Metropolitan Neurological Hospital, Tokyo, Japan

Kerry H. Levin, M.D.
Department of Neurology, Cleveland Clinic Foundation, Cleveland, Ohio

Alan J. McComas, F.R.C.P.(C)
Professor of Medicine and Neurosciences, Faculty of Health Sciences, McMaster University, Hamilton, Ontario, Canada

Robert G. Miller, M.D.
Clinical Professor of Neurology, University of California San Francisco Medical Center; Chairman, Department of Neurology, California Pacific Medical Center, San Francisco, California

Viggo Kamp Nielsen, Dr. Med.
Associate Professor, Department of Neurology, University of Aarhus; Chairman, Department of Clinical Neurophysiology, University Hospital of Aarhus, Aarhus, Denmark

José Ochoa, M.D., D.Sc.
Professor of Neurology and Neurosurgery, Department of Neurology and Neurosurgery, Oregon Health Sciences University; Director of Neuromuscular Disease Unit, Department of Neurology, Good Samaritan Hospital–Medical Center, Portland, Oregon

Bram W. Ongerboer de Visser, M.D.
Professor and Chairman of Clinical Neurophysiology, Academic Medical Center, University of Amsterdam, Amsterdam, The Netherlands

Jack H. Petajan, M.D., Ph.D.
Professor of Neurology, University of Utah School of Medicine; University of Utah Medical Center, Salt Lake City, Utah

David C. Preston, M.D.
Instructor, Department of Neurology, Harvard Medical School; Director of Neuromuscular Service, Department of Neurology, Brigham and Women's Hospital, Boston, Massachusetts

Michael H. Rivner, M.D.
Associate Professor of Neurology, Department of Neurology, Medical College of Georgia; Associate Professor and Director, EMG Laboratory, Department of Neurology, Medical College of Georgia, Augusta, Georgia

Mark Sivak, M.D.
Assistant Professor, Department of Neurology, Mt. Sinai School of Medicine; Director of ALS and Myasthenia Gravis Clinics, Department of Neurology, Mt. Sinai Medical Center, New York, New York

John D. Stewart, M.B.B.S., M.R.C.P., F.R.C.P.(C)
Associate Professor, Department of Neurology and Neurosurgery, McGill University; Neurologist, Department of Neurology, Montreal Neurological Institute, Montreal, Quebec, Canada

Thomas R. Swift, M.D.
Professor and Chairman of Neurology, Department of Neurology, Medical College of Georgia, Augusta, Georgia

P. K. Thomas, C.B.E., M.D., D.Sc.
Emeritus Professor of Neurological Science, Royal Free Hospital School of Medicine and Institute of Neurology, London, England

Asa J. Wilbourn, M.D.
Director, EMG Laboratory, Department of Neurology, The Cleveland Clinic Foundation; Associate Professor of Neurology, Case-Western Reserve University, School of Medicine, Cleveland, Ohio

Douglas W. Zochodne, M.D., F.R.C.P.(C)
Assistant Professor, Department of Clinical Neurosciences, University of Calgary; Neurologist, Department of Clinical Neurosciences, Foothills Hospital, Calgary, Alberta, Canada

Preface

The neurophysiological examination is but an extension of the neurological and neuromuscular examinations. Clinical neurophysiologists must have a comprehensive and thorough knowledge of neuromuscular diseases. Each patient must be examined before any neurophysiological testing to localize the lesion(s) properly, establish a working diagnosis and differential diagnosis, and map a plan for the most appropriate electrophysiological testing to help further localize the lesion(s) and characterize any pathophysiological abnormalities.

It was the editors' original intention to discuss electromyography and other electrodiagnostic procedures in their clinical context so that readers can better understand the proper place of electrodiagnostic tests in the overall management of their patients. We have been fortunate to present in one text the cumulative knowledge of physicians of sound clinical acumen and established knowledge and skills in clinical electrophysiology. The authors do not always agree. Differences in perspective, view, and opinion emerge from a careful reading of the text. We respect these differences and believe they reflect the "real world," where even the experts disagree. Such differences in emphasis and opinion simply reflect the incompleteness of our shared knowledge.

This volume is about a third larger than the 1987 edition. This expansion reflects the inclusion of new chapters: "Central Electromyography" by Tetsuo Komori and W. F. Brown, "The Autonomic Nervous System" by Douglas Zochodne and Mikihiro Kihara, "Ischemic Neuropathy" by Asa Wilbourn and Kerry Levin, "Atypical Motor Neuron Diseases" by David Preston and John Kelly, "Pediatric Electromyography" by Royden Jones, and "Electromyography in the Critical Care Unit" by Charles Bolton.

Some chapters from the first edition have changed authorship. We thank Bram Ongerboer de Visser and Giorgio Cruccu for their chapter on the brainstem and cranial nerves, Asa Wilbourn and Michael Aminoff for the chapter "Radiculopathies," Andrew Eisen for his chapter on the plexopathies, John Stewart for "Mononeuropathies of the Lower Extremities," Henry Berry for "Traumatic Peripheral Nerve Lesions," Alan McComas and Andrew Eisen for "Motor Neuron Disorders," and Micheal Rivner and Tom Swift for their chapter on diseases of neuromuscular transmission. We were saddened by the death of John Humphrey who contributed the chapter "Disorders of Neuromuscular Transmission" in the 1987 edition.

All of the other chapters have been updated from the first edition, and we thank all the authors for their very fine work.

As we emphasized in the preface to the 1987 edition, our objective is to marry the clinical analysis of neuromuscular disorder with the most appropriate electrophysiological techniques currently available. We believe that all of the contributors have been successful in this regard and hope that our readers find this second edition a worthy successor to the first.

W.F.B.
C.F.B.

Acknowledgments

I would like to thank my colleagues in neuromuscular disease here in London, including my co-editor Charles Bolton, Angelika Hahn, Sally Stewart, Michael Strong, Arthur Hudson, Joseph Gilbert, and David Munoz for their support and encouragement as we face the day-to-day challenges of neuromuscular disease. Thomas Feasby was a very important strength in the neuromuscular unit in London and has taken on new challenges as the Chair of Clinical Neurological Sciences at Calgary University, Calgary, Alberta.

For any success I have attained in neuromuscular disease in London, I owe a great deal to the support of my EMG technologists, Brad Watson, Jim Veitch, and Erin Kendrick, as well as to the support and encouragement of Mark Davis, Glen Smelzer, and Rob Snow from the Clark Davis Company and, most recently, Daniel Stashuk of Waterloo University. Only my secretary, Nola McGregor, knows how many manuscript drafts of mine and others have passed through her hands, and she is not telling. I could not have done this job without her patience and thoroughness.

Finally, I would like to thank my wife, Janet, and our children, Timothy and Martha, for their support.

W.F.B.

For their help and support over the years, I thank my wife, Margaret, and our children, David, Katherine and Nancy. My co-editor, Bill Brown, has been a valued colleague in electromyography. I am indebted to my "staff" at Victoria Hospital, Betsy Toth, Secretary, Tony Parkes, Hussein Remtulla, and Linda Bernardi, Electromyography Technologists, and Kevin Power, Biomedical Technician. Angelika Hahn, Tom Feasby, and Wilma Koopman in the Victoria Neuromuscular Clinic and my colleagues in Clinical Neurological Sciences are a constant inspiration. I have relied heavily on the advice and help of Bryan Young in pursuing our interests in neurocritical care. Finally, I wish to acknowledge the assistance of Chris Davis and his associates at Butterworth-Heinemann as well as Tom Conville and his associates at Ruttle, Shaw & Wetherill.

C.F.B.

Introduction

Electrophysiologic tests are an extension of the neuromuscular examination and provide important clues to the location, character, and severity of neuromuscular disorders. Coupled with the findings from nerve and muscle biopsies and the results of immunological, biochemical, and, most recently, powerful molecular biological studies, available diagnostic tools powerfully enhance our understanding of the pathogenesis and pathophysiology of neuromuscular disorders and allow more effective and specific therapy for these diseases.

Electrophysiologic tests embrace a wide repertoire of tools. These include newer methods for quantifying the results of needle electromyographic studies, motor unit estimates, assessments of motor cortical excitability and central motor and sensory conduction, detecting conduction block, and direct assessment of conduction across the roots and adjacent plexuses. Ever more sophisticated techniques for assessing neuromuscular transmission and disorders of the muscle fiber membrane and methods for assessing the contractile responses of muscles are additional improvements. These newer techniques and embellishments of older techniques considerably enhance our capacity to locate and determine the pathophysiology of neuromuscular diseases. Many of the newer techniques would not have been possible without the introduction of the computer to electromyography.

The future for electrodiagnosis of neuromuscular disease is bright and secure. As always, however, the choice of techniques and their proper interpretation will be best understood in the context of all the relevant clinical and other supporting laboratory evidence. This book, now in its second edition, was written to enhance the understanding of clinical electrophysiologists, electromyographers, neurologists, and physiatrists, as well as orthopedists and plastic surgeons, regarding the power and limitations of clinical electrophysiology in the study of neuromuscular diseases.

W.F.B.
C.F.B.

I

Approaches to the Nervous System in Electromyography

1

Central Electromyography

Tetsuo Komori
William F. Brown

CONTENTS

LIST OF ACRONYMS

CMCT	Central motor conduction times
CST	Corticospinal tract
DCM	Direct cortical motor neuron system
D wave	Direct wave
EPSP	Excitatory postsynaptic potential
IPSP	Inexcitatory postsynaptic potential
I wave	Indirect wave
MEP	Motor evoked potential
MN	Motor neuron
M potential	Supramaximal compound muscle action potential
MTL	Motor terminal latency
MU	Motor unit
PTN	Pyramidal tract neuron
SR	Spinal roots
TES	Transcranial electrical stimulation
TMS	Transcranial magnetoelectrical stimulation

In the 1930s, Penfield and Boldrey[1] mapped the human sensorimotor cortex with electrical stimulation at operation. Their celebrated homunculus was based on stimulation at relatively few points per subject, simple observation of the pattern of movements, and combining observations from many subjects. Milner-Brown et al.[2] stimulated the motor cortex directly at the time of temporal lobectomy for epileptic surgery and were able to evoke responses readily from the smaller sized motor unit (MU) action potentials from the thenar muscles as well as defining the time course of the excitability changes produced by motor cortical stimulus on the spinal motor neurons (MNs) (Figures 1.1 and 1.2). Merton and Morton,[3] however, were the first to devise a practical means for transcranially electrically stimulating the motor cortex. Their study opened a whole new chapter in clinical electrophysiology because for the first time electrophysiologists were presented with opportunities to assess transmission in the cortical spinal pathway and more easily assess motor conduction in the plexus and roots.

The introduction of the magnetic coil as a means of more painlessly stimulating the motor cortex led to widespread adoption of this technique for assessing central motor conduction and proximal conduction in the peripheral nervous system. Assessing central motor conduction, however, is obviously more complex than assessing conduction in the peripheral nervous system. The various neural elements in the cortex are affected in different ways by the different types of stimulation as well as changes in the stimulus intensity. Fortunately the essential groundwork for understanding transcranial stimulus evoked muscle responses was laid down in basic studies of motor cortical stimulation by Patton and Amassian,[4] Phillips and Porter,[5] and Amassian et al.[6] Their pioneering studies have made the task of interpreting the results of transcranial electrical and magnetoelectrical stimulation in health and disease much easier.

The techniques of high-voltage electrical and magnetoelectrical stimulation have also made it possible to stimulate components of the peripheral nervous system and to assess more directly conduction in the proximal segments of the peripheral nervous system.

BASIC PHYSIOLOGY

In the motor cortex, pyramidal tract neurons (PTNs) are oriented radially with respect to the cortical surface. There are about 20,000 to 30,000 of the largest PTNs in humans. Most of the latter project monosynaptically to spinal motor neurons (MNs) and compose the direct cortical motor neuronal (DCM) system. The density of the DCM system increases in high primates and is probably most dense in humans.[7] The DCM system is probably the most important, if not exclusive, mediator of the transcortical stimulus evoked motor responses in humans. PTNs are known to send collaterals to some brain stem neurons and spinal MNs at several levels sometimes many segments away from their primary target MNs. Other corticifugal neurons project to the basal ganglia, brain stem reticular formation, and the red nucleus, although the last system is probably much less important in humans. Some lateral medullary reticulospinal neurons transmit rapidly and project monosynaptically to spinal MNs.[7–9] The latter constitute therefore another rapidly transmitting corticospinal system in addition to the DCM system.

STIMULATION OF THE MOTOR CORTEX IN MONKEYS

Electrical stimulation of the motor cortex may excite PTNs both directly and indirectly.[4,6] In response to a single cortical shock, one or more volleys may be recorded from the pyramid or lateral corticospinal tract (CST). The earliest such volley has a relatively stable latency and is resistant to hypoxia or injury of the motor cortex. This direct or D wave is probably the result of direct stimulation of PTNs at their initial segments or nearby nodes of Ranvier. Following the D wave are a series of later waves that recur at relatively regular intervals, the so-called indirect or I waves. These successive volleys or waves are readily lost in the face of cortical hypoxia or injury and probably represent repetitive presynaptic excitation of the PTNs through stimulation of excitatory interneurons in the cortex or tangentially arranged fibers projecting to the PTNs. Not all interneurons in the motor cortex, however, are excitatory: Some are GABAergic and inhibitory.[10]

Phillips and others in a series of experiments characterized the responses of the motor cortex to surface anodal and cathodal stimulation.[5,11] They showed that lowest threshold responses as recorded from the CST or intracellularly directly from the MNs occurred in response to surface anodal stimulation. Such anodal shocks might be expected to evoke an outward depolarizing current in the region of the

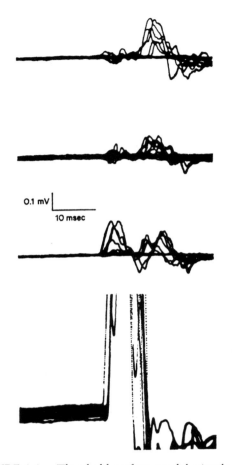

FIGURE 1.1.   *Threshold surface anodal stimulation of the exposed precentral motor cortex in a human. The stimulating electrode was a silver ball electrode whose position was adjusted to evoke with the least stimulus intensity in an all or nothing response from a few of the contralateral thenar motor units. The weakest stimuli evoked motor unit discharges of relatively longer latency (top) as compared with stronger stimuli (below). The shorter latency responses perhaps represent direct stimulation of corticospinal neurons monosynaptically projecting to the thenar motor neurons, whereas the larger latency discharges could represent indirect presynaptic excitation of the same or similar corticospinal neurons, although this cannot be proved in this type of study. Incidentally, the size of the motor unit action potentials, here recorded with surface electrodes, is based on their relatively small size and has probably been generated by lower threshold type I motor neurons (and units).*

initial segment and adjacent several nodes of Ranvier of the PTNs and a corresponding inward hyperpolarizing current in the dendritic tree near the surface. Weak anodal shocks produced a short-latency stable CST volley, able to follow stimulus frequencies as high as 500 c/s. This volley clearly corresponded to the D wave and was rapidly conducted. Further increases in the intensity of the surface anodal stimulus produced later waves, the intervals between which were relatively fixed and corresponded to repetitive, relatively well-synchronized volleys in the CST or I waves. Weak surface cathodal stimulation evoked only I waves, although if the intensity of the stimulus was increased sufficiently, a D wave could be obtained. The required stimulus intensity for the latter, however, was always much higher as compared with surface anodal stimulation.

In the baboon, stimulation at the best motor cortical point for various cervical MNs revealed that maximum DCM excitatory postsynaptic potentials (EPSPs) were of the order of 3 to 4 mV, being largest for the intrinsic hand muscles and extensor digitorum communis muscle and much smaller for proximal muscles; indeed for some MNs, no EPSP could be shown.[5,11] Maximum EPSPs of 3 to 4 mV and minimal EPSPs of the order of 0.1 to 0.2 mV suggest that as many as 15 to 20 PTNs may project monosynaptically to the same MN. Intracortical microstimulation studies in monkeys suggest that cortical regions containing PTNs projecting to the same MNs are characteristically composed of several loci overlapping with other loci projecting to synergistic or even antagonistic MNs.[12]

One unique property of DCM EPSPs identified by Phillips was a progressive increase in the size of successive EPSPs in response to repetitive corticospinal volleys.[11] This property of potentiation was not present in segmental group IA EPSPs. They also observed mixed effects on some cervical MNs, including inhibitory postsynaptic potentials (IPSPs) or EPSPs terminated by IPSPs. Repetitive corticospinal volleys and temporal summation of successive EPSPs at the MN level were often necessary to discharge the MN.[5]

That responses to motor cortical stimulation may not be exclusively mediated by the CST is shown by the ability to evoke motor responses by cortical stimulation following section of the pyramidal tract.[13] Repetitive and stronger cortical stimuli, however, were required to evoke a delayed motor response. The latter could have been mediated through corticoreticulospinal or other cortically originating extrapyramidal pathways.

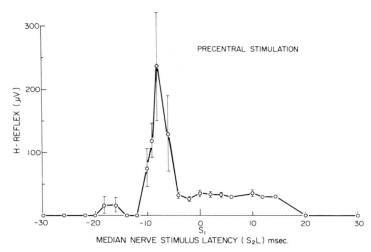

FIGURE 1.2.   *Study of the effect of motor cortical stimuli on the excitability of spinal motoneurons in a 45-year-old patient with focal motor seizures. The precentral motor cortex was stimulated by single 0.5-ms anodal pulses delivered directly to the exposed motor cortex at the best location for evoking threshold responses from the thenar muscles at the least stimulus intensity. Thenar responses were recorded with surface electrodes. The cortical (S₁) test stimulus was delivered at time 0 and conditioning (S₂) stimuli to the median nerve at the wrist at various times relative to S₁. The median nerve stimulus intensity was adjusted to just exceed motor threshold. At that intensity, successive stimuli evoked all or nothing discharges in a few motor units, occasional F waves from the latter but never H waves. The cortical stimulus was set to evoke all or nothing responses from a few thenar motor units, or, in some cases, there was no thenar response. At each S₁–S₂ interstimulus period, 10 stimuli were delivered, and the mean ± 1 SD values of the late H waves were calculated. Median nerve stimuli of an intensity employed here could be expected to excite thenar muscle afferents, including the primary spindle afferents monosynaptically projecting to thenar motor neurons. The expected time for generation of the primary spindle excitatory postsynaptic potentials (EPSPs) might be expected to be 10 to 14 ms following the median nerve stimulus based on a mean late response latency of 28 ms and a motor terminal latency of 4 ms. The minimum time from delivery of the motor cortical stimulus to arrival of the most rapid corticospinal volley at the level of the thenar motor neurons was estimated to be 4 ms, based on a latency from the cortical stimulus to thenar motor unit discharges of 20 ms and at time from spinal motoneurons to the thenar muscles of 16 ms (12 ms plus 4 ms for the motor terminal latency). Combined S₁ and S₂ evoked large H waves; the maximum H waves being evoked when S₂ was delivered somewhere between 4 and 10 ms before the cortical stimulus, a time when maximum summation of segmental spindle primary and direct cortical motoneuronal EPSPs might be expected (FAC I). A later period of facilitation (FAC II) was revealed by progressively delaying S₂ with respect to S₁. FAC II may be a result of repetitive firing of pyramidal tract neurons. Voluntary contraction of the thenar muscles greatly potentiated the size of the H wave (about 10 times), less potentiation being seen with finger flexion and none with elbow flexion.*

High-Voltage Electrical Stimulation

Cortical stimulation

Transcranial electrical stimulation (TES) was made possible by the development of a special high-voltage stimulator designed to deliver brief pulses through low-output impedance and large surface area electrodes to reduce the current density.[3,14] The methods employed to deliver high-voltage electrical stimuli through the scalp and skull vary. The earliest studies employed an anode positioned over the appropriate motor area—usually 7 cm lateral on a line from the vertex to the external meatus for the hand, with the cathode positioned anteriorly[3,15,16] or at the vertex.[17–22] For lower limb muscles, the anode was positioned at the vertex and the cathode anteriorly[16,23] or 7 cm lateral on a line between the vertex and the external meatus,[22] the reverse of the arrangement for preferential stimulation of distal hand muscles.

The required stimulus intensity may be reduced by employing a wide band cathode wrapped around the head like a crown[24] or similar band-like electrodes composed on multiequidistant and connected electrode plates[25,26] wrapped around the head about 2 cm above the inion-nasion plane. The anode was positioned similarly over the hand or foot area. Such crown-like cathodes may reduce the required stimulus intensity by as much as 200 to 500 volts, possibly because the lines of current flow follow better the radial orientation of the PTNs and penetrate more deeply as compared with employing a focal cathode positioned 4 to 6 cm ahead or central to the anode, as described by Merton and Morton[3] and Marsden et al.[15] Others tried positioning the cathode on the hard palate, but the stimuli were judged too uncomfortable for alert subjects, although they were found to be acceptable for intraoperative use.[27]

Normal motor cortical evoked potentials. The threshold for motor responses to TES is lowest for the intrinsic hand and forearm extensor muscles and highest for proximal arm muscles; leg muscles have a higher threshold than arm muscles. Increasing the intensity of the anodal cortical stimulus increases the peak to peak size of the motor evoked potential (MEP) to a maximum. Further increases in the stimulus may, however, more than double the duration of the MEP relative to the maximum M potential evoked by supramaximal stimulation of the peripheral nerve. For both arm and leg muscles, the average latency in response to maximal cortical stimuli may be up to 4 ms shorter as compared with threshold TES.[17,28] The progressively shorter latencies may reflect, in part at least, recruitment of higher threshold, larger MNs with faster conduction velocities,[21] a phenomenon in keeping with the size principle.[29,30]

Similar to the MEP, however, the twitch evoked by cortical stimulation may greatly exceed the twitch evoked by supramaximal stimulation of the peripheral nerve.[28] Twitches and M potential sizes exceeding those evoked by supramaximal peripheral nerve stimuli strongly suggest the presence of repetitive firing of spinal MNs in response to the single cortical shock. Such repetitive firing has been clearly shown by collision experiments.[28] For example, cortical stimulation continues to evoke a potential from the hypothenar muscles despite supramaximal stimulation of the ulnar nerve delivered at the same time as the cortical shock. The residual TES evoked electromyographic activity can be explained only by repetitive discharges of MNs, only the first efferent volley of which would be blocked by the antidromic volley in the ulnar nerve. As expected, these residual electromyographic discharges have a somewhat longer latency (by about 4 ms) as compared with the minimal TES evoked electromyographic discharge.

Burke et al.[31] have shown that anodal stimulation at the vertex evokes multiple waves recordable by epidural electrodes in the thoracic region that are entirely analogous to the D and I waves. Stronger cortical stimuli shortened the latency of the D wave, however, suggesting that stronger stimuli may actually activate corticospinal axons at subcortical levels possibly as deeply as the internal capsule or cerebral peduncle. The latter suggestion is in line with earlier studies in the monkey, in which strong electrical stimulation on the scalp shifted the presumed site of activation of corticospinal fibers to as deeply as the pyramid in the medulla.[32]

Other muscles activated by transcranial stimulation of the motor cortex. Although most applied studies using TES concentrated on motor responses from intrinsic hand or biceps muscles in the arm or tibialis anterior in the leg, muscles of the trunk, diaphragm, and rectal sphincter may be activated by TES. For example, motor responses to TES of the brain may readily be recorded from the pectoralis major and latissimus dorsi,[33] diaphragm,[34] neck,[35] and even the weakly contracted external sphincter ani muscles.[14] The short latencies to all the foregoing muscles except the external rectal sphincter strongly suggest that these responses are mediated by fast monosynaptic or perhaps disynaptic corticospinal pathways.[33]

To elicit MEPs from the diaphragm, intercostal muscles, and external anal sphincter muscle, the anode was best positioned near the vertex and the cathode either anteriorly or lateral to the anode.[33,34] For neck muscles, the anode was best positioned at 6 cm lateral to the vertex with the cathode anterior to the anode.[35]

Central motor conduction times (CMCTs) for the diaphragm are of the order of 4 to 4.4 ms and similar to CMCTs for the deltoid muscle. Both are short enough to suggest transmission by rapidly conducting monosynaptic projections to their respective spinal MNs. The amplitude of the diaphragmatic response is greatly increased and the latency reduced during inspiration. Facilitation of the diaphragmatic response to magnetoelectrical stimulation has also been shown to occur in response to inhalation of carbon dioxide as well as voluntary ventilation.[36]

MEPs may be readily evoked from the sternocleidomastoid muscle bilaterally, but the latency to the contralateral sternocleidomastoid muscle is approximately one-half that to the ipsilateral sternocleidomastoid muscle. In contrast to the sternocleidomastoid muscle, only contralateral responses may be evoked from trapezius and splenius capitis muscles.[35] TES also readily evokes MEPs from the intercostal muscles—the relatively short latencies also suggesting monosynaptic corticospinal projections to these MNs—and, as with the diaphragm, the size of the electromyographic response is changed by respiration.[33]

Responses of single motor units to magnetic stimulation. By applying weak magnetoelectrical stimuli, it is possible to activate single MUs in limb muscles.[37–40] The latencies of such MUs as recorded with needle electrodes from intrinsic hand muscles vary widely from unit to unit (22 to 32 ms) and diminish by as much as 1.5 ms with stronger stimuli.

If single intrinsic hand MUs are recruited using weak voluntary contraction, randomly delivered magnetoelectrical stimuli increase the probability of firing single MUs somewhere between 20 and 31 ms (the primary peak) following the stimulus depending on the MU. In some MUs, the probability of discharge increases again between 56 and 90 ms (the secondary peak) following the stimulus. The primary peak in the peristimulus frequency histogram is further divisible for most MUs into two or three subpeaks, with an interpeak latency of 1.4 ± 0.4 ms.

The subpeaks probably correspond to the arrival of successive corticospinal volleys, subsequent EPSPs and MN discharges.[40,41] The latency at which a given MU fires following the cortical stimulus depends on the excitability of the MN, which, in turn, is governed by the cycle of initial hyperpolarization and subsequent depolarization that follows each voluntary discharge of the MN. Corticospinal volleys timed to arrive at the MN during the period of hyperpolarization as a consequence will evoke a discharge in the voluntarily discharging MN at a longer latency than would be the case for a corticospinal volley arriving while the MN was partially depolarized. It is this natural cycle of excitability changes in the MN, following each voluntary discharge, that determines which corticospinal volley in the train of two or three set up by a single cortical stimulus will cause the MN to fire.[40]

Stimulation of the spinal roots

High-voltage electrical stimuli delivered over the surface of the vertebral column may also be used to stimulate the roots and is capable of evoking supramaximal M potentials from limb muscles with appropriate positioning of the cathode: the C-6 spine for C-7–T-1 muscles and the L-1 spine for lumbosacral muscles (Figure 1.3). For cervical stimulation, the anode may be positioned either rostral or caudal to the cathode, or for stimulation at L-1, over the iliac crest or caudal to L-1.

In the cervical region, the actual site of stimulation is 20 to 30 mm distal to the cervical enlargement based on a latency shorter by 1.0 to 1.5 ms, as compared with the latency for intrinsic hand muscles derived from studies of F latencies or direct electrical stimulation through needle electrodes positioned in close proximity to the spinal roots.[42] For the lower limb, based on comparisons with F latencies, high-voltage electrical stimulation over the L-1 spine probably stimulates the ventral roots close to the conus medullaris. In keeping with such an extramedullary site for stimulation of the roots, for both the cervical and lumbosacral regions, is the absence of any potentiation of the resulting muscle responses by voluntary recruitment.

Stimulus intensities greatly exceeding those required for supramaximal stimulation of the roots in the cervical region may also evoke muscle potentials in lower limb muscles. This suggests that such intense stimuli are also capable of direct stimulation of descending long motor tracks in the cervical cord.[42]

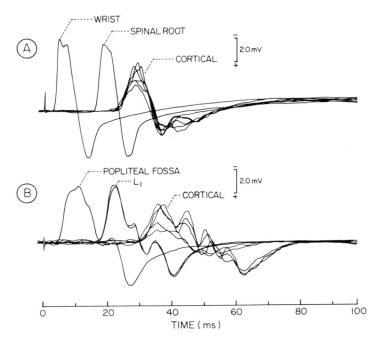

FIGURE 1.3.   *Peripheral and central motor conduction to hypothenar (A) and anterior and lateral compartment (AL) muscles (B). Recordings were carried out with surface electrodes. In the case of the hypothenar muscles, the ulnar nerve was stimulated supramaximally at the wrist and axilla and the respective C-8–T-1 spinal roots using a DEVICES D-180 stimulator. For AL muscles, the common peroneal nerve was supramaximally stimulated at the fibular head (FH), popliteal fossa (PF), and the respective ventral roots at L-1 with the D-180 stimulator. Magnetoelectrical stimulation at or just ahead of the vertex (Cadwell ME-10) in combination with modest voluntary contraction of the muscles evoked motor evoked potentials (MEPs) of normal latency and size. The central motor conduction time was calculated by latency to cortical stimulus − latency to supramaximal root stimulation (ms) and incorporates an important peripheral component, including conduction in the intraspinal and intraforaminal roots in the case of cervical stimulation. The size of the MEPs in normal subjects is at least one-third to one-half of the size of the maximum M potential evoked by root stimulation.*

In our experience, there is little, if any, change in latency of the M potentials from hand muscles over the range of stimulus intensities between 100% and 130% of that required to evoke maximal M potentials. Others, however, have reported an apparent distal advance of the site of stimulation with excessive increases in the stimulus intensity.[43] High-voltage electrical stimulation in the cervical region is quite capable of evoking maximal M potentials, an important criterion if the technique is to be used to assess conduction block over the roots and plexus (see Chapter 20).

Facilitation of the motor cortical evoked potentials.   One important property of both high-voltage electrical and magnetoelectrical stimulation is the ability of the test subject to potentiate the electromyographic response greatly by voluntary conduction of the targeted muscles.[17,21,28] The resultant transcortical MEPs and twitches may well exceed the maximum M potentials evoked by supramaximal stimulation of peripheral nerves and may be explained only by repetitive firing of MNs.

Not only does weak to moderate voluntary contraction of the targeted muscles increase the size of the MEPs, but also shortening of the latency of the MEPs, often by several milliseconds, also occurs. Indeed, simply directing the test subject to focus attention on the targeted muscle, or MU, without any ongoing electromyographic activity is capable of facilitating MEPs. Such potent potentiation of MEPs probably takes place at the level of the spinal cord, although the mechanism remains unestablished.[28,44]

Transcranial magnetoelectrical stimulation (TMS) evoked MEPs may also be facilitated by contraction of the same muscles on the side ipsilateral to the stimulus. The latter may reflect intracortical facilitation, whereas contralateral facilitation probably reflects facilitation at the spinal level.[45]

MEPs evoked by TES and TMS may also be facilitated by any of several other methods, such as transcallosal stimulation, vibration of the tendon of the target muscle, conditioning stimuli delivered to peripheral nerves, and cerebellar stimulation. TES of the ipsilateral cerebral hemisphere 8 to 24 ms before the TES of the contralateral motor cortex facilitates the latter, an effect probably mediated through transcallosal facilitation.[47] Indeed, a transcallosal potential may be recorded from the hand area of one hemisphere in response to an anodal stimulus delivered to the opposite hand area with a latency difference of 9 to 14 ms.[46]

The size of transcranial stimulus MEPs may also be increased by continuous vibration of the tendon of the target muscle. This effect may be mediated by the facilatory effect of Ia muscle afferents on spinal MS.[47]

Subthreshold motor stimuli delivered to the median nerve 30 to 50 ms before motor cortical stimulation has also been shown to increase the size of the MEPs, perhaps as a result of the facilatory effect of Ia muscle afferents on the excitability of PTNs[48–50] (Figure 1.4). Such median nerve stimulation may increase MEP size by close to 200%.[51] Even direct stimulation of the cerebellar hemisphere ipsilateral to the target muscle increases MEPs when the cerebellar stimulus is delivered 3 to 7 ms before the cortical stimulus.[51]

TES has several advantages such as direct excitation of PTNs and the ability to stimulate roots supramaximally and therefore assess proximal conduction block. The main disadvantage of TES is the attendant discomfort, although the level of discomfort may be reduced appreciably by distributing the cathode in a ring about the head and careful positioning of the anode over the desired cortical region.

Magnetoelectrical Stimulation

Cortical stimulation

A practical technique using a brief current pulse passed through a coil to induce a short time-varying

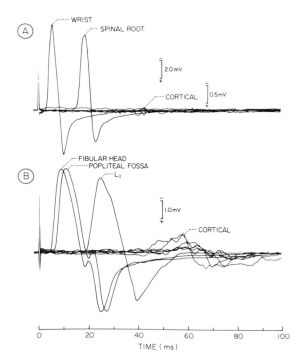

FIGURE 1.4. *Patient with primary lateral sclerosis. (A) Surface hypothenar muscle recordings in response to supramaximal stimulation of the ulnar nerve at the wrist and the C-8–T-1 spinal roots, the latter using a DEVICES D-180 stimulator and magnetoelectrical stimulation of the motor cortex at the vertex. Note the absent response to the cortical stimulus despite the higher gain for the latter recording. (B) Surface electromyographic recordings from the anterior and lateral compartment muscles. The common peroneal nerve was stimulated supramaximally at the fibular head and popliteal fossa and the respective ventral roots at the L-1 spinous process level, using in the latter case the DEVICES D-180 stimulator. Note the small motor evoked potential and the greatly prolonged central motor conduction time here (over 23 ms).*

magnetic field and a current in the underlying tissues has been developed.[52–55] The magnetic field passes freely through air, the scalp, and bone to induce a current parallel but opposite in direction to the inducing current in the coil. The induced current is of maximal intensity beneath and in the immediate vicinity of the coil. When the coil is tangentially applied to the skull, the induced cortical currents are primarily tangential to the cortical surface and probably preferentially excite horizontally disposed intracortical interneurons and axonal elements with the cortex.

The fact that the magnetic field passes freely through the scalp explains why the technique is able to stimulate the underlying cortex without accompanying pain from stimulation of pain receptors in the scalp, periosteum, and dura. The main advantage of TMS is the apparent painlessness of the stimulus, although some subjects find the unexpected jerks and movements of tensed limbs disconcerting.

The latencies of TMS MEPs are characteristically delayed by several milliseconds by comparison with TES MEPs. Current evidence suggests the reason for the longer latencies is that TMS currents excite PTNs indirectly, perhaps because the induced currents are tangentially disposed relative to the cortical surface and more likely to excite presynaptic elements oriented in the same plane rather than PTNs oriented at right angles to the cortical surface. Such presynaptic stimulation results in I waves but not a D wave.

One important disadvantage of magnetoelectrical stimulation is the inability to evoke maximum M potentials when used to stimulate roots in the cervical or lumbosacral region. Also because TMS appears to excite PTNs preferentially indirectly, TMS may not be as useful as TES for monitoring CST function in the operating room, where responses to indirect stimulation of PTNs are more readily suppressed by inhalation anesthetics.

Attempts have been made to modify the design of the magnetic coil to focus the induced current more precisely.[56–61] As well, the direction of the inducing current in the coil may be an important determinant of the size of the evoked muscle responses in coils such as the original Sheffield and Digitimer models, in which the inducing current was a monophasic pulse. The more recent Cadwell model delivers a biphasic pulse and the size of MEP is possibly more independent of the direction of the inducing current.[61]

Stimulation of the roots and peripheral nerves

Magnetoelectrical stimulation over the cervical spine evokes maximum M responses in first dorsal interosseus (FDI) with the coil centered over C-3 and biceps-brachialis with the coil centered over C-5. The latencies are constant regardless of the exact position of the coil but are 1.0 ± 0.7 ms shorter than estimated latencies using F waves. M potentials are always submaximal regardless of the stimulus intensity and the exact location of the coil. The latter is an important point because it means that magnetoelectri-

cal stimulation cannot be used to assess conduction block in the proximal segments. Latencies with magnetoelectrical and high-voltage electrical stimulation in the cervical region are nearly identical, and the presumed site of stimulation in both cases is probably the spinal roots 30 to 60 mm distal to the appropriate cord segment.[62]

In the lumbosacral region, M potentials evoked by magnetoelectrical stimulation seldom exceed 70% of maximum, the form of the M potential is often dissimilar to that evoked by peripheral nerve stimulation, and the latencies remain constant within a wide range of coil positions. M potentials were maximum in quadriceps with the coil centered over L-1 and in extensor digitorum brevis (EDB) with the coil centered over S-3. As mentioned with respect to the latter, however, latencies were constant whatever the exact position of the coil between T-12 and L-2. As in the upper limb, latencies were always shorter than expected from F wave latencies, in the case of EDB, shorter by 3.0 ± 1.1 ms 1 SD, the longer latency corresponding to the latency of the EDB M potential evoked by high-voltage electrical stimulation at T-12. The much shorter latency to EDB in response to magnetoelectrical stimulation suggested that the actual site of stimulation of EDB motor fibers was at the S-1 level. Indeed, the latency of which closely corresponded to the latency to high-voltage electrical stimulation at the S-1 level.

Magnetic coils are impractical methods for stimulating peripheral nerve for the most part because stimulus currents cannot be readily confined to single nerve trunks.[63,64] On the other hand, the coil is able to excite deep nerve trunks or plexuses such as the sciatic nerve or brachial plexus, which may be inaccessible to surface electrical stimulation because the required stimulus intensities are painful or the regions are covered by bandages.

Applications of Electrical and Magnetoelectrical Stimulation in Humans—Normal Findings

Physiologic studies in humans have revealed findings entirely analogous to what might be anticipated from the earlier direct cortical stimulation studies in lower primates.[41] Thus despite the infolding of the motor cortex in humans, the lowest threshold TES MEPs were found when single-surface anodal stimuli were delivered to the appropriate region in the cortex.[65,66] Further, such stimuli were soon shown to evoke volleys corresponding to D and I waves readily detectable by electrodes inserted into the epidural space.[31,67,68] Further evidence for D and I waves has come from analysis of poststimulus histograms of voluntarily recruited single MUs in humans.[28,69] These latter studies have shown that the shortest latency response has a relatively stable latency and is easiest to evoke with high-voltage surface positive electrical stimulation. The same stimulus at higher intensities evokes later electromyographic discharges whose latencies tended to be grouped and that probably corresponded to successive I waves. In the same study, magnetoelectrical stimulation was shown to evoke electromyographic discharges preferentially best corresponding to successive I waves. In keeping with the latter, presynaptic activation of PTNs, benzodiazepines, which potentiate GABAergic interneurons, block electromyographic responses to TMS but not so readily responses to TES.[70]

Summary of normal studies of high-voltage electrical and magnetoelectrical stimulation in normal subjects

Studies have shown the following:

1. There is somatotopic localization and preferential excitability of certain regions of the motor cortex. This was best shown for TES.[65,66] Even so, the somatotopic localization is crude.
2. The size, latency, and duration of the MEPs are critically dependent on the type, intensity, and localization of the stimulus as well as the state of the cortical and spinal MNs. The most important of these factors include:
   a. The type of stimulus, whether magnetoelectrical, which preferentially indirectly excites PTNs, or high-voltage electrical stimulation, which is capable of both direct and indirect stimulation of PTNs.
   b. The polarity of the high-voltage electrical stimulus. The lowest threshold and shortest latency responses are observed with surface-positive stimulation.
   c. The intensity of the stimulus. The intensity of the stimulus determines the extent of the horizontal and vertical spread of the currents, vertical currents preferentially exciting PTNs directly and horizontal currents presynaptic elements in the cortex. Increasing the stimulus intensity increases the size and shortens the latency of MEPs.
   d. The excitability of the MN. The excitability of MNs may be greatly increased by weak voluntary contraction of the muscle(s).
   e. The excitability of the cortical neurons may be increased by conditioning afferent stimuli, especially from muscle afferents.

Assessment of Central Motor Conduction

For clinical studies, the most useful measures of central motor conduction are the CMCT between cortical stimulus and discharge of the MNs and the size and shape of the resultant electromyographic response in the target muscle.[71] In practice, the actual time between activation of PTNs and the time the CST volley arrives at the appropriate spinal segment or the actual times when MNs fire cannot be measured. What constitutes the CMCT of necessity therefore includes whatever time for temporal summation may be required for CST volley-induced EPSPs to exceed MN threshold and the short peripheral conduction time between the MN and the presumed sites where high-voltage electrical or magnetoelectrical pulse stimulated the respective roots or adjacent plexus (Figure 1.5).

CMCT may be calculated by subtracting the latency in response to spinal root stimulation from the latency in response to cortical stimulation.[72,73] Alternatively, CMCTs may be calculated by using the F wave latency.[16]

$$CMCT = \text{Latency cortex to muscle (ms)}$$
$$- \frac{\text{F Latency (ms)} - (\text{MTL [ms]} + 1 \text{ [ms]})}{2}$$

Because F waves must traverse the spinal and central roots, CMCTs calculated using F waves generally exceed those based on high-voltage electrical or magnetoelectrical stimulation of the roots, which stimulate peripheral motor axons distal to the ventral roots, at least in the cervical region. Factors affecting the CMCT operate at several levels, including:

1. The activation time of PTNs. PTNs may be directly activated at their initial segments or even as deep as the white matter depending on the intensity of the stimulus.[32] Indirect stimulation of the same neurons, as with magnetoelectrical stimulation, necessarily increases the latency of the response by at least one or more synaptic delays and the requisite conduction times of the various presynaptic elements in the cortex. The intensity of the stimulus determines the numbers of PTN cells excited and the extent to which they repetitively fire.

2. The transmission time between motor cortex and spinal motor neurons. The latencies of cortical stimulus evoked electromyographic responses are of such an order that the central pathway must be mediated by the most rapidly conducting pyramidal tract fibers or probably DCM axons.

3. The activation time of MNs. This time depends in part on the relative excitability of different

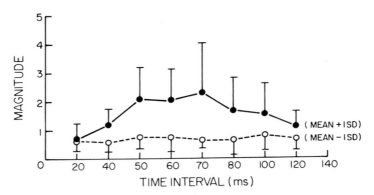

FIGURE 1.5. *Effects of conditioning percutaneous electrical stimulation of the median nerve at the wrist (closed circles) and the index and middle fingers (open circles) on the size of the thenar motor evoked potential (MEP) (recorded with surface electrodes) evoked by magnetoelectrical stimulation at the vertex. Stimulus trains of 50 stimuli were delivered at intervals from 20 to 120 ms before the test cortical stimuli. The intensity of the stimulus to the median nerve just exceeded motor threshold, whereas that delivered to the middle and index fingers was supramaximal. No significant change in MEP size, shown as a multiple of the control size, occurred in response to stimulation of the digits, whereas stimulation of the median nerve clearly facilitated the MEP size, especially for conditioning to test intervals of 50 to 100 ms.*

MNs. Excitability depends on both influence of other conditioning stimuli on the MN and the specific biophysical properties of the MN. MNs differ in their input resistance and relative threshold—smaller MNs possessing the lowest thresholds for recruitment, whereas the recruitment thresholds for larger MNs with lower input resistances and more rapidly conducting motor axons are characteristically higher.[30] The precise time MNs discharge depends in some instances on temporal summation of successive DCM EPSPs in response to successive CST volleys. In other instances, a single CST volley may generate EPSPs sufficiently large to discharge the MN without the need for subsequent CST volleys and temporal summation of EPSPs.

4. The size of unitary EPSPs. The number of PTNs, and specifically DCMs, excited by a single cortical stimulus, repetitive CST volleys, subsequent temporal summation of EPSPs, and size of unitary EPSPs are probably all important determinants of whether MNs discharge or not. Although never shown, dysfunctional DCM neurons could generate smaller unitary EPSPs, which, coupled with losses of DCM neurons, might greatly increase the need for repetitive firing of the remaining DCM fibers and perhaps other corticospinal systems if sufficient temporal summation of excitatory inputs is to occur to discharge the MNs.

5. The time between MN discharge and the site of stimulation of the motor root. This time is a function of the conduction velocities of the proximal

portion of the motor axons and the distance between the ventral horn and the site at which the high-voltage electrical or magnetoelectrical stimulus excites the ventral or spinal roots or perhaps adjacent plexus.

Factors affecting the size of electromyographic responses to cortical stimulation include the type of cortical stimulus, whether high-voltage electrical or magnetoelectrical, and most importantly the stimulus intensity. The latter determines the size of the corticifugal volley and the extent of repetitive firing of the DCM neurons and other corticospinal systems. The size of the electromyographic discharge, in turn, depends on the number of spinal MNs recruited by the CST volleys and the extent to which these MNs fire.

Volume conduction of electrical activity from muscles activated by root or cortical stimulation, but not supramaximal stimulation of the peripheral nerve, greatly influences the relative sizes of maximum M potentials evoked by supramaximal stimulation of a particular motor nerve and supramaximal root or cortical stimulation. For this reason it is best to choose recording sites that see very little, if any, volume-conducted electromyographic activity from stimulation of other peripheral nerves or roots if maximum M potentials to peripheral nerve and root stimulation are to be compared with both one another and the size of the MEP. One recording site meeting the aforementioned criteria is the hypothenar site when there is little appreciable volume conduction of electrical activity from median-supplied hand or forearm muscles or ulnar-supplied forearm muscles.

Activation of other muscles can also influence the size of the twitch recorded from intrinsic hand muscles unless very special care is taken to fix the arm and hand in such a way as to preclude any significant distortions of the twitch produced by activation by forearm and other intrinsic hand muscles.

Factors that probably increase central motor conduction time and reduce sizes of motor evoked potentials

Factors are as follows:

1. At the cortical level, reduced excitability of the motor cortex from:
   a. Losses of DCM and other PTNs.
   b. Losses of cortical interneurons.
   c. Changes in the dendritic trees of intracortical neurons and DCM and other PTNs.
   d. Intracortical synaptic failures as a result of hypoxia, ischemia, or drugs.
   e. Enhanced GABAergic activity with resulting inhibition of PTNs.
   f. Reduced capacities for repetitive firing of PTNs, possibly as a result of *d* and *e*.
2. Slowed conduction between the motor cortex and spinal MNs from:
   a. Demyelination, remyelination, and possibly axonal shrinkage of DCM and other pyramidal axons.
   b. Transmission by normally slower conducting pyramidal tract axons.
   c. Activation of longer latency cortico-fugal systems.
3. At the MN level:
   a. Reduced size of corticospinal excitatory volleys from losses of DCM and other PTNs.
   b. Increased temporal dispersion of DCM and other corticifugal EPSPs.
   c. Reduced sizes of unitary EPSPs.
   d. Reduced excitabilities of MNs perhaps through loss of facilitory inputs.
   e. Pharmacologic blockade of synaptic transmission at the MN level.
   f. Increased requirement for temporal summation of EPSPs.
   g. Loss of the more rapidly conducting motor axons.
4. Reduced conduction velocities in motor axons.
5. Displacement of the site of excitation of the roots distally because of stimulus lead through the use of too high a stimulus intensity.

CLINICAL APPLICATIONS OF HIGH-VOLTAGE ELECTRICAL AND MAGNETOELECTRICAL STIMULATION

Multiple Sclerosis

Cowan et al.[72] clearly showed increased CMCTs to biceps in thenar muscles, CMCTs sometimes exceeding four to six times the normal values. There was often a poor correlation between CMCT and the clinical findings. Similar abnormalities were reported by Mills and Murray in 1985, again using TES. In 1986, Hess et al.[45] applied TMS to the cortex together with high-voltage electrical stimulation in the cervical region to study CMCTs in multiple sclerosis patients. They reported increased CMCTs in the majority of limbs and sometimes in limbs with apparently normal power. In 1988, Ingram et al.[75] examined CMCT to the thenar, biceps brachialis, and tibialis anterior muscles employing magnetoelectrical stimulation at the cortical, cervical, and lumbosacral levels. CMCT was increased in the majority of the patients. Absent MEPs were most common in those with marked clinical disabilities. Increases in CMCT were often accompanied by dispersed and reduced sizes of MEPs, but there was no correlation between CMCT and the duration of the disease. Sometimes CMCT was greatly increased in limbs with normal power.

Hess et al. in 1987,[76] using a combination of high-voltage electrical stimulation in the cervical region and TMS, showed that CMCTs were abnormal in 79% of definite and 55% of probable multiple sclerosis cases. Often there was only a moderate increase in latency, but latencies could be very prolonged. Prolonged CMCTs correlated well with abnormally brisk tendon reflexes, and there was good concordance with changes in somatosensory evoked potentials. Prolonged CMCTs were considered to reflect several factors, including slowed conduction in pathologic fibers because of demyelination, conduction in normally smaller and more slowly conducting CST fibers, greatly increased temporal summation times for EPSPs at the spinal MN level, and possibly transmission through other corticifugal systems.

Maximum conduction velocities in descending motor pathways in the spinal cords of multiple sclerosis patients were shown by Snooks and Swash[77] to be slowed in five patients with multiple sclerosis and one patient with a radiation myelopathy. These studies were carried out employing high-voltage electrical stimulation at the C-6, L-1, and L-4 levels while recording the electromyographic responses from the pelvic floor muscles and tibialis anterior. More recently, greatly prolonged latencies in single MUs and indirect evidence of incremental temporal dispersion of DCM EPSPs has been shown in multiple sclerosis.[40]

Amyotrophic Lateral Sclerosis

Several studies of central motor conduction in amyotrophic lateral sclerosis have shown prolonged CMCTs or absent MEPs in a majority of patients.[73,78,79] In some cases, the CMCTs exceeded control upper limit values by two to three times.[73] The preceding studies all used high-voltage electrical stimulation of the cortical, cervical, and lumbosacral levels, but similar results were shown by Eisen et al.[80] using magnetoelectrical stimulation at the cortical and cervical levels. The latter study showed modest increases in CMCT to biceps brachialis, extensor digitorum communis, or thenar muscles as well as reductions in the sizes of MEP responses relative to the sizes of maximum M potentials evoked by cervical or lumbosacral stimulation.

A subgroup of patients with primary lateral sclerosis has been studied, with most exhibiting absent MEPs, whereas in the remainder MEPs were greatly prolonged.[81,82]

Stroke

In baboons, Bentivoglio et al.[83] demonstrated slowed conduction in the pyramidal fibers through the ventral pons in response to reductions in brain stem blood flow below 30% of control values. Magnetoelectrical cortical and cervical stimulation have also been applied to the study of central motor conduction in patients with hemispheric infarctions.[84] In a study of 20 patients, 11 of whom had hemispheric infarctions and nine of whom had capsular infarctions, MEPs were absent in six of the nine capsular infarctions and nine of the hemispheric infarctions. MEPs may also be abolished by precentral infarctions (Figure 1.6). In some cases, the electromyographic responses were delayed. Absent MEPs were most characteristic of cortical-subcortical infarctions, whereas prolonged CMCTs were sometimes seen in subcortical infarctions.[85] Abnormalities in central motor conduction proved a better indicator of outcome than somatosensory evoked potentials in at least one study.[85]

Parkinson's Disease

Central motor conduction in Parkinson's disease is normal.[86]

Spondylitic Myelopathy

High-voltage electrical stimulation of the motor cortex and cervical cord with spondylitic cervical myelopathy have shown delayed central motor conduction,[23,87] and where cervical radiculopathies were present as well as the cervical myelopathy, delays in response to stimulation of the cervical roots were also present.[23] Absent MEPs in lower limb muscles as well as delayed central motor conduction to the same muscles were common in cervical spondylitic myelopathies.[23]

Cerebellar Ataxia

Delayed central motor conduction and temporal dispersion of MEPs were found in 10 of 11 patients with Friedreich's ataxia and were most normal in

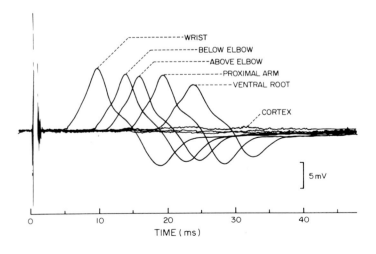

FIGURE 1.6. *Patient with small precentral infarction showing absent MEP despite 100% maximal magnetoelectrical stimulation at and just ahead of the vertex. Surface electromyographic recordings were carried out and the respective hypothenar motor fibers supramaximally stimulated at the wrist, below and above the elbow, axilla (proximal arm), and ventral roots (or more probably spinal roots). The last was carried out using a DEVICES D-180 stimulator.*

patients with early onset of Friedreich's ataxia and more common in patients with early-onset as compared with late-onset cerebellar degeneration.[88]

Hereditary Motor Sensory Neuropathies

TMS combined with high-voltage electrical stimulation in the neck has been applied to studies of central motor conduction in hereditary motor sensory neuropathies and hereditary spastic paraplegia by Claus et al.[89] Delayed CMCTs were most evident in patients with hereditary motor sensory neuropathy type I neuropathy with upper motor neuron findings clinically, the mean CMCT being approximately twice that in controls. More modest increases in CMCT were seen in hereditary motor sensory neuropathy type II neuropathies accompanied by upper motor neuron findings, but CMCTs were normal in hereditary spastic paraplegia. Central motor conduction was normal in hereditary motor sensory neuropathy I and II cases without clinically apparent signs of upper motor neuron involvement.

Radiculopathies

Cervical root stimulation, through a needle electrode inserted just lateral to the spinous process, has been applied to the diagnosis of cervical radiculopathies by Berger et al.[90] These studies revealed reductions in M potentials in 100% and increases in latency in 61%, of muscles supplied by the appropriate root, of cases in which one or more clinical signs indicative of a radiculopathy were present. Even in cases in which there were no clinical signs of a radiculopathy and the presentation was primarily characterized by pain, latency increases were found in a quarter of the cases and reductions in amplitude in over one-half of the cases. This study suggested that high-voltage electrical or magnetoelectrical stimulation might be helpful in the diagnosis of cervical and possibly lumbosacral radiculopathies, although the site of stimulation in the case of Berger's study was probably proximal to the intervertebral foramen, whereas high-voltage electrical and magnetoelectrical stimulation probably stimulate roots distal to the intervertebral foramen in the case of the cervical region. Chokroverty et al.[91] applied magnetoelectrical stimulation to four cases of lumbosacral radiculopathy. Their studies showed delayed latencies on the affected side of tibialis anterior or soleus.

A comparison of magnetoelectrical and high-voltage electrical stimulation of the cervical and lumbosacral roots was reported by Britton et al.[62] Their study showed that magnetoelectrical stimulation in the cervical region evoked the maximum response in the first dorsal interosseus muscle (FDI) with the coil centered around C-3 and from the biceps with the coil centered around C-5. Latencies were constant regardless of the precise position of the coil, the M potentials were always submaximal, and the latencies always shorter by 1.3 ± 0.7 ms 1 SD as compared to latencies derived using the F wave techniques. The last observation suggested that the actual site of stimulation using magnetoelectrical stimulation was actually 20 to 30 mm distal to the spinal cord. In the lumbosacral region, M potentials never exceeded 70% of maximum; again onset latencies were constant, but unfortunately the form of M potentials elicited with magnetoelectrical stimulation over the lumbosacral spine were often dissimilar to those evoked by supramaximal stimulation of peripheral nerves. Maximum M responses from quadriceps were obtained with the coil centered around L-1 and from extensor digitorum brevis muscle (EDB) with the coil centered over S-3. The latency of the electromyographic responses from EDB, however, were the same whatever the position of the coil between S-2 and L-2, and the latencies were always shorter than would be predicted from F studies from EDB by 3.0 ± 1.1 ms. The latter F latencies were very similar to latencies for this muscle in response to high-voltage electrical stimulation over L-1. This observation suggests that high-voltage electrical stimulation is capable of stimulating the ventral roots supplying EDB very close to the cord, but that magnetoelectrical stimulation, whatever the position of the coil, stimulates the same motor fibers just distal to the intervertebral foramen. The foregoing studies would suggest that magnetoelectrical stimulation may have little practical place in the study of lumbosacral radiculopathies. High-voltage electrical stimulation may turn out to be beneficial in the detection of lumbosacral radiculopathies, but in the cervical region, both magnetoelectrical and high-voltage electrical stimulation, because they apparently stimulate the roots distal to the intervertebral foramen, may not turn out to be useful detectors of cervical radiculopathies.

Chronic Inflammatory Demyelinating Polyneuropathy with Multifocal Lesions in the Central Nervous System

Delayed central motor conduction in chronic inflammatory demyelinating polyneuropathy with multifocal lesions in the central nervous system found by magnetic resonance imaging has been shown by Thomas et al.[92] (see Figure 17, Chapter 20).

Cranial Nerve Studies

TMS may be used to stimulate the facial nerve by applying the coil tangentially across the occipital-parietal region. Such painless, relatively low-intensity stimuli evoke maximum M potentials in various facial muscles nearly identical to those elicited by supramaximal stimulation of the facial nerve in the stylomastoid fossa using conventional bipolar surface electrical stimulation. The latency difference between the two potentials represents the conduction time between the exit of the facial nerve from the brain stem and the stimulus site in the stylomastoid fossa.[93,94] Central motor conduction in corticofacial pathways may be assessed by magnetoelectrical stimulation of the contralateral motor cortex by centering the coil 3 to 6 cm lateral to the vertex on the contralateral side.

In one series of 26 patients with various lesions affecting the facial nerve, there was no response to transcranial stimulation of the VII nerve in all 16 patients with Bell's palsy, conduction was delayed in seven patients with demyelinating neuropathies, and a reduced electromyographic response was seen in one patient with a pontine glioma and no electromyographic response was seen in two patients with trauma affecting the facial nerve.[95]

Epilepsy

In a study of 58 patients with partial or generalized epilepsy, magnetoelectrical stimulation resulted in no short-term changes in the electroencephalogram or induction of seizures and no change in the overall frequency of seizures in the long term.[96] Hufnagel et al.,[97] however, in the study of 13 patients with partial complex seizures, in whom their anticonvulsants had been reduced deliberately preoperatively, showed that TMS using either single or serial stimulation could activate a known epileptic focus but induced no epileptiform activity outside this focus.

Influence of Anesthetic Agents on Cortical Stimulus Evoked Motor Responses

Nitrous oxide, in the rat, has been shown to suppress MEPs by TES.[98] The presumed site of the block was at the spinal interneuron or neuronal level because there was no accompanying block in neuromuscular transmission and the size of the electromyographic response was the same whether the motor pathway was stimulated at the cortical or midcervical cord levels. In humans, nitrous oxide has also been shown to reduce the size of MEPs to TES,[98,99] but fentanyl, flunitrazepam, and thiopental produced no changes in the sizes of MEPs. Benzodiazepines such as midazolam have been shown to reduce the size of MEPs to TMS. These agents produce no change in peripheral nerve trunk stimulus evoked M potentials or F waves, but infusion of midazolam results in progressive reduction in the size of MEPs to TMS, the longest latency components of the electromyographic discharge being the first to go. GABAergic interneurons are known to be densely represented in cortex.[10] These interneurons are inhibitory, and benzodiazepines are potent enhancers of GABA-mediated inhibition. Because TMS is thought to be mediated presynaptically, the action of this family of compounds in reducing the sizes of MEPs to TMS could result from enhanced presynaptic inhibition of the PTNs. It is important to note, however, that the same compound also produced some reduction in MEP size to TES, although, as pointed out earlier, part of the MEP response to the latter may also include indirect presynaptic excitation of PTNs.

Zentner[100] suggests that monitoring motor conduction is a useful indicator of the integrity of the central motor pathways during neurosurgical operations. In his studies, the motor cortex was stimulated by means of high-voltage electrical stimulation and recordings carried out from the thenar and tibialis anterior muscles. Changes in latency were not as helpful an indicator as reductions in the sizes of the electromyographic response, reductions exceeding 50% providing a useful indicator of dysfunction in the spinal cord in the course of surgery. Reduction in amplitude exceeding 50% were necessary because of the known effects of anesthetic agents on neuromuscular and spinal synaptic transmission. Haghighi and Oro[101] compared the value of somatosensory evoked potentials and cortical stimulus evoked motor responses as monitors of spinal cord function in the presence of hypotension. Hypovolemic hypotensive shock increased the latencies and reduced the sizes of both somatosensory evoked potentials and cortical stimulus evoked motor responses but were more sensitive than the former to hypotension.

Volleys may readily be recorded by epidural or even surface electrodes in the spinal region in response to motor cortical stimulation.[27] Monitoring changes in the latter D and I waves[102] from the spinal cord as well as MEPs has proved to be a helpful monitoring tool in conditions such as spinal cord compression,[27] trauma,[103–105] ischemia of the central nervous system including the spinal cord,[106,107] hypotension,[101] or direct operative invasion of the spinal cord.[27,67]

Safety

With two exceptions to date, no significant adverse effects have been reported in response to supramaximal electrical or magnetoelectrical stimulation of the brain, spinal cord, or peripheral nerve trunks. Kandler[108] has reported the rare induction of seizures following magnetoelectrical stimulation of the brain in stroke and epilepsy cases. In the case of high-voltage electrical stimulation using voltages as high as 750 volts with very short time constants of 150 μs or less, the energy delivered is simply too small to injure neural tissue directly. Trains of high-voltage electrical stimulation maintained over several hours may, however, be sufficient to injure neuronal tissue.[109] No changes in the electroencephalogram have been observed following as many as 250 electrical stimuli of the order of 750 volts and of 100 μs

duration,[110] and no histopathologic changes have been observed under the light microscope in neural tissues subjected to repeated direct cortical stimulation of the human brain.[111] Similarly, studies of the safety of magnetoelectrical stimulation in cats[112] have shown no systematic changes in sensory evoked potentials, the electroencephalogram, blood pressure, blood rate, or cerebral blood flow. In humans, no kindling effect has been shown in response to stimulus frequencies of less than 3 c/s.[54] Bridgers and Deleney[113] were unable to show any changes in the electroencephalogram or cognitive functions following repeated magnetoelectrical stimulation at the vertex. A small reduction in serum prolactin level was sometimes observed, but the level did not correlate with the number of stimuli. Estimates of maximum charge densities covered by magnetoelectrical stimuli suggests that the charge density is $\frac{1}{100}$ or less of the threshold charge density required for neural injury by direct electrical stimulation of the brain.[109,114,115]

REFERENCES

1. Penfield W, Boldrey E. Somatic motor and sensory representation in the cerebral cortex of man as studied by electrical stimulation. Brain 1937; 60:389–443.
2. Milner-Brown HS, Girvin JP, Brown WF. The effects of motor cortical stimulation on the excitability of spinal motoneurons in man. Can J Neurol Sci 1975; 2:245–253.
3. Merton PA, Morton HB. Stimulation of the cerebral cortex in the intact human subject. Nature 1980; 285:227.
4. Patton HD, Amassian VE. The pyramidal tract: Its excitation and function. In: Magoun HW, ed. Handbook of physiology. Section 1, Neurophysiology. Washington D.C.: American Physiological Society, 1960:837–861.
5. Phillips CG, Porter R. Corticospinal neurones. Monographs of the Physiological Society No. 34. London: Academic Press, 1977.
6. Amassian VE, Stewart M, Quirk GJ, Rosenthal JL. Physiological basis of motor effects of a transient stimulus to cerebral cortex. Neurosurgery 1987; 20:74–93.
7. Kuypers HGJM. Anatomy of the descending pathways. In: Brooks VB, ed. Handbook of physiology. VII Motor Control, Part 1. Washington D.C.: American Physiological Society, 1981:597–666.
8. Wilson VJ, Peterson BW. Vestibulospinal and reticulospinal systems. In: Brooks VB, ed. Handbook of physiology. VII Motor Control, Part 1. Washington D.C.: American Physiological Society, 1981:667–702.

9. Asanuma H. The pyramidal tract. In: Brooks VB, ed. Handbook of physiology. VII Motor Control, Part 1. Washington D.C.: American Physiological Society, 1981:703–733.
10. Krnjevic K. Transmitters in motor systems. In: Brooks VB, ed. Handbook of physiology. VII Motor Control, Part 1. Washington D.C.: American Physiological Society, 1981:107–154.
11. Phillips CG. Motor apparatus of the baboon's hand. Proc R Soc B 1969; 173:141–174.
12. Asanuma H. The motor cortex. New York: Raven Press, 1989.
13. Wiesendanger M. The pyramidal tract. Recent investigations on its morphology and function. Ergebn Physiol 1969; 61:72–136.
14. Merton PA, Hill DK, Morton HB, Marsden CD. Scope of a technique for electrical stimulation of human brain, spinal cord, and muscle. Lancet 1982; 2:597–600.
15. Marsden CD, Merton PA, Morton HB. Direct electrical stimulation of corticospinal pathways through the intact scalp in human subjects. Adv Neurol 1983; 39:387–391.
16. Robinson LR, Jantra P, Mackan IC. Central motor conduction times using transcranial stimulation and F wave latencies. Muscle Nerve 1988; 11:174–180.
17. Rothwell JC, Thompson PD, Day BL, et al. Motor cortex stimulation in intact man. 1. General characteristics of EMG responses in different muscles. Brain 1987; 110:1173–1190.
18. Rossini PM, Caramia M, Zarola F. Mechanisms of nervous propagation along central motor pathways: Non-invasive evaluation in healthy subjects and in patients with neurological diseases. Neurosurgery 1987; 20:183–191.

19. Rossini PM, Gigli GL, Marciani MG, et al. Non-invasive nervous propagation along 'central' motor pathways in intact man: Characteristics of motor responses to 'bifocal' and 'unifocal' spine and scalp non-invasive stimulation. Electroencephalogr Clin Neurophysiol 1987; 66:88–100.

20. Rossini PM, Caramia M, Zarola F. Central motor tract propagation in man: Studies with non-invasive, unifocal, scalp stimulation. Brain Res 1987; 415:211–225.

21. Calancie B, Nordin M, Wallin U, Habbarth K. Motor unit responses in human wrist flexor and extensor muscles to transcranial cortical stimuli. J Neurophysiol 1987; 58:1168–1185.

22. Benecke R, Meyer BU, Gohmann M, Conrad B. Analysis of muscle responses elicited by transcranial stimulation of the cortico-spinal system in man. Electroenceph Clin Neurophysiol 1988; 69:412–422.

23. Abbruzzese G, Dall'agata D, Morena M, et al. Electrical stimulation of the motor tracts in cervical spondylosis. J Neurol Neurosurg Psychiat 1988; 51:796–802.

24. Hassan NF, Rossini PM, Cracco RQ, Cracco JB. Unexposed motor cortex activation by low voltage stimuli. In: Morocutti C, Rizzo PA, eds. Evoked potentials. Neurophysiological and clinical aspects. Amsterdam: Elsevier, 1985:107–113.

25. Rossini PM, Di Stefano E, Stanzione P. Nerve impulse propagation along central and peripheral fast conduction motor and sensory pathways in man. Electroencephalogr Clin Neurophysiol 1985; 60:320–334.

26. Rossini PM, Marciani MG, Caramia M, et al. Nervous propagation along "central" motor pathways in intact man: Characteristics of motor responses to "bifocal" and "unifocal" spine and scalp non-invasive stimulation. Electroencephalogr Clin Neurophysiol 1985; 61:272–286.

27. Levy WJ, York DH, McCafferey M, Tanzer F. Motor evoked potentials from transcranial stimulation of the motor cortex in humans. Neurosurgery 1984; 15:287–302.

28. Day BL, Rothwell JC, Thompson PD, et al. Motor cortex stimulation in intact man. 2. Multiple descending volleys. Brain 1987; 110:1191–1209.

29. Henneman E, Somjen G, Carpenter DO. Functional significance of cell size in spinal motoneurons. J Neurophysiol 1965; 28:460–580.

30. Henneman E, Mendell LM. Functional organization of motoneuron pool and its inputs. In: Brooks VB, ed. Handbook of physiology. VII Motor Control, Part I. Washington D.C.: American Physiological Society, 1981:423–507.

31. Burke D, Hicks RG, Stephen JPH. Corticospinal volleys evoked by anodal and cathodal stimulation of the human motor cortex. J Physiol 1990; 425:283–299.

32. Edgley SA, Eyre JA, Lemon RN, Miller S. At what level is the corticospinal pathway excited by electromagnetic and percutaneous electrical stimulation of the brain? Evidence from the anaesthetized macaque monkey. J Physiol 1990; 420:47p.

33. Gandevia SC, Plassman BL. Responses in human intercostal and truncal muscles to motor cortical and spinal stimulation. Resp Physiol 1988; 73:325–338.

34. Gandevia SC, Rothwell JC. Activation of the human diaphragm from the motor cortex. J Physiol 1987; 384:109–118.

35. Gandevia SC, Applegate C. Activation of neck muscles from the human motor cortex. Brain 1988; 111:801–813.

36. Murphy K, Mier A, Adams L, Guz A. Putative cerebral cortical involvement in the ventilatory response to inhaled CO_2 in conscious man. J Physiol 1990; 420:1–18.

37. Hess CW, Mills KR. Low threshold motor units in human hand muscles can be selectively activated by magnetic brain stimulation. J Physiol 1986; 380:62p.

38. Hess CW, Mills KR, Murray NMF. Responses in small hand muscles from magnetic stimulation of the human brain. J Physiol 1987; 388:397–419.

39. Zidar J, Trontelj JV, Mihelin M. Percutaneous stimulation of human corticospinal tract: A single fiber study of individual motor unit responses. Brain Res 1987; 422:196–199.

40. Boniface SJ, Mills KR, Schubert M. Responses of single spinal motoneurons to magnetic brain stimulation in healthy subjects and patients with multiple sclerosis. Brain 1991; 114:643–662.

41. Mills KR. Magnetic brain stimulation: A tool to explore the action of the motor cortex on single human spinal motoneurones. Trends Neurosci 1991; 14:401–405.

42. Mills KR, Murray NMF. Electrical stimulation over the human vertebral column: Which neural elements are excited? Electroenceph Clin Neurophysiol 1986; 63:582–589.

43. Plassman BL, Gandevia SC. High voltage stimulation over the human spinal cord: Sources of latency variation. J Neurol Neurosurg Psychiat 1989; 52:213–217.

44. Berardelli A, Cowan JMA, Day BL, et al. The site of facilitation of the response to cortical stimulation during voluntary contraction in man. J Physiol 1985; 360:52p.

45. Hess CW, Mills KR, Murray NMF. Magnetic stimulation of the human brain: Facilitation of motor responses by voluntary contraction of ipsilateral and contralateral muscles with additional observation on an amputee. Neurosci Lett 1986; 71:235–240.

46. Amassian VE, Cracco RQ. Human cerebral cortical responses to contralateral transcranial stimulation. Neurosurgery 1987; 20:148–155.

47. Rossini PM, Caramia M. Methodological and phys-

iological considerations on the electric or magnetic transcranial stimulation. In: Rossini PM, Marsden CD, eds. Non-invasive stimulation of brain and spinal cord: Fundamentals and clinical applications. New York: Alan R. Liss, 1988:37–65.

48. Deletis V, Dimitrijevic MR, Sherwood AM. Effects of electrically induced afferent input from limb nerve on the excitability of the human motor cortex. Neurosurgery 1987; 20:195–197.

49. Troni W, Cantello R, De Mattei M, Bergamini L. Muscle responses elicited by cortical stimulation in the human hand: Differential conditioning by activation of the proprioceptive and exteroceptive fibers of the median nerve. In: Rossini PM, Marsden CD, eds. Non-invasive stimulation of brain and spinal cord: Fundamentals and clinical applications. New York: Alan R. Liss, 1988:73–83.

50. Komori T, Watson BV, Brown WF. Influence of peripheral afferents to cortical and spinal motoneuron excitability. Muscle Nerve 1992; 15:48–51.

51. McCaffrey M, Erickson JP. Modulation of cat motor evoked potential by prior cerebellar or somatosensory stimulation. Neurosurgery 1987; 20:193–195.

52. Polson MJR, Barker AT, Freeston IL. Stimulation of nerve trunks with time varying magnetic fields. Med Biol Engineer Comput 1982; 20:112–124.

53. Barker AT, Jalinous R, Freestone IL. Non-invasive magnetic stimulation of human motor cortex. Lancet 1985; 1:1106–1107.

54. Barker AT, Freeston IL, Jalinous R, Jarratt JA. Clinical evaluation of conduction time measurements in central motor pathways using magnetic stimulation of human brain. Lancet 1986; 1:1325–1326.

55. Barker AT, Freeston IL, Jalinous R, Jarratt JA. Magnetic stimulation of the human brain and peripheral nervous system: An introduction and the results of an initial clinical evaluation. Neurosurgery 1987; 20:100–109.

56. Nai-Shin Chu. Motor evoked potentials with magnetic stimulation: Correlations with height. Electroencephalogr Clin Neurophysiol 1989; 74:481–485.

57. Rosler KM, Hess CW, Heckmann R, Ludin HP. Significance of shape and size of the stimulating coil in magnetic stimulation of the human motor cortex. Neurosci Lett 1989; 100:347–352.

58. Amassian VE, Cracco RQ, Maccabee PJ. Focal stimulation of human cerebral cortex with the magnetic coil: A comparison with electrical stimulation. Electroencephalogr Clin Neurophysiol 1989; 74:401–416.

59. Epstein CM, Schwartzberg DG, Davey KR, Sudderth DB. Localizing the site of magnetic brain stimulation in humans. Neurology 1990; 40:666–670.

60. Cohen LG, Bradley JR, Nilsson J, et al. Effects of coil design on delivery of focal magnetic stimulation. Technical considerations. Electroencephalogr Clin Neurophysiol 1990; 75:350–357.

61. Claus D, Murray NMF, Soitzer A, Flugel D. The influence of stimulus type on the magnetic excitation of nerve structures. Electroencephalogr Clin Neurophysiol 1990; 75:342–349.

62. Britton TC, Meyer BU, Herdmann J, Benecke R. Clinical use of the magnetic stimulator in the investigation of peripheral conduction time. Muscle Nerve 1990; 13:396–406.

63. Evans BA, Litchy WJ, Daube JR. The utility of magnetic stimulation for routine peripheral nerve conduction studies. Muscle Nerve 1988; 11:1074–1078.

64. Chokroverty S. Magnetic stimulation of the human peripheral nerves. Electromyogr Clin Neurophysiol 1989; 29:409–416.

65. Cohen LG, Hallett M. Methodology for non-invasive mapping of human motor cortex with electrical stimulation. Electroencephalogr Clin Neurophysiol 1988; 69:403–411.

66. Cohen LG, Hallett M. Non-invasive mapping of human motor cortex. Neurology 1988; 38:904–909.

67. Katayama Y, Tsubokawa T, Maejima S, et al. Corticospinal direct response in humans: Identification of the motor cortex during intracranial surgery under general anaesthesia. J Neurol Neursurg Psychiat 1988; 51:50–59.

68. Inghilleri M, Berardelli A, Cruccu G, et al. Corticospinal potentials after transcranial stimulation in humans. J Neurol Neurosurg Psychiat 1989; 52:970–974.

69. Day BL, Dressler D, Maertens de Noordhout A, et al. Electric and magnetic stimulation of human motor cortex: Surface guide and single motor unit responses. J Physiol 1989; 412:449–473.

70. Schonle PW, Isenberg C, Crozier TA, et al. Changes of transcranially evoked motor responses in man by midazolam, a short acting benzodiazepine. Neurosci Lett 1989; 101:321–324.

71. Claus D. Central motor conduction: Method and normal results. Muscle Nerve 1990; 13:1125–1132.

72. Cowan JMA, Rothwell JC, Dick JPR, et al. Abnormalities in central motor pathway conduction in multiple sclerosis. Lancet 1984; 2:304–307.

73. Hugon J, Lubeau M, Tabaraud F, et al. Central motor conduction in motor neuron disease. Ann Neurol 1987; 22:544–546.

74. Mills KR, Murray NMF. Corticospinal tract conduction time in multiple sclerosis. Ann Neurol 1985; 18:601–605.

75. Ingram DA, Thompson AJ, Swash M. Central motor conduction in multiple sclerosis: Evaluation of abnormalities revealed by transcutaneous magnetic stimulation of the brain. J Neurol Neurosurg Psychiat 1988; 51:487–494.

76. Hess CW, Mills KR, Murray NMF, Schriefer TN. Magnetic brain stimulation: Central motor conduction studies in multiple sclerosis. Ann Neurol 1987; 22:744–752.

77. Snooks SJ, Swash M. Motor conduction velocity in the human spinal cord: Slowed conduction in multiple sclerosis and radiation myelopathy. J Neurol Neurosurg Psychiat 1985; 48:1135–1139.

78. Berardelli A, Inghilleri M, Formisano R, Accornero N. Stimulation of motor tracts in motor neuron disease. J Neurol Neurosurg Psychiat 1987; 50:732–737.

79. Ingram DA, Swash M. Central motor conduction is abnormal in motor neuron disease. J Neurol Neurosurg Psychiat 1987; 50:159–166.

80. Eisen A, Shytbel W, Murphy K, Hoirch M. Cortical magnetic stimulation in amyotrophic lateral sclerosis. Muscle Nerve 1990; 13:146–151.

81. Pringle CE, Hudson AJ, Munoz DG, et al. Primary lateral sclerosis. Brain 1992; 115:495–520.

82. Brown WF, Ebers GC, Hudson AJ, et al. Motor evoked responses in primary lateral sclerosis. Muscle Nerve 1992; 15:626–629.

83. Bentivoglio P, Branston NM, Symon L. Changes in pyramidal tract conduction with brain-stem ischaemia in baboons. J Physiol 1986; 380:57.

84. Berardelli A, Inghilleri M, Manfredi M, et al. Cortical and cervical stimulation after hemispheric infarction. J Neurol Neurosurg Psychiat 1987; 50:861–865.

85. Macdonell RAL, Donnan GA, Bladin PF. A comparison of somatosensory evoked and motor evoked potentials in stroke. Ann Neurol 1989; 25:68–73.

86. Dick JPR, Cowan JMA, Day BL et al. The cortico motoneurone connection is normal in Parkinson's disease. Nature 1984; 310:407–409.

87. Thompson PD, Dick JPR, Asselman P, et al. Examination of motor function in lesion of the spinal cord by stimulation of the motor cortex. Ann Neurol 1987; 21:389–396.

88. Claus D, Harding AE, Hess CW, et al. Central motor conduction in degenerative ataxic disorders: A magnetic stimulation study. J Neurol Neurosurg Psychiat 1988; 51:790–795.

89. Claus D, Waddy HM, Harding AE, et al. Hereditary motor and sensory neuropathy and hereditary spastic paraplegia: A magnetic stimulation study. Ann Neurol 1990; 28:43–49.

90. Berger AR, Busis NA, Logigian EL, et al. Cervical root stimulation in the diagnosis of radiculopathy. Neurology 1987; 37:329–332.

91. Chokroverty S, Sachdeo R, Dilullo J, Duvoisin RC. Magnetic stimulation in the diagnosis of lumbosacral radiculopathy. J Neurol Neurosurg Psychiat 1989; 52:767–772.

92. Thomas PK, Walker RWH, Rudge P, et al. Chronic demyelinating peripheral neuropathy associated with multifocal central nervous system demyelination. Brain 1987; 110:53–76.

93. Maccabee PJ, Amassian VE, Cracco RQ, Cracco JB. Intracranial stimulation of facial nerve in humans with the magnetic coil. Electroencephalogr Clin Neurophysiol 1988; 70:350–354.

94. Haghighi SS, Estrem SA. Estimation of facial central motor delay by electrical stimulation of the motor cortex of the dog. Electroencephalogr Clin Neurophysiol 1990; 75:82–87.

95. Schriefer TN, Mills KR, Murray NMF, Hess CW. Evaluation of proximal facial nerve conduction by transcranial magnetic stimulation. J Neurol Neurosurg Psychiat 1988; 51:60–66.

96. Tassinari CA, Michelucci R, Plasmati R, et al. Transcranial magnetic stimulation in epileptic patients: Usefulness and safety. Neurology 1990; 40:1132–1133.

97. Hufnagel A, Elger CE, Durmen HF, et al. Activation of the epileptic focus by transcranial magnetic stimulation of the human brain. Ann Neurol 1990; 27:49–60.

98. Zentner J, Ebner A. Nitrous oxide suppress the electromyographic response evoked by electrical stimulation of the motor cortex. Neurosurgery 1989; 24:60–62.

99. Zentner J, Kiss I, Ebner A. Influence of anesthetics —nitrous oxide in particular—on electromyographic response evoked by transcranial electrical stimulation of the cortex. Neurosurgery 1989; 24:253–256.

100. Zentner J. Noninvasive motor evoked potential monitoring during neurosurgical operations on the spinal cord. Neurosurgery 1989; 24:709–712.

101. Haghighi SS, Oro JJ. Effects of hypovolemic hypotensive shock on somatosensory and motor evoked potentials. Neurosurgery 1989; 24:246–252.

102. Boyd SG, Rothwell JC, Cowan JMA, et al. A method of monitoring function in corticospinal pathways during scoliosis surgery with a note on motor conduction velocities. J Neurol Neurosurg Psychiat 1986; 49:251–257.

103. Fehlings MG, Tator CH, Linden RD, Piper IR. Motor evoked potentials recorded from normal and spinal cord-injured rats. Neurosurgery 1987; 20:125–130.

104. Simpson RK, Baskin DS. Corticomotor evoked potentials in acute and chronic blunt spinal cord injury in the rat: Correlation with neurological outcome and histological damage. Neurosurgery 1987; 20:131–137.

105. Levy WJ, McCafferey M, Hagichi S. Motor evoked potential as a predictor of recovery in chronic spinal cord injury. Neurosurgery 1987; 20:138–142.

106. Konrad E, Taaker WA, Levy WJ, et al. Motor evoked potentials in a dog: Effect of global ischemia on spinal cord and peripheral nerve signals. Neurosurgery 1987; 20:117–124.

107. Simpson RK Jr, Baskin DS. Early component changes in corticomotor evoked potentials following experimental stroke. Stroke 1987; 18:1141–1147.

108. Kandler R. Safety of transcranial magnetic stimulation. Lancet 1990; 1:335:469–470.

109. Agnew WF, McCreery DB. Considerations for safety in the case of extracranial stimulation for motor evoked potentials. Neurosurgery 1987; 20:143–147.

110. Cohen LG, Hallet M. Cortical stimulation does not cause short-term changes in the electroencephalogram. Ann Neurol 1987; 21:512:513.

111. Gordon B, Lesser RP, Rance NE, et al. Parameters for direct cortical electrical stimulation in the human: Histopathologic confirmation. Electroencephalogr Clin Neurophysiol 1990; 75:371.

112. Eyre JA, Flecknell PA, Kenyon BR, et al. Acute effects of electromagnetic stimulation of the brain on cortical activity, cortical blood flow, blood pressure and heart rate in the cat: An evaluation of safety. J Neurol Neurosurg Psychiat 1990; 53:507–513.

113. Bridgers SL, Deleney RC. Transcranial magnetic stimulation: An assessment of cognitive and other cerebral effects. Neurology 1989; 39:417–419.

114. Yuen TGH, Agnew WF, Bullara LA, et al. Histological evaluation of neural damage from electrical stimulation: Considerations for the selection of parameters for clinical application. Neurosurgery 1981; 9:292–299.

115. Agnew WF, Yuen TGH, McCreery DB. Morphologic changes after prolonged electrical stimulation of the cat's cortex at defined charge densities. Exper Neurol 1983; 79:397–411.

2

Tremor

Jack H. Petajan

CONTENTS

LIST OF ACRONYMS

AT	action tremor
CNS	central nervous system
CPT	corticopallidothalamic
EEG	electroencephalogram
EMG	electromyography
ET	essential tremor
FDI	first dorsal interosseous
IT	intention tremor
OC	olivocerebellar
PT	physiologic tremor
RS	reticulospinal
RT	resting tremor
SMU	single motor unit
SND	striatonigral degeneration
ST	spasmodic torticollis
VS	vestibulospinal

The clinical electromyographer will often encounter patients with tremor during the course of investigations of neuromuscular disorders. Tremor may be detected for the first time in this manner, so some knowledge of tremor can be useful to the electromyographer. Further, tremor occurring at minimal muscle contraction can mimic an altered recruitment pattern suggestive of a pathologic process resulting in a decreased number of motor units (MUs). Thus a knowledge of how tremor can influence electromyography (EMG) is essential to an accurate and reliable interpretation of findings. An analysis of MU behavior during tremor can provide important information regarding tremor mechanisms. The application of chemical lesioning, stereotactic lesions, and receptor blockade techniques in the central nervous system has added new insights to the understanding of tremor mechanisms.

DEFINITION OF TREMOR AND ITS MEASUREMENT

Tremor is a rhythmic oscillation of a body part. The term *rhythm* is defined as an event (movement, in this case) that occurs with a *regular recurrent pattern*. Casual exposure to a patient with tremor compels one to press this definition further. How is *regular* defined, since tremor frequency varies? Are tremor frequency and variability the same in all body parts? If tremor is present in the hands, do they move synchronously? Are there factors that alter frequency and amplitude of tremor, such as posture or effort? The confusion in terminology can be reduced by attending to such factors as the conditions under which tremor is observed.

Tremor is reported and measured in a variety of ways. EMG records the rhythmic MU activation that may be associated with tremor, but without a description of the mechanical characteristics of the tremor, the electromyographic findings may be misleading. For example, assume that fast flexor and slow extensor muscles are synchronously activated at 20 c/s. This rate is above the natural resonating frequency at the wrist of 9 c/s.[1] The rise time and peak force of contraction of muscles acting around the joint will determine whether or not movement occurs. Thus tremor cannot be defined completely on the basis of the rhythmic discharge of MUs or by measurement of the frequency of movement alone.

Using accelerometry, the dominant tremor rate recorded in the outstretched upper extremity is 10 c/s.[2] The term "rate" refers to the average periodicity of a recurring event that varies. "Frequency" is the term applied to an event that occurs precisely at the same time interval such as the output of an electrical signal generator. The derivative of the acceleration of a sinusoidal movement in millimeters per second squared (mm/s^2) emphasizes the higher frequency components because the acceleration increases as the square of tremor frequency in cycles per second.[3] Movement must accelerate more rapidly to accommodate more rapid tremor.

Complex movements can occur during tremor. Accelerometers measure movements in a given plane. An adequate mechanical description of the *pill rolling* hand tremor of Parkinson's disease would require measurements in three planes.[4] Other techniques of measurement have included the use of variable-capacitance transducers,[5] photo cells,[6] and force transducers, usually combined with surface recording of EMG.[7]

The rhythmic discharge of MUs constitutes only one aspect of the tremor phenomenon. The literature contains relatively few descriptions of single MU behavior in tremor, probably because such studies are quite difficult when tremor is vigorous. The recruitment pattern of MUs and their respective rates of firing are often impossible to discern when recruitment is full during a tremor burst. When tremor is less vigorous, such observations can be made. Sometimes tremor can be reduced by adjusting posture and promoting relaxation. Finally, the electromyographer will encounter patients who have a tendency to group MU potentials during minimal or moderate muscle contraction. These patients usually do not complain of tremor, yet their electromyograms do not differ significantly from those of patients with essential tremor (unpublished observations). This emphasizes that tremor is likely a common phenomenon and would support the view that essential tremor may be simply an amplification of physiologic tremor.

The resonating frequency of an object is inversely proportional to its mass. As inertia increases, more force is required to vibrate an object at any given frequency. If force is below a critical level sufficient to produce movement and the force is applied in an alternating sinusoidal fashion, no tremor occurs. Thus the electromyographer may detect MUs firing in rhythmic bursts in proximal muscles in the absence of apparent tremor. These findings may be present within the context of a movement disorder or other associated neurologic findings and can contribute to diagnosis. At other times, the findings may be present in relative isolation, unassociated with the pathology being examined but adding confusion to the diagnosis of a neuromuscular disorder.

ELECTRODIAGNOSTIC APPROACH TO TREMOR

Because the electromyographer may encounter tremor during examination of a patient, he or she should have a systematic approach to further evaluation of the tremor. Some suggestions follow:

1. Place the limb at complete rest and determine whether tremor is present. Record well-focused MU potentials on a strip chart at a speed of approximately 50 cm per second. Determine the time interval between tremor bursts and the pattern of MU recruitment from burst to burst. Obtain a surface recording from the same muscle.
2. Have the patient initiate minimal muscle contraction. Determine its influence on tremor frequency and amplitude. Assess the ease with which single MUs can be activated and recruited.
3. Determine the distribution of muscles participating in the tremor. Record from flexor and extensor muscles simultaneously at the same speed as given previously. This will allow measurement of the degree of synchrony between flexor and extensor tremor discharges. Records can also be made from the contralateral limb or muscle remote from those obviously involved, such as the tongue or diaphragm.
4. Posture and limb position can influence tremor. The patient should be examined in lying, sitting, and standing positions. Specific postures may elicit tremor; a semiflexed posture may bring out parkinsonian tremors.
5. A crude mechanical record of tremors can be made with a photocell or strain gauge. Accelerometers are also available but are usually not present in most EMG laboratories.
6. When appropriate, tremor should be measured while the subject performs an activity such as writing that may enhance tremor. For example, a digitizing tablet that quantifies tremor during writing has been used.[8]

DIFFERENT TYPES OF NORMAL PHYSIOLOGIC TREMORS

The discussion of different types of tremor consists first of a description of the tremor and the conditions under which it has been observed. Next the mechanisms responsible for the tremor are considered under the following headings: (1) central nervous system and, where possible, the results of chemical "lesioning" of the brain and neurotransmitters; (2) reflex—involving primarily spinal reflex mechanisms; (3) anatomic and mechanical factors; and (4) interactions between factors.

Physiologic Tremor

Definition

This tremor is not present in a completely relaxed extremity. A microtremor can be recorded from the limb exclusive of ballistocardiac effect and respiration. Its frequency is approximately 10 c/s, which is also that of earth vibration.[9] MU activity is required for the appearance of physiologic tremor. It appears when a limb is maintained in space against gravity. In the fingers, this tremor is 8 to 12 c/s in young adults but decreases in frequency in children and the elderly.[1,2] In some individuals, the tremor is so fine that it can just be detected with the naked eye. In others, especially following exercise, under conditions of emotional excitement, or use of β_2-receptor agonists such as those used in the treatment of asthma,[149] tremor of the outstretched hands is easily seen. The tremor is seen in the distal extremities where resonance with the 10 c/s muscle contraction is possible.

Electromyographic features

At low levels of tremor, an orderly recruitment of MUs is seen, with some units firing repetitively at high rates (greater than 60 c/s) when tremor amplitude increases. Firing in agonist-antagonist muscles is not synchronous, but tremor bursts often overlap.

Central nervous system

Physiologic tremor depends on the maintenance of posture, with the tremor increasing in amplitude and decreasing in frequency with slow movement. Participation of suprasegmental motor control systems is suggested by the influence of voluntary movement on these tremor characteristics and the observation that tremors in the range of 5 c/s are generated from such central nervous system structures as the basal ganglia and may use long loop reflexes (see later). Tremor is present, however, in the limbs of patients with spasticity associated with decorticate, decerebrate, and spinal postures, not including clonus.

Tremor is also present in muscles caudal to the level of spinal transection in cats.[10] Detailed electromyographic studies of tremor under these conditions need to be done.

In normal control subjects, physiologic tremor can be enhanced by slight voluntary muscle contraction and the Jendrassik maneuver (forceful isometric muscle contraction) remote from the region of interest. Other factors that enhance physiologic tremor include increased metabolic rate, fatigue, anxiety, alcoholism, and the administration of epinephrine.[3] Central catecholamine mechanisms, most likely involving noradrenaline, may play a role in physiologic tremor. The wide distribution of these systems emanating from the locus ceruleus and lateral tegmental systems makes them good candidates for involvement in such generalized motor phenomena.[11]

The basic rhythm of electroencephalography (EEG) is in a range identical to that of physiologic tremor. There is a poor correlation, however, between alpha rhythm and physiologic tremor; also physiologic tremor is not synchronous between various body parts.[12-14] On the other hand, photic stimulation provided at a frequency close to the subject's alpha rhythm (10 cycles per second ± 0.35 SD) and physiologic tremor of the finger (10.3 cycles per second ± 0.68 SD) reveals a positive correlation coefficient of 0.49 ± 0.14 SD and, under the spontaneous condition 0.13 ± 0.16 SD, an effect considered significant at the P <0.05 level.[15] These results were interpreted as supporting the hypothesis of a functional relationship between the two mechanisms.

Spinal reflex and other mechanisms

Experiments involving muscle contraction and tremor recording against compliant and fixed resistances and tendon vibration support the concept that spindle Ia afferents play a role in physiologic tremor.[16] Such techniques permit experimental manipulation of muscle length and tension during tremor recording or direct activation of Ia afferents by tendon vibration. Instability in the spindle Ia servomechanism can elicit tremor.[17-20] Physiologic tremor is absent in tabes dorsalis,[21] presumably because this disorder selectively interrupts afferent input to the spinal cord; Ia afferents are disconnected. Contrary to the spindle servomechanism concept is the observation that tremor frequency is the same regardless of muscle location and length of reflex pathway.[22] Some observers have reported persistence of physiologic tremor in deafferented limbs[23] or with interruption of the stretch reflex.[22,24] The completeness of deafferentation has been questioned in these cases.[11]

Patients have been examined under a variety of experimental conditions. When maintaining the foot in a position of sustained plantar flexion, a tremor of 6 to 9 c/s was recorded.[25] When slowly raising and lowering the heel, the tremor frequency changed to 4 to 8 c/s.[25] The latter tremor has been termed a *physiologic action tremor*. Flexion of the elbow against a compliant resistance (spring) has been found to yield a peak tremor frequency determined by analysis of force and surface electromyographic oscillations, both of which were highly correlated. High force levels were associated with high tremor amplitude. When flexing the elbow against an unyielding resistance, no peak tremor frequency was found.[7] The results were believed to support the view that the tremor present with compliant loading of the arm is due to the stretch reflex. Compliant loading would permit a physical amplification of the length changes in muscle when it is sustaining load. In further experiments using elbow flexion against a compliant resistance, tendon vibration of agonist or antagonist leading to greater Ia afferent activity increased tremor amplitude. Tremor bursts recorded by EMG were 180 degrees out of phase. The stretch reflex, dynamic Ia afferents using a spinal dissynaptic inhibitory pathway, was believed to be the best explanation for the phenomenon. The influence of voluntary muscle contraction, that is, a corresponding increase in Ia afferent activity, on stretch reflex amplitude was believed to be a similar phenomenon.[7]

Recordings of single MUs during slowly increasing muscle contraction have revealed increased synchronization of MU firing that may be very prominent in some subjects in the absence of obvious tremor. In proximal flexor muscles, recruitment or the addition of other MUs participating in contraction occurs when firing rates reach nearly 10 c/s. Examination of all the MUs firing as the limb is held against gravity (position of function) reveals each to be firing at or very near physiologic tremor frequency.[26] In extensor muscles, recruitment frequency was slightly higher. The probability of synchronization is statistically increased when all MUs participating in maintaining the antigravity posture within a given muscle are firing at or near the same frequency. This frequency is at the upper limit of the primary range of firing.

Single studies have also disclosed interesting interactive aspects of MU firing. At the moment of recruitment or when several MUs fire closely together, as in the production of a small ballistic con-

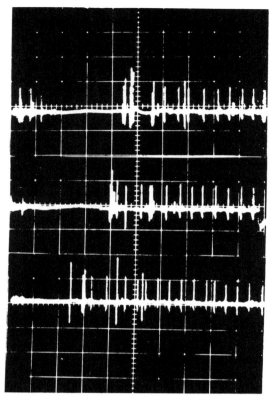

"CLICK" OFF - ON

NORMAL SUBJECT

DOUBLE BALLISTIC RESPONSE
IN I.D.I.

200 ms/cm

FIGURE 2.1.   *Single motor units (MUs) recorded from first dorsal interosseous are shown. The subject is attempting to maintain firing in first recruited single MU during recruitment of a second, higher threshold single MU. He is instructed to reduce effort instantaneously when recruitment occurs and to continue firing the first recruited unit. A pause in firing consistently occurs in all subjects, such that the next expected first recruited single MU does not appear. The* microballistic *activation of two or more single MUs resulting in a silent period is seen during which single MUs cannot be voluntarily activated.*

traction (a rectangular increase in force), an inhibition of MU firing is observed.[27] This was most easily seen when only two MUs were firing. This phenomenon is likely analogous to the silent period following sudden loading of a muscle during sustained contraction. When unit two fired immediately following unit one, the next firing of unit one was delayed. The nearly synchronous firing of two or more MUs and the resultant delay are identical to a *microballistic* activation of MUs followed by a silent period (Figure 2.1). The recruitment of larger MUs and their temporal proximity of firing are even more likely to produce synchronization and tremor. Possible mechanisms include spinal recurrent inhibition, interruptions of spindle afferent discharge, and activation of

Ib tendon organ afferents. All of these systems could be sites for β-adrenergic receptor activation, which could make the tremor susceptible to adrenergic influence.

In a detailed study of the outstretched "pointing" finger, Lippold[20] concluded that "physiological tremor in the 8 to 12 cycles per second band is due to the oscillation in the stretch reflex servo-loop." In his experiments, the outstretched finger was set into oscillation by a brief stepwise displacement. The sinusoidal movements that followed in the range of physiologic tremor, were accompanied by an appropirate burst of EMG, and did not dampen as expected if the oscillation occurred purely on a mechanical basis. In addition, the tremor produced was influenced in exactly the same manner as physiologic tremor by temperature change and ischemia. Ischemia has been reported by some investigators not to interrupt physiologic tremor. Ischemia was sufficient to interrupt the stretch reflex arc. Again, such experiments may not result in complete spindle deafferentation.

Physiologic tremor and intention tremor amplitude have been shown to increase under conditions of increased barometric pressure. Adaptation to the condition was noted for physiologic tremor by day 8, but no adaptation occurred for intention tremor.[28] It has been proposed that high atmospheric pressure reduces muscarinic recurrent Renshaw inhibition, leaving the motoneurons hyperexcitable.[10]

Synchronization of MUs in wrist extensor muscles was determined for physiologic tremor, enhanced physiologic tremor following administration of terbutaline, and voluntary wrist flexion-extension movement. Increased synchronization was found for enhanced physiologic tremor and still greater synchronization for voluntary tremor. For enhanced physiologic tremor, the increased synchronization was believed to result from increased muscle spindle afferent activity from both flexor and extensor muscles. For voluntary tremor, supraspinal and segmental common synaptic input onto motoneurons was believed to be at or near maximum.[29] The data fit best the model of transmembrane current generating repetitive firing in motoneurons first at low inherent levels of repetitive firing, then at progressively higher levels with some montoneurons firing at very high rates, resulting from failure to repolarize. According to the model, synchronization in firing also occurred when collaterals from supraspinal neurons contacted two or more different motoneurons in the same pool.

Mechanical and other factors

Physiologic tremor is most apparent in the distal extremities because of the higher resonating frequencies of their parts, such as the fingers. With advancing age, tremor frequency slows and may be observed in more proximal muscles, including the head. Phonation may be influenced by tremor.

The heartbeat has been considered an energy source for physiologic tremor. Body parts such as the fingers can resonate at 8 to 12 c/s under conditions of complete denervation as a result of mechanical vibration transmitted from other parts of the body.[1] An analysis of tremor in multiple body parts using cross-correlation analysis for detection of tremor coherence has led investigators to conclude

that less than 10% of tremor results from the heartbeat.[15]

Summary and interaction of factors

Inertial properties of the limb and the tendency for MUs to group or fire more synchronously at or about the recruitment frequency during sustained minimal or moderate muscle contraction are responsible for physiologic tremor. Spinal reflex mechanisms with positive feedback, the dynamic spindle servoloop, and conduction delays of reciprocal inhibition and as yet poorly understood connections between motoneurons may be responsible for the synchronization of MU firing. Physiologic tremor and the slight reduction in frequency of tremor that occurs with intention, physiologic action tremor, varies somewhat from subject to subject and in its most intense form may become essential tremor.

Shivering

Human subjects exposed to cold experience involuntary tonic muscle contraction that favors a flexed posture. This muscle contraction has been termed *thermomuscular tone*.[30] There is cocontraction of flexor and extensor muscles. As cooling progresses, bursts of more forceful muscle contraction occur that produce the tremor of shivering. The most effective cooling stimulus for shivering is direct cooling of the skin by evaporation, with shivering occurring rapidly when large areas of skin are cooled. The threshold for activation of shivering, however, is lowered by reduced core temperature. During administration of epidural anesthesia, shivering was observed to occur when tympanic membrane temperature fell by 0.5°C. Vasoconstriction preceded shivering, and there was no sensation of cold.[31] Epidural injectate temperature did not influence response.

Bursts of shivering last seconds and are noted first in the muscles of the head (masseter), neck, and shoulders, before appearing elsewhere. Basic tremor rate varies but is in the range of 5 to 10 c/s. As the tremor becomes more vigorous, the amplitude of the tremor increases, while the rate decreases.[30,32]

Motor unit behavior during shivering

Thermomuscular tone appears as the tonic firing of MUs that is no different from gradually increasing voluntary muscle contraction. When shivering occurs, bursts of large or high threshold, rapidly firing MUs are seen (Figure 2.2). Action potentials recorded from MUs participating in such bursts are usually of higher amplitude than those involved in

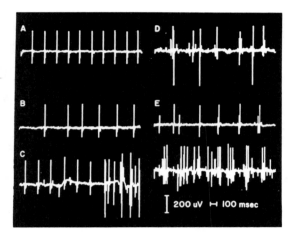

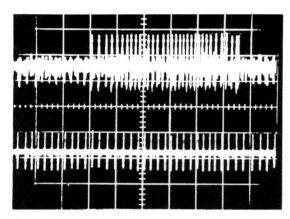

FIGURE 2.2. *(A) Preshivering tone in biceps. (B) Irregular firing in biceps motor unit just before shivering tremor. (C) Recruitment of motor units during shivering burst, which occurs at low stable frequency of primary unit in biceps. (D) Primary unit fires at slow rhythmic rate during recruitment, which accompanies the onset of shivering in biceps. (E) Biceps (upper record) and triceps (lower record) preshivering tone and shivering tremor develop earlier in triceps.*

FIGURE 2.3.   *Single motor unit recording of tonic preshivering tone and high-frequency burst are shown during the initiation of shivering tremor in triceps of human subject exposed to evaporative cooling. Sweep speed is 5 ms per division.*

thermomuscular tone, suggesting either a nearer signal generator or larger muscle fibers. Bursting units also require higher force levels for voluntary activation and fire more rapidly. Simultaneous recordings from biceps and triceps reveal that this bursting activity occurs first in triceps. The bursting units fire at or above the recruitment frequency. Tonic MUs already firing are recruited into the tremor bursts and appear to be paced by the larger units that initiate the tremor (Figure 2.3). As the tremor becomes more vigorous, the *pacer* units appear first in extensor muscles, which oppose the flexed posture.[33] Ideally shivering must permit some shortening of muscle that releases heat more effectively than isometric contraction but must not allow large movements of the limb, which would dissipate heat to the environment. The low-amplitude flexion-extension tremor of shivering, most apparent in proximal muscles, achieves this goal.[34]

Role of central nervous system

Shivering depends on the integrity of the posterolateral hypothalamus. The *shivering pathway* projects via the median forebrain bundle through the tegmentum of midbrain and pons, close to the rubrospinal tract to end on spinal motoneurons. Control is mediated through both corticospinal and reticulospinal pathways. Motoneurons under tonic control may have different connections from those responsible for shivering bursts. The noradrenergic system of the lateral tegmental tract and possibly the locus ceruleus may play a role in thermal regulation. Beta blockade, however, can abolish nonshivering thermogenesis, which is usually associated with an increase in shivering. Shivering persists following bilateral pyramidotomy.[35]

Spinal mechanisms

Direct cooling of the spinal cord causes increased motoneuron excitability and shivering. In the guinea pig, shivering is controlled by the temperature of C-6–T-1 spinal cord that in turn receives blood draining from interscapular areas of brown fat, which is a major source of nonshivering thermogenesis. Brown fat is an exceptionally large source of heat in the infant animal before the development of shivering. In the guinea pig, when nonshivering thermogenesis is inhibited by beta blockade, shivering then ensues.[35]

Thermomuscular tone can develop on exposure to cold following experimental dorsal rhizotomy, but shivering does not occur.[36] Hypothermia and failure to shiver have been demonstrated in the Lewis rat with hyperacute experimental allergic encephalomyelitis. No lesions were found in the hypothalamus incriminating spinal cord or peripheral nerves as responsible.[37] Muscle spindles themselves are sensitive to temperature,[38] with a maximum frequency of tonic firing occurring in the range of 25 to 30°C. Bursting phasic MUs may provide the perturbation necessary to activate the spinal servomechanism important for involving and sustaining the majority of tonic MUs in the shivering tremor. Bursts of large MUs scattered throughout the muscle would result in shortening of muscle spindles within the region of contraction, which in turn would influence the excitability of motoneuron maintaining local thermomuscular tone. As is the case with physiologic tremor, the filtering properties imposed by the mass of the limb determine the amplitude and rate of limb movements.

Interactive factors

The central nervous system controls tremor at suprasegmental and spinal levels. Shivering is initiated by high-frequency bursts of MUs, which may serve as the pacers for the development of tremor. Spinal servomechanisms, very likely, are responsible for maintaining the tremor activity that is initiated by the pacer units. Mechanical properties of the limb determine the tremor frequency and amplitude.

Tremor Resulting from Fatigue

During sustained muscle contraction, such as when maintaining the index finger in extension or the hand extended at the wrist for a period of minutes, a tremor develops. Following vigorous exercise that produces muscle fatigue, it is difficult to perform skilled movements because of increased tremor.

Accelerometric and electromyographic analysis of such tremors reveals that the amplitude of physiologic tremor (10 to 12 c/s) increases as a consequence of fatigue. The electromyographic power (integral of voltage versus time) at all physiologic tremor frequencies increases. As isometric muscle contraction is maintained over a period of minutes (15 to 45 minutes), a second peak in the 4 to 6 c/s range develops associated with a marked synchronization of MU firing. Surface electromyographic recordings reveal high-amplitude slow waves (W waves) with an appearance similar to the M wave resulting from supramaximal stimulation of motor nerve. The W waves result from essentially 100% synchronization of MU firing, which occurs following prolonged muscle contraction.[39]

Another interesting phenomenon that may bear on the development of tremor following prolonged contraction of muscle is that a slowing of firing rate of MUs occurs despite maintenance of maximal effort (Figure 2.4). This slowing is especially apparent in patients with corticospinal tract disease. The slowing in normal subjects occurs in conjunction with activation failure that most likely is related to slowed relaxation of muscle fibers and reduced conduction along muscle fiber sarcolemma or impaired action potential as fatigue develops. In other words, MU firing rate declines as the ability of the neuromuscular transmission-activation and contraction system to respond to the nerve impulses decreases. High-frequency direct stimulation of muscle results in rapid loss of tension that can be partially restored if the frequency of stimulation is reduced. The reduction in normal MU firing rate as muscle fatigue develops results in greater ability to maintain muscle tension. Following maximal voluntary contraction of biceps brachii and elbow flexed 45 degrees against gravity, few if any MU action potentials can be recorded.[40] This interesting central phenomenon has been termed the *wisdom* of the neuromuscular control system by Marsden.[41]

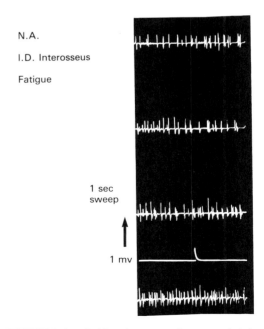

N.A.

I.D. Interosseus

Fatigue

1 sec sweep

1 mv

FIGURE 2.4. *Subject is attempting to maintain maximal effort in first dorsal interosseous muscle. Reduction in firing rate can be seen as effort is maintained.*

Central nervous system mechanisms

The great synchronization of MU firing resulting in the 4 to 6 c/s tremor during prolonged muscle contraction is in the frequency range of tremor generated from the basal ganglia, and oscillation in long loop reflexes may be involved. Experiments involving perturbations applied to the outstretched fingers demonstrate that the 4 to 6 c/s tremor results from oscillation in a long servoloop, probably involving basal ganglia, motor cortex, or both.[39]

Spinal reflex mechanisms

The enhanced 10 to 12 c/s tremor seen early during sustained muscle contraction is enhanced physiologic tremor dependent on the same spinal servoloop mechanisms as physiologic tremor. This fatigue tremor is influenced in an identical manner to physiologic tremor in response to mechanical perturbation, deafferentation, and limb cooling. The increased tremor is identical to that seen with adrenergic stimulation and may have an identical mechanism that results in increased MU recruitment in tremor bursts. The motoneuron facilitation resulting from the Jendrassik maneuver produces identical changes in physiologic tremor.

Interaction of factors and summary

Limb inertia influences the expression of fatigue tremor so the appearance of the 4 to 6 c/s tremor results in a higher amplitude tremor and the possibility for tremor in larger body parts when they are involved. The possibility that muscle properties are altered by sustained muscle contraction in a manner that could lead to slow oscillations has been investigated. Muscle twitch times were not changed following 1 hour of submaximal muscle contraction causing 4 to 6 c/s tremor.[39]

Spinal reflex mechanisms that cause physiologic tremor and responsive in an identical manner to adrenergic stimulation are responsible for the 10 to 12 c/s tremor seen in early stages of fatigue. The 4 to 6 c/s tremor appearing later may involve oscillations in long loop reflexes. The factors responsible for this central fatigue may be relevant to an understanding of pathologic tremors as well as fatigue seen in patients with pyramidal tract disease.

Pathologic Tremors

Essential tremor

Definition, prevalence, and clinical features. Essential tremor is not present at rest and appears under the same conditions as physiologic tremor. Its frequency is 8 to 10 c/s, with lower frequencies being present in the young and elderly. If intense, it can interfere with fine motor performance in a young person. On physical examination, the tremor is most easily detected in the outstretched fingers. It can be seen in the protruded tongue or heard in the voice. Handwriting or drawing a straight line may record a fine oscillation. In the elderly with tremor at lower frequency, more proximal muscles become involved, and the tremor is called *senile tremor*. It is sometimes confused with parkinsonian tremor, and some investigators believe that the two conditions may coexist more frequently than would be expected on a random basis.[42] Essential tremor is inherited as an autosomal dominant trait, which is one of the factors that accounts for its wide variability from person to person. It is likely that an electromyographic study of family members would disclose many with tremor, which is not of functional significance.

Electromyographic recording of essential tremor is best accomplished by a needle electrode in first dorsal interosseous during gentle abduction of the finger. Simultaneous recording from forearm flexors and extensors when the arm is held against gravity will also record characteristic tremor bursts.

Virtually all of the factors that make physiologic tremor worse also increase essential tremor, such as activation of the noradrenergic system. Conversely, conditions that decrease emotional excitement, such as the ingestion of antianxiety drugs, reduce the severity of tremor. Patients with disturbing essential tremor often learn that the ingestion of ethyl alcohol will substantially reduce the severity of tremor or even abolish it. As a consequence, the rate of alcoholism among patients with essential tremor is significantly higher than in a sex-matched and age-matched population.[43] These results emphasize the importance of treating disturbing and apparent tremor in a young person.

Prevalence of essential tremor has been investigated in a study of a rural biracial Mississippi county (Copiah County). Persons over 40 years of age were surveyed and included residents of households and institutions. An overall prevalance rate of 414.6 per 100,000 inhabitants was determined, with higher rates for women than men and for whites than blacks.[44] In a similar study of a rural Finnish population, a prevalence of 55.5% was determined on the basis of clinically established cases. The disease was more common in older age groups. In younger patients, the condition was more common in men than in women.[45] In a Chinese study of 258 cases of tremor, 46 patients had essential tremor: 65.8%

were male, 34.2% female. Mean age was 36 years (range 14 to 89 years). Hands were involved in all patients, with varying involvement of other muscles, such as orbicularis oris, muscle of phonation, etc. Thirty-two percent were familial.[46] The highly differing prevalence rates in these studies, and especially the high prevalence of tremor, strongly point toward a diagnosis of essential tremor in patients with an intense physiologic tremor. The results lend support to the view that physiologic tremor and essential tremor blend together and may in fact represent varying degrees of the same phenomenon.

In a Chinese study, essential tremor has been reported as associated with a variety of pathologic states, including parkinsonism,[47] Charcot-Marie-Tooth disease,[48] Tourette's syndrome,[49] buccolingual facial dyskinesia,[50] manic depressive illness associated with Klinefelter's syndrome,[51] dystonia with torticollis,[52] writing tremor,[114] spastic dysphonia,[53,54] and orthostatic tremor.[55] Unilateral essential tremor following limb trauma has been reported. A patient having vocal cord nodules and essential tremor has been described.[56] The authors suggest that some patients may receive recurrent laryngeal nerve resection for a disorder that is actually essential tremor and may respond to appropriate treatment.

The most effective treatment of essential tremor is beta blockade. Both nonspecific β-blockers such as propranolol and specific cardiac blockers such as atenolol suppress essential tremor (see later). The effectiveness of propranolol therapy decreases with time, and in 3 to 6 months the dose must be increased.[57] Primidone has been reported to be effective treatment.[58,59]

Role of central nervous system. In studies of physiologic tremor, Marsden et al.[23] have demonstrated that intraarterial isoproterenol infusion of the involved limb accentuates tremor, whereas intraarterial propranolol infusion suppresses physiologic tremor. In similar experiments by Young et al.[60] on essential tremor, infusion of propranolol was found to have no effect on the tremor. These results suggest that the role of β-adrenergic receptors in these two types of tremors is different. The magnitude of enhanced motoneuron excitability associated with essential tremor might be such that the effects of peripheral beta blockade could not be detected. The strong parallel between essential tremor and physiologic tremor cannot be ignored and suggests a common cause. Cerebellar blood flow is increased in patients with essential tremor.[61]

Reflex and spinal mechanisms. The frequency and amplitude of essential tremor can be reset by the same peripheral mechanical perturbations that alter physiologic tremor.[62] This strongly suggests that peripheral mechanisms play a role in tremor genesis.

Electromyographic features. In proximal and distal muscles, the EMG needle electrode records clusters of MUs firing at approximately the same rate: 8 to 10 c/s. It has been reported that tremor bursts occur synchronously in flexor and extensor muscles in essential tremor and that the order of recruitment of MUs in the tremor bursts is random[63] (Figure 2.5). Computer analysis of individual MU firing rates has demonstrated stable firing rate for individual MUs firing at near the mean tremor rate.[29]

In normal subjects, MUs are recruited in an orderly manner in both slow and fast voluntary muscle contractions. In general, small MUs are recruited before larger ones. In addition, the first recruited unit increases its firing rate to a given level, usually >10 c/s, before recruitment of a second unit. Increased firing rates in single MUs are associated with pathologic processes that reduce the number of units available for recruitment or cause spatial reorganization of the MU, such as reinnervation and the phenom-

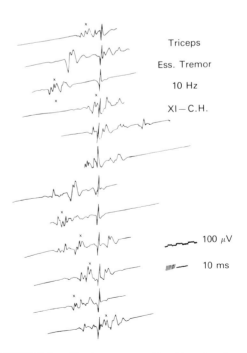

FIGURE 2.5. *Single motor units appearing in tremor bursts of triceps muscle are shown. Disordered recruitment is shown or indicated by varying position of x unit.*

enon of fiber type grouping.[64] In recordings from normal subjects imitating essential tremor, there is an orderly pattern of MU recruitment that is usually duplicated in each tremor burst. During very rapid contraction, single MUs may fire repetitively at high rates (>60 c/s).

The behavior of tremor bursts and the recruitment pattern are a function of the frequency and amplitude of the tremor. In general, tremors of lower frequency, most often seen in elderly patients, are more likely to exhibit alternating flexor and extensor tremor bursts and orderly recruitment of MUs. As the tremor amplitude increases, it becomes more vigorous. MUs may fire as in a ballistic contraction. Under these circumstances, single MUs will fire repetitively at high rates (>60 c/s), and the appearance of orderly recruitment within a tremor burst is lost.

Electrical stimulation of motor nerves producing muscle twitch in extensor indicis and tibialis anterior muscles causes an inhibition and synchronization of tremor with stimulation in essential tremor and Parkinson's disease. The duration of inhibition was 92.1 ± 6.8 ms for essential tremor and 183 ± 6.0 ms for Parkinson's disease. In parkinsonism, the inhibitory phase lasted longer if the muscle twitch was induced during the second half of the tremor cycle. The effect of voluntary contraction and unloading suggested that inhibition and resetting of the tremor cycle resulted from autogenic mechanisms mediated by Ib afferent discharge.[65]

Interaction of factors. Both central nervous and peripheral reflex mechanisms seem important in the genesis of essential tremor. The ability to reset essential tremor by peripheral mechanical perturbation is the strongest evidence for a peripheral reflex mechanism. The similarities between physiologic tremor and essential tremor with respect to the various factors that modify tremor frequency and amplitude cannot be ignored. More investigation of the role of β-adrenergic receptors and essential tremor must be done. The basic tremor frequency involving essentially all muscles studied by EMG expresses itself in movement of the limbs as a feature of limb mass, that is, resonating frequency, and in this respect does not differ from physiologic tremor.

Intention tremor: action tremor, rubral tremor, cerebellar tremor, terminal tremor, postural tremor, titubation

Definition and clinical features. The primary feature of this tremor is its presence during movement or intention. Goal-directed movement of the upper extremity toward a target, such as the hand reaching for an object, results in a slow (3 to 7 c/s) tremor that increases in amplitude as the target is approached.[2,3] The tremor may involve one side of the body or one limb. Finally the effort to stand to reach the fully erect posture may produce a slow (2 to 3 c/s) up and down bobbing of the trunk.[66] This may be so prominent as to be designated *orthostatic tremor.*[55] On physical examination, tremor is present on finger to nose or finger-nose-finger and heel to shin testing with the eyes open. In its most severe form, seen most often in patients with generalized or diffuse multiple sclerosis, the slightest voluntary movement of a limb or the head stimulates a high-amplitude, waving-bobbing tremor. Lesions involving the dentatorubrospinal tract produce this (rubral) tremor. Most commonly lesions are in the anterior medullary velum or midbrain. Examples reported include toxoplasma abscess of midbrain[67] and vascular hamartoma (radiated) of pineal region.[68]

Role of central nervous system. A lesion involving the cerebellum and its efferent connections is associated with intention tremor. Although data permitting pathophysiologic correlations are limited, it is likely that the extent, medial-lateral, or rostral caudal location of the lesion influences the body distribution of tremor as well as such features as frequency and amplitude. The cerebellum is a regulator or governor of posture and movement (for an excellent overview of cerebellar function, see Brooks and Thach[69]). Stimulation of the cerebellum can result in altered posture but does not produce specific movements. Through its connections with proprioceptors and modulation of the gamma efferent system intentional movement is continuously adapted to conform to conditions of posture. The isolated movement of the hand to pick up an object is associated with postural adjustments throughout the body that support this primary movement.

Lesions of the cerebellum result in errors of force, timing, and velocity during intended movement. Electromyographic recordings of agonist and antagonist muscles during intended movements are useful in documenting these errors.

Movements have been classified as follows: (1) Simple movements—the movement occurs across a single joint and requires only agonist activity. One kind of simple movement is a ballistic movement during which there is sudden unrestrained contraction of agonist, causing the body part to move freely until striking an object. Skilled ballistic movements are required in such activities as playing the piano.

In this instance, the movement must be self-terminated and involves agonist-antagonist-agonist firing in sequence. (2) Compound movements—movements result in a change in posture across two or more joints. Agonists and antagonists with synergists must act in an appropriately timed manner to achieve a smoothly flowing, continuous movement (a golf swing).

Electromyographic studies of muscles participating in simple movements in human subjects with cerebellar lesions or in monkeys during cooling of dentate nucleus have disclosed delays in initiating activity and prolongation of agonist discharge. In compound movements, a fragmentation or degradation of movement occurs. In reaching the target, the limb moves in multiple directions, each followed by an exaggerated correction. The velocity of movement varies in a similarly abnormal manner. Electromyographic records reveal an overlap of agonist and antagonistic activity in addition to activity in excess of that normally required to reach the target.

The cerebellum receives information from the cerebral cortex, where intended movements stored as complex programs, or plans for movement probably originate as well as the spinal cord and vestibular system. The ratio of input to output is 40:1. Purkinje cells, which are the primary recipients of all input to the cerebellum, maintain a high tonic discharge, as do cells in the dentate, interpositus, and fastigial nuclei. Purkinje cells exert an inhibitory influence on nuclear cells and continually adjust their firing rates during ongoing movement. Most studies indicate a relatively wide distribution of Purkinje-nuclear cell influence on individual limb movement. A somatotopic organization of cerebellar cortex and nuclei exists. This organization is duplicated for movements generated by cerebral cortex via pontine nuclei to posterior lobe to dentate nuclei and for movements under postural control mediated by spinal cord (spinocerebellar tracts) to anterior lobe to interpositus nuclei. Afferents from labyrinth for dynamic and static head control project directly to the flocculonodular lobe.

The dentate nucleus consists of a dorsomedial part, which along with fastigial, globose, and emboliform nuclei project to vestibular nuclei, medullary reticular formation, large cells of the red nucleus, and tegmentum of midbrain and pons. These connections are *paleocerebellar* and are considered to be phylogenetically "older" than the ventrolateral portion of the dentate nucleus and its connections. Head on body and, to a lesser extent, truncal stability are mediated through the paleocerebellar system. The large ventrolateral *neocerebellar* portion of the

dentate nucleus projects to the small-celled portion of the red nucleus, which then projects to nucleus ventralis lateralis of the thalamus and frontal cortex.[70]

Because of the importance of the lower extremities and truncal antigravity muscles in maintaining the erect posture, the anterior lobe (spinocerebellum) receives most of its input from these regions. Correspondingly, the upper extremities and control of distal limb movements project predominantly to posterior lobe (*cortical* cerebellum). There is also a medial, intermediate, and lateral organization corresponding to trunk, proximal, and distal extremities.

The cerebellum receives information from a variety of sensory systems, including touch and pain receptors, vestibular apparatus, and visual system. Physiologic data strongly support proprioceptive input, but this has been less well documented anatomically. An important component of proprioceptive input is the modulation of muscle tone in a manner appropriate to ongoing motor activity. Patients with cerebellar disorders do better than those with parkinsonism when relying only on proprioceptive input to make postural corrections.[71] Hypotonia resulting from cerebellar lesions most probably occurs as a result of decreased gamma motoneuron activity. Reduced tonic vibration reflex on the side of cerebellar lesions supports this conclusion. Hypotonia is most prominent immediately following cerebellar lesioning, following which there is gradual recovery of tone. Normal proprioception and alpha motoneuron activation depend on a continuous adjustment of gamma activity, which permits optimum measurement of muscle length during all phases of movement.

It has been demonstrated that long loop reflexes are delayed as well as enhanced in patients with cerebellar atrophy. The tibial nerve was stimulated while electromyographic recordings were made from tibialis anterior and gastrocnemius muscles. A synchronized discharge occurred in tibialis anterior at 120 ms in both patients and controls; a stretch reflex was produced in tibialis anterior. A long loop response occurred synchronously in gastrocnemius and tibialis anterior 90 to 120 ms later in controls. The latency of this latter response was prolonged in the patient group. The cerebellar tremor could be synchronized by this stimulation. The tremor frequency declined with progression of cerebellar atrophy, and the long loop latency increased. These results associate a delay in the long loop reflex connection with the presence of tremor. The circumstantial evidence of cerebellar atrophy implies that cerebellar connections are important in the long loop reflex as well as the tremor.[72] Muscle spindle afferent, most likely secondaries, may convey information to cerebellum as one limb of the reflex. Cooling or lesioning of the anterior lobe results in a slow tremor (3 to 4 c/s) involving lower extremity flexor and extensor muscles and results in truncal bobbing.[72] In a study of cortical cerebellar degeneration, truncal bobbing at 2.5 to 3.5 cycles per second was found to be associated with pronounced atrophy of the superior cerebellar vermis.[73]

The cerebellum seems to function as a switching and timing device with a structural organization not unlike that of a computer. Purkinje cells of the cerebellar cortex and neurons of the dentate and interpositus nuclei became active before and during quick wrist movements.[74] The earliest activity occurred in dentate nuclei, followed by motor cortex and interpositus nucleus activation.[75,76] Local cooling of the dentate nucleus prolonged reaction times, supporting the view that the dentate nucleus is important to the initiation of movements.[77] Some investigators have suggested that gamma motoneurons are activated by nucleus interpositus via the rubrospinal tract.[78] The rubrospinal system, however, projects monosynaptically to alpha motoneurons as well.[79] Thus the cerebellum is involved in the appropriate timing of alpha motoneuron activity and in the adjustment of fusimotor tone, which in turn ensures an accurate ongoing assessment of static and dynamic changes in muscle length. Miller, Oscarsson,[80,81] and Lundberg[82] have proposed that the cerebellum acts as a comparator, which measures the error between the ideal template of motoneuron activation that is stored in memory and that movement which actually occurs. Although not responsible for originating or planning movement, the cerebellum may play an important role in motor learning because it constantly receives information on the status of ongoing motor performance as well as input from cerebral cortex concerning motor intention.

Electromyographic features. Electromyographic recordings from flexor and extensor muscles reveal alternating discharges in the range of 3 to 5 c/s. Tremor bursts and overlapping agonist and antagonist discharge found in patients with cerebellar disease can be mimicked by normal subjects. Low amplitude tremor bursts in which single MUs can be discriminated exhibit normal recruitment patterns.

Intention tremor worsens as effort increases. Dysmetria or failure to bring the finger or other part accurately to a target is characterized by an oscillatory movement that increases as the target is approached. Thus intention tremor, dysmetria, and even pendular reflexes might be viewed as resulting from a mismatch between outflow and proprioceptive input.

Spinal and reflex mechanisms. The spinal cord is a conveyor of information to the cerebellum and the site of alpha and gamma motoneurons. The order of MU recruitment is probably normal in disorders of the cerebellum, but levels of facilitation of both tonic and phasic motoneurons are probably reduced, resulting in both hypotonia and apparent weakness; that is, the contribution of the stretch reflex to maintenance of muscle force is absent.

In spinocerebellar degeneration associated with a severe loss of proprioception, the patient is unaware of the level of motor output or effort. Using audiovisual feedback of MU action potentials to establish control, patients were able to maintain and adjust firing rate of single MUs in a normal manner. When feedback was interrupted, MU firing ceased immediately. The results suggest that when audiovisual feedback substitutes for the defective proprioceptive input, motor control becomes normal, as defined in this limited condition.[1]

Interactive and mechanical factors. Intention tremor is influenced by psychic arousal and posture. The amplitude of the tremor is a function of the degree of movement required. Limiting the effort required to produce a movement, such as unweighting the limb, and increasing limb inertia by weighting the limb have both been used to reduce tremor severity. The resonating frequency of the body part determines the extent to which the tremor is manifested in movement. Lower tremor frequency is capable of producing movement of the entire body, as in truncal titubation. Low level tonic electrical stimulation of antagonist muscles during movement can suppress intention tremor.

Resting Tremor

Definition

Resting tremor is best typified by parkinsonian tremor.[2,3] This tremor occurs when the body part is at rest but may be accentuated by alterations in posture, such as flexing the arms or leaning forward, or by slight muscle contraction. In the hands, a typical flexion-pronation-supination movement called *pill rolling* is seen. Tremor can also be accentuated by emotional excitement. The tremor usually is detected first in one upper extremity and is most commonly caused by Parkinson's disease. Gradually over months or years, tremor becomes more generalized. It is usually associated with rigidity and bradykinesia. In some patients, the common signs of parkinsonism are preceded by signs of unilateral dystonia in the leg or arm. These signs may be present for months or even years before the development of parkinsonism. Other symptoms of parkinsonism include sialorrhea, increased seborrheic secretion, heat intolerance, cold tolerance, and a variety of dysautonomic symptoms.

Role of central nervous system

Resting tremor can occur in Parkinson's disease, in which there is a degeneration of the pigmented cells of the substantia nigra[3] and other catecholamine-containing neurons as well. Intoxication, such as by manganese associated with loss of pallidal neurons[83] and chronic use of phenothiazines,[84] can result in a parkinsonian syndrome. In the former condition, dementia and dystonic states (torticollis) are common, whereas in the latter, tremor is uncommon. These conditions involve the dopaminergic system projecting to the striatum but each in a different manner. It has been demonstrated that this system is topographically organized,[11] which accounts for tremor being present in various regions of the body as well as unilateral involvement. It is also well known that signs of tremor, rigidity, and akinesia all vary independently of one another, some patients manifesting only akinesia with little or no tremor and rigidity. This variation is especially apparent early in the disease. In addition, some patients may manifest a high-frequency tremor in the range of physiologic tremor, that is, 8 to 10 c/s, associated with a high degree of rigidity.[22,85]

The discovery of Parkinson's disease in young people using a "designer" amphetamine containing 1-methyl-4-phenyl-1,2,3,6-tetrahydrophridine (MPTP) has resulted in the ability to induce parkinsonian signs in primates. In addition, a new drug, selegiline, a monoamine oxidase B inhibitor, has also been developed that inhibits the action of MPTP and slows the progression of Parkinson's disease.

One view of the pathophysiology of Parkinson's disease is that the loss of dopaminergic neurons in the substantia nigra results in increased inhibitory output from the basal ganglia to the thalamus. Because there are two populations of striatal output neurons that are influenced differently by dopamine, loss of dopamine causes different effects. There is a decrease in inhibitory activity of neurons projecting to the internal division of the globus pallidus (GPi) and an increase in the inhibitory activity projecting to the external division of the globus pallidus (GPe). Increased inhibition in GPe results in decreased inhibition of subthalamic nucleus (STN). Lesions placed in STN of two African green monkeys made parkinsonian by MPTP resulted in marked improvement in all signs of the disease—tremor, rigidity, and bradykinesia.[86] The findings support the concept of a neuronal generator of regular spontaneous discharge, which is modulated for purposes of postural support of automatic movements. The results suggest that STN may be an important component of the generator.

Studies of cerebral glucose utilization in MPTP-treated primates have revealed decreased utilization in substantia nigra, pars compactas, and ventral tegmentum but increased utilization in areas innervated by these regions: postcommissural putamen and dorsolateral caudate nucleus. Significant increases were also found in globus pallidus (+40%) and pedunculopontine nucleus (+15%). Utilization, however, was decreased in STN (−17%). Findings were abnormal on the side of MPTP infection.[130] These results would seem to contradict the hypothesis of increased activity in STN as a primary factor in the generation of parkinsonian signs.[87]

In a review article comparing the pathophysiology of petit mal epilepsy with that of parkinsonism, release of *GABAergic burst promoting systems* resulting in *rhythmic network oscillation of thalamocortical neurons* by decreased striatal dopamine levels was proposed as a common feature of both conditions. It was further proposed that drugs effective in the treatment of petit mal epilepsy might also be effective in Parkinson's disease and vice versa.[88]

In striatonigral degeneration, rigidity and akinesia are present in association with striatal atrophy not present in parkinsonism and atrophy of substantia nigra. Striatonigral degeneration is believed to be one of the multisystem atrophies in which striatum, pigmented nuclei, pontine nuclei, inferior olives, and cerebellar Purkinje cells are all at risk for involvement. On the basis of histopathology, parkinsonism is a distinctly different entity.[89] Tremor is common in parkinsonism, whereas in striatonigral degeneration pill-rolling tremor is not seen. Electromyographic recordings from flexor or extensor muscles in patients with striatonigral degeneration, however, reveal rigidity to be associated with rapid bursts of activity occurring at 10 c/s and responsible for the ratchet-like resistance to passive movement (unpublished observations). This may be misinterpreted as tremor activity.

Diffuse Lewy body disease[90] can emulate parkinsonism, but a prominent early feature is dementia, not common in early classic Parkinson's disease. The disease can be differentiated from Alzheimer's disease because of the hypokinetic rigid syndrome that is present early in the course.

Electromyographic features

The tremor frequency is 4 to 7 c/s, generally with alteration between flexor and extensor muscles. MU recruitment is orderly in each tremor burst, and single MUs can be found firing at tremor frequency in the absence of obvious limb movement. In some patients with minimal rest tremor, tonic single MUs that initiate muscle contraction are seen to fire evenly without tremor but begin to fire at tremor frequency and to recruit other MUs in tremor bursts as effort increases, indicating that facilitation may be necessary to elicit tremor in some patients[91] (Figure 2.6).

Patients with Parkinson's disease have great difficulty initiating single MU activity and in adjusting the firing rate of single MUs in the presence of adequate audiovisual feedback. At the level of single

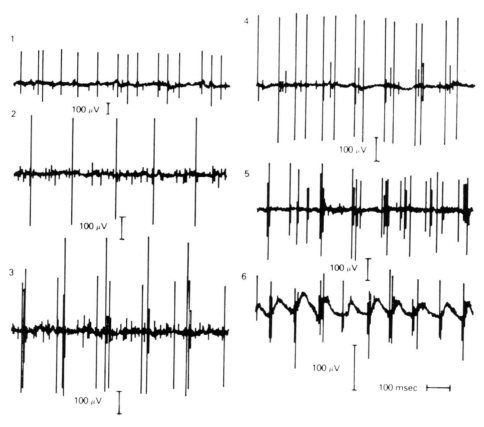

FIGURE 2.6.   *(1) Units shown were activated during minimal contraction (first dorsal interosseous) in a patient with tremor (identified by bursts of activity with intervals of silence). (2) The first unit activated during minimal contraction (biceps) fired at tremor frequency. (3) Units recruited at higher levels of effort also fire at tremor frequency. First unit activated is that shown in (B) (biceps). (4) Minimal contraction activated a unit firing at essentially normal frequency, which then lapsed into tremor as effort was increased (biceps). (5) Tremor seen as a clustering of several units firing in bursts with differing basic frequency of each unit (first dorsal interosseous). (6) Visible tremor was not present in this patient, but single units firing at a fixed and unusually high frequency were found.*

MU control, akinesia is manifested as an inability to modulate frequency. In the absence of frequency control, there is a constant free-running MU discharge in the form of resting tremor. How the striatum and its connections free of dopaminergic influence produce tremor, rigidity, and akinesia is unknown.[91]

Cogwheel rigidity may be synchronized with a tremor in the range of physiologic tremor (10 c/s), as stated earlier, or occur at a slower rate in time with resting tremor. Even an action tremor has been reported in Parkinson's disease.[22,92] Resting tremor does not always disappear with intention. Facilitation supported by limb movement may actually make tremor visible when it is nearly absent at rest. Mechanical perturbation can reset these higher frequency tremors in patients with Parkinson's disease, which has led some investigators to conclude that parkinsonian resting tremor depends to some extent on peripheral mechanisms.[93] In contrast to essential tremor, however, resting tremor cannot be reset by mechanical perturbation, suggesting that central generators are an important source of the tremor.[62] Recordings from Ia afferents in Parkinson's patients with resting tremor have revealed rhythmic discharges during muscle contraction and relaxation.[94]

Neurons in motor cortex and thalamus have been reported to fire in rhythm with tremor in primate models of parkinsonism.[95] Lesions of nucleus ventralis lateralis intermedius of thalamus and globus pallidus stop resting tremor.[96–98] The role of these structures in resting tremor is unknown, but disturbance in a servomechanism involving these structures produces an oscillation resulting in resting tremor.

Spinal and reflex mechanisms

Studies of peripheral mechanisms involved in parkinsonian tremor have generally concluded that the myotatic reflex is not involved in the genesis of the tremor. For example, rhythmic forces applied to the wrists of patients with parkinsonian tremor did not produce alterations in the tremor rate but only beats, which depend on the difference in rate between the tremor and the applied rhythm. The conclusion of these studies was that there was no electromyographic evidence for servodriving or servoassistance in the genesis of tremor.[98] In comparative studies of action tremor, postural tremor, and clonus and Parkinson's disease, it was found that 80% of patients with Parkinson's disease manifest a tremor at 4, 5, and 6 c/s. These authors concluded that this combination of tremor frequencies is the strongest objective criterion for the diagnosis of basal ganglia disease.[99]

Interation of factors and summary

The 4 to 8 c/s slow resting tremor of parkinsonism is generated centrally and may involve oscillations in long loop reflexes. The tremor manifested depends on the resonating frequency of the parts involved. Patients with high-frequency tremor, in the range of 10 c/s, may manifest little typical resting tremor, and some patients have intention tremor as well. The mechanisms for the latter two tremors may be different from the usual resting tremor and be more dependent on peripheral mechanisms.

Resting tremor of parkinsonism appears to be generated by failure of suprasegmental control at the level of the basal ganglia. How single MU frequency modulation is controlled by the striatum and its connections is unknown. Perhaps spontaneous discharge of pallidal neurons is rhythmic when the inhibiting influence of striatum is removed. Different effects of altered inhibition on external pallidum (increased inhibition) and internal pallidum (decreased inhibition) with resultant increase in activity in STN may play a large role in the genesis of parkinsonian signs.[86] The ability of patients with Parkinson's disease to produce sudden ballistic contractions involving recruitment of large numbers of MUs indicates that spatial recruiting mechanisms, mediated by thalamocortical pathways, are relatively intact.

Other Tremors

Neurogenic tremor and tremor in association with neurogenic atrophy

An *irregular* tremor called *neurogenic tremor* has been reported in patients with chronic relapsing-remitting polyneuropathy.[100] It varies from 6 to 8 c/s and also in amplitude. A tremor is often also present in patients with moderately severe neurogenic atrophy. A large reduction in the number of MUs in a muscle and an increase in their size consequent to collateral reinnervation results in a failure to produce smooth graded muscle contraction or to sustain steady contraction. Large MUs present in such disorders as amyotrophic lateral sclerosis may fire irregularly and with sustained contraction fire more slowly. These irregular muscle contractions do not conform precisely to the definition of tremor stated earlier but may be misinterpreted as tremor of other origin (Figure 2.7).

In a study of 14 patients with tremor resulting from different acquired peripheral neuropathies, the only common finding was weakness. The tremor associated with neuropathy was believed to be weak-

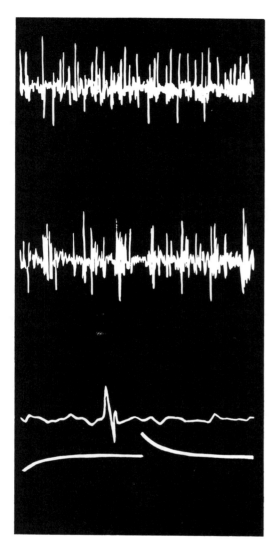

FIGURE 2.7.   *Needle electrode recording from biceps brachii (1 mV calibration and 100 ms sweep) reveals tremor-like irregular bursts of firing of large motor units as maximal isometric contraction is sustained (middle trace).*

ness-enhanced physiologic tremor. Slowing was demonstrated in Ia fibers as well.[101] Tremor as a consequence of altered sensory input cannot be excluded in such cases.

Needle electrode examination of single MU action potentials in severe neurogenic atrophy may reveal that tremor movement in a digit occurs synchronously with the discharge of the MU. Such tremor is quite common in patients recovered from poliomyelitis.

Spasmodic torticollis

Inclusion of torticollis in a discussion of tremor arises from the fact that tremor may initiate muscle spasm, or the abnormal movement may consist entirely of a slowly repeating muscle contraction. The sternocleidomastoid muscle is most commonly the site of such tremors, which begin as clustered firing of MUs at a few cycles per second, which then fuse into sustained contraction that does not differ in any way from contraction that may be initiated voluntarily (Figure 2.8).

A pattern of muscle activation is usually seen that results in a stereotyped abnormal rotation, flexion, or extension of the head on the neck. Also seen are associated movements of the shoulder, extremities, trunk, and even lower extremities, indicating the presence of a more generalized dystonia. The central pathway for head rotation involves efferent connections from vestibular nucleus to interstitial nucleus of Cajal in the midbrain via median longitudinal fasciculus. Interstitial nucleus then projects to contralateral thalamus, which then projects to motor cortex, the *head turning area*, Brodman area 8.[102] The nucleus also gives off fibers to the spinal cord (the interstitiospinal tract), the vestibular nuclei, the perihypoglossal nuclei, and the paramedian reticular formation. Disinhibition of nuclei in this system by deafferentation and irritative lesions of the motor pathway, that is, thalamocortical system to spinal accessory nerve, could result in the syndrome of spasmodic torticollis.

In most patients, EMG reveals widespread neck muscle activity, with a variety of maneuvers being briefly effective in reducing the spasm. These include touching the face, either to counteract the movement or to promote a voluntary *nuzzling* motion in the direction opposite that of the head-turning. In some cases, the direction of gaze influences the movement. No consistent effects of lifting weights or opening and closing the eyes have been found. In 30 patients reported by Mathews et al.,[103] 12 turned to the right, 15 turned to the left, one had retrocollis, and two turned in both directions. In this group of patients, six had additional neurologic findings. One had writer's cramp, one had torsion dystonia, and one had essential tremor. The patients were psychologically normal. Only one patient ultimately recovered. An

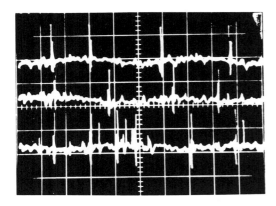

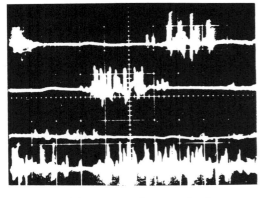

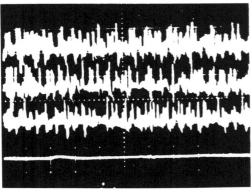

TORTICOLLIS
SCM

START

SPASM
CLONIC

SPASM
TONIC

50 ms
200 mv

FIGURE 2.8. *Tremor and clonus tonic spasm in sternocleidomastoid muscle in patient with spasmodic torticollis.*

association of torticollis and writer's cramp has been recognized.[104]

Opinion is divided between psychologic and organic causes of spasmodic torticollis. In two cases of my own, the torticollis began within a few days of the unexpected death of a spouse. In one instance, a woman discovered her husband dead when he did not return from emptying the trash. In other cases, a vascular loop has been found at surgery that impinges on spinal accessory nerve, or an acute event such as neck injury or ear infection has preceded the development of torticollis.

Torticollis can be produced in cats following midbrain lesions.[105] Pneumoencephalography has disclosed atrophy in frontal and parietal regions in 10 of 13 patients with spasmodic torticollis in the absence of other neurologic signs or symptoms.[106] One case of myopathy in sternocleidomastoid and accessory neuropathy has been reported.[107]

The causes of the abnormal head movements may be classified into (1) primary—resulting from irritation of the spinal accessory nerve itself, or (2) secondary—conditions causing excitation of the spinal accessory nerve by activation of the motor or sensory nerve by activation of the motor or sensory pathways that lead to head turning. Primary causes include tumors such as meningioma in the region of the foramen magnum, vascular loops, and other sources of mechanical irritation to the nerve. Among secondary causes are hyperthyroidism or hypothyroidism, encephalitis, Wilson's disease, ocular muscle imbalance, maldevelopment of neck muscles, "fragment" of torsion dystonia, colloid cyst of III ventricle, and phenothiazine intoxication. Still for the greater majority of cases, the cause is unknown.

The electromyographer can be of assistance in the analysis of spasmodic torticollis when surgical treatment is being considered. For example, one or two muscles may initiate and sustain the abnormal movement, with other muscles becoming active as a consequence of excessive shortening. Spinal accessory nerve section to sternocleidomastoid muscle operating as prime mover may significantly reduce the severity of the spasm. Further, in contrast to the usual pattern of left sternocleidomastoid activation followed by later right trapezius contraction, left sternocleidomastoid and left trapezius may contract in synchronous bursts, suggesting a common irritation to left spinal accessory nerve produced by tumor or abnormal blood vessel.

The surgical treatment of spasmodic torticollis has focused attention on the afferent and efferent innervation of sternocleidomastoid and trapezius muscles. In rabbits, cats, and monkeys, the efferent innervation to sternocleidomastoid and trapezius is carried in the spinal accessory nerve, whereas the afferent fibers, mainly proprioceptive, are carried in C-2, C-3, and C-4. These afferents subsequently join the spinal accessory nerve.[108]

Writing tremor

Writing tremor is an action tremor precipitated by the act of writing. Usually there is a pronation-supination tremor; sometimes finger flexion-extension occurs. The frequency is from 5 to 7 c/s. If the effort to write continues, a spasm in flexion may occur. A background of cocontraction leading to dystonic posturing is commonly present.[109] In many cases of writing tremor, a history of a prolonged period of writing under stressful conditions may be obtained. The tremor has been defined as a selective action tremor not responding to propranolol but benefited by centrally acting anticholinergic agents.[110] In some cases, however, essential tremor is also present, and treatment of essential tremor by propranolol may concomitantly benefit writing tremor. In a single case report, a patient was described with a pronator teres muscle excessively sensitive to stretch. Beats of pronation-supination tremor occurred on attempts to write. Motor point block of the pronator teres muscle temporarily abolished the tremor.[111] Selective thalamotomy of ventralis intermedius nucleus successfully treated three patients with progressive 5 to 7 c/s tremor during writing.[112]

The modal frequency of postural tremor for the hand is 7 c/s. The dominant tremor frequency is highly dependent on the passive resonant properties of hand tissues.[113] The overlap of this frequency with that of writing tremor suggests that writing tremor may be an enhanced postural tremor. The influence of fatigue on postural tremor in increasing the amplitude of the dominant frequency may be a factor. Sustained effort could result in structural changes in muscle and nerve that maintain the tremor characteristic of excessive fatigue.

The term *writer's cramp* refers to the cocontraction of forearm, wrist, and finger flexor and extensor muscles that may develop during the act of writing. In some cases, muscle contraction may be more extensive and even include the lower extremities. The muscle activity is not a cramp as usually defined because MU action potentials firing as in voluntary activation are recorded. A dystonic reaction seems unlikely because other motor activities requiring the writing hand are performed normally. A *writer's cramp* can also develop in conjunction with the performance of other skilled motor activities such as typing or playing a musical instrument. This fact and the spread of muscle activation to the entire extremity and other limbs as well *do* support a more generalized dystonic state.

Myoclonus

Myoclonus is defined as an abrupt contraction of an entire muscle that results in a visible jerk of a body part. Thus myoclonic jerks usually produce movement about a joint, whereas *palatal myoclonus* produces movement of the palate. In myoclonus of the extremities or trunk, sudden irregular jerking movements are produced. This bursting irregular muscle activity does not qualify as tremor. Palatal myoclonus, however, is seen as a regular 100 to 180 per minute contraction of the palate. Of considerable interest is that other muscles innervated by cranial motor nerves and the diaphragm may contract in synchrony with the palatal movements or independently. Other muscles involved include pharyngeal constrictors, larynx, tongue, extraocular muscles (usually rotatory nystagmus), and muscles of the upper extremities. The abnormal movements persist during sleep and under barbiturate anesthesia. Speech and breathing are often affected by the tremor.[114]

A lesion of the central tegmental tract, which is the major connection between inferior olive and red nucleus, is believed to be responsible for palatal myoclonus.[115] In three autopsied cases in which neoplasm was involved, a lesion of the dentate nucleus with secondary hypertrophy and demyelination of the contralateral olive were demonstrated.[114] In general, a lesion involving the "triangle" of fibers connecting the dentate nucleus with the contralateral olivary nucleus by way of the central tegmental tract passing in the vicinity of the red nucleus will result in palatal myoclonus and its associated features.[116,117] In unilateral cases, palatal myoclonus occurs ipsilateral to the olivary nucleus involved. A lesion of the superior cerebellar peduncle (dentatorubral tract) will not cause palatal myoclonus, but rather a slower action tremor as described earlier. One view is that the crucial lesion is an olivary hypertrophy with proliferation of dendrites and terminal endings secondary to deafferentation involving reticulo-olivary fibers in the central tegmental tract or dentato-olivary fibers from contralateral dentate nucleus.[118] Postdenervation hypersensitivity has been proposed as a mechanism for palatal myoclonus based on an analysis of the time of its occurrence following brain stem infarction.[119] Causes of lesions producing palatal myoclonus include progressive bulbar palsy, syringobulbia, encephalitis, glioma, angioma, demyelination, trauma, and infarction of the brain stem, usually involving the central tegmental tract.[120] In one report, rest tremor of upper extremities not attributable to Parkinson's disease was associated with palatal myoclonus and brain stem infarction.[121]

Electromyographic recordings from involved muscles reveal rhythmic ballistic discharge. Simultaneous recording and observation of multiple muscles, including eye muscles paced by the same tremor mechanism, often reveal synchronous discharge, but independent oscillations also occur.

Asterixis

Asterixis is not tremor, but rather an irregular loss of postural tonus in the outstretched extremity that is recovered so quickly that the extremity appears to flap.[122] If the patient is asked to hold the hands straight out in front with fingers maximally extended, the irregular dropping movements with quick recovery are easily seen. The movement has been described as an act of flexion at the wrist without the assistance of electromyographic recording. When occurring frequently, at rates approaching one per second, the limb may appear to be involved by an irregular slow *tremor*. The usual rate of occurrence is every 2 to 30 seconds. Asterixis can be demonstrated also in the dorsiflexed foot or the protruded tongue.

Asterixis is usually seen in association with increased postural tremor and multifocal myoclonus accompanying toxic or metabolic brain disease of diverse types. Asterixis is an important early sign of toxic encephalopathy. Unilateral or focal asterixis has been reported in association with *acute midbrain dysfunction* in the absence of encephalopathy,[123] in the presence of thalamic hemorrhage,[124] and in midbrain infarction.[125] These findings suggest that asterixis may result from some kind of mesodiencephalic dysfunction resulting in impaired ability to sustain motor activity and attention.

Clonus

Clonus is not spontaneous rhythmic contraction; rather it is elicited by rapid stretch of a muscle. Muscles vary with respect to the ease with which clonus can be produced. For example, it is easily elicited in soleus muscle by rapid dorsiflexion of the foot and appears as a repetitive 5 to 7 c/s waning discharge as the foot is held passively in dorsiflexion. By contrast, rapid stretch of the tibialis anterior muscle does not result in clonus.

Clonus is generally present when there is an impairment of motor pathways to spinal cord from brain stem or motor control regions of the cerebrum.[3] It is usually found in association with hyperreflexia and in those conditions in which antigravity posture is accentuated, that is, decorticate, decerebrate, and spinal postures. The phrase *pyramidal sign* is used by the clinician to designate the presence of an extensor plantar response, weakness, and hyperreflexia. This suggests that these changes, including clonus, result from a lesion of those fibers passing through the medullary pyramids. Isolated lesions of the medullary pyramids result in weakness, reduction in deep tendon reflexes, hypotonia, increased flexion withdrawal response (Babinski's response), and appearance of other *pathologic reflexes*. Thus the hyperreflexia present in the patient with spinal cord transection or infarction of the internal capsule results from involvement of other motor pathways controlling motoneuron excitability and sensitivity of the muscle to stretch.

Vestibulospinal and reticulospinal systems important in the control of body posture are involved when hyperreflexia and clonus are present. These brain stem regions may be separated from cerebral control by midbrain intercollicular transection and become disinhibited as in decerebrate posture, subjected to abnormal control from basal ganglia–thalamic control systems (decorticate posture), or separated entirely from the motoneuron and myotatic servomechanisms by spinal transection.

A variety of circumstances can theoretically lead to the development of clonus, usually associated with hyperreflexia. Denny-Brown[126] proposed an increased excitability of the muscle stretch receptors as the essential pathophysiologic mechanism. Sudden shortening of the muscle results in a volley of impulses to the homonymous motoneuron pool, which then fires synchronously, following which the muscle relaxes. This lengthening results in a second contraction, somewhat less forceful than the preceding one, so the periodic contraction wanes in amplitude.

Application of the concepts of servocontrol to the mechanism of clonus discloses that it is necessary only to eliminate the spindle bias adjustment by gamma efferent neurons to establish a condition leading to clonus. The gamma system mediates differential, integral, and anticipatory control of the myotatic loop. The gamma system represents the only peripheral representation of vestibulospinal and reticulospinal systems. In the simplest case, if the spindle is the receptor component of an on/off servomechanism, clonus will occur as predicted from the usual oscillatory output of this system. The rhythmic Ia afferent discharge associated with muscle lengthening recorded in clonus supports this cncept.[94] An additional factor is the level of tonic bias applied to the spindle. Group II (trail) endings, static receptors that respond primarily to length rather than changes in length, as the Ia afferents do, may set the spindle tonic afferent discharge at various levels. Needle electrode recordings from antigravity muscles, such as soleus, in patients with spasticity frequently record ongoing tonic MU discharge. The rate of this discharge can often be set by slow passive stretch of the muscle. Also, tonically firing

MUs are found that may not respond to stretch (unpublished observations). These units may be functionally disconnected from the myotatic loop. Under these circumstances of *independent* and hyperexcitable motoneurons, the condition of *alpha rigidity* exists. By the variable operation of the gamma system, the level of muscle tone, posture, rigidity, resistance to passive movement (spasticity), and hyperreflexia can be set. For this reason, clonus may be present in an individual without spasticity. Studies of spastic paresis support the view that increased resistance to passive muscle stretch results from decreased threshold of the myotatic reflex, leading to increased reflex-induced stiffness.[127]

Increases in motoneuron excitability and an increase in gamma tonus may result in transient clonus in a normal person in an excited state. Studies of clonus involving the soleus muscle have revealed patterns of clonus that are best explained by the presence of background muscle tone on which the clonus is superimposed.

The electromyographer will have the opportunity to examine the responses of single MUs to passive slow and rapid stretch in patients with spasticity. In general, an orderly recruitment of MUs occurs during bursts of clonus, but the interval between discharges will vary[128] (Figure 2.9). Sometimes individual units will fire repetitively during more vigorous contractions. The findings of tonic firing in antigravity muscles and the length-dependent change in firing rate may assist in the diagnosis of suprasegmental disorders.

Tremor resulting from intoxication

Enhanced physiologic tremor can occur as a result of the administration of sympathomimetic drugs, such as those used in the treatment of asthma.[129] Similarly ingestion of caffeine, amphetamine, and related drugs also increases physiologic tremor. A tremor similar to essential tremor or enhanced physiologic tremor is seen in patients on tricyclic antidepressants,[130] sodium valproate,[131,132] and lithium.[133] Cigarette smoking has been shown to increase physiologic tremor amplitude over all frequencies from 1 to 25 c/s.[134] A tremor, possibly enhanced physiologic tremor, has been reported as a result of industrial exposure to metallic mercury.[135] Action or rubral tremor is found in alcoholics[136–138] and may be present in patients with cerebellar involvement resulting from other causes, such as the chronic use of diphenylhydantoin.

Clonus Bursts - Soleus

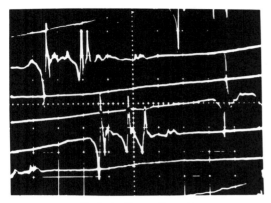

Orderly Recruitment

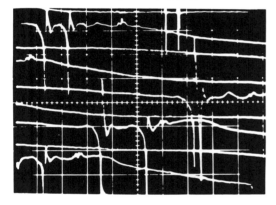

FIGURE 2.9.   *Orderly recruitment of single motor units (upper trace) but varying interspike intervals (lower trace) are shown in soleus muscle during bursts of clonus.*

PHYSICAL FACTORS INVOLVED IN TREMOR

The reader is referred to several excellent reviews of tremor that discuss in detail the physical and mathematical aspects of tremor.[3,139,140,141] In this section, several relevant basic physical concepts are reviewed, with emphasis on aspects relevant to the electromyographer.

Inertia and Limb Oscillation

Any part of the body that tremors can be represented as a mass (*M*) to which a force is being applied. Newton's second law of motion states that the net accelerating force equals the product of mass and acceleration (a) in the direction of force, or:

$$F(t) = M\, a(t) = M\frac{dv}{dt}$$

The equation is expressed as a function of time (t) because both accelerating force and acceleration change with time. The transfer function indicates that force *(F(t))* is transformed into a velocity *(V(t))*. By rearranging and integrating the equation, the following is obtained:

$$\int a(t)dt = \frac{1}{M} = \int F(t)dt$$

$$V(t) - V_1 = \frac{1}{M}\int_{t_1}^{t} F(t)dt$$

which states that the changes in velocity that occurred over time *(t − t₁)* are a function of the integral of accelerating force divided by the mass. In simpler form:

$$V(t) = \frac{1}{M}\int F(t)dt$$

which simply omits the stated initial condition. The right side of the equation is defined as inertia (*H*) and in summary as a transfer function is expressed as $\frac{V}{F} = H$.

Considering this relation alone, it can be seen that to initiate oscillation in any body part with high inertia requires proportionately high levels of force. Rhythmically applied forces sufficient to produce oscillation or movement around a joint (torque) must be applied over a time interval that permits acceleration of the part to develop. Attempting to rock a car out of a snowbank at periodicity too high to permit movement is analogous to a high-frequency tremor of muscle applied to the proximal limb. The tremor transmitted to the body by the heart (ballistocardiac tremor) occurs at a frequency of approximately 1 c/s, low enough to "accommodate" the inertial properties of the entire body and large body parts. Body movement produced by breathing is in the same category.

The standard example given of an oscillating system is a spring with stiffness (*K*) expressed in units of force or mass required to produce a unit of strain (force per unit of extension of muscle under isometric conditions) connected to a mass (*M*), which is damped by internal friction represented as a shock absorber or dash-pot. The amplitude of oscillation (*y*) of the system is:

$$y(t) = A \sin(2 \, \text{II} \, f_n t)$$

where f_n represents the natural reasonating frequency of the system, the frequency requiring the least accelerating force, or the frequency at which the maximal amplitude of oscillation occurs.

Taking into consideration the stiffness of the spring:

$$f_n = \frac{1}{2 \, \text{II}} - \sqrt{\frac{-K}{M}}$$

or the natural frequency increases as the square root of stiffness and inversely as the square root of mass.

Because of internal friction or viscosity (*D*) of the dash-pot (shock absorber), the amplitude of oscillation (*y*) declines over time following an initial perturbation.

$$f_n = \frac{1}{2\pi} - \sqrt{\frac{-K}{M}}$$

The rate of decline can be expressed as if an opposing force applied at frequency f_d (damping frequency) were operating:

$$y(t) = Ae^{pt} \sin(2 \, \text{II} \, f_d t)$$

where *A* is a constant depending on the size of the initial perturbation and f_d is defined in relation to the natural frequency of f_n as:

$$f_d = f_n - \sqrt{1 - \delta^2}$$

or

$$\delta^2 = 1 - \sqrt{\frac{f_d}{f_n}} \quad \text{where } \delta \text{ is the damping ratio.}$$

Damping declines to 0 as f_d approaches the value of f_n. The rate constant for decay is *p*, where $p = 2 \, \text{II} \, f_n$, which reveals that when the natural frequency of vibration is high, oscillations decay rapidly. The damping ratio is related to mass and stiffness in this system by the equation:

$$\delta = \frac{1}{2} \left(\frac{D}{KM} \right)$$

It is a large step from this analogy to an idealized limb (Figure 2.10). The limb is a heterogeneous structure with respect to properties of stiffness and contains centers of mass that decrease in proportion to the forces applied; that is, the muscle moving a part is progressively smaller as the mass of the part moved decreases. Muscle stiffness increases with ac-

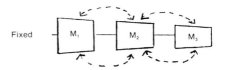

FIGURE 2.10.   *The idealized limb is shown as a series of interconnected masses M_1, M_2, and M_3, each subjected to force or torque capable of producing motion around the point of connection. The net movement of each component mass can be seen to be a function of level of force, frequency of force application, spatial arrangement of force and mass, and size of each mass.*

tive contraction and with increasing length. Connective tissue, especially the joints around which the motion occurs, contributes stiffness, which must become appreciable with advancing age. Stiffness of all tissues is affected by limb core temperature, which declines exponentially from proximal to distal locations.

The movement around the joint involves torque rather than force and inertial properties of the limb being moved. The stiffness of large muscles is greater than that of a small muscle, so empiric measures of tremor amplitude are required to ascertain movement produced at any given tremor frequency. Further, the model of muscle as an elastic element in series with an elastic element and in parallel with a viscous element is not linear as length changes. Finally, elastic damping (viscous) and stiffness properties are influenced by the nature of the contractile mechanism itself, the myofibrillar content of muscle fibers and the extent to which play exists in cross-linkages between myofilaments and the rate at which they are broken and remade. Fortunately, the net influence of MU activity on the movement produced in tremor can be determined empirically. Physical factors permit a *window* of 4 to 8.5 c/s (resonating frequency of the human forearm).[19] Tremor present in this range not associated with rhythmic activation of MUs is necessarily of mechanical origin.

PHYSIOLOGIC MECHANISM IN TREMOR GENESIS

Motor Unit Behavior

Maintenance of the modest effort required to hold a limb in space against the forces of gravity causes activated MUs to fire at a frequency near the upper limit of the primary range or at the recruitment frequency (the frequency existing just before recruitment of a second MU), which is approximately 10 c/s. If the majority of MUs are firing at 10 c/s, synchronization will result in tremor. Added to this are several mechanisms that serve to promote synchronization. These include Renshaw cell activity as well as muscle spindle and tendon organ input. Synchronization can be observed quite easily in the normal subject attempting to sustain steady firing of a single MU using audiovisual feedback to maintain control. If a small ballistic contraction is initiated in first dorsal interosseous as a result of passive perturbation of the finger or by an involuntary or voluntary jerk, a silent period of approximately 100 ms in length appears, then a second, third, or more small ballistic responses occur, each separated by the same 100-ms interval. This was observed in a study of control subjects and patients with Huntington's disease, who produced numerous small jerking movements called *microchorea* (Figure 2.11).[27] These results are consistent with those of Lippold[20] and Halliday and Redfearn,[17] discussed earlier in their studies of physiologic tremor. What has not been appreciated is that the nearly synchronous firing of even two or three MUs may result in a silent period and a brief period of MU synchronization. Autogenic inhibition at the spinal level, most likely mediated by Renshaw and other interneurons, seems the logical source of this synchronization because physiologic tremor frequency does not vary significantly with the length of the myotatic loop. This does not, however, exclude the myotatic loop as capable of resetting or responding to the initiation of tremor.

A silent period or double interval has been observed following the occurrence of a doublet MU discharge. This nearly synchronous double discharge of the same MU occurs on a peripheral basis.[142] Double or greater numbers of discharges occurring at high rates of firing are seen in ballistic contractions. Such contractions are consistently followed by a pause lasting around 100 ms in limb muscles. The silent period following double discharge and the pause following ballistic contraction may occur on the same basis. The factors responsible for MU synchronization are responsible for physiologic tremor, and an *enhancement* of synchronization, still not fully understood, is the most likely cause of essential tremor.

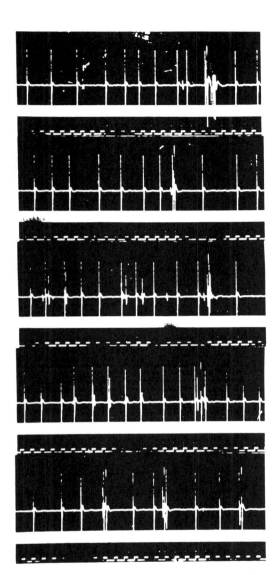

FIGURE 2.11. *A patient with Huntington's disease but no clinically apparent chorea attempts to maintain stable firing in single motor unit of the first dorsal interosseous using audiovisual feedback of needle electrode recorded action potential to establish control. Brief bursts of motor unit potentials followed by pause are seen. This represents the phenomenon of* microchorea. *Time marker indicates 10-ms interval.*

Reflex Mechanism in Tremor

There is marked variability in normal persons in the ease with which deep tendon reflexes can be elicited and an overall positive correlation between the amplitude of physiologic tremor or the severity of essential tremor and the degree of hyperreflexia. These semiquantitative clinical observations suggest that the gain of the stretch reflex plays some role in the amplitude of physiologic tremor and possibly essential tremor.[143] Gain is defined as the ratio of system output to input, and with regard to the myotatic static receptors, it is usually defined as the force recorded per unit of muscle extension under defined conditions. Spinal reflex gain will affect the amplitude and tendency for oscillations to occur. For example, the amplitude of the action potential of extensor indicis proprius muscle activated in response to perturbation of the finger when it is held in extension is proportional to the degree of reflex gain. In other words, the number of MUs recruited into the response to peripheral limb perturbation is proportional to reflex gain.

The frequency of a tremor is dependent not only on the mechanical factors described earlier, but also on delays in the oscillatory circuits involved. The phenomenon of clonus is the best example of the role of delay as a function of pathway length in regulating tremor frequency. The clinical observation of ankle clonus occurring at 4 to 7 c/s and biceps brachii clonus, occurring at a significantly faster rate, supports this concept. Cooling of an extremity slows conduction speed, the rate of muscle contraction, and the rate of physiologic tremor. These observations support a spinal reflex basis for physiologic tremor.

Theoretically *long loop* reflexes, requiring travel to brain stem or higher levels as the mechanism for tremor, would result in lower tremor frequencies. There is overlap in tremor rates between clonus and the resting tremor of parkinsonism. Resting tremor of Parkinson's disease, however, cannot be reset as can essential tremor by peripheral perturbation.[62] Long loop reflexes have been suggested as a physiologic basis for pathologic tremors,[144] but as yet their pathways have not been defined, and their role in disease states has not been elucidated.

Central Oscillators

Central oscillators or drives for tremor are apparently present in the resting tremor of Parkinson's disease, palatal myoclonus, and the tremor induced by harmaline, a monoamine oxidase inhibitor.[145,146] In Parkinson's disease resting tremor, Ia afferent discharge occurs during both contraction and relaxation phases of the tremor strongly indicating periodic gamma efferent activity during muscle contraction.[94] Section of dorsal roots in experimental resting tremor results in either no change or enhancement of resting tremor.[147] Finally, microelectrode recordings from thalamus, motor cortex, and motoneurons following curarization have revealed rhythmic motoneuron discharge at expected tremor frequency.[95]

The drug harmaline induces rhythmic firing of neurons in the inferior olive that continues following complete deafferentation.[148] The complex interaction of this system with the dentato-rubro-olivary *triangle* has been discussed in relation to the periodic disinhibition of spinal interneurons that occurs.[149]

Action tremor mechanisms seem to require both spinal-dependent and cerebellar-dependent loops. The pendular reflex in the hypotonic patient with a cerebellar lesion is probably the clinical parallel of the phase lag in response to sinusoidal stretch seen in the decerebellate cat.[150] In experiments in which the cerebellum was reversibly cooled, some degree of peripheral resetting of tremor frequency could be accomplished.[151] A damping or regulation of motoneuron recruitment by the cerebellum occurring in response to intention that interacts with spinal reflex mechanisms requires further elucidation.

TREATMENT

General Aspects

Most patients with pathologic tremor note a strong association of tremor amplitude or intensity and the degree of psychic arousal. A tremor that is quite tolerable within the confines of home may become unbearable and embarrassing in public. As a consequence, some patients learn to use anxiolytic or sedating drugs in preparation for public apperance. Correspondingly, nearly all patients benefit from learning relaxation techniques such as meditation, self-hypnosis, and *guided imagery*. The presence of tremor, especially at the frequency of physiologic tremor and essential tremor, suggests nervousness to the observer. Presenting the appearance of being "nervous" over a period of many years can influence human relations to a point that psychotherapy may be required.

A variety of mechanical techniques have been used in the treatment of tremor. These include the use of support-restraint devices, weights applied to the limb to increase inertia,[152] and devices designed to limit effort in performing skilled movements. The last of these seems to be the most useful, especially in the treatment of action tremor. As mentioned earlier, tonic electrical stimulation of antagonist muscle can reduce action tremor. Physical therapy designed to improve strength and range of motion may result in better motor control, even without influencing the tremor.

Surgical approaches to the treatment of tremor have ranged from neurectomy to lesion-making in the central nervous system. Thalamotomy involving nucleus ventralis lateralis or nucleus ventralis intermedius has been reported to abolish parkinsonian rest tremor, postural tremor, intention tremor, and tremor involving the head and neck (spasmodic torticollis).[153–156] Action tremor in patients with multiple sclerosis has been reported to respond to electrical stimulation of contralateral midbrain and basal ganglia.[157] In all of the tremors studied, phase-locked bursting discharge of neurons in the relevant regions was recorded. The relatively universal effectiveness of these surgeries and the variety of tremors treated suggest interruption of a common thalamocorticomotor oscillating pathway; the cortical motor *interneuron* responsible for the movement is disconnected.

Specific Therapies

Essential tremor

Patients with essential tremor have known for a long time that ethyl alcohol benefits the tremor in contrast to other means of sedation, which accounts for a high rate of alcoholism among patients with this disorder. Fortunately, with the introduction of β-blockers, such as propranolol, a new mode of therapy was discovered. Propranolol is effective therapy for essential tremor in the dose range from 120 to 240 mg daily.[158–161] The therapeutic response appears to be independent of the serum level of the drug.[162,163] Therapeutic trials with d-propranolol, which has membrane-stabilizing properties but does not produce beta blockade, revealed that it had no influence on tremor in comparison to the d-1-propranolol, which produces beta blockade and is effective treatment.[164] A comparison of the effectiveness of beta$_1$ blockade using atenolol and beta$_1$ plus beta$_2$ blockade using timolol on isoproterenol-induced tremor and essential tremor revealed a significantly greater effect of beta$_2$ blockade.[165] Only a temporary effect on essential tremor was found for beta$_1$ plus beta$_2$ blockade. Comparison of propranolol and metoprolol revealed that over time the effect of metoprolol on essential tremor disappeared.[166]

Therefore beta$_2$ blockade appears to be the essential mechanism of action for effective treatment of essential tremor. Both central and peripheral sites of action may be important.

Other drugs, such as primidone, have been reported to be successful in the treatment of essential tremor[151,167,168] and may be tried in patients such as those with asthma, who cannot be treated with propranolol. Over time (3 to 6 months), the dose of propranolol required to control tremor may have to be increased.[169]

Action tremor

Methods for reducing the effort applied in performance of skilled movement are the physical therapy of choice in the treatment of action tremor. This can be done by unweighting the extremity, either by spring support or by resting the part (elbow, for example) on a foam pad when eating or brushing the teeth.

Action tremor has been reported to be responsive to thalamotomy and electrical stimulation of midbrain and basal ganglia. Although case reports of successful treatment of this kind appear, it seems unlikely that this therapy will find wide usage because such patients usually have a variety of concurrent severe neurologic and medical problems that complicate their management.

In general, the medical therapy of action tremor has been uniformly unsuccessful. Considerable spontaneous variability in the severity of action tremor exists, which impedes reliable assessment of the effects of therapy. It should be noted that the use of such drugs as baclofen and diazepam, both of which reduce the muscle tonus associated with spasticity, may actually enhance action tremor in some patients because the damping influence of increased muscle tone on the tremor is reduced. At the same time, the anxiolytic action of diazepam may help the patient function under conditions of stress.

In a small series of patients with multiple sclerosis, isoniazid was reported to benefit action tremor.[170] It is necessary to give vitamin B$_6$ at the same time. Isoniazid must be used with extreme caution in patients with preexisting neurologic disease, especially those with mild organic brain syndrome. Isoniazid is a common cause of dementia. Although the action tremor is improved, it is replaced by a fine tremor that may be accompanied by asterixis as signs of dementia develop. In doses effective for treatment of tremor, isoniazid may cause worsening of other manifestations of such disorders as multiple sclerosis.

Action tremor has also been treated with l-dopa.[171] The tremor is *suppressed*. Double-blind control studies have not been carried out.

Writing tremor

Writing tremor, in contrast to writer's cramp, which may be a component of a dystonic syndrome, has been shown in a number of cases to be clonic activity, presumably on the basis of muscle spindle hypersensitivity in muscles such as pronator teres. Motor point anesthetic block of the offending muscles has resulted in complete but temporary relief of the tremor.[111] Repeated blockade with long-acting local anesthetics has not been tried. Beta blockade is of no use, but anticholinergic drugs, muscle relaxants and spasmolytic drugs are of modest help. Botulinum toxin injection into selected muscles may prove to be the most effective therapy.[111a] Most treatments reduce the intensity of the tremor but do not abolish it.

Most patients with writer's cramp will require psychotherapy. They become anxious and fearful even on anticipating the act of writing. Physical therapy is directed at placing the patient in control of hand and forearm muscle contraction-relaxation through the use of writing and finger exercises practiced in a relaxed atmosphere. Daily practice and positive reinforcement are necessary. In many respects, the patient must learn to write all over again. If essential tremor is associated with writing tremor, propranolol should be tried.

Spasmodic torticollis

Spasmodic torticollis may be symptomatic of a number of underlying diseases, including hyperthyroidism, hypoparathyroidism, Wilson's disease, ocular muscle imbalance, congenital maldevelopment, injury to neck muscles, postencephalitic manifestation, reaction to drugs (especially phenothiazines), irritative phenomena resulting from tumor or abnormal blood vessels, and as a *fragment* of torsion dystonia. Treatment of the underlying disease process may produce dramatic relief of the torticollis. In the majority of patients, however, no specific cause is identified. Sometimes the history may disclose that the patient's work requires repetitive rotation of the head or continuous readjustment of head position. The repetitive movement may result in *habit spasms* that usually occur whenever the original stimulus is presented, such as tucking a violin under the chin.

Drugs reported to have been successful in the treatment of spasmodic torticollis include diazepam,

haloperidol, amantadine, baclofen, and amitriptyline.[172–174] Isoniazid, pyridoxine, and l-glutamine have been used in combination.[175] The mechanism of action of each of these drugs is quite different, and some are potentially quite toxic. A regimen for treatment of a patient with newly developed spasmodic torticollis might include amitriptyline, which often reduces the severity of muscle spasm, possibly on the basis of its central anticholinergic action. Doses as high as 200 mg daily may be necessary. Subsequently baclofen might be added, with the dose ranging from 60 to 100 mg daily. The purpose of the therapy is to diminish the severity of spasm to tolerable levels. There seems to be little further improvement by the addition of still another drug, such as diazepam. Drug therapy is accompanied by the use of behavioral techniques, such as promoting head turning by touching the face contralateral to the movement, the use of an earphone speaker to promote orientation of the head toward a sound, and range of motion exercises. It is probably a reasonable idea to avoid the use of haloperidol, which of itself can produce dystonia in some patients.

Pain in the suboccipital region on one or both sides is common. Physical therapy is directed at stretching cervical muscles and maintaining a range of motion. Neck pain can be reduced by having the patient assume a prone position with several pillows beneath the chest, so the head can hang forward. Hot moist towels or a cooling gel pad are placed on the back of the neck during this *head hanging* traction.

The therapeutic response with spasmodic torticollis overall has not been encouraging. In a series of patients reported by Sorenson and Hamby,[176] 61 of 71 patients stated that they had received no benefit from medical therapy, and only 39 were satisfied with their postoperative condition. Perhaps the outlook at present is somewhat brighter. The earlier emphasis on stereotactic thalamotomy has been replaced by the use of selective peripheral denervation with heavy reliance on electromyographic recordings. Using this approach, Bertrand et al.[177] have reported results on 35 patients; 88% had good to excellent results, 9% had a fair result, and 3% had poor results. The authors suggest the use of peripheral denervation as the first procedure of choice. Botulinum toxin injections into selected muscles may be as effective as neurectomy.[111a] EMG was helpful in selecting muscles involved and also revealed *inhibited* antagonists that require biofeedback for retraining of function after surgery.

In our own experience, selection of the primary

muscle responsible for the abnormal head rotation and section of the nerve to that muscle or use of botulinum toxin does result in marked reduction in the degree of abnormal movement. Microsurgery with concomitant electromyographic recording from muscle during electrical stimulation of rootlets of the spinal accessory nerve has been an effective method for reduction of abnormal muscle activity and preservation of function. Patient perception of the degree of improvement, however, may be another matter. Despite head position in the midline, some patients still "feel" that position is abnormal and may attempt to correct it by assuming abnormal postures. Retraining of muscles immediately after surgery would seem to be mandatory. More experience with this procedure in a clearly defined group of patients is needed. It must be understood that nerve section is not a cure for spasmodic torticollis but a procedure that may make life more tolerable.

Improvement has been reported using various electromyographic and other biofeedback techniques.[178,179] Improvement usually occurs, but it will disappear unless the patient uses the technique on a daily basis. Most patients will not persist in the long-term use of this technique.

Palatal myoclonus

Drugs used in the general treatment of myoclonus, including clonazepam, tetrabenazine, valproic acid, and carbamazepine, may be helpful in treating palatal myoclonus.[172,180,181] Palatal myoclonus, however, seems more resistant to treatment than other forms of myoclonus. On the other hand, it can disappear spontaneously.[182]

Inasmuch as some patients with palatal myoclonus may be unaware of it, treatment must be adapted to the patient's complaint. A clicking noise resulting from opening and closing of the eustachian tubes may be disturbing to the patient and others. Section of the levator palatini muscles has not been successful in treating this symptom.

Resting tremor of parkinsonism

Centrally acting anticholinergic drugs such as trihexyphenidyl have been used for many years to treat Parkinson's disease. Theoretically these drugs reduce the influence of the disinhibited pallidum on the thalamocortical motor system. More recently l-dopa has been used to substitute for the impaired dopaminergic influence from substantia nigra on the striatum. Direct action of dopamine on cholinergic neurons in the striatum reactivates the inhibitory modulation of the striatum on the pallidum and thereby modifies the signs and symptoms of parkinsonism.

NEUROCHEMICAL ANATOMY AND TREMOR

Two primary central generators of tremor have been proposed. These are the corticopallidothalamic (CPT) loop and the olivocerebellar system.[3,183] More recently, an important influence of the STN on the CPT loop has been suggested.[86]

Corticopallidothalamic loop

In this model, resting tremor is generated in the CPT loop as a result of repetitive activity in globus pallidus that is no longer under the inhibitory influence of the striatum. The normal inhibitory function of the striatum mediated by its cholinergic neurons is lost as a consequence of degeneration of dopaminergic neurons in the substantia nigra. Coupled with the repetitive activity in pallidal neurons is an impairment of frequency control in spinal motoneurons, possibly in cortical motoneurons as well. As a consequence of CPT loop dysfunction, rate coding of motoneurons is lost. As mentioned previously, a revised view of the altered inhibitory input from striatum to globus pallidus has been proposed, the net effect of which is to increase subthalamic nucleus activity. Decreased inhibition of internal globus pallidus and increased inhibition of external globus pallidus result in increased subthalamic nucleus activity.

The CPT loop and the striatum that regulates it are topographically organized. In normal function, it has the capacity to activate individual motoneurons selectively anywhere in the spinal cord. When diseased, the involvement is usually manifested first on one side of the body, sometimes in one extremity. Dystonia may precede the features of parkinsonism. The neurotransmitter of importance in this system is dopamine, present in and represented by the mesotelencephalic system, which consists of the nigrostriatal and mesocortical projections[10] acting on dopamine receptors that have been classified into multiple subtypes.

The olivocerebellar system

Tremors present on action (action tremor) or maintenance of posture (physiologic tremor) and possibly essential tremor are generated from this system. Palatal myoclonus is generated from lesions in the lateral tegmental tract or from deafferentation of the olivary nucleus, whereas action tremor results from involvement of the dentatorubral tract. The noradrenergic system is strongly represented in the brain stem as the lateral tegmental system and locus ceruleus. The lateral tegmental system projects to the dorsal, medial, and lateral reticular formation, then to the hypothalamus and other brain regions, including basal ganglia and the spinal cord. The locus ceruleus projects to hypothalamus, isocortex, cerebellar cortex, and thalamus.[11]

The essential feature of the noradrenergic system is its diffuse representation and its intimate relationship with arousal and recruitment mechanisms. The *amplitude* of responses is disordered when this system is involved. Recruitment of motoneurons is excessive in proportion to the executive command for a specific movement. If essential tremor is caused by a lesion in this system, even the orderly recruitment of motoneurons may be disrupted. The tremors generated from this system are usually diffuse and made worse by adrenergic stimulation. The association of central dysautonomia and such disorders as olivopontocerebellar degeneration and essential tremor add further support to the association between these central noradrenergic systems and the genesis of tremor.[184–187] Although the modeling given here is a crude and grossly oversimplified attempt at conceptualizing neurochemical mechanisms for the generation of tremor, it clearly demonstrates the framework on which improved understanding of tremor pathophysiology can be established.

SUMMARY

Tremor is rhythmic oscillation of a body part that occurs with a regular recurrent pattern. Physical properties of a body part that define its inertia will determine whether or not rhythmic forces applied to it will result in tremor.

Tremor may result from physical factors even remote from a body part or by the rhythmic and synchronized firing of MUs. The physiologic mechanisms by which this process may occur at the spinal level include the myotatic servoloop, recurrent inhibition of motoneurons, and tendon organ activation. Physiologic tremors and essential tremor are mediated by spinal mechanisms and occur at the same rate, 8 to 12 c/s. Tremor rhythm can be reset by mechanical perturbation. The tremor is activated by maintenance of posture. Physiologic tremor and essential tremor are both increased by sympathetic stimulation, but essential tremor may result from factors causing increased MU recruitment within the

spinal cord. Peripheral beta$_2$ blockade does not suppress essential tremor, suggesting that the central nervous system plays a role in tremor genesis.

Intention tremor occurs at 3 to 7 c/s and results from lesions involving efferent cerebellar connections. The body distribution of the tremor is probably related to the specific portion of cerebellar outflow that is involved. The integrating motor pathway includes connections from dentate nucleus to red nucleus, thalamus, and motor cortex. The ratio of input to output neurons for cerebellum is 40:1. The olivocerebellar system regulates the amplitude of motor responses. Tremor results from a mismatch between proprioceptive input and motor output produced by an abnormal gain.

The resting tremor of parkinsonism results from rhythmic discharges in pallidal neurons no longer under the inhibitory influence of striatal cholinergic neurons. Decreased inhibition of STN by external globus pallidus may be important in the genesis of the signs of parkinsonism. Besides tremor, the frequency modulation of motoneurons is impaired, resulting in akinesia. Resting tremor results from a central oscillation. The rhythm of tremor cannot be reset by peripheral perturbation. The motor outflow pathway includes thalamus and motor cortex. The 4 to 6 c/s tremor may result from oscillation in long loop reflexes.

Other tremors arise from a variety of causes. Neurogenic tremor results from activation of spatially disordered MUs; tremor in spasmodic torticollis from oscillations in the vestibulointerstitial-thalamocortical *head turning* mechanism; writing tremor from increased sensitivity to muscle stretch in such muscles as pronator teres or as a fragment of dystonia; palatal myoclonus from a deafferented olivary nucleus, possibly resulting in postdenervation hypersensitivity and hypertrophy; asterixis from intermittent loss of postural tonus; clonus from increased muscle spindle sensitivity with absence of servocontrol resulting in sinusoidal oscillation. Treatment of pathologic tremor consists of propranolol or primidone for essential tremor and l-dopa for resting tremor. Other pathologic tremors respond only partially to treatment.

Pathologic tremors result from an uncovering and amplification of rhythmic neuronal discharges that are inherent properties of neurons and their circuits required for normal movement. The essential motor control features are (1) selection of the part to be moved, (2) selection of the speed of movement, and (3) selection of the amplitude of movement. The pallidothalamocortical system is required for selection of the part and its speed of movement. It is topographically organized. Dopamine is a crucial neurotransmitter in this system. The amplitude of the movement may be controlled by noradrenergic systems. A portion of this system involves cerebellar outflow connections.

As knowledge of noradrenergic and other trans-mitter systems increases, through application of chemical lesioning and blockade techniques, under-standing of tremor mechanisms can also be expected to improve. Also required will be the elucidation of neurophysiologic and neuroanatomic factors requir-ing opportunistic studies of pathologic tremor in the clinic.

REFERENCES

1. Marsden CD. The mechanisms of physiological tremor and their significant in pathological tremors. In: Desmedt JE, ed. Progress in clinical neurophys-iology. Physiological tremor, pathological tremors and clonus. Basel: Karger, 1978:1–16.
2. Marshall J. Tremor. In: Vinken PJ, Bruyn GW, eds. Handbook of clinical neurology. Amsterdam: North Holland, 1970:809–825.
3. Stein RB, Lee RG. Tremor and clonus. In: Brook-hart JM, Mountcastle VB, Brooks VB, Geiger SR, eds. Motor control handbook of physiology—the nervous system. American Physiological Society, Betheseda, MD. 1981:325–343.
4. Frost JD Jr. Triaxial vector accelerometry: A method for quantifying tremor and ataxia. IEEE Trans Biomed Eng 1978; 25(1):17–27.
5. Sinclair KG, Honour AJ, Griffiths RA. A simple method of measuring tremor using a variable-ca-pacitance transducer. Age Ageing 1977; 6(3):168–174.
6. Petajan JH, Watts N. Effects of coiling on the tri-ceps surae reflex. Am J Phys Med 1962; 41:240–251.
7. Mathews PB, Muir RB. Comparison of electro-myogram spectra with force spectra during human elbow tremor. J Physiol (Lond) 1980; 302:427–441.
8. Elble RJ, Sinha R, Higgins C. Quantification of tremor with a digitizing tablet. J Neurosci Methods 1990; 32(3):193–198.
9. Rohracher H. Standige muskel aktivitat (Mikrovi-bration), tonus and konstanz der korpertemperatur. 2. Biol 1959; III:38–53.
10. Hugon M, Fugui L, Seki K. Deep sea diving: Hu-man performance and motor control under hyper-baric conditions with inert gas. In: Desmedt JE, ed. Advances in neurology. Motor control mechanisms in health and disease. New York: Raven Press 1983:829–849.
11. Moore RY. Catecholamine neuron systems in brain. Ann Neurol 1982; 12:321–327.
12. Lippold OCJ. The origin of the alpha rhythm. Edin-burgh: Churchill Livingstone, 1973.
13. Jasper HH, Andrews HL. Brain potentials and vol-untary muscular activity in man. J Neurophysiol 1938; 1:87–100.
14. Marsden CD, Meadows JC, Lange GW, Watson RS. The role of the ballistocardiac impulse in the genesis of physiological tremor. Brain 1969; 92:647–662.
15. Isokawa M, Komisaruk BR. Convergence of finger tremor and EEG rhythm at the alpha frequency induced by rhythmical photic stimulation. Elec-troenceph Clin Neurophysiol 1983; 55(5):580–585.
16. Cussons PD, Mathews PB, Muir RB. Enhancement by agonist or antagonist muscle vibration of tremor at the elastically loaded human elbow. J Physiol (Lond) 1980; 302:443–461.
17. Halliday AM, Redfearn JWT. An analysis of the frequency of finger tremor in healthy subjects. J Physiol (Lond) 1956; 134:600–611.
18. Henatsch HD. Instability of the proprioceptive length servo: Its possible role in tremor phenomena. In: Yahr MD, Purpura DP, eds. Neurophysiological basis of normal and abnormal motor activation. New York: Raven Press, 1967:75–89.
19. Joyce GC, Rack PMH. The effects of load and force on tremor at the normal human elbow joint. J Physiol (Lond) 1974; 240:375–396.
20. Lippold OCJ. Oscillation in the stretch reflex arc and the origin of the rhythmical 8–12 c/s compo-nent of physiological tremor. J Physiol (Lond) 1970; 206:359–382.
21. Halliday AM, Redfearn JWT. Finger tremor in ta-betic patients and its bearing on the mechanism producing the rhythm of physiological tremor. J Neurol Neurosurg Psychiat 1958; 21:101–108.
22. Lance JW, Schwab RS, Peterson EA. Action tremor and the cogwheel phenomenon in Parkinson's dis-ease. Brain 1963; 86:95–110.
23. Marsden CD, Foley TH, Owen DAL. Peripheral beta-adrenergic receptors concerned with tremor. Clin Sci 1967; 33:53–65.
24. Andrews CJ, Neilson PD, Lance JW. The compar-ison of tremors in normal, Parkinsonian, and ath-etotic man. J Neurol Sci 1973; 19:53–61.
25. Pozos RS, Iaizzo PA, Petry RW. Physiological action tremor of the ankle. J Appl Physiol 1982; 52(1):226–230.
26. Petajan JH. Antigravity posture for analysis of mo-tor unit recruitment: The "45 degree test." Muscle Nerve 1990; 13:355–359.
27. Petajan JH, Jarcho LW, Thurman DJ: Motor unit

control in Huntington's disease: A possible pre-symptomatic test. Adv Neurol 1979; 23:163–175.

28. Spencer J, Findling A, Brachrach AJ, et al. Tremor and somatosensory studies during chamber He-O₂ compression to 13.1, 25.2, 37.3, and 49.4 ATA. J Appl Physiol 1979; 47(4):804–812.

29. Logigian EL, Wierzbicka MM, Bruyninakx F, et al. Motor unit synchronization in physiologic, enhanced physiologic and voluntary tremor in man. Ann Neurol 1988; 23:242–250.

30. Burton AC, Bronk D. The motor mechanism of shivering and thermal muscular tone. Am J Physiol 1937; 119:284.

31. Sessler DI, Ponte J. Shivering during epidural anesthesia. Anesthesiology 1990; 72(5):816–821.

32. Kawamura Y, Kishi K, Fujimoto J. Electromyographic analysis of the shivering movement. Jap J Physiol 1953; 15:676–686.

33. Petajan JH, Williams DM. Behavior of single motor units during pre-shivering tone and shivering tremor. Am J Phys Med 1972; 51:16–22.

34. Stuart D, Ott K, Ishikawa K, Eldred E. The rhythm of shivering: I. General sensory contributions. Am J Phys Med 1966; 45:61–74.

35. Hensel H. Neural processes in thermoregulations. Physiol Rev 1973; 53:948–1017.

36. Perkins JF Jr. The role of the proprioceptors in shivering. Am J Physiol 1945; 145:264–271.

37. Hansen LA, Pender MP. Hypothermia due to an ascending impairment of shivering in hyperacute experimental allergic encephalomyelitis in the Lewis rat. J Neurol Sci 1989; 94:231–240.

38. Cooper S. Muscle spindles and other muscle receptors. In: Bourne SH, ed. The structure and function of muscle. New York: Academic Press, 1960: 379.

39. Lippold O. The tremor in fatigue. In: CIBA Foundation Symposium '82. Human muscle fatigue: Physiological mechanisms. London, 1981:234–248.

40. Gooch JL, Newton BY, Petajan JH. Motor unit spike counts before and after maximal voluntary contraction. Muscle Nerve 1990; 13:1146–1151.

41. Marsden CD, Meadows JC, Merton PA. "Muscular wisdom" that minimizes fatigue during prolonged effort in man: Peak rates of motoneuron discharge and slowing of discharge during fatigue. In: Desmedt JE, ed. Motor control mechanism in health and disease. New York: Raven Press, 1983:169–211.

42. Growdon JH, Young RR, Shahani BT. The differential diagnosis of tremor in Parkinson's disease. Trans Am Neurol Assoc 1975:100.

43. Schroeder D, Nasrallsh HA. High alcoholism rate in patients with essential tremor. Am J Psychiatry 1982; 139(11):1471–1473.

44. Haerr AF, Anderson DW, Schoenberg BS. Prevalence of essential tremor. Results from the Copiah county study. Arch Neurol 1982; 39(12):750–751.

45. Rautakorpi I, Takala J, Marttila RJ, et al. Essential tremor in a Finnish population. Acta Neurol Scand 1982; 66:58–67.

46. Hsu YD, Chang MK, Sung SC, et al. Chung-Hua-I-Hsueh-Tsa-Chih 1990; 45(2):93–99.

47. Schwab RS, Young RR. Non-resting tremor in Parkinson's disease. Trans Am Neurol Assoc 1971; 96:305–307.

48. Salisachs P, Codina A, Gimenez-Roldan S, Sarranz JJ. Chacot-Marie-Tooth disease associated with 'essential tremor' and normal and/or slightly diminished motor conduction velocity. Report of 7 cases. Eur Neurol 1979; 18(1):49–58.

49. Ziegler DK. Tourette's syndrome and essential tremor in a septuagenarian (letter). Arch Neurol 1982; 39(2):132.

50. Martinelli P, Gabellini AS. Essential tremor and buccolinguofacial dyskinesias. Acta Neurol Scand 1982; 66(6):705–708.

51. Lesage J, Chouinard G. Manic-depressive illness associated with Klinefelter's syndrome and essential tremor (letter). Am J Psychiatry 1978; 135(6):757–758.

52. Baxter DW, Lal S, Rasminsky M. Essential tremor and dystonic syndromes. Can J Neurol Sci 1979; 6:74.

53. Rosenfield DB, Donovan DT, Sulek M, et al. Neurologic aspects of spasmodic dysphonia. J Otolaryngol 1990; 19(4):231–236.

54. Whyte S, Darveniza P. A review of 20 cases of spastic dysphonia. Clin Exp Neurol 1989; 26:177–181.

55. Gabellini AS, Martinelli P, Gulli MR, et al. Orthostatic tremor: Essential and symptomatic cases. Acta Neurol Scand 1990; 81(2):113–117.

56. Hartman DE, Overholt SL, Vishwanat B. A case of vocal cord nodules masking essential (voice) tremor. Arch Otolaryngol 1982; 108(1):52–53.

57. Calzetti S, Sasso E, Baratti M, Fava R. Clinical and computer-based assessment of long-term therapeutic efficacy of propranolol in essential tremor. Acta Neurol Scand 1990; 81(5):392–396.

58. Sasso E, Perucca E, Fava R, Calzetti S. Primidone in the long-term treatment of essential tremor: A prospective study with computerized quantitative analysis. Clin Neuropharmacol 1990; 13(1):67–76.

59. Koller WC, Vetere-Overfield B. Acute and chronic effects of propranolol and primidone in essential tremor. Neurology 1989; 39(12):1587–1588.

60. Young RR, Growdon JH, Shahani BT. Beta-adrenergic mechanisms in action tremor. N Engl J Med 1975; 293:950–953.

61. Colebatch JG, Findley LJ, Frackowiak RS, et al. Preliminary report: Activation of the cerebellum in essential tremor. Lancet 1990; 336(8722):1028–1030.

62. Lee RG, Stein RB. Resetting of tremor by mechanical perturbations: A comparison of essential tremor and parkinsonian tremor. Ann Neurol 1981; 10(6):523–553.

63. Shahani BT, Young RR. Action tremors: A clinical neurophysiological review. In: Desmedt JE, ed. Progress in clinical neurophysiology. Physiological tremor, pathological tremors and clonus. Basel: Karger, 1978:129–137.

64. Petajan JH, Thurman DJ. EMG and histochemical findings in neurogenic atrophy with electrode localisation. J Neurol Neurosurg Psychiat 1981; 44:1050–1053.

65. Bathien N, Rondot P, Toma S. Inhibition and synchronisation of tremor induced by a muscle twitch. J Neurol Neurosurg Psychiat 1980; 43(8):713–718.

66. Taly AB, Nagaraja D, Vasanth A. Trunkal tremor: Orthostatic or essential? J Assoc Physicians India 1989; 37(8):539–541.

67. Koppel BX, Daras M. "Rubral" tremor due to midbrain *Toxoplasma* abscess. Mov Disord 1990; 5(3):254–256.

68. Pomeranz S, Shalit M, Serman Y. "Rubral" tremor following radiation of a pineal region vascular hamartoma. Acta Neurochir Wien 1990; 103:79–81.

69. Brooks, VB, Thach WT. Cerebellar control of posture and movement. In: Brookhart JM, Mountcastle VB, Brooks VB, Geiger SR, eds. Handbook of physiology. The nervous system. Baltimore: Williams & Wilkins, 1981:877–948.

70. Brodal A. Neurological anatomy in relation to clinical medicine, ed. 3. New York: Oxford University Press, 1981.

71. Bronstein AM, Hood JD, Gresty MA, Panagi C. Visual control of balance in cerebellar and parkinsonian syndromes. Brain 1990; 113:767–779.

72. Mauritz KH, Schmitt C, Dichgans J. Delayed and enhanced long latency reflexes as the possible cause of postural tremor in late cerebellar atrophy. Brain 1981; 104:97–116.

73. Silfverskiold BP. Cortical cerebellar degeneration associated with a specific disorder of standing and locomotion. Acta Neurol Scand 1977; 55(4):257–262.

74. Thach WT. Discharge of cerebellar neurons related to two maintained postures and two prompt movements. J Neurophysiol 1970; 33:527–547.

75. Thach WT. Single unit studies of long loops involving the motor cortex and cerebellum during limb movements in monkeys. In: Desmedt JE, ed. Progress in clinical neurophysiology. Vol. 4. Cerebral motor control in man: Long loop mechanism. Basel: Karger, 1978:94–106.

76. Thach WT. Correlation of neural discharge with pattern and force of muscular activity, joint position, and direction of intended next movement in motor cortex and cerebellum. J Neurophysiol 1978; 41:654–676.

77. Lamarre Y, Spidalieri G, Lund JP. Patterns of muscular and motor cortical activity during a simple arm movement in monkey. Can J Physiol Pharmacol 1981; 59:748–756.

78. Schieber MH, Thach WT. Alpha-gamma dissociation during slow tracking movements of the monkey's wrist: Preliminary evidence from spinal ganglion recording. Brain Res 1980; 202:213–216.

79. Shapalov AI. Neuronal organization and synaptic mechanisms of supraspinal motor control in vertebrates. Rev Physiol Biochem Pharmacol 1975; 72:1–54.

80. Miller S, Oscarsson O. Termination and functional organizations of spino-olivo-cerebellar paths. In: Fields WS, Willis WD, eds. The cerebellum in health and disease. St. Louis: Green, 1970:172–200.

81. Oscarsson O. Functional organization of spinocerebellar paths. In: Iggo A, ed. Handbook of sensory physiology, somatosensory system. Berlin: Springer-Verlag, 1973:339–380.

82. Lundberg A. Function of the ventral spinocerebellar tract: A new hypothesis. Exp Brain Res 1971; 12:317–330.

83. Mema I, Marvin O, Fuenzalida S, Cotzias G. Chronic manganese poisoning. Neurology 1967; 17:18.

84. Ayd FJ. A survey of drug induced extrapyramidal syndromes. JAMA 1961; 175:1054.

85. Garfinkel VS, Osovets SM. Mechanisms of generation of oscillations in the tremor form of parkinsonism. Biofizika 1973; 18:731–738.

86. Bergman H, Wichmann T, Delong MR. Reversal of experimental parkinsonism by lesions of subthalamic nucleus. Science 1990; 249:1436–1437.

87. Palombo E, Prrino LJ, Bankiewicz KS, et al. Local cerebral glucose utilization in monkeys with hemiparkinsonism induced by intracarotid infusion of the neurotoxin MPTP. J Neurosci 1990; 10(3):860–869.

88. Buzsaki G, Smith A, Berger S, et al. *Petit mal* epilepsy and parkinsonian tremor: Hypothesis of a common pacemaker. Neuroscience 1990; 36(1):1–14.

89. Bannister R, Oppenheimer D. Parkinsonism, system degenerations and autonomic failure. In: Marsden DC, Fahn S, eds. Movement disorders, neurology 2. Butterworth Int'l Medial Reviews, London, Boston, 1981:174–190.

90. Crystal HA, Dickson DW, Lizardi JE, et al. Antemortem diagnosis of diffuse Lewy body disease. Neurology 1990; 40(10):1523–1528.

91. Petajan JH, Jarcho LW. Motor unit control in Parkinson's disease and the influence of levodopa. Neurology (Minn) 1975; 25(9):866–869

92. Teravainen H, Calne DB. Action tremor in Par-

kinson's disease. J Neurol Neurosurg Psychiat 1980; 43(3): 257–263.

93. Stiles RB, Pozos RS. A mechanical-reflex oscillator hypothesis for parkinsonian hand tremor. J Appl Physiol 1976; 40:990–998.

94. Hagbarth KG, Wallin G, Lofstett L, Awuilonius SM. Muscle spindle activity in alternating tremor of parkinsonism and in clonus. J Neurol Neurosurg Psychiat 1975; 38:636–641.

95. Joffroy AJ, Lamarre Y. Rhythmic unit firing in the precentral cortex in relation with postural tremor in a deafferented limb. Brain Res 1971; 27:386–389.

96. Narabayashi H, Ohye C. Parkinsonian tremor and nucleus ventralis intermedius (VIM) of the human thalamus. In: Desmedt JE, ed. Progress in clinical neurophysiology. Physiological tremor, pathological tremors and clonus. Basel:Karger, 1978:165–182.

97. Cooper IS. Motor functions of the thalamus with recent observations concerning the role of the pulvinar. Int J Neurol 1971; 8:238–259.

98. Walsh EG. Beats produced between a rhythmic applied force and the resting tremor of parkinsonism. J Neurol Neurosurg Psychiat 1979; 42(1):89–94.

99. Findley LJ, Gresty MA, Halmagyi GM. Tremor, the cogwheel phenomenon and clonus in Parkinson's disease. J Neurol Neurosurg Psychiat 1981; 44(6):534–546.

100. Adams RD, Shahani BT, Young RR. Tremor in association with polyneuropathy. Trans Am Neurol Assoc 1972; 97:44–48.

101. Said G, Bathien N, Cesaro P. Peripheral neuropathies and tremor. Neurology (NY) 1982; 32(5):480–485.

102. Bertrand C, Molina-Negro P, Martinez SN. Combined stereotactic and peripheral surgical approach for spasmodic torticollis. Appl Neurophysiol 1978; 41:122–133.

103. Mathews WB, Beasky P, Parry-Jonos W, Garland G. Spasmodic torticollis: A combined study. J Neurol Neurosurg Psychiat 1978; 41:485–492.

104. Meares R. An association of spasmodic torticollis and writer's cramp. Br J Psychiat 1971; 119:441–442.

105. Mizawa I. Experimental spasmodic torticollis in the cat. Arch J Chir 1963; 32:597–624.

106. Kuste M, Iivanainen M, Juntunen J, Setala A. Brain involvement in spasmodic torticollis. Acta Neurol Scand 1981; 6:373–380.

107. Sarnat HB. Idiopathic torticollis: Sternocleido-mastoid myopathy and accessory neuromyopathy. Muscle Nerve 1981; 4(5):374–380.

108. Henry AK. Extensile exposure, ed 2. New York: Churchill Livingstone, 1973:81.

109. Elble RJ, Moody C, Higgins C. Primary writing tremor. A form of focal dystonia? Mov Disord 1990; 5(2):118–126.

110. Klawans HL, Glantz R, Tanner CM, Goetz CG. Primary writing tremor: A selective action tremor. Neurology (NY) 1982; 32(2):203–206.

111. Rothwell JC, Traub MM, Marsden CD. Primary writing tremor. J Neurol Neurosurg Psychiat 1979; 42(12):1106–1114.

111a. Jankovic J, Brin MF. Drug Therapy: Therapeutic uses of botulinum toxin. NEJM 1991; 324(17):1186–1194.

112. Ohye C, Miyazaki M, Hirae T, et al. Primary writing tremor treated by stereotactic selective thalamotomy. J Neurol Neurosurg Psychiat 1982; 45(11):988–997.

113. Wade P, Gresty MA, Findley LJ. A normative study of postural tremor of the hand. Arch Neurol 1982; 39(6):358–362.

114. Nathanson M. Palatal myoclonus: Further clinical and pathophysiological observations. Arch Neurol Psychiat (Chic) 1956; 75:285.

115. Hermann C Jr, Brown JW. Palatal myoclonus: A reappraisal. J Neurol Sci 1967; 5:473–492.

116. Lapresle J. Rhythmic palatal myoclonus and the dentato-olivary pathway. J Neurol 1979; 220(4):223–230.

117. Guillain G, Mollaret P. Deux cas de myoclonies synchrones et rhthmees velopharyugo-laryngo-oculo-diaphragmatique. Le probleme anatomique et physiologique. Rev Neurol 1931; 11:545.

118. Alajouanine T, Hornet T. Myoclonies de desafferentation olivaire. In: Bonduelle M, Gastant H, eds. Les Myoclonies. Paris: Masson et cie, 1968:143–146.

119. Matsuo F, Ajax ET. Palatal myoclonus and denervation supersensitivity in the central nervous system. Ann Neurol 1979; 5(1):72–78.

120. Swanson PD, Luttrell CN, Magladery JW. Myoclonus—a report of 67 cases and review of the literature. Medicine 1962; 41:339.

121. Masucci E, Kurtzke J. Palatal myoclonus associated with extremity tremor. J Neurol 1989; 236(8):474–477.

122. Shahani BT, Young RR. Asterixis—a disorder of the neural mechanisms underlying sustained muscle contraction. In: Manik S, ed. The motor systems: Neurophysiology and muscle mechanisms. New York: Elsevier Scientific, 1976:301–313.

123. Tarsy D, Lieberman B, Chirico-Posst J, Benson F. Unilateral asterixis associated with a mesencephalic syndrome. Arch Neurol 1977; 34(7):446–447.

124. Donat JR. Unilateral asterixis dur to thalamic hemorrhage. Neurology (NY) 1980; 30(1):83–84.

125. Bril V, Sharpe JA, Abby P. Midbrain asterixis. Ann Neurol 1979; 6:362–364.

126. Denny-Brown D. The basal ganglia and their relation to disorders of movement. London: Oxford University Press, 1961.

127. Powers RK, Marder-Meyer J, Rymer WZ. Quantitative relations between hypertonia and stretch

reflex threshold in spastic hemiparesis. Ann Neurol 1988; 23:115–124.

128. Petajan JH. Motor unit control in spasticity. In: Feldman RG, Young RR, Koella WP, eds. Spasticity: Disordered motor control. Chicago: Symposia Specialists, Inc., Medical Books, Year Book, 1979:233–247.

129. Marsden CD, Meadows JC, Lowe RD. The influence of noradrenaline, tyramine, and activation of sympathetic nerves on physiological tremor in man. Clin Sci 1969; 37:243–252.

130. Marsden CD, Tarsy D, Baldessarini RJ. Spontaneous and drug-induced movement disorders in psychotic patients. In: Benson F, Blumer D, eds. Psychiatric aspects of neurologic disease. New York, Grune & Stratton, 1975:219–265.

131. Karas BJ, Wilder BJ, Hammond EJ, Bauman AW. Valproate tremors. Neurology (NY) 1982; 32(4):428–432.

132. Hyman NM, Dennis PD, Sinclair KG. Tremor due to sodium valproate. Neurology (Minneap) 1979; 29:1177–1180.

133. Besch P, Thomsen J, Prytz S, et al. The profile and severity of lithium-induced side effects in mentally healthy subjects. Neuropsychobiology 1979; 5(3):160–166.

134. Lippold OC, Williams EJ, Wilson CG. Finger tremor and cigarette smoking. Br J Clin Pharmacol 1980; 10(1):83–86.

135. Fawer RF, de Ribaupierre Y, Guillemin MP, et al. Measurement of hand tremor induced by industrial exposure to metallic mercury. Br J Ind Med 1983; 40(2):204–208.

136. Bajada S, Fisher A. Resting tremor in alcoholic brain disease. Proc Aust Assoc Neurol 1977; 14:15–23.

137. Freed E. Alcohol-triggered neuroleptic-induced tremor, rigidity and dystonia (letter). Med J Aust 1981; 2(1):44–45.

138. Rosenhamer H, Silfverskiold BP. Slow tremor and delayed brain stem auditory evoked responses in alcoholics. Arch Neurol 1980; 37(5):293–296.

139. Rack DMH. Limitations of somatosensory feedback in control of posture and movement. In: Brookhard JM, Mountcastle VB, Brooks VB, Geiger SR, eds. Handbook of physiology, Section I. The nervous system. Vol II. Motor control. Bethesda, MD: American Physiological Society, 1981: 229–256.

140. Houk JC, Rymer WZ. Neural control of muscle length and tension. In: Brookhard JM, Mountcastle BV, Brooks VB, Geiger SR, eds. Handbook of physiology, Section I. The Nervous System. Vol II. Motor control, Part 1. Bethesda, MD: American Physiological Society, 1981:257–324.

141. Milsum JH. Biological Control systems analysis. New York: McGraw-Hill, 1966:16–18.

142. Halonen JP, Lang ATT, Partanen VSJ. Change in motor unit firing rate after double discharge: An electromyogram study in man. Exp Neurol 1977; 55:538–545.

143. Young RR, Habarth K. Physiological tremor enhanced by maneuvers affecting the segmental stretch reflex. J Neurol Neurosurg Psychiat 1980; 43:248–256.

144. Stein RB, Oguztoreli MN. Tremor and other oscillations in neuro-muscular systems. Biol Cybern 1976; 22:147–157.

145. Llinas R, Volkind RA. The olivo-cerebellar system: Functional properties as revealed by harmaline-induced tremor. Exp Brain Res 1973; 18:69–87.

146. Weiss MJ. Rhythmic activity of spinal interneurons in harmaline treated cats. A model for olivo-cerebellar influence at the spinal level. J Neurol Sci 1982; 54(3):341–348.

147. Ohye C, Bouchard R, Larochelle L, et al. Effect of dorsal rhizotomy on postural tremor in the monkey. Exp Brain Res 1970; 10:140–150.

148. Lamarre YU, Jaffroy AJ, Dumont M, et al. Central mechanisms of tremor in some feline and primate models. J Can Sci Neurol 1975; 2:227–233.

149. Lamarre Y, Demontiguy C, Dumont M, Weiss M. Harmaline induced rhythmic activity of cerebellar and lower brain stem neurons. Brain Res 1971; 32:246–250.

150. Jansen JKS, Matthews PBC. The central control of the synaptic response of muscle spindle receptors. J Physiol (Lond) 1962; 161:357–378.

151. Broks VB, Kozlovskaya IB, Atkin A, et al. Effects of cooling dentate nucleus on tracking task performance in monkeys. J Neurophysiol 1973; 36:974–995.

152. Hewer RL, Cooper R, Morgan MH. An investigation into the value of treating intention tremor by weighting the affected limb. Brain 1972; 95:579–590.

153. Narabayashi H, Ohye C. Importance of microstereoencephalotomy for tremor alleviation. Appl Neurophysiol 1980; 43:222–227.

154. Mimura Y, Bekku H, Miyamoto T, et al. VL thalamotomy for the treatment of tremor in patients with thalamic syndrome. Appl Neurophysiol 1975–1977; 39(3–4):199–201.

155. Andrew J, Fowler CJ, Harrison MJ. Tremor after head injury and its treatment by stereotaxic surgery. J Neurol Neurosurg Psychiat 1982; 45(9):815–819.

156. Andrew J, Fowler CJ, Harrison MJ, Dendall BE. Post-traumatic tremor due to vascular injury and its treatment by stereotactic thalamotomy. J Neurol Neurosurg Psychiat 1982; 45(6):560–562.

157. Brice J, McLellan L. Suppression of intention tremor by contingent deep-brain stimulation. Lancet 1980; 1:1221–1222.

158. Calzetti S, Findley LJ, Gresty MA, et al. Effect of

a single oral dose of propranolol on essential tremor: A double-blind controlled study. Ann Neurol 1983; 13(2):165–171.

159. Baruzzi A, Procaccianti G, Martinelli P, et al. Phenobarbital and propranolol in essential tremor: A double-blind controlled clinical trial. Neurology (NY) 1983; 33(3):296–300.

160. Jefferson D, Jenner P, Marsden CD. Relationship between plasma propranolol concentration and relief of essential tremor. J Neurol Neurosurg Psychiat 1979; 42(9):831–837.

161. Teravainen H, Larsen A, Fogelholm R. Comparison between the effects of pindolol and propranolol on essential tremor. Neurology (Minneap) 1977; 27(5):439–442.

162. McAllister RG Jr, Markesbery WR, Ware RW, Howell SM. Suppression of essential tremor by propranolol: Correlation of effect with drug plasma levels and intensity of beta-adrenergic blockade. Ann Neurol 1977; 1(2):160–166.

163. Sorensen PS, Paulson OB, Steiness E, Jansen EC. Essential tremor treated with propranolol: Lack of correlation between clinical effect and plasma propranolol levels. Ann Neurol 1981; 9(1):53–57.

164. Larsen TA, Ter "av" Ainen H. Propranolol and essential tremor: Role of the membrane effect. Acta Neurol Scand 1982; 66(3):289–294.

165. Dietrichson P, Espen E. Effects of timolol and atenolol on benign essential tremor: Placebo-controlled studies based on quantitative tremor recording. J Neurol Neurosurg Psychiat 1981; 44(8):677–683.

166. Calzetti S, Findley LJ, Perucca E, Richens A. Controlled study of metoprolol and propranolol during prolonged administration in patients with essential tremor. J Neurol Neurosurg Psychiat 1982; 45(10):893–897.

167. Young RR. Essential-familial tremor and enhanced physiological tremors. In: Johnson RT, ed. Current therapy in neurologic disease. Philadelphia: BC Decker, 1985:270–275.

168. Winkler GF, Young RR. Efficacy of chronic propranolol varieties. N Engl J Med 1974; 290:984–988.

169. Young RR, Shahani BT. Pharmacology of tremor. Clin Neuropharmacol 1979; 4:139–156.

170. Sabra AF, Hallett M, Sudarsky L, Mullally W. Treatment of action tremor in multiple sclerosis with isoniazid. Neurology (NY) 1982; 32(8):912–913.

171. Findley LJ, Grestly MA. Suppression of "rubral" tremor with levodopa. Br Med J 1980; 281:1043.

172. Klawans HL, Weiner WJ. Textbook of Clinical Neuropharmacology. New York: Raven Press, 1981.

173. Gildenberg PL. Comprehensive management of spasmodic torticollis. Appl Neurophysiol 1981; 44(4):233–243.

174. Gilbert GJ. The medical treatment of spasmodic torticollis. Arch Neurol 1972; 27:503–506.

175. Korein J, Lieberman A, Kupersmith M, Levidow L. Effect of L-glutamine and isoniazid on torticollis and segmental dystonia. Ann Neurol 1981; 10(3):247–250.

176. Sorenson BF, Hamby WB. Spasmodic torticollis: Results in 71 surgically treated patients. Neurology 1966; 16:867–878.

177. Bertrand C, Molina-Negro P, Martinaz SN. Technical aspects of selective peripheral denervation of spasmodic torticollis. Appl Neurophysiol 1982; 45:326–330.

178. Cleeland CS. Behavioral techniques in the modification of spasmodic torticollis. Neurology 1973; 23:1241–1246.

179. Martin PR. Spasmodic torticollis: A behavioral perspective. J Behav Med 1982; 5(2):249–273.

180. Ferro JM. Palatal mycoclonus and carbamazepine. Ann Neurol 1981; 10(4):402.

181. Sakai T. Palatal myoclonus responding to carbamazepine. Ann Neurol 1981; 9(2):199–200.

182. Aberfeld DC. Disappearing palatal myoclonus. Neurology 1982; 32(3):372–378.

183. Lamarre Y. Tremorgenic mechanisms in primates. In: Meldrum B, Marsden CD, eds. Advances in neurology. New York: Raven Press, 1975:23–24.

184. Song JH, Mastri AR, Segal E. Pathology of Shy-Drager syndrome. J Neuropath Exp Neurol 1979; 38:353–368.

185. Ziegler MC, Lake CR Kopin IO. The sympathetic nervous system defect in primary orthostatic hypotension. N Engl J Med 1977; 296:293–297.

186. Lindval O, Bjorkland A, Skagorberg G. Dopamine-containing neurons in the spinal cord: Anatomy and some functional aspects. Ann Neurol 1983; 14:255–260.

187. Galass G, Nemni R, Baraldi A, et al. Peripheral neuropathy in multiple systems atrophy with autonomic failure. Neurology 1982; 32:1116–1121.

3

Neurophysiologic Examination of the Trigeminal, Facial, Hypoglossal, and Spinal Accessory Nerves in Cranial Neuropathies and Brain Stem Disorders

Bram W.
Ongerboer de Visser
Giorgio Cruccu

CONTENTS

LIST OF ACRONYMS

BAEP	brainstem auditory evoked potential
MEP	motor evoked potential
MIR	masseter inhibitory reflex
M-wave	direct motor response
N	negative scalp potential
P	positive scalp potential
R1	first or early blink reflex response
R2	second or late blink reflex response
R1/D ratio	ratio between R1 latency and latency of the direct response obtained by facial nerve stimulation
SEP	somatosensory evoked potential
SP1	first or early silent period
SP2	second or late silent period
TMD	temporomandibular joint dysfunction
VEP	visual evoked potential
W	early waves of the trigeminal nerve SEP

Testing reflexes passing through the trigeminal system is an important part of a routine neurologic examination. The clinical observer cannot, however, assess the latencies or, even, absent responses and recovery characteristics of these reflexes; these data could provide additional diagnostically useful information. Some aspects of the trigeminal reflexes, such as reflex inhibition of muscle activity, cannot be observed by the clinician at all. Electrophysiologic studies therefore offer the clinician valuable diagnostic and prognostic information. Lesions affecting the V and VII nerves of the brain stem can be localized and their evolution monitored throughout the course of a disease. Electrophysiologic testing of cranial nerves and brain stem function does not rely on trigeminal reflex recording alone. Muscle innervated by the trigeminal, facial, hypoglossal, and spinal accessory nerves is readily accessible to needle electromyography (EMG). Nerve conduction studies, at one time confined to the facial nerve, can now be performed on other cranial nerves as a result of the introduction of magnetic transcranial stimulation. Finally, this chapter discusses the much debated problem of trigeminal evoked potentials. Electrophysiologic assessment of other cranial nerves, such as brain stem auditory evoked potentials for the acoustic nerve, visual evoked potentials for the optic nerve, and eye movement recordings for the oculomotor system, is not dealt with here.

ORBICULARIS OCULI REFLEXES

Blink Reflex and Corneal Reflex

The *blink reflex* elicited by tapping one side of the forehead or the glabella has long been used in neurology. It was first described by Overend in 1896.[1] Kugelberg, in 1952,[2] was the first to study electromyographically the blink reflex evoked by electrical stimulation of the supraorbital nerve. Kugelberg showed that the reflex consisted of two responses (Figure 3.1). The first or early reflex, R1, is a brief response that occurs at a latency of about 10 ms ipsilateral to the side of the stimulation. The second or late response, R2, has a latency of about 30 ms and is more prolonged and bilateral. The common afferent limb of the reflex components is mediated via ophthalmic division of the trigeminal nerve mainly through medium myelinated (A-beta) cutaneous fibers.[2–4] The facial nerve is the common efferent limb.

Clinicoelectrophysiologic correlation and electrocoagulation experiments in cats suggest the R1 is

mediated through the pons.[5–8] Electrophysiologic and anatomic studies in humans strongly suggest that the early reflex is exteroceptive and not proprioceptive in nature.[6,8] It is relayed through an oligosynaptic arc including one to three interneurons, probably located in the vicinity of the main sensory nucleus of the trigeminal nerve (Figure 3.1). R1 is not visible clinically but may have a preparatory function, by shortening the late blink reflex delay.[9]

The R2 blink reflex correlates with closure of the eyelids. Nerve impulses responsible for R2 are conducted through the spinal tract in the dorsolateral region of the pons and medulla oblongata before they reach the most caudal area of the spinal trigeminal nucleus.[10,11] From there, impulses are relayed through polysynaptic medullary pathways ascending both ipsilaterally and contralaterally to the stimulated side of the face, before connecting to the facial nuclei. The crossing of impulses takes place in the caudal medullary region, and the trigeminofacial connections are thought to pass through the lateral reticular formation and lie medial to the spinal trigeminal nucleus[11] (Figure 3.1). R1 and R2 share the same motoneurons.[9]

The *corneal reflex* is evoked by a light mechanical stimulus to the surface of the cornea and consists of a bilateral contraction of the orbicularis oculi muscles, closing the eyelids. The reflex is typically nociceptive and serves to protect the eye.

The cornea is innervated by unmyelinated (C) and small myelinated (A-delta) fibers.[12] After penetrating the cornea, the latter axons lose their myelin sheath. Both types of axons terminate in the stroma and epithelium as free nerve endings. They constitute the receptive part of the reflex arc. The A-delta fibers, which constitute the afferent units of the corneal reflex,[4,13] pass through the long ciliary nerves and the ophthalmic division of the trigeminal sensory root, to reach the pons.[8,14] The central pathway is similar to the R2 of the blink reflex[14] (Figure 3.2). Afferent impulses descend along the spinal trigeminal tract, reach below the obex at the level of the trigeminal subnucleus caudalis, and ascend through a multisynaptic chain of interneurons in the lateral reticular formation before projecting to facial motoneurons.

Despite similar medullary pathways and motoneurons, the corneal and late blink hibit important differences.[13–16] Co bers are smaller than the affere and form a small fiber bur and descending tract blink reflex probably

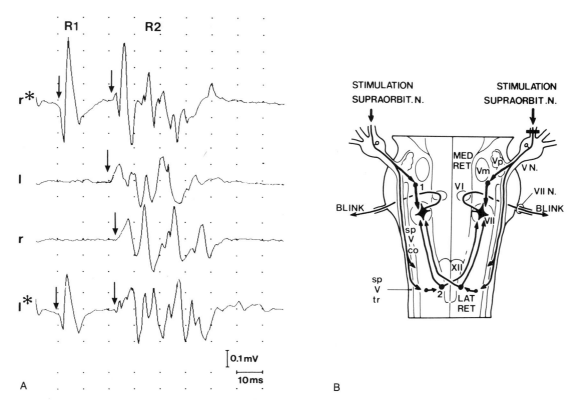

FIGURE 3.1. *(A) Normal early (R1) and bilateral late (R2) blink reflex. Upper two traces show responses from the right (r) and left (l) lower eyelids to right (r*) and lower to left (l*) supraorbital nerve stimulation. (B) Diagram showing the presumed location of the bulbar interneurons subserving the two components of the blink reflex: (1) interneurons subserving the ipsilateral early components; (2) interneurons subserving the bilateral late component. (Vm, Trigeminal motor nucleus; Sp V Co, spinal trigeminal complex; Sp V Tr, spinal trigeminal tract; VI, abducens nucleus; VII, facial nucleus; VII N, facial nerve; V N, ophthalmic trigeminal sensory root; XII, hypoglossal nucleus; LAT RET, lateral reticular formation; MED RET, medial reticular formation.)*

No early response precedes the corneal reflex, and the latency and duration of the blink response are both greater and habituate less to repetitive stimulation as compared with the R2. On the other hand, the R2 is more secure than the corneal reflex. These dissimilarities explain why the blink reflex cannot be equated with the corneal reflex and why clinical disorders may affect the two reflexes separately.

nique and Normal Blink Reflex Responses

cording of the electrical blink reflex, the
upine on a bed with the eyes open. The
rve is stimulated transcutaneously.
aced over the supraorbital notch
le is placed about 2 cm higher

and rotated laterally at an oblique angle to avoid spread of current to the contralateral supraorbital nerve (Figure 3.3). If the second trigeminal division is to be examined, the infraorbital nerve is stimulated by placing the cathode over the nerve as it exits through the infraorbital foramen at the inferior rim of the orbit and the anode about 2 cm below the cathode.

To minimize habituation, shocks should be delivered at intervals of 7 seconds or more, while the subject is kept alert.[17] Low-intensity shocks are used initially and the intensity gradually increased until at the optimal stimulus intensity, maximal and nearly stable responses with repeated trials occur. Even in normal subjects, R1 is sometimes difficult to obtain. To facilitate the response, the patient is asked to

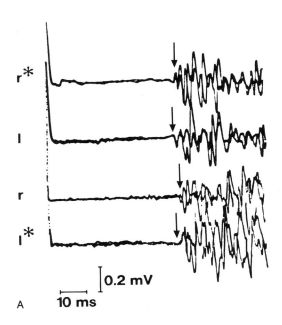

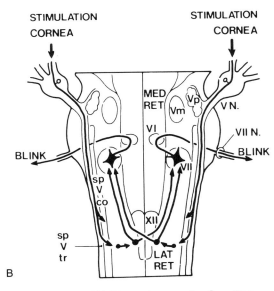

A

B

FIGURE 3.2. *(A) Normal corneal reflex. Upper two traces show responses from the right (r) and left (l) lower eyelid to mechanical stimulation of the right (r*) cornea. Lower two traces are the responses to stimulation of the left (l*) cornea. (B) Diagram showing the presumed location of the bulbar interneurons subserving the corneal reflex. (For key abbreviations, see legend to Figure 3.1.)*

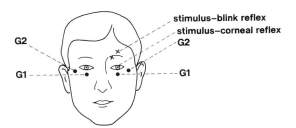

FIGURE 3.3. *Electrode placements for recording responses to supraorbital nerve and corneal stimulations. (G1 = active electrode and G2 = reference electrode in this and other figures.)*

close the eyes, or stimuli are given in pairs at a short time-interval (5 ms).[18] Reflex responses from the inferior portion of both orbicularis oculi muscles are recorded simultaneously by surface electrodes. The active surface electrode is placed on the mid-third of the inferior orbital rim and the reference electrode on the lateral surface of the nose or the temple (Figure 3.3). A ground electrode is taped under the chin or placed around the upper arm. The pass band extends from 30 to 1600 c/s. The optimal time to stimulate is between spontaneous blinks.

After a stimulation of each supraorbital nerve (see Figure 3.1), three latency times should be measured: (1) from stimulus artifact to the initial deflection of R1, (2) to the earliest deflection of the ipsilateral R2, and (3) to the earliest deflection of the contralateral R2. In adult subjects, the mean latency of R1 is 10 ms and that of R2 is 30 ms. R1 and R2 are delayed if they exceed 13 ms and 41 ms.[19,20] A difference between the two sides greater than 1.5 ms for R1 and 8 ms for R2 is considered abnormal. In addition, the difference between the ipsilateral and contralateral R2 should not exceed 5 ms[19] or 8 ms.[20] Amplitudes vary considerably from one subject to the next. The normal values (mean ± SD) are 0.38 ± 0.23 mV for R1, 0.53 ± 0.24 mV for ipsilateral R2, and 0.49 ± 0.24 mV for contralateral R2.[19] Stimulation of the infraorbital nerve always evokes an R2 response but not necessarily an R1. When R1 is not present, it is difficult to evaluate R2 because of the wide range of latencies. An absent R2, however, is certainly abnormal. In most normal subjects, stimulation of the third, mandibular, trigeminal division at the mental nerve elicits no blink reflex at all.

Technique and Normal Corneal Reflex Responses

During recording of the corneal reflex responses, the subject lies supine on a bed or sits in a reclining chair. Responses are recorded simultaneously with surface electrodes positioned as for the blink reflex (see Figure 3.3). Again the best time to stimulate the cornea is between spontaneous blinks. The cornea may be stimulated mechanically or electrically (Figure 3.3). For mechanical stimulation, blink reflexes may be evoked by successive manual application of a small metal sphere, 2 mm in diameter, to the cornea.[21] The examiner holds the upper eyelid up with one finger. When the sphere touches the cornea, contact is made between the subject and an electronic trigger circuit; this circuit delivers a pulse, which triggers the sweep of a dual trace oscilloscope on the EMG apparatus (band width 30 to 1600 c/s).

When the corneal reflex is studied by *electrical stimulation,* the cornea is touched lightly with a thin, saline-soaked cotton thread connected to the cathode of a constant-current stimulator. The anode is placed on the earlobe or forearm.[22] Square pulses, 1 ms duration, 0.1 to 3 mA are delivered manually, and the oscilloscope is triggered by the stimulus. Electrical shocks excite A-delta nerve fibers directly. To measure the reflex threshold and study the recovery curve with the double-shock technique, it is necessary to use electrical stimulation, which provides a controlled and reproducible stimulus.

Mechanical stimulation provides a more natural type of stimulus and activates first receptors and then nerve fibers. In some pathologic conditions, it is easier to perform. Three pairs of latency times should be assessed from stimulus artifact to onset of the electromyographic response (see Figure 3.2). Normally when the cornea is touched mechanically, the latency of the direct (ipsilateral) response does not exceed the contralateral or consensual response latency by more than 8 ms. The latencies of the direct responses evoked by successive stimulation of the two corneas should not differ by more than 10 ms. This applies also to the consensual response latencies.[21]

With an electrical stimulus, the difference between the direct and consensual response never exceeds 5 ms, whereas the difference between the responses evoked from the two corneas never exceeds 8 ms. The reflex threshold in normal subjects rarely exceeds 0.5 mA.[22] Mechanical and electrical stimuli elicit reflex responses with similar latencies. Absolute latency values range from 36 ms to 64 ms with mechanical stimulation and from 35 ms to 50 ms with electrical stimulation. This wide range of latencies narrows if patients are divided into age groups, to account for the influence of age. The restricted intraindividual latency difference and its high degree of constancy make the corneal reflex recording of great value in unilateral lesions.

Corneal and blink reflex studies may be useful in three pathologic groups: disorders affecting the reflex arcs directly; disorders affecting the reflex arcs indirectly by compression; and lesions, such as hemispheric lesions, outside the primary reflex arcs. Another area where corneal and blink reflex recordings are of undoubted diagnostic value is in the assessment of the functional state of brain stem interneuronal activity, which may be examined by repetitive stimulation. Aberrant reinnervation of the facial nerve and increased excitability of facial nucleus motoneurons may also be investigated if the presence of the corneal and blink reflexes is examined in facial muscles other than the orbicularis oculi muscles. Late blink and corneal reflex disorders do not necessarily show the same type of abnormality.

Recovery Curves

Because of passive mechanisms (e.g., after-hyperpolarization potential) or the intervention of negative feedback circuits, the excitability of some reflex circuits is depressed following the initial reflex volley. The excitability of the reflex may be assessed by measuring the size of the reflex response to a second stimulus delivered at progressively longer intervals following the initial conditioning stimulus. From such a study, a recovery curve (or excitability cycle) for the reflex may be constructed to measure the excitability of the reflex circuit.[23]

Stimulus intensity and position of the stimulating and recording electrodes are the same as for blink reflex study. Electrical stimuli of equal intensity are delivered in pairs, at varying interstimulus intervals. The response to the first shock is called the *conditioning response* and the response to the second stimulus the *test response* (Figure 3.4). The sizes (amplitude, duration, or area) of the two responses are measured, and the size of the test response is expressed as a percent of the conditioning response. For each interstimulus time-interval, several trials must be repeated and the responses or the measures averaged. Between successive trials rest periods (of at least 20 s) are indispensable if habituation of the polysynaptic responses (R2) is to be avoided. The recovery curve is drawn by plotting the size of the test response, as a percent of the conditioning response, on the Y-axis and the time-interval on the X-axis (Figure 3.4).[13,23]

The useful range of interstimulus time-intervals varies from reflex to reflex. A complete excitability cycle of the orbicularis oculi reflexes examines the time-intervals between 10 ms and 100 ms at 10 ms intervals and those between 100 ms and 1500 ms at

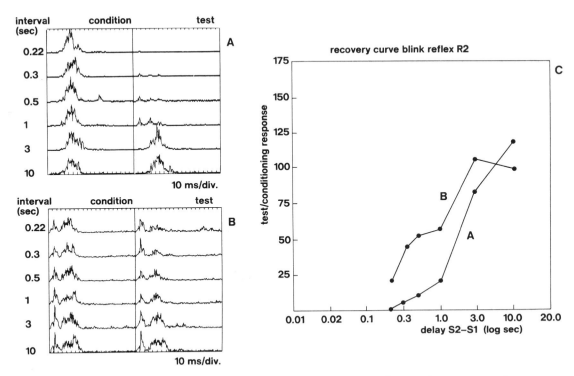

FIGURE 3.4. *Recovery cycle of the blink reflex. Rectified and averaged (6×) electromyographic responses are presented at intervals from 220 ms up to 10 seconds between conditioning and test stimuli, in a control subject (A) and patient with blepharospasms (B). (C) Complete recovery curves for the late component (R2) of the blink reflex in the same control subject and patient. The patient shows significantly less suppression at intervals smaller than 1 second (S1, Conditioning stimulus; S2, test stimulus).*

100 ms intervals. Not all of these time-intervals, however, need be checked.

The test R1 summates with the conditioning R1 or R2 at short time-intervals of up to 60 to 70 ms (the apparent facilitation may reach 250% at 30 to 40 ms intervals). At longer intervals, R1 is changed little by the conditioning shock except for a slight reduction of the order of 80% at an interval of 100 ms and slowly recovers to 90% to 100% of the conditioning response as the interval reaches 200 to 500 ms.[23,24] The test R2 is usually completely lost when the interval reaches 200 to 300 ms after which it slowly recovers, reaching about 40% to 50% of single shock values at an interval of 500 ms and 70% to 90% at an interval of 1500 ms.

The recovery of the corneal reflex parallels but is more rapid than that of R2. The test corneal reflex already measures about 30% at an interval of 200 ms (when R2 of the blink reflex is still abolished) and reaches 90% to 100% at the 1500 ms interval.[13,23]

Because the same motoneurons are shared by the

various orbicularis oculi reflexes, the difference in recovery times (progressively longer for R1, corneal reflex, and R2) are commonly attributed to the difference in the interneuronal net. The R2 of the blink reflex response is most susceptible to changes in excitability, and the R2 recovery curve provides valuable information for research and clinical settings.

The recovery of R2 of the blink reflex is facilitated (i.e., the recovery curve is shifted up) in several movement disorders: Parkinson's disease, dystonia, and tics. In these diseases, the enhanced recovery of R2 may be attributed to hyperactivity of the medullary interneurons, in turn secondary to suprasegmental dysfunction. In patients with Parkinson's disease, the R2 recovery curve changes during "on" and "off" periods and correlates with l-dopa fluctuations. The R2 recovery curve also helps in the diagnosis of dystonia. In patients with generalized, segmental, or even focal dystonias without any clinical involvement of facial muscles, the curve is enhanced. It is normal usually only in focal arm dystonias, such as writer's cramp. Finally, the R2 recovery curve has been reported to be bilaterally enhanced in patients with essential hemifacial spasm.[24] This finding, demonstrating an intraaxial dysfunction, may help to differentiate essential from postparalytic spasms.

Light Stimulus–Evoked Blink Reflex

Yates and Brown[25] studied orbicularis oculi reflex responses evoked by light stimuli given by a photic stimulator. In a control group, they obtained the optimal response and the shortest latency (50.0 ms ± 9.0 ms [2 SD]), with the stimulator held at a distance of 200 mm in front of the eyes. In a large group of patients with multiple sclerosis, abnormalities of the light-blink reflex and the electrical blink reflex together were 15% more common than the corresponding percentages of pattern visual evoked potentials and brain stem auditory evoked potentials (both 69%). For both types of blink reflexes, Yates and Brown confirmed the frequencies of abnormalities reported earlier by Lowitzsch et al.[26] Interestingly, the light-blink reflex was found to be abnormal in patients who had recovered from an attack of optic neuritis long before the investigation and already had normal visual fields and acuity. In contrast, none of the patients with definite multiple sclerosis and a history of optic neuritis had a normal light-blink reflex.

Light-blink reflex testing appears to be quite acceptable to patients and requires little time to carry out. When it is combined with the electrical blink, large areas of the brain stem can be tested with commonly available equipment.[25–27] It is therefore surprising that the light-blink reflex test has not yet been introduced to more EMG laboratories.

Further research is needed to trace the central circuit mediating the light-blink reflex. Afferent optic fibers probably enter the brain stem in the pretectum, and impulses are then conveyed to the facial nuclei in the pons.[28]

JAW REFLEXES

Jaw-Jerk Reflex

The *jaw-jerk* induced by a tap on the chin was first described in 1886 by de Watteville[29] and has also been called *jaw reflex, mandibular reflex,* and *masseter reflex.* Its clinical value is generally confined to the distinction between normal and brisk reactions. The latter may indicate upper motoneuron pathol-

ogy. A reduced or even an absent jaw-jerk is not clinically significant because these findings can also be observed in healthy subjects. On clinical examination, a unilateral interruption of the reflex arc may not be detectable. Electromyographic recording of the jaw-jerk still evoked by tapping the chin with a reflex hammer allows the study of these features (Figure 3.5).[30,31]

Persistence of the human jaw-jerk after ipsilateral sensory rhizotomy of the V nerve as reported by McIntyre and Robinson[32] demonstrated that its afferent and efferent fibers pass through the so-called trigeminal motor root. By estimating the length of peripheral pathways, the diameter of the largest fibers, and the mean latency, these authors also deduced that the jaw-jerk is a monosynaptic reflex. More recently, other authors have reported absent or delayed reflexes ipsilateral to lesions of the trigeminal sensory root, in patients with no electromyographic evidence of masseter denervation.[33,34] Although these observations do not exclude a small lesion of the motor root with involvement of muscle spindle afferents, they do suggest that A-alpha proprioceptive fibers of the jaw-jerk pass through the trigeminal sensory root (Figure 3.5). The observation of an absent reflex response in selective lesions of the mandibular root in the face of a normal masseter electromyographic study implies that the jaw-jerk is mediated by a unilateral reflex pathway through the brain stem.[35] Abnormal jaw-jerks have been described ipsilateral to midbrain lesions.[30,36] These observations have now been verified neuroanatomically in midbrain lesions involving the mesencephalic tract and nucleus of the trigeminal nerve, sparing the trigeminal motor nucleus and fibers in the pons.[8,34] As in the cat,[37] the cell body of origin for the afferent limb of the reflex arc therefore appears to be the trigeminal mesencephalic nucleus (Figure 3.5). The ipsilateral trigeminal motor nucleus in the pons is activated monosynaptically causing contraction of the masseter muscle.

Masseter Inhibitory Reflex

The electromyographic *silent period* (SP) refers to a transitory relative or absolute reduction in electromyographic activity evoked in the midst of an otherwise sustained contraction.[38] The SP in human masseter muscles was first described by Hoffman and Tonnies in 1948[39] as the inhibitory component of the tongue-jaw reflex seen after electrical stimulation of the tongue.

The wealth of literature about inhibition of masseter muscle activity confirms that mechanical or

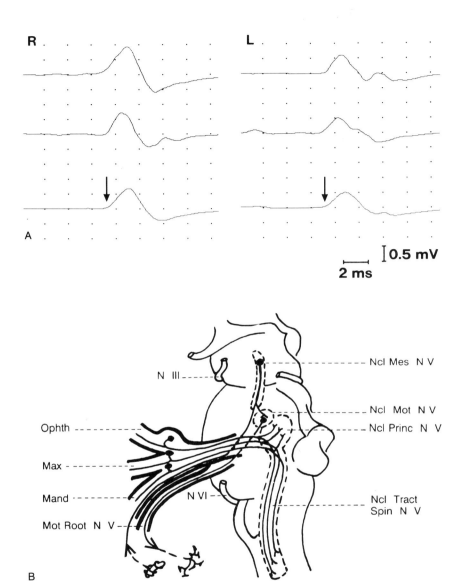

FIGURE 3.5.   *(A) Normal jaw jerk responses from the right (R) and left (L) masseter muscle. The lower traces are made by averaging, and the arrows mark the latency times. (B) Diagram showing the reflex arc subserving the jaw jerk. (Ncl Mes N V, Mesencephalic nucleus of the trigminal nerve; Ncl Mot N V, motor nucleus of the trigeminal nerve; Ncl Princ N V, principal sensory nucleus of the trigeminal nerve; Ncl Tract Spin N V, nucleus of the trigeminal spinal tract; N III, oculomotor nerve; Ophth, ophthalmic trigeminal root; Max, maxillary trigeminal root; Mand, mandibular trigeminal root; Mot Root NV, trigeminal motor root; N VI, abducens nerve.*

electrical stimulation anywhere within the mouth or on the skin of the maxillary and mandibular trigeminal divisions evokes a reflex inhibition in the jaw-closing muscles. These reflexes probably play a role in the reflex control of mastication, by preventing intraoral damage that could occur with uncontrolled contraction of jaw-closing muscles, and in jaw movements during speech. The masseter inhibitory reflex (MIR), also called the *cutaneous SP or exteroceptive suppression,* is evoked by electrical stimulation of the mental or infraorbital nerve and consists of early and late phases of electrical silence (SP1 and SP2), interrupting the voluntary electromyographic activity in the ipsilateral and contralateral masseter muscle[38,40,41] (Figure 3.6). After stimulation of the mental or infraorbital nerve, impulses reach the pons via the sensory mandibular or maxillary root of the trigeminal nerve.[41]

The SP1 response (10 to 15 ms latency) is probably mediated by medium-size myelinated afferents (A-beta)[4,42] and by one inhibitory interneuron, located close to the ipsilateral trigeminal motor nucleus (Figure 3.6). The inhibitory interneuron projects onto jaw-closing motoneurons bilaterally. The whole circuit lies in the midpons.[43]

The SP2 response (40 to 50 ms latency) as well is probably mediated by afferents in the A-beta fiber range,[4] although some authors regard it as a nociceptive reflex. In their intraaxial course, the afferents for SP2 descend in the spinal trigeminal tract and connect with a polysynaptic chain of excitatory interneurons, probably located in the lateral reticular formation, at the level of the pontomedullary junction[43] (Figure 3.6). The last interneuron of the chain is inhibitory and gives rise to ipsilateral and contralateral collaterals that ascend medial to the right and left spinal trigeminal complexes, to reach the trigeminal motoneurons.[43]

Brain stem inhibitory reflexes cannot be tested by clinical procedures alone. In some patients, no signs of trigeminal impairment are visible clinically, and other trigeminal reflex responses are even normal, yet MIR testing reveals trigeminal abnormalities.

Technique and Normal Jaw-Jerk Responses

To elicit the jaw-jerk, the examiner holds one finger on the subject's chin and taps it with a reflex hammer held in the other hand; this action triggers with a microswitch the sweep of the oscilloscope.[20,30,31] Electromyographic responses are recorded simultaneously from the two sides (see Figure 3.5) by surface electrodes. The active electrode is placed on the masseter muscle belly, in the lower third of the distance

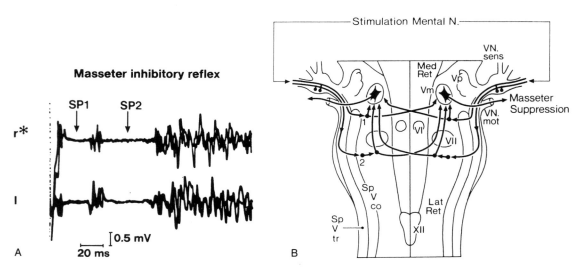

FIGURE 3.6. *(A) Normal early (SP1 = first silent period) and late (SP2 = second silent period) phase of the masseter inhibitory reflex. (r* = stimulation of the right mental nerve with responses from the right [r] masseter muscle and responses from the left [l] masseter.) (B) Diagram showing the presumed location of the bulbar interneurons subserving (1) the early (SP1) and (2) the late (SP2) phase of the masseter inhibitory reflex. (For key abbreviations, see legend to Figure 3.1.)*

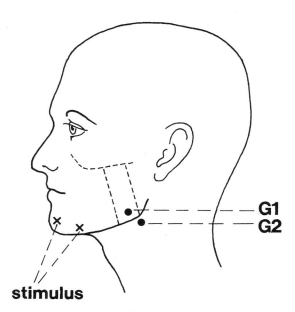

stimulus

FIGURE 3.7. *Electrode placements for recording the jaw-jerk and masseter inhibitory reflex with electrode placements for stimulating the mental nerve.*

between the zygoma and the lower edge of the mandible, and the reference electrode is placed below the mandibular angle (Figure 3.7). Reflex responses can also be picked up by a small-diameter concentric needle electrode inserted into each masseter. In this case, a ground electrode is taped onto the forehead, neck, or upper arm. To ensure a constant latency, taps should be delivered at intervals of 5 seconds or more. The latency, which is the most useful parameter, must be evaluated in several trials or measured on the averaged signal[27,31] (see Figure 3.5).

The mean latency in healthy subjects is 7.6 ms, with a SD of 1.3 ms and a range of 6.4 to 9.2 ms. A wider range of latency increases the mean latency at older ages.[20] Comparison between the latencies simultaneously recorded on the two sides in one subject is of great value. A R/L difference of more than 0.5 ms and a consistent unilateral absence of the reflex are pathologic findings. A bilaterally absent reflex at advanced ages has no definite clinical significance because this may also occur in healthy subjects.

Technique and Normal Masseter Inhibitory Reflex Responses

The MIR is recorded bilaterally with the same electrode position described for the jaw-jerk: the active electrode over the lower third of the masseter muscle belly and the reference just below the angle of the mandible (see Figure 3.7). The optimal filter bandwidth is 20 to 5000 c/s. Subjects are seated upright in a chair and instructed to clench the teeth as hard as possible for periods of 2 to 3 seconds, with the aid of auditory feedback. The reflex can be measured properly only if the patient maximally clenches the teeth. It may be necessary to use a concentric needle electrode because surface recordings may be contaminated by activity in the facial muscles.

Single electrical shocks 0.2 ms in duration are delivered to the mentalis or infraorbital nerves, through surface electrodes placed over the respective foramina. The stimulus must be of sufficient intensity (usually 20 to 50 mA or about two to three times the reflex threshold) to evoke clear evidence of both the SP1 and SP2. Such stimuli are well tolerated by subjects.

Measurements of reflex latency, duration, depth, or area of suppression (see Figure 3.6) are more difficult than for excitatory reflexes, as the reflexes are "read" as periods of reduced or arrested voluntary activity, which is often asynchronous. The higher the firing frequency and numbers of motor units recruited, the greater the accuracy of measurements. Subjects should therefore clench their teeth maximally. Several trials must be studied, usually eight to 16, allowing 10 to 30 seconds of rest between the contractions. Some authors measure latencies to the last electromyographic peak, others to the last crossing of the isoelectric line, and others to the beginning of the electrical silence. Each is satisfactory if the same criterion is maintained and intraindividual differences between right and left stimulations are examined. A latency difference greater than 2 ms for SP1 or 6 ms for SP2 is abnormal.[4,43]

In a few subjects, little or no electromyographic activity occurs between the two SPs. SP1 and SP2 merge into a single long-lasting SP, even when the strength of contraction is maximum. In this case, the latency to the recurrence of electromyographic activity is taken as a measure of SP2. Latency differences between ipsilateral and contralateral stimuli for unilateral muscle recordings should not exceed 8 ms.

If full-wave rectification of the electromyographic signal is possible, eight to 16 trials should be averaged; latency and duration may be measured from the intersection of the rectified averaged signal and 80% of the background electromyographic level.[4,44] In 50 normal subjects (aged 16 to 60 years), the mean latency was 11.4 ms (SD 1.3) for SP1 and 47 ms (SD 6) for SP2; the duration was 20 ms (SD 4) for SP1 and 40 ms (SD 15) for SP2.[45]

As for blink reflex studies, the pattern of abnormality the MIR provides information on the site of the lesion. An *afferent* abnormality (absent or delayed direct and crossed responses to unilateral stimulation) indicates a lesion along the afferent paths—intraaxial or extraaxial—before the site of crossing of impulses.[43] SP1 is more susceptible than SP2 to extraaxial lesions, such as trigeminal neuropathy.[4] A *mixed* type of abnormality consisting of an afferent delay or block to unilateral stimulation as well as abnormalities of crossed responses to contralateral stimulation or abnormalities in the latter in response to stimulation of either side indicates a brain stem lesion. The lesion involves the dorsal pontine tegmentum at the level of the midpons if both SP1 and SP2 are affected and the lower pons or the pontomedullary junction if SP2 alone is affected.[43] An *efferent* type of abnormality (absent or delayed responses confined to the muscle on one side, regardless of the side of stimulation) is extremely rare except in unilateral masticatory spasm.[45]

Recovery Curves

The recovery cycle of the MIR may be studied by delivering paired stimuli at interstimulus time-intervals of 100 ms, 150 ms, 250 ms, and 500 ms (Figure 3.8). For each time-interval, a series of 8 to 16 rectified and averaged trials are repeated, with the same low rate of stimulation and alternation of *clench* and *rest* phases as described for the assessment of the reflex values and the addition of a rest period of at least 3 minutes following each series. The latter precaution is necessary to avoid fatigue or habituation. The recovery curve is drawn by plotting the time-intervals on the X-axis and plotting on the Y-axis the size (area or duration) of the response to the second shock (test) as a percentage of the size of the response to the first shock (conditioning) (Figure 3.8).

The recovery of SP1 in normal subjects is 86% (SD 19), 88% (SD 15), 93% (SD 19), and 96% (SD 10), for time-intervals of 100 ms, 150 ms, 250 ms, and 500 ms. For the same time-intervals, the recovery of SP2 is 24% (SD 29), 54% (SD 30), 75% (SD 23), and 79% (SD 20). The correlation between time-interval (milliseconds) and size of the test response (percent) is linear for SP1 ($Y = 0.02 X + 85$) and logarithmic to the base 10 for SP2 ($Y = 75 \log X - 120$).[45] Recovery can also be evaluated, however, by simply measuring the duration of SP1 and SP2 in nonrectified recordings, and for clinical use, measuring the recovery of SP2 at the 250 ms interval may be sufficient.

A study of the recovery curves of the masseter inhibitory reflex is useful to quantify some of the pathophysiologic features in movement disorders. The recovery of SP2 at the 250-ms interval may reach 80% to 100% in dystonia or Parkinson's disease (Figure 5.8), whereas in Huntington's chorea, it is within normal limits (about 60%).[45]

Corneomandibular Reflex

The corneomandibular reflex is elicited clinically by touching the cornea with a dry wisp of cotton wool.[46,47] The reflex response is a slight protrusion and a contralateral deviation of the mandible from contraction of the inferior head of the lateral pterygoid muscle. The corneomandibular reflex must not be confused with the corneomental reflex.[48,49] The latter seen as a subtle movement of the skin over the chin, is caused by contraction of the mental muscle and occurs in many healthy subjects. Opinions differ as to whether the corneomandibular reflex response can be elicited in health as well as pathologic conditions.[46,47,50–54] The reflex has been observed mostly in cases of severe brain disease with dementia. The suggestion that the corneomandibular reflex is one of the few clinical signs reflecting a structural lesion of the corticobulbar tract[47] has been verified and studied in greater detail with electrophysiologic methods.[55] When tested electrophysiologically, some of the clinical corneomandibular reflexes turned out to be corneomental reflex responses. In many patients, electromyographic recordings disclose corneomandibular reflexes not visible clinically. Electromyographic studies have also shown the corneomandibular reflex to be absent in controls.

To elicit the corneomandibular reflex, the cornea is touched with a 2-mm diameter metal sphere, connected to an electronic trigger circuit using the same setup as used for recordings of the corneal reflex (see Figure 3.3). Electromyographic activity from the lateral inferior pterygoid muscle is studied best with single fine polytef (Teflon)-coated wire electrode 0.1 mm in diameter, threaded into the tip of a 4-cm disposable needle. About 3 mm of the Teflon coating is stripped off the recording end of the wire, the end of which is bent backwards at an acute angle after it emerges from the tip of the needle. The needle is positioned in the mandibular notch, just ahead of the condylar head, about 1 cm below the zygomatic arch, and perpendicularly to the surface before being advanced to a depth of about 4 cm. The needle is then gently removed, leaving the wire electrode in place. The free ends of the electrode are then connected to a preamplifier lead through a tightly coiled

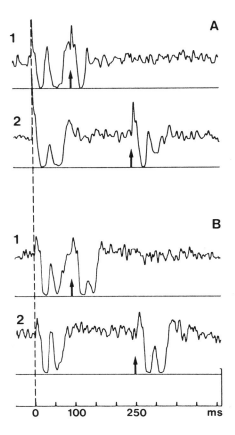

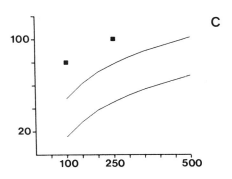

FIGURE 3.8. *Recovery curves of the masseter inhibitory reflex. (A) Recording from the masseter muscle in a healthy subject. Rectified and averaged signal (eight trials). Paired stimuli are delivered to the ipsilateral mental nerve. The first (conditioning) shock is indicated by the dashed line. The second (test) shock is indicated by the arrows. The first shock always evokes an early and a late silent period (SP1 and SP2). After a second shock with an interstimulus interval of 100 ms, the test SP2 is almost abolished (A1) and partly recovers with an interval of 250 ms (A2). (B) The same as in (A) in a patient with Parkinson's disease. The test SP2 is only slightly suppressed at the interstimulus interval of 100 ms (B1) and completely recovers at the interval of 250 ms (B2). (C) Recovery curve of the SP2 component of the masseter inhibitory reflex. X-axis: interstimulus interval (ms); Y-axis: area of the test response expressed as percentage of the conditioning response. The two curves are ± standard errors of the estimate in 20 healthy subjects. The two squares indicate the recovery value for the 100-ms and 250-ms intervals measured in (B). Note that the recovery of SP2 was enhanced in the patient with Parkinson's disease.*

steel spring. An inactive surface electrode is positioned over the posterior zygoma. Placement of the electrode within the pterygoid muscle may be checked by recording electromyographic activity during downward and contralateral mandible movement. A pair of surface electrodes placed ipsilaterally over the lateral half of the chin will allow simultaneous examination of reflex discharges from the mentalis muscle.

In suprabulbar lesions involving the corticobulbar tract,[55] several types of reflex contraction can be observed: bilateral responses after touching each cornea (Figure 3.9), a response ipsilateral to each stimulated cornea, bilateral contraction after stimulation of the cornea on one side combined with a crossed response on stimulation of the other cornea, or an ipsilateral response to stimulation of one cornea but no response to stimulation of the other cornea.

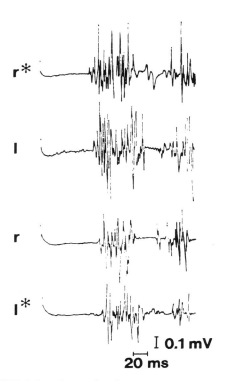

FIGURE 3.9.   *Example of corneomandibular re-*
flex responses. Upper two traces, responses from
the right (r) and left (l) inferior head of the lateral
pterygoid muscle obtained by stimulation of the
right (r*) cornea. The lower two traces show the
responses evoked by stimulation of the (l*) cornea.

Following mechanical stimulation of the cornea, the average latency is 73.3 ms ± 7.4 SD, and the R/L difference is 5 ms (range 0 to 12 ms). The long latency suggests multiple intramedullary synaptic connections. Afferent impulses for the corneomandibular reflex and afferent impulses for the corneal reflex pass along similar fibers, whereas ascending trigeminotrigeminal interneuronal connections probably run in the bulbar lateral reticular formation. Efferent impulses to the lateral inferior pterygoid muscle are mediated through the trigeminal motor root.

NEEDLE ELECTRODE EXAMINATION

The muscles of the tongue; face, such as the frontalis, the orbicularis oculi, or oris; and the neck, including the sternocleidomastoid or trapezius, are easily ac-

cessible to concentric needle electrode examination. Masticatory muscles, including the masseter and the temporalis, are also readily accessible. More difficult to approach is the medial pterygoid which is attached to the posterior border of the ramus of the mandible. Even more difficult to examine is the lateral ptery-goid muscle, a method for which has already been described. Electromyographic examination of the extraocular or laryngeal muscles is complicated and requires the assistance of an ophthalmologist or an otolaryngologist. These muscles are not discussed in this chapter.

Except for the trapezius, muscles supplied by the cranial nerves are characterized by more numerous, shorter duration, smaller amplitude motor unit potentials than is the case for limb muscles. The motor unit action potentials are more difficult to analyze because their higher firing rates make it difficult to distinguish normal motor unit potentials from myopathic potentials and even from the fibrillation potentials and positive sharp waves seen in axonal degeneration. In the latter situation therefore, the muscle under study must be completely relaxed. As in limb muscle, evidence of reinnervation is demonstrated electrically by polyphasic wave forms and increases in duration and amplitude.

Needle electrode recording is also useful for evaluating patients with involuntary facial movements. The clonic twitches seen in hemifacial spasm appear as high-frequency bursts of synchronized potentials. In contrast, dystonic movements are characterized by multiunit asynchronous activity of varying duration. In patients with blepharospasm, the bursts of involuntary activity are sometimes semirhythmic (Figure 3.10A), whereas facial myokymia is characterized electromyographically by regularly recurring bursts of three to ten motor units, each burst firing independently of the others (Figure 3.10B).[74]

Trontelj et al.[56] have described a single fiber electromyographic technique for measuring motor end plate jitter in the orbicularis oculi muscle, as a diagnostic test for neuromuscular transmission disorders such as myasthenia gravis. The technique causes patients little discomfort. A small monopolar needle electrode for stimulation is inserted into the extramuscular facial nerve branches at the point where they traverse the zygomatic arch. Single muscle fiber action potentials are picked up by a single-fiber electromyographic electrode inserted into the orbital portion of the orbicularis oculi muscle. Higher stimulus rates can be used with extramuscular nerve fiber stimulation than with the intramuscular stimulation commonly used in jitter studies in limb muscle. In-

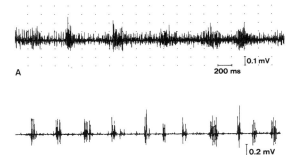

FIGURE 3.10. *(A) An illustration of electromyographic activity recorded from the orbicularis oculi muscle in a patient with prolonged spasms and bursts of semirhythmic eye closure. (B) Facial myokymia. Spontaneous activity showing regularly recurring bursts of motor unit potentials in the right orbicularis oris muscle in a patient who appears to have multiple sclerosis.*

dividual fiber potentials show greater jitter values and latencies as compared with limb muscles. The major reason for this may be the smaller diameters of facial muscle fibers. The observation that smaller muscle fibers tend to have a longer latency and jitter supports the reported relationship between muscle fiber diameter and motor unit size.[57]

CRANIAL NERVE CONDUCTION STUDIES AND MAGNETIC TRANSCRANIAL STIMULATION (FACIAL, TRIGEMINAL, AND ACCESSORY NERVES)

The spinal nerves are now routinely investigated by stimulating the nerve along its course in the limb and recording the direct motor response (M wave) from the target muscles. Measurement of the latency and amplitude of the M wave provides quantitative information on nerve function and possible demyelination or axonal loss.

Of the cranial nerves, only the facial nerve was commonly studied with this method because stimulation of the other nerves—lying for most of their course in the depth of craniofacial structures—was difficult. By means of magnetic transcranial stimulation, however, the intracranial root of most cranial nerves may be excited painlessly and the motor responses recorded from the target muscles.

Facial Nerve Conduction Studies

Electrical stimuli are delivered to the *facial nerve* (Figure 3.11) through surface electrodes placed near the stylomastoid foramen, that is, just below and anterior to the mastoid bone. In some conditions (e.g., in hemifacial spasm), selective stimulation of upper (zygomatic) or lower (mandibular) branches of the nerve is useful. Surface recording electrodes are placed over the orbicularis oculi, nasalis, orbicularis oris, or mentalis muscles. The reference electrode is placed either over the nasal bone or the same muscle of the opposite side. The position of the ground electrode is not critical; it is often placed on the lip, chin, or wrist.

The main problem with surface recordings from facial muscles is that signals from nearby muscles may be volume conducted to the recording electrode, often altering the M wave and making the assessment of latencies and amplitudes difficult. To obtain a M wave with an initial negative inflection and maximum amplitude, it is sometimes necessary to move the active and reference electrodes because the optimal position varies slightly between subjects. Some investigators prefer recording from a concentric needle-electrode placed at the corner of the mouth or the lateral epicanthus of the eye. Needle recordings are more selective with much less pickup from nearby muscles, whereas only a proportion of motor units contribute to the signal. Measurements of latency and amplitude are therefore less accurate for needle recordings as compared with surface recordings.

Normal latencies, as measured for surface recordings from 150 facial muscles of adult subjects, range from 2.5 ms to 5 ms, with a mean of 3.2 ms (SD 0.7). Amplitudes vary widely between muscles and individuals and may be usefully compared only between sides.

Studies of facial M waves may reveal a subclinical facial nerve impairment or in the presence of a manifest facial dysfunction, help define the site of lesion and degree of axonal loss. In Bell's palsy, an amplitude reduction to 50% of the contralateral response indicates distal degeneration.

Magnetic Transcranial Stimulation of Cranial Nerves

Magnetic stimulators work by discharging a capacitor through a circular wire coil. A large current flows transiently, and a large magnetic field of up to 2 Tesla is generated about the coil. Because the magnetic field changes rapidly, electrical currents may be

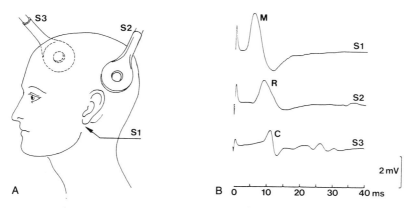

FIGURE 3.11.　*Nerve conduction in the proximal and distal facial nerve pathways. (A) Site of stimulation. S1: Electrical stimulation of the left facial nerve near its exit from the stylomastoid foramen. S2: Placement of the magnetic coil for transcranial stimulation of the left facial nerve root. S3: Placement of the magnetic coil for transcranial stimulation of the face area of the right motor cortex. (B) Surface recordings from the left mentalis muscle. M wave after stimulation of the nerve (M) at 3-ms latency. Motor evoked potential after stimulation of the intracranial root (R) at 5-ms latency. Motor evoked potential after stimulation of the contralateral motor cortex (C) at 9-ms latency. This last potential must be recorded during voluntary contraction.*

induced as an annulus underneath the coil in underlying tissues. For clinical neurophysiology, the advantage of the technique is that the magnetic field passes through the skull with little attenuation, and the induced currents can excite the brain or intracranial nerve roots without pain. Commercially available stimulators with concentric coils range from 6 cm to 10 cm in diameter. Large coils inevitably produce less focal stimulation but have the advantage of greater depth of stimulation.

Low-intensity (30% to 50% of the stimulator output) magnetic stimulation on the side of the skull excites the cranial nerves in their proximal course. For *facial nerve* stimulation,[58] the coil is positioned flat over the parieto-occipital surface, behind and above the ear (Figure 3.11). The position of the coil is not critical; the induced electrical field excites nerve root fibers near their entry into the petrous bone. Responses are recorded from the same facial muscles and with the same electrode position used to study the M wave evoked by electrical stimulation at the stylomastoid foramen (see earlier). The amplitude is similar or only slightly smaller than that of the M wave. The latency (about 5 ms) varies slightly, according to the conduction distance to a given facial muscle, as does the latency of the M wave. The transosseous conduction time (latency difference between transcranial stimulation of the root

and peripheral stimulation at the stylomastoid foramen) is fairly constant, averaging 1.25 ms (SD 0.2) in 58 subjects; the intraindividual side difference is very small: 0.2 ms (SD 0.2).[59] In patients with Bell's palsy in the acute stage, the M wave is usually normal, whereas the response to transcranial stimulation of the root is absent.

The *trigeminal motor root* may be readily stimulated by positioning the coil either in the same position as for facial root stimulation or just superior and anterior to the ear. Whatever the position of the coil, the nerve fibers are preferentially excited near the foramen ovale. Responses are recorded from the masseter with the same electrode position used in jaw-jerk recordings (see earlier). The mean latency is 2.1 ms (SD 0.3).[60] For *accessory nerve* stimulation, the coil is positioned below the ear, just posterior to the insertion of the sternocleidomastoid muscle on the mastoid. The nerve fibers are excited at their exit from the skull. Surface recordings are taken from the sternocleidomastoid muscle. The active electrode is placed between the upper two-thirds and the lower third of the muscle belly and the reference electrode on the distal tendon. For trapezius muscle stimulation, the active electrode is placed over the upper margin of the muscle, midway between the neck and the shoulder, and the reference electrode over the spinous process of the C-6. The mean latency is 2.3

TCS

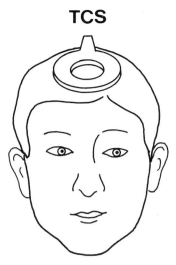

FIGURE 3.12. *Magnetic transcranial stimulation (TCS) of the facial motor cortex performed with a large (10 cm) coil placed flat over the vertex.*

ms (SD 0.4) in the sternomastoid and 3.7 ms (SD 0.5) in the trapezius muscles.[61]

Magnetic transcranial stimulation of the facial motor cortex is performed with a large (10 cm) coil placed flat over the vertex (Figure 3.12) or a small (6 cm) coil centered 3 to 4 cm lateral to the vertex and slightly anterior to the biauricular line (see Figure 3.11). Magnetic shocks of medium intensity (40% to 80% of the stimulator output) activate the corticobulbar neurons directed to the motor nuclei of the trigeminal, facial, and accessory nerves. The responses are called *motor evoked potentials* (MEPs). In contrast to responses to root or nerve stimulations, the responses to cortical stimulations, even at maximum intensity, are commonly absent in relaxed cranial nerve muscles. The patient must voluntarily contract the target muscles. In surface recordings and during contraction, the mean reported latency of MEPs is 9.7 ms (SD 0.9) in *facial* muscles,[59,62] 6 ms (SD 0.4) in *masseter* muscles,[60] 6.9 ms (SD 0.7) in *sternocleidomastoid* muscles, and 9 ms (SD 0.5) in *trapezius* muscles.[63] The amplitude of MEPs is far smaller than that of the corresponding M waves (20% to 40%) and varies widely.

In hemispheric lesions, responses to stimulation of the contralateral cortex may be absent or delayed, whereas responses to stimulation of the intracranial roots are always normal. This may also occur in patients with a lesion directly involving the brain stem nuclei if nerve axons are intact.

TRIGEMINAL SOMATOSENSORY EVOKED POTENTIALS

The Problem of Myogenic Artifacts with Surface Stimulations

Continued efforts to find a satisfactory way of recording trigeminal evoked potentials have been hampered by several difficulties. The first difficulty is that with both stimulating and recording electrodes positioned on the surface of *sphere* presented by the head, conditions are ideal for the pickup of artifact from the electrical shock by the recording electrodes. Second, scalp recording electrodes easily pick up any muscular activity evoked at the site of stimulation. Third, stimuli delivered over the face readily evoke cranial reflexes (such as the early blink reflex in the orbicularis oculi muscles or the reflex inhibition in temporal muscles), which contaminate or even hide the genuine neural activity.

The simplest method for obtaining trigeminal evoked potentials is to stimulate trigeminal afferents electrically by surface electrodes. The technique is identical to that commonly employed to evoke somatosensory evoked potentials (SEPs) from upper or lower limbs. Two main sites for surface stimulation have been described: one on the lips as proposed by Stohr and Petruch[64] and the other on the gums as proposed by Bennett and Jannetta.[65] The former authors describe scalp responses named N1 (12.5 ± 0.87 ms), P1 (18.5 ± 1.51 ms), and N2 (26.9 ± 2.23 ms); the latter report other scalp responses, occurring at later latencies, called N20 (20 ± 1.8 ms), P34 (34 ± 4.0 ms), and N51 (51 ± 6.6 ms). Although a number of papers have discussed the clinical applications of these evoked responses, their neural origin has never been proved. Evidence suggests that direct activation of the muscles underlying lip electrodes and reflex contraction of various cranial muscles, in response to lip or gum stimulation, may contaminate the scalp potentials.

Using lip or gum stimulation in anesthetized and curarized subjects, Leandri et al.[66] were indeed unable to record scalp responses, whereas cortical SEPs from median nerve stimulation were readily obtained. Caution should therefore be exercised in the interpretation and use of trigeminal responses evoked by surface stimulation.

Early Waves of Scalp Potential Evoked by Percutaneous Infraorbital Nerve Stimulation

Trigeminal afferents may also be stimulated selectively by employing two fine needle electrodes, intro-

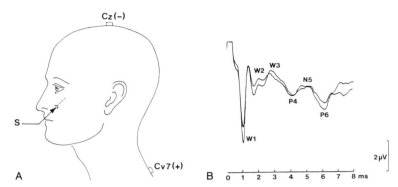

FIGURE 3.13.   *Early waves of the trigeminal evoked potentials. (A) Placement of stimulating and record-ing electrodes. Electrical stimulation of the infraorbital nerve through two fine needle electrodes inserted into the infraorbital foramen (S). The active recording electrode is placed over the vertex (Cz) and the reference electrode over the spinous process of the seventh cervical vertebra (Cv7). (B) Two averaged signals (500 trials each) are superimposed, to check reproducibility of the waves. The first three waves (W1, W2, and W3) originate from the maxillary nerve, the trigeminal sensory root, and presynaptic afferents in the pons. The later waves (P4, N5, and P6) are postsynaptic and sometimes less stable and reproducible.*

duced into the infraorbital foramen to stimulate the nerve trunk (Figure 3.13). This provides a massive, purely sensory input without simultaneous activation of muscles. The two needles, about 35 mm long and 0.35 mm in diameter, should be Teflon insulated with 1 to 2 mm bare tips. Electrical pulses 0.05 ms in duration, and intensity four to five times the sensory threshold (0.05 to 0.3 mA), are delivered every 0.3 second. A scalp derivation (vertex) with noncephalic reference (neck) is employed to record the responses; a series of 500 to 1000 trials should be averaged.

The scalp potentials (Figure 3.13) consist of a series of early far-field potentials named W1 (0.9 ± 0.1 ms), W2 (1.8 ± 0.1 ms), W3 (2.5 ± 0.2 ms), P4 (3.9 ± 0.2 ms), N5 (4.8 ± 0.3 ms), P6 (5.8 ± 0.3 ms), and N7 (6.9 ± 0.3 ms).[67] Because these waves all occur earlier than any reflexes, they cannot be explained by volume pickup of any reflex activity. When recorded with an overall bandwidth of 20 to 5000 c/s (3 db points), the amplitude of these waves ranges from a mean value of 4.9 μV for W1 to 0.4 μV for N5. The first three components are remarkably constant and can be recorded readily in all individuals, provided that the infraorbital stimulating electrodes are positioned correctly. According to intraoperative recordings, W1 originates from the proximal part of the maxillary nerve, W2 from the retrogasserian root, and W3 from the intrapontine portion of the trigeminal fibers directed toward the

brain stem nuclei. Although direct proof of the exact origin of the subsequent waves is lacking, they are believed to arise from the trigeminal nuclei (P4), trigeminal lemniscus (N5), thalamus (P6), and thalamic radiation (N7).

Because of their constancy and demonstrated origin, the first three waves are the most useful. We recommend measuring the interpeak intervals and side to side differences rather than the actual latency of each peak. The three SD upper *limits of normality* are 1.2 ms for W1–W2 and 2.2 ms for W1–W3. R/L latency differences should not exceed 0.13 ms for W1–W2 and W1–W3.

Using this method, conduction can be reliably assessed between the maxillary nerve and the brain stem, a tract that may be involved in a variety of pathologic processes of the base of the skull. Trigeminal evoked potentials are capable of detecting subclinical lesions affecting the V cranial nerve.[67]

Later waves, including those probably arising from the cortex, have been recorded after stimulation of the infraorbital nerve but only in anesthetized and curarized subjects[66] and then of much lower amplitude than the median nerve SEPs. In awake subjects, the search for these later responses (from 10 ms on) is clinically fruitless.

Eliciting trigeminal evoked potentials by percutaneous stimulation of the infraorbital nerve is undeniably invasive. Nevertheless, insertion of the two needles into the infraorbital foramen is no more painful than many electromyographic procedures. We believe that evoked potentials elicited by surface stimulation are unreliable and therefore initially assess trigeminal function by means of reflex recordings. If the application of evoked potential techniques is judged to be potentially useful, percutaneous stimulation of the infraorbital nerve is used to evoke the potentials.

Some investigators have attempted "natural" types of stimulation, using taps or air puffs directed to the skin of the face innervated by the three divisions of the trigeminal nerve. All the responses described have latencies over 10 ms and are therefore liable to be contaminated by muscular reflex activity. Apart from the theoretical interest of these responses from selective mechanical stimulation, at the moment too little evidence exists either of their origin or of their possible clinical utility.

CLINICAL APPLICATIONS

Trigeminal Neuropathy

In trigeminal nerve lesions, when the affected side is stimulated, either the afferent impulses to the brain stem are slowed, or in severe lesions, totally obstructed, resulting in an afferent delay or a block of the reflex responses (Figure 3.14, 1). Stimulation of the unaffected side produces a normal ipsilateral (direct) and contralateral (consensual) reflex response. In the *blink reflex,* R1 is usually delayed or absent, with an afferent delay of R2. In slight first branch lesions, corneal and to a some lesser extent early blink reflexes are generally more exposed than the late blink reflex.[4,15,16] Thus R1 may be delayed when R2 is bilaterally normal and the *corneal reflex* may show an afferent delay, whereas the two blink reflex components are normal. In more severe cases, an afferent block of the corneal reflex response may occur with an afferent delay of R2 of the blink reflex.

In the *MIR,* the following combinations of abnormality may be found, according to the degree of severity of nerve damage.[4,15,18,41,68] Mild to moderate lesions affecting afferent fibers sometimes cause an afferent delay of SP1 alone. With more severe interruption of afferent fibers, bilateral absence of SP1 may be seen with a bilateral delay of SP2.

The blink reflex can be abnormal with a lesion of the supraorbital nerve branch or, more proximally, the ophthalmic division of the trigeminal nerve. An abnormal corneal reflex may reflect damage to the long ciliary nerves or, more proximally, the oph-

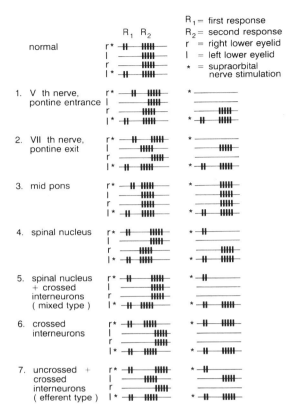

FIGURE 3.14. *Diagram of blink reflex responses in normal subjects and patients (see text). Patterns of abnormality found in the second blink reflex responses also apply to corneal reflex responses evoked by mechanical or electrical corneal stimulation.*

thalmic division where the ciliary nerves join the ophthalmic root. Blink and corneal reflexes are not necessarily both affected because they are mediated by different sets of afferents and different central circuits.[15,16] Further, the corneal reflex is more sensitive because it is mediated by fewer afferents than the blink reflex. In lesions of the infraorbital nerve or, more proximally, the maxillary root, the blink reflex and the MIR may be abnormal in response to infraorbital nerve stimulation. Injury to the mental nerve or the mandibular root may result in abnormalities of the MIR. Features of denervation or reinnervation or both in masseter EMG indicate a lesion of the masseter nerve or, more proximally, the trigeminal motor root. Electromyographic abnormalities may occur with or without an abnormal jaw-jerk, that is, a delay or absence on the involved side; the reverse is also true.[20,35] To localize the site of lesion, it is helpful to study trigeminal reflexes evoked from all three divisions. Abnormalities in all divisions suggest a proximally located nerve lesion. An abnormality in one division suggests only a more peripherally sited lesion.

Disorders of the various reflexes passing through the trigeminal system have been reported in a number of distinct peripheral trigeminal lesions, such as traumatic injury,[20,69] infectious diseases,[35] tumors affecting the facial bones or the intracranial portion of the V nerve,[35,69–71] surgical damage to the trigeminal nerve,[4,33,35] and trigeminal sensory neuropathy associated with scleroderma or mixed connective tissue disease.[68,72]

Trigeminal Pain

For patients reporting pain in the trigeminal territory, neurophysiologic testing of trigeminal function by blink and corneal reflex, MIR, and trigeminal evoked potential recordings may offer the clinician useful information. Abnormalities may be shown in divisions that appear clinically unaffected. Objective assessment is also helpful for patients with facial pain associated with trigeminal neuralgia, postherpetic neuralgia, vascular malformations in the posterior fossa, benign tumors of the cerebellopontine angle, multiple sclerosis, and even patients with no clinical signs or complaints other than pain.

Reflex and evoked responses are more markedly affected if the pain is constant rather than paroxysmal and agrees with the common notion that a dysfunction of only a few fibers may be necessary to provoke paroxysmal pain, whereas much more extensive lesions are not usually associated with paroxysmal pain; indeed, neuralgic pain is relieved by surgical deafferentation, whereas constant pain is often worsened by the latter procedure.

In *symptomatic trigeminal pain,* the trigeminal reflex studies are often very sensitive as they test all three divisions (blink reflex for the first and second divisions and MIR for the second and third divisions). The most sensitive reflexes are the early blink reflex (R1) and early masseter inhibitory period (SP1).[73] The scalp potentials evoked by percutaneous infraorbital stimulation are also abnormal in most cases because the maxillary division is most often involved.[73]

In the majority of patients with *idiopathic trigeminal neuralgia (tic douloureux)*, all neurophysiologic tests are normal. In a few cases,[20,73,74] however, mild reflex abnormalities have been reported. The early waves obtained by infraorbital nerve stimulation, and in particular the 3-ms wave (W3), are abnormal in 20% to 30% of patients with idiopathic trigeminal neuralgia,[73,75] a proportion decidedly less than that reported in studies based on late waves evoked by surface stimulations.[64,65]

Diagnostic protocols for patients with trigeminal pain should rely primarily on trigeminal reflexes. These techniques are less invasive as compared with trigeminal evoked potentials, and the finding of any abnormality implies an underlying structural lesion. In patients with paroxysmal pain, the presynaptic waves of the evoked potential are more sensitive, possibly because slight reductions in conduction velocities or the loss of a few axons may not be sufficient to produce significant changes in reflex responses, which are influenced by the temporospatial summation at each synapse. Although the early waves of the evoked potential may be abnormal in some cases of idiopathic trigeminal neuralgia, any abnormality should prompt further investigation to search for a cause that may require surgical attention; this holds particularly true in young subjects.

A possible lesion of the afferent branch can be located by finding an abnormal early SEP in response to infraorbital nerve stimulation. Wave W1, originating from the maxillary nerve, is altered in patients with lesions affecting this segment of the trigeminal pathway, examples of which include Tolosa-Hunt syndrome, maxillary bone fracture, and postherpetic neuralgia. Of course, in these cases the subsequent waves are altered also. Lesions at more proximal sites, including tumors in the cerebellopontine angle, vascular malformations of the brain stem, and multiple sclerosis, may alter wave W3, which originates from inside the pons.[73,75]

The most commonly reported causes of *symptomatic* neuralgia are vascular anomalies in the posterior fossa and benign tumors of the cerebellopontine angle, both of which affect the proximal portion of the trigeminal root, and multiple sclerosis with a plaque in the root entry zone.[76] As in cases of neuralgia secondary to well-documented lesions, altered conduction in *idiopathic trigeminal neuralgia* appears to take place between the sites of origin of W2 and W3, that is, in the region of the root entry into the pons.[73] Some authors believe that the neuralgic pain in these patients is caused by benign lesions such as vascular anomalies compressing or irritating the root close to the pons. These anomalies may be otherwise asymptomatic and undetected by radio-

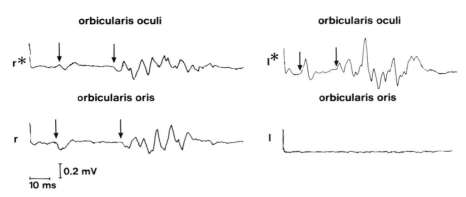

FIGURE 3.15.   *Example of synchronic early and late reflex responses in the orbicularis oculi and oris muscles on the right (r) side, evoked by stimulation of the right supraorbital nerve (r*) in a patient with chronic Bell's palsy. Stimulation of the left supraorbital nerve (l*), on the unaffected side, elicited normal reflex responses only in the left (l) orbicularis oculi muscle. Responses on the right side were slightly delayed.*

logic examination and found only at surgery or autopsy.[76,77] Trigeminal evoked potential recordings may therefore be useful in selecting patients suitable for microsurgical decompression in the posterior fossa.

Facial Neuropathy

Facial nerve conduction studies and blink reflex recordings help in the evaluation of facial neuropathies. In *Bell's palsy,* the facial nerve is affected in its intraosseous portion by an acute inflammatory process. Conduction block is immediate. Focal demyelination is common, and distal degeneration occurs in about one-fourth of cases.

In the first 4 to 5 days after onset of the palsy, the M wave is normal, whereas the response to magnetic stimulation of the intracranial root is absent,[59] showing that the site of lesion is in the intraosseous canal. If distal degeneration occurs, the amplitude of the M wave drops by the end of the first week. From this stage, the amplitude ratio between M waves on the affected and contralateral side provides a prognostically valuable estimate of axonal loss.[74] Needle EMG recordings may reveal fibrillation potentials after 3 weeks or more.

The blink reflex, which examines the whole course of the facial nerve, may provide valuable information from the onset of the palsy. Almost all patients reveal abnormalities of both the R1 and R2 components in the ipsilateral orbicularis oculi muscle, regardless of the side of the stimulation (efferent

type of abnormality) (Figure 3.14, 2). Although most patients show a complete absence of responses, some show a delay and reduction in size of the blink responses. The latter findings, or the reappearance of previously absent responses, indicate a conduction defect without substantial axonal loss, from which the patient will completely—or almost completely—recover.

In patients without distal degeneration, the latency of R1 is usually delayed by a few milliseconds (2 ms in the series reported by Kimura et al.[78]) and returns to normal in 2 to 4 months. In patients with substantial degeneration, R1 is absent and the M wave markedly reduced in amplitude for several months and in some cases even a few years. Recovery is nearly always unsatisfactory because of facial synkinesis as a result of aberrant regeneration. Aberrant R1 and R2 responses may appear in lower facial muscles, such as the orbicularis oris or the mentalis (Figure 3.15). Recording of blink reflex responses of single motor unit potentials from upper and lower facial muscles may reveal remarkably synchronous discharges in these muscles.

Hemifacial Spasm

Hemifacial spasm is characterized by involuntary, paroxysmal bursts of clonic or tonic contractions of the facial muscles on one side. It is termed *idiopathic* or *primary* when it does not follow Bell's palsy and *postparalytic* or *secondary* when it does.[79]

Although there is no general agreement, the most

commonly reported cause of *primary facial spasm* is a compression by a vascular malformation or an artery—often a cerebellar artery—impinging on the facial nerve at its exit from the pons.[80] Several types of posterior fossa tumors have also been reported in association with hemifacial spasm.[80]

Needle EMG shows neither denervation potentials nor abnormal motor unit potentials but paroxysmal bursts of high-frequency discharges (up to 300 c/s) of motor units. The firing pattern varies, with short bursts of one or a few motor units, lasting from 10 to 100 ms, or prolonged spasms of several synchronized motor units, lasting even some seconds. Simultaneous recordings from an upper and a lower facial muscle often show this paroxysmal activity to be perfectly synchronous in the two muscles.

If by chance spontaneous activity is scarce or absent at the moment of recording, it may be induced by a 2 to 3 minute hyperventilation. Hyperventilation presumably causes respiratory alkalosis, which reduces the ionizable calcium level, in turn triggering ectopic excitation.[81]

Nerve conduction studies in hemifacial spasm reveal normal M potentials from the facial muscles. Selective stimulation of the mandibular branch of the facial nerve, however, sometimes evokes a delayed (7 to 10 ms) response in the orbicularis oculi muscle, whereas stimulation of the zygomatic branch may conversely evoke a delayed response in the lower facial muscles. Further, both the M wave and the synkinetic responses are sometimes followed, immediately or after a pause of electric silence, by afteractivity. This is highly variable and best recorded with needle electrode studies. Findings include discharges of single motor unit potentials or a doublet or trains of potentials lasting 50 ms or more. In any event, the interspike frequency is very high, as it is for the spontaneous activity.

Regardless of the presence of paroxysmal spontaneous activity, *blink reflex* studies are useful for evaluating hemifacial spasm. In recordings from the orbicularis oculi muscle, R1 and R2 are sometimes slightly delayed on the ipsilateral side, although not all investigators agree with this finding. Stimulation of the supraorbital nerve also evokes anomalous responses, which resemble the blink reflex in lower facial muscles (Figure 3.16), such as the orbicularis oris or mentalis, a helpful diagnostic sign.[82] An R2-like response occasionally appears in lower facial muscles of normal subjects, but R1 never does. In hemifacial spasm, the latency of the synkinetic R1-like response in lower facial muscles is similar to the latency of the orbicularis oculi R1 response. Stimu-

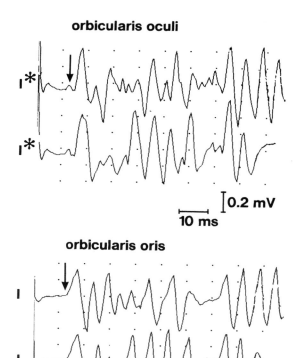

orbicularis oculi

[0.2 mV

10 ms

orbicularis oris

FIGURE 3.16. *Example of repetitive discharges in synchronic reflex responses in the left (l) orbicularis oculi and oris muscles after stimulation of the left supraorbital nerve (l*) in a patient with idiopathic hemifacial spasms on the left side. Responses were picked up by the surface electrodes and two responses were recorded below each other.*

lation of facial nerve branches as well as stimulation of the supraorbital nerve may also evoke high-frequency discharges that are synchronous in both upper and lower facial muscles (Figure 3.16).

Several investigators agree that the spontaneous or evoked high-frequency discharges represent ectopic excitation occurring at a point along the nerve where the membrane resting potential is unstable, possibly because of a demyelination.[81] Cross-talk between upper and lower facial motor axons is more controversial. Most authors believe the spasm is fully explained by ephaptic transmission between the nerve fibers.[81] Some still believe in aberrant regeneration, similar to that complicating Bell's palsy. Finally, others propose a combination of primary damage to the nerve with a secondary nuclear dysfunction (*kindling* model).[83] The recovery curve of the R2 response of the blink reflex has been reported to be enhanced in hemifacial spasm, which suggests the presence of hyperexcitability of facial motoneurons and brain stem interneurons.[24]

The *postparalytic hemifacial spasm,* although infrequent, must be differentiated from the primary spasm as well as from synkinesis owing to aberrant regeneration after Bell's palsy. In all three conditions, synkinesis between upper and lower facial muscles is clinically evident. Similarly, synkinetic responses are often evoked by selective stimulation of facial nerve branches or the supraorbital nerve. Unlike responses in the primary spasm, facial muscle M waves and motor unit potentials may be abnormal in postparalytic spasm, as they are in Bell's palsy. Conversely, the main difference between synkinesis owing to aberrant regeneration and postparalytic spasm is that needle recordings in the latter reveal spontaneous high-frequency discharges of motor unit action potentials and high-frequency after-activity evoked by facial or supraorbital nerve stimulations, in a manner similar to primary spasm.

Polyneuropathy and Motor Neuron Disease

Kimura[18,84] has reported that *blink reflex* studies applied in an appropriate clinical setting may provide clinically useful information in diabetic neuropathy, Guillain-Barré syndrome, chronic inflammatory neuropathy, and hereditary motor and sensory neuropathy type I and II. Cranial nerve involvement was demonstrated best by measuring the latency of R1. The latency of R2 varies widely and depends more than R1 on the state of interneuronal excitability. This may explain why individual R2 latencies were commonly within the normal range despite the finding that the average latency for R2 in the patients was significantly increased. Kimura[18] has further suggested that a ratio of the latency of R1 to the latency of the direct response (D) obtained by stimulation of the facial nerve just anterior to the mastoid process (R1/D ratio) might be useful for comparing the distal segment of the facial nerve to the remainder of the reflex arc, including the trigeminal nerve, pontine relay, and proximal segment of the facial nerve. A reduced R1/D ratio suggests that the facial nerve conducted more slowly in the distal segment. Pronounced slowing in the proximal segment would increase the ratio, provided that the trigeminal nerve and the pontine relay are intact.

In motoneuron disease and particularly in amyotrophic lateral sclerosis, progressive muscular atrophy and the adult and juvenile types of progressive bulbar palsy, the most commonly affected motor nuclei in the brain stem are those of the vagal, glossopharyngeal, and hypoglossal nerves. Motor nuclei of other cranial nerves are less frequently affected. Of the muscles supplied by the former nerves, those of the tongue are most easily accessible by *needle EMG.* The finding of fibrillation potentials or positive sharp waves or both, with or without fasciculation potentials, demonstrates bulbar involvement. The patient must be asked to relax the tongue as much as possible during recording because spontaneous activity may be confused with the numerous motor unit potentials that are usually present. A proper diagnosis occasionally depends on demonstrating involvement of the corticobulbar tract. In such cases, recording of the *corneomandibular reflex* or *magnetic transcranial stimulation* of the corticobulbar tract might be of great value.

Brain Stem Lesions

Lesions affecting the lower pons and the dorsolateral medulla oblongata (or both) cause seven types of *blink reflex* abnormalities. These are schematically presented in relation to the site of the central lesion by Figure 3.14 (see also Figures 3.1 and 3.2). The figure may serve as a guide to relate a specific abnormality to the location of the causal lesion in the central reflex arc. In Figure 3.14, abnormalities are shown as delayed responses, but of course a complete interruption of impulses produces absent responses.

In principle, all the abnormal R2 features occurring in the *blink reflex* also occur in *corneal reflex* responses. The first two abnormalities in the figure are due to central impairment of ingoing sensory trigeminal or outgoing facial nerve fibers and resemble the features caused by a more peripheral trigeminal or facial nerve lesion. A medullary lesion causing the mixed type 5 (see Figure 3.14), extends more medially than the lesion causing type 4. In type 6, the lesion is located centrally in the dorsal medullary region and affects the medial part of the lateral reticular formation mediating crossed impulses. Type 7 suggests the presence in the lateral bulbar reticular formation of a lesion interrupting the ipsilateral and contralateral impulses that ascend to the facial nucleus on the side of the lesion.

Changes in *jaw-jerk, blink reflex, light stimulus–evoked blink,* and *corneal reflex* have been reported in *multiple sclerosis.*[7,25–27,30,36,85] Kimura[7] demonstrated that the R1 of the blink reflex was abnormal in the majority of a group of 260 patients with multiple sclerosis (see Figure 3.14, type 3). In 40% of patients, a delayed or absent R1 (Figure 3.17) occurred even in the absence of clinical signs of brain stem damage. In multiple sclerosis patients, silent lesions have also been disclosed by changes in corneal, blink, and jaw reflexes.[85] It is useful therefore to study the trigeminal reflexes in multiple sclerosis patients without clinical symptoms of brain stem damage (Figure 3.18). A combination of trigeminal reflex abnormalities, in particular an abnormal jaw-jerk accompanied by a disorder of one of the other reflexes, reflects damage to different levels of the trigeminal system and may contribute to the diagnosis.

The lateral medullary *syndrome of Wallenberg* is commonly associated with an abnormality of the corneal reflex and R2 of the blink reflex, whereas R1 is spared.[8,10,11,14,15] In most patients, type 4 abnormality (see Figure 3.14) occurs with a bilateral delay or in more severe cases with a bilateral loss of the two reflexes following stimulation of the affected side. Such findings are explained by a lesion involving the descending trigeminal spinal tract, and in these cases stimulation of the unaffected side elicits bilaterally normal responses. Type 5 abnormality,

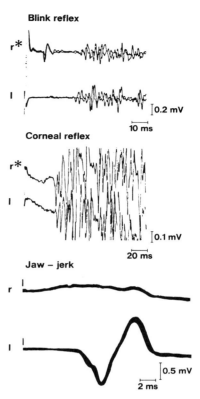

FIGURE 3.18.   *Example of a jaw-jerk with an absent response on the right (r) and a normal response on the left (l) side found unexpectedly in a patient with multiple sclerosis. The blink and corneal reflexes were normal (r* = stimulation of the right supraorbital nerve [blink reflex] or cornea [corneal reflex]).*

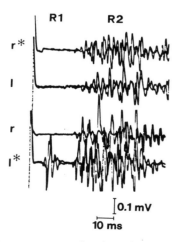

FIGURE 3.17.   *Example of an absent early blink reflex (R1) with normal late blink reflex (R2) responses on the right (r) and left (l) side after stimulation of the right supraorbital nerve (r*) in a patient with multiple sclerosis. The absent R1 indicates a pontine lesion. Stimulation of the left supraorbital nerve (l*) elicited normal R1 and R2 responses in the left and right orbicularis oculi muscles.*

the mixed type, occurs in fewer patients, in whom an afferent delay or block is seen after stimulation of the affected side. Stimulation of the normal side elicits normal direct responses, but consensual responses are delayed or absent because of a delay or complete obstruction of impulses through crossed interneurons. Although type 7 (see Figure 3.14) is very rarely seen in Wallenberg's syndrome, it is of special clinical importance (Ongerboer de Visser BW, unpublished data). After stimulation of either side, the corneal reflex response or R2 is delayed or lost on the side of the infarction (efferent impairment). Reflex responses on the unaffected side are normal, no matter which side is stimulated. R1 is normal on either side. The efferent abnormality on the affected side points to a lesion in the bulbar lateral reticular formation cranial to the crossing of impulses. Because R1 can only be studied by electromyographic recordings, on a merely visual inspection of the reflex, the type 7 abnormality is easily confused with a facial nerve lesion.

Wallenberg's syndrome is usually recognizable without difficulty on clinical grounds alone, although some cases are hard to identify on the clinical evidence alone. In such cases, blink and corneal reflex recordings may provide the clinician with valuable information about the extent of the medullary infarction. When the infarction extends medially beyond the spinal tract and its nucleus (see Figure 3.14, type 5) the symptoms often last a long time, and the majority of patients never recover completely.

Conversely, an afferent delay or loss of the R2 or corneal reflex responses with stimulation on the affected side (see Figure 3.14, type 4) coincides in most patients with a more rapid and complete recovery of symptoms. The corneal reflex apparently is more likely to be affected than the late blink reflex with ischemic lesions.[15]

The trigeminal reflex abnormalities seen in multiple sclerosis or Wallenberg's syndrome can also occur in degenerative diseases, such as olivopontocerebellar atrophy or intraaxial brain stem tumors and even extraaxial tumors that compress the lower brain stem. In the last case, electrical blink or corneal reflex abnormalities may point to extension of the lesion beyond the trigeminal complex (see Figure 3.14, type 5) suggesting growth of the tumor into the medulla oblongata or secondary infarction of the medulla. If stimulation on the affected side (see Figure 3.14, type 4) reveals delays only, the responses may return to normal in short order if the brain stem is decompressed. Such a normalization may occur after an operation for a tumor involving the foramen magnum or after successful traction for dislocation of the dens epistrophei within the foramen magnum in patients with severe rheumatoid arthritis (unpublished data).

Disorders of the *lower two-thirds of the pons* may cause a range of *MIR* abnormalities similar to those already described for the blink reflex.[43] A combined study of the various trigeminal reflexes and the MIR in these disorders can be revealing. The MIR is sometimes abnormal in patients with no clinical signs of trigeminal system impairment and even in those without abnormalities of other trigeminal reflexes. Further, analysis of SP1 and SP2 components helps to localize the site of damage within the trigeminal pathways. Extrinsic lesions rarely affect SP2 alone, whereas intrinsic lesions rarely affect SP1 alone. Abnormalities found after stimulation of one or the other side are common in intrinsic pontine lesions. If the abnormalities involve the crossed responses only or are of the mixed type (similar to type 6 or 5 of the blink reflex [see Figure 3.14]), they are undoubtedly produced by an intrinsic lesion. If both SP1 and SP2 are affected, the lesion involves the dorsal pontine tegmentum at the level of the midpons, whereas if SP2 alone is affected, the lesion involves the lower pons or pontomedullary junction.

In *upper brain stem disorders,* as in vascular and neoplastic lesions, the finding of an abnormal *jaw jerk* with normal electromyographic features from the masseter muscles suggests a midbrain lesion involving structures adjacent to the aqueduct.[31,34] Spontaneous activity in the masseter muscle suggests involvement of the trigeminal motor nucleus in the lateral rostral pons.

Hemispheric Lesions

When blink reflexes are recorded to study structural lesions in the cerebral hemispheres, it is important to keep the subject alert. Reduced alertness or sleep reduces the size and increases the latencies of the R2 and to a lesser extent R1 responses.[86–90] In comatose patients, late reflexes may even disappear.[91]

Ischemia, hemorrhage, and tumors in the cerebral hemispheres may alter some components of the corneal reflex and MIR responses.[15,92–95] Studying patients in the early phase after a stroke, Fisher et al.[96] reported delayed R1 responses, which subsequently returned to normal. During chronic states, however, changes in R2 may persist for several weeks or even longer. In hemispheric disorders, corneal and late blink reflex responses may be absent or diminished bilaterally when the affected side of the face is stimulated (similar to type 4 in Figure 3.14). Stimulation of the normal side often reveals an additional absence or diminution of the consensual response (similar to type 5 in Figure 3.14). Because the polysynaptic R2 is more profoundly inhibited than the oligosynaptic R1, interruption of descending pathways to the bulbar reflex system is more likely to reduce facilitation of interneurons. This idea is further supported by similar corneal and late blink reflex abnormalities in patients with the lateral medullary syndrome involving the lateral reticular network.[11,15] The descending facilitory influence on the bulbar pathway probably originates in wide areas of the cortex, but the most common site of origin is the lower postcentral area, which corresponds to the sensory representation of the face.[15,92,94] In contrast to suppression of the R2, the R1 may slightly be facilitated on the paretic side in chronic pyramidal tract lesions. This facilitation may be explained by removal of pyramidal inhibitory influences on facial motoneurons as they impinge on spinal motoneurons.

The electromyographer should realize that supratentorial lesions may change corneal and blink reflex features. Changes in sizes and latencies of facial reflexes must therefore be interpreted with caution.

In hemiplegia from hemispheric infarction, magnetic transcranial stimulation of the face area in the motor cortex often shows delayed or absent motor evoked potentials in facial, masticatory, or tongue muscles.[62,97]

Movement Disorders

Of the electrophysiologic tests described in this chapter, the study of the late blink reflex and its recovery curve (see Figure 3.4) is the most sensitive for movement disorders such as Parkinson's disease, Huntington's chorea, and dystonia involving the craniofacial muscles.

In these diseases, facial reflexes with short latencies (jaw-jerk, R1 of the blink reflex, and SP1 of the MIR) are unaltered, as they are in hemiplegia. This observation indicates that the afferent and efferent fibers of the reflex arc and the brain stem monosynaptic or oligosynaptic circuits are not directly affected by these diseases. Transcranial stimulation of the corticobulbar tracts or cranial nerve roots yields normal results as well.[62] In contrast, reflexes with longer latencies and polysynaptic pathways, which undergo a strong suprasegmental influence, are often altered.

In *Parkinson's disease,* the duration of the R2 is characteristically increased, habituates less,[98,99] and recovers more rapidly than in control subjects,[23,100] probably because of an increased excitability of the interneuronal pool secondary to the basal ganglia dysfunction. Recovery of R2 at the 500-ms interval, for instance, may be greater than 50%, as compared with the far slower recovery (20% to 30% at same interval) usually seen in control subjects (see Figure 3.4). Further, in patients with "on-off" fluctuations, the abnormalities of R2 duration and recovery are significantly higher in "off" than in "on" periods,[100] which indicates that the reflex abnormalities are related to the level of dopamine depletion along the nigrostriatal pathway. Habituation of R2 is consistently increased by treatment with l-dopa and dopaminergic agonists.[98]

Similar to R2 of the blink reflex, SP2 of the MIR shows a great enhancement of the recovery curve (see Figure 3.8) in patients with Parkinson's disease.[45] Because the reflex latency and duration are normal, it would appear that the mechanisms that regulate the recovery of SP2 are selectively perturbed. The basal ganglia dysfunction, probably responsible for the lack of habituation in Parkinson's disease, might also cause the hypoactivity of an inhibitory control on the pontomedullary interneuronal net, control that presumably regulates the recovery of SP2.

Although electrical stimulation of the striatum facilitates and inhibits a variety of trigeminal reflexes,[101] there are no known direct projections from the basal ganglia to the lateral reticular formation at caudal brain stem levels.[102] A primary basal ganglia dysfunction may nonetheless secondarily perturb corticoreticular or rubroreticular projections.

In *dystonia,* abnormalities of the orbicularis oculi reflexes are similar to those found in Parkinson's disease. In patients with blepharospasm, R1 may be increased in amplitude, but its recovery cycle is unchanged.[103,104] R2 is increased in amplitude and decidedly prolonged in duration. The corneal reflex is also increased, although to a lesser degree.[103] The recovery curves of R2 (see Figure 3.4), as measured with the paired-stimulation technique, are enhanced in blepharospasm and in oromandibular dystonia.[103,104] An interesting point is that similar results have been observed in some patients with spasmodic torticollis and spasmodic dysphonia. The size of R1 and duration of R2 are increased only in those patients whose dystonia directly involves the orbicularis oculi muscle, whereas the recovery curve of R2 may be enhanced in patients whose dystonia does not involve the orbicularis oculi muscle.[105] Normal recovery curves are usually seen in dystonia limited to the arm.[104,106]

Berardelli et al.[103] found that the masseter SPs evoked by infraorbital stimulation were absent in some patients with blepharospasm and oromandibular dystonia. Thompson et al.[107] found a normal masseter SP in patients with focal dystonia of the jaw. Measuring the maximum suppression (or "depth") of the masseter SP evoked by supraorbital stimulation, Nakashima et al.[108] found similar values in patients with torticollis and normal subjects; the suppression in the sternocleidomastoid muscle, however, was reduced in these patients. Because of the variable findings, the behavior of the MIR has not been agreed on.

The recovery curves of the SP2 component of the MIR, however, have been found to be greatly enhanced in a group of dystonic patients (with and without facial dystonia); the mean recovery at the 250-ms stimulus interval was almost double than that in normal subjects.[45] This enhancement, similar to that found in patients with Parkinson's disease, is possibly secondary to similar mechanisms.[45] The recovery of SP2 was facilitated in patients with and without direct involvement of the jaw muscle,[45,105] as was the recovery of the R2 component of the blink reflex, which was facilitated in patients with and without strict involvement of eye-closing muscles.[106]

The behavior of the blink reflex in *Huntington's chorea* is similar to that in hemiplegia, although the abnormalities are less severe. R1 is normal.[109,110] R2 shows an enhanced habituation[111,112] and an increased latency.[109–111] Agostino et al.[109] have also found a significant correlation between the severity of involuntary facial movements and the latency of R2 and the corneal reflex.

The suppression of the R2 component of the blink reflex in Huntington's chorea as well as in hemiplegia is thought to be secondary to the loss of tonic facilitation from the postcentral cortical region on the brain stem interneuronal pool.

In contrast, the MIR, including recovery curves of SP1 and SP2, is normal.[45,110] The different behavior of R2 (suppressed) and SP2 (unaffected) suggests that in Huntington's chorea some interneurons of the lateral reticular formation are differentially affected; alternatively, a possible hypoexcitability of the SP2 interneuronal net is compensated by the pyramidal activation, since the MIR is recorded during strong voluntary contraction.[45,105]

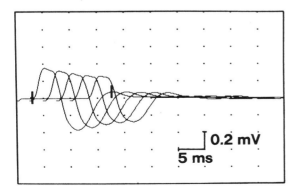

FIGURE 3.19. *Pathologic decrement (amplitude, 26%; area, 24%) of the fifth compared with the first potential evoked by repetitive 5 per second stimulation of the accessory nerve in a patient with myasthenia gravis.*

Hemimasticatory spasm is a rare condition, often associated with hemifacial atrophy and characterized by painful involuntary contractions of the masseter or temporal muscles on one side. The involuntary movements are paroxysmal and may appear as brief twitches or long-lasting spasms, as in hemifacial spasm. Needle EMG of masticatory muscles reveals typical high-frequency discharges of synchronized potentials, as in hemifacial spasm, and the jaw-jerk is absent on the affected side. Study of the MIR during the spasm shows an efferent block, that is, SP1 and SP2 are completely absent in the affected muscle, regardless of the side of stimulation; the SPs are absent probably because the motor potentials are ectopically generated along the nerve and cannot be suppressed by the reflex inhibitory input on the motoneuron.[45] Hemimasticatory spasm is probably secondary to trigeminal neuropathy.[107]

Myasthenia Gravis

Because neck and proximal limb muscles are more frequently involved in the disease,[113] *repetitive stimulation of the accessory nerve* (Figure 3.19) has a higher diagnostic yield in myasthenia gravis than repetitive stimulation of the ulnar or median nerve at the wrist. Moreover, because the accessory nerve is mainly a motor nerve, stimulation is less painful than it is in the mixed median or ulnar nerve. With a 5 per second stimulation after a 1-minute period of exhaustion of tetanic (40 per second) submaximal nerve stimulation just behind the sternocleidomastoid muscle, Schumm and Stohr[113] found a significant decrement (more than −8%) of the fifth compared with the first potential in 87% of trapezius recordings as compared with 60% of abductor pollicis brevis recordings. Only a few patients with slight symptoms or in remission showed no significant decrement.

In patients with mild generalized myasthenia gravis or those in remission,[56] *single-filber eletromyographic* measurement of motor end plate jitter is probably more sensitive in the orbicularis oculi muscle than in the frontalis muscle. On the other hand, jitter in the frontalis muscle has a markedly higher diagnostic yield than jitter in limb muscles. This difference is even more pronounced in the ocular form of myasthenia gravis.[114] In mild neuromuscular transmission disorders, the diagnostic yield of jitter measurement in the orbicularis oculi muscle can be improved by raising the stimulation rate to 20 c/s. At this frequency, normal jitter may worsen dramatically and even be associated with blockings. As yet it is not known whether single-fiber electromyographic measurements in the orbicularis oculi muscle are more useful for detecting defects in myasthenic neuromuscular transmission than looking for pathologic decrements in the trapezius muscle using posttetanic accessory nerve stimulation.

Temporomandibular Dysfunction

Temporomandibular joint dysfunction is a condition characterized by pain in the orofacial region (in muscles and joints), joint sounds, limited mouth opening, and difficulty in chewing. The cause of the disease is still controversial. Most authors agree on a multifactorial etiology, with muscle hyperactivity and changes in the peripheral input from periodontal mechanoreceptors and muscle spindles as the key mechanisms, although the question remains whether this muscle hyperactivity or the unbalanced proprioceptive input is a cause or a consequence of the dysfunction.[115]

Electromyographic studies in patients with temporomandibular dysfunction show an asymmetry in the recruitment of motor unit potentials from the masticatory muscles on the two sides. For example, there may be differences in the size of the *jaw-jerk* and in some patients its latency between sides. These differences, however, can be abolished by either opening or closing the mouth, an improbable finding with a structural lesion of the reflex pathways.

The neurophysiologic test most studied in temporomandibular dysfunction is the *masseter SP to chin tap (tap-SP)*. This SP is obtained by tapping the patient's chin with a triggered hammer (as described in the jaw-jerk technique) while the patient clenches the teeth, thus providing an interferential electromyographic pattern. In these conditions, the jaw-jerk is followed by a period of electrical silence in the jaw-closing muscles. Normal mean latency and duration of the tap-SP, as measured from 50 masseter muscles of adult subjects, are 10 ms (SD 1.3) and 28 ms (SD 8 ms).[116,117] The measurement of the tap-SP, however, entails the same difficulties as described for the MIR evoked by electrical stimulation. Further, the duration of this SP not only depends on the strength of the voluntary contraction and amplitude of the background electromyographic activity,[118] but also on the strength of the chin taps, which cannot be as controlled and reproducible as electrical shocks.

Despite the shortcomings of the technique, many authors, however, agree that the duration of the tap-SP is significantly longer in patients with temporomandibular dysfunction.[116,119,120] A survey of the literature shows that the mean duration of the tap-SP is 40 ms (SD 18 ms, 290 masseter muscles) in patients and 27 ms (SD 7 ms, 190 muscles) in normal subjects. It is important to know that the late silent period (SP2) of the MIR evoked by stimulations of the oral region is, in contrast, ill-defined and often reduced in duration in patients with TMD. All the reflex abnormalities (jaw-jerk asymmetries, duration of the SP) have been reported to improve markedly or even return to normal after occlusal therapy.[116,119]

REFERENCES

1. Overend W. Preliminary note on a new cranial reflex. Lancet 1896; 1:619.
2. Kugelberg E. Facial reflexes. Brain 1952; 75:385–396.
3. Shahani BT. The human blink reflex. J Neurol Neurosurg Psychiatry 1970; 33:792–800.
4. Cruccu G, Inghilleri M, Fraioli B, et al. Neurophysiologic assessment of trigeminal function after surgery for trigeminal neuralgia. Neurology 1987; 37:631–638.
5. Tokunaga A, Oka M, Murao T, et al. An experimental study on facial reflex by evoked electromyography. Med J Osaka Univ 1958; 9:397–411.
6. Shahani BT, Young RR. Human orbicularis oculi reflexes. Neurology 1972; 22:149–154.
7. Kimura J. Electrical elicited blink reflex in diagnosis of multiple sclerosis. Review of 260 patients over a seven-year period. Brain 1975; 98:413–426.
8. Ongerboer de Visser BW. Anatomical and functional organization of reflexes involving the trigeminal system in man: Jaw reflex, blink reflex, corneal reflex and exteroceptive suppression. Adv Neurol 1983; 39:729–738.
9. Dengler R. Rechl F, Struppler A. Recruitment of single motor units in the human blink reflex. Neurosci Lett 1982; 34:301–305.
10. Kimura J, Lyon LW. Orbicularis oculi reflex in Wallenberg syndrome: Alteration of the late reflex by lesions of the spinal tract and nucleus of the trigeminal nerve. J. Neurol Neurosurg Psychiatry 1972; 35:228–233.
11. Ongerboer de Visser BW, Kuypers HGJM. Late blink reflex changes in lateral medullary lesions. An electrophysiological and neuroanatomical study of Wallenberg's syndrome. Brain 1978; 101:285–294.
12. Lele PP, Wedell G. Sensory nerves of the cornea and cutaneous sensibility. Exp Neurol 1959; 1:334–359.
13. Cruccu G, Agostino R, Berardelli A, et al. Excitability of the corneal reflex in man. Neurosci Lett 1986; 63:320–324.
14. Ongerboer de Visser BW, Moffie D. Effects of brainstem and thalamic lesions on the corneal reflex. An

electrophysiological and anatomical study. Brain 1979; 102:595–608.

15. Ongerboer de Visser BW. Comparative study of corneal and blink reflex latencies in patients with segmental or with central lesions. Adv Neurol 1983; 39:757–772.

16. Berardelli A, Cruccu G, Manfredi M, et al. The corneal reflex and R2 component of the blink reflex. Neurology 1985; 35:797–801.

17. Boelhouwer AJW, Brunia CHM. Blink reflexes and the state of arousal. J Neurol Neurosurg Psychiatry 1977; 40:58–63.

18. Kimura J. Conduction abnormalities of the facial and trigeminal nerves in polyneuropathy. Muscle Nerve 1982; 5:139–144.

19. Kimura J, Powers JM, Van Allen MW. Reflex response of orbicularis oculi muscles to supraorbital nerve stimulation. Study in normal subjects and in peripheral facial paresis. Arch Neurol 1969; 21:193–199.

20. Ongerboer de Visser BW, Goor C. Electromyographic and reflex study in idiopathic and sympatomatic trigeminal neuralgias: Latency of the jaw and blink reflexes. J Neurol Neurosurg Psychiatry 1974; 37:1225–1230.

21. Ongerboer de Visser BW, Mechelse K, Megens PHA. Corneal reflex latency in trigeminal nerve lesions. Neurology 1977; 27:1164–1167.

22. Accornero N, Berardelli A, Cruccu G, et al. Corneal reflex elicited by electrical stimulation of the human cornea. Neurology 1980; 30:782–785.

23. Kimura J. Disorders of interneurons in parkinsonism. The orbicularis oculi reflex to paired stimuli. Brain 1973; 96:87–96.

24. Valls-Sole J, Tolosa ES. Blink reflex excitability cycle in hemifacial spasm. Neurology 1989; 39:1061–1066.

25. Yates SK, Brown WF. Light-stimulus-evoked blink reflex: Methods, normal values, relation to other blink reflexes, and observations in multiple sclerosis. Neurology 1981; 32:272–281.

26. Lowitzsch K, Kuhnt U, Sakmann C, et al. Visual pattern evoked responses and blink reflexes in assessment of MS diagnosis. J Neurol 1976; 213:17–32.

27. Yates SK, Brown WF. The human jaw jerk: Electrophysiologic methods to measure the latency, normal values, and changes in multiple sclerosis. Neurology 1981; 31:632–634.

28. Tavy DL, van Woerkom TCAM, Bots GTAM, et al. Persistence of the blink reflex to sudden illumination in a comatose patient. Arch Neurol 1984; 42:323–324.

29. De Watteville A. Note on the jaw-jerk, or masseteric tendon reaction, in health and disease. Brain 1886; 8:518–519.

30. Goodwill CJ, O'Tuama L. Electromyographic recording of the jaw reflex in multiple sclerosis. J Neurol Neurosurg Psychiatry 1969; 32:6–10.

31. Ongerboer de Visser BW, Goor C. Jaw reflexes and masseteric electromyograms in mesencephalic and pontine lesions. An electrodiagnostic study. J Neurol Neurosurg Psychiatry 1976; 39:90–92.

32. McIntyre AK, Robinson RG. Pathway for the jaw jerk in man. Brain 1959; 82:468–474.

33. Ferguson IT. Electrical study of jaw and orbicularis oculi reflexes after trigeminal nerve surgery. J Neurol Neurosurg Psychiatry 1978; 41:819–823.

34. Ongerboer de Visser BW. Afferent limb of the human jaw reflex: Electrophysiologic and anatomic study. Neurology 1982; 32:536–546.

35. Goor C, Ongerboer de Visser BW. Jaw and blink reflexes in trigeminal nerve lesions. Neurology 1976; 26:95–97.

36. Hufschmidt HJ, Spuler H. Mono- and polysynaptic reflexes of the trigeminal muscles in human sclerosis. J Neurol Neurosurg Psychiatry 1962; 25:332–335.

37. Jerges DR. Organization and function of the trigeminal mesencephalic nucleus. J Neurophysiol 1963; 26:379–392.

38. Shahani BT, Young RR. Studies of the normal human silent period. In: Desmedt JE, ed. New development in electromyography and clinical neurophysiology. Basel: Karger, 1973: 589–602.

39. Hoffman P, Tonnies JF. Nachweis des vollig konstanten vorkommens des zungen-kiefer-reflexes beim menschen. Pflugers Archiv 1948; 250:103–108.

40. Godeaux E, Desmedt JE. Exteroceptive suppression and motor control of the masseter and temporalis muscles in normal man. Brain Res 1975; 85:447–458.

41. Ongerboer de Visser BW, Goor C. Cutaneous silent period in masseter muscles: A clinical and electrodiagnostic evaluation. J Neurol Neurosurg Psychiatry 1976; 39:674–679.

42. Cruccu G, Agostino R, Inghilleri M, et al. The masseter inhibitory reflex is evoked by innocuous stimuli and mediated by A beta afferent fibres. Exp Brain Res 1989; 77:447–450.

43. Ongerboer de Visser BW, Cruccu G, Manfredi M, et al. Effects of brainstem lesions on the masseter inhibitory reflex. Functional mechanisms of reflex pathways. Brain 1990; 113:781–792.

44. Cruccu G, Agostino R, Fornarelli M, et al. Recovery cycle of the masseter inhibitory reflex in man. Neurosci Lett 1984; 49:63–68.

45. Cruccu G, Pauletti G, Agostino R, et al. Masseter inhibitory reflex in movement disorders. Huntington's chorea, Parkinson's disease, dystonia, and unilateral masticatory spasm. Electroenceph Clin Neurophysiol 1991; 81:24–30.

46. Guiot G. Valeur localisatrice et pronostique du reflexe corneo-pterygoidien. Le phenomene de la diduction lente du maxillaire. Sem Hopital Paris 1946; 22:1368–1396.

47. Guberman A. Clinical significance of the corneomandibular reflex. Arch Neurol 1982; 39:1368–1372.

48. Benedek L, Von Angyal L. Ueber die palmomentalen und corneomentalen reflexe. Z ges Neurol Psychiat 1941; 172:632–638.

49. Wieser ST, Muller-Fahlbusch H. Ueber nociceptive reflexe des gesichtes. Dtsch Z Nervenheilk 1962; 183:530–543.

50. Troemner E. Der pterygo-corneal-reflex. Z ges Neurol Psychiat 1922; 78:306–309.

51. Von Soelder F. Ueber den corneo-mandibular-reflex. Z ges Neurol Psychiat 1904; 23:13–15.

52. Wartenberg R. Winking-jaw phenomenon. Arch Neurol Psychiat 1948; 59:734–753.

53. Ansink BJJ. Physiological and clinical investigations into 4 brainstem reflexes. Neurology 1962; 12:320–328.

54. Gordon RM, Bender MB. The corneomandibular reflex. J Neurol Neurosurg Psychiatry 1971; 34:236–242.

55. Ongerboer de Visser BW. The recorded corneomandibular reflex. Electroenceph Clin Neurophysiol 1986; 63:25–31.

56. Trontelj JV, Khuraibet A, Mihelin M. The jitter in stimulated orbicularis oculi muscle: technique and normal values. J Neurol Neurosurg Psychiatry 1988; 51:814–819.

57. Andreassen S, Arendt-Nielsen L. Muscle fibre conduction in motor units of the human anterior tibial muscle: A new size principle parameter. J Physiol (Lond) 1987; 391:561–571.

58. Maccabee PJ, Amassian VE, Cracco RQ, et al. Intracranial stimulation of the facial nerve in humans with the magnetic coil. Electroenceph Clin Neurophysiol 1988; 70:350–354.

59. Roesler KM, Hess CW, Schmid UD. Investigation of facialmotor pathways by electrical and magnetic stimulation: Sites and mechanisms of excitation. J Neurol Neurosurg Psychiatry 1989; 52:1149–1156.

60. Cruccu G, Berardelli A, Inghilleri M, et al. Functional organization of the trigeminal motor system in man. A neurophysiological study. Brain 1989; 112:1333–1350.

61. Priori A, Berardelli A, Inghilleri M, et al. Electrical and magnetic stimulation of the accessory nerve at the base of the skull. Muscle Nerve 1991; 14:477–478.

62. Cruccu G, Inghilleri M, Berardelli A, et al. Cortico-facial and cortico-trigeminal projections. A comparison by magnetic brain stimulation in man. In: Rossini PM, Mauguiere F, eds. New trends and advanced techniques in clinical neurophysiology (EEG suppl. 41). 1990, New York, Elsevier Science Publishers, 1990:140–144.

63. Berardelli A, Priori A, Inghilleri M, et al. Cortico-bulbar and corticospinal projections to neck muscle motoneurons in man. Exp Brain Res 1991; 87:402–406.

64. Stohr M, Petruch F. Somatosensory evoked potentials following stimulation of the trigeminal nerve in man. J Neurol 1979; 220:95–98.

65. Bennett MH, Jannetta PJ. Evoked potentials in trigeminal neuralgia. Neurosurgery 1983; 13:242–247.

66. Leandri M, Parodi CI, Zattoni J, et al. Subcortical and cortical responses following infraorbital nerve stimulation in man. Electroenceph Clin Neurophysiol 1987; 66:253–262.

67. Leandri M, Parodi CI, Favale E. Normative data on scalp responses evoked by infraorbital nerve stimulation. Electroenceph Clin Neurophysiol 1988; 71:415–421.

68. Auger RG, McManis PG. Trigeminal sensory neuropathy associated with decreased oral sensation and impairment of the masseter inhibitory reflex. Neurology 1990; 40:759–763.

69. Kimura J, Rodnitzky RL, Van Allen WM. Electrodiagnostic study of trigeminal nerve: Orbicularis oculi reflex and masseter reflex in trigeminal neuralgia, paratrigeminal syndrome, and other lesions of the trigeminal nerve. Neurology 1970; 20:574–583.

70. Eisen A, Danon J. The orbicularis oculi reflex in acoustic neuromas: A clinical and electro-diagnostic evaluation. Neurology 1974; 24:306–311.

71. Lyon LW, Van Allen WM. Alteration of the orbicularis oculi reflex by acoustic neuroma. Arch Otolaryngol 1972; 95:100–103.

72. Ashworth B, Tait GBW. Trigeminal neuropathy in connective tissue diseases. Neurology 1971; 21:609–614.

73. Cruccu G, Leandri M, Feliciani M, et al. Idiopathic and symptomatic trigeminal pain. J Neurol, Neurosurg Psychiatry 1990; 53:1034–1042.

74. Kimura J. Electrodiagnosis in disease of nerves and muscles. Principles and practice, ed 2. Philadelphia: FA Davis, 1989.

75. Leandri M, Parodi CI, Favale E. Early trigeminal evoked potentials in tumours of the base of the skull and trigeminal neuralgia. Electroenceph Clin Neurophysiol 1988; 71:114–124.

76. Selby G. Diseases of the fifth cranial nerve. In: Dick PJ, Thomas PK, Lambert EH, Bunge E, eds. Peripheral neuropathy. Vol 2. Philadelphia: WB Saunders, 1984:1224–1265.

77. Jannetta PJ. Arterial compression of the trigeminal nerve at the pons in patients with trigeminal neuralgia. J Neurol Neurosurg Psychiatry 1967; 26:159–162.

78. Kimura J, Giron LT, Young SM. Electrophysiological study of Bell's palsy. Electrically elicited blink reflex in assessment of prognosis. Arch Otolaryngol 1976; 102:140–143.

79. Zulch KJ. Idiopathic facial paresis. In: Vinken PJ, Bruyn GW, eds. Handbook of clinical neurology. Vol 8. Amsterdam: Elsevier, 1970:241–302.

80. Digre K, Corbett JJ. Hemifacial spasm: Differential diagnosis, mechanism, and treatment. Adv Neurol 1988; 49:151–176.

81. Nielsen VK. Pathophysiology of hemifacial spasm:

I. Ephaptic transmission and ectopic excitation. Neurology 1984; 34:418–426.

82. Auger RG. Hemifacial spasm: Clinical and electrophysiologic observations. Neurology 1975; 25:989–993.

83. Moller AR, Jannetta PJ. On the origin of synkinesis in hemifacial spasm: Results of intracranial recording. J Neurosurg 1984; 61:569–576.

84. Kimura J. An evaluation of the facial and trigeminal nerves in polyneuropathy: Electrodiagnostic study in Charcot-Marie-Tooth disease, Guillain-Barre syndrome, and diabetic neuropathy. Neurology 1971; 21:745–752.

85. Sanders EACM, Ongerboer de Visser BW, Barendswaard EC, Arts RJHM. Jaw, blink and corneal reflex latencies in multiple sclerosis. J Neurol Neurosurg Psychiatry 1985; 48:1284–1289.

86. Shahani B. Effects of sleep on human reflexes with a double component. J Neurol Neurosurg Psychiatry 1968: 31:574–579.

87. Shahani B. The human blink reflex. J Neurol Neurosurg Psychiatry 1970; 33:792–800.

88. Ferrari E, Messina C. Blink reflexes during sleep and wakefulness in man. Electroencephalogr Clin Neurophysiol 1972; 32:55–62.

89. Kimura J, Harada O. Excitability of the orbicularis oculi reflex in all night sleep: Its suppression in non-rapid eye movement and recovery in rapid eye movement sleep. Electroencephalogr Clin Neurophysiol 1972; 33:369–377.

90. Kimura J, Harada O. Recovery curves of the blink reflex during wakefulness and sleep. J Neurol 1976; 213:189–198.

91. Kimura J. The blink reflex as a test for brainstem and higher central nervous system functions. In: Desmdet JE, ed. New developments in electromyography and clinical neurophysiology. Basel: Karger, 1973:682–691.

92. Ongerboer de Visser BW. Corneal reflex latency in lesions of the lower postcentral region. Neurology 1981; 31:701–707.

93. Berardelli A, Accornero N, Cruccu G, et al. The orbicularis oculi response after hemispheral damage. J Neurol Neurosurg Psychiatry 1983; 46:837–843.

94. Kimura J, Wilkinson T, Damasio H, et al. Blink reflex in patients with hemispheric cerebrovascular accident (CVA). Blink reflex in CVA. J Neurol Sci 1985; 67:15–28.

95. Cruccu G, Fornarelli M, Manfredi M. Impairment of masticatory function in hemiplegia. Neurology 1988; 38:301–306.

96. Fisher MA, Shahani B, Young RR. Assessing segmental excitability after acute rostral lesions: II. The blink reflex. Neurology 1979; 29:45–50.

97. Benecke R, Mayer BU, Schoenle P, et al. Transcranial magnetic stimulation of the human brain: Responses in muscles supplied by cranial nerves. Exp Brain Res 1988; 71:623–632.

98. Penders CA, Delwaide PJ. Blink reflex studies in patients with parkinsonism before and during therapy. J Neurol Neurosurg Psychiatry 1971; 34:674–678.

99. Messina C, Di Rosa AE, Tomasello F. Habituation of blink reflexes in parkinsonism patients under levodopa and amantadina treatment. J Neurol Sci 1971; 17:141–148.

100. Agostino R, Berardelli A, Cruccu G, et al. Corneal and blink reflexes in Parkinson's disease with "on-off" fluctuations. Mov Disord 1987; 2:227–235.

101. Labuszewski T, Lidsky TI. Basal ganglia influences on brain stem trigeminal neurons. Exp Neurol 1979; 65:471–477.

102. Carpenter MB. Anatomy of the corpus striatum and brain stem integrating systems. In: Brookhart JM, Mountcastle VB, eds. Handbook of physiology. The nervous system II. Bethesda, MD: American Medical Association, 1981:947–955.

103. Berardelli A, Rothwell JC, Day BL, et al. Pathophysiology of blepharospasm and oromandibular dystonia. Brain 1985; 108:593–608.

104. Tolosa E, Montserrat L, Bayes A. Blink reflex studies in focal dystonias: Enhanced excitability of brainstem interneurons in cranial dystonia and spasmodic torticollis. Mov Disord 1988; 3:61–69.

105. Cruccu G. Pathophysiological aspects of cranial movement disorders. In: Berardelli A, Benecke R, Manfredi M, Marsden CD, eds. Motor disturbances II. London, Academic Press, 1990:203–216.

106. Nakashima K, Rothwell JC, Thompson PD, et al. The blink reflex in patients with idiopathic torsion dystonia. Arch Neurol 1990; 47:413–416.

107. Thompson PD, Obeso JA, Delgado G, et al. Focal dystonia of the jaw and the differential diagnosis of unilateral jaw and masticatory spasm. J Neurol Neurosurg Psychiatry 1986; 49:651–656.

108. Nakashima K, Thompson PD, Rothwell JC, et al. An exteroceptive reflex in the sternocleidomastoid muscle produced by electrical stimulation of the supraorbital nerve in normal subjects and in patients with spasmodic torticollis. Neurology 1989; 39:1354–1358.

109. Agostino R, Berardelli A, Cruccu G, et al. Correlation between facial involuntary movements and abnormalities of blink and corneal reflexes in Huntington's chorea. Mov Disord 1988; 3:281–289.

110. Bollen E, Arts R, Roos R, et al. Brainstem reflexes and brainstem auditory evoked responses in Huntington's chorea. J Neurol Neurosurg Psychiatry 1986; 49:313–315.

111. Esteban A, Gimenz-Roldan S. Blink reflex in Huntington's corea and Parkinson's disease. Acta Neurol Scand 1975; 52:145–157.

112. Ferguson IT, Lenman JAR, Johnston BB. Habituation of the orbicularis oculi reflex in dementia and dyskinetic states. J Neurol Neurosurg Psychiatry 1978; 41:824–828.

113. Schumm F, Stohr M. Accessory nerve stimulation in

the assessment of myasthenia gravis. Muscle Nerve 1984; 7:147–151.

114. Sanders DB, Howard JF, Johns TR. Single-fiber electromyography in myasthenia gravis. Neurology 1979; 21:68–76.

115. Van Steenberghe D, De Laat A, eds. Electromyography of jaw reflexes in man. Leuven, Leuven University Press, 1989.

116. Bayley JO Jr, McCall WD Jr, Ash MM Jr. Electromyographic silent periods and jaw motion parameters: quantitative measures of temporomandibular joint dysfunction. J Dental Res 1977; 56:249–253.

117. McCall WD Jr, Hoffer M. Jaw muscle silent periods by tooth tap and chin tap. J Oral Rehab 1981; 8:91–96.

118. Bessette RB, Duda L, Mohl ND, et al. Effect of biting force on the duration of the masseteric silent period. J Dental Res 1973; 52:426–430.

119. Skiba TJ, Laskin DM. Masticatory muscle silent periods in patients with MPD syndrome before and after treatment. J Dental Res 1981; 60:699–706.

120. Widmalm SE. The silent period in the masseter muscle of patients with TMJ dysfunction. Acta Odont Scand 1976; 34:43–52.

4

Negative Symptoms and Signs
of Peripheral Nerve Disease   William F. Brown

CONTENTS

LIST OF ACRONYMS

M	muscle compound action
MTL	motor terminal latency
MU	motor unit
MUAP	motor unit action potential
S-MUAP	surface record motor unit action potential

CLINICAL MANIFESTATIONS OF NEUROMUSCULAR DISEASE

The clinical manifestations of peripheral nerve disease vary with the functions of the affected nerve fibers, the underlying pathophysiologic changes in these nerve fibers, and the speed with which a neuropathy develops. Generation of ectopic impulses at various sites in nerve fibers, or possibly the neurons themselves, is the principal cause of the *positive* manifestations of peripheral nerve disease. The latter include paresthesia, dysesthesia, pain, various other sensory symptoms, fasciculation, neuromyotonic phenomenon, myotonia, and other disorders of hyperexcitability covered in Chapter 5. In this chapter, attention is directed to the negative somatic manifestations of peripheral nerve disease, with the emphasis on weakness and wasting. Autonomic disturbances, another important source of abnormal manifestations in peripheral nervous system disease, are discussed in Chapter 6.

ASSESSMENT OF STRENGTH AND MUSCLE BULK

The two chief negative signs of disease affecting the somatic motor system are weakness and wasting, the general causes of which are outlined in Tables 4.1 and 4.2. Clinical assessment of power is clearly semi-quantitative, the most commonly applied standard being the Medical Research Council (MRC) scale. The latter scale discriminates well between various grades of severe paralysis but is less helpful where weakness is mild or moderate. Clinical assessments of power should be based, therefore, on the quality as well as the force of a contraction. For example, maximal contractions in healthy cooperative subjects are usually characterized by a prompt and smooth increase in the strength of the contraction to peak effort evident as well in the full attention given the task by the subject. Such maximal contractions can usually be maintained with little fluctuation or decay for the brief periods required by an examiner to make assessments.

The sense of what constitutes a full and normal contraction depends on the experience of the examiner and takes into account the subject's size, age, physical fitness, occupation, and the strength of other apparently unaffected muscles as well as examiner's own strength. Such assessments are necessarily subjective, but experienced examiners are more than

TABLE 4.1.   Causes of weakness in neuromuscular disease

Central dysfunction
Incomplete or disorderly recruitment of motor units
Lack of effort because of
Misunderstanding of task
Anxiety, fear
Pain
Hysteria, malingering
Lesions affecting
Sensorimotor cortex
Cerebellar lesions, acute
Corticospinal lesions
Peripheral nervous system
Loss of motor neurons/axons
Rate-limited firing frequencies of motor neurons, axons
Conduction block
Neuromuscular transmission disorders
Muscle fiber disorders

capable of defining the pattern of weakness in various muscles and grading strength sufficiently well to serve for serial examinations and identifying changes heralding progression or resolution of motor deficits. Although maximum twitch tensions and maximum voluntary contractions can be satisfactorily measured for a few muscles, these studies are time-consuming and are not without their own technical limitations. Problems encountered by examiners in the assessment of power often begin with a failure of the examiner to communicate to the patient precisely what is expected. On the other hand, patients may not put out a full effort for fear the contraction will bring on pain or in some way injure the muscles or nearby joints.

In cases in which patients fail, for whatever reason, to exert a full effort, it might be helpful sometimes to compare the force generated by a maximum voluntary contraction with that evoked by either direct supramaximal tetanic stimulation of the muscle or the motor nerve. If the subject is making a full effort, the forces generated should be similar by

TABLE 4.2.   Causes of wasting in neuromuscular disease

Disuse
Malnutrition
Motoneuronal or axonal degeneration
Muscle fiber atrophy in primary myopathies
Wasting—more apparent than real
? Wasting in long-lasting conduction block

either of the latter two methods. Delivery of a single supramaximal direct or indirect stimulus in the course of the maximum voluntary contraction may add additional helpful information as to the completeness of a voluntary contraction.[1] Such an *interpolated* twitch coming in the midst of an apparently maximal effort on the part of the subject tests the completeness of the recruitment of all motor units (MUs). If all the MUs have been recruited, the interpolated twitch should be absent, but the less complete the recruitment, the larger the interpolated twitch. The interpolated twitch may be usefully applied for assessing power in patients with hysterical paralysis and some central motor disorders.

The introduction of magnetoelectrical stimulation as a means of assessing central motor conduction when combined with maximal peripheral nerve stimulation provides yet another means of assessing the intactness of the motor system when there is a question of hysterical paralysis or malingering (see Chapter 11). In such cases, magnetoelectrical stimuli characteristically evoke normal sized M responses from apparently paralyzed muscles.

Weakness in neuromuscular transmission disorders may have some special features (see Chapter 23). For example, in myasthenia gravis, power may trail off with sustained or repetitive maximal voluntary contraction despite continued full effort and may noticeably improve following 5 to 10 mg of edrophonium chloride delivered intravenously. The ptosis and sometimes even weakness of the extraocular muscle at times improves following application of a cold pack to the orbit for a few moments, perhaps as a result of the improved safety factor for neuromuscular transmission induced by the cooling of the underlying muscles. It is unusual, however, for any increment in power to be detected in the Lambert-Eaton syndrome probably because the increment usually is fully developed by the first 10 to 50 impulses, and because the latter takes only a few seconds, any improvement in strength would probably be missed by the examiner. Absent or hypoactive tendon reflexes may, however, return or be enhanced following a brief period of voluntary contraction in this disease. Weakness, exercise intolerance, the second wind phenomenon, and contractures are variously seen in some of the glycogen storage and mitochondrial myopathies and myotonia and paralysis in the myotonic and periodic paralysis disorders, all of which are considered in Chapter 23.

The pattern of muscles affected can be quite characteristic, as in cases of fascioscapulohumeral dystrophy, myotonic dystrophy, and acid maltase deficiency.[2,3] In addition, other features, such as the associated cutaneous lesions in dermatomyositis, provide important clues to the specific diagnosis.

It is well to remember that power and muscle bulk may be sustained in the face of sometimes severe losses of MUs. For example, McComas et al. have shown that maximum twitch tensions may be normal despite the loss of up to 90% of the MUs in chronic neurogenic disorders.[4] The correspondence between strength and the quantitative extent of MU losses is probably best for acute neurogenic disorders. In healthy older subjects (>60 years), the maximum twitch tension, maximum voluntary contraction, and maximum voluntary contraction, and maximum M potential size in biceps brachialis decline by about one-third in the face of losses of about 50% of the motor units as compared with young adults (20 to 40 years) (Table 4.3).[5]

CLINICAL PATTERNS IN NEUROMUSCULAR DISEASE

The pattern of muscles involved in various neuromuscular diseases provides one of the most important clues as to the type of neuropathy or muscle disease. Neuropathies or axonopathies often manifest earliest at the distal extremities of the longest fibers and advance centripetally. For example, the motor manifestations often begin with wasting and weakness in the intrinsic foot muscles. Centripetal advance leads to the appearance of weakness and wasting in the anterolateral muscles below the knee

TABLE 4.3. Comparison of various electrical and mechanical parameters in the biceps-brachialis muscles of young (20–40 years of age) and older (60 years of age and older) subjects

	Young (n = 24)	Older (n = 20)
Maximum M potential peak to peak amplitude (mV)	14.5 ± 4.0	9.6 ± 2.8*
Motor unit estimate	357 ± 97	189 ± 77*
Maximum twitch contraction (Nm)	4.8 ± 2.6	3.2 ± 1.8†
Maximum voluntary contraction (Nm)	63.1 ± 26.6	42.5 ± 17.1*

Entries are mean ± 1 standard deviation.
* $P < 0.01$.
† $P < 0.05$.

and, to a lesser extent, the calf muscles, at which time the intrinsic hand muscles often become affected. Involvement of the thigh muscles is usually accompanied by extension to the forearm muscles. Still later, the pelvic muscles, proximal arm, and sometimes the abdominal muscles become affected. In sensory or sensorimotor neuropathies, an equivalent distal to proximal advance of sensory loss occurs. The preceding pattern is characteristic of the so-called distal symmetric dying back neuropathies. Experimental acrylamide neuropathy, for example, begins with the earliest functional failures at the receptor end-organs of sensory afferents and neuromuscular junctions and is followed by a centripetal advance of loss of excitability in the axons.[6,7]

Symmetric distal dying back neuropathies may be mimicked by multifocal neuropathies.[8] The latter may be suspected by either a history or findings suggestive of a multifocal neuropathy with selective cutaneous, motor nerve, or root involvement usually at the onset of the neuropathy. Progression of the neuropathy is accompanied by extension to nearby nerves, producing a more confluent picture superficially similar to a symmetric distal centripetally advancing neuropathy. Careful history taking, meticulous examination, and electrophysiologic studies usually reveal the true nature of such neuropathies by disclosing their multifocal nature, and this may be confirmed in some cases by a nerve and muscle biopsy that shows evidence of a vasculitis or other cause for a multifocal neuropathy.

The clinical examination supported by electrophysiologic studies helps to identify the more obvious multiple mononeuropathies and asymmetric and proximal patterns of neuropathies as well as something of the types of the fibers affected. Neuropathies affecting the larger myelinated sensory fibers are characterized by impairments in touch, pressure, localization, two-point discrimination, and vibratory and position sense losses, whereas losses of small myelinated and unmyelinated fibers are often characterized by defects in sweating, thermal sensibility, and nociceptive sensations.[9]

Overall, the clinical examination remains the single best tool for establishing the pattern of a neuropathy or myopathy. Most of the somatic musculature can be tested, including the oculomotor, trigeminal, facial, pharyngeal, laryngeal, and tongue muscles as well as the muscles of the shoulder and pelvic girdle, many of the trunk muscles, and most of the limb muscles. Muscle bulk, however, cannot be assessed for some deep inaccessible muscles such as iliacus and the psoas without the aid of computed

tomography or magnetic resonance imaging. Even modest obesity may also mask severe wasting, especially in the thigh muscles. Substantial infiltration of muscle by fat is a common accompaniment of aging.

Motor neuronopathies and axonopathies are often accompanied by wasting with two important exceptions. First, 3 to 10 weeks may pass before wasting becomes apparent in acute neuronopathies or axonopathies. Second, if progression of the neuronopathy or axonopathy is slow or arrested, wasting and weakness may be surprisingly minimal or even absent despite moderate and sometimes severe losses of MUs and markedly reduced recruitment patterns in needle electromyographic studies. Such findings attest to the remarkable capacity for collateral reinnervation of denervated muscle fibers by surviving motor axons and explains the relative preservation of the maximum twitch in the face of severe losses of MUs in chronic neurogenic disorders alluded to earlier.

MOTOR NEURONAL-AXONAL DEGENERATION

Experimental studies of wallerian degeneration such as that which follows transection or crush of peripheral nerves as well as various models of axonal neuropathies have been reviewed.[9–16] The chief electrophysiologic findings of importance to the electromyographer are summarized in Table 4.4, and are further considered in other reviews.[17,18]

CONSEQUENCES OF NERVE TRANSECTION

The consequences of crush or section of peripheral nerve are considered here because of their clinical importance and because they provide such a good model for studying other motor neuronal and axonal disorders. The consequences of nerve crush or section may be divided into the *degenerative phase,* within the first weeks following the injury, and the subsequent *regenerative phase,* which begins almost immediately after the injury and continues for many months. Following crush or section of a nerve trunk, the axons and the myelin sheath distal to the site of injury begin to break down almost immediately. For the electrophysiologist, the most important changes are the loss of excitability of nerve fibers in the distal nerve trunk, failures of neuromuscular transmission,

TABLE 4.4.   Indicators of neuronal-axonal degeneration

Loss of nerve fibers
  Motor
    Decreased maximum M potential amplitude (area)
    Decreased recruitment
    Decreased motor unit estimates
  Sensory
    Decreased amplitude of compound nerve action
      potential
Denervation of muscle (no equivalent for sensory fibers)
  Fibrillation potentials
  Positive sharp waves
Reinnervation (no equivalent for sensory fibers)
  Increased M potential amplitude
  Increased fiber density
  Increased amplitude and duration of motor unit potentials
  ± increased territory of motor unit (potential)
  Increased incidence of linked potentials
  Neuromuscular increased jitter ± blocking
  Axonal blocking
Conduction velocities
  Normal or only minimally reduced

---

and appearance of fibrillation activity in the denervated muscles.[19–21]

In humans, within 100 hours of the crush or section, nerve fibers begin to lose their excitability distal to the injury. This is signaled in affected nerves by progressive reductions in the size of compound nerve action potentials and in motor nerves by a steady decline in the size of the muscle twitch and maximum M potentials elicited by supramaximal stimuli delivered distal to the site of injury. The progressive reduction in M potential size reflects conduction block affecting more and more of the axons in the distal stump and failures of neuromuscular transmission at the distal end of the motor axons. The time interval to the loss of end plate and miniature end plate potentials varies more or less linearly with the length of the nerve distal to the site of injury, with failures in neuromuscular transmission usually preceding the loss of excitability in the motor axons themselves.[22] This observation is in keeping with the fact that the earliest degenerative changes are seen in the motor axon terminals. In most instances, maximum motor conduction velocities distal to the site of injury remain normal or close to normal up to the point of complete loss of the M potential.

Fibrillation potential activity appears in denervated muscles after a latent period proportional to the length of the nerve distal to the site of injury.

Thus in cases in which the VII cranial nerve or spinal ventral roots have been interrupted or crushed, fibrillation activity may appear as early as 7 to 10 days following the lesion in the respective facial and paraspinal muscles and 3 to 4 weeks for distal limb muscles supplied by the same affected roots.

Within a few days of the breakdown of motor axons distal to the site of injury, sprouts from surviving motor axons appear and subsequently reinnervate some of the denervated muscle fibers. A second burst of reinnervation activity may follow the arrival in the muscle of regenerated axons from the proximal stump. The time taken for the latter varies, being shortest for muscles supplied closest to the injury site and longest for those furthest away, because of the relatively slow rate of regeneration (1 to 4 mm a day).

The appearance of fibrillation potential activity in a denervated muscle is often preceded by an increase in insertional activity and positive sharp waves in association with needle insertion and movement. Conduction velocities may be somewhat reduced for several centimeters proximal to the site of injury, a phenomenon well explained by reductions in axonal diameter and paranodal and internodal demyelination in the nerve trunk in the proximal stump.[23,24]

From the distal end of the proximal stump, axonal sprouts appear as early as 24 hours following the crush or section. Some of these sprouts subsequently make their way successfully across the gap and enter the distal nerve trunk. Under the best of circumstances, as when the nerve trunk has been surgically sectioned and the ends immediately reopposed, regenerating axons may cross the site of a nerve section as early as 3 to 4 days following the section. In humans, however, even where section of the nerve trunk is clean, the time taken for even a few axons to enter the distal stump is somewhat longer (at least 7 to 10 days) and probably takes much longer where the site of section is rough and irregular, the cut ends are poorly opposed, the wound is infected, or excessive scarring develops. In the latter cases, crossing the site of a crush may take several weeks or even fail completely, especially if the injury was extensive and the connective tissue framework of the nerve trunk disrupted. Studies in our laboratory of the cat sciatic nerve have shown that even where the nerve was cleanly cut and immediately sutured together, no more than 40% to 60% of the nerve fibers succeeded in crossing the site of the section. Further, many of the latter fibers would probably have failed to establish terminal connections appropriate to their normal functions.

Regenerating nerve fibers, at first, are entirely de-

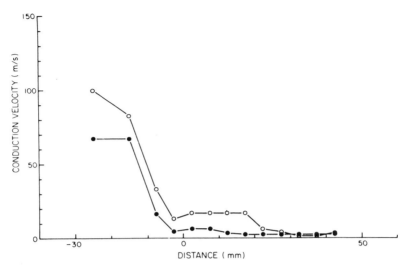

FIGURE 4.1. *Changes in the conduction velocities of two afferents in the cat, one a group I afferent (open circles) and the other a group II afferent; both had been sectioned 3 weeks previously.*[9] *Note the reduction in their conduction velocities just proximal to the transection (10 to 20 mm) and the very low conduction velocities at their distal extremities beyond the transection, where the velocities were on the order of 1 to 2 m/s. The latter indicates that the fibers at this point must have been unmyelinated or, at the most, very poorly myelinated. Their axons were probably very thin as well at this level. The actual axon tips probably extend a short distance beyond the distal limits shown here because to demonstrate the distal extremity of axons by these techniques requires that not only the impulse be generated by the electrical stimulus delivered to the nerve, but also that the impulse, once initiated, must be able to conduct without interruption all the way to the dorsal root recording site. Continuous conduction in the most distal extremities of such axons seems likely and has been demonstrated experimentally.*[27] *(Reprinted with permission from Brown WF. The Physiological and Technical Basis of Electromyography. Boston: Butterworths, 1984.)*

void of any myelin sheath. This and their smaller diameter readily explain the very slow conduction velocities (less than 5 m per s) so characteristic of these fibers[25–27] (Figure 4.1). Thresholds of such immature fibers to electrical stimulation may be very high and exceed by 20 to 100 times the thresholds of the same fibers 20 to 30 mm proximal to the site of the injury (Figure 4.2).[28] Conduction in the unmyelinated growing ends of the regenerating fibers is probably continuous, but saltatory conduction probably follows when the concentrations of sodium channels at future nodes of Ranvier are sufficiently high and myelination has proceeded far enough to sustain dys-continuous (or saltatory) conduction.

Behind the growing tips of the axons, myelination begins and advances centrifugally with the growth of the axons. Further maturation is accompanied by an increase in the number of myelin lamellae laid down and progressive increases in the diameters of the axons. These maturational changes explain the accompanying reductions in the thresholds of the regenerating fibers to electrical stimulation as well as the accompanying increases in the conduction velocities of the fibers. Conduction velocities may reach values commensurate with those of the parent neuron and type of fiber, provided that the fibers are able to reach an appropriate end-organ and sufficient time elapses for full maturation. In humans, the conduction velocities of motor and sensory fibers following nerve section may reach 80% to 100% of normal values.[29–32]

The functional outcome following suture of sectioned nerves likely depends on the number of nerve fibers crossing the site of the section and successfully reaching appropriate muscles or sensory end-organs. Central remodeling of the inputs to motoneurons and the central projections of sensory afferents may also help to compensate for errors in the regenerative patterns within the nerve trunk.

In humans, recovery may be surprisingly good.

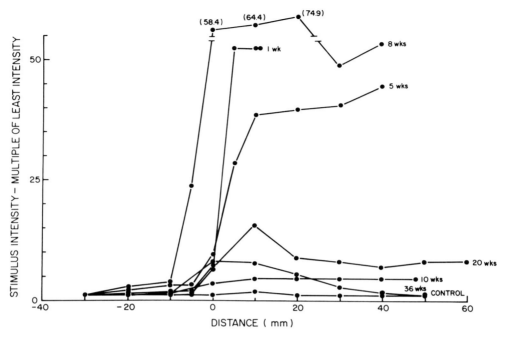

FIGURE 4.2.   *Plot of the changes in stimulus intensity required to evoke a maximum dorsal root potential (DRP) at various distances proximal and distal to the site of a previous transection and immediate resuture.*[9] *Studies were carried out at intervals from 1 to 36 weeks following the experimental transection. Intensities are plotted as multiples of the least current required to elicit a maximum DRP between 0 and 30 mm proximal (−) to the transection site. Note that in the early period (1 to 8 weeks posttransection), stimulus intensities were sometimes 10 × 100 those required to excite the nerve proximal to the transection. By 10 or more weeks, the intensities necessary were much closer to normal. (Reprinted with permission from Brown WF. The Physiological and Technical Basis of Electromyography. Boston: Butterworths, 1984.)*

For example, Buchthal and Kuhl[32] reported that compound sensory nerve action potentials were first detectable using near-nerve recording techniques proximal to the section site in response to stimulation of individual digits by 4 to 5 months following section and resuture. These compound sensory nerve action potentials subsequently increased in size, amplitude, and area, although the potentials themselves were very temporally dispersed and composed of many components. The latter finding no doubt reflects the wide range of the conduction velocities of the immature regenerated nerve fibers. At about the same time, and preceded to a degree by reductions in the amount of fibrillation potential activity seen in the respective intrinsic hand muscles, voluntary recruited MU potentials make their appearance. The conduction velocities of motor axons at this point are characteristically quite low (less than 10 m/s),

and the thresholds of the fibers to direct electrical stimulation distal to the original section site are usually high.

The earliest detectable motor unit action potentials (MUAPs) are often composed of several separate and distinct spike components, as recorded with intramuscular electrodes[33] (Figure 4.3). High jitter values and impulse blocking are common. The latter reflect the reduced safety factors at newly formed neuromuscular junctions and conduction in as yet immature axon collaterals within the network of MU terminal and preterminal branches.

Thereafter the number of MUAPs voluntarily recruitable by the subject or by indirect electrical stimulation increases. Individual MUAPs recorded with intramuscular needle electrodes or surface electrodes increase in amplitude, often reaching values many times normal, while at the same time the durations

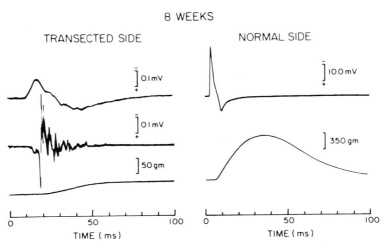

FIGURE 4.3. *Comparison of the surface-recorded maximum M potentials and maximum twitch contractions of the tibialis anterior muscle of the cat following transection of the lateral division of its sciatic nerve 8 weeks previously (left) and the corresponding potential and twitch on the normal side (right).[9] Note that at 8 weeks, the maximum M potential on the transected side was not only much more reduced in amplitude, but also more dispersed and its duration much more prolonged with respect to the normal M potential. The longer duration of the surface-recorded potential was matched by an equally dispersed intramuscularly recorded potential (left middle trace). The twitch contraction time was very prolonged and was much smaller in size compared with the normal twitch at this stage. The prolongation of the twitch is partly explained on the basis of the greatly desynchronized actions of the muscle fibers contributing to the twitch.*

of the MUAPs progressively fall to more normal values. These increased amplitudes no doubt reflect the increased numbers of muscle fibers supplied by the same motor neuron and lying within the pickup territory of the electrode as well as possibly compensatory hypertrophy of some muscle fibers. The progressively shorter durations probably reflect the improved synchronization between the discharges of muscle fibers within the MU as the preterminal and terminal axons mature in size and degree of myelination, and the conduction velocities of the muscle fibers within the MU become more uniform. In addition, there may well be increases in the number of muscle fibers supplied by each motor neuron. In contrast to controls, however, in whom MUs are recruited in an orderly manner, characteristically MU recruitment is disorderly following section and repair of a peripheral nerve trunk.[34] Where a nerve trunk has been severed proximally, muscles receive their innervation in an orderly manner, beginning with the nearest muscle, the most distal receiving its innervation last.

The closer the site of the transection to the muscles supplied by the nerve, the earlier and more complete the recovery. The reasons for this are not altogether clear. Possibly the shorter the distance, the greater the possibility the original end plates and sensory organs will survive and the less the chance that collagen deposition and endoneural shrinkage will impede successful regeneration of the axons in the distal stump.[35]

The greater mingling of nerve fibers destined for widely separate muscles and other end-organs within the same fascicle in proximal nerve trunks makes the task of reaching appropriate end-organs much more difficult for axons as compared with more distal injuries, in which axons destined for similar targets in the periphery are much more likely to occupy the same fascicle. The poorer outcome from proximal transection of peripheral nerve trunks may also reflect the reduced capabilities of parent cell bodies to survive insults so close to the cell bodies themselves.

NEURONOPATHIES AND AXONOPATHIES

The pathophysiologic features of these neuropathies are considered elsewhere in this book and in other sources. Whatever the specific type of motor neuronopathy or axonopathy, however, the electrophysiologic features depend on the tempo of the disorder. Acute motor neuronopathies or axonopathies are characteristically accompanied by moderate to abundant indications of denervation, instabilities of axonal and neuromuscular transmission, abnormal excitabilities of motor fibers, and maximum M potential sizes bearing a reasonably close relation to the numbers of viable motor neurons and axons than would be the case for more slowly progressive motor neuronal or axonal disorders (Table 4.5). The latter may exhibit little or no abnormal insertional or fibrillation potential activity or evidence of instabilities of axonal or neuromuscular transmission. Maximum M potentials in these cases may be relatively preserved, even in the face of severe motor axon losses, presumably because reinnervation is able to keep pace with the rate of axonal loss until the final stages when the normal complement of motor axons is all but lost. Examples of such chronic motor neu-

ronal or axonal disorders include the hereditary motoneuronal and axonal neuropathies (see Chapter 15). In some of the very chronic motor neuronopathies or axonopathies, maximum motor conduction velocities may be reduced to as little as half of the lower limit of normal. In such cases, invariably five or fewer MUs remain, and conduction velocities measured in motor nerves with greater complements of motor fibers are much more normal.[36]

CONDUCTION BLOCK

Occurrence and Underlying Basis

Normally when there is sufficient temporal and spatial convergence of excitatory inputs to motoneurons, an action potential is triggered at the initial segment of the motoneuron. The latter impulse travels in a saltatory fashion centrifugally to reach the network of intramuscular branches before ending in

TABLE 4.5. Neuronopathies and axonopathies

Muscle Fibers	Acute	Chronic
Increased insertional activity Fibrillation potential Positive sharp waves	Common, may be abundant	May be little or none
Motor Unit Action Potentials *(intramuscular (IM) recorded)*		
Recruitment	Reduced	Reduced
Linked potentials	Common, often blocking	Uncommon
Blocking, axonal neuromuscular	Common	Uncommon
Fluctuations in sizes and shapes of MUAPs	Common	Uncommon
Repetitive firing	Common	Uncommon
Fiber density	Variable	Increased, may be striking

Abnormally large amplitude
  MUAPs
	Uncommon in acute-subacute	Characteristic of well-
		  established mature
		  reinnervation patterns

Decrements in MUAPs in
  response to repetitive
  stimulation
	Maybe	No

Maximum M potential	Decreased in proportion to
	  number of motor axons
	  (neurons, units) lost
		Relatively preserved even in
		  face of severe losses of
		  motor axons

Maximum motor conduction
  velocities
	Normal or nearly so	Usually within normal range
		  but may be slowed to ½ the
		  normal lower limit if only 1
		  or 2 motor units remain

MUAP, motor unit action potential.

the prejunctional axon terminals of a few muscle fibers, as in the case of the extraocular or facial muscles, and to hundreds of muscle fibers in the case of much larger muscles. At each of hundreds of successive nodes of Ranvier between the initial segment to the distal axon terminals, impulses are faithfully regenerated, membrane currents at successive nodal regions well exceeding the requirements for regeneration of the action potential, with some reduction in safety factor for transmission at branch points and the junction of the last myelinated segment and the prejunctional amyelinated terminal.

Full power requires that most or all MUs be recruited and their respective firing frequencies reach whatever frequencies are necessary to produce the maximum tension possible for each MU. Reductions in the maximum force of contractions could result from losses of motor axons or motoneurons or blocking of transmission of centrifugally conducted impulses at one or more sites throughout the course of the motor axons in the case of the latter. The site(s) of the conduction block could be situated anywhere within the ventral roots, plexuses, main nerve trunks, or preterminal and terminal network of branches ending within the muscle itself. The last-mentioned sites could block activity in a variable fraction of the MU, depending on how proximally sited the conduction block was within the terminal network. Conduction block in terminal branches may be recognized by single fiber electromyography. Failure of transmission of the impulse, of course, also occurs at one or more sites in axons undergoing wallerian or axonal degeneration just before total loss of excitability in the fiber(s). Such *axonal conduction block,* although occasionally recognizable clinically if serial electrophysiologic studies are carried out distal to the site of breakdown within the 5 to 10 days following the onset of the illness or injury, is not discussed in this chapter (see Chapter 20). Conduction block in intact axons is most commonly seen in the acute-subacute primary demyelinating neuropathies and focal compressive mononeuropathies such as those affecting the ulnar, median, common peroneal, and radial nerves as well as the cervical or lumbosacral roots.

In demyelinating neuropathies, conduction block usually results from paranodal or internodal demyelination.[9] The latter need affect no more than two to three successive nodes of Ranvier to block transmission of the impulse and, in the case of motor fibers, the contribution of the affected axon's MU to a maximal contraction. In nerve fibers containing typically hundreds of nodes of Ranvier, therefore,

demyelination could affect fewer than 1% of the total number of nodes of Ranvier (or internodal segments) for conduction block to occur. In such minimally affected nerve fibers the conduction velocities in the remaining sections of the nerve fibers could well be normal. Only where demyelination affects many more nodes and internodes (short of conduction block) would the conduction velocity be expected to fall to as much as one-half of the normal maximum values accompanied by corresponding prolongation of the motor distal latency. Such degrees of slowing when they do occur suggest that the demyelination is longitudinally extensive. An apparent reduction in conduction velocity may also be seen proximal to a region of conduction block affecting the larger and more rapidly conducting fibers, the reduced conduction velocity proximal to such a site of conduction block representing normal conduction in the remaining smaller and more slowly conducting fibers in which transmission remained intact.

The electromyographic assessment of conduction block is fraught with technical problems (Table 4.6). These problems are most readily understood and appreciated in motor fibers. As recorded by surface electrodes situated over the innervation zone (reference electrode over the tendon or suitable other site), single surface-recorded (S-MUAPs) are usually biphasic, with total durations that range from 5 to 15 ms in most human muscles. If all S-MUAPs had similar conduction velocities, shapes, and sizes, maximum M potentials representing the compound sum of all the component S-MUAPs would be identical whether the respective motor axons were stimulated at the motor point or at the level of the ventral roots. Such is not the case, however. For example, the maximum hypothenar M potential as elicited by a stimulus delivered to the roots often shows some reduction in amplitude and to a lesser extent negative peak as well as a modest increase in negative peak dura-

TABLE 4.6. Factors affecting changes in maximum M potential as an indicator of conduction block in human peripheral neuropathies

The relative numbers of S-MUAPs of different sizes (amplitude and area), shapes, and conduction velocities in a muscle (group)
The distance between the motor point and site of stimulation
The temperature of the muscle
The band pass of the recording system
Any changes in the relationships between S-MUAP size and conduction velocities.

tion when compared with the M potential elicited by stimulation at the wrist. Even these small reductions in amplitude and area and increases in duration bespeak progressive temporal dispersion in the summation of the component S-MUAPs because of differences in the conduction velocities of their axons and shapes and sizes of the component S-MUAPs. The result is that as the site of stimulus is moved proximally, S-MUAPs of more slowly conducting axons are increasingly dispersed in time with respect to S-MUAPs of more rapidly conducting motor axons to the point where the after positive phases of the latter overlap with the initial negative phases of the more slowly conducting fibers. It is this phase cancellation that accounts for the reduction in the area of the negative peak of the maximum M potential. Such progressive temporal dispersion and interpotential phase cancellations no doubt account for the reductions in substantial peak amplitude and negative peak area in control nerves, where the range of conduction velocities ranges between 20% and 30% and probably even more so in demyelinating neuropathies.

In demyelinating neuropathies, the relative contributions of interpotential phase cancellation and conduction block to any observed reductions in M potential size is difficult to ascertain. Some authors have suggested that up to 50% reductions in M potential size may be explained by interpotential phase cancellation and as a consequence, reductions in M size of less than 50% must be considered as no more than suggestive of conduction block.[37,38] The criteria for conduction block, however, must take into account the acuteness of the demyelinating neuropathy, the presence or absence of any evidence of increased temporal dispersion, and the specific normative values for the group of motor fibers being examined. For example, more than 80% of median-thenar MUs are simple negative-positive biphasic potentials and the range of their conduction velocities of the order of 20% to 25%.

One way of resolving the problem of distinguishing conduction block from the effects of interpotential phase cancellations and enhanced temporal dispersion is to compare maximum twitch tensions and maximum M potentials as the site of stimulation of a motor nerve is moved proximally. In the case of the adductor pollicis muscle, we have shown that in most instances there is a reasonably good correlation between the size (area) of the maximum M potential and the size of the maximum twitch (Figure 4.4). That is, a reduction in the maximum M potential is paralleled by a roughly equivalent reduction in max-

imum twitch tension as the stimulus site was moved proximally in Guillain-Barré polyneuropathy and in some instances other demyelinating peripheral neuropathies. Single MU and maximum whole muscle twitches are monophasic and hence not subject to intertwitch phase cancellations. Unfortunately, however, such twitch recordings may be distorted through the actions of other, sometimes much more powerful, muscles even when special precautions are taken to ensure rigid fixation of the limb. In adductor pollicis twitch recordings, for example, it is important to fix the hand and forearm in such a way as to prevent the flexor carpi ulnaris from distorting and adding to the adductor twitches when the ulnar nerve is stimulated about the elbow and upper arm.

Over the short distances (10 to 40 mm) characteristic of the lesions in most focal compressive and entrapment neuropathies, enhanced temporal dispersion and interpotential phase cancellations are probably not major factors accounting for the reductions in the maximum M potential size (area or amplitude), and reductions in the latter in excess of 20% can, therefore, be taken as strong evidence for conduction block.

Even though enhanced temporal dispersion and interpotential phase cancellations among component MUAPs are important factors governing the shape and size of maximum M potential over conduction distances of 200 mm or more, these are not the only important factors to consider. For example, if all MUAPs were of an equal size, the proportion of motor axons (0 to 100%) in which conduction is blocked could be deduced simply from comparing the sizes of maximum M potential elicited by stimuli delivered close to the motor point at some more proximally situated site of stimulation along the nerve trunk. If there were a 50% reduction in the maximum M potential, it might be assumed that conduction was blocked in one-half of the motor axon population. MUAPs, however, are not uniform in size. They vary widely in amplitude and area as well as in the tension they generate (Figure 4.5), and although there seem to be relatively few large-amplitude MUAPs, these dominate the maximum M potential such that loss of only a few of the largest MUAPs could reduce the size of the maximum M potential well in excess of what might result from conduction block affecting much larger numbers of small sized MUAPs (Figure 4.6). Therefore without some knowledge of which MUs (axons) are blocked, it is impossible to infer, solely from measurements of the maximum M potential, the proportion of the MU pool whose fibers are blocked.

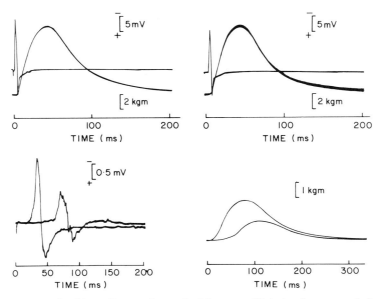

FIGURE 4.4. *Top: Normal subject. Comparison of adductor pollicis (surface-recorded) maximum M potentials and twitches as elicited by just supramaximal stimuli delivered to the ulnar nerve at the wrist and just proximal to the elbow. Note that although there was a small reduction in the amplitude of the maximum M potential, there was no change in the size of the twitch elicited by the more proximally applied two stimuli. Bottom: Patient with chronic demyelinating polyneuropathy. Here the reduction in the maximum M potential is paralleled by an equivalent reduction in the twitch of the adductor pollicis muscle. The reductions may not necessarily indicate the true proportions of adductor pollicis alpha motor axons in which transmission was blocked between the wrist and elbow. For example, conduction block preferentially affecting the larger sized (twitch and amplitude) adductor pollicis motor units could have an impact on the M potential and twitch equivalent to that of conduction block affecting far larger numbers of the smaller amplitude and twitch-producing adductor pollicis motor units.*

Conduction Block in Demyelinating Neuropathies

Conduction block is undoubtedly the major cause of weakness in Guillain-Barré polyneuropathy, although a mild or moderate degree of axonal degeneration is common and in a few patients seems to be the dominant histopathologic change (see Chapter 20). Conduction block, where present, may appear to be more or less uniformly distributed along the length of motor axons, based on the finding of progressive reductions in the maximum M potential size as the site of the stimulus is moved proximally. In other patients, the site of conduction block appears to be proximally or distally situated or both. In yet other patients, conduction block is concentrated at entrapment sites. The last condition suggests a local compressive factor, for example, in the case of the ulnar nerve, at the elbow, or for the common peroneal nerve at the fibular head.

In slowly progressive or relapsing inflammatory polyneuropathies, conduction block is harder to assess because of the greatly increased temporal dispersion sometimes evident in the much greater than normal durations of the maximum M potentials as the stimulus sites are moved proximally. Sometimes, however, conduction block can be unequivocally shown as a clear reduction in maximum twitch tension when the twitch is elicited by a stimulus delivered at the proximal site, as compared with a more distal site along the same motor nerve trunk. Even in acute Guillain-Barré polyneuropathy, once the first 2 to 3 weeks are over, temporal dispersion often becomes more apparent, and for the reasons outlined earlier, this makes it hazardous to assess conduction block based solely on the analysis of changes in the maximum M potential.

Sometimes there seems to be little correlation between the degree of weakness and the conduction

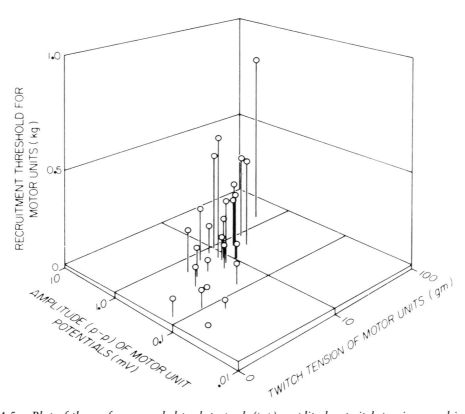

FIGURE 4.5. *Plot of the surface-recorded peak to peak (p-p) amplitudes, twitch tensions, and isometric recruitment thresholds at which 25 first dorsal interosseous motor units were recruited in a healthy young man.*[9]

block as assessed electrophysiologically. There are several possible explanations for these discrepancies. First, as pointed out earlier in this section, reduction in the size of the maximum M potential (amplitude and area) as the site of the stimulation of the motor nerve trunk is displaced proximally reflects the numbers of motor axons blocked, the sizes of the respective MUAPs, and the influence of interpotential phase cancellation on the shape and size of the maximum M potential. Second, the site(s) of conduction block may lie proximal to the most proximal stimulation site in the study, for example, in the arm proximal to the spinal roots (see Figure 20.9) and in the leg proximal to popliteal fossa or sciatic notch. In the lower limbs, it is possible to stimulate the ventral roots directly by either needle electrodes inserted into the subarachnoid space or high-voltage electrical stimulation on the surface at L-1, using a DEVICES D-180 stimulator (Figure 4.7). We no longer employ needle stimulation because the D-180

high-voltage stimulator works very well as a means of stimulating the lumbosacral ventral roots from the surface and is well tolerated by most subjects.

Third, the muscles chosen for electrophysiologic studies are most often situated in the hand or foot because of their accessibility and the long lengths of motor nerve they offer for study. The strength, however, of some of these muscles, for example, the extensor digitorum brevis, cannot be assessed clinically. In contrast, the major motor disabilities affecting standing, walking, getting up, sitting, or lifting the arms depend much more on the proximal and intermediate limb muscles as well as on the muscles of the trunk. The latter groups of muscles along with the bulbar musculature are readily assessed clinically, but conduction block affecting their respective motor nerves is often not tested. For this reason, we now routinely assess conduction to the anterior and lateral compartment muscles as well as the extensor digitorum brevis, in both instances stim-

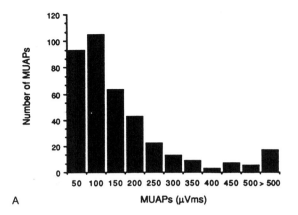

A

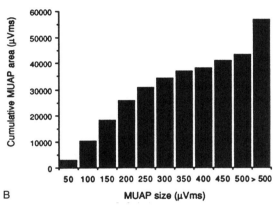

B

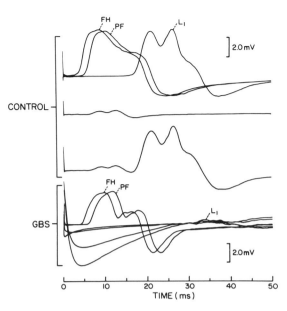

FIGURE 4.7. *Shown are the maximum anterior and lateral compartment M potentials as recorded with surface electrodes in response to supramaximal stimulation at L-1, the popliteal fossa (PF), and fibular head (FH) from a control subject. In the middle of the three control traces, the posterior tibial nerve was supramaximally stimulated at the level of the popliteal fossa and the volume-conducted response to the anterior and lateral compartment surface electrodes recorded. In the bottom of the three control traces, supramaximal stimulation at L-1 and the posterior tibial nerve in the popliteal fossa was carried out together to exclude any volume-conducted activity from the calf muscles from the record recorded in response to L-1 stimulation. In this case, there was little significant contribution from the calf muscles to the anterior and lateral compartment recording. In the bottom tracing, equivalent M potentials were recorded from the anterior and lateral compartment muscles in response to supramaximal stimulation at L-1, popliteal fossa, and fibular head. Striking conduction block and conduction slowing were evident between the L-1 and popliteal fossa stimulus sites, but in this case, no conduction block was present between the fibular head and popliteal fossa and which stimulus sites the maximum M potentials were of equivalent size to control values.*

FIGURE 4.6. *(A) Plot of numbers of surface-recorded thenar motor unit action potentials (MUAPs) of different sizes (negative peak areas in mVms) for controls under the age of 40. Ten to 15 single MUAPs were collected per subject by stimulating the nerve at various sites between the wrist and axilla and collecting the first MUAP excited in an all or nothing manner above threshold. (B) Cumulative sum of the above MUAPs beginning with the smallest and ending with the largest MUAPs. Note the relative abundance of the smaller sized MUAPs, which despite their relatively larger numbers, made little contribution to the sum of all MUAPs.*

ulating at L-1 using the DEVICES D-180 high-voltage stimulator.

Conduction Block in Entrapment Neuropathies

Ulnar nerve

In the case of entrapment neuropathies, conduction block is much more readily assessed because of the relatively short conduction distances involved. This is especially so for the ulnar nerve, for by stimulating the nerve just supramaximally at 20-mm intervals, beginning distal to the cubital tunnel and extending proximally as much as 40 to 60 mm proximally to the tip of the medial epicondyle, conduction block can often be precisely quantitated and localized. In 111 successive ulnar neuropathies studied at our center, conduction block was found in 10% of the affected ulnar nerves and was most commonly found in the 20- to 40-mm segment of the nerve as it passed behind the medial epicondyle (Figure 4.8). In a smaller number of nerves, the conduction block and corresponding maximum slowing of conduction centered about the cubital tunnel. Percent reductions in the maximum M potential were usually similar for the adductor pollicis, first dorsal interosseous, and hypothenar muscle groups but were usually much less pronounced for ulnar motor fibers supplying more proximal muscles, such as the flexor carpi ulnaris and ulnar component of the flexor digitorum profundus muscles, from which similar surface recordings can be made of the maximum M potential. In keeping with the appreciably greater percentage reduction in the maximum M potential recorded from ulnar-supplied intrinsic hand muscles as compared with the flexor carpi ulnaris and flexor digitorum profundus, the weakness and frequency of fibrillation potential activity was also greater in the intrinsic hand muscles. The segments of the ulnar nerve exhibiting the greatest decline in maximum M potential size also corresponded in most patients to the segment demonstrating the slowest conduction velocity. The site of the major conduction abnormalities demonstrated by surface stimulation corresponds very well with the most abnormal sites using direct intraoperative recordings and stimulation (Figure 4.9). As well, more recent studies in our laboratory have shown what we believe to be evidence of continuous conduction as well as conduction block in ulnar nerve fibers across the elbow in a case of postcondylar ulnar neuropathy (see Figure 4.11).

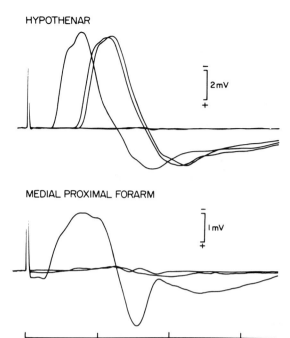

FIGURE 4.8. *Preoperative electrophysiologic study of the ulnar nerve from a patient with a severe weakness in ulnar-supplied intrinsic hand and forearm muscles. On the top are shown successive surface recordings from the hypothenar muscles in response to supramaximal stimulation of the ulnar nerve proximal to the medial epicondyle, just distal to the medial epicondyle, distal to the cubital tunnel, and at the wrist. In the bottom traces, surface recordings were made from the proximal medial forearm in response to supramaximal stimulation of the ulnar nerve just proximal to the medial epicondyle, distal to the medial epicondyle, and distal to the cubital tunnel. In this case, there was striking evidence of conduction block in both muscle groups with almost no response to stimulation proximal to the elbow.*

Median nerve

In normal subjects, there is seldom more than a 10% and never more than a 20% reduction in the size of the maximum thenar M potential as elicited by supramaximal stimulation of the median nerve just proximal to the carpal tunnel compared with the M potential elicited by stimulation just distal to the

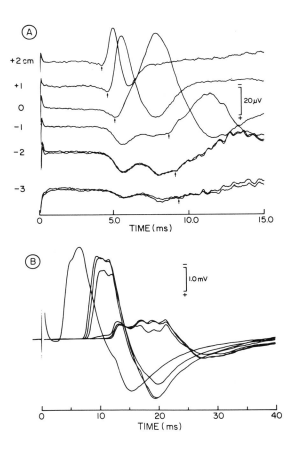

FIGURE 4.9. *The corresponding intraoperative compound nerve action potential recordings (A) and hypothenar muscle recordings (B) with the case illustrated in Figure 4.8 are shown here. In (B), the ulnar nerve was just supramaximally stimulated at 1-cm intervals, beginning 3 cm proximal to the tip of the medial epicondyle and ending 2 cm distal to the tip of the medial epicondyle. The most striking conduction block and conduction slowing were in the 1-cm segment just proximal to the tip of the medial epicondyle. In (A), the ulnar nerve was supramaximally stimulated at the wrist and the compound nerve action potentials recorded from the ulnar nerve, monopolarly, at 1 cm intervals across the elbow. Note the striking increase in the negative peak amplitude and area of the compound nerve action potential noticeable, especially at the 0, −1, and −2 recording sites. This striking increase in the negative peak area strongly suggests the presence of continuous conduction block, a conclusion supported by the presence of very slow conduction between the 0 and −1 recording sites (less than 5 m/s). The initial positive deflections at the −1, −2, and −3 recording sites probably represent volume-conducted activity seen by the reference electrode inserted into the subcutaneous tissue a few centimeters away.*

carpal tunnel. In carpal tunnel entrapments, reductions greater than 20% were present in about one-quarter of these neuropathies (Table 4.7), but in most instances the reductions were less than 50% (Figure 4.10).

The presence or absence of conduction block, as judged by these criteria, bore no apparent relationship to the maximum motor conduction velocity proximal to the entrapment site—here across the forearm—or the duration of the symptoms. The same was true in the ulnar nerve entrapments at the elbow, where the maximum motor conduction velocity proximal to the entrapment site at the elbow was usually normal. Where the conduction velocity proximal to the entrapment site was slower than normal, the degree of slowing of the conduction velocity bore no relation to the completeness of the conduction block. Hence our studies suggest that for most patients conduction block did not preferentially affect the more rapidly conducting motor nerve fibers. In a manner similar to the ulnar neuropathies, fibrillation potential activity was more common in the thenar muscles supplied by the median nerve in those neuropathies in which there was clear evidence of conduction block across the entrapment site, fibrillation potential activity being present in about 40% of the latter as compared with 13% of neuropathies without conduction block. The positive correlation betwen fibrillation potential activity and conduction block probably reflects the severity of the pathologic changes in the underlying nerves (Table 4.7). That is, where demyelination is sufficiently severe to produce conduction block in some fibers, there is usually evidence of wallerian degeneration in other nerve fibers. There was a positive correlation between the degree of conduction block assessed by the reduction in maximum M potential size across the carpal tunnel and the motor distal latency, those nerves with a greater reduction in maximum M potential amplitude exhibiting longer MTLs.

TABLE 4.7.   The incidence of conduction block and fibrillation potential activity in entrapment neuropathies of the median and ulnar nerves*

Nerve	Number	Percent Nerves with Conduction Block	Percent Reduction in Maximum M Potential Peak to Peak Amplitude			Neuropathies with Fibrillation Potentials, Percent Reductions in Peak to Peak Amplitude	
			10–49%	50–89%	90% and over	Less than 10%	Over 10%
Median	59	24	86	14	0	13	40
Ulnar	111	10	63	37	0	33	82

* Conduction block was judged to be present where there was a greater than 20% reduction in the peak to peak amplitude (and area) of the maximum M potential, accompanied by less than a 10% increase in the negative peak duration of the maximum M potential measured across the carpal tunnel in the case of the median nerve and in the case of the ulnar nerve between a stimulus site 20 to 40 mm distal to the cubital tunnel and a second site 40 to 60 mm proximal to the tip of the medial epicondyle.

Peroneal nerve

In 30 acute peroneal neuropathies, the incidence of conduction block was much higher (Table 4.8) and the degree of the conduction block more complete.[39] As in the ulnar neuropathies, the completeness of the block, based on the magnitude of the reduction of the maximum M potential amplitude, was greater in motor fibers supplying distal muscles—here the extensor digitorum brevis as compared with the more proximal muscles such as the anterior and lateral compartment muscles (Figure 4.11). Clinical disability in peroneal palsies is a function of the degree of weakness in the dorsiflexors and evertors of the foot. As was the case for the ulnar nerve, it was common for the degree of conduction block for distal muscles, in the case of the peroneal nerve, as assessed by the magnitude of the reduction in the M potential size for the extensor digitorum brevis muscle to exceed, and in some patients to exceed greatly, the extent of the former proximal muscles supplied by the same nerve, here by the degree of block in the anterior and lateral compartment muscles. By comparing maximum M sizes on the affected and unaffected sides and the changes in M size across the fibular head, it is possible to estimate the relative contribution of conduction block and axon loss in peroneal neuropathies. Fibrillation potential activity was common in both the extensor digitorum brevis and the anterior and lateral compartment muscles, developing within 3 weeks in all acute peroneal neuropathies in which there was electrophysiologic evidence of conduction block of the common peroneal nerve, and the degree of fibrillation potential tended to correlate with the extent of the block, at least to extensor digitorum fibers (Table 4.9). There is no clear experimental evidence to prove that conduction block alone can produce fibrillation potential in muscles. The problem, however, with many of the experimental models designed to test the latter question is that the mechanical devices, toxins, or other agents used to produce the long-term experimental conduction block were all capable of directly causing axonal damage.

Conduction Block in Acute Radial Neuropathies

Similar techniques to those applied to the peroneal nerve may also be applied to other focal neuropathies, including the radial nerve as in the case of the so-called Saturday night palsy[40] (Figure 4.12). These neuropathies, similar to the acute peroneal palsies, exhibit striking conduction block usually localized to the spiral groove.

Conduction block may last many months without apparently much change in the case of entrapment and compressive neuropathies. Nerve fibers whose axons are intact may not remyelinate sufficiently to restore saltation. Failing this, continuous conduction may develop in the more severely demyelinated segments, as one way of restoring conduction to the affected fibers (see Figure 4.11). As in the ulnar and median entrapment neuropathies, there was a good correlation between the magnitude of the reduction in the maximum M potential and the degree of conduction slowing measured across the most affected segment in the nerve in these acute peroneal neuropathies.

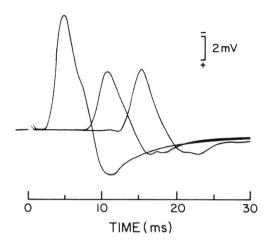

2 mV

TIME (ms)

FIGURE 4.10. *Conduction block in the median nerve beneath the flexor retinaculum. Shown are the surface-recorded maximum thenar M potentials elicited by just supramaximal stimuli delivered to the median nerve just distal to the flexor retinaculum, just proximal to the flexor retinaculum, and at the elbow. Note the one-half reduction in area and peak to peak amplitude of the maximum M potential across the carpal tunnel, here unaccompanied by any increase in the duration (total or negative peak) of the maximum M potential across the carpal tunnel. Here there was no wasting of thenar muscles, but there was readily detectable clinical weakness in the action of the abductor pollicis brevis muscle. There was no slowing of conduction across the forearm to suggest that the faster conducting motor fibers were blocked at the site of the entrapment, even though the conduction velocity across the carpal tunnel itself was very slow, here 5.2 m/s. The latter value is an average value throughout the carpal tunnel; the actual conduction velocity measured across the most abnormal segment could be much lower.*

Reversibility of Conduction Block

In some cases of demyelinating peripheral neuropathy, it is possible to show that reducing the temperature of the nerve can restore conduction to a small fraction of blocked fibers. Reducing the temperature prolongs the transmembrane currents accompanying the action potential. This allows the internal longitudinal currents in nodal regions proximal to the block to flow long enough to overcome the greatly increased transverse leakage currents in the demyelinated region, while leaving sufficient internal longitudinal current to depolarize nodal regions beyond the block to beyond threshold level and generate an action potential, thereby restoring transmission of the impulse through the formally blocked region. This effect is similar to that postulated to account for the reversibility of signs in central demyelinating diseases such as multiple sclerosis when the central body temperature is reduced.

An example of reversible conduction block is illustrated by Figure 4.13. In this subject a series of thenar maximum M potentials were recorded using surface electrodes in response to stimulation at the elbow (A-C). In this normal subject, the temperature of the forearm and therefore the median nerve was altered by means of a continuous coil of tubing wrapped around the forearm from wrist to elbow and through which warm or cool water could be passed. The forearm intramuscular temperature was continuously recorded by a thermistor electrode. The temperature of the thenar muscle group was kept constant throughout the study. Note that in the control subject as the temperature was progressively reduced from 35 to 25°C, there was a progressive increase in latency but no change in the area, shape, or amplitude of the thenar potential elicited by stimulation at the elbow. (B) and (C) Similar studies were carried out from a patient with acute Guillain-Barré polyneuropathy. (C) shows that not only is the max-

Table 4.8. Incidence of conduction block and fibrillation activity in acute peroneal neuropathies*

| | | Percent Nerves with Conduction Block | Percent Reduction in Maximum M Potential Peak to Peak Amplitude | | | Neuropathies with Fibrillation Potentials, Percent Reductions in Peak to Peak Amplitude | |
Nerve	Number		10–49%	50–89%	90% and over	Less than 10%	Over 10%
Peroneal	30	90	23	42	35	66	96

* Criterion for conduction block similar to that used in the median and ulnar nerves; see Table 4.7.

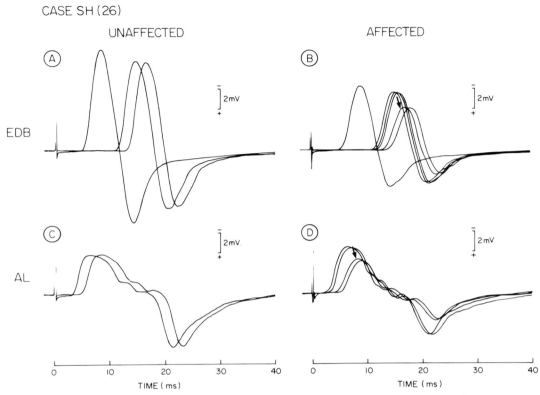

FIGURE 4.11.   *Electrophysiologic studies on the unaffected (A and C) and affected (B and D) sides in a 26-year-old patient with an acute peroneal neuropathy. The peroneal nerve was supramaximally stimulated at the ankle, just distal to the fibular head and popliteal fossa while recording with surface electrodes over the extensor digitorum brevis (EDB) muscle (A and B). In (C) and (D), the peroneal nerve was supramaximally stimulated at the fibular and popliteal fossa, while recordings were made with surface electrodes from the anterior and lateral compartment (AL) muscles. The first recorded potentials on the affected side illustrate a greater amount of axon loss for EDB (35.4%) than for AL (4.9%) when compared with the unaffected side.[39] Arrows indicate conduction block 20 mm proximal to the midfibular head in both the EDB and the AL motor fibers. The amount of conduction block is greater in AL (39%) than in EDB (18.9%) fibers. In (B) and (D), the peroneal nerve was supramaximally stimulated at 20-mm intervals beginning just distal to the fibular head and moving proximally in an attempt to localize the site of maximal conduction slowing and block.*

imum thenar M potential elicited by stimulation at the wrist about one-half of that in normal subjects (see (A)) but also the potential elicited by elbow stimulation was half the size of that elicited at the wrist. This reduction is size strongly suggested the presence of conduction block affecting as many as three-quarters of the median motor fibers supplying these muscles—if fibers were affected without regard to their size. In addition, the conduction block is distributed throughout the length of the nerve be-

tween the elbow and the motor point. Portions of the nerve proximal to the elbow may well have been affected, of course, but were not studied here. In this patient, unlike the normal subject shown in (A), as the forearm was cooled from 35 to 25°C, there was an abrupt increase in the area and amplitude of the thenar M potential, the increase in this subject first developing at about 31°C. This increase in area of the M potential suggests that conduction has been restored to a few of the motor fibers in the median

TABLE 4.9. Fibrillation potential activity in the extensor digitorum brevis muscle

Percent Reductions in Maximum EDB M Potential Amplitude (Peak to Peak)	Number	0*	+†	++‡	+++§
Less than 10%	3	1	1	0	1
10–49%	6	0	1	3	1
50–89%	10	0	2	4	4
90% and over	9	0	3	5	1

EDB, Extensor digitorum brevis (muscle).
* 0 = no fibrillation potentials.
† + = occasional fibrillation potential.
‡ ++ = moderate number of fibrillation potentials.
§ +++ = abundant fibrillation potentials.

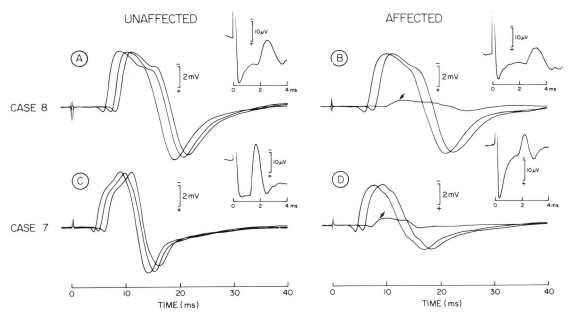

FIGURE 4.12. *Electrophysiologic studies on the unaffected (A and C) and affected (B and D) sides in two cases of acute (Saturday night) radial nerve palsy.*[40] *Arrows indicate the degree of conduction block across the spiral groove in the extensor and abductor pollicis longus motor fibers (91% and 68%). Superficial radial compound nerve action potentials are shown in the upper right-hand corner for each of the unaffected and affected sides. Note the reduction in negative peak amplitude relative to the unaffected side of the superficial peroneal compound sensory nerve action potential (surface recorded) was 33% and 58% in the affected limbs.*[40] *In these studies, surface recordings were made from the extensor and abductor pollicis longus muscles with surface electrodes and the radial nerve supramaximally stimulated at the elbow and just distal and proximal to the spiral groove. Surface-recorded antidromic superficial radial compound sensory nerve action potentials are also shown in the wrists for the unaffected and affected sides.*

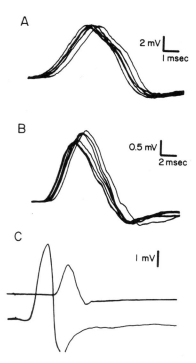

FIGURE 4.13.   *Reversible conduction block in median nerve fibers.*

nerve, whose motor unit potentials contribute to the maximum thenar M potential.

Conduction Block in Radiculopathies

Cervical and lumbosacral radiculopathies often cause pain and paresthesia and may also be accompanied by numbness and weakness. The latter may sometimes be present without any sign of wasting clinically or electrophysiologic evidence of denervation or reinnervation, even when sufficient time has elapsed for these signs of wallerian degeneration to appear. Such weakness and numbness must be caused, in some patients at least, by focal demyelination sufficient to produce conduction block with little if any accompanying axonal degeneration in neighboring nerve fibers in the root. Conduction block or even focal conduction slowing across the sites of compression in cervical or lumbosacral roots is difficult to demonstrate using electrophysiologic techniques except where the roots and adjacent spinal nerves and plexus can be directly studied by positioning electrodes near the nerves. The latter techniques are difficult to apply even when the roots

are exposed at operation. Investigators using traditional techniques must be content with recognizing the reduced recruitment patterns that accompany conduction block or fiber loss in looking for fibrillation potential activity and other electrophysiologic indications of denervation and reinnervation in muscles receiving a major part of their innervation from the affected root.

Conduction Block in Sensory Fibers

Conduction block can sometimes be satisfactorily shown in sensory fibers, especially when conduction is studied over successive short intervals (10 to 20 mm) (Figure 4.14) or, rarely, when the conduction block is complete, as a wholly positive wave without a following negativity when recordings are made just beyond the conduction block. In most recordings from nerve trunks, however, conduction block is much more difficult to prove compared with motor studies, where recordings are made from muscles rather than nerve trunks. This is because MUAPs have relatively long durations and are biphasic, as recorded over the innervation zone, whereas single nerve fiber potentials are triphasic, much shorter in duration, and considerably smaller in size (about $\frac{1}{1000}$ of the amplitude of MUAPs even when recorded with near-nerve electrodes). Even single MUAPs exceed the noise level of the recording system by 10 to 500 times and are easily detected, whereas single nerve fiber potentials recorded from a nerve trunk are rarely detectable above the noise level of the recording system except when high-gain electronic averaging techniques are employed together with the use of needle recording electrodes optimally positioned close to the nerve. The compound nerve action potential is the sum of the component single-fiber potentials. Because of the short durations of single nerve fiber action potentials, their triphasic nature, and differences among their conduction velocities, which are at least of an order similar to or greater than that of alpha motor axons, however, there is a much greater reduction in the size of a compound nerve action potential as compared with the maximum compound muscle action potential, as recorded from muscle with surface electrodes, when both are compared over equivalent conduction distances. The much greater reduction in the compound nerve action potential no doubt reflects the comparatively much greater impact of interpotential phase cancellations on the area of the compound nerve action potential as compared with

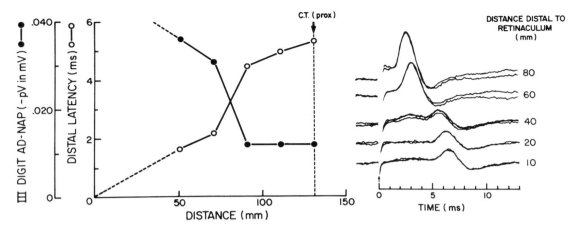

FIGURE 4.14.   *Example of a focal conduction delay and block in median sensory fibers toward the distal end of the carpal tunnel. Shown are the antidromic distal compound sensory nerve action potentials recorded by a pair of ring electrodes about the third digit. They were elicited by percutaneous stimulation of the median nerve at 20-mm intervals, beginning in this patient at the proximal border of the carpal tunnel. Note the increase in size, area, and amplitude of the potential between 40 and 60 mm distal to the proximal border of the flexor retinaculum. This patient reported intermittent paresthesia and numbness that awakened her at night for several months; there was persistent numbness in the median distribution as well. (AD-NAP, Antidromic–nerve action potential; −pV, negative peak voltage.)*

the compound muscle action potential. Conduction block in recordings from nerve trunks can be reliably appreciated only when studied with monophasic recording techniques, in which both the compound nerve action potentials are monophasic and interpotential phase cancellations do not occur.

REFERENCES

1. McComas AJ, Kereshi S, Quinlan J. A method for detecting functional weakness. J Neurol Neurosurg Psychiatry 1983; 46:280–286.
2. Engel AG, Banker BQ, eds. Myology. New York: McGraw-Hill, 1986.
3. Walton J: Disorders of voluntary muscle. New York: Churchill Livingstone, 1988.
4. McComas AJ, Sica REP, Campbell MJ, Upton ARM. Functional compensation in partially denervated muscles. J Neurol Neurosurg Psychiatry 1971; 34:453–460.
5. Doherty TJ, Vandervoort AA, Taylor AW, Brown WF. Effects of aging on the estimated number of functioning human motor units. Proceedings of the Society for Neuroscience, New Orleans, 1991:1392.
6. Sumner AJ, Asbury AK. Physiological studies of the dying-back phenomenon. Brain 1975; 98:91–100.
7. Sumner AJ. The physiology of peripheral nerve disease. Philadelphia: WB Saunders, 1980.
8. Kissel JT, Slivka AP, Warmolts JR, Mendell JR. The clinical spectrum of necrotizing angiopathy of the peripheral nervous system. Ann Neurol 1985; 18:251–257.
9. Brown WF. The physiological and technical basis of electromyography. Boston: Butterworths, 1984.
10. Gilliatt RW. Physical injury to peripheral nerves. Physiologic and electrodiagnostic aspects. Mayo Clin Proc 1981; 56:361–370.
11. Brown WF. The place of electromyography in the analysis of traumatic peripheral nerve lesions. In: Brown WF, Bolton CF, eds. Clinical electromyography, ed. 1. Boston: Butterworths, 1987:159–175.
12. Selzer M. Regeneration of peripheral nerve. In: Sumner AJ, ed. The physiology of peripheral nerve disease. Philadelphia: WB Saunders, 1980:358–431.
13. Miller RG. Injury to peripheral motor nerves. Muscle Nerve 1987; 10:698–710.
14. Lundborg G. Nerve injury and repair. London: Churchill Livingstone, 1988.
15. Sunderland S. The anatomy and physiology of nerve repair. Muscle Nerve 1990; 13:771–784.
16. Seckel BR. Enhancement of peripheral nerve regeneration. Muscle Nerve 1990; 13:785–800.

17. Dorfman LJ. Quantitative clinical electrophysiology in the evaluation of nerve injury and regeneration. Muscle Nerve 1990; 13:822–828.

18. Stalberg E. Use of single fiber EMG and macro EMG in the study of reinnervation. Muscle Nerve 1990; 13:804–813.

19. Erlanger J, Schoepfle GM. A study of nerve degeneration and regeneration. Am J Physiol 1946; 147:550–581.

20. Gilliatt RW, Taylor JC. Electrical changes following section of the facial nerve. Proc R Soc Med 1959; 52:1080–1083.

21. Wilbourn AJ. Serial conduction studies in human nerve during wallerian degeneration. Electroencephalogr Clin Neurophysiol 1977; 43:616.

22. Miledi R, Slater CR. On the degeneration of rat neuromuscular junctions after nerve section. J Physiol 1970; 207:507–528.

23. Cragg BG, Thomas PK. Changes in conduction velocity and fiber size proximal to peripheral nerve lesions. J Physiol 1961; 157:315–327.

24. Dyck PJ, Lais AC, Karnes JL, et al. Permanent axotomy, a model of axonal atrophy and secondary demyelination and remyelination. Ann Neurol 1981; 9:575–583.

25. Berry CM, Grundfest H, Hinsey JC. The electrical activity of regenerating nerves in the cat. J Neurophysiol 1944; 7:103–115.

26. Devor M, Govrin-Lippman R. Maturation of axonal sprouts after nerve crush. Exp Neurol 1979; 64:260–270.

27. Feasby TE, Bostock H, Sears TA. Conduction in regenerating dorsal root fibers. J Neurol Sci 1981; 49:439–454.

28. Brown WF, Hurst LN, Routhier C. Regeneration following nerve experimental transection and microneural repair. Fifth International Congress on Neuromuscular Disease, Marseille, France, 1982.

29. Struppler A, Huckauf H. Propagation velocity in regenerated motor nerve fibers. Electroencephalogr Clin Neurophysiol 1962; 22(suppl 22):58–60.

30. Ballantyne JP, Campbell MJ. Electrophysiological study after surgical repair of sectioned human peripheral nerves. J Neurol Neurosurg Psychiatry 1973; 36:797–805.

31. Donoso RS, Ballantyne JP, Hansen S. Regeneration of sutured human peripheral nerves: An electrophysiological study. J Neurol Neurosurg Psychiatry 1979; 42:97–106.

32. Buchthal F, Kuhl V. Nerve conduction, tactile sensibility, and the electromyogram after suture or compression of peripheral nerve: A longitudinal study in man. J Neurol Neurosurg Psychiatry 1979; 42:436–451.

33. Jasper HH. The rate of reinnervation of muscle following nerve injuries in man as determined by the electromyogram. Trans R Soc Can 1944–47; 38–41 (Sec 5):81–91.

34. Milner-Brown HS, Stein RB, Lee RG. Pattern of recruiting human motor units in neuropathies and motor neuron disease. J Neurol Neurosurg Psychiatry 1974; 37:665–669.

35. Sunderland S. Nerves and nerve injuries, ed. 2. Edinburgh: Churchill-Livingstone, 1978.

36. Hahn AF, Brown WF, Koopman WF, Feasby TE. X-linked dominant hereditary motor and sensory neuropathy. Brain 1990; 113:1511–1525.

37. Kimura J, Sakimura Y, Machida M, et al. Effect of desynchronized inputs on compound sensory and muscle action potentials. Muscle Nerve 1988; 11:694–702.

38. Rhee EK, England JD, Sumner AJ. A computer simulation of conduction block: Effects produced by actual block versus interphase cancellation. Ann Neurol 1990; 28:146–156.

39. Brown WF, Watson BV. Quantitation of axon loss and conduction block in peroneal nerve palsies. Muscle Nerve 1991; 14:237–244.

40. Watson BV, Brown WF. Quantitation of axon loss and conduction block in acute radial nerve palsies. Muscle Nerve 1992; 15:768–773.

5

Positive Manifestations of Nerve Fiber Dysfunction: Clinical, Electrophysiologic, and Pathologic Correlates

Mark Sivak
José Ochoa
José M. Fernández

CONTENTS

LIST OF ACRONYMS

AAEE	American Association of Electromyography and Electrodiagnosis
ALS	amyotrophic lateral sclerosis
ATPase	adenosine triphosphatase
CBZ	carbamazepine
CPA	cerebellopontine angle
EMG	electromyography
gK	potassium conductance
gL	leakage conductance
gNa	sodium conductance
INMS	intraneural microstimulation
MCNG	microneurography
PHT	phenytoin
PTR	posttetanic repetitive (activity)
RT	radiotherapy
2,4D	dichlorophenoxy acetic acid

The manifestations of positive character emanating from nerve impulse dysfunction of peripheral nerve fibers are many. On the motor side, they rarely produce physical discomfort or impede function and often have only cosmetic relevance for the patient. Positive motor phenomena are powerful diagnostically and can be readily recorded by conventional electromyography (EMG). On the other hand, positive sensory symptoms may be crippling, but their electrophysiologic documentation is arduous, invasive, and often impossible to achieve. In this chapter, we correlate clinical presentation, descriptive electrophysiology, and associated nerve fiber pathology for a variety of such positive phenomena of neuropathic origin, while discussing abnormal mechanisms that may underlie their generation.

POSITIVE MOTOR PHENOMENA OF PERIPHERAL NERVE FIBER ORIGIN

Fasciculation

Until the late 1930s, the terms *fibrillation* and *fasciculation* were often used interchangeably, leading to much confusion in the literature. Their delineation as separate entities paralleled the development of clinical EMG. Denny-Brown and Pennybacker[1] defined fasciculation as the spontaneous activity of an entire motor unit (MU), which they based on electrical potential amplitude and configuration criteria. They further postulated the anterior horn cell to be the site of origin of fasciculations. This idea, although logical in the light of the disease states associated with these positive motor phenomena, has not been proved by subsequent work to be necessarily correct. In fact, the weight of accumulated data against the anterior horn cell as the sole site of generation was so compelling that a decade later Denny-Brown[2] revised his conjecture. He suggested that since associated disease processes clearly affected the entire motor neuron, fasciculations might have multiple sites of origin. Years later, Richardson[3] in his review redefined fasciculations closer to the modern concept but categorized several subtypes that are no longer in use. Although cumulative evidence progressively clarified factors pertinent to the genesis of fasciculations, the interpretations tended to separate proponents of various generators into two main camps: those placing the site of origin proximally (proximal axon and anterior horn cell) and those favoring a distal axonal site.[4,5] Further, with increasing knowledge of operant generator mechanisms

(generator site, potential amplitude and wave form, and the characteristics of the nerve responses), the conceptual boundaries between such phenomena as fasciculation, cramp, and myokymia became less clear.

The currently accepted definition of a fasciculation potential is: "The electric potential often associated with the spontaneous discharge of a single MU. Most commonly these potentials occur sporadically and are termed *single fasciculation potentials.* Occasionally the potentials occur as grouped discharge and are termed a *brief repetitive discharge.* The occurrence of repetitive firing of adjacent fasciculation potentials, when numerous, may produce an undulating movement of muscle.[7]

Clinically the presence of fasciculations may be helpful in establishing peripheral nervous system disease. Fasciculations have several characteristic features observable when visible on physical examination. They often produce a brief muscle twitch in a small ribbon of muscle and are usually random in distribution and discharge pattern, seeming to jump from place to place. When involving large, more proximal muscles, the twitch is especially visible. In small distal muscles, particularly of the hands, they may produce actual joint movement resembling myoclonus. Fasciculation tends to be exaggerated by cold exercise or muscle percussion and may be induced or enhanced by hyperventilation as well as with a variety of drugs, including acetylcholinesterase inhibitors. Fasciculations rarely induce a patient to seek medical consultation but are rather a sign of motor neuron involvement observed or elicited on examination.

On electromyographic examination, fasciculation potentials have several characteristics that make them distinguishable from other types of spontaneous activity. They are the size of MU potentials, their amplitude generally reflecting the condition of the voluntary MUs of that muscle.[8] Like MUs in various states of disease, their configuration lies on a continuum from simple to complex and polyphasic, with differing durations. Each fasciculation potential usually shows a uniform and repeating wave form but under some conditions, as in a fluctuating distal generator,[11] may show a changing configuration. Usually fasciculations, like other forms of spontaneous activity, are not under voluntary control, but more recent evidence suggests that a significant proportion of fasciculating MUs (at least 10%) may be activated voluntarily.[12–14] Evidence that the fasciculation potential is not under voluntary control includes the inability to activate waveforms identical to the fasciculating units on volition. Because distally generated fasciculations may be triggered via an axon reflex-like pathway, however, the wave form would necessarily be distinct and not reproducible by voluntary contraction.[11,15] The firing rate of fasciculations is quite variable, from 1 to 50 per minute.[3]

Fasciculation in normal subjects

Fasciculations need not reflect disease of the MU. The occurrence of fasciculations in apparently normal individuals is well known. Their surprising ubiquity was demonstrated in a study conducted by Reed and Kurland,[16] who questioned a large number of healthy volunteers about the incidence and character of fasciculations they may have experienced. Seventy percent of people reported the occurrence of fasciculations. They noted the onset before the age of 30 and persistence of fasciculations on an intermittent basis thereafter. Two major patterns were reported by this population. The first was characterized by episodes of slow undulating activity correlating with an electromyographic picture of irregular discharges of differing MUs. The second much more common pattern was a rapid twitching of one part of a muscle, reflected on EMG as a single, rapidly discharging, often polyphasic MU. The muscles most commonly involved were those about the eyes, hands, and calves, but the phenomenon could occur anywhere. These fasciculations were usually rapid, up to 50 per min.[3]

Fasciculation as a pathologic sign

Both spontaneous fasciculations and contraction fasciculations may occur in patients. Contraction fasciculations were described by Denny-Brown and Pennybacker[1,2]; however, because these fasciculations are induced volitionally, the term does not refer to a true fasciculation as defined today. True fasciculations, occurring spontaneously, characteristically display random recurrence rates, whereas contraction fasciculations are more regular. Contraction fasciculations are produced by the recruitment of large MUs early in voluntary effort in a partially denervated and reinnervated muscle. On contraction, the visible muscle activity is characterized by coarse twitches.[2] There has been discussion regarding the source of these large MU potentials. They may represent either surviving units that have become enlarged by collateral sprouting or the uncovering of the largest MUs now recruited in isolation following denervation and atrophy of smaller ones. Although

the exact nature of this response remains unresolved, the term has largely disappeared from the literature.

The *first major class* of clinically significant spontaneous fasciculations is associated with a spectrum of disorders with pathology ranging from the anterior horn cell to the muscle itself.[11] The MU potentials here are usually, but not exclusively, polyphasic[2,3] and although still random in recurrence, may be either generalized in distribution, as in motor neuron disease, or localized, as in root disease. The discharge frequency is usually low, less than 20 per minute,[8] and unaffected by sleep.[9] Some semantic confusion surrounds the classification of these fasciculations. The term *malignant* has been reserved for those fasciculations associated with progressive anterior horn cell diseases, particularly amyotrophic lateral sclerosis (ALS). Fasciculations reflecting other disease states are referred to as *benign*. Numerous attempts to establish criteria for the differentiation of malignant and benign fasciculations have been made. Trojaborg and Buchthal[8] systematically studied fasciculations in patients with a spectrum of motor neuron diseases, including ALS, as well as in normal subjects. The potentials were compared for configuration, duration, polyphasia, amplitude, and frequency of discharge. Of these parameters, only frequency was found to be significantly different between groups. The average frequencies were one per 3.5 seconds for malignant and one per 0.8 second for benign potentials; however, marked intergroup overlap renders this differential parameter nearly valueless. Amplitude was noted to be 30% lower in patients with ALS, but this reflected a change equally apparent in voluntary MUs, whereas the incidence of polyphasic configuration was between 10% and 20% in both groups. Using single fiber techniques, Stålberg and Trontelj[10,11] and Janko et al.[12] classified fasciculations on the basis of differences in jitter (variation of the interval between muscle fiber potentials of the same MU), blocking (failure of one of these potentials to occur), and fiber density (number of recorded potentials greater than 200 µV). In motor neuron disease, fasciculation potentials always have abnormal jitter, many of the components (75%) show intermittent blocking, and most have increased fiber density (mean 4.3). These abnormalities reflect active collateral reinnervation with functional instability of the new axonal twigs and end plates. The highest degree of reliability is achieved by the concurrence of (1) other signs of organic dysfunction, that is, fibrillation potentials, and so forth; (2) progressive dysfunction (clinical and electrical); and (3) diffuse anatomic distribution.

The *second major class* of true fasciculations are those that may be induced by various maneuvers. As these fasciculations may blend into other phenomena (neuromyotonia, myokymia, cramp), however, they tend to test the limit of the specific definition of fasciculation. One group of such fasciculations are those associated with ischemia. During an experimental ischemic period, there is usually little motor activity, but during the ensuing period of 15 minutes or longer, abundant spontaneous activity of the MU is induced.[17] This activity begins as individual potentials of multiple MUs that quickly fuse, yielding repetitive discharges of gradually diminishing frequency terminating after a series of interrupted bursts.[11,17] This period of spontaneous activity is proportional to the duration of ischemia and may be augmented by hyperventilation or applied electrical stimuli.[17] Fasciculations may also be induced or exaggerated in both normal and diseased muscle by pharmacologic manipulation. It has long been known that myasthenic patients may experience fasciculation potentials as a side effect of anticholinesterase medication. Carbamates, and ammonium phenolates in general[18] may induce fasciculations when used systemically. Neostigmine, physostigmine, and succimethonium[18,19] as well as other unrelated drugs such as penicillin may induce fasciculations when applied at the myoneural junction in mammalian muscle preparations.[20] Further, marked electrolyte imbalance and tetanic electrical nerve stimulation may induce fasciculations.[17]

Site of origin of fasciculation

The first major challenge to the concept of the anterior horn cell as the generator of fasciculations came in 1946 with the experiments of Forster et al.[21] These experiments showed the persistence of fasciculations in muscles of patients with ALS 11 to 12 days following complete motor nerve section. Although spontaneous discharges are a well-recognized early consequence of nerve section, the prolonged persistence of the fasciculatory activity, terminating only with wallerian degeneration, (as signaled by the onset of fibrillations) favors a distal neuronal site of origin.

Although compelling, this evidence has been countered by other observations. Fasciculations have been demonstrated in leg muscles of patients with pathology limited to the cervical cord owing to local spondylosis with compression. The activity may disappear following decompressive surgery.[22,23] Other evidence indicating proximal origin includes the observation of synchronous fasciculations in antagonist as well as homologous muscles,[24] making their origin unlikely anywhere but at the spinal cord. Numerous doubts, however, have been expressed about the ability to verify true synchrony.[2] Similarly, spinal anesthesia, although not completely effective, may temporarily eradicate 50% to 65% of benign fasciculations.[4] Some fasciculation potentials studied physiologically have features that suggest origin in the spinal cord, presumably related to collateral sprouts between neurons.[25]

Although there is now general agreement that fasciculation reflects abnormal impulse generation in the motor neuron, controversy continues as to whether the major site of impulse generation is proximal or distal. Wettstein,[4] using collision techniques, demonstrated that 26% of fasciculations were of proximal origin, with the majority of potentials being of variable origin. Stålberg and Trontelj[11] reported fasciculations apparently of proximal origin because they were slow and irregular in discharge pattern. These potentials had no effect on the latency of the next occurring discharge and caused no compensatory pause, suggesting a nerve cell origin. They are analogous to extradischarges (discussed under Extradischarge, later), which are also known to occur commonly in ALS and neuropathy (Figure 5.1).

Calvin[26] has proposed that the initial segment of motor axons may act as a site for the generation of extra impulses. Indeed, the initial segment resembles in many ways the distal myelinated–nonmyelinated junction found in motor terminal arborization branches. The density of sodium channels is high and the recovery phase is rapid in the initial segment, properties that enhance the integrative functions of this region. Impulses generated at the initial segment, through antidromic invasion of the dendritic tree, can possibly trigger a second impulse at the initial segment because of its shorter recovery cycle in the initial segment relative to the dendritic region. Such a postulated mechanism for fasciculation remains hypothetical.[26]

Conversely, much of the experimental work on fasciculations tends to favor a distal axonal site of origin. Again, work by Forster et al.[21] showed the persistence of fasciculation 11 to 12 days after complete nerve section. The phenomenon terminated with the onset of fibrillation potentials.

Using collision techniques, Roth[5] was able to demonstrate an overwhelming preponderance of fasciculations arising in terminal axons. In a parallel fashion, the previously cited pharmacologic triggering agents act distally. Physostigmine applied exclu-

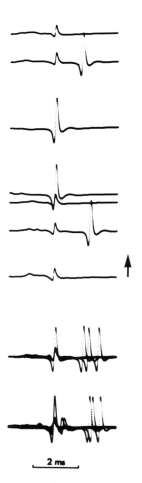

FIGURE 5.1. *Fasciculations recorded (single-fiber electromyography) in a patient with amyotrophic lateral sclerosis. Upper part, with moving film to show the rather rapid and irregular discharge rate. Below, two groups of 10 superimpositions. The two fibers appear independently or jointly, with variable interpotential intervals and in changing order. (Reprinted with permission from Stålberg E, Trontelj JV. Single fiber electromyography. Working, Surrey, U.K.: Miravalle Press, 1979: 190.)*

sively to the terminal axon can elicit back-discharges, which may be detected as high as nerve roots,[27] making the genesis of fasciculations possible via an axon reflex.[28] Other drugs are also capable of eliciting and augmenting similar discharges in peripheral nerves.[18-20] This response and the resulting fasciculation persist despite peripheral nerve block.[2,4,19] Similarly, repetitive activity in the motor axon

persists[20] at a time when muscle activity has been abolished by curare.[19,20] The site of drug application is crucial: Only the motor point, the area of the terminal axonal arborization, and not the parent axon or other muscle loci, is capable of inducing back-discharges.[20] This evidence strongly supports presynaptic elements of the myoneural junction or terminal arborization branches as the generator site.

In some situations, the wave form of the fasciculation potentials may vary from one discharge to another. This finding is most consistent with an axon reflex-like propagation from generators of fasciculations,[11,28] arising in variable distal sites. Similarly, although single-fiber components of fasciculation potentials with constant configuration usually show normal jitter, this is not always true. The observed jitter abnormalities are thought to arise from subnormal and supernormal membrane excitability persisting postdischarge in terminal axonal branches.[11,18] Owing to their small caliber and poor myelination, distal axonal branches have repolarization cycles that are relatively longer than the rest of the axon.[26] Locally persistent negative afterpotentials, with the attendant heightened excitability in contiguous repolarized nerve segments, is thought to be the mechanism of potential generation. The negative current then is propagated proximally (antidromically) and eventually reaches the parent axon, which may become depolarized orthodromically.[11] The observed jittering and blocking components are thought to be due to persistent relative or absolute refractoriness of the terminal branches.[11] Although the intact axon itself is markedly resistant to spontaneous impulse generation,[26] the distal myelinated–nonmyelinated junctions are particularly vulnerable sites.[5,18,29] Here are found the steepest resting membrane potential gradients.[18] Increased excitability and reduced accommodation further typify this area,[5,18] thus facilitating ectopic impulse generation induced by transient membrane potential fluctuations.*

Although the axon reflex concept fits much of the experimental data (especially the pharmacologically induced fasciculations), not all clinically observed and physiologically studied fasciculations are consistent with this type of impulse propagation. Indeed, fasciculations occurrng in the context of root or

---

* The term *accommodation* is used to describe responses of excitable membranes to slow depolarizing currents without generation of an action potential. A more complete explanation may be sought in standard physiology texts such as Mountcastle VB, ed. Medical physiology; ed 14. St. Louis: Mosby, 1980.

nerve compressive lesions would logically be of proximal origin. These potentials were formerly referred to as *compression fasciculations* by Richard[3] and were suggested to be due to changes induced by nerve ischemia.[17] Demyelination, which is a significant pathologic change in nerve compression lesions, causes changes in membrane capacitance, conductance, and resistance (to be discussed later) and has been shown to be an important predisposing mechanism leading to ectopic impulse generation. Demyelination may also foster ephaptic cross-talk.[26] On the other hand, postischemic MU discharges occurring independent of demyelination are well documented. The mechanism thought responsible for postischemic discharges is the rapid return of nerve excitability from 0.5 to 1 minute postischemia, with a slower recovery of accommodation.[11,17,30] These excitability changes seem to be related to a reduction of sodium channel inactivation and possibly to an alteration in potassium ion kinetics.[26] The combination of normal or increased excitability with reduced accommodation predisposes the fiber to spontaneous discharge. Thus, mechanical nerve compression in one way or another induces excitability changes in nerves sufficient to cause fasciculation.[3]

The final locus of fasciculation generation possibly resides in the muscle itself.[11] This site has been particularly stressed in benign fasciculation. The proposed mechanism is one of ephaptic transmission by depolarizing current flow arising from synchronous activity in populations of adjacent muscle fibers. Single-muscle fiber electromyographic studies of these potentials reveal blocking despite low jitter, a finding inconsistent with neuromuscular transmission abnormalities.[11] The firing rate of myogenic fasciculations varies up to eight to 10 per second.[31] Clinically these fasciculations are large and coarse and unaffected by neuromuscular junction manipulations such as blockade with curare or augmentation with acetylcholine.[31] It is proposed that a muscle fiber with a partially depolarized resting potential spontaneously discharges and induces depolarization currents in surrounding fibers, which also have a resting membrane potential abnormally close to threshold. This type of fasciculatory activity would correlate with the more or less continuous quivering activity reported by Reed and Kurland's subjects.[16]

Thus there is sufficient experimental and clinical evidence that fasciculations may arise at several sites. Of the conditions associated with fasciculations, most tend to involve either the anterior horn cell or the proximal root. These include ALS, progressive muscular atrophy, poliomyelitis, syringomyelia, and root compression. Somewhat more distally focused pathologies, however, associated with fasciculation include nerve compression, peroneal muscular atrophy, and polyneuropathy.[3,22] Given this wide diversity of clinical abnormalities, multiple generator sites for fasciculations seem likely.

Just as fasciculations reflect spontaneous muscle activity triggered by electrical impulses generated at varying loci along peripheral nerve fibers, an assortment of other spontaneously occurring phenomena have similar sites of origin. These include myokymia, neuromyotonia, cramp, tetany, and the electrically observed double discharge. The clinical phenomenology of these disorders is diverse, but the basic pathophysiologic mechanisms, although not fully elucidated, appear to be related. Although some of these phenomena have definite pathologic significance, as for example, myokymia, cramp is most often observed in normal subjects, and tetany may be seen in both normal and pathologic conditions. In light of this, it seems reasonable to begin with a discussion of the proposed underlying pathophysiology that binds these various states together and then proceed to a discussion of their differences.

Extradischarge

The simplest form of repetitive activity and perhaps the most commonly encountered in routine EMG is the *double discharge, extradischarge,* or *doublet.*[15,29,32,33] It consists of a pair of discharges of a MU instead of a single response to ectopically generated or volitionally evoked stimulation. When the repeating discharge is further multiplied, it is called a *triplet* (three potentials) or even *multiplet.*[32] Although sometimes observed in normal subjects at the onset of voluntary activation,[33] the double discharge is distinctly more common in pathological states, usually chronic in course. The observed lesions, combining axonal compromise with focal demyelination, are localized to the more proximal segments of nerves.[15,33] Conditions in which double discharges are found include proximal neuropathies, hereditary polyneuropathies, chronic idiopathic polyradiculoneuropathy, and, curiously, myotonic dystrophy,[15,33] polymyositis, and muscular dystrophies.[34]

The doublet is often found in association with other spontaneous activities of nerve fiber origin, such as myokymia, neuromyotonia, tetany, and cramp. The component potentials of the doublet have the amplitude, duration, and configuration of MU potentials and are identical except that the second potential of the pair is of somewhat smaller amplitude[11,15] when the interpotential interval is shorter than 10 ms.[9,11,15] This possibly reflects recurrence during the period of diminished excitability. Because the second discharge, as monitored with single-fiber EMG, contains all the components of the original potential without evidence of terminal arborization branch block, and it changes in amplitude and shape in parallel with the original potentials on repositioning the recording electrode (Figure 5.2), the generator is most likely in the peripheral axon.[11] Double discharges induce a compensatory pause of 50% or more in the interpotential interval, a further expression of their axonal origin.[9,15,29] The potentials occur at a fairly fixed interpotential interval and recur regularly. The interval is most commonly of 9 ms duration[15] but occurs within a range of 2 to 20 ms. By definition, if the interval of the discharge is long, between 20 and 80 ms, the group, which is in all other ways identical to a doublet, is called a *paired discharge*.[32] Double discharges with an unusually short interpotential latency are occasionally noted; their generator mechanism remains obscure.[29]

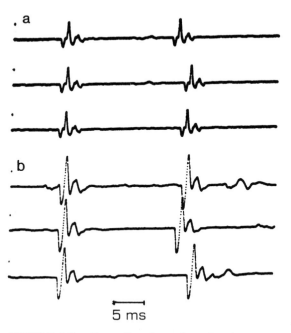

FIGURE 5.2.   *Recording from the orbicularis oculi muscle of a patient with facial myokymia owing to multiple sclerosis. The late potentials (extradischarges of the firsts) have the same shape and amplitude and changes in parallel on slight electrode movement from a to b.*

Although the component potentials of the doublet occur at a relatively constant interpotential interval, the single-fiber components of each potential may show considerable jitter, from 0.5 ms to 4 ms, probably as a result of discharge-related changes in excitability in distal nerve fiber branches.[11,29] By combining techniques of collision and blocking induced with paired stimuli and F wave studies, the site of recurrence may sometimes be identified and has suggested varying sites of origin.[11,29]

Ectopic generation of extradischarge

Among the possible sites of ectopic impulse generation, portions of axons exhibiting changes in myelination and spatial inhomogeneities are favored.[35,36] As previously discussed, myelinated–unmyelinated junctions are particularly likely candidates.[26,29] Such structural characteristics occur in normal nerves at the initial segment and the terminal axonal branches as well as at sites of focal demyelination in diseased nerve.[26] The physiologic mechanisms for ectopic impulse generation in these regions may depend on the distribution of sodium channels in the membrane. As noted by Ritchie,[37] sodium channels are normally found in high concentrations at the nodes of Ranvier, with very few occurring in internodal axolemma. Further, in regions where abrupt transitions in axonal diameter or myelin thickness normally occur,[26,36] changes are also observed in both nodal and internodal lengths. These *compensatory* alterations are thought to function as current boosters, insuring conduction through otherwise insecure segments of nerve.[26] This same process has been described at axonal branch points that have matching structural features.[26,36]

In areas of focal demyelination, similar changes occur (Figure 5.3). Initially the loss of myelin insulation of the internodal axolemma effectively decreases transmembrane resistance. The decrease in thickness of high-resistance material separating axoplasm from the external fluid medium, effectively increasing membrane capacitance.[26] It is important to note that not only is there more membrane exposed, but also the nature of that newly exposed surface is intrinsically different from the normal nodal structure, specifically in regard to the density of sodium channels. The net effect of these early changes is to increase the actual sodium ion transmembrane impedance of the entire exposed membrane[26,38] as well as to elevate total membrane capacitance.[39] Therefore more charge is required to drive a more sluggishly reactive membrane, leading

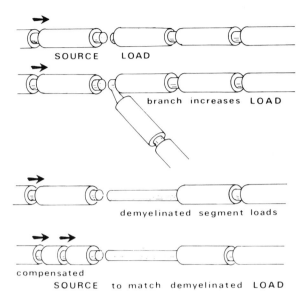

SOURCE LOAD

branch increases LOAD

demyelinated segment loads

compensated
SOURCE to match demyelinated LOAD

FIGURE 5.3. *Source-load relationships for a propagating impulse in a myelinated axon. Inward net current is assumed for the source's nodes; the region labeled LOAD is still passive, being just in front of the active region. A side branch or a demyelinated region will increase the load. If the source conductance is inadequate to drive such increased loads, compensation might occur via closely spaced nodes (as at bottom; see Waxman and Brill, 1978), increased sodium channel density, or increased nodal ara. (Reprinted with permission from Calvin WH. To spike or not to spike? Controlling the neurons rhythm preventing the ectopic beat. In: Culp WJ, Ochoa J, eds. Abnormal nerves and muscles as impulse generators. New York: Oxford University Press, 1982). Waxman SG, Brill MH: Conduction through demyelinated plaques in multiple sclerosis: Computer simulations of facilitation by short internodes. J. Neurol, Neurosurg. & Psychiat. 41; 408–16 1978.*

to excitation-conduction failure.[26,38] The subsequent combination of internodal segment shortening proximal to the demyelinated area and a postulated deposition of new sodium channels[38] effectively causes an increase in potential current density,[26] which stabilizes impulse propagation. The longer stretches of membrane surface through which ion flux occurs,[26,35] the slower continuous conduction along the unsheathed membrane,[38] and the relative persistence of open sodium channels all tend to enhance excitability and thus increase the likelihood of ectopic

impulse generation.[38] Further, with an area of slowed conduction adjacent to normally conducting membrane, imbalances in the depolarization and repolarization cycles may occur, increasing the chances of retrograde impulse propagation. Such potentials are known as *back-discharges*.[26]

A small hump has been noted immediately preceding the second action potential component of a double discharge. This is thought to represent retrograde impulse propagation.[26,40,41] It is postulated that this antidromic potential arises at the axon hillock and spreads to the somadendritic segment, inducing changes in the resting potential of the traversed membrane.[26,35] Dendrites containing the more slowly reactive potassium channels as well as sodium channels develop a prolonged state of depolarization. This wave of depolarization may travel back to the axon hillock, reaching it after excitability has recovered, and thus generate a second discharge.[26,35] Because of the refractoriness of the somadendritic membranes, a second wave of retrograde propagation is not induced[26] (Figure 5.4).

Matters complicate still further. Calvin[26] has noted that as the applied current is increased, the frequency of extradischarges increases, and at a fiber-specific critical frequency, the discharge rate may double or triple, eventually leading to perpetuation of discharges. The mechanism of this multiplication phenomenon is not known but possibly relates to spontaneous oscillations in membrane potential, combined with an activity-enhanced m-state–h-state overlap.*

Activity-dependent increases in extracellular potassium ion concentration may also cause recurrent discharges or multiplets.[26] If, along the course of an axon, several sites of demyelination or configurational changes occur, sequences of reverberating orthodromic and antidromic discharges may arise, which become manifest as repetitive activity.[39]

Calcium ions have long been known to be fundamental to excitable membranes. Calcium has an apparent membrane surface effect, but its role remains unclear.[42] Closely allied to the calcium ion kinetics are alterations in membrane excitability associated with fluctuations of pH and carbon dioxide.

---

* The terms *m* and *h* are state functions related to sodium conductance introduced in the Hogkin-Huxley model of nerve excitation. For details the interested reader is referred to appropriate texts, for example, Excitation and conduction in nerve fibers. In: Mountcastle VB, ed. Medical physiology, ed. 14. Vol. 1. St. Louis: Mosby, 1980:46–81.[35]

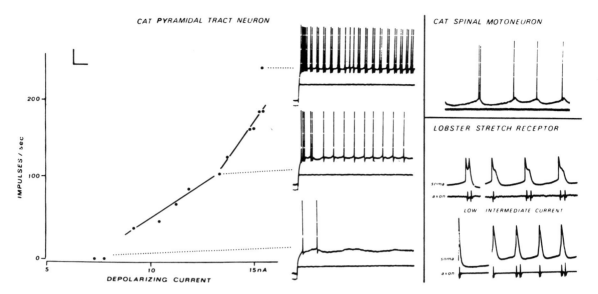

FIGURE 5.4.   *Repetitive firing with extra spikes: examples from a fast pyramidal tract neuron, a spinal motor neuron, and two lobster stretch receptor neurons. Extra spikes are associated with postspike humps in most cases; however, in the lower right corner is a case where delayed retrograde invasion of the somal dendritic region allowed the initial segment to be reexcited. (Reprinted with permission from Calvin WH. Reexcitation in normal and abnormal repetitive firing of CNS neurons. In: Chalafonitis N, Boisson, eds. Abnormal neuronal discharges. New York: Raven Press, 1978.)*

These factors again seem to have little direct action but rather work through changes in calcium ion concentrations.[35,43] During the alkalosis induced by hyperventilation, calcium ion becomes protein bound, causing an apparent hypocalcemia, which if maintained will lead to marked spontaneous activity in both sensory and motor nerves.[44] This induced activity, which normally subsides as ion equilibrium is restored, may be reversed with intravenous calcium infusion.[45] Once the hyperventilation-induced spontaneous discharges have subsided, they may be reinitiated with electrical nerve stimulation.[46] Conversely, with prolonged high-frequency electrically induced nerve activity, the intracellular calcium and sodium concentrations increase, with eventual membrane hyperpolarization and cessation of spontaneous activity.[35] Hypomagnesemia produces changes similar to and exaggerating those seen with hypocalcemia, further enhancing excitability. This leads to increased spontaneous activity discharge rates and prolongs the duration of the responses, probably by inducing or accentuating hypocalcemia rather than through independent action.[43] Compared with calcium infusion, magnesium has a similar, but less marked, membrane-stabilizing effect.[43] Early work on human nerve excitability changes, induced by

hyperventilation, described spontaneously generated single MU potentials and more commonly doublets, which initially increased in frequency and then persisted for 10 to 15 minutes after hyperventilation had been discontinued.[44] This was accompanied by carpopedal spasm and tetany.[47,48] The smallest fibers were the first recruited.[44] Ischemia induced with a blood pressure cuff further prolonged the neural spontaneous activity, particularly in the proximal segment, and made it more sensitive to electrical stimulation,[44] accommodation being more easily perturbed here than in distal segments.[41,48]

Ectopic generation of ongoing discharges

All the aforementioned mechanisms most commonly produce doublets, although they may produce multiple discharges. We now consider mechanisms that tend to produce multiple burstings or ongoing discharges. These are the types of activity seen in most states of nerve pathology. In his classic study, Adrian[49] cut mammalian nerves and recorded prolonged sensory and motor ongoing activity, somewhat more marked in sensory nerve. Three patterns of activity were noted, consisting of regular high-frequency discharges at 150 c/s, irregular low-frequency ongoing activity, and finally high-frequency activity occurring in bursts that repeated at low frequencies (20 to 50 c/s). The frequency of activity was manipulable by drying or cooling the preparations, changing the constituents of the bathing medium to unphysiologic degrees, or recutting the nerve. Conversely, activity could be reduced by stripping the nerve sheaths, introducing procaine hydrochloride (Novocain) into the bath, or adding 0.01% calcium chloride. Wall et al.[50] repeated these same experiments using more modern techniques. They were unable to duplicate Adrian's results when the entire nerve was cut but obtained similar results when small branches of the nerve were allowed to remain in contact with muscle. It thus appears that ongoing nerve activity requires some degree of nerve continuity.

Early investigations of the genesis of muscle fibrillation activity noted that physostigmine placed at the myoneural junction in nerve-muscle preparations induced bursts of tetanic muscle contractions associated with repetitive discharges of nerve terminals, which could be monitored as high as the ventral roots.[27,41] Similar responses were obtained with anti-acetylcholinesterase and quaternary ammonium phenolate compounds,[11,41] suggesting a presynaptic action of acetylcholine. This may be the mechanism of repetitive discharges noted in patients treated with antiacetylcholinesterase medication.[41] These pharmacologic manipulations resulted in increased nerve excitability by the induction of a depolarizing negative afterpotential and reduced membrane resistance. The persistent mild membrane depolarization makes repetitive activity more likely.[41] Prolonged high-frequency electrical stimulation induces a drop in the nerve responses thought to reflect a block of presynaptic acetylcholine receptors.[41] With very high-frequency nerve discharges, the capacity of myoneural junction and muscle to follow may be exceeded, such that manifest muscle activity becomes an inaccurate reflection of the neural events.[40]

The *ischemic* and *postischemic* periods are also associated with marked changes in both sensory and motor nerve activity. This may vary from the commonly encountered brief postischemic paresthesias commonly referred to as a limb "going to sleep," to the full-blown picture of postischemic repetitive activity in motor and sensory fibers. During early stages of ischemia,[30] paresthesias are normally induced together with rare, isolated motor action potentials.[11,17] In the ischemic period, accommodation actually increases slightly and then gradually returns to normal.[27,41,48] The first 30 seconds of the postischemic period are characterized by the rapid return

of volitional activity.[11] During the ensuing 30 seconds, the onset of spontaneous sensory and motor nerve fiber discharge is first noted.[11] The discharges begin with single potentials and doublets recurring at low frequencies (20 to 80 c/s). These then become irregular and over several minutes evolve into a high-frequency bursting pattern (2 to 30 spikes at 100 to 180 c/s).[17] Gradually there is a shortening of burst duration and a prolongation of the interburst interval, until the activity ceases altogether.[11,17] As observed with posthyperventilation repetitive activity, electrical stimulation may reinstate bursting. The mechanism of this repetitive activity seems to be a postischemic fall in accommodation, which is again more marked proximally.[17,41,48,51] Several theories have been advanced to account for the observed changes in accommodation. The often-cited view that unopposed increased potassium leak during ischemia results in an increase in extracellular potassium is not confirmed by observation.[30] An alternate theory proposes that during ischemia there is an alteration of the sodium pump with leakage of both sodium and potassium because the pump energy is dependent on oxidative metabolism. Once energy metabolism is restored, the ion shifts may render the membrane hyperexcitable.[30]

Repetitive electrical stimulation of a nerve induces a period of increased membrane excitability, or reduced threshold, followed by a somewhat more protracted period of reduced excitability commencing immediately after the absolute and relative refractory periods. With very strong stimulation, a third brief period of reduced threshold may be produced. The periods of increased and decreased membrane electrical excitability are called *supernormal* and *subnormal periods*. By increasing the number and frequency of conditioning stimuli, the excitability recovery curves may be altered. With increased number of stimuli in the range of 8 to 12, the initial supernormal period may be enhanced in amplitude, but there is no significant change in either the duration or magnitude of the subnormal period.[41] Bergmans[30] has labeled the subnormal period the H_1 *period,* and its duration is about 150 ms, the first 50 ms of which is the period of supernormal excitability. The induced H_1 period probably reflects the slower kinetics of the repolarizing potassium current, which reestablishes the resting membrane voltage.[30] With more prolonged stimulation of the same preparation, such as 300 c/s for 30 seconds, the supernormal and subnormal periods become more protracted, lasting up to 1 second. The long-lasting subnormal period, designated the H_2 *period* by Bergmans, was initially thought to be a manifestation of endoneurial potassium accumulation, but it probably reflects the induced operation of the sodium–potassium pump mechanism.[30] During these subnormal or H_1 and H_2 periods, the latency between stimulation and electrical response is slightly prolonged, and the stimulus threshold is variably increased.[30] Under these conditions, one would predict a delay in electrical signal transmission. Some controversy, however, exists as to whether there is actual conduction slowing in this situation.[52] Because of their different responses to manipulation by applied anodal and cathodal currents, and resistance to ischemia, the H_1 period is probably passive, whereas the H_2 period is active and energy dependent.[30] The earlier supernormal periods probably correspond to intervals of increased sodium channel availability induced by an increase in intracellular sodium concentration.[52]

With short-duration tetanic stimulation, for instance, 10 seconds of 150 to 500 c/s, a period of posttetanic repetitive activity (PTR-I) is induced in the MUs. When the conditioned nerve is restimulated, repetitive activity is induced. This may be enhanced and prolonged with critically timed double stimuli and may persist for up to 45 minutes.[41] The repetitive activity is thought to be initiated by a presynaptic effect of acetylcholine and spread by an axon reflex mechanism.[41] When the tetanizing stimulus is longer (300 c/s for 30 min or more), the induced activity (PTR-II) is manifest by continuous and bursting activity, which may be electrically triggered for hours.[41] Ischemia will depress PTR-II, implicating an active energy-requiring mechanism, again possibly the electrogenic sodium pump.[41] The exact clinical significance of these phenomena is unknown.

The final mechanism underlying ectopic impulse generation to be discussed is that of *ephaptic transmission*. Early evidence of its existence was presented by Granit et al.,[53] who demonstrated the short-term existence of sensory root responses when stimulating ventral roots in cats with cut nerves. Rasminsky[54] showed ephapses to exist on a long-term ongoing basis in a genetically determined demyelinating neuropathy in rats. Demyelinated areas may have a large outward current flow[38] and may be in close proximity to demyelinated segments in neighboring fibers,[53] conditions favoring ephaptic transmission (cross-talk) (Figure 5.5). What makes this ephaptic transmission effective for subsequent generation of repeated discharges is the fact that accommodation is significantly reduced in demyelinated membrane.[26,54] Demyelination noted in a variety of clinical states, such as nerve compression, chronic

idiopathic polyradiculoneuropathy, and Charcot-Marie-Tooth disease, may thus predispose to long-term impulse generation.

With this understanding of possible types of ectopic generators, we now focus attention on a resulting spectrum of clinical presentations of muscle activity generated in the neural elements of the MU.

Myokymia

Myokymia is a somewhat unusual phenomenon noted in a distinct group of clinical settings. The activity is usually most prominent in proximal muscles but may be ubiquitous. The movements are undulating and frequently described as worm-like movements of muscle, or "live flesh." The actual movement is produced by nonuniform discharges of various parts of the involved muscle, thus yielding little directed movement.[55,56] The first description was by Kny in 1888[57] followed closely by Schultze in 1895,[58] who first used the term *myokymia*. Since then, myokymia has been reported in the French, German, Spanish, and English literature. The currently accepted definition of myokymia is "a continuous quivering or undulating movement of surface and overlying skin and mucous membrane associated with spontaneous, repetitive discharge of MU potentials.."[7] This is only a little different from the definition proposed by Denny-Brown and Foley in 1948.[59] The electrical correlation is myokymic discharge; these discharges may be defined as MU potentials that fire spontaneously repetitively and may be associated with clinical myokymia. Two firing patterns have been described. Commonly the discharge involves a brief, repetitive firing of single units for a short period (up to a few seconds) at a uniform rate (2 to 60 c/s) followed by a short period (up to a few seconds) of silence, with repetition of the same sequence for a particular potential. Less commonly, the potential recurs continuously at a fairly uniform firing rate (1 to 5 c/s). Myokymic discharges are a subclass of grouped discharges and repetitive discharges.

Some points in the definitions given here are contested; for example, some propose firing frequency ranges to be faster (40 to 60 c/s[60] or 25 to 100 c/s[11]). The degree of clinical expression may vary from time to time, so the myokymia may be more evident at one examination than another.

Myokymia is a peripheral process as opposed to a central process, such as has been suggested for stiff man syndrome.[61,62] Myokymia may be further clas-

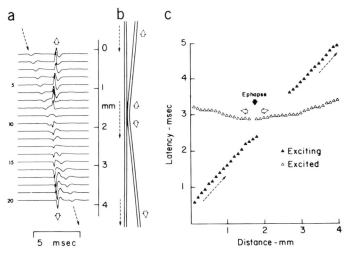

FIGURE 5.5. *Ephaptic transmission between two single fibers in a systrophic mouse ventral root. (A) Computer-averaged records (32 sweeps) of external longitudinal current at intervals of 200 μm from proximal (top) to distal (bottom). The impulse in the exciting fiber propagates away from the spinal cord, giving rise to a downward deflection at a progressively greater latency at successive positions along the root over the almost 4 mm illustrated (dashed arrow). An impulse arises in a second fiber in midroot and is propagated toward the spinal cord (upward deflections in records 108) and away from the spinal cord (downward deflections in records 10 to 20) (open arrows). At record 9, the recording electrodes straddle the site of origin of this impulse, and no clear-cut initial upward or downward deflection is seen. See Rasminsky (1980) for details of recording technique. (B) Diagrammatic indication of the site of ephaptic interaction near record 9. (C) Latency to the peak of external longitudinal current versus distance along the root for the exciting and excited fibers. The distance scale corresponds to (A); zero time is arbitrary. (Reprinted with permission from The Physiological Society from Rasminsky M. Ephaptic transmission between single nerve fibers in the spinal nerve roots of dystrophic mice. J Physiol 1980; 305:151–169.*

sified into two main categories: (1) generalized myokymia, usually symmetric in limb muscles, and (2) focal myokymia, often asymmetric and noted in particular neural or segmental distributions (e.g., facial myokymia).

Generalized myokymia

Generalized myokymia is part of the syndrome of continuous muscle fiber activity (Isaacs' syndrome).[56,64] It usually has its onset in the second decade, affecting males predominantly.[64] The first symptoms include muscle cramps[65–68] and muscle stiffness,[69] with a marked delay in relaxation after muscle contraction.[55,56,67,68] The initial abnormalities may be focal[65] but gradually generalize over time. Consequent to the stiffness, there may be some compromise of fine movements. Patients commonly report that with a "warm-up" period of muscle activity, there is a significant reduction in the prolonged postcontraction relaxation phase,[67] making movements more fluent. Characteristically the muscle activity persists during sleep.[64] Because of the constant contractions, the affected muscles may be hypertrophied, although a large number of patients have distal muscular atrophy as part of the syndrome.[55,67,68] In some instances, the continuous muscle activity may lead to joint deformity, although this is more common with neuromyotonia. Most often the tendon reflexes are absent or diminished throughout, possibly as a result of the constant muscle activity, since they may return when therapy effectively reduces the myokymia.[66,67] Hyperhydrosis frequently accompanies myokymia[65] and is thought to be a response to heat generated by the constant muscle activity,[68] rather than a release of reflex sweating.[68]

Several etiologic classes of generalized myokymia exist: A common one is symptomatic myokymia associated with diseases of peripheral nerves as seen with Guillain-Barré syndrome,[71] with metabolic derangements such as uremia and thyrotoxicosis,[69] and with gold toxicity.[70] Myokymia is mostly seen as an idiopathic phenomenon, and occasionally it may be hereditary, affecting either sex, and may be expressed in families over several generations.[64,105] In one family reported, it appeared associated to kinesigenic ataxia.[72] On the whole, this condition is rare.

Clinical observations and pharmacologic manipulation of myokymia are useful in localizing the site of origin of this abnormal activity. As mentioned earlier, myokymia persists at rest and during sleep.[64] Attempts to suppress the activity with spinal and general anesthesia are unsuccessful.[65,67] Drugs with primary action on the central nervous system, such as diazepam, are notoriously ineffective in modifying myokymia.[66] The activity is, however, blocked with curare and related drugs,[65,67] thus eliminating muscle as the site of origin. Peripheral nerve blocks are variably effective,[65] and ischemia induced with a sphygmomanometer reduces the activity,[65] only to be followed by markedly exaggerated activity in the postischemic period.[67,69]

The above-mentioned observations strongly suggest that the generator sites are in large myelinated peripheral nerve fibers and dependent on oxidative metabolism. There is ambiguity concerning the location along the peripheral nerve where the generator was most likely to lie. Evidence provided by an unusual case of myokymia induced by intoxication with an insecticide, dichlorophenoxy acetic acid (2,4D), indicated a proximal generator.[66] Other studies suggest the terminal arborization branches of the peripheral motor nerves as the site of generation.[56,69] Several investigators have demonstrated that the myokymic activity may indeed have multiple and varying sites of origin, the greater percentage of activity being abolished with distal than with proximal local anesthetic nerve blocks.[65,66,68,73] One study showed that a 53% reduction of activity was induced with ulnar nerve block performed at the level of the elbow and that the efficacy of the procedure could be increased to 90% when the block was carried out at the wrist.[66]

Focal demyelination seems to be an important pathologic process at the background of myokymia. As previously discussed, areas with focal demyelination may be sites of ectopic impulse generation and, if multiple, may generate reverberating discharges, thus producing self-sustained reexcitation.[26,36,38,39,44] Two other possible causative mechanisms have also been proposed: disease within the spinal cord involving Renshaw cells or physiologic deafferentation of alpha motor neurons with the re-

sultant exaggeration of spontaneous resting membrane voltage oscillations.[78–80] These latter sites may be most relevant in certain forms of focal myokymia, especially facial myokymia, to be discussed later under Focal Myokymia.

The electromyographic picture of myokymia is quite distinctive. When the activity is not associated with obvious nerve disease, the motor nerve conduction velocities are usually normal to only slightly slowed, but moderate slowing or absence of conducted sensory nerve action potentials has been reported.[66] The myokymic activity observed during needle EMG is made up of spontaneous recurrent potentials, each of which resembles a normal MU (*fractional* units, meaning small MUs, have been reported;[66] their nature is unclear); these occur as single potentials, doublets, triplets, or multiplets.[56] The activity is quasirhythmic[71] and tends to wax and wane in amplitude.[72] During voluntary effort or with electrical activation, the myokymic discharges may initially increase followed by prominent afterdischarges when activation has been discontinued.[56,65] With cessation of voluntary activity, a brief silent period follows.[65,71] Fasciculations are often noted, but myotonic discharges are not observed either electrically or clinically.[55,64,66] The activity described here shows marked improvement with therapy using such agents as phenytoin and carbamazepine.

Focal myokymia

Facial myokymia and segmental myokymia are two major subgroups of focal myokymias. *Segmental myokymia* may be found incidentally during electromyographic examination for other problems. In one series, only about half of the patients had clinically observable myokymia.[71] Most of these patients developed their problems after a course of radiotherapy (RT) to the brachial plexus. Being quite specific of RT plexopathy, the presence of myokymia in the electromyographic examination is of great help in the differential diagnosis between neoplastic and RT-induced brachial plexopathy.[74–76] Widely variable intervals between RT and symptom onset were reported, with a range of 4 months to 21 years, the average being 6.5 years. Total radiation dose varied between 1600 and 6600 rad, with an average of 4500 rad.[71] Those patients with focal myokymia but never treated with RT usually had long-standing peripheral nerve problems such as chronic radiculopathies,[69,71] carpal tunnel syndromes,[71,81] and nerve injuries.[69,82] Another group of patients not having undergone RT had multiple sclerosis.[71] A few cases of short-lived myokymia associated with acute neuropathic disorders have been reported in patients with vasculitis, ischemic neuropathy, and acute Guillain-Barré syndrome.[71]

In contrast to generalized myokymia, the focal activity in post-RT patients was not significantly influenced by 10 minutes of ischemia.[71] The bursts tended to be longer (21.9 spikes per burst versus 10.6 spikes per burst) and recurred less frequently.[71] The frequency range of recurrence of potentials within each burst was wide (5 to 62 c/s), the average being 28 c/s.[71] Like all myokymia, the activity exhibited diverse discharge patterns and the termination of discharges was preceded by a decline in the intraburst spike frequency.[71] Attempts to alter the bursting patterns by direct nerve stimulation were effective only when stimuli were delivered during the burst proper[71] (Figure 5.6).

The second subclass of focal myokymia, *facial myokymia,* was initially reported and named by Op-

penheim in 1916 and Kino in 1928.[83,84] Facial myokymia is currently defined as "rhythmic or semi-rhythmic fine worm-like motion of one or more facial muscles, usually unilateral. They do not usually produce much clinically evident contraction, and are not influenced by voluntary activity, sleep, or reflex activity."[32,85,86] The onset is abrupt, producing a sensation of tension in the involved part of the face.[90] Several disease states are associated with this type of activity, the most common being multiple sclerosis.[85,86] Facial myokymia in this setting is usually a transient, early sign, often associated with other manifestations of brain stem dysfunction, some degree of facial nerve palsy being the most common. It is interesting to note that myokymia spares the frontalis muscle.[86] The second most common disease state associated with facial myokymia is pontine glioma.[86] The myokymia here may occur at any stage of disease, usually in conjunction with prominent facial muscle paralysis. Myokymia associated with

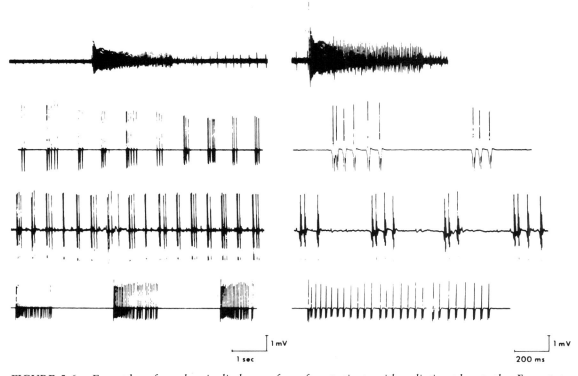

FIGURE 5.6. *Examples of myokymic discharges from four patients with radiation plexopathy. From top to bottom: biceps muscle, vastus lateralis muscle, biceps muscle, and pronator teres muscle. Note that each discharge is shown at a faster sweep speed on the right. (Reprinted with permission from Albers JW, Allen AA, Bastron AA, et al. Limb myokymia. Muscle Nerve 1981; 4:494–504. Copyright 1981 John Wiley & Sons, Inc.)*

pontine tumor is usually marked and progressive, involving any facial muscle, including the frontalis. Facial myokymia is less commonly seen with brain stem vascular disease, atypical trigeminal neuralgia, ALS, rarely Guillain-Barré syndrome,[86] syringobulbia,[87] and basilar invagination,[88] but it has been reported to be frequent in facial (Bell's) palsy.[89]

Generator sites associated with facial myokymia appear to be either central or peripheral.[91] A peripheral generator seems to apply most convincingly to the myokymia associated with Guillain-Barré syndrome[92] and facial palsy[89] (Figures 5.7 and 5.8). Facial nerve stimulation eliciting antidromic neural activity induces no compensatory pause in the myokymia firing rate; this as well as the coincidental involvement of taste suggests a peripheral generator.[92] In fact, focal demyelination of the facial nerve with normal brain stem has been documented in one fatal case of Guillain-Barré syndrome associated with facial myokymia.[93] An intraaxial generator site seems more likely in the more common disease state associations, such as multiple sclerosis, pontine glioma, and large cerebellopontine angle (CPA) tumor with attendant brain stem compression.[86] In these conditions, the myokymia may be obliterated with high peripheral nerve blocks. Central demyelination is a major feature of these lesions.[86,92] Significantly, facial

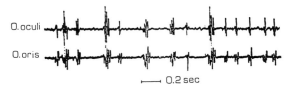

FIGURE 5.8. *Hemifacial spasm. Involuntary synchronous contractions of upper and lower facial muscles.*

myokymia is not observed in smaller CPA tumors unassociated with brain stem compression.[95]

Proposed central mechanisms behind the generation of facial myokymia include loss of interneuronal inhibition,[95,96] somewhat akin to the pathophysiology presumed for segmental myokymia,[79,80] or a combination of factors that may induce or exaggerate steady membrane depolarizing oscillations.[85]

Electromyographic examination reveals two possible patterns of myokymic activity that correspond to the clinically observed phenomena. Both patterns produce asynchronous MU activity of different frequencies that vary from place to place within the same muscle.[85,90] The individual component potentials are single, doublet, or triplet groups.[91,96] One pattern consists of continuous, high-frequency, 30-

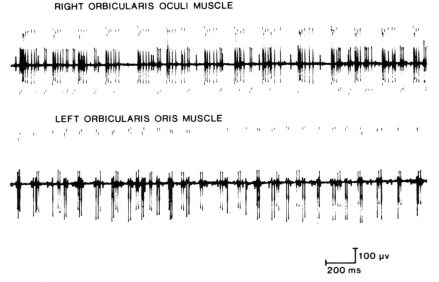

RIGHT ORBICULARIS OCULI MUSCLE

LEFT ORBICULARIS ORIS MUSCLE

100 µv
200 ms

FIGURE 5.7. *Recordings of myokymic discharges in facial muscles on needle electromyography. (Reprinted with permission from Daube JR, Kelly JJ, Martin RA. Facial myokymia with polyradiculoneuropathy. Neurology 1979; 29:662–669.)*

to 100-c/s bursting recurring at 2 to 10 c/s, usually found in myokymia associated with multiple sclerosis.[86,91,92] The second pattern, discontinuous discharges at low frequency,[91] is usually found in the tumor-related cases.[86,91] These bursts have a spike frequency of 27 to 300 c/s, a duration of 0.3 to 2.5 seconds and recur at a frequency of 0.2 to 1.9 c/s.[86] A postburst silent period is associated with the activity.[90] The underlying pathologies and patterns of myokymia show substantial group overlap.

Hemifacial spasm

Although apparently related on clinical grounds, hemifacial spasm is intrinsically different from facial myokymia. Hemifacial spasm may be confined to only a few facial muscles, and mild cases may outwardly resemble facial myokymia. In contrast to facial myokymia, many of these cases are idiopathic, and gross facial nerve palsy is uncommon.[97,100] The syndrome usually begins in the orbicularis oculi muscle with brief twitching, which gradually increases in frequency and extends to involve other facial muscles.[97] The duration of the episodes lengthens and gradually develops into tonic-clonic activity with varying degrees of synkinesis.[97] The entire syndrome displays two basic patterns of activity. The first has been designated the *blink burst* by Willison[96] and consists of a rapid twitch of several facial muscles after a blink. Small blinks induce minor spasms in eye muscles only, whereas large blinks induce activity in a much wider muscular distribution.[99] Electrical induction of the activity produces patterns identical to those seen with volitional activation of these muscles.[99] The second form of spontaneous activity is a long-lasting slow contraction that is not easily induced by voluntary blink or electrical stimulation.[99]

As opposed to the more common central pathologic substrates associated with facial myokymia, hemifacial spasm is proposed to arise from a peripheral nerve demyelinating lesion.[100–102] If true, such pathologic changes may favor the combination of ectopic impulse generation and ephaptic transmission.[38,97] Abnormal local circumstances promoting ephaptic transmission include local nerve compression, reduction of extraaxonal space, and an increase in interstitial resistance.[97] Equally important is the slowing of conduction through the demyelinated area.[97] Following impulse activity, autoexcitation in the demyelinated area may persist for several seconds,[26,39,97] further fostering ephaptic transmission. Thus the requirements of ephaptic conduction, increased interstitial resistance,[101] and conduction

slowing in contiguous fibers[97] would be satisfied in the pathologic setting of hemifacial spasm.

Ephapses transmit excitation from the slower conducting fiber to the faster one, but electromyographic studies have shown that the observed ephaptically transmitted responses are bidirectional, traversing the divisions of the facial nerve, implying differential involvement of many fibers.[97] The bidirectionality renders a pure nuclear mechanism unlikely because synaptic conduction is essentially unidirectional.[97] Moreover, a single-fiber electromyographic study of hemifacial spasm showed that electrical stimulation of peripheral branches of the facial nerve may elicit low jitter responses in muscles innervated by other branches of the nerve. These responses disappeared after facial nerve decompression, strongly suggesting reversible ephaptic transmission between the axons at the site of compression.[98]

EMG in hemifacial spasm as in facial myokymia again reveals two patterns corresponding to the two clinical manifestations. The *blink burst* or rapid twitch pattern is composed of sudden-onset, high-frequency bursts (200 to 400 c/s) made up of 2 to 40 potentials.[96,99] The slower contraction pattern consists of ongoing activity of 20 to 48 c/s,[99,102] once again not easily evoked by volition or electrical nerve stimulation.[99] The synkinetic activity may be demonstrated by electrical stimulation of one branch of the facial nerve, to evoke responses in muscles supplied by the other divisions of the facial nerve.[97,103] This probably occurs via an ephapse, and the latency measurements of synkinetically evoked muscle responses suggest conduction slowing, possibly reflecting demyelination.[97,103] Electrically induced blink reflex studies produce muscle responses of increased amplitude as compared with normal subjects, in both upper and lower facial muscles, suggesting lateral spread of the signal.[103,104] Late-occurring afterdischarges also suggest delayed conduction with possible reexcitation and reflection of no nerve action potentials owing to a persistently depolarized membrane segment. Two types of late afterdischarges have been characterized. The first, *after-activity*, represents extradischarges occurring immediately after an electrically evoked response. The second, *late activity*, is used to describe similar discharges occurring after a period of variable latency and persisting for 50 to 100 ms. Both late activity and after-activity are synchronous in different muscles, beginning as single discharges and becoming bursts of identical wave forms recurring at 250- to 300-c/s frequency.[97] Hemifacial spasm may be increased with hyperventilation and may evolve into tonic-clonic spasm lasting 30 to 50 seconds.[97] When fully developed, this activity produces large facial movements and bears no resemblance to facial myokymia.

Neuromyotonia

Much confusion exists in the literature about this term, coined by Mertens and Zschoche,[63] which has been variably associated with Isaacs' syndrome, the syndrome of continuous muscle fiber activity, neurotonia, and so on. The American Association of Electromyography and Electrodiagnosis (AAEE) *Glossary* defined *neuromyotonia* as "a clinical syndrome of continuous muscle fiber activity manifested as continuous muscle rippling and stiffness. The accompanying electric activity may be intermittent or continuous. Terms used to describe related clinical syndromes are continuous muscle fiber activity, Isaacs' syndrome, Isaacs-Mertens syndrome, quantal squander syndrome, generalized myokymia, pseudomyotonia, normocalcemic tetany and neurotonia."[7] Neuromyotonic discharge, the electrical correlate of the observed activity is defined as "bursts of motor unit potentials, which originate in the motor axons firing at high rates (150 to 300 [c/s]) for a few seconds and which often start and stop abruptly. The amplitude of the response typically wanes. Discharges may occur spontaneously or be initiated by needle movement, voluntary effort and ischemia or percussion of a nerve"[7] (Figure 5.9).

Neuromyotonia shares many features with myokymia (including apparently common pathogenetic mechanisms) while showing significant differences as well (e.g., the firing rate of afterdischarges is much higher in neuromyotonia). The clinical settings of neuromyotonia are quite varied but share some major features. Muscle stiffness and cramps are usual manifestations.[64,105]

The neuromyotonia syndromes may be divided between those that are and those that are not associated with neuropathy.[55] A second classification, perhaps more useful, is based on heredity. Sporadic cases, the most common, tend to be the most severe and are often associated with diffuse weakness and distal atrophy.[55,105,106] Although the familial cases resemble the sporadic ones clinically, their expression is usually milder.[55,105]

Of the clinical manifestations, focal muscle stiffness, which may be progressive and become generalized with time, is the most common.[105,111] Again, as in myokymia, the stiffness may be initially relieved with exercise.[55,106] When marked, the muscle spasms and stiffness with the associated slow relaxation and the persistent muscle hyperactivity may be so severe

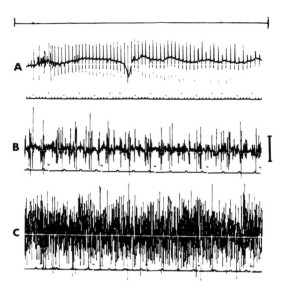

FIGURE 5.9. *(A) Electromyographic activity in the right tibialis anterior muscle illustrating some of the last rapidly firing motor units to switch off as involuntary activity ceases several seconds after a voluntary contraction of the muscle. The larger unit is firing at 100/s. Scale: 10 ms per division. (B) Rapid bursts of electromyographic activity recorded from an external intercostal muscle. Scale: 10 ms per division. (C) Large numbers of rapidly firing motor units in the abductor digiti minimi muscle during voluntary contraction. Scale: 10 ms per division. Vertical bar: 1 mV. (Reprinted with permission from the British Medical Journal from Walsh JC: Neuromyotonia: An unusual presentation of intrathoracic malignancy. J Neurol Neurosurg Psychiatry 1976; 39:1086–1091.)*

as to produce permanent joint deformity.[55,62] Most patients show diminished or absent tendon reflexes, often secondary to the muscle activity.[62,106,111] Electrical or clinical myotonia is not usually present.[62,73,106] In approximately 80% of patients, onset is between the ages of 15 and 25,[62] whereas about 75% of patients have clinically evident myokymia (usually generalized) and fasciculations.[62,105,106] Hyperhydrosis is noted in 50% of patients,[62,106] and 25% of cases are associated with distal limb atrophy.[55,62,105]

Muscle activity in neuromyotonia characteristically persists during sleep[62] and is not blocked with general or spinal anesthesia[106] or diazepam.[62] Phenytoin, carbamazepine, and tocainide have been found to be strikingly effective either alone or in combination.[55,62,105-108,111] The effect of these drugs varies from complete elimination of the activity to marked amelioration of the muscle stiffness and related phenomena. As the stiffness and activity diminish, the previously absent deep tendon reflexes may return,[109] suggesting ongoing activity rather than neuropathy as the relevant factor. Some patients may show continuing symptomatic relief and a diminishing requirement for the drugs.[65,108]

Muscle biopsy has shown a variety of changes suggestive of denervation and reinnervation with atrophy and grouping of both type 1 and type 2 fibers.[71,73,107] Nerve biopsies, although sometimes reported as abnormal, are to date not comprehensively characterized.[55,71,73,106]

Clinical EMG in neuromyotonia reveals an associated neuropathy in some patients, which is indicated by generally abnormal conduction studies or by prolonged distal latencies only with normal conduction velocities.[55,67,73] Needle examination demonstrates virtually constant MU activity characterized by rhythmic high-frequency (150 to 300 c/s) bursts of from 2 up to 200 potentials recurring irregularly at 0.5 to 4 c/s and occasionally up to 10 c/s.[11,62,105-107] The component units may be complex or simple, with normal jitter between component spikes.[11] The bursts may fatigue with activity,[55] possibly reflecting the clinically observed "warm-up" phenomenon.[55,106] Electrical or voluntary activation produces prominent afterdischarges,[73,105,106] which persist for up to 30 seconds after stimulation and are followed by a relatively quiet period of variable duration (3 to 15 s).[106] This persistent afteractivity is the logical electrical equivalent of the observed delayed relaxation after effort.[73] Abnormal activity induced by volition occurs as either single, doublet, or multiplet potentials and does not interfere with the bursting rate.[105] Further, the fibers that are involved with bursting can also be activated volitionally.[11] Similar to the clinical neuromyotonia, the bursting and repetitive activity are not influenced with either general or spinal anesthesia[105,106] and may be variably reduced with peripheral nerve blocks,[62,73,80] whereas all activity is stopped by curare and related drugs.[53,55] Temperature changes are strikingly influential, with bursts disappearing altogether with cooling[105] and doubling in frequency with warming.[73] Ischemia produces a variable effect, causing increase in activity in some patients[11,55] and a reduction in others.[67,105]

It has been repeatedly shown that both phenytoin and carbamazepine have a profound effect on blocking the electrophysiologic events in neuromyotonia.[55,62,105-107] Phenytoin is known to reduce PTR

without blocking normal impulse transmission in both nerve and MU preparations.[47,55,110,112] Phenytoin also normalizes the incidence of miniature end plate potentials induced by elevated potassium concentrations in bathing solutions.[113] Detailed studies of the mechanism of action of phenytoin reveal that it may reduce the sodium ion conductance (gNa) without affecting the resting membrane potential or changing the potassium conductance (gK) or leakage conductance (gL).[114,115] Phenytoin has some effect in blocking calcium channels,[116] but the calcium dynamics are apparently normal.[108] Carbamazepine is also highly effective,[55,105] and its main action seems to be the reduction of gNa and gK (gNa 20% more than gK)[114] as well as reducing the gL and the resting membrane potential.[114] By the combination of laboratory and clinical data, changes in gNa must be fundamental to generation of neuromyotonia.

Several observations in combination suggest a peripheral localization of the generator of neuromyotonia. These include normal jitter, spontaneous activity that is variably abolished with peripheral nerve block and persists during sleep, and lack of effect of diazepam but complete abolition of muscle activity with curare and related drugs.

These conditions are essentially fulfilled with Bergmans' PTR II, that is, long-duration tetanic stimulation inducing marked distal hyperpolarization in axons, possibly owing to induced overactivation of the electrogenic sodium pump[41] and possible interaction of induced anodal break current and spontaneous membrane oscillation. Bergman[41] emphasizes that although the sodium pump is dependent on oxidative metabolism and its operation ceases with ischemia, pump activity may be actually increased by other mechanisms in the early stages of anoxia. The observed abrupt cessation of bursts[41] may be due to activity-related changes in the intracellular and extracellular ionic concentrations. Further, the variable effect of peripheral nerve block[73] may suggest multiple generator sites. This hypothesis is consistent with the observed responses of neuromyotonia to manipulation.

Microneurography performed in a few patients showed a marked increase in activity in sensory fibers,[55] possibly reflecting a more generalized nerve membrane disorder.

Cramp

Cramp is associated with visible contraction of an entire muscle or part of it and is a frequent phenomenon in normal as well as in pathologic conditions. Nocturnal cramps occur in 16% of normal subjects.[117] Cramp thus differs from most of the previously discussed spontaneous motor phenomena because it may be a common normal occurrence, like fasciculations. There are several clinical classes of cramp. They are spontaneous night cramps; cramps occurring while awake without apparent stimulus; or cramps occurring as a result of voluntary effort, as in *associated cramp*.[118] Cramp may be fairly reliably reproduced by forcefully volitionally contracting a passively shortened muscle.[117] It may be terminated with forceful stretching of the contracted muscle or by activation of antagonist muscles, but it cannot be affected by attempted use of cramped muscles.[61,118]

There are numerous states of altered physiologic balance as well as frank pathology associated with cramp. Its occurrence is increased in pregnancy,[61,118] dehydration, and sweating (possibly owing to sodium loss,[61,118]) and in metabolic alterations, such as thyrotoxic myopathy, hypothyroidism, uremia, or hypomagnesemia.[62,118] The incidence of cramp associated with hemodialysis has been shown to be reducible by increasing the sodium content of the dialysate.[118] Cramp also occurs in partially denervated muscles, for example, in ALS and radiculopathy.

Work by Kugelberg[48] and by Layzer strongly suggests that cramp is of peripheral nerve origin (see also reference 118). The exact mechanism of cramp remains obscure, and perhaps it is a common expression of several mechanisms, as its clinical settings are so diverse. Local anesthetic peripheral nerve block is sometimes effective in stopping activity, but spinal anesthesia, general anesthesia, and diazepam do not affect cramp.[118] Following severe cramp, the marked pain, which may persist for days, is stopped by a peripheral nerve block.

Electromyographically, cramp consists of high-frequency (200 to 300 c/s) repetitive MU potentials, usually beginning with single potentials and then with doublets. The activity gradually spreads out to involve enlarging areas of a muscle in synchronous discharges. The muscle may further display several different discharge sites activated simultaneously or sequentially.[51,59,117] The activity waxes and wanes and may continue for several minutes. With cramp termination by muscle stretch, the discharges become interrupted and asynchronous and then stop altogether.[59] Thereafter the muscle may remain irritable with spontaneous fasciculations for several minutes.[59] In some individuals, cramp may be electrically induced by nerve stimulation at 10 to 40 c/s for 1 to 4 seconds.[118]

Tetany

Tetany is defined as "a clinical syndrome manifested by muscle twitching, cramps, and carpal and pedal spasm. These clinical signs are manifestations of peripheral nerve and central nervous system irritability from several causes. In these conditions, repetitive discharges (double discharge, triple discharge, multiple discharge) occur frequently with voluntary activation of MU potentials, or may appear as spontaneous activity, and are enhanced by systemic alkalosis or local ischemia."[7] Tetany is usually the result of low serum levels of ionized calcium or, exceptionally, magnesium. Causes of this syndrome include hyperventilation, hypothyroidism, rickets, and uremia.[61,118] In the French and German literature, patients with normocalcemic tetany are referred to as *spasmophilia*.[118,120] A rare form of normocalcemic tetany, inherited as an autosomal dominant trait, has been described.[121,122] Despite normal concentrations of total and ionized calcium, these patients respond to intravenous infusion of calcium.

Here we are concerned only with that part of the syndrome associated with changes in the peripheral nervous system. The symptoms usually begin with distal tingling paresthesias, which gradually spread proximally. Next, fasciculations begin distally and become repetitive and long-lasting, evolving into carpopedal spasms and eventual opisthotonus. The spasmodic activity frequently involves the laryngeal muscles, producing a stridulous voice, but eye muscles are never involved.[81] Between episodes of spasm, the nerves remain very irritable and respond to percussion with repetitive activity (Chvostek's sign). Hyperventilation is another effective way of inducing muscle spasms.

The generators for the activity mostly reside in the peripheral nerve, although some may be of myogenic origin.[11] This preponderance of a neural generator location is reflected in the fact that curare blocks most but not all of the spasm.[61] The spontaneous MU activity of tetany is not terminated with nerve block, suggesting that the generator site is distal.[61] With a reduction of extracellular calcium concentration, the excitability of the axonal membrane increases, whereas accommodation decreases, with similar changes being observed during as well as after hyperventilation and following ischemia. Some forms of tetany are thought to reflect calcium-independent mechanisms.[81]

On EMG, the component potentials are the size of MUs and often occur as doublets and triplets,[11,81,118] separated by an interval of 4 to 20 ms in bursts of 5 to 25 c/s[118] (Figure 5.10). To avoid false-positive results, the electromyographic test under ischemia should not be prolonged for more than 10 minutes. Even when normal subjects may show doublets or triplets, however, normocalcemic tetany may be assumed if multiplets occur lasting for more than 2 minutes.[120]

Other Unrelated Spontaneous Muscle Movements

Contracture

This is a cramp-like rigid contraction of muscles seen in phosphorylase deficiency (McArdle's disease), phosphofructokinase deficiency, and some unusual muscle diseases (e.g., Brody syndrome[123]). The last-mentioned condition results from an abnormality of calcium reuptake owing to a lack of calcium ATPase in sarcoplasmic reticulum of type II muscle fibers.[123] The resultant defect prevents contraction deactivation, producing a rigid state.[61,123] The electromyogram is silent.[61,118,123]

Stiff man syndrome

The stiff man syndrome, again associated with painful muscle cramp and stiffness, is apparently of central origin.[110,118] The syndrome usually begins in patients in their forties, with rigidity and significant muscle pain[68] precipitated by voluntary activity.[106] It

is usually most marked proximally,[106] especially in the neck and trunk muscles.[61] The jaw muscles are spared,[106] and the tendon reflexes are brisk.[68] The rest of the neurologic examination is normal.[66] Ectopic generation is thought to be due to abnormal function in spinal interneurons, causing depolarization of the anterior horn cells.[11] The potentials resemble MUs, but they occur during rest.[66] This spontaneous activity is blocked with sleep, diazepam, and spinal and general anesthesia,[61,66] a behavior that clearly separates it from activity that arises from peripheral nerves.

POSITIVE SENSORY PHENOMENA OF PERIPHERAL NERVE FIBER ORIGIN

Unfortunately for clinicians and investigators of sensation, normal and abnormal impulse activity in sensory pathways, in contrast to similar activity in alpha motor axons, produces no obvious externally visible signs to the observer. We are forced, as a consequence, to rely on the subjective sensory experiences reported by the subject and any accompanying change in expression or autonomic activity, as, for example, may be associated with activity in pain fibers.

Abnormal sensations communicated by patients with nerve fiber disease are common and share a

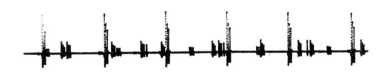

A   ┡━━━┥ 0.2 sec

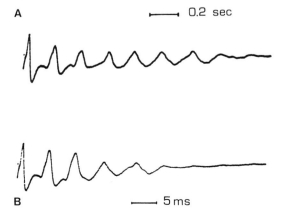

B   ┝━━ 5 ms

FIGURE 5.10. *(A) Electromyographic recording in a case of tetany after 10 minutes of ischemia showing triplets and multiplets. (B) One of the complexes (multiplets) of (A) shown in greater detail. Note that all the potentials are extradischarges of the first potential to the left. Because of the short interpotential interval (about 5 ms), there is progressive distortion of the subsequent potentials.*

number of characteristic features. Together with their occurrence in the absence of adequate stimulus or as an inadequate response to receptor stimulation, they have a "perverted" subjective quality: tingling, pins and needles, buzzing, pricking, burning, cold, itching, and so on, plus a spectrum of pains (see under Paresthesias, following). Sometimes they are called paresthesias only when nonpainful, which assumes, probably fallaciously, that the basic mechanisms for paresthesias and neuropathic pains should be necessarily different.

Methodologic advances have made it possible to investigate somatosensory mechanisms better by monitoring neural activity in single sensory units in awake human subjects. Indeed, much of what we know today about normal and abnormal electrophysiology of the human sensory unit has been contributed through application of microneurography.[124–126] More recently, intraneural microstimulation[127,128] of microneurographically identified sensory units has allowed us to question directly the human brain on how it reads the upcoming messages administered to classified peripheral nerve fibers, in terms of subjective quality, magnitude, and localization. For example, subjective quality is normally decoded specifically from particular kinds of afferent channels; thus there is now conclusive evidence in favor of *specificity,* as in the classic proposals. The magnitude of somatic sensation can be resolved in the total absence of spatial summation; that is, the contents of afferent messages in single units do carry information that the brain assesses quantitatively. The cortical localization function (locognosia) is also precise, to the millimeter level, again in the absence of spatial summation. Indeed, the brain "knows" the skin map of the hand at the single-unit level of resolution.[127–129]

Paresthesias

It is only on the basis of the knowledge just described that one can begin to understand what determines the abnormal subjective attributes of certain positive sensory phenomena commonly described by patients suffering from dysfunction of the sensory pathways. Indeed, paresthetic sensations may have aberrant qualities, absurd magnitudes, and chaotic projected localizations. The basis for these sensations could be investigated by comparing the activity in various single sensory fibers with the subjective sensory experiences reported by the subject. Athough there are limited opportunities to introduce electrodes into the nerves of neuropathic patients, it is easy to provoke reversibly paresthesias in normal nerves, for example, in the postischemic state.[130–135] Unitary afferent impulses generated ectopically from nerve fibers previously subjected to ischemia can be recorded in volunteers.[136,137] After some 20 minutes of ischemia provoked by a sphygmomanometer cuff inflated around the forearm above systolic pressure, the cuff is released and the cold hand becomes reddish and then feels hot; this is followed by a predictable sequence of paresthesias that features "buzzing," "pricking," "pseudocramp," and ultimately "tingling." There is no pain or itching. There is only a brief period of muscle twitching, probably reflecting the fact that motor nerve fibers retain better accommodation than sensory fibers.[138]

Encouragingly, isolated examples continue to be documented of ectopic impulse generation correlated to positive sensory phenomena symptomatic to disease of the primary sensory unit. Ochoa et al.[139] reported unitary discharges of abnormal bursting character recorded from fascicles innervating skin in humans experiencing spontaneous paresthesias projected to the appropriate nerve territory. Figure 5.11 illustrates paroxysmal unitary discharges recorded at upper arm level from a skin fascicle to the median nerve in one of those authors. This kind of discharge was observed on different occasions for weeks and months after mild mechanical injury to the nerve in the upper arm, leading to spontaneous and mild stimulus-induced pain. In contrast to electrode injury discharge, electrode movement did not influence the frequency of these discharges.

Although spontaneous afferent activity in slowly adapting type II (SA-II), as well as cold afferent and unmyelinated C sympathetic efferent unitary activity is a normal event in human sensory fascicles, the physiologic character of such activity is unmistakable by several criteria and distinct from the abnormal bursts that repeat relentlessly, independent of natural afferent or reflex stimulation. The fact that it has been consistently impossible to influence these paroxysmal discharges by natural stimulation of the cutaneous territory of the nerve indicates that the protagonist fibers are functionally or anatomically disconnected from the periphery. This circumstance unfortunately precludes classification of the fiber types.

In a thoroughly documented series of five patients, the ectopically generated impulses were recorded antidromically from skin nerve fascicles.[140] Ectopic multiunit nerve activity that correlated in amount and time with the positive sensory symptoms was recorded when paresthesias were provoked by elevation of the arm in a patient with symptoms

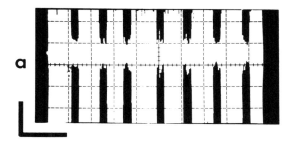

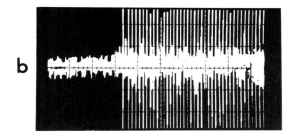

FIGURE 5.11. *Sample of ectopic discharges recorded from a median nerve fascicle supplying paresthetic skin in a human subject (JO, November 26, 1980). Single fiber is engaged in abnormal spontaneous activity—relatively long bursts of sudden onset and termination repeated at fairly regular intervals. The sequence was followed for almost 2 hours. Paroxysmal activity was obviously going on at the time of electrode insertion because the signals were audiomonitored from a distance well before becoming discernible from noise in the oscilloscope screen (on further penetration of the electrode toward the spike source). Signal amplitude, but not discharge frequency, changed appropriately when the electrode gently approached or withdrew. (A) Prolonged bursts displayed at low sweep speed (calibration = 10 μV and 10 s). (B) Faster sweep shows abrupt onset, regularity, and relatively high impulse frequency (40 per s) during a 1-second fraction of a burst shown in (A). (Reprinted with permission from Ochoa J, Torebjork HE, Culp WJ, Schady W. Abnormal spontaneous activity in single sensory nerve fibers in humans. Muscle Nerve 1982; 5:574–577. Copyright 1982 John Wiley & Sons, Inc.)*

consistent with a thoracic outlet syndrome (Figure 5.12). In the same article, antidromically conducted nerve impulses, for all intents and purposes generated in a dorsal nerve root (or ganglion), were recorded from the sural nerve in a patient with radiculopathy caused by lumbosacral disc disease. Again

there was excellent correlation between the amount and time course of abnormal neural activity and positive sensory symptoms, as illustrated in Figure 5.13. Dramatically, abnormal activity generated in the central branch of primary sensory units in the spinal cord was recorded antidromically from the peripheral branch, in a skin nerve fascicle, in a patient with multiple sclerosis and sign of Lhermitte.

Powerful as it obviously is, this technique cannot at this point in time be recommended as a routine clinical electrodiagnostic test. Demanding great care and skill in both application and interpretation, intraneural microstimulation and microneurography currently remain clinical research tools.

Sign of Tinel

"Le signe du fourmillement"[141] has legitimately but indirectly been attributed to abnormal mechanosensitivity and afferent discharge from regenerating nerve sprouts.[142,143] Evidence on development of mechanosensitivity at the level of the demyelinated fibers in the peripheral and central nervous systems[144,145] calls for the amplification of our concepts regarding the possible pathologies underlying the clinical sign of Tinel.

Figure 5.14 illustrates slow unitary ascending volleys recorded from a skin nerve fascicle terminating in an amputation neuroma of the superficial peroneal nerve. The volleys were triggered by tapping on the neuroma and appeared at much shorter latency than sympathetic reflexes. Concomitantly the patient reported a painful "electrical" sensation projecting within the peroneal nerve territory. Clearly abnormal nerve fibers terminating in the neuroma, not in sensory end-organs, had developed mechanoreceptive properties and generated ectopic impulses when stimulated mechanically.

The series mentioned earlier, by Nordin et al.,[140] includes recording of the electrical correlates of the sign of Tinel in a patient with ulnar nerve entrapment at the elbow. In that patient, the locally injured nerve fibers responsible for the abnormal mechanosensitive behavior were obviously not anatomically interrupted because the activity was recorded antidromically from a site distal to the elbow. Conduction velocity measurement demonstrated that most fibers were of large diameter and myelinated.

Pain as a Symptom of Nerve Fiber Disease

Although strictly speaking, pain as a manifestation of nerve fiber disease is a legitimate positive sensory phenomenon that implies abnormal activity in sen-

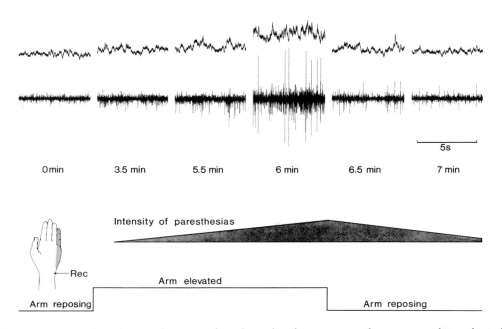

FIGURE 5.12.   *Recording from a skin nerve fascicle in the ulnar nerve at the wrist supplying the indicated receptive field. The lower trace shows the multiunit activity, and the upper trace is the mean voltage neurogram. The intensity of paresthesias provoked by holding the arm elevated for 6 minutes is schematically presented. The nerve activity is increased and decreased in parallel with the paresthesias. (Reprinted with permission from Elsevier Biomedical Press from Nordin M, Nystrom B, Wallin U, et al. Ectopic sensory discharges and paresthesiae in patients with disorders of peripheral nerves, dorsal roots and dorsal columns. Pain 1984; 20:231–245.)*

sory pathways, its pathophysiology remains evasive, and its electrophysiologic correlates may never become accessible to routine clinical EMG. Chronic pain as a sequela of nerve injury deserves special discussion in view of its prevalence and crippling consequences. Several theories presupposing different anatomic substrates have been advanced to explain this aberration. For example, Noordenbos[146] proposed that pain from nerve disease is a release phenomenon owing to damage to large-caliber afferents. This theory, inspired by Henry Head's ideas of sensation, was based on studies with Graham Weddell on the pathology of postherpetic neuralgia. Such is the *fiber dissociation theory,* which led to the *gate control theory* of pain mechanisms.[147]

Another theory incriminates artificial synapses or ephapses, resulting in cross-excitation of "pain" fibers at the site of injury by ascending or descending impulses. Since Granit's group[53] discussed the ephapse in the context of neuralgia, there has been much debate about its real role. Rasminsky[54,148] conclusively restored credit to the ephapse in a natural

animal model, but its relevance to neuritic pain remains unclear. Ephaptic phenomena in rats have also been confirmed in traumatic neuromas as a long-term feature, with possible implications in the pathophysiology of abnormal sensation.[149,150]

A more recent theory proposes spontaneous impulse generation from immature sprouts in small-diameter afferents, through very convincing reports based on electrophysiologic or behavioral studies in amputation neuromas in rodents.[151–154] Again, it is assumed, but there can be no certainty, that those animals experienced pain. Similar studies in humans are not available.

Possible Histopathologic Correlates for Positive Sensory Nerve Fiber Phenomena

The spectrum of pathologic deviations in the structure of human nerve fibers, as displayed by light-microscopy and electron-microscopy, are well described in standard publications, and it is likely that more than one kind of pathologic deviation can pro-

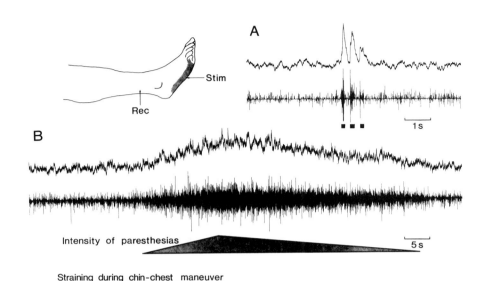

FIGURE 5.13. *Multiunit recording from the sural nerve with receptive field indicated. Afferent discharges evoked by tactile stimuli (marked by bars) in the receptive field are shown in (A), with neurogram in the lower trace and mean voltage neurogram in the upper trace. In (B) is shown the waxing and waning nerve activity correlating to the schematically presented intensity of paresthesias evoked by straining during chin-chest maneuver. (Reprinted with permission from Elsevier Biomedical Press from Nordin M, Nystrom B, Wallin U, et al. Ectopic sensory discharges and paresthesiae in patients with disorders of peripheral nerves, dorsal roots and dorsal columns. Pain 1984; 20:231–245.)*

duce ectopic generation of nerve impulses. Immature axon sprouts in experimental animals have established properties as mechanosensitive and chemosensitive structures and also as spontaneous generators of nerve impulses. The evidence for a similar behavior in humans is strong but indirect. In the example of sign of Tinel illustrated in Figure 5.14, it is assumed that the mechanosensitive generators are indeed axon sprouts because the nerve ended in a neuroma after unambiguous neurosurgical transection with excision of several centimeters of distal nerve stump. Thus in this particular patient, injured axons in continuity are out of the question as possible sources. Further, in a quantitative light-microscopic and electron-microscopic study of human neuromas (in continuity) from patients with chronic pain and sign of Tinel, the common denominator was the presence of a population of immature nerve fibers trapped at the site of neuroma and sign of Tinel.[155] The findings are well summarized by the case of Mr. C. He was hit by a bullet in 1944, suffering an injury to the superficial radial nerve in the forearm. Shortly thereafter he developed spontaneous pain referred to the hand, in association with

perverted sensation in the cutaneous territory of the injured nerve. While the region felt numb and had diminished ability to sense stimuli, at the same time there was an abnormally exaggerated sensitivity to noxious stimuli. Further, innocuous stimuli would induce painful sensation (hyperalgesia). In addition, the patient was aware of a mechanosensitive trigger point (sign of Tinel), which was stationed at the original site of injury, where gentle tapping elicited painful electrical sensations shooting down the limb. Mr. C lived with his symptoms until 1977, when he sought medical advice owing to a declining tolerance. As anticipated, diagnostic nerve blocks using local anesthetics injected proximal to the site of injury temporally suppressed pain and Tinel sign, while rendering the hypersensitive skin analgesic.

The offending nerve was excised from Mr. C early in 1977. It was possible to obtain counts and caliber spectra to include all the myelinated fibers in the nerve trunk at three levels, at the site of neuroma and proximal and distal to it. To the best of the authors' knowledge, this had not been done before with human nerves. The histogram from the neuroma level showed an exaggerated disproportion be-

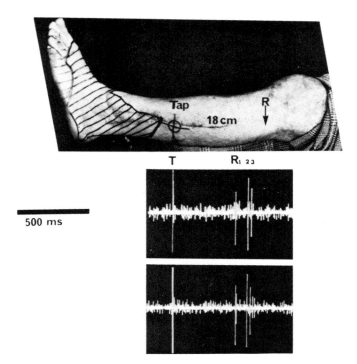

FIGURE 5.14. *Traumatic injury to the superficial peroneal nerve of a patient, leading to chronic pain and hyperalgesia referred to the foot. Surgical excision of a segment of injured nerve eventually led to the development of a painful sign of Tinel at the point of nerve section. Tapping the sensitive spot (T) elicited abnormal sensations referred to the dorsum of the foot. Microneurographic recording (R) from the superficial peroneal nerve near the head of the fibula picked up ascending volleys of impulses during elicitation of the sign of Tinel. Five unitary signals with consistent latencies were recorded in various combinations in successive recordings. Three of these ($R_{1,2,3}$) are shown in two sweeps following mechanical artifact T. Velocities in the region of 0.4 meters per second would indicate conduction in extremely thin, unmyelinated axons. Distal delay along sprouts of small myelinated fibers also is possible (Reprinted with permission from Ochoa J, Torebjörk HE, Culp WJ, et al. Abnormal spontaneous activity in single nerve fibers in humans. Muscle Nerve 1982; 5:574–577. Copyright © 1982 John Wiley & Sons, Inc.)*

tween large and small fibers consistent with either a dropout of large fibers or a proliferation of small fibers. That there was an actual increase in total numbers of small fibers at the site of neuroma and Tinel sign was obvious from comparing total fiber counts at all levels. From their spatial arrangement in clusters, it was clear that many small fibers were immature sprouts rather than surviving fibers originally of small diameter.

The typical picture at the neuroma site consists of focal disintegration of the perineurium with regrowth of nerve fibers outside main fascicles and the formation of minute new fascicles. Most immature fibers occur in these new fascicles, and it is amazing that in Mr. C, after more than three decades, these

sprouts did not mature. This probably reflects lack of reconnection with peripheral targets.[156–159] Presumably, fibers cannot regrow into the mainstream, perhaps because the *minifascicles* may be blind-ended. Unmyelinated fibers also show evidence of sprouting. Again, sprouting is mostly confined to the level of injury, emphasizing the failure of the abortive sprouts to advance into the distal portion of the nerve.

Locally demyelinated nerve fibers have also, more recently, established a reputation as ectopic impulse generators. The human electrophysiologic evidence from Nordin et al.[140] strongly indicates that the substrates for the antidromically conducted sensory nerve impulses and the paresthesias evoked, in parallel in their patients, must be myelinated nerve fibers with local lesions in continuity. As mentioned earlier, in experimental animals, morphophysiologic evidence was raised by Smith and McDonald,[144,145] clearly indicating that locally demyelinated fibers in posterior columns behave both as spontaneous and mechanosensitive generators. These findings obviously establish a common pathophysiologic basis for some forms of Tinel and Lhermitte's signs and for neuropathic and myelopathic paresthesias.

As an addendum to conventional demyelinating pathology, a particular aberration of the myelin sheath—the myelin balloon—has been implicated as a probable ectopic generator.[160]

REFERENCES

1. Denny-Brown D, Pennybacker JB. Fibrillation and fasciculation in involuntary muscle. Brain 1938; 61:311–334.
2. Denny-Brown D. Interpretation of the electromyogram. Arch Neurol Psych 1949; 61:99–128.
3. Richardson AT. Muscle fasciculation. Arch Phys Med Rehab 1954; 35:281–286.
4. Wettstein A. The origin of fasciculations in motorneuron disease. Ann Neurol 1979; 5:295–300.
5. Roth G. The origin of fasciculations. Ann Neurol 1982; 12:542–547.
6. Roth G. Fasciculations and their F-response. Localization of their axonal origin. J Neurol Sci 1984; 63:299–306.
7. Jablecki CK, Bolton CF, Bradley WG, et al. AAEE glossary of terms in clinical electromyography. Muscle Nerve 1987; 10 (No. 8S).
8. Trojaborg W, Buchthal F. Malignant and benign fasciculations. Acta Neurol Scand 1965; 41(suppl 13):251–254.
9. Montagna P, Liguori R, Zucconi M, et al. Fasciculations during wakefulness and sleep. Acta Neurol Scand 1987; 76:152–154.
10. Stålberg E, Trontelj JV. Single fibre electromyography. Old Woking, Surrey, U.K.: The Mirvalle Press Ltd, 1979.
11. Stålberg E, Trontelj JV. Abnormal discharges generated within the motor unit as observed with single-fiber electromyography. In: Culp WJ, Ochoa J, eds. Abnormal nerves and muscles as impulse generators. New York: Oxford University Press, 1982: 443–474.
12. Janko M, Trontelj JV, Gersak K. Fasciculations in motor neuron disease: Discharge rate reflects extent and recency of collateral sprouting. J Neurol Neurosurg Psychiatry 1989; 52:1375–1381.
13. Guiloff RJ, Modarres-Sadeghi. Voluntary activation and fibre density of fasciculations in motor neuron disease (abstr.). J Neurol Sci 1990; 98(suppl):75.
14. Conradi S, Grimby L, Lundemo G. Pathophysiology of fasciculations in ALS as studied by electromyography of single motor units. Muscle Nerve 1982; 5:202–208.
15. Partanen VSJ. Lack of correlation between spontaneous fasciculations and double discharges of voluntarily activated motor units. J Neurol Sci 1979; 42:261–266.
16. Reed DM, Kurland LT. Muscle fasciculations in a healthy population. Arch Neurol 1963; 9:363–367.
17. Kugelberg E. "Injury activity" and "trigger zones" in human nerves. Brain 1946; 69:310–324.
18. Werner G. Neuromuscular fasciculation and antidromic discharges in motor nerves: Their relation to activity in motor nerve terminals. J Neurophysiol 1960; 23:171–187.
19. Meadows JC. Fasciculation caused by suxamethonium and other cholinergic agents. Acta Neurol Scand 1971; 47:381–391.
20. Noebels JL, Prince DA. Presynaptic origin of penicillin afterdischarges at mammalian nerve terminals. Brain Res 1977; 138:59–74.
21. Forster FM, Borkowski WJ, Alpers BJ. Effects of denervation on fasciculations in human muscle. Arch Neurol Psychiatry 1946; 56:276–283.
22. King RB, Stoops WL. Cervical myelopathy with fasciculations in the lower extremities. J Neurosurg 1963; 20:948–952.
23. Kasdon DL. Cervical spondylitic myelopathy with reversible fasciculations in the lower extremities. Arch Neurol 1977; 34:774–776.
24. Norris FH. Synchronous fasciculation in motor neuron disease. Arch Neurol 1965; 13:495–500.
25. Borg J. Refractory period of single motor nerve fibers in man. J Neurol Neurosurg Psychiatry 1984; 47:344–348.
26. Calvin WH. To spike or not to spike? Controlling the neuron's rhythm, preventing the ectopic beat. In: Culp WJ, Ochoa J, eds. Abnormal nerves and muscles as impulse generators. New York: Oxford University Press, 1982:295–321.
27. Masland RL, Wigton RS. Nerve activity accompanying fasciculation produced by prostigmin. J Neurophysiol 1940; 3:269–275.
28. Stålberg E, Trontelj JZ. Demonstration of axon reflexes in human motor nerve fibers. J Neurol Neurosurg Psychiatry 1970; 33:571–579.
29. Roth G. Double discharges of distal origin. J Neurol Sci 1980; 47:35–48.
30. Bergmans J. Modifications induced by ischemia in the recovery of human motor axons from activity. In: Culp WJ, Ochoa J, eds. Abnormal nerves and muscles as impulse generators. New York: Oxford University Press, 1982; 419–442.

31. Harvey AM, Kuffler SW. Synchronization of spontaneous activity in denervated human muscle. Arch Neurol Psychiatry 1944; 52:495–497.

32. Kraft GH, Daube JR, DeLisa JA, et al, eds. A glossary of terms used in clinical electromyography. Rochester MN: Nomenclature Committee of the American Association of Electromyography and Electrodiagnosis, 1980.

33. Partanen VSJ. Double discharges in neuromuscular diseases. J Neurol Sci 1978; 36:377–382.

34. Stålberg E. Electrogenesis in human dystrophic muscle. In: Rowland LP, ed. Pathogenesis of human muscular dystrophies. Amsterdam: Excerpta Medica, 1977:570–587.

35. Diamond J, Ochoa J, Culp WJ. An introduction to abnormal nerves and muscles as impulse generators. In: Culp WJ, Ochoa J, eds. Abnormal nerves and muscles as impulse generators. New York: Oxford University Press, 1982:3–26.

36. Howe JF, Calvin WH, Loeser JD. Impulses reflected from dorsal root ganglia and from focal nerve injuries. Brain Res 1976; 116:139–144.

37. Ritchie JM. Sodium channel density in excitable membrane. In: Culp WJ, Ochoa J, eds. Abnormal nerves and muscles as impulse generators. New York: Oxford University Press, 1982:168–190.

38. Bostock H, Sears TA. The internodal axon membrane: Electrical excitability and continuous conduction in segmental demyelination. J Physiol 1978; 280:273–301.

39. Calvin WH, Howe JF, Loeser JD. Ectopic repetitive firing in focally demyelinated axons and some implications for trigeminal neuralgia. In: Anderson DJ, Matthews B, eds. Pain in trigeminal region. Amsterdam: Elsevier/North Holland Biomedical Press, 1977:125–136.

40. Bergmans J. Physiological observations on single human nerve fibers. In: Desmedt JE, ed. New developments in electromyography and clinical neurophysiology. Vol. 2. Basel: Karger, 1973:89–127.

41. Bergmans J. Repetitive activity induced in single human motor axons: A model for pathological repetitive activity. In: Culp WJ, Ochoa J, eds. Abnormal nerves and muscles as impulse generators. New York: Oxford University Press, 1982:393–418.

42. Burchiel KJ. Ectopic impulse generation in demyelinated axons: Effects of $PaCO_2$, pH and disodium edetate. Ann Neurol 1981; 9:378–383.

43. Orchardson R. The generation of nerve impulses in mammalian axons by changing the concentrations of the normal constituents of extracellular fluid. J Physiol 1978; 275:177–189.

44. Kugelberg E. Activation of human nerves by hyperventilation and hypocalcemia. Arch Neurol Psychiatry 1948; 60:153–164.

45. Brick JF, Gutmann L, McComas CF. Calcium effect on generation and amplification of myokymic discharges. Neurology 1982; 32:618–622.

46. Burchiel KJ. Abnormal impulse generation in focally demyelinated trigeminal roots. J Neurosurg 1980; 53:674–683.

47. Morrell F, Bradley W, Ptashne M. Effect of diphenylhydantoin on peripheral nerve. Neurology 1958; 8:140–144.

48. Kugelberg E. Neurologic mechanisms for certain phenomena in tetany. Arch Neurol Psychiatry 1946; 56:507–521.

49. Adrian ED. The effects of injury on mammalian nerve fibers. Proc R Soc B 1930; 106:596–618.

50. Wall PD, Waxman S, Basbaum AI. Ongoing activity in peripheral nerve: Injury discharge. Exp Neurol 1974; 45:576–589.

51. Denny-Brown D. Clinical problems in neuromuscular physiology. Am J Med 1953; 15:368–390.

52. Raymond SA, Lettvin JY. After effects of activity in peripheral axons as a clue to nervous coding. In: Waxman SG, ed. Physiology and pathobiology of axons. New York: Raven Press, 1978:203–225.

53. Granit R, Leksell L, Skoglund CR. Fiber interaction in injured or compressed region of nerve. Brain 1944; 67:125–140.

54. Rasminsky M. Ectopic generation of impulses and cross-talk in spinal nerve roots of "dystrophic" mice. Ann Neurol 1978; 3:351–357.

55. Lance JW, Burke D, Pollard J. Hyperexcitability of motor and sensory neurons in neuromyotonia. Ann Neurol 1979; 5:523–532.

56. Gardner-Medwin D, Walton JN. Myokymia with impaired muscular relaxation. Lancet 1969;1:127–130.

57. Kny E. Ueber ein den paramyoclonus multiplex (Friedreich) nahestehendes Krankheitshild. Arch Psychiatry Nervenkr 1888; 19:577–590.

58. Schultze F. Beitrag zur Muskelpathologie. Deutsch Z Nervenheilk 1895; 6:65–70.

59. Denny-Brown D, Foley JM. Myokymia and the benign fasciculation of muscular cramps. Trans Assoc Am Phys 1948; 61:88–96.

60. Daube JR. Needle examination in clinical electromyography. In: Course A. Fundamentals of EMG. Sixth Annual Continuing Education Course of American Association of Electromyography and Electrodiagnosis. Rochester, MN, 1983:3–14.

61. Rowland LP. Cramps, spasms and muscle stiffness. Rev Neurol (Paris) 1985; 141:261–273.

62. Lütschg J, Jerusalem F, Ludin HP et al. The syndrome of "continuous muscle fiber activity." Arch Neurol 1978; 35:198–205.

63. Mertens HG, Zschocke S. Neuromyotonie. Klin Wochenschr 1965; 43:917–925.

64. Welch LK, Appenzeller O, Bicknell JM. Peripheral neuropathy with myokymia, sustained muscular contraction, and continuous motor unit activity. Neurology 1972; 22:161–169.

65. Irani PF, Purohit AV, Wadia NH. The syndrome of continuous muscle fiber activity. Evidence to suggest

proximal neurogenic causation. Acta Neurol Scand 1977; 55:273–288.

66. Wallis WE, Van Poznak, Plum F. Generalized muscular stiffness, fasciculations, and myokymia of peripheral nerve origin. Arch Neurol 1970; 22:430–439.

67. Lublin FD, Tsairis P, Streletz LJ, et al. Myokymia and impaired muscular relaxation with continuous motor unit activity. J Neurol Neurosurg Psychiatry 1979; 42:557–562.

68. Hughes RC, Matthews WB. Pseudo-myotonia and myokymia. J Neurol Neurosurg Psychiatry 1969; 32:11–14.

69. Harman JB, Richardson AT. Generalized myokymia in thyrotoxicosis. Lancet 1954; 2:473–474.

70. Caldron PH, Wilbourn AJ. Gold neurotoxicity and myokymia (letter). J Rheumatol 1988; 15:528.

71. Albers JW, Allen AA, Bastron JA, et al. Limb myokymia. Muscle Nerve 1981; 4:494–504.

72. Brunt ERP, Van Werden TW. Familial paroxysmal kinesigenic taxia and continuous myokymia. Brain 1990; 113:1361–1382.

73. Warmolts JR, Mendell JR. Neurotonia: Impulse-induced repetitive discharges in motor nerves in peripheral neuropathy. Ann Neurol 1980; 7:245–250.

74. Lederman RJ, Wilbourn AJ. Brachial plexopathy: Recurrent cancer or radiation? Neurology 1984; 34:1331–1335.

75. Harper CM, Thomas JE, Cascino TL, Litchy WJ. Distinction between neoplastic and radiation-induced brachial plexopathy, with emphasis on the role of EMG. Neurology 1989; 39:502–506.

76. Roth G, Magistris MR, Le Fort D, et al. Plexopathie brachiale post-radique. Blocs de conduction persistants, Décharges myokymiques et crampes. Rev Neurol (Paris) 1988; 144:173–180.

77. Esteban A, Traba A. Plexopatía braquial postradiación. Estudio clínico y neurofisiológico. Arch de Neurobiol 1990; 53:23–32.

78. Carnevale NT, Wachtel H. "Subthreshold" oscillations underlying burst firing patterns. In: Culp WJ, Ochoa J, eds. Abnormal nerves and muscles as impulse generators. New York: Oxford University Press, 1982:273–294.

79. O'Connor PJ, Wynn Parry CB, Davis R. Continuous muscle spasm in intramedullary tumors of the neuraxis. J Neurol Neurosurg Psychiatry 1966; 29:310–314.

80. Walsh JC. Neuromyotonia: An unusual presentation of intrathoracic malignancy. J Neurol Neurosurg Psychiatry 1976; 39:1086–1091.

81. Adams RD, Victor M. Principles of neurology. New York: McGraw-Hill, 1981:999–1000.

82. Medina JL, Chokroverty S, Reyes M. Localized myokymia caused by peripheral nerve injury. Arch Neurol 1976; 33:587–588.

83. Oppenheim H. Zeitungen und Fortschritte aus dem Gebiet der Neurologie und Psychiatrie 1916; 20:14–18.

84. Kino F. Muskelwogen (myokymie) als Fruhsymptom der multiplen Sklerose. Deutsche Z Nervenheilk 1928; 104:31–41.

85. Andermann F, Cosgrove JBR, Lloyd-Smith DL, et al. Facial myokymia in multiple sclerosis. Brain 1961; 84:31–44.

86. Radu EW, Skorpil V, Kaeser HE. Facial myokymia. Eur Neurol 1975; 13:499–512.

87. Riaz G, Campbell WW, Carr J, Ghatak N. Facial myokymia in syringobulbia. Arch Neurol 1990; 47:472–474.

88. Chalk CH, Litchy WJ, Ebersold MJ, Kispert DB. Facial myokymia and unilateral basilar invagination. Neurology 1988; 38:1811–1812.

89. Bettoni L, Bortone E, Ghizzoni P, Lechi A. Myokymia in the course of Bell's palsy. An electromyographic study. J Neurol Sci 1988; 84:69–76.

90. Matthews WB. Facial myokymia. J Neurol Neurosurg Psychiatry 1966; 29:35–39.

91. Wasserstrom WR, Starr A. Facial myokymia in the Guillain-Barré syndrome. Arch Neurol 1977; 34:567–577.

92. Daube JR, Kelly JJ, Martin RA. Facial myokymia with polyradiculoneuropathy. Neurology 1979; 29:662–669.

93. Van Zandycke M, Martin JJ, Vande Gaer L, Van den Heyning P. Facial myokymia in the Guillain-Barré syndrome: A clinicopathologic study. Neurology 1982; 32:744–748.

94. Oda K, Fukushima N, Shibasaki H, Ohnishi A. Hypoxia-sensitive hyperexcitability of the intramuscular nerve axons in Isaacs' syndrome. Ann Neurol 1989; 25:140–145.

95. Tenser RB, Corbett JJ. Myokymia and facial contraction in brain stem glioma. An electromyographic study. Arch Neurol 1974; 30:425–427.

96. Willison RG. Spontaneous discharges in motor nerve fibers. In: Culp WJ, Ochoa J, eds. Abnormal nerves and muscles as impulse generators. New York: Oxford University Press, 1982; 383–392.

97. Nielsen VK. Pathophysiology of hemifacial spasm. I. Ephaptic transmission and ectopic excitation. Neurology 1984; 34:418–426.

98. Sandors DB. Ephaptic transmission in hemifacial spasm: A single-fiber EMG study. Muscle Nerve 1989; 12:690–694.

99. Hjörth RJ, Willison RG. The electromyogram in facial myokymia and hemifacial spasm. J Neurol Sci 1973; 20:117–126.

100. Digre K, Corbett JJ. Hemifacial spasm: Differential diagnosis, mechanism, and treatment. Neurol 1988; 49:151–175.

101. Nielsen VK, Jannetta PJ. Pathophysiology of hemifacial spasm III. Effects of facial nerve decompression. Neurology 1984; 34:891–897.

102. Alvarez-Sabin J, Fernándoz JM, Matias-Güiu J,

Codina A. Espasmo hemifacial en el síndrome de Guillain-Barré. Rev Neurol (Barcelona) 1986; 14:81–85.

103. Nielsen VK. Pathophysiology of hemifacial spasm II. Lateral spread of the supraorbital nerve reflex. Neurology 1984; 34:427–431.

104. Estéban A, Molina-Negro P. Primary hemifacial spasm: A neurophysiological study. J Neurol Neurosurg Psychiatry 1986; 49:58–63.

105. Auger RG, Daube JR, Gomez MR, et al. Hereditary form of sustained muscle activity of peripheral nerve origin causing generalized myokymia and muscle stiffness. Ann Neurol 1984; 15:13–21.

106. Isaacs H. A syndrome of continuous muscle-fiber activity. J Neurol Neurosurg Psychiatry 1961; 24:319–325.

107. Jackson DL, Satya-Murti S, Davis L, et al. Isaacs syndrome with laryngeal involvement: An unusual presentation of myokymia. Neurology 1979; 29:1612–1615.

108. Isaacs H, Heffron JJA. The syndrome of "continuous muscle fiber activity" cured: Further studies. J Neurol Neurosurg Psychiatry 1974; 37:1231–1235.

109. Zisfein J, Sivak M, Aron A, et al. Isaacs syndrome with muscle hypertrophy reversed with phenytoin therapy. Arch Neurol 1983; 40:241–242.

110. Isaacs H. Continuous muscle fiber activity in an Indian male with additional evidence of terminal motor fiber abnormality. J Neurol Neurosurg Psychiatry 1967; 30:126–133.

111. Hahn AF, Parkes AV, Bolton CF, Stewart SA. Neuromyotonia in hereditary motor neuropathy. J Neurol Neurosurg Psychiatry 1991; 54:230–235.

112. Raines A, Standaert FG. Pre and postjunctional effects of diphenylhydantoin at the cat soleus neuromuscular junction. J Pharmacol Exp Ther 1966; 153:361–366.

113. Su PC, Feldman DS. Motor nerve terminal and muscle membrane stabilization by diphenylhydantoin administration. Arch Neurol 1973; 28:376–379.

114. Schauf CL, Davis FA, Marder J. Effects of carbamazepine in the ionic conductance of myxicola giant axons. J Pharmacol Exp Ther 1974; 189:538–543.

115. Lipicky RJ, Gilbert DL, Stillman IM. Diphenylhydantoin inhibition of sodium conductance in squid giant axon. Proc Nat Acad Sci USA 1972; 69:1758–1760.

116. Greenberg DA, Cooper EC, Carpenter CL. Phenytoin interacts with calcium channels in brain membranes. Ann Neurol 1984; 16:116–117.

117. Norris FH, Gasteiger EL, Chatfield PO. An electromyographic study of induced and spontaneous muscle cramps. Electroencephalogr Clin Neurophysiol 1957; 9:139–147.

118. Layzer RB. Motor unit hyperactivity states. In: Vinken PJ, Bruyn GW, eds. Handbook of clinical neurology. Vol 41, Part 2. Amsterdam: North Holland, 1979:295–316.

119. Bonciocat C, Stoicescu N, Vacariu A, et al. Electrical activity induced by ischemia in the skeletal muscle of patients of spasmophilia. Physiologie 1988; 25:35–41.

120. Deecke L, Müller B, Conrad B. Zur Standardisierung des elektromyographischen Tetanietests in der Diagnostik der normokalzämischen Tetanie: 10 minütiger Trousseau bei Patienten und Gesunden. Arch Psychiatr Nervenkr 1983; 233:23–37.

121. Isgreen WP. Normocalcemic tetany—a problem in erethism. Neurology 1976; 26:825–834.

122. Day JW, Parry GJ. Normocalcemic tetany abolished by calcium infusion. Ann Neurol 1990; 27:438–440.

123. Karpati G, Charuk J, Carpenter S, et al. Myopathy caused by a deficiency of Ca^{++} adenosimetriphosphatase in sarcoplasmic reticulum (Brody's disease). Ann Neurol 1986; 20:38–49.

124. Vallbo AB, Hagbarth KE. Activity from skin in mechanoreceptors recorded percutaneously in awake human subjects. Exp Neurol 1968; 21:270–289.

125. Vallbo AB, Hagbarth KE, Torebjörk HE, et al. Somatosensory, proprioceptive and sympathetic activity in human peripheral nerves. Physiol Rev 1979; 59:919–957.

126. Hagbarth KE. Exteroceptive, proprioceptive and sympathetic activity recorded with microelectrodes from human peripheral nerves. Mayo Clin Proc 1979; 54:353–365.

127. Torebjörk HE, Ochoa JL. Specific sensations evoked by activity in single identified sensory units in man. Acta Physiol Scand 1980; 18:145–156.

128. Ochoa JL, Torebjörk HE. Sensation evoked by intraneural microstimulation of single mechanoreceptor units innervating the human hand. J Physiol 1983; 342:633–654.

129. Schady WJL, Torebjörk HE, Ochoa JL. Cerebral localization function from the input of single mechanoreceptive units in man. Acta Physiol Scand 1983; 119:277–285.

130. Lewis T, Pickering GW, Rothschild P. Centripetal paralysis arising out of arrested blood flow to the limb. Including notes on a form of tingling. Heart 1948; 16:1–32.

131. Zotterman Y. Studies in peripheral nervous mechanism of pain. Acta Med Scand 1933; 80:185–242.

132. Kugelberg E. Accommodation in human nerves and its significance for the symptoms in circulatory disturbances and tetany. Acta Physiol Scand 1944; 8 (suppl 24).

133. Weddell G, Sinclair DC. "Pins and needles"; observations on some of the sensations aroused in limbs by application of pressure. J. Neurol Neurosurg Psychiatry 1947; 10:26–46.

134. Gordon G. "Pins and needles." Nature 1948; 162:742–743.

135. Merrington WR, Nathan PW. Study of post-ischemic paresthesiae. J Neurol Neurosurg Psychiatry 1949; 12:1–18.

136. Torebjörk HE, Ochoa JL, McCann FV. Paresthesiae: Abnormal impulse generation in sensory nerve fibers in man. Acta Physiol Scand 1979; 105:518–520.

137. Ochoa J, Torebjörk HE. Paresthesiae from ectopic impulse generation in human sensory nerves. Brain 1980; 103:835–853.

138. Culp WJ, Ochoa J, Torebjörk HE. Ectopic impulse generation in myelinated sensory nerve fibers in man. In: Culp WJ, Ochoa J, eds. Abnormal nerves and muscles as impulse generators. New York: Oxford University Press, 1982; 513–532.

139. Ochoa J, Torebjörk HE, Culp WJ, et al. Abnormal spontaneous activity in single nerve fibers in humans. Muscle Nerve 1982; 5:S74–S77.

140. Nordin M, Nyström B, Wallin V, et al. Ectopic sensory discharges and paresthesiae in patients with disorders of peripheral nerves, dorsal roots and dorsal columns. Pain 1984; 20:231–245.

141. Tinel J. Le signe du "fourmillement" dans les lesions des nerfs périphériques. Presse Med 1915; 23:388–389.

142. Konorski J, Lubinska L. Mechanical excitability of regenerating nerve fibers. Lancet 1946; 250:609.

143. Brown AG, Iggo A. The structure and function of cutaneous "touch corpuscles" after nerve crush. J Physiol 1963; 165:28.

144. Smith KJ, McDonald WI. Spontaneous and mechanically evoked activity due to a central demyelinating lesion. Nature 1980; 286:154.

145. Smith KJ, McDonald WI. Spontaneous and evoked electrical discharges from a central demyelinating lesion. J Neurol Sci 1982; 55:39.

146. Noordenbos W. Pain. Amsterdam: Elsevier North Holland Biomedical Press, 1959.

147. Wall PD. The gate control theory of pain mechanisms: A re-examination and a restatement. Brain 1978; 101:1–18.

148. Rasminsky M. Ectopic excitation, ephaptic excitation and autoexcitation in peripheral nerve fibers of mutant mice. In: Culp WJ, Ochoa J, eds. Abnormal nerves and muscles as impulse generators. New York: Oxford University Press, 1982:344–362.

149. Seltzer Z, Devor M. Ephaptic transmission in chronically damaged nerves. Neurology 1979; 29:1061–1064.

150. Devor M, Bernstein J. Abnormal impulse generation in neuromas: Electrophysiology and ultrastructure. In: Culp WJ, Ochoa J, eds. Abnormal nerves and muscles as impulse generators. New York: Oxford University Press, 1982; 363–380.

151. Wall PD, Gutnick M. Properties of afferent nerve impulses originating from a neuroma. Nature 1974; 248:740–743.

152. Govrin-Lippman R, Devor M. Ongoing activity in several nerves: Source and variation with time. Brain Res 1978; 159:406–410.

153. Wall PD, Devor M. Consequences of peripheral nerve damage in the spinal cord and in neighboring intact peripheral nerves. In: Culp WJ, Ochoa J, eds. Abnormal nerves and muscles as impulse generators. New York: Oxford University Press, 1982:588–603.

154. Scadding JW. Ectopic impulse generation in experimental neuromas: Behavior, physiological and anatomical correlates. In: Culp WJ, Ochoa J, eds. Abnormal nerves and muscles as impulse generators. New York: Oxford University Press, 1982:533–552.

155. Ochoa J, Noordenbos W. Pathology and disordered sensation in local nerve lesions: An attempt at correlation. In: Bonica JJ, Liebeskind JC, Albe-Fessard DG, eds. Advances in brain research and therapy. New York: Raven Press, 1979:67–90.

156. Sanders FK, Young JZ. Effects of peripheral connections in diameter of nerve fibers. Nature 1945; 155:237–238.

157. Weiss P, Edds MV Jr, Cavanaugh M. Effects of terminal connections on caliber of nerve fibers. Anat Rec 1945; 92:215–233.

158. Aitken JT, Sherman M, Young JZ. Maturation of regenerating nerve fibers with various peripheral connections. J Anat 1947; 81:1–22.

159. Evans DHL, Murray JG. A study of regeneration in a motor nerve with unimodal fibre diameter distribution. Anat Rec 1956; 126:311–333.

160. Ochoa J. Some aberrations of nerve repair. In: Gorio A, Millesi H, Mingrino S, eds. Posttraumatic peripheral nerve regeneration; experimental basis and clinical implications. New York: Raven Press, 1981; 147–155.

6

The Autonomic Nervous System

Douglas W. Zochodne
Mikihiro Kihara

CONTENTS

LIST OF ACRONYMS

HMSN	hereditary motor and sensory neuropathy
HSAN	hereditary sensory and autonomic neuropathy
QSART	quantitative sudomotor axon reflex test
SIT	silastic imprint test
SSR	sympathetic skin response
TST	thermoregulatory sweat test
Ach	acetylcholine
GBP	Guillain-Barré polyneuropathy (syndrome)
ANS	autonomic nervous system
BP	blood pressure

The autonomic nervous system (ANS) is the least explored segment of the nervous system in most clinical neurophysiologic laboratories. This does not mean, however, that it is the least relevant because we now recognize that abnormalities of the ANS are common and important. In diabetes, for example, autonomic dysfunction occurs early and may precede other symptoms and signs of diabetic polyneuropathy. Selective study of sudomotor fibers permits the electromyographer to access indices of unmyelinated fiber function not generally available. These types of studies are important because in some neuropathies, such as that associated with amyloidosis, unmyelinated fiber involvement may be predominant. In Guillain-Barré polyneuropathy (GBP), autonomic abnormalities may be life-threatening.

The list of autonomic tests described in this chapter is inclusive, and it is unlikely that most laboratories would use all of them in their repertoire. It is necessary, however, to have a background for interpreting the clinical ANS literature and to be able to choose what tests from each category one's laboratory might wish to emphasize. In laboratories with limited resources, competence in performing the *Ewing battery* (described later) combined with sudomotor testing may be a reasonable way to assess autonomic function in many patients.

ANATOMIC OVERVIEW

The ANS is divided into a craniosacral parasympathetic and paravertebral sympathetic outflow. Cranial parasympathetic outflow includes pupilloconstrictor fibers traveling with the third cranial nerve, fibers traveling with the seventh and ninth cranial nerves to the salivary glands, fibers traveling with the seventh cranial nerve to the lacrimal glands, and the outflow from the vagus. Vagal output includes cardioinhibitory fibers, bronchoconstrictor fibers, and fibers subserving upper and middle gastrointestinal tract motility. Sacral fibers (S-2, S-3, S-4) innervate the lower gastrointestinal tract, the detrusor muscle of the bladder, and smooth muscles of erectile tissue vasculature. The parasympathetic neurotransmitter is acetylcholine.

The sympathetic primary order neurons arise in the hypothalamus and descend in the lateral white matter of the brain stem and spinal cord. At cord levels T-1–L-2, these fibers innervate second order neurons in the gray matter of the intermediolateral horn of the spinal cord. Second order fibers exit the spinal cord through the ventral roots then may take one of three pathways. Some fibers branch off to paravertebral ganglia (through white rami communicans) then synapse. Third order fibers leave the ganglia and rejoin the mixed spinal nerves through the gray rami communicans. Other third order fibers travel directly from the ganglia to end organs. Some second order fibers travel to ganglia at other segmental levels before synapsing by traveling through the sympathetic chain connecting paravertebral ganglia. Still others travel cephalad into the lower (stellate) middle or superior sympathetic ganglia or caudad into the superior, middle, and inferior splanchnic nerves to synapse in celiac, superior mesenteric, and inferior mesenteric ganglia. Third order fibers are distributed widely to innervate resistance arterioles, sweat glands, and other organs. Piloerection, or *goose flesh,* is also mediated by sympathetic fibers. The neurotransmitter of third order neurons is norepinephrine except for sudomotor fibers that contain acetylcholine.

The oculosympathetic second order neuron supply exits the cord at T-1 traveling upward through the lower and middle cervical sympathetic ganglia and cervical sympathetic chain to synapse in the superior cervical sympathetic ganglion. From here, third order fibers innervate the eye. Unfortunately, we now know that this classic anatomic profile is further confused by mingling of second and third order fibers in the rami, chain, and splanchic nerves.

A diversity of action is mediated by subclasses of cholinergic and adrenergic receptors and frequent colocalization of peptides in final order autonomic fibers. Purinergic transmission is also probably important but is not discussed further in this chapter. Figure 6.1 is a simplified illustration of the relevant anatomy of autonomic nervous testing.

AUTONOMIC TESTING

Bedside Evaluation

A thorough neurologic and ANS bedside examination should precede specialized testing. Relevant questions are included in Table 6.1. There should be a cardiovascular and neurologic bedside examination with supine and upright measurements of blood pressure and pulse. The examination should include pupillary testing to light and accommodation, attention to pupillary size and shape, and notation of obvious sweating abnormalities (i.e., is there localized absence of sweating [anhidrosis] or excessive sweating [hyperhidrosis]). Patients with lower limb

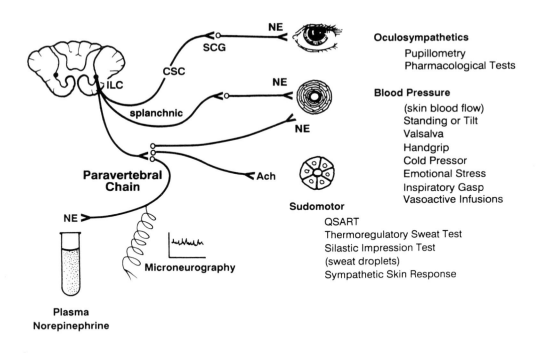

A

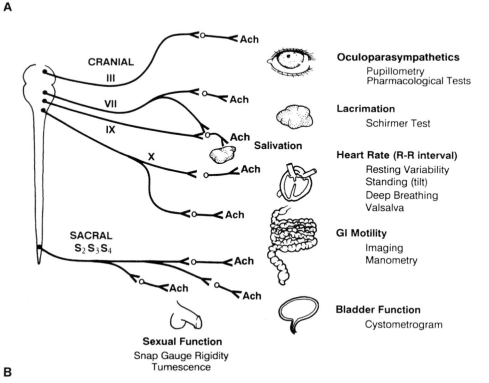

B

FIGURE 6.1.   *Simplified illustration and summary of the relevant anatomy of selected autonomic sympathetic (A) and parasympathetic (B) tests.*

TABLE 6.1. Bedside evaluation of the autonomic nervous system

Question	Possible Significance
Dizzy spells or fainting (? heart disorder)	Possible cardiac arrhythmia, postural hypotension
Palpitations	As above
Postural or postprandial dizziness, lightheadedness, or fatigue	Postural hypotension from adrenergic failure
Inability to sweat	Sudomotor dysfunction
Heat intolerance	As above
Nocturnal diarrhea, constipation, bowel incontinence	Abnormal lower gastrointestinal motility
Bladder retention or incontinence	Bladder denervation
Bloating, heartburn, nausea, excessive belching	Gastric atony
Impotence	Erectile dysfunction from autonomic denervation
Visual blurring or photophobia	Accommodation/pupillary dysfunction

anhidrosis have dry socks. The extremities should be examined for trophic changes including ulceration. Rectal examination may be helpful to assess striated muscle function sharing the sacral root supply (S-2, 3, 4) with parasympathetic fibers. Also, an anorectal motility disorder may include fecal soiling, suggesting incontinence, or impaction if there is severe constipation.

Cardiovascular Function

Testing batteries

Several methods have been used to test autonomic cardiovascular function.[1] There is a confusing array of available methods to choose from, but some investigators[2,3] have recommended a basic battery, the *Ewing battery* listed in Table 6.2. The R-R interval used is the reciprocal of heart rate derived

TABLE 6.2. Ewing battery

R-R interval change with Valsalva
Heart rate change with deep breathing
R-R interval change after standing (*30:15* ratio)
BP change (systolic) with standing
BP change (diastolic) with sustained handgrip

BP, Blood pressure.

from the R wave of the electrocardiogram (ECG). It provides more accurate dynamic short-term variability than analysis of heart rate over fixed time periods. Newer software has made its analysis simpler.[3] Continuous intraarterial blood pressure and ECG telemetry monitoring in an intensive care–like setting may be required in some circumstances (as in GBP).

Valsalva ratio

The Valsalva maneuver requires forced expiration against a resistance (30 to 40 mm Hg) for 15 to 20 seconds. Table 6.3 describes the phrases of the Valsalva maneuver and their significance. Figure 6.2 illustrates the changes with the influence of posture and preceding rest. R-R interval analysis during the Valsalva maneuver reflects the integrity of the afferent baroreflex pathway (see later), central connections, and efferent R-R control mediated by the vagus nerve. Investigators recommend three con-

TABLE 6.3. Valsalva maneuver

Phase	R-R Interval (heart rate)	Blood Pressure	Mechanism
I	↑ (rate ↓)	↑	Increased left atrial return increases cardiac output with compensatory bradycardia
II	↓ (rate ↑)	↓	Increased intrathoracic pressure reduces right atrial venous return—cardiac output falls with compensatory cardiac acceleration
III	↓ (rate ↑)	↓ ↓	Sudden reduction in intrathoracic pressure reduces left atrial return, reducing cardiac output
IV	↑ ↑ (rate ↓ ↓)	↑ ↑	Cardiac output returns to normal, but reflex peripheral vasoconstriction has occurred in II and III, increasing blood pressure

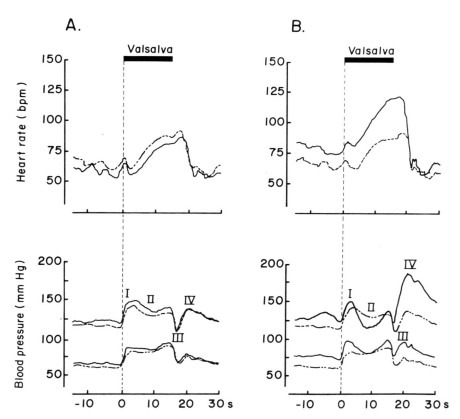

FIGURE 6.2.   *Effects of Valsalva maneuver on heart rate and blood pressure. Phases I through IV of the Valsalva response are indicated. (A) Influence of preceding rest (solid line, 1 minute of preceding rest; dashed line, 5 minutes of preceding rest). (B) Influence of posture (solid line, after 20 minutes of standing; dashed line, after 5 minutes supine). (Modified with permission from Ten Harkel ADJ, Lieshout JJV, Liesh-out EJV, et al. Assessment of cardiovascular reflexes: Influence of posture and period of preceding rest. J Appl Physiol 1990; 68(1):147–153.)*

secutive Valsalva maneuvers with determination of the maximum/minimum R-R interval ratio (normal patients have a ratio greater than 1.21; abnormal is classified as 1.2 or less).[4] Patients with proliferative retinopathy may be at risk of retinal hemorrhage from the Valsalva and should avoid it.[2]

Deep breathing

The afferent and efferent pathway loops for this test are similar to those of the Valsalva maneuver. Six breaths are taken in and out evenly over 60 seconds (5 s for inspiration and 5 s for expiration). The patient should be instructed to breathe deeply, and the examiner should time the breaths. The mean of the differences between the minimum and maximum

heart rate during three consecutive breaths is taken (normal persons have a variation of greater than 15 beats per minute, and abnormal is classifed as a change of 10 beats per minute or less[4]).

Standing

Standing results in sudden dependent venous pooling. There is an initial fall in blood pressure with cardiac acceleration. Later blood pressure returns to normal (from peripheral vasoconstriction), and there is cardiac deceleration. The R-R interval normally shortens at or around the fifteenth heart beat and is longest around the thirtieth beat. The 30:15 ratio thus compares the longest/shortest R-R interval after standing and is normally 1.04 or greater (abnormal classified as 1.00 or less).[4] The blood pressure should be taken 1 minute after standing, and the systolic reading should not fall more than 10 mm Hg in normal persons (an abnormal fall is classified as >30 mm Hg fall in systolic blood pressure).[4]

Handgrip

This test measures sympathetic vasoconstriction that results from effort. A handgrip is continued at 30% of the maximum voluntary contraction for up to 5 minutes using a dynamometer. By the end of contraction, the diastolic pressure should rise 16 mm Hg or more from the mean of three pressures recorded before the test (abnormal classified as 10 mm Hg or less).[2]

Resting *heart rate variability*

Normally the R-R interval shortens during inspiration and lengthens during expiration (normal sinus arrhythmia). R-R intervals with quiet breathing vary with heart rate, age, sympathetic activity, and other factors (meals, coffee, medications). Preferably the test is done in a quiet relaxed atmosphere in the morning after an overnight fast, and the aforementioned complicating factors are eliminated where possible.[1] Variability has been described by the difference between minimum and maximum R-R interval or its standard deviation.[5,6] At least two methods of accounting for changes in R-R variability as a function of heart rate have been described.[1,7] The simplest method is to express variability as a percentage of the mean R-R interval.[7] Investigators have used short periods of recording (e.g., 10 minutes)[7] or ambulatory 24-hour records.[6]

Baroreflex testing

The baroreflex maintains blood flow to vital organs when there is a sudden fall in mean arterial pressure. The afferent loop has receptors (sensitive to transmural pressure) in the carotid sinus and aortic arch (less important) with innervation by the glossopharyngeal and vagus nerves. The efferent portion of the reflex includes inhibition of vagal cardiac slowing, sympathetic cardioacceleration, and vasoconstrictive output to resistance vessels. Most R-R interval tests require an intact baroreflex.

Two methods have been used for specific testing.[8] Infusion of an intravenous pressor agent, such as phenylephrine (50 to 150 μg) increases blood pressure and the R-R interval. Bolus injection may be

the most useful route. The slope of the relationship between the R-R interval (*Y* axis) and blood pressure (*X* axis) is described as *baroreflex sensitivity*.[8] For example, a greater (steeper) slope implies that for a given change in pressure, the R-R interval response is greater (more sensitive). Reciprocal responses from a reduction in blood pressure after nitroprusside and amyl nitrate have also been studied, but no standardized protocols exist. A second method was described by Eckberg et al.[9] A neck suction chamber device was constructed and molded to the anatomy of the subject with rubber seals to isolate the anterior and lateral neck (including that portion with carotid baroreceptors). The chamber pressure was altered through its attached tubing, interpreted by carotid baroreceptors as a change in arterial pressure (because they are sensitive to transmural pressure). An ECG and arterial catheter were used to record an increase in the R-R interval and fall in blood pressure in response to suction. With this setup, brief suctions may be delivered timed to a specific portion of the R-R interval because the response varies depending on the portion of the cycle suction is applied.

Other tests

Other tests of autonomic cardiovascular function are less standardized. The inspiratory gasp[10] can be used to measure R-R interval changes (reduction followed by an increase). Blood pressure also rises from increased sympathetic adrenergic outflow. The stimulus is sudden lung inflation and the afferent loop mediated by lung and airway mechanoreceptors. The patient is asked to inspire as quickly and deeply as possible and to hold it for 10 seconds.[11]

The cold pressor test, a test of adrenergic sympathetic output, measures the change of blood pressure after immersion of the upper limb into cold water (4°C for 90 s).[10] The *face into cold water* and mental stress tests (e.g., mental arithmetic) measure changes in efferent sympathetic activity (blood pressure) and in the R-R interval under vagal control. The immediate heart rate response to lying[12] is a small immediate decrease in R-R interval over three to four beats. This is followed by an increase over the standing level in the next 25 to 30 beats. A brief cough produces an immediate shortened R-R interval over 2 to 3 seconds followed by a lengthening over 18 to 20 seconds.[4,13]

Provocative pharmacologic tests are reviewed in detail by Bannister and Mathias.[10] In postganglionic autonomic denervation, receptor suprasensitivity results in excessive pressor responses to dilute intravenous norepinephrine infusions (these tests require careful medical monitoring). Other drugs used to test for adrenergic denervation supersensitivity have included methoxamine and antidiuretic hormone.[14,15] A loss of the pressure response to tyramine identifies postganglionic sympathetic loss because tyramine releases norepinephrine from nerve terminals. Atropine induces cardiac acceleration in normal subjects but fails to do so in patients with vagal dysfunction. Intravenous infusions of clonidine have been used to assess the integrity of the central alpha-adrenergic system by provoking release of growth hormone (in normals). This response may be absent in patients with autonomic failure.[16]

Assessment of regional sympathetic function may be accomplished using laser Doppler flowmetry of skin blood vessels. This method records the changes in local blood flow that occur from reflex alterations in sympathetic output. An abrupt fall in flow is recorded in normal subjects in the finger or toe following inspiratory gasp, standing, cold pressor testing, and phases II through IV of the Valsalva maneuver.[11] The responses decline with age and have significant variability, reduced by careful control of the testing environment including temperature.

In the venoarteriolar reflex, local arteriolar constriction (and a fall in blood flow) occurs because of an increase in venous transmural pressure.[17] The change in blood flow may be measured by lower limb laser Doppler flowmetry of skin before and after lowering the limb.[18] The laser Doppler probe is attached to the skin over the extensor digitorum brevis. After obtaining baseline data, the leg is lowered >40 cm below the heart by flexing the knee, recording for 2 minutes, then reextending the leg. A reduction in blood flow represents reflex vasoconstriction. This test is less useful than the quantitative sudomotor axon reflex test (QSART), or R-R interval studies, as a test of autonomic function in patients with neuropathy.[18]

The effects of lower body suction are similar to those of standing. Application of 40 mm Hg negative pressure to the lower body below the iliac crests normally lowers systolic pressure by less than 12 mm Hg, decreases forearm blood flow, and increases plasma norepinephrine (see later).[19–22]

Thermography measures regional alterations in skin temperature as an indirect measure of skin blood flow. It has been used to localize focal peripheral neuropathies, plexopathies, or radiculopathies. The usefulness of thermography has been seriously questioned.[23] It provides no information about general autonomic function.

Sudomotor Function

There are two types of sweat glands. Apocrine glands mediate emotional sweating. Eccrine glands receive sympathetic cholinergic innervation and are important for thermoregulation in humans. Surrounding the secretory cell of eccrine glands are myoepithelial cells that receive central drive from the thermoregulatory center and contract to expel sweat droplets. Clinical tests of sudomotor function (Table 6.4) include the QSART, the sympathetic skin response (SSR), the thermoregulatory sweat test (TST), and the Silastic imprint test (SIT).

Quantitative sudomotor axon reflex test

The QSART is a quantitative, sensitive, and reliable test of postganglionic sudomotor function. Acetylcholine (10%) iontophoresis (a method of enhancing skin penetration of a pharmacologic agent by providing an electrical gradient) with a constant current generator stimulates two populations of sweat glands: one directly and a second by a reflex mechanism. Reflex stimulation passes along sympathetic C fibers antidromically to fiber branch points. At these points, the impulses are reflected back now orthodromically in the peripheral branches to stimulate the second population of sweat glands by a reflex mechanism. Only reflex sweating is quantitated using a sudorometer chamber, and it has a latency of 1 to 2 minutes. This chamber employs a low-humidity stream of nitrogen at a constant tem-

TABLE 6.4.   Tests of sudomotor function

Test	Stimulus	Result	Reference
QSART	Iontophoresis of acetylcholine	Humidity change detected in chamber	24
SSR	Shock, startle, inspiration	Skin bioelectric potential recorded by electrodes	25
TST	Warming	Indicator turns color	28
SIT	Iontophoresis of pilocarpine or acetylcholine	Soft impression mold showing sweat droplet imprint	35
			34

QSART, Quantitative sudomotor axon reflex test; SSR, sympathetic skin response; TST, thermoregulatory sweat test; SIT, Silastic imprint test.

perature to evaporate the sweat droplets permitting analysis and recording of changes in humidity. The information is converted to absolute sweat volumes using a calibration equation.[24] Figure 6.3 illustrates the sudorometer chamber and sweat output tracings.

Sympathetic skin response

The sympathetic skin response is an electrical potential recorded over palmar or plantar skin thought to originate in synchronous activity of eccrine sweat glands.[25–27] The galvanic skin response is related but reflects a change in the electrical resistance of the skin with sudomotor activation. The recording electrodes for the SSR are applied to the ventral and dorsal surfaces of the foot, hand, upper arm, or thigh. The stimulus might include an electrical stimulation, pain, startle, cough, or deep inspiration. When the responses are reflexly evoked, they are synchronous and symmetric. The potentials have the same morphology when evoked by electrical stimulation at different sites (e.g., median versus peroneal nerve remote from recording electrodes). While maintaining the position of the stimulating and recording electrodes, repeated stimulations may change the amplitude or morphology of the response, but the latency from the onset of stimulation is generally preserved. The advantage of the method is its simplicity, but it is of limited value because of its variability and tendency to habituate.[25] Shahani et al.[25] did not find a close correlation between an abnormal SSR and symptoms of dysautonomia. The responses were more often absent in axonal than demyelinating neuropathy and correlated with decreased numbers of unmyelinated fibers on a sural nerve biopsy. Thus the SSR may be more useful as a test of C fiber function than autonomic abnormality.[25] Figure 6.4 illustrates a normal SSR in the palm evoked by electrical stimulation of the peroneal nerve and inspiration.

Thermoregulatory sweat test

TST is a sensitive qualitative test of sudomotor function that provides important information about the distribution of sweat loss. Quantitative tests such as QSART and SIT (see next) record small areas and may suffer from sampling bias. The method by Guttmann[28] involved the application of quinizarin indicator on dry skin. The presence of sweating causes a change in the indicator from brown to a violet color. Thermal stimulation using heat cradles or sweat cabinets can be used to induce a rise in oral temperature of 1°C if (1) the resting core temperature

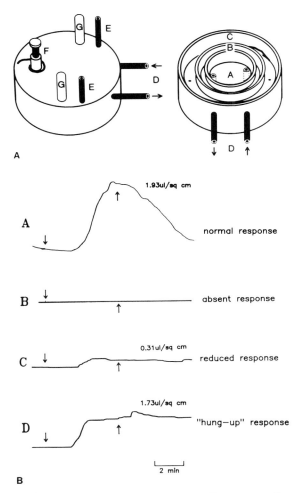

FIGURE 6.3. *QSART testing. (A) The sweat cell is strapped to the skin and has multiple compartments: A central recording compartment (A), air-gap (B), circumferential stimulus moat filled with aceytylcholine (C) filled by a cannula (E). Nitrogen gas (D) is taken in and out of the sweat recording chamber, and anodal current (F) is passed into the stimulus moat. Attachment posts (G) are for straps. (B) Patterns of sweat output: Normal (A), absent (B), reduced (C), and persistent (D). (Reprinted with permission from Low PA, Fealey RD. Sudomotor neuropathy. In: Dyck PJ, Thomas PK, Asbury AK, et al, eds. Diabetic neuropathy. Philadelphia: WB Saunders, 1987:140–145.)*

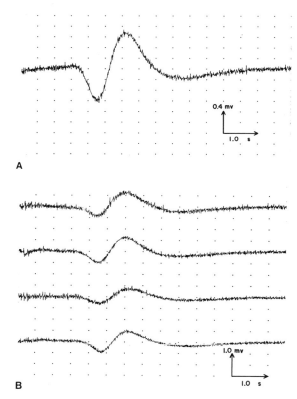

FIGURE 6.4.   *Sympathetic skin response recorded over the palm with stimulation of the deep peroneal nerve (A) or with deep inspiration (B). The morphology (and latency) of the response with inspiration is variable.*

is above 36.5°C, and (2) the subject is not dehydrated. It is essential that the subject has not taken anticholinergic agents including antihistamines or antidepressants for 48 hours before the test.[29] The disadvantages of the TST are its inability to distinguish between postganglionic and preganglionic lesions, the qualitative nature of the information obtained, and the staining of clothing. Global anhidrosis may be preganglionic (as in Shy-Drager syndrome, Parkinson's disease) or postganglionic (as in acute panautonomic neuropathy).[30,31] Hemianhidrosis or a hemicorpal sweating abnormality may be seen in a complete interruption of sympathetic efferent pathways from the hypothalamus to the intermediolateral column of spinal cord as a result of syringomyelia, spinal cord neoplasms, or cerebral infarction.[32,33] Distal anhidrosis may be seen in polyneuropathy.

Silastic imprint test

In this test, Silastic impression material is spread over the surface of the skin, stimulated by acetylcholine or pilocarpine iontophoresis. With hardening of the Silastic, each sweat droplet leaves an imprint, the size of which reflects the quantity of sweat released at that site. Hence the imprint may be used to count the number of sweat glands, the amount of sweat released by each gland, and the total sweat volume in a given skin surface area. The sweat imprint can be photographed, magnified, and digitized, and a sweat histogram can be constructed.[34,35]

Bladder, Gastrointestinal, and Sexual Function

Bladder function

The mainstay of bladder function testing is the cystometrogram. The bladder is filled with measured amounts of water or carbon dioxide, and reflex detrusor contraction pressure waves are recorded. Sitting, standing, and walking help activate detrusor reflexes. This test also can be used to detect the threshold of sensation to bladder filling or may be combined with electronically integrated sphincter electromyography (EMG)[36] of the urethra or perianal sphincter. Simultaneous recording of bladder and intraurethral pressure can be used to assess the relationship between detrusor and sphincter action. Specialized techniques also permit continuous ambulatory recording.[37] Sample radiologic studies may be useful[38]; for example, atonic bladder visualized by an intravenous pyelogram and quantitative measure of urine flow may provide an index of detrusor (urine expulsion) function.[39] Bradley and Lin[40] have also studied evoked anal sphincter responses to bladder or urethral stimulation to assess the bladder/urethra-sacral cord-anal sphincter loop. The characteristics of these somatic reflexes are given in greater detail elsewhere.[40]

Gastrointestinal function

Several methods are available for testing gastrointestinal function. Although these include radiologic assessment of barium gastric emptying or accumulation, other tests are more sensitive. Radioscintigraphic measures may be used to distinguish abnormalities in solid or liquid phase gastric emptying. Radioactive iodine (^{131}I) fiber and technetium (^{99m}Tc) sulfur colloid are useful solid phase isotope markers, the latter prepared in eggs.[41] For the liquid phase, indium (^{111}In) diethylenetriaminepenta-acetic acid (DTPA) stabilized with 1% albumin has been recommended.[41] Manometry is particularly useful in assessing esophageal function but also may be used to assess gastric motility, intestinal motility, and anorectal function.[42,43] De Ponti et al.[44] review these and other methods of evaluating gastrointestinal function.

Sexual function

Assessment of sexual function is generally available only in men. Several methods can measure erection. Snap-gauge fasteners measure maximum penile rigidity by recording the force required to break an applied strip at the penis tip or shaft or both.[45] Portable devices are also available to measure nocturnal penile rigidity and circumferential expansion (tumescence) continuously.[46] Finally sexual dysfunction can be indirectly studied by measurements of conduction velocity in the dorsal nerve of the penis,[47] the latency of the bulbocavernosus reflex from urethral stimulation,[48] and the latency of the cortical pudendal evoked response.[40,49]

Pupillary Testing

Pupillary diameter depends on the balance between competing sympathetic (largely alpha-adrenergic[50]) noradrenergic dilatation and parasympathetic cholinergic constriction. In darkness, parasympathetic input is limited,[51] and pupillary size is particularly determined by the adrenergic input. Pupillary size normally declines with age.[52] The amplitude of pupillary constriction to light is determined by the integrity of the afferent light-efferent parasympathetic pathway as well as adrenergic activity.[50] It is also dependent on the pretesting pupillary diameter[53] because smaller pupils constrict less, but age has no effect on pupillary constriction, provided that diameter is accounted for.[51] The light reflex latency is also dependent on diameter, cholinergic activity and adrenergic activity.[50] The velocity of pupillary redilatation is independent of diameter.[51] The first or rapid phase of pupillary redilatation depends on cancellation of parasympathetic constriction, and the second half requires active adrenergic driving.[54,55] Assessment of pupillary redilatation is illustrated in Figure 6.5. Pupillary cycling time has largely been applied toward assessing afferent pupillary reflex dysfunction.[56]

Accurate assessment of the pupils requires a pupillometer. For simple darkness pupillary diameters, a modified Polaroid camera may suffice.[52] For dynamic measurements, however, sophisticated continuous recording devices are required. Smith and Smith[51] use an infrared TV pupillometer from which the light source is narrower than the pupil (to avoid an effect from the pretest pupillary size). By a forced-choice method, the threshold of light detection is ascertained, and light intensity is provided at 6 log units above this. Some workers block the parasympathetic component pharmacologically to assess darkness diameter.[50]

Provocative pharmacologic testing of the pupil is also of value. To identify the oculosympathetic paralysis of Horner's syndrome, 5% or 10% cocaine instillation indicates whether norepinephrine levels at the nerve terminal-pupillodilator muscle junction are normal.[54] Cocaine blocks the reuptake of norepinephrine and induces mydriasis in the normal eye. In the Horner's syndrome eye, norepinephrine levels are low regardless of the site of pathology, and the pupil fails to dilate. Hydroxyamphetamine (1%) causes release of norepinephrine from the adrenergic pupillary nerve terminal.[54] If the lesion is in this nerve (i.e., third order or postganglionic), the pupil does not dilate. A first or second order sympathetic pathway lesion causes excessive mydriasis from suprasensitivity. In parasympathetic failure (e.g., Adie's pupil), the pupil is suprasensitive to dilute cholinergic agents such as pilocarpine (0.125%) that do not normally cause miosis.[55]

Microneurography

This method relies on direct recordings of nerve traffic within human peripheral nerve trunks (e.g., median, peroneal, or tibial nerves) to measure efferent sympathetic activity at rest or during autonomic reflexes. Detailed reviews of the techniques have been published.[57–59] The test requires specialized training and is likely inappropriate for routine clinical work. Fascicles are impaled with tungsten microelectrodes that have tip diameters of a few microns. At rest, these record spontaneous bursts of sympathetic discharge. In fascicles of cutaneous nerves supplying skin, these bursts include both vasoconstrictor and sudomotor output.[59] Activity declines with vasodilatation following moderate heating but increases when sudomotor activity ensues with sweating. There are bursts following arousal, emotional excitement, and deep breathing.[59] In fascicles of nerves supplying muscles, the bursts are time-locked with the cardiac cycle (diastole), and further activity accompanies the vasoconstriction of hypotension.[59] Maneuvers that increase muscle sympathetic output[59] include standing, Valsalva, handgrip, emo-

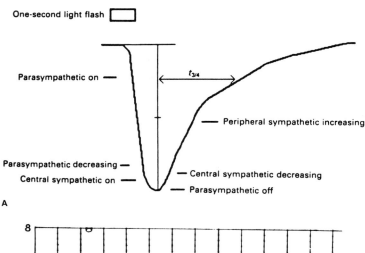

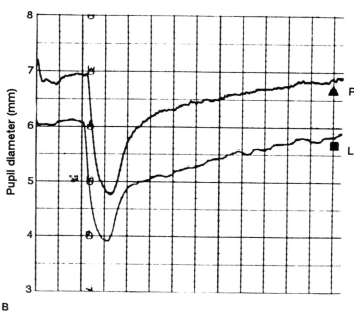

FIGURE 6.5. *Pupillograph tracings (infrared television). (A) The postulated autonomic mechanisms active in various parts of the response. (B) The effect of the left Horner's syndrome in a patient with cluster headaches. The +3/4 is the time to three-fourths pupillary redilatation. In the upper tracing (normal eye), +3/4 measures 3.1 seconds, but the result is prolonged at 6.4 seconds in the lower Horner eye (one vertical bar = 1 second). This is appreciated as a reduced slope of recovery in the lower tracing of (B). The test is not used to localize the level of involvement. (Reprinted with permission from Smith SA. Pupillary function in autonomic failure. In: Bannister R, ed. Autonomic Failure, ed 2. Oxford: Oxford University Press, 1988:393–412.)*

tional stress,[60] and the cold pressor test.[61] Infusion of vasoactive drugs also changes this measurement.[62] The differences in muscle nerve and skin nerve sympathetic activity reflect the differences in their normal physiologic role. Muscle blood flow may be a more important buffer of changes in systemic blood pressure.

Biochemical Tests

Plasma norepinephrine levels are an indirect measurement of adrenergic nerve terminal activity. Levels change in response to posture, emotion, blood volume, hypoglycemia, and other factors. They decline rapidly after collection,[63] necessitating strictly standardized collection and processing methods. Arterial levels are higher than venous levels and rise with age.[63] Low supine levels may suggest postganglionic adrenergic terminal loss because they indicate a lower basal level of norepinephrine release.[64] Failure of norepinephrine to rise with standing implies that norepinephrine is not released from the terminals in reflex fashion as a result of a lesion anywhere along the efferent sympathetic arm.[19,64] Other biochemical studies are less useful: urinary and cerebrospinal fluid norepinephrine metabolites, plasma renin, dopamine hydroxylase, hypoglycemic counterregulatory hormones, epinephrine, and others.[19,63,65]

DISORDERS OF THE AUTONOMIC NERVOUS SYSTEM

Diabetic Autonomic Neuropathy

The high prevalence of autonomic neuropathy in diabetes provided much of the original impetus to develop standardized autonomic testing. In experimental animals, deficits in autonomic conduction are demonstrated as early as 4 months after the onset of hyperglycemia.[66] In humans, autonomic tests may be abnormal within 2 years of onset, without specific symptoms.[67,68] The first detectable abnormality is loss of *resting* R-R interval variability. Figure 6.6 illustrates early loss of R-R variation in diabetic patients. In an unselected series of 500 insulin-dependent diabetic patients, 17% had abnormal heart rate variation,[69] and the incidence of abnormality increased with age. Orthostatic hypotension occurs somewhat later and is present in 10% to 13% of diabetics.[69,70] The presence of somatic neuropathy increases the prevalence of abnormalities. In a series of 73 patients with documented diabetic neuropathy studied by Low et al.,[31] 67% had abnormal R-R interval responses to deep breathing or the Valsalva maneuver, and 58% had abnormal foot QSART testing. Frequent autonomic symptoms are constipation, diarrhea, sweating abnormalities, hypoglycemic unawareness, and impotence. Postural dizziness may be less common.[71–73] Ewing et al.[6] also recorded 24-hour ECGs in 64 diabetics and found higher heart rates from loss of vagal cardioinhibition and a reduction in diurnal variation. Diabetic patients have poor exercise tolerance and may have a reduction of supine venous norepinephrine, arterial norepinephrine, and tissue norepinephrine.[1,74] This correlates with the absence or reduction of sympathetic activity recorded by microneurography in diabetes.[75] Total cardiac denervation, as in a transplanted heart, was reported by Lloyd-Mostyn and Watkins.[76] The patient was 28 years old and had been diabetic for 16 years with 67 hospital admissions. There was no change in heart rate with any attempt to stimulate, inhibit, or pharmacologically block autonomic nerves to the heart.

Using the Ewing battery in 543 selected patients with diabetes,[77] 61% had at least one abnormal test, whereas 43% had two abnormal tests. The relative rate of abnormalities (see earlier for definitions of abnormal results) in this population is illustrated in Figure 6.7. Results of abnormal cardiovascular testing methods in diabetes are summarized in Table 6.5.

Distal anhidrosis is common in diabetes.[78] Heat intolerance may be associated with anhidrosis.[79] Diabetics may have gustatory sweating, which may occur as a result of aberrant regeneration of sympathetic cholinergic fibers.[80] Abnormalities in QSART and SIT are likely due to postganglionic denervation.[31] Figure 6.3(B) illustrates QSART changes in diabetes. Men with mild autonomic involvement may have enlarged direct and indirect

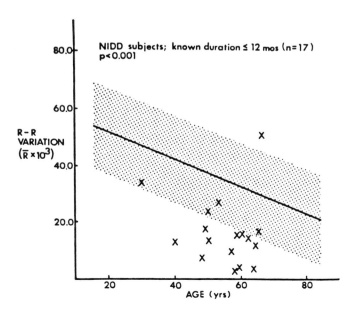

FIGURE 6.6.   *Illustration of the presence of R-R interval variability loss in noninsulin-dependent diabetics (NIDD) with hyperglycemia of recent onset. The bold regression line is derived from normal subjects, and the shading reflects 70% confidence bands. (Reprinted with permission from Pfeifer MA, Weinberg CR, Cook DL, et al. Autonomic neural dysfunction in recently diagnosed diabetic subjects. Diabetes Care 1984; 7:447–453.)*

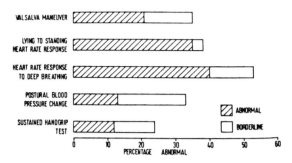

FIGURE 6.7. *Relative prevalence percentages of abnormal autonomic tests in a selected population of 543 diabetic subjects. (Reprinted with permission from Ewing DJ, Martyn CN, Young RJ, Clarke BF, et al. The value of cardiovascular autonomic function tests: 10 years experience in diabetes. Diabetes Care 1985; 8:491–498.)*

sweat droplet size by SIT. This may be a result of multiple reinnervation of sweat glands or alterations in receptor function.[34] The findings of Kennedy et al.[35] were that diabetics had smaller, less numerous, and more irregularly distributed sweat droplets measured by SIT. The density and total area of sweating with axon-reflex mediation are lower.[34]

Gastrointestinal syndromes associated with diabetes mellitus have been summarized by DePonti et al.[44] and Feldman and Schiller.[81] In the upper gastrointestinal tract, esophageal motor abnormalities have been reported with nonspecific symptoms of reflux and dysphagia.[44,82,83] Gastric stasis (gastroparesis) is frequent in diabetes and may occur radiologically in up to 22% of asymptomatic patients.[84] Symptoms include dyspepsia, bloating, nausea, and vomiting. Imaging studies have identified slow emptying, often more marked with solids. Manometry has disclosed hypomotility.[42,85] Pylorospasm and intestinal *burst* patterns may lead to pseudo-obstructive symptoms.[44,86] In the lower gut, diarrhea, often nocturnal, and constipation are common.[72,81,87] The latter may lead to a megasigmoid syndrome.[88] Fecal incontinence may be associated with or separate from diabetic diarrhea.[81]

Diabetic bladder involvement is largely a result of afferent sensory dysfunction with a delay in the detrusor reflex and later areflexia.[39,40] Urine flow rate may be reduced or interrupted.[40] The symptom of impotence in diabetic men is common, with a reported prevalence of 35%,[73] but several other factors, particularly atherosclerosis, may contribute to this figure.[89] Tests of sexual function in diabetes have

TABLE 6.5. Autonomic system abnormalities in diabetes mellitus*

Cardiovascular Function
Abnormal Valsalva ratio (71, 77, 94, 95)
Abnormal heart rate response to deep breathing (1, 77, 96, 97)
Loss of R-R interval variation at *rest* (6, 68, 76, 96, 98)
Abnormal *30:15* ratio or equivalent (77, 99, 100)
Postural hypotension (77, 99, 100, 101)
Abnormal response to sustained handgrip (77, 100, 102)
Loss of sympathetic activity recorded by microneurography (75)

Sudomotor Function
Abnormal QSART response (31)
Abnormal TST pattern (72, 78, 79, 103, 104, 105)
Abnormal SIT method (34, 35)
Abnormal SSR method (26)

Gastrointestinal, Bladder, and Sphincter Function
Esophageal incoordination (44, 82, 83)
Gastroparesis (42, 81, 84, 85)
Nocturnal diarrhea (44, 72, 81)
Pseudo-obstruction (44, 86)
Loss of bladder detrusor reflex (39, 40)
Impotence (73)

Pupillary Function
Decreased darkness pupillary diameter (92)
Decreased pupillary light reflex amplitude and abnormal redilatation (51, 53, 93)

* Numbers in parentheses are appropriate references.
QSART, Quantitative sudomotor axon reflex test; TST, thermoregulary sweat test; SIT, Silastic imprint test; SSR, sympathetic skin response.

not been extensively documented. The conduction velocity of the dorsal nerve of the penis may be reduced in impotent diabetic men[90] and bulbocavernosus or anal reflex latencies delayed.[48,91]

The darkness diameter of the pupil in diabetes is reduced, particularly as the duration of diabetes increases.[50,92] This may be secondary to defective adrenergic mydriasis.[92] Diabetic patients also have a reduced pupillary light reflex amplitude (corrected for diameter) and abnormal sympathetic light reflex recovery (see Figure 6.5).[92,93]

Abnormalities of the venoarteriolar reflex have been described in diabetes, but this testing method is less useful.[18]

Autonomic Involvement in Guillain-Barré Polyneuropathy

Acute autonomic dysfunction now rivals respiratory failure and thromboembolism as an important cause of death in patients with GBP. Prospective evaluation has indicated that one or more features of autonomic neuropathy develop in the majority of GBP patients. The neuropathy may involve afferent or autonomic efferent fibers. Most early reports of GBP, however, such as that of Haymaker and Kernohan,[106] preceded the advent of intensive respiratory care, and it was argued that most vasomotor disturbances in GBP were secondary to hypoxia. In these reports, respiratory mortality likely preceded clinically significant autonomic disease. Singh et al.[107] provide prospective information suggesting that autonomic dysfunction occurs in the majority of GBP patients. Of 24 patients evaluated, 16 (66.7%) had involvement. Tachycardia, hypertension, and postural hypotension were each observed in approximately one-third of patients. In this study, autonomic dysfunction was not life-threatening, but several other series claim otherwise. Truax[108] noted some evidence of autonomic dysfunction in 65% (cardiovascular in 59%) of 169 retrospectively reviewed patients from the Massachusetts General Hospital. Lichtenfeld[109] reports on 12 prospective and 16 retrospective cases of GBP. Over 60% had hypertension, and a similar proportion had ECG abnormalities. Autonomic dysfunction was closely related to sudden death in four among the six fatalities in this series. Several case reports attest to the intensive management autonomic disturbances may require.[110–114]

Alterations in resting and reflex blood pressure measurements in GBP imply sympathetic dysfunction. Clinical manifestations have included extreme lability in continuous blood pressure recordings with unpredictable episodes of hypertension and hypotension and *cardiovascular collapse*. Truax[108] reported hypertension in 27% of his series that was paroxysmal in 24% and sustained in 3%. Paroxysmal hypertension correlated with quadriplegia and respiratory failure. In GBP patients, hypertensive episodes may be associated with subarachnoid hemorrhage[115,116] and pulmonary edema.[116] They may also be followed by abrupt hypotension or sudden death.[106,109,117] The reports of McQuillan and Bullock[112] and Lichtenfeld[109] are particularly illustrative of the difficulties that may occur. In the former case, systolic pressure fluctuations over 3 minutes exceeded 50 mm Hg despite sedation and antihypertensives. Extreme sensitivity to antihypertensive agents also occurs in GBP.

Most reports indicate that GBP patients with ANS involvement have an outpouring of vasoactive catecholamines with elevated plasma norepinephrine levels[111,118–120] and elevated urinary catecholamine

assays[115,118,120–123] that were either correlated with autonomic involvement or fell with recovery. The microneuronographic recordings of Fagius and Wallin[124] in three patients with GBP identified excessive sympathetic outflow during the acute phase with hypertension and tachycardia.

Sympathetic hypofunction also may occur in GBP. In 43% of Lichtenfeld's[109] patients and 19% of Truax's[108] patients, there was postural hypotension. Birchfield and Shaw[125] reported three of six GBP patients in whom postural hypotension was a presenting feature. Postural hypotension alone does not distinguish between an afferent baroreflex pathway lesion or a lesion of sympathetic output fibers. The bedridden state, with poor muscle tone, could account for some degree of postural hypotension. In two of the patients, however, an excessive pressor response to phenylephrine indicated denervation supersensitivity of resistance vessels. This suggested an efferent sympathetic lesion. In the prospective GBP series of Singh et al.,[107] postural hypotension was present in 35%, impaired responses to sustained handgrip in 25%, and an abnormal cold immersion test in 36% of patients. Bansal et al.[126] supported these findings by identifying abnormal cold immersion tests in six of 15 patients studied. The most suggestive evidence of sympathetic hypofunction is that of anhidrosis, noted in 12.5% of Singh's series[107] and in all seven patients tested by Tuck and McLeod.[127]

Excessive unregulated vagal activity generated by ectopic activity in diseased nerve may be responsible for instances of sudden bradyarrhythmia and asystole, sometimes requiring a pacemaker.[110,114,128–130] These *vagal spells* occur following tracheal suctioning or Valsalva-like maneuvers.[108] Acute vagal deficits could be responsible for tachyarrhythmias with sinus tachycardia most frequently reported.[107,116,129] In the Massachusetts General Hospital series, sustained sinus tachycardia was present in 37% of patients and correlated with the degree of weakness, respiratory failure, and bulbar involvement.[108] Truax[108] argued against a vagal cause of the tachycardia because its rate was faster and more sustained than that seen in parasympathetic blockade. In addition, the response to carotid sinus massage was intact. In contrast, Lichtenfeld[109] described tachycardia that was unresponsive to carotid sinus stimulation. Persson and Solders[130a] observed a reduction in R-R variation in six GBP patients with an improvement accompanying clinical recovery. Similar R-R variation reduction was reported by Frison et al.[131] Singh et al.[107] reported abnormal heart rate ratios to deep breathing in 31.6% and an abnormal Valsalva heart rate ratio in 28.6 of 24 patients with GBP. Bansal et al.[126] noted a reduced mean heart rate acceleration to atropine in their series of 15 patients with GBP, with recovery in five patients. Abnormalities of baroreceptor afferents also could account for sinus tachycardia or diminution of the R-R interval with deep breathing. Tuck and McLeod[127] assessed baroreflex sensitivity to pharmacologic manipulation of blood pressure and noted abnormalities in four of seven patients tested.

Other arrhythmias and ECG changes have been frequently noted in GBP patients.[109,115,116,122,123,129, 130,132,133] These have included atrial tachyarrhythmias, such as fibrillation, flutter and paroxysmal tachycardia, ventricular tachycardia, elevated or depressed ST segments, flat or inverted T waves, Q-T interval prolongation, axis deviation, and various forms of conduction block.[108]

Urinary retention has occurred in about one-third of GBP patients.[108,109,134,135] A number of other autonomic abnormalities are less frequent. These have included constipation, present in 14% of the MGH series[108]; fecal incontinence (two patients of the latter series), ileus, and gastroparesis reported by Lichtenfeldt,[109] Crozier and Ainley,[136] and in 9% of the MGH series; diarrhea[137]; sexual dysfunction[138,139]; and pupillary abnormalities.[140,141] Litchtenfeld[109] also described episodes of facial flushing, chest tightening, and bradycardia, attributed to parasympathetic overactivity and duplicated with intravenous edrophonium chloride. Gecow and Pawela[142] described bronchial smooth muscle paresis in 15% of 83 children with GBP.

Pandysautonomia

Acute primary affliction of the ANS variably described as autonomic neuropathy, pandysautonomia, or acute panautonomic neuropathy, has been considered a *forme-fruste* autonomic variant of GBP. Although Young et al.[143] described *pure* pandysautonomia, there have been other reports with variable involvement of sensory fibers as well as autonomic fibers.[144-146] Some forms appear to involve cholinergic neurons selectively.[147]

The patient of Young et al.,[143] a 49-year-old man, had a 1-month history of lethargy, lightheadedness, visual blurring, photophobia, and dry eyes among other complaints. He also complained of loss of sweating, constipation, urinary incontinence, and sexual dysfunction. Cerebrospinal fluid showed albuminocytologic dissociation. Detailed investiga-

tions during several hospital admissions documented unreactive pupils inappropriately reactive to dilute methacholine and unreactive to cocaine; loss of pain, piloerection, and flare to intradermal histamine; hypersensitivity to infused norepinephrine; postural hypotension; loss of phase IV blood pressure overshoot with the Valsalva maneuver; anhidrosis; constancy of heart rate with hypotension; loss of gastrointestinal motility; and atonicity and poor emptying of the bladder. Recovery occurred over approximately 2 years.

Pandysautonomia was also described by Low et al.[30] in two patients. The first patient was a 46-year-old woman who developed postural lightheadedness, blurred vision, and urinary retention over a few days. Predominant postganglionic involvement was suggested by an impaired intradermal methacholine response, suprasensitivity to phenylephrine, loss of sural nerve unmyelinated and small myelinated fibers, and inappropriate pupillary constriction to dilute pilocarpine. Cerebrospinal fluid protein was normal. Persistent abnormalities were present 5 years later. The second patient was a 73-year-old woman who developed postural lightheadedness, urinary retention, constipation, dry eyes, and a dry mouth after an influenza-like illness. Paresthesias were reported, and cerebrospinal fluid protein was elevated. Studies disclosed an inappropriate pupillary response to dilute pilocarpine, an impaired pupillary response to light, and patchy hypohidrosis.

Summers and Harris[148] describe a 43-year-old woman with malaise and other complaints 2 weeks following a viral infection, likely rubella. Autonomic findings included postural hypotension, loss of sinus arrhythmia, anhidrosis of the limb and trunk, and failure of pupillary dilation with 4% cocaine. Plasma supine norepinephrine was low and did not rise with tilting. There was albuminocytologic dissociation. At 38 months, her deficits persisted.

Other Autonomic Neuropathies

Patients with botulism have acute cholinergic autonomic dysfunction that usually but not always accompanies weakness.[149,150] Cholinergic or more widespread dysautonomia also occurs in Lambert-Eaton myasthenic syndrome.[151] Symptoms may include dry mouth and reduced potency. Testing may identify impairment of sweating, lacrimation, salivation, pupillary function, and other abnormalities.[152,153] A paraneoplastic pandysautonomia has also been described,[145,154] may be associated with somatic neuropathy, and may accompany a variety of tumor types, especially oat cell carcinoma. The Riley-Day syndrome,[155] also classified as hereditary sensory and autonomic neuropathy (HSAN) type III,[156] is an autosomal recessive disorder usually afflicting Jewish children. Autonomic symptoms include defective lacrimation, abnormal temperature control, skin blotching, excessive salivation, perspiration, hypertension, and postural hypotension. Esophageal motility abnormalities associated with vomiting and other gastrointestinal changes are also reported.[156] Two other inherited conditions labeled HSAN types I and II have acral anhidrosis, but generalized autonomic dysfunction is not a feature.[156] HSAN types IV and V are rare, have sudomotor abnormalities, and may have abnormal temperature regulation (in type IV). Ross's syndrome[157] is segmental anhidrosis with Adie's pupil. The cause is unknown and may overlap with the eight patients described by Low et al.[158] with chronic idiopathic anhidrosis. Of the latter group, all had complete or incomplete anhidrosis, three had pupillary abnormalities (sympathetic lesion in two, combined lesion in one), five had skin vasomotor abnormalities, and none of the seven patients tested had R-R interval abnormalities or postural hypotension. Half were judged to have a preganglionic lesion and the rest to have a postganglionic lesion.

Reflex sympathetic dystrophy is a chronic limb pain syndrome characterized by localized hyperpathia, allodynia, hyperhidrosis, swelling, temperature changes, and trophic alterations. The diagnosis is clinical, but relief in some patients with regional guanethidine has suggested that localized sympathetic overactivity is an important feature.[159,160]

Autonomic Involvement in Other Polyneuropathies

McLeod[150,161] divided autonomic dysfunction associated with peripheral neuropathy into two groups: clinically important autonomic involvement and clinically unimportant involvement. The former group included diabetes and GBP, as described earlier, and the rarer conditions of amyloidosis, acute intermittent porphyria, familial dysautonomia (Riley-Day syndrome; see earlier) and finally chronic sensory and autonomic neuropathy.

Autonomic involvement is early and prominent in polyneuropathy associated with amyloidosis because of particular involvement of unmyelinated and small myelinated fibers.[162] Detailed clinical, pathologic, and genetic features have been reviewed by Cohen and Rubinow.[162] Symptoms in both acquired and familial forms include postural hypotension, impotence, anhidrosis, constipation, fecal and urinary incontinence, and nocturnal diarrhea. Some autonomic dysfunction may occur because of direct amyloid deposition in the gastrointestinal tract or heart. Esophageal manometry has identified abnormal tracings in 63% of patients,[162] and secondary malabsorption from stasis and bacterial overgrowth may develop.[162,163] Orthostatic hypotension reportedly portends a poor prognosis[162] and may be associated with sudden syncope. Scalloped pupils in type I (Portuguese, Adrade) probably result from involvement of the ciliary body[164,165] and usually develop in later disease.[162] Autonomic testing in patients with amyloid neuropathy[11] has identified reduced vasoconstriction to cold, standing, Valsalva maneuver, and inspiratory gasp. Falco de Freitas et al.[166] studied patients with familial amyloid polyneuropathy and observed postural hypotension; decreased supine and standing plasma norepinephrine; and blunted R-R interval responses to atropine, isoprenaline, and Valsalva maneuver. Atrioventricular and ventricular conduction abnormalities have also been reported (67% in one series), necessitating permanent cardiac pacing in a significant number of patients.[167] Autonomic involvement in secondary amyloidosis may be rare but has also been reported.[168]

Autonomic symptoms are prominent in porphyria and have been reviewed by Gorchein.[169] The porphyrias associated with neurologic manifestations include acute intermittent porphyria, variegate porphyria, and hereditary coproporphyria. Gastrointestinal features attributed to (although not proved) autonomic neuropathy in acute porphyria include severe attacks of abdominal pain, nausea, vomiting, constipation, and perhaps diarrhea. Gorchein[169] described three patients with acute intermittent porphyria and abdominal pain. Upper gastrointestinal motility studies identified duodenal atony and abnormally spaced gastric migrating complexes. Tachycardia and hypertension may be prominent during acute porphyric attacks and have been attributed to vagal dysfunction and deafferented baroreceptors.[169-171] Autonomic testing during acute attacks has identified abnormalities more frequently than between attacks.[169] Various authors have identified absence of bradycardia with the Valsalva maneuver,[172-174] an abnormal 30:15 ratio,[173,174] reduced heart rate variability to deep breathing,[174] impaired blood pressure response to sustained handgrip,[174] and postural hypotension.[172,175]

Ingall et al.[176] performed autonomic testing in 14 patients with chronic inflammatory demyelinating polyneuropathy. Abnormalities in the 30:15 ratio in only three patients and an abnormal thermoregulatory sweat test in five patients indicated only mild autonomic involvement. Low et al.[177] studied autonomic involvement in alcoholic (nutritional) neuropathy. There was stocking and glove pattern anhidrosis in all eight patients tested. Abnormal Valsalva ratios were identified in 22% of the group, but postural hypertension and denervation hypersensitivity were absent. Baroreflex studies were normal. Vagal neuropathy has been identified by others in alcoholism.[178,179] Autonomic abnormalities have been reported in toxic neuropathies due to vincristine,[180] thallium,[181] perhexiline maleate,[182] and arsenic.[183] Several reports have documented autonomic neuropathy in uremia.[184–186] Autonomic reflexes have also been tested in hereditary motor and sensory neuropathy (HMSN) type I by Jammes,[187] who observed an abnormal pattern of skin temperature, abnormalities in reflex cardiovascular changes to tilting, distal anhidrosis, reduction in tear formation, and abnormal pupillary dilatation with darkness or cocaine. Brooks[188] studied vascular reflexes in 17 adult patients with HMSN type I and identified blunted Valsalva ratios in five patients, reduced R-R responses to standing in two patients, and postural hypotension in two patients. Solders et al.[189] identified severe but transient vagal dysfunction in diphtheria with normal sympathetic function. Other sporadic reports of autonomic involvement in neuropathies have been summarized in the report by McLeod and Tuck.[150]

Central *Autonomic Disorders*

McLeod and Tuck[150] divided *central* autonomic disorders into progressive autonomic failure (PAF) and other central disorders with autonomic involvement. PAF has been reviewed in detail elsewhere.[150,190] It may be divided into a *pure* category without other signs of neurologic disease, PAF with parkinsonian features, and PAF with multiple system atrophy (Shy-Drager syndrome[191]). Bannister and Oppenheimer[190] described four patients with PAF and multiple system atrophy. Symptoms and signs of autonomic dysfunction included urinary frequency, urinary incontinence, impotence, blurred vision, postural hypotension, and pupillary abnormalities. Autonomic testing abnormalities included abnormal Valsalva, blood pressure, and heart rate responses; anhidrosis; and abnormalities of limb vasoconstriction to lower body suction, heating, ice, emotion, and infusion of adrenergic agonists. Similar findings were described by Mathias et al.[192] Kirby and Fowler[38] describe results of bladder testing: Bladder contractions were involuntary (with leakage) or absent (atonic) later in the disease. There was also loss of urethral tone. Loss of preganglionic fibers from the intermediolateral cell column of the spinal cord has been a prominent pathologic feature of PAF.[193–195]

Low and Fealey[196] evaluated 38 PAF patients and 59 patients with PAF plus multiple system atrophy at Mayo Clinic over a 3.5-year period.[194,197] All had orthostatic hypotension, anhidrosis as assessed by the thermoregulatory sweat test, and abnormalities of R-R intervals to deep breathing and Valsalva. An interesting finding in some patients was a normal QSART test in areas of anhidrosis (judged by the thermoregulatory sweat test), suggesting that these patients had a preganglionic sudomotor lesion. Most patients had combined preganglionic and postganglionic disorders. Postganglionic abnormalities were less severe in PAF than in pandysautonomia.[147] Supine norepinephrine levels (reflecting postganglionic norepinephrine nerve terminal integrity) were reduced in PAF without multiple system atrophy. Standing norepinephrine levels (reflecting the integrity of the adrenergic efferent relay at all levels) were reduced in both groups. Ziegler et al.[64] reported similar findings.

Other *central* disorders with autonomic involvement have been reported. In Parkinson's disease (exclusive of the PAF variety), orthostatic hypotension and abnormal R-R interval studies have been reported.[198,199] Spinal cord lesions above T-6 impair descending vasomotor and sudomotor control. This results in postural hypotension and anhidrosis below the level of the lesion.[32,150,200,201] Cutaneous stimuli or bowel or bladder distention may evoke inappropriate sympathetic mediated hypertension and vasoconstriction.[200,202,203] Tracheal suctioning may cause bradycardia and cardiac arrest.[150] Autonomic abnormalities (absent baroreflex in acute disorders) have also been reported in cerebrovascular disease,[204] brain stem tumors,[205,206] tabes dorsalis,[207] and multiple sclerosis.[208] Hypertension and cardiovascular abnormalities were reported in poliomyelitis.[209–211] The mechanism was uncertain, but hypoxia, myocarditis, and central disease were considered. Hypertension appeared to be more severe in bulbospinal disease.

Cohen and Laudenslager[212] tested autonomic function in 10 human immunodeficiency virus (HIV)–infected patients. Five had abnormalities, four of whom had acquired immunodeficiency syndrome (AIDS) (Center for Disease Control IV). One had postural hypotension, four had blunted R-R intervals with deep breathing, five had reduced R-R interval responses to Valsalva, and four had an absent QSART response. All but one had other signs of neurologic dysfunction, but definite peripheral nerve involvement was not present.

Elderly patients have abnormalities in autonomic function, but the most prominent is orthostatic hypotension.[147,213] Normal age-related loss of intermediolateral cell column neurons may be the cause.[214]

ACKNOWLEDGMENTS

We acknowledge the helpful comments of Dr. Phillip A. Low. Ms. Barbara S. Proksa, Dr. Robert Semmler, and Mr. James D. Schmelzer also made useful editorial suggestions. Mrs. Lisa Fregeau provided expert secretarial and library assistance.

REFERENCES

1. Pfeifer MA, Peterson H. Cardiovascular autonomic neuropathy. In: Dyck PJ, Thomas PK, Asbury AK, et al., eds. Diabetic neuropathy. Philadelphia: WB Saunders, 1987:122–133.
2. Ewing DJ, Clarke BF. Diagnosis and management of diabetic autonomic neuropathy. Br Med J 1982; 285:916–918.
3. Ewing DJ. Which battery of cardiovascular autonomic function tests? Diabetologia 1990; 33:180–181.
4. Ewing DJ. Recent advances in the investigation of diabetic autonomic neuropathy. In: Bannister R, ed. Autonomic failure, ed 2. Oxford: Oxford University Press, 1988:667–689.
5. Ewing DJ, Borsey DQ, Bellavere F, Clarke BF. Cardiac autonomic neuropathy in diabetes: Comparison of measures of R-R interval variation. Diabetologia 1981; 21:18–24.
6. Ewing DJ, Borsey DQ, Travis P, et al. Abnormalities of ambulatory 24 hour heart rate in diabetes mellitus. Diabetes 1983; 32:101–105.
7. Persson A, Solders G. R-R variations, a test of autonomic dysfunction. Acta Neurol Scand 1983; 67:285–293.
8. Jones JV. Cardiovascular baroreflex control in man. In: Bannister R, ed. Autonomic failure, ed 2. Oxford: Oxford Press, 1988:129–141.
9. Eckberg DL, Cavanaugh MS, Mark AL, Abboud FM. A simplified neck suction device for activation of carotid baroreceptors. J Lab Clin Med 1975; 85:167–173.
10. Bannister R, Mathias C. Testing autonomic reflexes. In: Bannister R, ed. Autonomic failure, ed 2. Oxford: Oxford University Press, 1988:289–307.
11. Low PA, Neumann C, Dyck PJ, et al. Evaluation of skin vasomotor reflexes by using laser doppler velocimetry. Mayo Clin Proc 1983; 58:583–592.
12. Bellavere F, Ewing DJ. Autonomic control of the immediate heart rate response to lying down. Clin Sci 1982; 62:57–64.
13. Cardone C, Bellavere F, Ferri M, Fedele D. Autonomic mechanisms in the heart rate response to coughing. Clin Sci 1987; 72:55–60.
14. Parks VJ, Sandison AG, Skinner SL, Whelan RF. Sympathomimetic drugs in orthostatic hypotension. Lancet 1961; 1:1133–1136.
15. Mohring J, Glanzer K, Maciel JA Jr, et al. Greatly enhanced pressor response to antidiuretic hormone in patients with impaired cardiovascular reflexes due to idiopathic orthostatic hypotension. J Cardiovasc Pharmacol 1980; 2:367–376.
16. Da Costa DF, Bannister R, Landon J, Mathias CJ. Growth hormone response to clonidine is impaired in patients with central sympathetic degeneration. Clin Exp Hypertension 1984; 6:1843–1846.
17. Henriksen O. Local sympathetic reflex mechanism in regulation of blood flow in human subcutaneous adipose tissue. Acta Physiol Scand 1977; 450(suppl):1–48.
18. Moy S, Opfer-Gehrking TL, Proper CJ, Low PA. The venoarteriolar reflex in diabetic and other neuropathies. Neurology 1989; 39:1490–1492.
19. Bannister R, Sever P, Gross M. Cardiovascular reflexes and biochemical responses in progressive autonomic failure. Brain 1977; 100:327–344.
20. Bennett T, Hosking DJ, Hampton JR. Cardiovascular responses to graded reductions of central blood volume in normal subjects and in patients with diabetes mellitus. Clin Sci 1980; 58:193–200.
21. Goldsmith SR, Francis GS, Cowley AW, Cohn JN. Response of vasopressin and norepinephrine to lower body negative pressure in humans. Am J Physiol 1982; 243:H970–H973.
22. Johnson JM, Rowell LB, Niederberger M, Eismann MM. Human splanchnic and forearm vasoconstrictor responses to reduction in right atrial and aortic pressures. Circ Res 1974; 34:515–524.
23. So YT, Olney RK, Aminoff MJ. Evaluation of thermography in the diagnosis of selected entrapment neuropathies. Neurology 1989; 39:1–5.
24. Low PA, Caskey PE, Tuck RR, et al. Quantitative sudomotor axon reflex test in normal and neuropathic subjects. Ann Neurol 1983; 14:573–580.
25. Shahani BT, Halperin JJ, Boulu P, Cohen J. Sympathetic skin response—a method of assessing unmyelinated axon dysfunction in peripheral neuro-

pathies. J Neurol Neurosurg Psychiatry 1984; 47:536–542.

26. Knezevic W, Bajada S. Peripheral autonomic surface potential. A quantitative technique for recording sympathetic conduction in man. J Neurol Sci 1985; 67:239–251.

27. Uncini A, Pullman SL, Lovelace RE, Gambi D. The sympathetic skin response: Normal values, elucidation of afferent components and application limits. J Neurol Sci 1988; 87:299–306.

28. Guttmann L. The management of the quinizarin sweat test (QST). Postgrad Med J 1947; 23:353.

29. Fealey RD, Low PA, Thomas JE. Thermoregulatory sweating abnormalities in diabetes mellitus. Mayo Clin Proc 1989; 64:617–628.

30. Low PA, Dyck PJ, Lambert EH, et al. Acute panautonomic neuropathy. Ann Neurol 1983; 13:412–417.

31. Low PA, Zimmerman BR, Dyck PJ. Comparison of distal sympathetic with vagal function in diabetic neuropathy. Muscle Nerve 1986; 9:592–596.

32. Guttmann L. Spinal cord injuries. In: Disturbances of vasomotor control, ed 2. Oxford: Blackwell, 1976:295–330.

33. Kihara M, Watanabe H, Tomita T, et al. Disturbance of sweating in patients with infarction of cerebral cortex. Auton Nerv Syst 1987; 24:434.

34. Kihara M, Opfer-Gehrking TL, Low PA. Comparison of directly stimulated with axon reflex-mediated sudomotor responses in human subjects. Ann Neurol 1989; 26:169.

35. Kennedy WR, Sakuta M, Sutherland D, Goetz FC. Quantitation of the sweating deficiency in diabetes mellitus. Ann Neurol 1984; 15:482.

36. Bradley WE. Cystometry and sphincter electromyography. Mayo Clin Proc 1976; 51:329–335.

37. Bhatia NN, Bradley WE, Haldeman S, Johnson BK. Continuous ambulatory urodynamic monitoring. Br J Urol 1982; 54:357–359.

38. Kirby RS, Fowler CJ. Bladder and sexual dysfunction in diseases affecting the autonomic nervous system. In: Bannister R, ed. Autonomic failure, ed 2. Oxford: Oxford University Press, 1988:413–431.

39. Bradley WE. Diagnosis of urinary bladder dysfunction in diabetes mellitus. Ann Intern Med 1980; 92:323–326.

40. Bradley WE, Lin JT. Assessment of diabetic sexual dysfunction and cystopathy. In: Dyck PJ, Thomas PK, Asbury AK, et al., eds. Diabetic neuropathy. Philadelphia: WB Saunders, 1987:146–154.

41. Thomforde GM, Brown ML, Malagelada J-R. Practical solid and liquid phase markers for studying gastric emptying in man. J Nucl Med Tech 1985; 13:11–14.

42. Malagelada J-R, Stanghellini V. Manometric evaluation of functional upper gut symptoms. Gastroenterology 1985; 88:1223–1231.

43. Read NW, Haynes WG, Bartolo DCC, et al. Use of

anorectal manometry during rectal infusion of saline to investigate sphincter function in incontinent patients. Gastroenterology 1983; 85:105–113.

44. DePonti F, Fealey RD, Malagelada J-R. Gastrointestinal syndromes due to diabetes mellitus. In: Dyck PJ, Thomas PK, Asbury AK, et al., eds. Diabetic neuropathy. Philadelphia: WB Saunders, 1987.

45. Ek A, Bradley WE, Krane RL. Snap-gauge band: New concept in measuring penile rigidity. Urology 1983; 21:63.

46. Bradley WE, Timm GW, Gallagher JM, Johnson BK. New method for continuous measurement of nocturnal penile tumescence and rigidity. Urology 1985; 26:4–9.

47. Bradley WE, Lin JTY, Johnson B. Measurement of the conduction velocity of the dorsal nerve of the penis. J Urol 1984; 131:1127.

48. Sarica Y, Karacan I. Bulbocavernosus reflex to somatic and visceral nerve stimulation in normal subjects and in diabetics with erectile impotence. J Urol 1987; 138:55–58.

49. Haldeman S, Bradley WE, Bhatia NN, Johnson BK. Pudendal evoked responses. Arch Neurol 1982; 39:280–283.

50. Pfeifer MA, Cook D, Brodsky J, et al. Quantitative evaluation of sympathetic and parasympathetic control of iris function. Diabetes Care 1982; 5:518–528.

51. Smith SA, Smith SE. Assessment of pupillary function in diabetic neuropathy. In: Dyck PJ, Thomas PK, Asbury AK, et al., eds. Diabetic neuropathy. Philadelphia: WB Saunders, 1987:134–139.

52. Smith SA, Dewhirst RR. A simple diagnostic test for pupillary abnormality in diabetic autonomic neuropathy. Diabetic Med 1986; 3:38–41.

53. Smith SA, Smith SE. Reduced pupillary light reflexes in diabetic autonomic neuropathy. Diabetologia 1983; 24:330–332.

54. Thompson HS. Diagnosing Horner's syndrome. Trans Am Acad Ophthamol Otolaryngol 1977; 83:840–842.

55. Smith SA. Pupillary function in autonomic failure. In: Bannister R, ed. Autonomic failure, ed 2. Oxford: Oxford University Press, 1988:393–412.

56. Miller SD, Thompson HS. Pupil cycle time in optic neuritis. Am J Ophthalmol 1978; 85:635–642.

57. Vallbo AB, Hagbarth KE, Torebjork HE, Wallin BG. Somatosensory, proprioceptive and sympathetic activity in human peripheral nerves. Physiol Rev 1979; 59:919–957.

58. Wallin BG, Fagius J. The sympathetic nervous system in man—aspects derived from microelectrode recordings. Trends Neurosci 1986; 9:63–67.

59. Wallin BG. Intraneural recordings of normal and abnormal sympathetic activity in man. In: Bannister R, ed. Autonomic failure, ed 2. Oxford: Oxford University Press, 1988:177–195.

60. Anderson EA, Wallin BG, Mark AL. Dissociation

of sympathetic nerve activity in arm and leg muscle during mental stress. Hypertension 1987; 9(suppl III):114–119.

61. Victor RG, Leimbach WN, Seals DR, et al. Effects of the cold pressor test on muscle sympathetic nerve activity in humans. Hypertension 1987; 9:429–436.

62. Eckberg DL, Andersson OK, Hedner T, et al. Baroreflex control of muscle sympathetic activity and plasma noradrenaline in man. J Hypertension 1986; 4(suppl 6):S718–S719.

63. Polinsky RJ. Neurotransmitter and neuropeptide function in autonomic failure. In: Bannister R, ed. Autonomic failure, ed 2. Oxford: Oxford University Press, 1988:321–347.

64. Ziegler MG, Lake CR, Kopin IJ. The sympathetic-nervous-system defect in primary orthostatic hypotension. N Engl J Med 1977; 296:293–297.

65. Polinsky RJ, Kopin IJ, Ebert MH, et al. Hormonal responses to hypoglycemia in orthostatic hypotension patients with adrenergic insufficiency. Life Sci 1981; 29:417–425.

66. Ward KK, Low PA, Schmelzer JD, Zochodne DW. Prostacyclin and noradrenaline in peripheral nerve of chronic experimental diabetes in rats. Brain 1989; 112:197–208.

67. Ewing DJ, Clarke BF. Diabetic autonomic neuropathy: Present insights and future prospects. Diabetes Care 1986; 9:648–665.

68. Pfeifer MA, Weinberg CR, Cook DL, et al. Autonomic neural dysfunction in recently diagnosed diabetic subjects. Diabetes Care 1984; 7:447–453.

69. O'Brien IAD, O'Hare JP, Lewin IG, Corrall RJM. The prevalence of autonomic neuropathy in insulin-dependent diabetes mellitus: A controlled study based on heart rate variability. Quart J Med 1986; 61:957–967.

70. Krolewski AS, Warram JH, Cupples A, et al. Hypertension, orthostatic hypotension and the microvascular complications of diabetes. J Chron Dis 1985; 38:319–326.

71. Ewing DJ, Clarke BF. Diabetic autonomic neuropathy: A clinical viewpoint. In: Dyck PJ, Thomas PK, Asbury AK, et al., eds. Diabetic neuropathy. Philadelphia: WB Saunders, 1987:66–88.

72. Rundles RW. Diabetic neuropathy. General review with report of 125 cases. Medicine 1945; 24:111–160.

73. McCulloch DK, Campbell IW, Wu FC, et al. The prevalence of diabetic impotence. Diabetologia 1980; 18:279–283.

74. Neubauer B, Christensen NJ. Norepinephrine, epinephrine and dopamine contents of the cardiovascular system in long-term diabetes. Diabetes 1976; 25:6–10.

75. Fagius J. Microneurographic findings in diabetic polyneuropathy with special reference to sympathetic nerve activity. Diabetologia 1982; 23:415–420.

76. Lloyd-Mostyn RH, Watkins PJ. Total cardiac denervation in diabetic autonomic neuropathy. Diabetes 1976; 25:748–751.

77. Ewing DJ, Martyn CN, Young RJ, Clarke BF. The value of cardiovascular autonomic function tests: 10 years experience in diabetes. Diabetes Care 1985; 8:491–498.

78. Goodman JI. Diabetic anhidrosis. Am J Med 1966; 41:831–835.

79. Martin MM. Involvement of autonomic nerve fibers in diabetic neuropathy. Lancet 1953; 1:560–565.

80. Watkins PJ. Facial sweating after food: A new sign of diabetic autonomic neuropathy. Br Med J 1973; 1:583–587.

81. Feldman M, Schiller LR. Disorders of gastrointestinal motility associated with diabetes mellitus. Ann Intern Med 1983; 98:378–384.

82. Hollis JB, Castell DO, Braddom RL. Esophageal function in diabetes mellitus and its relation to peripheral neuropathy. Gastroenterology 1977; 73:1098–1102.

83. Loo FD, Dodds WJ, Soergel KH, et al. Multipeaked esophageal peristaltic pressure waves in patients with diabetic neuropathy. Gastroenterology 1985; 88:485–491.

84. Kassander P. Asymptomatic gastric retention in diabetes (gastroparesis diabeticorum). Ann Intern Med 1958; 48:797–812.

85. Horowitz M, Harding PE, Chatterton PE, et al. Acute and chronic effects of domperidone on gastric emptying in diabetic autonomic neuropathy. Dig Dis Sci 1985; 30:1–9.

86. Faulk DL, Anuras S, Christensen J. Chronic intestinal pseudoobstruction. Gastroenterology 1978; 74:922–931.

87. Bargen JA, Bollman JL, Kepler EJ. The "diarrhea of diabetes" and steatorrhea of pancreatic insufficiency. Proc Staff Meet Mayo Clin 1936; 11:737–742.

88. Berenyi MR, Schwarz GW. Megasigmoid syndrome in diabetes and neurologic disease Am J Gastroenterol 1967; 47:311–320.

89. Kaiser FE, Korenman SG. Impotence in diabetic men. Am J Med 1988; 85(suppl 5a):147–152.

90. Lin JT, Bradley WE. Penile neuropathy in insulin-dependent diabetes mellitus. J Urol 1985; 133:213–215.

91. Andersen JT, Bradley WE. Early detection of diabetic visceral neuropathy. An electrophysiologic study of bladder and urethral innervation. Diabetes 1976; 25:1100–1105.

92. Smith SA, Smith SE. Evidence for a neuropathic aetiology in the small pupil of diabetes mellitus. Br J Ophthalmol 1983; 67:89–93.

93. Hayashi M, Ishikawa S. Pharmacology of pupillary responses in diabetics—correlative study of the responses and grade of retinopathy. Jpn J Ophthalmol 1979; 23:65.

94. Dyrberg T, Benn J, Christiansen JS, et al. Prevalence of diabetic autonomic neuropathy measured by simple bedside tests. Diabetologia 1981; 20:190–194.

95. Sharpey-Schafer EP, Taylor PJ. Absent circulatory reflexes in diabetic neuritis. Lancet 1960; 1:559–562.

96. Persson A, Solders G. R-R variations, a test of autonomic dysfunction. Acta Neurol Scand 1983; 67:285–293.

97. Sundkvist G, Almer L-O, Lilja B. Respiratory influence on heart rate in diabetes mellitus. Br Med J 1979; 1:924–925.

98. Bennett T, Riggott PA, Hosking DJ, Hampton JR. Twenty-four hour monitoring of heart rate and activity in patients with diabetes mellitus: A comparison with clinic investigations. Br Med J 1976; 1:1250–1251.

99. Beylot M, Haro M, Orgiazzi J, Noel G. Abnormalities of heart rate and arterial blood pressure regulation in diabetes mellitus. Relation with age, duration of diabetes and presence of peripheral neuropathy. Diab Metab (Paris) 1983; 9:204–211.

100. Fernandez-Castaner M, Mendola G, Levy I, et al. The prevalence and clinical aspects of the cardiovascular autonomous neuropathy in diabetic patients. Med Clin (Barc) 1985; 84:215.

101. Canal N, Comi G, Saibene V, et al. The relationship between peripheral and autonomic neuropathy in insulin dependent diabetes: A clinical and instrumental evaluation. In: Canal N, Pozza G, eds. Peripheral neuropathies. Amsterdam: Elsevier, 1978:247.

102. Hulper B, Willms B. Investigations of autonomic diabetic neuropathy of the cardiovascular system. Horm Metab Res 1980; suppl 9:77–80.

103. Odel HM, Roth GM, Keating FR Jr. Autonomic neuropathy simulating the effects of sympathectomy as a complication of diabetes mellitus. Diabetes 1955; 4:92–98.

104. Barany FR, Cooper EH. Pilomotor and sudomotor innervation in diabetes. Clin Sci 1956; 15:533–540.

105. Low PA, Walsh JC, Huang CY, McLeod JG. The sympathetic nervous system in diabetic neuropathy. A clinical and pathological study. Brain 1975; 98:341–356.

106. Haymaker W, Kernohan JW. The Landry-Guillain-Barré syndrome. A clinicopathologic report of fifty fatal cases and a critique of the literature. Medicine 1949; 28:59–141.

107. Singh NK, Jaiswal AK, Misra S, Srivastava PK. Assessment of autonomic dysfunction in Guillain-Barré syndrome and its prognostic implications. Acta Neurol Scand 1987; 75:101–105.

108. Truax BT. Autonomic disturbances in the Guillain-Barré syndrome. Semin Neurol 1984; 4:462–468.

109. Lichtenfeld P. Autonomic dysfunction in the Guillain-Barré syndrome. Am J Med 1971; 50: 772–780.

110. Narayan D, Huang MTC, Mathew PK. Bradycardia and asystole requiring permanent pacemaker in Guillain-Barré syndrome. Am Heart J 1984; 108:426–428.

111. Richards AM, Nicholls MG, Beard MEJ, et al. Severe hypertension and raised haematocrit: Unusual presentation of Guillain-Barré syndrome. Postgrad Med J 1985; 61:53–55.

112. McQuillan JJ, Bullock RE. Extreme labile blood pressure in Guillain-Barré Syndrome. Lancet 1988; 2:172–173.

113. Stapleton FB, Skoglund RR, Daggett RB. Hypertension associated with the Guillain-Barré syndrome. Pediatrics 1978; 62:588–590.

114. Guidon C, Granthil C, Djiane P, Francois G. Dysautonomie en deux temps au cours d'un syndrome de Guillain-Barré. Ann Fr Anesth Reanim 1986; 5:447–449.

115. Davies AG, Dingle HR. Observations on cardiovascular and neuroendocrine disturbance in the Guillain-Barré syndrome. J Neurol Neurosurg Psychiatry 1972; 35:176–179.

116. Bredin CP. Guillain-Barré syndrome: The unsolved cardiovascular problems. Irish J Med Sci 1977; 146:273–279.

117. Eiben RM, Gersony WM. Recognition, prognosis and treatment of the Guillain-Barré syndrome (acute idiopathic polyneuritis). Med Clin North Am 1963; 47:1371–1380.

118. Ventura HO, Messerli FH, Barron RE. Norepinephrine-induced hypertension in Guillain Barré syndrome. J Hypertension 1986; 4:265–267.

119. Yao H, Fukiyama K, Takada Y, et al. Neurogenic hypertension in the Guillain-Barré syndrome. Jpn Heart J 1985; 26:593–596.

120. Ahmad J, Kham AS, Siddiqui MA. Estimation of plasma and urinary catecholamines in Guillain-Barré syndrome. Jap J Med 1985; 24:24–29.

121. Davidson DLW, Jellinek EH. Hypertension and papilloedema in the Guillain-Barré syndrome. J Neurol Neurosurg Psychiatry 1977; 40:144–148.

122. Mitchell PL, Meilman E. The mechanism of hypertension in the Guillain-Barré syndrome. Am J Med 1967; 42:986–995.

123. Durocher A, Servais B, Caridroix M, et al. Autonomic dysfunction in the Guillain-Barré syndrome. Hemodynamic and neurobiochemical studies. Intens Care Med 1980; 6:3–6.

124. Fagius J, Wallin BG. Microneurographic evidence of excessive sympathetic outflow in the Guillain-Barré syndrome. Brain 1983; 106:589–600.

125. Birchfield RI, Shaw C-M. Postural hypotension in the Guillain-Barré syndrome. Arch Neurol 1964; 10:149–157.

126. Bansal BC, Sood AK, Jain SK. Dysautonomia in

Guillain-Barré syndrome. J Assoc Physicians India 1987; 35:417–419.

127. Tuck RR, McLeod JG. Autonomic dysfunction in Guillain-Barré syndrome. J Neurol Neurosurg Psychiatry 1981; 44:983–990.

128. Favre H, Foex P, Guggisberg M. Use of demand pacemaker in a case of Guillain-Barré syndrome. Lancet 1970; 1:1062–1063.

129. Greenland P, Griggs RC. Arrhythmic complications in the Guillain-Barré syndrome. Arch Intern Med 1980; 140:1053–1055.

130. Emmons PR, Blume WT, DuShane JW. Cardiac monitoring and demand pacemaker in Guillain-Barré syndrome. Arch Neurol 1975; 32:59–61.

130a. Persson A, Solders G. R-R variations in Guillain-Barré syndrome: a test of autonomic dysfunction Acta Neurol Scand 1983; 67:294–300.

131. Frison JC, Sanchez L, Garnacho A, et al. Heart rate variations in the Guillain-Barré syndrome. Br Med J 1980; 281:649.

132. Stewart IM. Arrhythmias in the Guillain-Barré syndrome (letter). Br Med J 1973; 2:665–666.

133. Palferman TG, Wright I, Doyle DV, Amiel S. Electrocardiographic abnormalities and autonomic dysfunction in Guillain-Barré syndrome. Br Med J 1982; 284:1231–1232.

134. Kogan BA, Solomon MH, Diokno AC. Urinary retention secondary to Landry-Guillain-Barré syndrome. J Urol 1981; 126:643–644.

135. Wheeler JS, Siroky MB, Pavlakis A, Krane RJ. The urodynamic aspects of the Guillain-Barré syndrome. J Urol 1984; 131:917–919.

136. Crozier RE, Ainley AB. The Guillain-Barré syndrome. N Engl J Med 1955; 252:83–88.

137. McCain MA. Guillain-Barré-associated diarrhea (letter). Dig Dis Sci 1985; 30:1112–1113.

138. McGuire EJ. Editorial. J Urol 1981; 126:644.

139. Guillain G. Radiculoneuritis with acellular hyperalbuminosis of the cerebrospinal fluid. Arch Neurol Psychiat 1936; 36:975–990.

140. Pinckney C. Acute infective polyneuritis with a report of five cases. Br Med J 1936; 2:333–355.

141. Williams D, Brust JCM, Abrams G, et al. Landry-Guillain-Barré syndrome with abnormal pupils and normal eye movements: A case report. Neurology 1979; 29:1033–1036.

142. Gecow A, Pawela I. Autonomic disturbances in the Guillain-Barré-Strohl syndrome in children. Pol Med J 1971; 10:1230–1235.

143. Young RR, Asbury AK, Corbett JL, Adams RD. Pure pan-dysautonomia with recovery. Description and discussion of diagnostic criteria. Brain 1975; 98:613–636.

144. Nass R, Chutorian A. Dysaesthesias and dysautonomia: A self-limited syndrome of painful dysaesthesias and autonomic dysfunction in childhood. J Neurol Neurosurg Psychiatry 1982; 45:162–165.

145. Fagius J, Westerberg C-E, Olsson Y. Acute pandysautonomia and severe sensory deficit with poor recovery. A clinical, neurophysiological and pathological case study. J Neurol Neurosurg Psychiatry 1983; 46:725–733.

146. Appenzeller O, Kornfeld M. Acute pandysautonomia. Arch Neurol 1973; 29:334–339.

147. Low PA. Autonomic Neuropathy. Semin Neurol 1987; 7:49–57.

148. Summers Q, Harris A. Autonomic neuropathy after rubella infection. Med J Aust 1987; 147:353–355.

149. Jenzer G, Mumenthaler M, Ludin HP, Robert F. Autonomic dysfunction in botulism B: A clinical report. Neurology 1975; 25:150–153.

150. McLeod JG, Tuck RR. Disorders of the autonomic nervous system: Part 1. Pathophysiology and clinical features. Ann Neurol 1987; 21:419–430.

151. Rubenstein AE, Horowitz SH, Bender AN. Cholinergic dysautonomia and Eaton-Lambert syndrome. Neurology 1979, 29:720–723.

152. Khurana RK, Koski CL, Mayer RF. Dysautonomia in Eaton-Lambert syndrome. Ann Neurol 1983; 14:123.

153. Mamdani MB, Walsh RL, Rubino FA, et al. Autonomic dysfunction and Eaton Lambert Syndrome. J Auton Nerv Syst 1985; 12:315–320.

154. Quinlan CD. Autonomic neuropathy in carcinoma of the lung. J Irish Med Assoc 1971; 64:430–431.

155. Riley CM, Day RL, Greeley DM, Langford WS. Central autonomic dysfunction with defective lacrimation. I. Report of five cases. Pediatrics 1949; 3:468–478.

156. Dyck PJ. Neuronal atrophy and degeneration predominantly affecting peripheral sensory and autonomic neurons. In: Dyck PJ, Thomas PK, Lambert EH, Bunge R, eds. Peripheral neuropathy, ed 2. Vol 2. Philadelphia: WB Saunders, 1984:1557–1600.

157. Ross AT. Progressive selective sudomotor denervation. A case with coexisting Adie's syndrome. Neurology 1958; 8:809–817.

158. Low PA, Fealey RD, Sheps SG, et al. Chronic idiopathic anhidrosis. Ann Neurol 1985; 18:344–348.

159. Schwartzman RJ, McLellan TL. Reflex sympathetic dystrophy. Arch Neurol 1987; 44:555–561.

160. Nathan PW. Pain and the sympathetic system. In: Bannister R, ed. Autonomic failure, ed 2. Oxford: Oxford University Press, 1988:733–747.

161. McLeod JG. Autonomic dysfunction in peripheral nerve disease. In: Bannister R, ed. Autonomic failure, ed 2. Oxford: Oxford University Press, 1988:607–623.

162. Cohen AS, Rubinow A. Amyloid neuropathy. In: Dyck PJ, Thomas PK, Lambert EH, Bunge R, eds. Peripheral neuropathy, ed 2. Vol 2. Philadelphia: WB Saunders, 1984:1866–1898.

163. French JM, Hall G, Parish DJ, Smith WT. Peripheral and autonomic nerve involvement in primary amyloidosis associated with uncontrollable diar-

rhea and steatorrhoea. Am J Med 1965; 39:277–284.

164. Andrade C. A peculiar form of peripheral neuropathy. Brain 1952; 75:408–426.

165. Lessell S, Wolf PA, Benson MD, Cohen AS. Scalloped pupils in familial amyloidosis. N Engl J Med 1975; 293:914–915.

166. Falco de Freitas A, Azevedo S, Maciel L. Defective cardiovascular autonomic responses in familial amyloidotic polyneuropathy. In: Glenner GG, Costa P, Freitas A, eds. Amyloid and amyloidosis. Amsterdam: Excerpta Medica, 1980:106.

167. Olofsson BO, Andersson R, Furberg B. Atrioventricular and intraventricular conduction in familial amyloidosis with polyneuropathy. Acta Med Scand 1980; 208:77–80.

168. Nordborg L, Kristensson K, Olsson Y, Sourander P. Involvement of the autonomous nervous system in primary and secondary amyloidosis. Acta Neurol Scand 1973; 49:31–38.

169. Gorchein A. Autonomic neuropathy in porphyria. In: Bannister R, ed. Autonomic failure, ed 2. Oxford: Oxford University Press, 1988:715–732.

170. Ridley A, Hierons R, Cavanagh JB. Tachycardia and the neuropathy of porphyria. Lancet 1968; 2:708–710.

171. Gibson JB, Goldberg A. The neuropathology of acute porphyria. J Pathol Bacteriol 1956; 71:495–509.

172. Stewart PM, Hensley WJ. An acute attack of variegate porphyria complicated by severe autonomic neuropathy. Aust NZ J Med 1981; 11:82–83.

173. Gupta GL, Saksena HC, Gupta BD. Cardiac dysautonomia in acute intermittent porphyria. Ind J Med Res 1983; 78:253–256.

174. Yeung Laiwah AAC, MacPhee GJA, Boyle P, et al. Autonomic neuropathy in acute intermittent porphyria. J Neurol Neurosurg Psychiatry 1985; 48:1025–1030.

175. Shirger A, Martin WJ, Goldstein NP, Huizenga KA. Orthostatic hypotension in association with acute exacerbations of porphyria. Proc Mayo Clin 1962; 37:7–11.

176. Ingall TJ, McLeod JG, Tamura N. Autonomic function and unmyelinated fibers in chronic inflammatory demyelinating polyradiculoneuropathy. Muscle Nerve 1990; 13:70–76.

177. Low PA, Walsh JC, Huant CY, McLeod JG. The sympathetic nervous system in alcoholic neuropathy. Brain 1975; 98:357–364.

178. Decaux G, Cauchie P, Soupart A, et al. Role of vagal neuropathy in the hyponatremia of alcoholic cirrhosis. Br Med J 1986; 293:1534–1536.

179. Duncan G, Johnson RH, Lambie DG, Whiteside EA. Evidence of vagal neuropathy in chronic alcoholics. Lancet 1980; 2:1053–1057.

180. McLeod JG, Penny R. Vincristine neuropathy: An electrophysiological and histological study. J Neurol Neurosurg Psychiatry 1969; 32:297–304.

181. Bank WJ, Pleasure DE, Suzuki K, et al. Thallium poisoning. Arch Neurol 1972; 26:456–464.

182. Fraser DM, Campbell IW, Miller HC. Peripheral and autonomic neuropathy after treatment with perhexiline maleate. Br Med J 1977; 2:675–676.

183. LeQuesne PM, McLeod JG. Peripheral neuropathy following a single exposure to arsenic. J Neurol Sci 1977; 32:437–451.

184. Solders G. Autonomic function tests in healthy controls and in terminal uraemia. Acta Neurol Scand 1986; 73:638–639.

185. Endre ZH, Perl SI, Kraegen EW, et al. Reduced cardiac beat-to-beat variation in chronic renal failure: A ubiquitous marker of autonomic neuropathy. Clin Sci 1982; 62:561–562.

186. Campese VM, Romoff MS, Levitan D, et al. Mechanisms of autonomic nervous system dysfunction in uremia. Kidney Int 1981; 20:246–253.

187. Jammes JL. The autonomic nervous system in peroneal muscular atrophy. Arch Neurol 1972; 27:213–220.

188. Brooks AP. Abnormal vascular reflexes in Charcot-Marie-Tooth disease. J Neurol Neurosurg Psychiatry 1980; 43:348–350.

189. Solders G, Nennesmo I, Persson A. Diphtheritic neuropathy, an analysis based on muscle and nerve biopsy and repeated neurophysiological and autonomic function tests. J Neurol Neurosurg Psychiatry 1989; 52:876–880.

190. Bannister R, Oppenheimer DR. Degenerative disease of the nervous system associated with autonomic failure. Brain 1972; 95:457–474.

191. Shy GM, Drager GA. A neurological syndrome associated with orthostatic hypotension. Arch Neurol 1960; 2:511–527.

192. Mathias CJ, Matthews WB, Spalding JMK. Postural changes in plasma renin activity and responses to vasoactive drugs in a case of Shy-Drager syndrome. J Neurol Neurosurg Psychiatry 1977; 40:138–143.

193. Bannister R, Ardill L, Fentem P. Defective autonomic control of blood vessels in idiopathic orthostatic hypotension. Brain 1967; 90:725–746.

194. Cohen J, Low PA, Fealey R, et al. Somatic and autonomic function in progressive autonomic failure and multiple system atrophy. Ann Neurol 1987; 22:692.

195. Kihara M, Takahashi A. Sweating disorder in Shy-Drager syndrome. Excerpta Medica International Congress Series, 1991; 517–519.

196. Low PA, Fealey RD. Structure and function of pre- and postganglionic neurons in pure autonomic failure and multisystem atrophy with autonomic failure. In: Bannister R, ed. Autonomic failure, ed 2. Oxford: Oxford University Press, 1988: 544–557.

197. Fealey RD, Schirger A, Thomas JE. Orthostatic hypotension. In: Spittell JA Jr, ed. Clinical medicine. Vol 7. Philadelphia: Harper & Row, 1985: 1–12.

198. Gross M, Bannister R, Godwin-Austen R. Orthostatic hypotension in Parkinson's disease. Lancet 1972; 1:174–176.

199. Kuroiwa Y, Shimada Y, Toyokura Y. Postural hypotension and low R-R interval variability in parkinsonism, spino-cerebeller degeneration, and Shy-Drager syndrome. Neurology 1983; 33:463–467.

200. Mathias CJ, Christensen NJ, Frankel HL, Spalding JMK. Cardiovascular control in recently injured tetraplegics in spinal shock. Q J Med 1979; 48:273–287.

201. Wallin BG, Stjernberg L. Sympathetic activity in man after spinal cord injury. Brain 1984; 107:183–198.

202. Guttmann L, Whitteridge D. Effects of bladder distension on autonomic mechanisms after spinal cord injuries. Brain 1947; 70:361–404.

203. Corbett JL, Frankel HL, Harris PJ. Cardiovascular reflex responses to cutaneous and visceral stimuli in man. J Physiol (Lond) 1971; 215:395–409.

204. Appenzeller O, Descarries L. Circulatory reflexes in patients with cerebrovascular disease. N Engl J Med 1964; 271:820–823.

205. Hsu CY, Hogan EL, Wingfield W, et al. Orthostatic hypotension with brain stem tumors. Neurology 1984; 34:1137–1143.

206. Wood JR, Camilleri M, Low PA, Malagelada J-R. Brainstem tumor presenting as an upper gut motility disorder. Gastroenterology 1985; 89:1411–1414.

207. Sharpey-Schafer EP. Circulatory reflexes in chronic disease of the afferent nervous system. J Physiol (Lond) 1956; 134:1–10.

208. Sterman AB, Coyle PK, Panasci DJ, Grimson R. Disseminated abnormalities of cardiovascular autonomic functions in multiple sclerosis. Neurology 1985; 35:1665–1668.

209. Weinstein L, Shelokov A. Cardiovascular manifestations in acute poliomyelitis. N Engl J Med 1951; 244:281–285.

210. Kemp E. Arterial hypertension in poliomyelitis. Acta Med Scand 1957; 157:109–118.

211. McDowell FH, Plum F. Arterial hypertension associated with acute anterior poliomyelitis. N Engl J Med 1951; 245:241–245.

212. Cohen JA, Laudenslager M. Autonomic nervous system involvement in patients with human immunodeficiency virus infection. Neurology 1989; 39:1111–1112.

213. Lipsitz LA. Orthostatic hypotension in the elderly. N Engl J Med 1989; 321:952–957.

214. Low PA. Quantitation of autonomic responses. In: Dyck PJ, Thomas PK, Lambert EH, Bunge R, eds. Peripheral neuropathy, ed 2. Philadelphia: WB Saunders, 1984: 1139–1165.

II

Diseases of the Peripheral Nervous System

7

Radiculopathies

Asa J. Wilbourn
Michael J. Aminoff

CONTENTS

LIST OF ACRONYMS

CMAP	compound muscle action potential
MUP	motor unit potential
NCS	nerve conduction studies
NEE	needle electrode examination
SEP	somatosensory evoked potential

In this chapter, the anatomical, clinical, thermographic, and, particularly, the electrodiagnostic aspects of radiculopathies are reviewed. The various electrodiagnostic techniques used in the detection of radiculopathies are discussed in some detail, with emphasis on their value and limitations and on certain technical aspects of clinical relevance.

HISTORICAL ASPECTS

Clinical

Root compression caused by disorders of the bones and supporting structures surrounding the spinal cord and cauda equina has been a source of human suffering and disability for centuries. Probably the earliest recorded instance of symptomatic root involvement appeared in the Edward Smith Surgical Papyrus, an Egyptian manuscript dated 2500 to 4500 years B.C.; it concerned a patient with back and leg pain that increased with leg elevation.[1-3]

Although its symptoms have been known for several thousand years, compressive radiculopathy was not recognized as a distinct clinical entity until this century. The link between lumbar intervertebral disc disorders and symptoms involving the back and lower extremities was not firmly established until the publication of Mixter and Barr's landmark article in 1934.[4] Until then and for some years afterwards, the lower limb symptoms of root compression were attributed to a variety of causes, the most common being sciatic nerve compromise by various conditions, such as scarring or piriformis muscle spasm.[5] (One legacy from those earlier times is the term *sciatica,* introduced by Hippocrates and used for centuries to describe, among other symptoms, the lower extremity pain experienced with L-5 or S-1 radiculopathies.[2,6])

Cervical intervertebral disc disorders were not generally recognized as a cause for neck and upper extremity symptoms until after the paper by Semmes and Murphey[7] on cervical radiculopathy was published in 1943. Before that time, such upper limb symptoms usually were attributed erroneously to lesions situated more distally along the peripheral neuraxis, particularly to brachial plexopathies resulting from compression by a hypertrophic anterior scalene muscle (scalenus anticus syndrome) or a vague inflammatory process (*brachial neuritis*).[5]

Beginning in the 1940s, a number of publications described compression of the spinal cord, cauda equina, and individual lumbosacral roots by degenerative changes of the spinal canal rather than solely by disc abnormalities; probably the most influential of these were the 1949 and 1954 articles by Verbiest,[8] concerned with narrowing of the lumbar canal, and the 1952 paper by Brain et al.[9] on cervical spondylosis. The current concepts of cervical and lumbar spondylosis causing secondary canal stenosis, sometimes superimposed on congenital stenosis, evolved over the following years. It is now appreciated that intervertebral disc protrusion is the most common cause for radicular symptoms only in adults less than 40 to 50 years of age. More complex degenerative changes of the spinal canal usually are responsible in older patients. Often multiple factors are involved, such as posterior osteophyte formation, facet subluxation, or hypertrophy owing to proliferative osteoarthritis and thickening or bulging of the ligamentum flava. Thus in patients older than 50 years, bone, rather than disc, material frequently is the source of root injury.[10-14]

It was not widely appreciated that root compression could result from thoracic disc disorders until after a series of papers appeared on the subject in the 1950s. The delay in recognition of thoracic radiculopathies probably stems from their relative infrequency and because they often are overshadowed by concomitant spinal cord compression.[11,15]

Electrodiagnosis

Electrodiagnostic examinations have been performed on patients with radiculopathies for almost 50 years. The first reported studies were those mentioned in 1944, by Weddell et al.[16] in their pioneering paper concerned with the electromyographic findings on needle electrode examination (NEE) in normal, denervated, and reinnervated muscles and in patients with certain *specific neurologic affections,* including facial nerve paralysis, spinal cord lesions and *sciatica.* Although they reported examining "the muscles of the lower extremities in over 50 cases of sciatica," as well as the upper extremity in at least one patient with a cervical radiculopathy, they did not perform the NEE primarily for diagnostic purposes. Instead they used it mainly to distinguish denervation atrophy from disuse atrophy in those patients who had limb muscle wasting and weakness. Thus many of the patients they studied probably had already undergone therapeutic laminectomies. Similarly, although they surveyed the paraspinal muscles in at least 50 patients (two series of 25 patients each), they studied them after laminectomy, to ascertain if the onset of fibrillation potentials was relatively constant in different individuals and to determine whether the paraspinal muscles were weak because of denervation or because of reversible ischemic conduction block. Weddell et al.[16] described the motor unit potential (MUP) firing pattern changes caused by nerve fiber injury as well as the biphasic spike form of fibrillation potentials. They also reported motor unit action potentials that appeared in *outbursts* on needle insertion and then fired repetitively, on an involuntary basis.[16] Presumably these were fibrillation potentials having a positive sharp wave form, which were not labeled as such until 1949.[17,18] In 1946, Brazier et al.[19] reported that they had identified cervical radiculopathies affecting the C-7 root in 12 patients using electrodiagnostic methods. They used surface rather than needle electrodes for recording, however, and primarily ink-writing oscillographs rather than cathode ray oscilloscopes for display. Moreover, for diagnosis, they relied on the presence of myotomal fasciculation potentials, rather than fibrillation potentials.[19]

The first article employing current methods to describe the value of the electromyographic examination in diagnosing radiculopathies appeared in 1950. Shea et al.[20] used the NEE to assess 75 consecutive patients with radiculopathies, 72 caused by disc disease and three by neoplasms. They reported a success rate of over 90% for detecting root damage, relying primarily on the presence of fibrillation potentials and suggestive reinnervational MUPs in an appropriate myotomal distribution (60 lumbosacral, 14 cervical, and one thoracic.)[20] In a subsequent paper, Woods and Shea[21] stressed the importance of NEE of the paraspinal muscles in the diagnosis of radiculopathy because those muscles are innervated by the posterior primary rami of the roots. By 1955, *root compression syndromes* merited an entire chapter in the first English-language book devoted solely to electromyography (EMG).[22] A number of other articles soon appeared, reporting the value of the electromyographic examination (i.e., the NEE) for diagnosing radiculopathies, particularly lumbosacral root lesions.[6,23–26] Several other electrodiagnostic procedures were added to the armamentarium of the electromyographer over the following years, including the late responses (H waves and F waves) and somatosensory evoked potentials (SEPs).

GENERAL ANATOMY

Thirty-one pairs of dorsal and ventral roots arise from the spinal cord, consisting of eight cervical, 12 thoracic, five lumbar, five sacral, and one coccygeal. Most of the fibers in the ventral roots originate from motor neurons in the anterior and lateral gray columns of the spinal cord. In contrast, the dorsal root axons arise from cells located outside the spinal cord, in the dorsal root ganglia (DRG). These collections of sensory cell bodies are situated very distally along the dorsal roots, immediately before they join the anterior roots to form the mixed spinal nerves (Figure 7.1). Consequently, the DRG usually are within the bony intervertebral foramina (i.e., they are intraforaminal rather than intraspinal). Just after leaving the intervertebral foramina, the spinal nerves terminate by dividing into small posterior and large anterior primary rami. The former supply the skin and deep intrinsic muscles of the posterior neck and trunk, whereas the latter supply the remaining portions of the trunk and, through intervening plexuses, the limbs.[11,27,28]

Except for C-8, the cervical roots exit cephalad to the vertebrae sharing their same numerical designations; for example, the C-6 root leaves the intraspinal canal by passing between the C-5 and the C-6 vertebrae. Because there are only seven cervical vertebrae but eight cervical roots, the C-8 root exits between the C-7 and T-1 vertebrae. Below that level, the roots exit caudal to the vertebrae with the same numerical designations; for example, the L-4 root passes between the L-4 and L-5 vertebrae.

In adults, the vertebral column is much longer than the spinal cord. Consequently, the various spinal cord segments are not at the same levels as the corresponding vertebral spinous processes. This

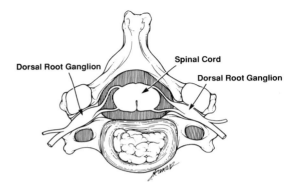

FIGURE 7.1.   *Cervical region, transverse section, showing the relationship of the spinal cord, spinal roots, and dorsal root ganglia to the surrounding bone structures. The dorsal root ganglia are within the intervertebral foramina.*

disparity increases from the neck caudally: "In the upper cervical region the cord level is approximately one segment above the spinous process of the same numerical designation, in the thoracic region there is typically a two-segment difference, and in the lumbar region the difference is almost three segments."[11] The spinal cord typically terminates at the L-1–L-2 disc level. Consequently, the more caudal spinal roots must descend beside and beyond it to reach their exiting foramina. Collectively these long intraspinal motor fibers and preganglionic sensory fibers compose the cauda equina[28–30] (Figure 7.2).

Referring physicians often view radiculopathies in terms of disc levels (e.g., L-4–L-5 lesion), whereas electromyographers refer to the specific root involved (e.g., L-4 root lesion). Such differences in viewpoint can lead to some misunderstanding regarding the root on which the electrodiagnostic examination should be focused. This can be a particular problem with lumbosacral radiculopathies because a lesion at a single disc level can compress roots derived from more than one segment; for example, a lesion at the L-4–L-5 level can injure the L-4, the L-5, or the S-1 root, depending on its size and location.[28,31,32]

The cutaneous region and muscles supplied by a specific spinal cord segment are referred to as a *dermatome* and a *myotome,* respectively. Consecutive dermatomes overlap; that is, a particular skin area generally is within the dermatomal field of two adjacent spinal nerves. Similarly, consecutive myotomes overlap, so almost all muscles are constituents of more than one myotome, receiving innervation from two or more contiguous roots.[31,33] Significant variation may occur between individuals in both the dermatomal fields and the muscles composing individual myotomes.[11,34] Further, dermatomes and myotomes of the same segment do not necessarily correspond anatomically, especially in the limbs. Thus the skin of the thenar eminence is in the C-6 dermatome, whereas the thenar muscles are components of the C-8 and T-1 myotomes.

ROOT ANATOMY AND PATHOPHYSIOLOGY

A number of factors at the root level directly bear on whether a particular electrodiagnostic study will help in the diagnosis of a radiculopathy and, if so, which component of it will be useful. The interplay of these same factors accounts for the fact that compression of the same root in different patients, or at different times in the same patient, may result in different clinical presentations.[28]

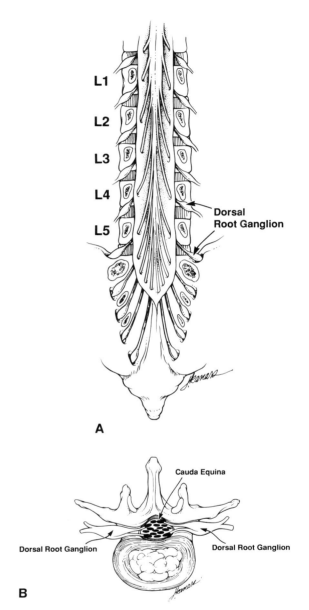

A

B

FIGURE 7.2. *(A) Lumbosacral region, coronal section, showing the relationship of the cauda equina and dorsal root ganglia to the surrounding bone structures. The sensory fibers of the cauda equina are preganglionic because their dorsal root ganglia are in the foramina. (B) Cauda equina and dorsal root ganglia, transverse section.*

Portions of the following material concerning various aspects of root compression are somewhat conjectural, based on various clinical, surgical, and electrophysiologic findings with radiculopathies and on extrapolation of known facts about the pathophysiologic effects of focal lesions affecting myelinated peripheral nerve fibers.[35-38] Little direct information is available regarding root pathophysiology because "the roots (are) a region over which conduction is not readily studied in man," a point McDonald[39] made a quarter-century ago.

Lesion Location

With compression from either disc herniation or spondylosis, the more distal segments of the roots typically are affected but at a site proximal to the DRG. Consequently, even when preganglionic sensory root fibers are so compromised that they undergo wallerian degeneration, the postganglionic peripheral sensory fibers are unaffected[28,40-42] (Figure 7.3). For this reason, sensory nerve conduction studies (NCS), which assess the peripheral sensory fibers only up to the DRG, show no abnormalities with radiculopathies.

Type of Fibers Affected

Roots are composed of smaller unmyelinated and larger myelinated axons; the myelinated fibers, in turn, are of various sizes. Fibers of all sizes presumably are injured with radiculopathies, but the large fibers may be more at risk from compression.[36] The most common symptom of root compression, pain within the dermatomal distribution or a portion

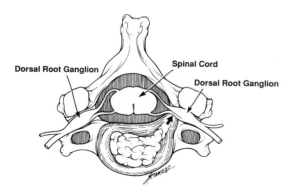

FIGURE 7.3. *Usual site of root injury with a compressive cervical radiculopathy. The sensory fibers are injured proximal to their dorsal root ganglia.*

Dorsal Root Ganglion
Spinal Cord
Dorsal Root Ganglion

thereof, is due to injury of the unmyelinated and smaller myelinated axons, whereas paresthesias, position and vibratory sense impairment, weakness, and changes in the tendon reflexes are indicative of large myelinated fiber dysfunction. Only damage of the larger myelinated fibers can be detected in the EMG laboratory because the function of only those fibers is assessed by the electrophysiologic procedures in use.[28]

Number of Fibers Affected

In compressive radiculopathies, only some, usually a minority, of the fibers in the affected root are injured. Moreover, only a fraction of the injured fibers typically undergo axon degeneration. Thus with relatively few exceptions, there is only partial axon loss, in contrast to root infarctions and surgical rhizotomies, which often cause virtually all the nerve root fibers to degenerate.[43-45]

Pathophysiology at Lesion Site

Focal lesions of myelinated root fibers typically cause axon degeneration, focal demyelination, or both. Which of these two pathophysiologic reactions is operative and the type and number of affected fibers are the major determinants of the electrophysiologic findings.[5,32,35,46]

Root compression beyond a certain degree destroys motor and sensory axons, and the axon segments separated from their cell bodies subsequently degenerate. Thus the motor fibers degenerate distal to the compression site, whereas the peripheral sensory fibers are spared, and only the central processes of the DRG cells are affected.

Mild root injury that is insufficient to cause axon degeneration may still damage myelinated fibers, producing focal demyelination that results in localized conduction abnormalities at the lesion site. Depending on its severity, focal demyelination causes conduction slowing or conduction block. Conduction slowing, in turn, can affect all the involved fibers to the same degree (focal synchronized slowing) or to different degrees (differential or desynchronized slowing). These various processes have different clinical and physiologic manifestations.[5,28]

Both axon loss and demyelinating conduction block prevent nerve impulses from traversing the lesion site. Consequently, when they affect a substantial number of fibers (which seldom occurs with single radiculopathies), they may cause identical clinical and electrophysiologic findings; these include a fixed sensory deficit, weakness, and deep tendon reflex abnormalities clinically as well as a neurogenic MUP firing pattern on NEE (see later), low amplitude/unelicitable H waves, and a decrease in the number of F waves obtainable with a particular number of stimuli. Certain electrophysiologic findings, however, are dissimilar. Thus when recorded from a clinically weak muscle during motor NCS, the compound muscle action potential (CMAP) obtained is low in amplitude or unelicitable if axon loss is the responsible process, but normal in amplitude if demyelinating conduction block is the cause of the weakness because the distal peripheral motor fibers are intact. Nonetheless, at least some fibrillation potentials typically will be found on NEE of the recorded muscle because severe conduction block lesions rarely occur in pure form; compression severe enough to cause focal demyelinating conduction block along a significant number of motor fibers almost invariably causes some fibers to degenerate.[47]

Conduction block affecting a minimal number of motor fibers probably causes no discernible clinical or electrophysiologic abnormalities. Mild motor axon loss at the root level similarly may have no clinical manifestations but does result in hundreds of individual muscle fibers fibrillating in at least some of the muscles of the affected myotome, the exact number reflecting the innervation ratios of the muscles. Because of its high sensitivity for detecting such minor axon loss, the NEE remains the premier method for diagnosing radiculopathies.[5,43]

In contrast to root lesions producing axon loss or conduction block, those causing conduction slowing via demyelination yield few clinical findings. Neither focal synchronized slowing nor differential slowing produce weakness or major sensory abnormalities because all nerve impulses ultimately reach their destinations. Differential slowing interferes with the transmission of discrete volleys of nerve impulses and therefore may cause impairment of deep tendon reflexes and vibratory appreciation, unelicitable H waves and increased scatter of F waves.[37,48] It is conceivable that transient conduction block may occur in association with focal conduction slowing at the root level in humans, but this has never been established.[38] Electrophysiologically, demyelinating focal conduction slowing may cause prolonged H wave latencies and delayed F waves if most or all of the fibers mediating these responses are affected; SEPs rarely are delayed, however, presumably because the region of conduction slowing is so small compared with the total length of the sensory pathway that is assessed.

ELECTRODIAGNOSIS OF RADICULOPATHIES

More patients are studied in North American EMG laboratories for suspected radiculopathies than for any other single cause, as Johnson et al.[49] first noted over a quarter-century ago. This is somewhat surprising when the following two points are considered. First, electrodiagnostic studies are not as sensitive for detecting radiculopathies as they are for detecting many other entities, such as carpal tunnel syndrome or generalized demyelinating polyneuropathies and polyradiculoneuropathies. There are several reasons for this lower sensitivity. (1) The very proximal location of the lesion severely compromises the value of the NCS portion of the examination: Focal conduction abnormalities (i.e., demyelinating and very early axon loss lesions) cannot be detected because the nerve fibers cannot be stimulated proximal to the lesion. (2) Compressive radiculopathies characteristically involve only a proportion of the root fibers. (3) A variety of pathophysiologic reactions occur at the lesion site, some of which—focal slowing, differential slowing, and all but severe conduction block—have no appreciable effect on any of the basic components of the electromyographic examination (NCS and NEE).[46] Second, despite numerous publications on the electrodiagnostic evaluation of radiculopathies, electromyographers disagree on a surprising number of important points concerning this topic (Table 7.1). These are discussed individually in the following sections.

TABLE 7.1. Electrodiagnostic assessment for radiculopathy*

Relative value of H wave; amplitude versus latency
Earliest time to perform NEE after onset of symptoms
Relative value of NEE of limb muscles versus paraspinal muscles.
Value of
  F waves
  Somatosensory evoked potentials
  NEE of paraspinal muscles after laminectomy
  Various NEE findings
    Insertional positive sharp waves
    Fasciculation potentials
    Complex repetitive discharges
    Neurogenic MUP firing pattern
    Polyphasic MUPs (early, late)

* Issues in dispute among electromyographers regarding the electrodiagnostic assessment for radiculopathy. Many of these are interrelated. See text for details.

NEE, Needle electrode examination; MUP, motor unit potential.

ELECTRODIAGNOSTIC PROCEDURES AVAILABLE

Conventional Nerve Conduction Studies

The motor and sensory NCS characteristically remain normal with monoradiculopathies, for different reasons.

Motor nerve conduction studies

Root lesions causing solely or predominantly focal demyelination never alter the findings because the nerve segments being assessed are distal to the lesion site, and conduction along them remains normal. Root lesions causing axon loss may affect the CMAP amplitude, which reflects the number of viable nerve fibers supplying the muscle. Consequently, the CMAP amplitude decreases as increasing numbers of motor fibers to the muscle degenerate. Even this component, however, usually is unaltered because the extent to which denervation occurs in myotomal muscles is limited, for two reasons: (1) With a typical radiculopathy, only a minority of the root fibers to individual muscles degenerate; (2) muscles are innervated by more than one segment, so involvement of one root leaves intact innervation from the unaffected root(s).[28] Moreover, the muscles used for recording during the basic upper and lower extremity motor NCS are innervated solely by the C-8 and T-1 roots and the L-5–S-2 roots, respectively, so motor axon loss involving any other roots, no matter how severe, will go undetected unless nonroutine motor NCS are performed.

With monoradiculopathies, low-amplitude CMAPs are seen only when the injured root is responsible for a substantial amount of the total innervation of the muscle under study and when an unusually high number of its fibers degenerate.[5,28] These two situations seldom coincide, so the CMAPs typically remain within the normal range. One major exception is the occasional patient with a severe axon loss L-5 radiculopathy: the CMAPs of the tibialis anterior and extensor digitorum brevis muscles following peroneal nerve stimulation usually are very low in amplitude.

By contrast, with multiradiculopathies, small or even unelicitable CMAPs frequently are recorded from muscles supplied by contiguous roots when the latter are injured. Concurrent involvement of adjacent roots indicates a more extensive lesion, often with more axon loss in each affected root than usual, and such lesions may compromise the entire inner-

vation of individual muscles. For the most part, multiradicular involvement is limited to the L-3 through S-2 roots and usually is secondary to cauda equina lesions; low-amplitude or even unelicitable CMAPs frequently are bilateral in these circumstances but are often asymmetric in degree. Whenever the CMAPs are small, the motor distal latencies and conduction velocities may be mildly slowed, owing to loss of the fastest conducting fibers. The lower extremity sensory NCS (sural; superficial peroneal sensory) remain normal in these patients, even when the CMAPs are of low amplitude or unelicitable, thereby suggesting the lesion is within the lumbar intraspinal canal.[28]

Sensory nerve conduction studies

The sensory NCS rarely are altered by radiculopathies, regardless of the pathophysiology and severity of the process, because only preganglionic sensory fibers are injured. The DRG and the peripheral sensory fibers derived from them, which are assessed by sensory NCS, are unaffected[40–42] (Figure 7.4).

Late Responses

F waves

First described by McDougall and Magladery in 1950, these responses were named *F waves* because they initially were recorded from the intrinsic foot muscles.[50] F waves are generated whenever the motor fibers of a peripheral nerve are stimulated. Nerve impulses travel not only toward the periphery along the stimulated fibers to produce the direct M response (CMAP), but also proximally to the spinal cord. When the antidromic impulses reach the spinal cord, a few of them cause motor neurons to discharge, thereby sending impulses back down the motor fibers to produce submaximal muscle activation, that is, small (F) responses that are variable in latency and configuration. Several different aspects of F waves can be assessed. The latency of the shortest response, the *minimal latency,* was the first parameter to be used and has been the most widely employed. It reflects conduction time along one of the largest diameter motor axons in the stimulated nerve.[50–58]

F wave studies assess the entire motor axon, from the anterior horn cell to the muscle fibers it supplies. They should, therefore, be quite useful in the assessment of very proximal neurogenic lesions, such as radiculopathies and plexopathies, because they can evaluate segments of the motor nerve that are more

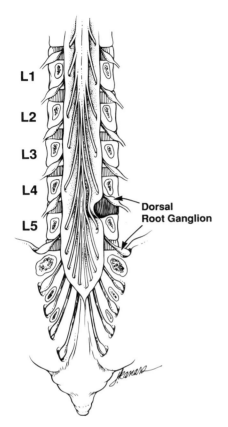

L1

L2

L3

L4

L5

Dorsal
Root Ganglion

FIGURE 7.4.   *One of the sites of root injury with a lumbosacral radiculopathy. The sensory root fibers are injured proximal to their dorsal root ganglia.*

proximal than those studied by conventional motor NCS. Unfortunately, however, most electromyographers have found F waves relatively useless for evaluating patients with radiculopathies. Usually they are normal, and even when abnormal they often are of little practical importance because changes of more localizing value are found on NEE.[28,46,59–61]

The low sensitivity of F waves for detecting compressive radiculopathies can be attributed to several factors. First, most criteria for F wave abnormalities require the lesion to cause focal slowing at the lesion site. This may not occur, or be detectable, for the following reasons: (1) The pathophysiology at the site of injury may be other than conduction slowing; that is, it may be solely axon loss or conduction block or a combination of the two. (2) Even if focal slowing is present, the affected segment is so short compared with the entire length of motor axon being

assessed that the slowing along it can easily be obscured. (3) F waves, being elicited by stimulation of the peripheral nerve supplying the recorded muscle, are mediated by motor fibers derived from more than one root; in patients with isolated radiculopathies, slowing affecting the fibers traversing the involved root can be concealed by the normal conduction along fibers traversing the uninvolved root(s). Second, even when F wave are prolonged, they do not localize the lesion to the root level. Instead, they merely indicate that conduction is slowed at one or more points along the motor axons, extending from the spinal cord distally. Slowed F waves, for example, do not distinguish radiculopathies from plexopathies, and in patients with proximal lesions, this is often the specific differential diagnosis. Third, F wave studies assess only the motor root fibers. This is probably an important limitation because radiculopathies cause sensory symptoms more often than motor, suggesting preferential involvement of the sensory fibers.[28]

H waves

The H reflex is a monosynaptic spinal reflex that, unlike the F wave test, assesses both motor and sensory fibers. It was first described by Hoffmann in 1918 and is named after him.[50] H waves are consistently obtained in adults only when the tibial nerve is stimulated in the popliteal fossa, and the response is recorded from the gastrocnemius/soleus muscle group. Thus in practical terms, the H response can be used only to assess the S-1 root. For the most part, H waves traverse the same nerve fiber pathways as impulses mediating the Achilles tendon reflex.[45] Consequently, when H waves and ankle jerks are elicited from the limb, the findings correlate highly with one another: In one study, the concordance was 86%.[62] Almost all electromyographers have found H responses to be very sensitive and therefore quite helpful for detecting S-1 radiculopathies. Rather surprisingly, however, these same electromyographers differ regarding which component of the H wave response is important for diagnostic purposes. Some consider only the H wave latency of value; they find it prolonged with S-1 radiculopathies,[63–68] indicating that focal slowing is the pathophysiology at the lesion site. In contrast, others consider the H wave amplitude alone to be important in S-1 radiculopathies: Either the response is unelicitable, or it is low in amplitude (less than 1 mV in amplitude, or less than 50% in amplitude of the contralateral H wave).[28,46] This suggests that axon loss, conduction block, or differential slowing is the pathophysiology responsible. In a study of 200 consecutive patients in whom H wave testing was performed bilaterally, H wave amplitudes were abnormal in 166 limbs, whereas the H latencies were abnormal (asymmetry of >2 ms) in only four limbs.[62] Reconciling these two markedly divergent views is difficult.

Among the various basic electrodiagnostic procedures, H wave studies have certain distinct advantages in assessing patients for radiculopathies. First, they are the only procedure that evaluates preganglionic sensory fibers. Second, like F waves, they theoretically become abnormal at the onset of root compression and remain abnormal until root integrity is restored. They therefore differ significantly from the NEE in this regard, as is noted subsequently. Third, they are extremely sensitive to compromise of the S-1 root fibers.[28]

Unfortunately, H wave studies also have significant limitations. First, because both the motor and sensory components of the H response traverse the S-1 root, they are of positive value only for assessing S-1 radiculopathies. Second, although their sensitivity for detecting S-1 radiculopathies is high, false-negative studies occasionally result, presumably because the particular S-1 root fibers mediating the response have been spared. Third, an abnormal H response does not localize pathology to the root level. Instead, the responsible lesion may be situated anywhere along the S-1 motor and sensory pathways being tested; that is, from the S-1 spinal cord segment through the motor and sensory roots, sacral plexus, sciatic nerve, and proximal portion of the tibial nerve. Fourth, H waves tend to remain unelicitable indefinitely once they are lost because of S-1 root compression. Hence their absence is of no value in establishing the development of an active S-1 radiculopathy in a patient with a previous S-1 lesion. Fifth, H waves are sensitive to other neurogenic processes besides radiculopathies. Bilaterally absent H waves are particularly vexing in this regard. They can be seen not only with bilateral S-1 radiculopathies, such as frequently occurs with cauda equina lesions, but also with generalized polyneuropathies (often as an early manifestation) and with some congenital spinal deformities; for example, spinal spondylolisthesis. Sixth, bilaterally absent H waves also are commonly found in two other circumstances: (1) in apparently normal patients over age 60 years of age; most often the lower extremity sensory responses are also unelicitable in these patients, but occasionally they are still present, and the resulting combination falsely suggests a lumbar intraspinal

canal lesion involving the S-1 fibers bilaterally; and (2) following conventional lumbar laminectomy, even when the surgery was performed for a unilateral lesion and for other than S-1 root compression; the reason for this is unknown, but in any patient, regardless of age, who has previously undergone a lumbar laminectomy, bilaterally unelicitable H responses must be interpreted with caution.[28,45]

Motor Nerve Root Stimulation

In this procedure, stimuli are applied to motor nerve fibers by means of a monopolar needle electrode inserted into the cervical paraspinal muscles, and the evoked CMAPs are recorded with surface electrodes from upper extremity muscles representative of the various cervical myotomes. These nerve root stimulations are performed bilaterally at different segmental levels, and the results are compared for differences in amplitude and latency.[69] This technique evolved from lumbosacral root stimulation techniques first described in the 1970s to evaluate the lumbosacral roots and plexus.[70,71] The cervical procedure has been used for both root and brachial plexus assessment, but its role in both contexts is controversial. At least one group of experienced electromyographers has reported that it is highly sensitive for detecting compressive cervical radiculopathies.[69] Others believe, however, that the motor fibers are being stimulated at the level of the mixed spinal nerve, or even the proximal brachial plexus, rather than within the intraspinal canal.[72,73] If the motor fibers are indeed being initially depolarized at either of the two extraforaminal sites, the segment of nerve being assessed is too distal to include that injured by root compression.

Somatosensory Evoked Potentials

SEPs are conveniently elicited by electrical stimuli that are delivered transcutaneously to a mixed or sensory nerve or, less commonly, to the skin in the territory of an individual nerve or nerve root.[74] Nerve stimulation excites particularly the large fast-conducting group Ia and group II afferent fibers. The stimuli, repeated at 3 or 5 Hz, should be monophasic rectangular pulses of short duration (100 to 300 μs) and at an intensity that is either slightly above motor threshold (if a mixed nerve is stimulated) or two or three times above sensory threshold. A contact impedance of 5000 ohms or less helps to reduce patient discomfort. For clinical purposes, the nerves most commonly stimulated are the median or ulnar at the wrist, the peroneal at the knee, and the posterior tibial at the ankle, but any accessible nerve can be stimulated. Responses are recorded with either surface or needle electrodes from the nerve proximal to the site of stimulation, and over the spine and scalp. A ground electrode placed on the stimulated limb reduces stimulus artifact. Guidelines have been published by the American Electroencephalographic Society concerning the optimal recording arrangements, but these are currently being revised.[75]

Computer averaging permits the SEPs to be extracted from background cerebral activity. The analysis time is governed by the SEP being recorded. The number of individual trials to be averaged depends on the size of the signal of interest, the quality of the recording, and the amount of background noise, but usually between 500 and 2000 individual trials are required when recording SEPs derived from stimulation of the upper limbs and between 1000 and 4000 responses to stimulation of the lower limbs. At least two averages should always be obtained to ensure that the findings are replicable. Noise relates most often to muscle and movement artifact and usually can be reduced by sedating the patient for the study. The optimal filter settings of the recording system depend on the purpose of the study, but in most clinical contexts a bandpass of 30 to 3000 Hz is satisfactory.[74]

The responses are characterized by their polarity at the active electrode with respect to the reference point and by their normal poststimulus mean latency in adults. In the SEPs derived by the stimulation of a nerve in the arm, it is generally possible to recognize consistently an Erb's point potential, an N13/P13-14 in recordings made between the cervical spine and the midfrontal scalp (FZ), and an N20 in the recording made between the contralateral "hand" area of scalp (C3'/C4') and FZ. Other early components are found less consistently in normal subjects. The cervical N13, which can be recorded referentially from the back of the neck, is derived predominantly from postsynaptic activity in the cord, whereas P14, which can be recorded over a wide area of the scalp, probably reflects activity in the medial lemniscus. The N20 probably is generated in the primary somatosensory cortex and is thus recorded using a bipolar derivation to eliminate far field activity recorded at the scalp. It is followed by a number of different peaks, depending on the site of recording over the scalp, and these probably have distinct cortical generators.[74]

Potentials generally can be recorded over the vertex (CZ) of the scalp with respect to a cephalic reference following stimulation of nerves in the lower extremity, such as the peroneal nerve at the knee, and P37 (sometimes designated P40) and N45 components are found following stimulation of the posterior tibial nerve at the ankle. In addition, with stimulation of a lower extremity nerve, a propagated negative potential can be detected over the cauda equina, and a widespread, nonpropagated negative lumbar potential can be recorded referentially over the thoracolumbar spine, which is related predominatly to postsynaptic activity in the lumbar cord.[76]

The SEPs are evaluated with regard to both component and intercomponent latency, in relation to height or limb length. Both absolute latency and interside latency difference are considered, and responses are judged to be abnormal if these exceed the mean value for control subjects by more than 2.5 or 3 standard deviations. Less stringent criteria for abnormality lead to an unacceptably high false-positive rate. The presence or absence of individual components of the response is also important in determining whether SEPs are abnormal. Changes in response amplitude and morphology are less useful when interpreting SEPs because of the normal wide variability in amplitude and the subjective nature of evaluating morphology.

On theoretical grounds, SEP studies should be important in the evaluation of suspected radiculopathies because they provide a means of determining function in the sensory root fibers. There are, however, a number of limitations to their use in this context. A discrete, compressive lesion may not cause a prolongation in latency of the SEP recorded over the spine or scalp because any slowing of conduction in the compressed segment of the nerve fibers traversing the involved root is masked by the normal velocity of conduction in the long pathway from the point of peripheral stimulation to the site at which the responses are generated. Moreover, when the SEP is elicited by stimulation of a multisegmental nerve trunk, any slowing of conduction caused by a lesion involving a single root will be obscured by the normal conduction speed in fibers traversing the adjacent, unaffected roots. Even if the lesion has caused focal conduction block in some fibers of the affected root, normal conduction in the remaining fibers—and the marked amplitude variation of SEPs between subjects and between sides in the same subject—usually prevents its recognition. Further, abnormal SEPs do not suggest either the age or nature of the underlying pathology and provide only limited information concerning the precise location of lesions proximal to the DRG.

Nerve trunk stimulation

With the aforementioned considerations in mind, it would be surprising if SEPs derived from nerve trunk stimulation provided information of any diagnostic value in patients with isolated radiculopathies. Indeed, we have found that in patients with isolated compressive lumbosacral root lesions, the peroneal-derived SEP is always normal.[59,77] Claims by some investigators of a high incidence of SEP abnormalities in such circumstances are difficult to evaluate because insufficient details usually are provided.[78]

In cervical spondylosis, patients without objective neurologic signs generally have normal median, ulnar, and radial SEPs; when radicular signs are present, the SEPs may be abnormal, regardless of whether there is an accompanying myelopathy.[79–81] An abnormal SEP, however, generally is accompanied by abnormalities on NEE, so little further is gained by the additional electrophysiologic study.

Cutaneous nerve stimulation

The cutaneous nerves segmentally are more specific than the nerve trunks from which they arise. Accordingly SEPs elicited by stimulating these nerves may reveal abnormalities caused by isolated radiculopathies when SEPs derived from nerve trunk stimulation are normal. Using this technique, Eisen et al.[82] reported that 57% of 28 patients with suspected cervical or lumbosacral root lesions had abnormal scalp-recorded SEPs, the abnormalities typically consisting of amplitude reductions or morphology alterations; latency abnormalities were uncommon. The diagnostic yield by NEE, however, was greater (75%).[82] Perlik et al.[83] subsequently used a similar technique to study 27 patients with low back pain, unilateral radicular symptoms, and abnormal computed tomography scans. They found that 21 of these patients had abnormal scalp-recorded SEPs. More importantly, only six had any other electrophysiologic abnormalities, and those six patients also had clinical abnormalities. The authors therefore suggested that SEPs elicited from cutaneous nerves were sensitive indicators of compressive radiculopathies.[83] Seyal et al.,[84] however, using the same technique, found scalp-recorded SEPs to be abnormal in only 20% of patients with appropriate radiologic abnormalities. Clearly, further clarification of the sensitivity of scalp-recorded SEPs derived from cutaneous nerve stimulation is required before the technique is used routinely to evaluate patients with suspected radiculopathies.

An approach that is more likely to reveal abnormalities involves recording the SEPs over the spine at the lumbar root entry zone, following stimulation of segmentally specific cutaneous nerves in the legs. In this regard, Seyal et al.[84] have studied 21 patients with lumbosacral radiculopathy by recording the responses over the spine as well as the scalp to stimulation of the saphenous, superficial peroneal, and sural nerves. They found that the SEPs recorded over the spine were abnormal in 10 patients, whereas the scalp-recorded responses were abnormal in only four. Spinal segmental SEPs thus appeared to be the more sensitive procedures. The most common abnormality was prolongation in latency of the spinal negative peak or its absence or attenuation relative to that elicited by stimulation of the asymptomatic limb. In three of their patients, segmental SEPs detected abnormalities when NEE failed to do so, but the complete extent of nerve root involvement as determined by clinical, radiographic, and electromyographic examination was predicted by SEPs in only one patient. There was, moreover, a poor correlation between the presence of SEP abnormalities and clinical sensory disturbance in a radicular distribution.[84]

Dermatomal stimulation

Another electrophysiologic approach to the diagnosis of radiculopathies has been to record the SEPs over the scalp to stimulation of the skin in a dermatomal distribution. This generally involves stimulation on the dorsum of the foot, between the first and second toes, for L-5, and on the lateral border of the foot, at the level of the fifth metatarsophalangeal joint, for S-1. Early investigators reported a remarkably high diagnostic yield in lumbosacral root entrapment syndromes, but these results have to be discounted because of the apparently arbitrary criteria selected for defining abnormality and the absence of data from control subjects.[85–87]

Aminoff et al.[59,77] found that in only about 25% of patients with clinically unequivocal L-5 or S-1 compressive root lesions could the diagnosis be confirmed, whereas NEE revealed signs of denervation in a myotomal pattern in 75%. Their experience therefore corresponds to that of Seyal et al., who detected abnormalities in the scalp-recorded SEPs (derived from cutaneous nerve stimulation) in only 20%.

Katifi and Sedgwick[88] used a technique similar to that of Aminoff et al. and obtained similar values from normal subjects. They reported, however, a much higher (95%) diagnostic yield for dermatomal

SEPs among patients with lumbosacral root disease. Unfortunately, many of their patients had widespread disease, which complicates the interpretation of the electrophysiologic findings, as also does the more generous criteria for abnormality that they used. Thus they regarded as abnormal any latency or interside latency values that exceeded the normal mean value by more than 2 (as opposed to 3) standard deviations, and they considered abnormal the absence of an initial positivity solely at the vertex of the scalp, whereas in occasional normal subjects, this peak may be absent or markedly attenuated at CZ but present at the ipsilateral C3'/C4' location.[89,90] They took the operative findings as their gold standard, and inspection of their data reveals that the dermatomal SEP findings suggested false-positive abnormalities of 12 roots, that is, roots that were found not to be involved at operation; indeed, in only four of their 21 patients were the operative findings accurately and completely predicted by the SEP studies, mirroring the experience of Aminoff et al. and again suggesting a very limited role for this approach.

The same conclusion seems justified with regard to cervical radiculopathy. In a study of 24 patients with radiologically verified cervical disc prolapse, 13 were evaluated with dermatomal SEP studies, and in 11 the results were abnormal.[91] In six of these 11 patients, however, the abnormality was at the wrong level. Thus a useful role for dermatomal SEPs in the diagnosis of cervical root lesions has not been demonstrated.

Needle Electrode Examination

Of all the electrodiagnostic methods used to assess patients with suspected radiculopathy, the NEE is by far the oldest, having been used first for that purpose in 1950,[20] and it still has the highest diagnostic yield.[28,59,77,82,92] For this reason, it remains the single most useful technique, and therefore it is emphasized in this chapter.

The NEE has a number of limitations when used to evaluate patients with root compression. First, it assesses only motor fibers. Second, it detects primarily only motor axon loss.[32,45] Although it may reveal an unusually severe demyelinating conduction block in motor root fibers, by demonstrating a neurogenic firing pattern of MUPs on NEE similar to that produced by equally severe axon loss lesions, this is infrequent with isolated compressive radiculopathies.[28] Third, when the findings are suggestive of a radiculopathy, they do not identify its cause; the NEE abnormalities caused by degenerative disc dis-

orders and spondylosis can be identical to those attributable to a number of other disorders, including osteomyelitis; neoplasms; arachnoid cysts; root lacerations; certain meningeal processes, for example, arachnoiditis and sarcoidosis; and various spinal nerve disorders, for example, those caused by diabetes mellitus, herpes zoster, and acquired immunodeficiency syndrome (AIDS).[11] Fourth, the findings on NEE may reveal the affected root but not the intervertebral level of the responsible pathology. This fact, as previously noted, has particular relevance with lumbosacral radiculopathies because the roots follow a rather long course within the intraspinal canal as components of the cauda equina, and those derived from more than one segment therefore are vulnerable to a single level lesion; for example, a disc herniation between the L-4 and L-5 vertebrae may compress the L-4 root, the L-5 root, or the S-1/S-2 roots, depending on whether it is far lateral, posterolateral, or midline, respectively.[31,45] Fifth, whenever NEEs are performed to evaluate patients with suspected radiculopathies, many muscles must be assessed for the study to be adequate. Some electromyographers are reluctant to do this. In a textbook concerned with neuromuscular disorders, for example, the authors state "it is rarely necessary to examine more than four muscles" in adults.[93] Such a parsimonious study is incompatible with the use of the NEE to diagnose radiculopathies. Several other limitations are discussed subsequently.

The basis for the NEE diagnosis of an isolated radiculopathy is the presence of abnormalities in at least two, and preferably more, limb muscles innervated by the involved root, coupled with the absence of such abnormalities in muscles innervated by other roots, including those adjacent to the affected one.[21,22] Thus the electrical abnormalities must be restricted to the distribution of a single myotome for the NEE to be indicative of an isolated radiculopathy.

A number of myotomal charts of the upper and lower extremities are available. Electromyographically determined myotomal charts, however, are more accurate than clinically determined ones because muscle strength testing is far less sensitive than the NEE for detecting minimal denervation.[28,33]

An additional stipulation for NEE diagnosis of a radiculopathy is that the affected muscles are innervated by different peripheral nerves.[28] This condition frequently is violated, without justification, with C-7 radiculopathies; often they are diagnosed whenever abnormalities are found in two or more C-7/radial-innervated muscles (e.g., triceps and extensor digitorum communis) without any attempt being made to find similar abnormalities in C-7/median-innervated muscles (e.g., pronator teres or flexor carpi radialis). This requirement, however, is too restrictive with many lumbosacral radiculopathies, because all the muscles distal to the knee, innervated by the L-5 and S-1 roots, receive intermediate innervation via the sciatic nerve. Consequently, with many chronic L-5 radiculopathies, in which the NEE abnormalities are detectable only in the more distal limb myotomal muscles, all the affected muscles are innervated by the sciatic nerve trunk. In this situation, it is sufficient to have the more distal nerve supply be derived from two different peripheral nerve branches, for example, the peroneal and tibial nerves. Also, detecting similar abnormalities in the appropriate paraspinal muscles is always helpful and sometimes (depending on the specific root involved) necessary for definite localization.

Several limb muscles and the appropriate paraspinal muscles must be surveyed for the NEE to be adequate. Muscles both within and outside the suspected myotome must be assessed. At least two or three muscles within the myotome must be studied, regardless of whether or not abnormalities are found. If they are, then they must be detected in this limited number of muscles to establish their myotomal distribution. Diagnosing a radiculopathy based on NEE changes in a single muscle is never justified because the responsible neurogenic lesion actually could be (1) located anywhere along the pathway extending from the anterior horn cells to the terminal nerve fibers supplying the muscle or (2) affecting the other root(s) that innervate the muscle, rather than the root arbitrarily designated as injured. Similarly, at least two or three muscles within a given myotomal distribution must be shown to be normal before it is reasonable to conclude that no NEE evidence of a radiculopathy is present because no single muscle innervated by a particular root invariably contains abnormalities when that root is compromised, particularly with incomplete lesions.

Whenever abnormalities have been demonstrated in a myotomal distribution, it is important to prove that they are restricted to that myotome by examining several other muscles in the same limb supplied by different roots. Failure to do this is one of the main reasons why diffuse neurogenic entities (e.g., motor neuron disease and polyradiculopathies) are misdiagnosed as monoradiculopathies in the EMG laboratory.

One method of assuring an adequate NEE is to perform a *general survey* or *root search,* by examining several proximal and distal limb muscles, including muscles from each myotome, plus the appropriate paraspinal muscles. Because of the pattern of paraspinal muscle innervation, muscles at and caudal to the suspected level are studied. If involvement of a specific root is suspected or if abnormalities are found in any of the muscles, additional muscles innervated by the root or roots in question are assessed. The specific muscles included in such a NEE evaluation vary from one electromyographer to another; the general surveys used by one of the authors to assess the upper and lower extremities are shown in Tables 7.2 and 7.3.

The question arises concerning which electrical *abnormalities,* when found in a myotomal distribution, are reliable for the diagnosis of a radiculopathy. Fibrillation potentials have been universally accepted for this purpose since the 1950 report by Shea et al.[20] Probably most electromyographers also would consider *chronic neurogenic MUP changes*—MUPs of increased duration, possibly increased amplitude, and usually polyphasic—as valuable indicators of a chronic (greater than 4 to 6 months duration) axon loss radiculopathy or the residuals of a remote, rather severe static lesion of that nature.

In the context of neurogenic lesions, fibrillation potentials are spontaneous, rhythmical action potentials generated by denervated muscle fibers. Because each motor unit consists of one neuron and all the muscle fibers it innervates, the loss of even a single motor root fiber can result in many individual muscle fibers fibrillating in at least some of the muscles of the myotome, and these minute potentials are readily detected on NEE.[43,94] For this reason, fibrillation potentials are the most sensitive indicator of motor axon loss, and demonstrating their presence in a root distribution has been the mainstay for the electromyographic diagnosis of a radiculopathy for over 40 years. This approach has significant disadvantages

TABLE 7.2.   General survey of upper extremity*

First dorsal interosseous (C-8, T-1)
Extensor indicis proprius (C-8)
Flexor pollicis longus (C-8, T-1)
Pronator teres (C-6, C-7)
Biceps (C-5, C-6)
Triceps (C-7)
Deltoid (C-5, C-6)
Cervical paraspinals

* Muscles included in the general survey (*root search*) of the upper extremity by one of the authors.

TABLE 7.3.   General survey of lower extremity*

Extensor digitorum brevis (L-5, S-1)
Abductor hallucis (S-1, S-2)
Tibialis anterior (L-4, L-5)
Flexor digitorum longus/tibialis posterior (L-5, S-1)
Medial gastrocnemius (S-1, S-2)
Vastus lateralis (L-2–L-4)
Gluteus medius/gluteus maximus (L-5; S-1, S-2)
Lumbar paraspinals

* Muscles included in the general survey (*root search*)
of the lower extremity by one of the authors.

as well, however, the most serious being related to the time of appearance and disappearance of fibrillation potentials following the onset of a static radiculopathy. Regarding the former, a lengthy delay occurs between the onset of denervation and the development of fibrillation potentials in the affected muscles. This time lag customarily is said to be 3 weeks, but in fact it is somewhat variable, relating to the length of the motor nerve segment interposed between the site of injury and the denervated muscle: The shorter the segment, the sooner fibrillation potentials appear. Thus they develop in a centrifugal distribution; for example, with L-5 or S-1 radiculopathies, fibrillation potentials may be detected as early as the second week after onset in the lumbar paraspinal muscles, by the third week in the midlimb muscles, and sometimes as late as the fifth week in the intrinsic foot muscles.[95] Moreover, in a relatively small percentage of patients (*late fibbers*), the appearance of fibrillation potentials is inexplicably delayed for 1 to 3 weeks beyond the customary time.

False-negative studies may result whenever NEEs are performed earlier than 21 days after the onset of symptoms; the earlier the study is performed, the more likely it is to be false-negative. The fact that fibrillation potentials do not develop at the onset of motor axon loss lesions is one of the main reasons that many clinicians relegate electrodiagnostic studies to a secondary role in assessing patients with suspected radiculopathies, failing to appreciate the important information that still can be gained from them. Nonetheless, this physiologic limitation is inherent to the procedure and cannot be circumvented.

A major misconception regarding fibrillation potentials and compressive radiculopathies is that root lesions causing motor axon degeneration will result in partial denervation throughout the myotome; that is, fibrillation potentials will be detectable in all the muscles innervated by the involved root. This erro-

neous theory originated with some early electromyographers, a few of whom went further and stipulated that fibrillation potentials had to be present not only in every muscle of the myotome, but also to the same degree in every muscle.[22] In practice, however, such total myotomal involvement is restricted to a relatively small number of patients studied: those with an unusually large amount of motor root axon loss, who are studied relatively early in their course, for example, between 3 weeks and 3 months following onset.

Fibrillation potentials seldom are found throughout the entire myotome with compressive monoradiculopathies for several reasons. First, the root innervation of individual muscles commonly varies among individuals. Consequently, in a given patient, a particular muscle may not be in the myotome to which it is customarily assigned. In most patients, for example, the tibialis anterior muscle receives a substantial amount of innervation from two roots: L-4 and L-5. In some limbs, however, it is innervated almost solely by either the L-4 or the L-5 root. Consequently, in some patients with L-5 radiculopathies, fibrillation potentials will not be detected in the tibialis anterior muscle, although they may be found in other muscles belonging to the L-5 myotome, whereas in other patients, they will be abundant in that muscle and accompanied by obvious MUP loss. Second, although each muscle is innervated by more than one root, it is not necessarily innervated to the same extent from each root. Instead, some muscles typically receive a preponderance of their innervation from a single root. These are designated *marker* muscles for that root because when the root is damaged they are far more likely to contain fibrillation potentials than are muscles receiving only a relatively small amount of their innervation from it. The marker muscles for the various cervical and lumbosacral roots, based on our experience, are shown in Figures 7.5 and 7.6. Third, as already noted, with compressive radiculopathies, usually only a portion of the root is affected, and typically only a portion of those fibers undergo axon loss. Hence some of the muscles of the myotome often are spared because the root fibers supplying them were not injured or not injured enough to degenerate. Fourth, fibrillation potentials typically are found more often in distal than proximal limb muscles with proximal partial axon loss lesions of any type. Fifth, an additional factor is introduced whenever static radiculopathies of several months duration are studied: the disappearance of myotomal fibrillation potentials in a proximodistal direction, as a result of collateral sprouting.[28] This

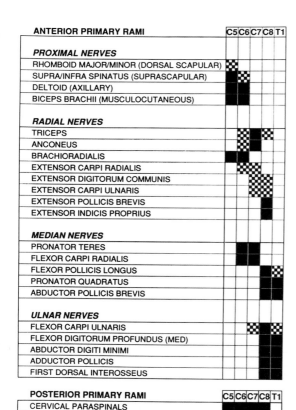

ANTERIOR PRIMARY RAMI	C5	C6	C7	C8	T1
PROXIMAL NERVES					
RHOMBOID MAJOR/MINOR (DORSAL SCAPULAR)	▨	▨			
SUPRA/INFRA SPINATUS (SUPRASCAPULAR)	■	▨			
DELTOID (AXILLARY)	■	■			
BICEPS BRACHII (MUSCULOCUTANEOUS)	■	■			
RADIAL NERVES					
TRICEPS			▨	■	▨
ANCONEUS			■	■	
BRACHIORADIALIS		■	■		
EXTENSOR CARPI RADIALIS			■	▨	
EXTENSOR DIGITORUM COMMUNIS				▨	
EXTENSOR CARPI ULNARIS				▨	▨
EXTENSOR POLLICIS BREVIS				■	
EXTENSOR INDICIS PROPRIUS				■	
MEDIAN NERVES					
PRONATOR TERES		■	■		
FLEXOR CARPI RADIALIS		■	■		
FLEXOR POLLICIS LONGUS				■	▨
PRONATOR QUADRATUS				■	■
ABDUCTOR POLLICIS BREVIS				■	■
ULNAR NERVES					
FLEXOR CARPI ULNARIS			▨	■	▨
FLEXOR DIGITORUM PROFUNDUS (MED)				■	■
ABDUCTOR DIGITI MINIMI				■	■
ADDUCTOR POLLICIS				■	■
FIRST DORSAL INTEROSSEUS				■	■

POSTERIOR PRIMARY RAMI	C5	C6	C7	C8	T1
CERVICAL PARASPINALS	■	■	■	■	
HIGH THORACIC PARASPINALS				■	■

ANTERIOR PRIMARY RAMI	L2	L3	L4	L5	S1	S2
PROXIMAL NERVES						
ILIACUS	■	▨				
ADDUCTOR LONGUS (OBTURATOR)	▨	■	■			
VASTUS LATERALIS/MEDIALIS (FEMORAL)		■	■			
RECTUS FEMORIS (FEMORAL)		■	■			
TENSOR FASCIA LATA (GLUTEAL)				■	▨	
GLUTEUS MEDIUS (GLUTEAL)				■	▨	
GLUTEUS MAXIMUS (GLUTEAL)				▨	■	▨
SCIATIC NERVES						
SEMI TENDINOSUS/MEMBRANOSUS (TIBIAL)				■	■	
BICEPS FEMORIS (SHT.HD) (PERONEAL)				■	■	▨
BICEPS FEMORIS (LONG HD) (TIBIAL)				■	■	
PERONEAL NERVES						
TIBIALIS ANTERIOR			▨	■		
EXTENSOR HALLUCIS				■	■	
PERONEAL LONGUS				■	■	
EXTENSOR DIGITORUM BREVIS				■	■	
TIBIAL NERVES						
TIBIALIS POSTERIOR			▨	■		
FLEXOR DIGITORUM LONGUS				■	■	
GASTROCNEMIUS LATERAL					■	▨
GASTROCNEMIUS MEDIAL					■	▨
SOLEUS					■	▨
ABDUCTOR HALLUCIS					■	■
ABDUCTOR DIGITI QUINTI PEDIS					■	■

POSTERIOR PRIMARY RAMI	L2	L3	L4	L5	S1	S2
LUMBAR PARASPINALIS	■	■	■	■		
HIGH SACRAL PARASPINALS					■	■

FIGURE 7.5.   *Chart of upper extremity muscles which authors have found useful in the electromyographic recognition of isolated cervical root lesions. Solid squares indicate "marker" muscles for the root, i.e., those that most often contain abnormalities. Checkered squares indicate muscles that, while also helpful for diagnosis, are abnormal less frequently. These charts are not intended to indicate the entire myotomal representation of the individual muscles.*

FIGURE 7.6.   *Chart of lower extremity muscles which authors have found useful in the electromyographic recognition of isolated lumbosacral root lesions. Solid squares indicate "marker" muscles for the root, i.e., those that most often contain abnormalities. Checkered squares indicate muscles that, while also helpful for diagnosis, are abnormal less frequently. These charts are not intended to indicate the entire myotomal representation of the individual muscles.*

important mechanism of reinnervation is discussed subsequently.

Another major misconception is that fibrillation potentials will always be present in the paraspinal muscles with a radiculopathy. In fact, NEE of the paraspinal muscles is unrevealing in many patients with proved root lesions. Thus in this regard, the paraspinal muscles must be viewed as any other muscle of the myotome; that is, they may or may not be partially denervated with a radiculopathy. Nonetheless, the value of finding paraspinal fibrillation potentials in patients with suspected radiculopathies

should not be minimized. Unless spinal surgery has been performed earlier through a midline posterior approach, NEE of the paraspinal muscles is always indicated. These muscles are innervated by the posterior primary rami, which are derived from the mixed spinal nerves almost as soon as the latter emerge from the intervertebral foramina; consequently, if paraspinal fibrillation potentials are found, the responsible lesion must be located very proximally, either within or close to the intraspinal canal.[32,44,96,97]

Assessment of the paraspinal muscles has definite

limitations, however, which often are not acknowledged. First, NEE of the paraspinal muscles usually is more difficult than of most limb muscles because achieving satisfactory muscle relaxation can be difficult, particularly in the thoracic, and sometimes the cervical, region.[46] (It is interesting to note that Weddell et al.,[16] in their 1944 report, contended that the cervical paraspinal muscles could not be examined by NEE because they were impossible to relax.) Second, because of extensive myotomal overlap, the particular root involved cannot be determined by the distribution of paraspinal fibrillation potentials.[28,32] Although some electromyographers believe that the deep paraspinal muscles are strictly segmentally innervated, whereas only the more superficial ones have marked segmental overlap, this concept has never been validated by systematic studies.[11] Third, with many unequivocal radiculopathies, fibrillation potentials simply cannot be found in the appropriate paraspinal muscles, no matter how extensive and exhaustive the search. There are two possible reasons for this: (1) The paraspinal muscles were never denervated because the motor root fibers innervating them were spared as a result of incomplete root involvement; (2) the paraspinal muscles were partially denervated for a relatively short period following the onset of root compression but were reinnervated, with the disappearance of the fibrillation potentials, before the NEE was performed.[28] Fourth, a number of entities in addition to typical compressive root lesions can produce focal paraspinal fibrillation potentials, including metastases to the motor roots and the posterior primary rami, arachnoiditis, various anterior horn cell disorders, necrotizing myopathies, and, especially, diabetes mellitus.[28] In diabetes, paraspinal fibrillation potentials most often are found bilaterally in the lower (lumbosacral) segments, but sometimes they are present bilaterally in a more widespread distribution. Fifth, the value of paraspinal muscle examination in patients who have undergone prior laminectomy via a midline posterior approach is controversial. It has been known since 1944 that fibrillation potentials can be seen in the paraspinal muscles after laminectomy because of retractor-related stretch injuries sustained by the posterior primary rami at the time of surgery.[16] For this reason, paraspinal fibrillation potentials found near the surgical scar in postlaminectomy patients are of uncertain etiology: local nerve injury versus recurrent radiculopathy. Because of this uncertainty, many electromyographers consider paraspinal muscle examination to be of no value in these patients. In contrast, a minority consider them beneficial in some instances, depending on the elapsed time since

surgery and on various aspects of needle placement (distance from surgical scar; depth of insertion).[33,45,95,97–99]

Just as NEEs can be performed too soon after the onset of a radiculopathy for fibrillation potentials to have developed, they can be performed too late, after myotomal fibrillation potentials have disappeared. With static radiculopathies, evidence of reinnervation—like changes of denervation—appears first in the most proximal muscles and proceeds distally. Reinnervation can occur via two different mechanisms: (1) progressive proximodistal regeneration from the injury site, which is the only process available if the muscle is totally denervated, and (2) collateral sprouting from surviving axons supplying the muscle[100]; this process is particularly effective in partially denervated muscles, such as is characteristic of radiculopathies, and is the predominant process for reinnervation of the distal limb muscles. Collateral sprouting occurs first in the proximal muscles and generally is more efficient in them.[43] For this reason, when NEEs are performed several months after the onset of static root injuries, fibrillation potentials frequently are limited to the more distal myotomal muscles, which have not yet been reinnervated. With many radiculopathies, the affected muscles are partially denervated to only a mild degree, and a minor amount of collateral sprouting restores full function. Consequently, within a few months, these muscles appear normal on NEE. Conversely, with other radiculopathies, denervation is severe enough that subsequent reinnervation via collateral sprouting leaves permanent MUP abnormalities, especially in the more distal muscles; such chronic neurogenic MUP changes are due to motor units containing more than their normal complement of muscle fibers, the additional muscle fibers having been adopted after the axons initially supplying them degenerated. Because the intact axons now each control substantially more muscle fibers than normal, they generate abnormal MUPs—chronic neurogenic MUPs—manifested by increased duration and sometimes increased amplitude. The latter change primarily is seen, in the context of radiculopathies, with chronic cervical root compression, most often caused by spondylosis.[44,95] Once such MUP changes have developed, they may persist indefinitely.

The distribution of fibrillation potentials and chronic neurogenic MUP changes within the myotome provides some information regarding the duration and activity of the denervating process. If fibrillation potentials are found throughout the myotome, in both proximal and distal limb muscles, unaccompanied by chronic neurogenic MUP changes, the radiculopathy is likely to be of relatively recent onset. Conversely, if only chronic neurogenic MUP changes are present, frequently restricted to the more distal muscles of the myotome, the radiculopathy is probably both static and remote in time. If both fibrillation potentials and chronic neurogenic MUP changes are present in a myotomal distribution, either an acute radiculopathy has been superimposed on a chronic one or a chronic progressive radiculopathy is present; which of these possibilities is most likely must be determined by the clinical history.[28,43]

Two points are noteworthy regarding myotomal fibrillation potentials and radiculopathies. First, the presence of fibrillation potentials throughout the root distribution several months after the onset of symptoms indicates that root compression is progressive rather than static in nature; that is, motor root fiber injury with subsequent axon degeneration must be ongoing to maintain fibrillation potentials in the proximal myotomal muscles. Second, with static radiculopathies, progressive muscle reinnervation occurs by collateral sprouting, independent of the status of the root fibers at the compression site. Consequently, fibrillation potentials may disappear from the myotome despite continued root compression (and the persistence of sensory symptoms)[28] (Figure 7.7). The fact that the NEE with static radiculopathies *normalizes with time* limits the ability of the procedure to detect chronic, nonprogressive radiculopathies.

Fibrillation potentials and chronic neurogenic MUP changes in a myotomal distribution are universally accepted as reliable evidence of present or prior root compromise, in the appropriate clinical situation. Whether other electrical abnormalities are similarly indicative of root compression is unclear, as is discussed next.

Insertional positive sharp waves are seen in several situations. They characteristically are found with very early axon loss lesions, preceding by a few days the development of spontaneous fibrillation potentials in denervated muscles. Based on this fact, some electromyographers perform NEEs earlier than 3 weeks after symptom onset, seeking to diagnose a radiculopathy by finding myotomal insertional changes alone. There are several serious problems with this approach. First, many muscles in the affected myotome may not contain insertional positive sharp waves so soon after the onset of root compression, although at a later time they may contain them. The fact that *some* patients may develop insertional positive sharp waves in some proximal limb myotomal muscles as early as the thirteenth day after onset[65] is irrelevant; unless *most* patients will do so, an unacceptably high incidence of false-negative studies will result if studies are performed that early. Second, insertional positive sharp waves should not be found throughout the myotome with a radiculopathy because they are transient phenomena, preceding the development of spontaneous fibrillation potentials. They may be seen in the proximal myotomal muscles alone with early lesions, but by the time they appear in the distal muscles, they should have been replaced by spontaneous fibrillation potentials more proximally. Consequently, whenever insertional positive sharp waves are present simultaneously in both proximal and distal myotomal muscles, a more extensive NEE is mandatory. Almost invariably it will

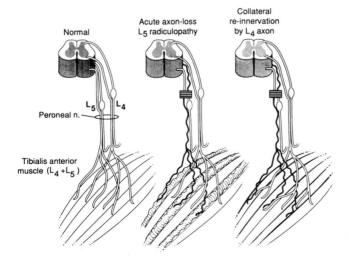

Normal

Acute axon-loss L5 radiculopathy

Collateral re-innervation by L4 axon

L5   L4

Peroneal n.

Tibialis anterior muscle (L4 +L5)

FIGURE 7.7.   *Muscle fibers denervated by a radiculopathy are reinnervated, by collateral sprouting from surviving motor axons supplying the muscle, despite persisting root compression. Reprinted with permission from RW Hardy (ed.) Lumbar disc disease, 2nd ed. New York: Raven Press, 1993:86.*

reveal that these insertional changes are widespread in distribution, rather than being restricted to a myotome as initially assumed. When widespread, these are referred to as *diffuse positive sharp waves* or *diffuse abnormal insertional activity;* they are genetically determined (autosomal dominant) incidental findings, and have no clinical significance other than that they are readily mistaken for evidence of early motor axon loss or brief myotonic discharges.[101–103] Moreover, if insertional positive sharp waves alone are used as criteria for the diagnosis of radiculopathy, other types of insertional activity, which can be mistaken for them, become potential sources for false-negative NEEs. The most common of these is *snap, crackle, and pop.* This type of abnormal insertional activity, named for its distinctive sound, is of no clinical significance. It is seen most often in young muscular men. Because some components of this activity have a positive sharp wave form and because it most often is found in the medial gastrocnemius and flexor digitorum longus muscles in the lower extremity, *snap, crackle, and pop* often erroneously is considered evidence of an S-1 radiculopathy.[104]

Neither fasciculation potentials nor complex repetitive discharges are seen in a root distribution often enough to be of any material value in diagnosing radiculopathies.[95] Typically fasciculation potentials that initially appear to be limited to a myotome are found, on more extensive NEE, to be widespread in distribution; usually they are evidence of *benign generalized fasciculations,* which are quite common in the adult population. Also, fasciculation potentials are seen so frequently in the abductor hallucis muscles as to justify being designated a normal variant. Complex repetitive discharges are indicative of a chronic lesion (i.e., one of at least 4 to 6 months duration) but are otherwise nonspecific in nature because they can be seen with both myopathic and neurogenic disorders. They are found so often in the iliacus muscles as to be considered a normal variant. With chronic root lesions, they occasionally are detected in one or two muscles—probably most often in the cervical paraspinal muscles—but only rarely are they seen in enough muscles of the myotome for diagnosis.[28]

 A neurogenic MUP firing pattern is one in which the MUPs in a muscle fire in decreased numbers but at a rapid rate. This is also known as *decreased recruitment.* The rapid firing rate of the motor units indicates that a substantial number of the motor fibers innervating the muscle being assessed cannot transmit nerve impulses to it, because of either axon loss or demyelinating conduction block. Root dysfunction with most radiculopathies is not severe enough to produce a neurogenic MUP firing pattern. Moreover, in the relatively few cases in which this pattern is seen, it usually is present in only one or two muscles of the myotome and therefore is too limited in distribution to be of diagnostic value. Further, it may be difficult, particularly for inexperienced electromyographers, to distinguish a reduced interference pattern in which the MUPs are firing in decreased numbers at a rapid rate from one in which they are firing in decreased numbers at a slow or moderate rate. Only the former, however, is evidence of a lower motor neuron lesion; the latter is seen with both incomplete voluntary effort and upper motor neuron lesions.[28,46]

Polyphasic MUPs are MUPs that contain more than four phases. Several different types of polyphasic MUPs can be seen with radiculopathies, and only one type is controversial. (1) In any muscle, 5% to 15% of the MUPs may normally be polyphasic.[46,94,105,106] Such MUPs are normal in their external configuration (i.e., amplitude and duration). (2) *Reinnervational* MUPs are seen early in the regenerative process, when the motor units are being functionally reestablished. These MUPs are not only highly polyphasic, but also are low in amplitude and prolonged in duration. They are transitional MUPs and will subsequently disappear as the motor units mature. (3) Almost all chronic neurogenic MUPs are polyphasic. This is of no significance, however, because the diagnostic importance of a chronic neurogenic MUP is determined by its amplitude and duration.

These different types of polyphasic MUPs can be seen with radiculopathies of varying duration. In addition to them, however, some electromyographers believe that another type of polyphasic MUP can be found in a myotomal distribution soon after the onset of a radiculopathy, that is, within the first week. This "early" polyphasic MUP appears too soon after symptom onset and lacks the external configuration to be either a *reinnervational* or a *chronic neurogenic* polyphasic MUP. The source of these early polyphasic MUPs with radiculopathies is unclear. Some attribute them to slowing along the small terminal nerve fibers, caused by demyelination; others consider them actually to be *pseudopolyphasic MUPs* the result of two motor units firing nearly simultaneously because of ephaptic transmission at the site of root compression.[65,107,108] To our knowledge, both of these theories are wholly speculative in nature, unsupported by substantive data. Similarly, some electromyographers believe that, with chronic radiculopathies, the only abnormalities on NEE may be an increased proportion of polyphasic MUPs, of normal amplitude and duration, in a myotomal distribution.[50,109–112]

Many electromyographers reject the concept that the NEE diagnosis of a radiculopathy can rest solely on the finding of polyphasic MUPs.[6,17,22,24,95] This approach is not only much more subjective in nature, but also, when performed correctly, it is very time-consuming because polyphasic MUPs must not only be found in the myotomal muscles, but also must be present in greater numbers than normal. To confirm the latter properly requires a quantitative approach, to prevent observer bias, rather than a subjective determination during the basic NEE. Otherwise, a great number of false-positive electromyographic examinations will occur.

Needle electrode examination findings with specific radiculopathies

Cervical radiculopathies constitute approximately 5% to 10% of all compressive radiculopathies.[113,114] Most cervical radiculopathies are single lesions involving one of the lower four cervical roots.[114,115,116] How often each specific cervical root is involved varies somewhat among the published series, but two reports, both concerned with 100 or more patients, noted very similar figures: C-7 radiculopathy, 69% to 70%; C-6, 19% to 25%; C-8, 4% to 10%; C-5, 2%.[116,118]

No cervical myotome extends throughout the upper extremity. Excluding C-8, all end no further distally than the midforearm. Because of the relatively short distances involved with most cervical radiculopathies, collateral sprouting usually is rather efficient. For this reason, fibrillation potentials are seldom seen with static cervical root lesions of more than 6 months duration.[28,112]

C-5/C-6 radiculopathies. Lesions of these two roots often are grouped together by electromyographers, not because both roots are necessarily affected together but because frequently it is difficult to distinguish one from another by NEE, owing to their extensive myotomal overlap. Abnormalities usually are found in the spinati, deltoid, biceps brachii, and brachioradialis muscles with both. Theoretically if the rhomboids are involved as well, the C-5 root should be the one compromised. Conversely, if the pronator teres and flexor carpi radialis are involved,

the C-6 root is affected. Unfortunately, in most patients the exact root injured remains uncertain because none of these other muscles contains abnormalities.[28] Finding mid or low cervical paraspinal fibrillation potentials with C-5/C-6 radiculopathies often is important for localization because the limb muscle abnormalities seen with them are equally consistent with an upper trunk brachial plexopathy, which frequently is in the differential diagnosis.

C-7 radiculopathies. Lesions of this root typically produce abnormalities in both C-7/radial-innervated muscles, especially triceps and anconeus, and in the C-7/median-innervated muscles: pronator teres and flexor carpi radialis. The particular combination of limb muscles involved with C-7 radiculopathies essentially can be caused only by lesions of the C-7 root and the middle trunk of the brachial plexus. Although C-7 radiculopathies are common, isolated middle trunk lesions are extremely rare.[28,44,119] For this reason, detecting paraspinal fibrillation potentials is less important for localization with C-7 radiculopathies than it is with lesions of the other cervical roots. Clinically, carpal tunnel syndrome rather commonly is confused with a C-7 root lesion; these are readily distinguished in the EMG laboratory. Also, radial mononeuropathies can be mistaken for C-7 radiculopathies and vice versa, if the NEE is limited to C-7/radial-innervated muscles and NCS are restricted.

C-8 radiculopathies. With lesions of this root, abnormalities typically are seen in many or all of the ulnar-innervated muscles, the C-8/radial-innervated muscles, for example, extensor indicis proprius and extensor pollicis brevis, and the C-8/median-innervated muscles, for example, abductor pollicis brevis and flexor pollicis longus. In our experience, the triceps muscle rarely shows NEE abnormalities with C-8 radiculopathies, although it is included in the C-8 myotome in many clinically determined myotomal charts.[28] C-8 radiculopathies, lower trunk brachial plexopathies, and ulnar mononeuropathies at the elbow frequently are confused with one another; not only may they all produce similar symptoms, but also often any one of them could result from the same clinical settings, for example, postoperatively. Consequently, both NCS (including median motor, ulnar motor, and ulnar sensory) and NEE of the lower cervical and upper thoracic paraspinal muscles frequently are important for accurate localization of C-8 radiculopathies.

Thoracic radiculopathies

Thoracic radiculopathies are rare, accounting for 2% or less of all radiculopathies.[113,115] This low incidence is fortunate for electromyographers because thoracic root lesions present particular difficulties in NEE assessment. Not only are the muscles in a thoracic myotome relatively few in number, but also most are difficult to examine for various reasons. Thus, obtaining adequate relaxation of the thoracic paraspinal muscles can be a frustrating task; assessing the abdominal muscles can be difficult in obese patients; and examining the intercostal muscles, because of their very close proximity to the pleural space, is avoided by most electromyographers. Moreover, even if fibrillation potentials are found in the paraspinal or the abdominal muscles, they do not allow localization to a specific thoracic root because of myotomal overlap.[28]

In many EMG laboratories, the majority of thoracic radiculopathies are diagnosed in elderly diabetic patients who have one, or frequently more, of their lower thoracic roots involved, often bilaterally. Most of these radiculopathies are due to root ischemia, rather than compression, although the exact cause cannot be proved by the NEE findings per se (see Chapter 18).

Lumbosacral radiculopathies

70-90% of compressive root lesions

Lumbosacral radiculopathies constitute the bulk of all radiculopathies that occur; out of every 10 patients with compressive root lesions, seven to nine of them have involvement of the lumbosacral roots, most particularly L-5 or S-1.[113,115]

Although the NEE findings with lumbosacral radiculopathies generally are similar to those seen with cervical radiculopathies, certain major differences are encountered. Most stem from the fact that the lumbosacral roots can be injured not only where they exit the intraspinal canal, as the cervical roots typically are, but also well within the intraspinal canal, where they are components of the cauda equina; also, because the roots are so compacted in the cauda equina, several may be injured by a single level lesion.[28,30] Consequently, the electrophysiologic demonstration that a specific lumbosacral root is damaged has less predictive value regarding the intervertebral level of the lesion than when a cervical radiculopathy is detected. Moreover, bilateral lesions are more common with lumbosacral than cervical radiculopathies. Accordingly, whenever electromyographic changes suggestive of a lumbosacral radic-

ulopathy are found in one lower extremity, at least a limited NEE should be performed on the contralateral lower limb, even if it is asymptomatic.[45,111,120] Because of their tendency to be bilateral, particularly in older patients, lumbosacral radiculopathies often are readily confused, both clinically and electrophysiologically, with polyneuropathies of the axon-loss type.

Another difference between the electromyographic presentation of cervical and lumbosacral root compression relates to the fact that the myotomes of both L-5 and S-1 have complete longitudinal limb representation, extending from the paraspinal muscles to the foot muscles. Consequently, the centrifugal appearance and disappearance of fibrillation potentials in the various muscles of the myotome are most apparent with lesions of these roots. With static radiculopathies of several months duration, fibrillation potentials often are restricted to L-5 and S-1-innervated muscles distal to the knee and usually persist in these muscles longer than the myotomal abnormalities caused by cervical and upper lumbar root lesions. This is because the more distal L-5 and S-1 myotomal muscles are further from the anterior horn cells that innervate them, and reinnervation therefore occurs later than it does in the more proximal myotomal muscles. Indeed, fibrillation potentials may be found in the more distal L-5 and S-1 myotomal muscles 12 to 18 months or more after onset of a nonprogressive lesion of these roots. Similarly, with very remote root lesions, these same muscles may be the only myotomal muscles in which chronic neurogenic MUP changes are seen.[28,45]

L-2, L-3, L-4 radiculopathies

Compressive lesions of the L-2, L-3, and L-4 roots occur much less frequently than do those of the L-5 and S-1 roots. Electromyographers consider this low incidence a blessing because the electrophysiologic assessment of these roots is difficult for several reasons. (1) The L-2, L-3, and L-4 myotomes overlap so extensively that it is often impossible to distinguish involvement of one root from another. Lesions of any of them can produce NEE abnormalities in the iliacus, the various quadriceps muscles, and the thigh adductor muscles. L-4 radiculopathies may also produce NEE changes in the tibialis anterior muscle, but the lack of such findings never excludes involvement of that root. (2) The L-2, L-3, and L-4 myotomes are composed of relatively few muscles compared with the L-5 and S-1 myotomes, and most of the accessible muscles in these myotomes are supplied by the same peripheral nerve, the femoral nerve. Consequently, because incomplete myotomal involvement occurs commonly with radiculopathies, L-2, L-3, and L-4 root lesions may occasionally show NEE abnormalities only in a femoral nerve distribution. (3) Almost all the muscles comprising the L-2, L-3, and L-4 myotomes are located in the proximal portion of the lower extremity (i.e., above the knee) and therefore are likely to reinnervate relatively soon after the onset of static root compression. (4) No sensory NCS have been devised for assessing the L-2 or L-3 fibers up to the DRG, and NCS of the lateral cutaneous nerve of the thigh and the saphenous nerve are not sufficiently reliable for assessing the sensory fibers derived from the L-4 DRG. As a result, even when axon loss is rather prominent in the L-2, L-3, and L-4 limb muscles, sensory NCS cannot be used to distinguish an intraspinal canal lesion (i.e., a radiculopathy) from a lumbar plexopathy.[28,119] Lumbar paraspinal fibrillation potentials are the only remaining differential feature, and unfortunately they are not always found. Because of these limitations, the electromyographic examination is more often false-negative with L-2, L-3, and L-4 root lesions than it is with those affecting the L-5 or S-1 roots. Moreover, even when NEE abnormalities are present, distinguishing an L-2, L-3, or L-4 radiculopathy from a lumbar plexopathy or femoral mononeuropathy may sometimes be impossible.[28]

In many EMG laboratories, most patients referred with suspected L-2, L-3, or L-4 radiculopathies are elderly, obese diabetics with unilateral or bilateral symptoms. In many of these patients, the root lesions are ischemic, rather than compressive, in etiology, representing the syndrome of diabetic amyotrophy (diabetic polyradiculopathy involving the L-2–L-4 roots). Just as is the case with lower thoracic radiculopathies in diabetic patients, however, the NEE findings cannot distinguish upper lumbar compressive lesions from those caused by ischemia (see Chapter 18).

L-5 radiculopathies

Lesions of the L-5 root are one of the most common radiculopathies encountered. Abnormalities are found in the peroneal-innervated muscles distal to the knee (e.g., tibialis anterior, extensor hallucis, peroneus longus, extensor digitorum brevis), all of which share L-5 innervation as well, but are not present in the short head of the biceps femoris, the only peroneal-innervated muscle proximal to the knee, because it is innervated mainly by the S-1 root. NEE abnormalities usually also are found in the flexor digitorum longus and tibialis posterior muscles and sometimes in the semimembranosus and semitendinosus; the tensor fascia lata; the gluteus medius and maximus (particularly the medius), and the low lumbar/high sacral paraspinal muscles. Excluding the L-5/common peroneal-innervated muscles, the flexor digitorum longus and tibialis posterior are the myotomal muscles that most often contain fibrillation potentials with L-5 root compression, because of their distal location. Hence at least one of them should be examined in every limb in which an L-5 root lesion is suspected.

Whenever an L-5 root lesion causes severe MUP dropout in the tibialis anterior muscle, either because of demyelinating conduction block or, far more often, because of axon loss, the clinical footdrop that results often is mistaken for that caused by a common peroneal mononeuropathy at the fibular head (CPM-FH). Although lesions along the peroneal fibers at these two widely separated points can produce a similar clinical picture, their electrodiagnostic features usually are strikingly different. Both the NCS and the NEE help in distinguishing them. The peroneal motor NCS readily demonstrates a CPM-FH caused by demyelinating conduction block and thus separates it from other lesions. The superficial peroneal NCS is usually unelicitable with CPM-FH in which there is axon loss but is normal with both L-5 radiculopathies and CPM-FH due to demyelinating conduction block. On NEE, the abnormalities are strictly limited to a common peroneal nerve distribution distal to the knee with CPM-FH, whereas they are characteristically more widely distributed with L-5 radiculopathies.[47] Although there are reports that L-5 radiculopathies may reproduce fibrillation potentials only in the L-5/common peroneal-innervated muscles distal to the knee, this rarely occurs in our experience.

S-1/S-2 radiculopathies

Lesions of the S-1 and S-2 roots frequently are discussed together because often they are difficult to distinguish from one another in the EMG laboratory due to myotomal overlap. Compression of either of these roots can produce abnormalities in the abductor hallucis and abductor digiti quinti pedis muscles in the foot as well as in the medial gastrocnemius and soleus muscles. S-1 root lesions may also produce abnormalities in the extensor digitorum brevis, flexor digitorum longus, lateral gastrocnemius, and several muscles proximal to the knee, including the long and short heads of the biceps femoris, the glutei (especially the maximus), and the high sacral paraspinal muscles. In addition, with S-1 radiculopathies, the H wave usually is abnormal.[28]

The sacral roots, being more medially situated in the cauda equina than the lumbar roots,[30] are more likely to be injured, often bilaterally, with midline lesions. Many patients with such bilateral involvement are referred to the EMG laboratory with the clinical diagnosis of *polyneuropathy* or *bilateral tarsal tunnel syndrome*. The results of the NCS, NEE, and sometimes the H wave test may help in determining which of these disorders actually is responsible for the patient's symptoms. Often the electromyographic examination must be extensive, encompassing at least two limbs and sometimes three.

S-2, S-3, S-4 radiculopathies

These roots may be involved with any midline cauda equina lesion. Isolated lesions of the S-2, S-3, and S-4 roots, however, in our experience, are rarely due to compression. Instead they are usually iatrogenic, the result of inadvertent injury during caudal anesthesia. Only limited abnormalities are seen with these lesions during the basic electrodiagnostic examination. The posterior tibial motor NCS are normal, as are H waves. The NEE of the limb muscles reveals no abnormalities or only mild changes in certain of the S-2-innervated muscles, particularly the soleus and abductor hallucis muscles. In these patients, NEE of the anal sphincter muscle should be performed. Both the right and the left portions of that muscle may be so severely denervated that MUP dropout is obvious and prominent enough that low-amplitude fibrillation potentials are readily detected. In all patients with bowel and bladder disturbances possibly caused by a lower motor neuron lesion, the S-2-innervated limb muscles should always be evaluated because, of the various limb muscles, they are the ones most likely to show abnormalities.[28]

Multiple lumbosacral radiculopathies

When two or more roots are compromised simultaneously, the lesion is more likely to be located in the lumbosacral region than in the cervical or thoracic areas. A disproportionate number of patients with multiple lumbosacral radiculopathies are elderly, and in most patients the roots are being injured within the cauda equina by either central disc herniations

or, more often, lumbar canal stenosis. These multiradicular lesions usually are bilateral, although frequently asymmetric, and typically they involve the lower lumbosacral roots, particularly S-1/S-2. Often these cause so much motor axon loss that the basic lower extremity NCS are abnormal; that is, the posterior tibial and peroneal motor NCS responses are low in amplitude or unelicitable. Characteristically with these lesions, the H waves are unelicitable bilaterally because of S-1 root compromise. As with other root lesions, the sensory fibers are injured proximal to the DRG, and the peripheral sensory NCS are not affected (although they may be unelicitable bilaterally because of advanced age) (see Figure 7.4).

Lumbar canal stenosis. This disorder is one of the major neurogenic causes for lower extremity disability in older patients. Clinically lumbar canal stenosis most often presents with *neurogenic intermittent claudication:* pain, paresthesias, and often weakness developing bilaterally in the buttocks and lower extremities, frequently in an ascending or descending fashion, after the patient walks a certain distance or stands for a certain period of time. These symptoms usually resolve promptly after the patient sits and sometimes after he or she just flexes the lumbar spine.

Lumbar canal stenosis has no characteristic electromyographic presentation. Instead the findings are extremely diverse, ranging from normal to severely, bilaterally abnormal. In approximately 50% of the patients, multiple lumbosacral radiculopathies are found, owing to cauda equina compromise. These often are severe in degree, chronic in nature, and slowly progressive. Consequently, chronic neurogenic MUP changes frequently dominate the findings on NEE; fibrillation potentials commonly are limited to the L-5- and S-1-innervated muscles distal to the knee, where they may be sparse in numbers. In the remaining 50% of patients with lumbar canal stenosis, various electromyographic patterns are found, including the followng:

1. Two distinct lumbosacral root lesions. These infrequently involve contiguous (or, less often, noncontiguous) roots on the same side (e.g., right L-5 and S-1 radiculopathy); more often a single root is damaged in each lower extremity, either symmetrically (e.g., bilateral S-1 radiculopathies) or asymmetrically (e.g., right L-5 radiculopathy and left S-1 radiculopathy).
2. An isolated radiculopathy, typically either an

L-5 or an S-1 root lesion, without side preference.

3. Definite but nondiagnostic abnormalities, such as unilateral or bilaterally absent H waves alone or fibrillation potentials or chronic MUP changes in one or two muscles of one or both lower extremities.

4. In the remaining patients, even very extensive electrodiagnostic studies of the lower extremity reveal no abnormalities.[45]

Because bilateral abnormalities are seen so often with lumbar canal stenosis owing to cauda equina compromise, both H wave measurements and NEE should be performed bilaterally whenever this disorder is clinically suspected.[45,120] Even when the contralateral limb is completely asymptomatic, at least a limited NEE should be performed on it (e.g., the tibialis anterior and medial gastrocnemius muscles sampled). In some patients, NEE abnormalities will be found only in the less symptomatic or asymptomatic limb.

What the electrodiagnostic examination will show in a patient with lumbar canal stenosis often can be predicted by considering the clinical presentation. Those patients who have bilateral fixed deficits (muscle weakness; sensory loss) are likely to have evidence of a cauda equina lesion on examination. Conversely, those who experience only intermittent symptoms and have no clinical deficits are likely to have normal or, at best, indeterminant electrodiagnostic studies.

Confounding factors

Advanced patient age. In many patients over the age of 60, neither H waves nor lower extremity sensory NCS responses can be elicited in either lower extremity, and the peroneal and tibial motor responses are borderline abnormal in amplitude and conduction velocity. Moreover, the older the patient, the more the MUPs in the distal lower extremity muscles become *chronic neurogenic* in appearance. All of these factors introduce an element of uncertainty in the interpretation of lower extremity assessments for lumbosacral radiculopathy.[28]

Polyneuropathy. Many patients with known axon loss polyneuropathies are referred to the EMG laboratory with suspected L-5 or S-1 radiculopathies. Detecting a superimposed radicular process in these patients can be difficult because some of the abnormalities typically found—for example, unelicitable

H waves, fibrillation potentials, or chronic neurogenic MUP changes in the more distal limb muscles —are common to both root lesions and polyneuropathies. Both lower extremities usually must be studied and often one of the upper extremities as well. The diagnosis of a radiculopathy in these instances frequently hinges on finding abnormalities in myotomal muscles proximal to the knee, for example, hamstrings, glutei, and paraspinal muscles.

Diabetes mellitus. Many patients with diabetes mellitus are evaluated for possible lumbosacral radiculopathies. Such studies often prove to be both time-consuming and frustrating for several reasons. First, most patients are elderly, and the confounding factors already mentioned regarding advanced patient age are operative. Second, many of them also have a generalized polyneuropathy, which causes additional problems. Finally, in many of them, fibrillation potentials can be found bilaterally in the lower lumbar paraspinal muscles, so their presence in diabetics is of little value for diagnosing a root disorder. For these reasons, the electrodiagnostic examinations typically must be more extensive than usual in these patients, and even then they are often inconclusive (see Chapter 18).

Remote poliomyelitis. Some middle-aged or elderly patients with suspected root compression had poliomyelitis in their youth. This neurogenic disorder frequently leaves conspicuous residual electrodiagnosis abnormalities, such as chronic neurogenic MUP changes and, less often, minimal fibrillation potentials, in a myotomal pattern. These NEE changes almost invariably are more widespread in distribution than any clinical deficit resulting from the poliomyelitis. Consequently, even when such changes are found in a limb that was clinically unaffected by poliomyelitis, they cannot be considered evidence of a superimposed radiculopathy. Moreover, the distribution of these abnormalities in any single limb is quite unpredictable; for example, they can be found in the C-7-innervated muscles in one upper extremity and in C-6 and C-8 distributions in the contralateral limb. Consequently, chronic radiculopathies cannot be diagnosed in patients with remote poliomyelitis, and acute radiculopathies can be suspected only whenever fibrillation potentials are found in rather abundant numbers in a myotomal distribution.

As can be seen, most of the confounding factors become operative under the same set of conditions: in older patients, with bilateral lower extremity symptoms. Unfortunately for many EMG laboratories, most of the patients referred for radiculopathy assessments are elderly, with suspected involvement of the lumbosacral roots, and in that age group the abnormalities are often bilateral, owing to lumbar canal stenosis. Hence in older patients, lower extremity electromyographic examinations for radiculopathies are far more likely to be inconclusive than when younger patients are assessed for lower extremity lesions or when patients of any age are assessed for cervical radiculopathies.

Differentiating root from plexus lesions

Many patients are studied electrophysiologically to determine whether their symptoms are due to a lesion at the root or plexus level. Neurogenic injuries at either of these two locations can affect most of the same fibers, so clinical findings are often similar. To compound the problem, the precipitating cause often can result in either a radiculopathy and/or plexopathy. Generally, the motor NCS, F waves, H waves, and NEE of the limb muscles do not help in making this distinction. The two procedures of benefit are the sensory NCS and NEE of the paraspinal muscles.[119] Unfortunately, both have their limitations. The sensory NCS are valuable because their amplitudes are not affected by axon loss radiculopathies, regardless of severity, but they are reduced by axon loss plexopathies of at least moderate severity. Their limitations include: (1) Appropriate studies are lacking to assess the sensory fibers derived from certain roots, that is, the C-5 root; the T-2 through T-12 roots; the L-1, L-2, and L-3 roots; and, for practical purposes, the L-4 root. (2) The sensory NCS amplitudes with mild axon loss plexopathies are either not affected or affected too mildly, to be considered abnormal. The NEE of the appropriate paraspinal muscles may be extremely helpful in this differentiation because the paraspinal muscles are innervated by the posterior primary rami, whereas the plexuses are a continuation only of the anterior primary rami. Thus paraspinal fibrillation potentials never are seen with plexopathies; unfortunately, however, they often cannot be found with radiculopathies either, for reasons stated earlier. Consequently, NEE of the paraspinal muscles is beneficial only when it shows changes suggestive of a root lesion.

Magnetic Stimulation

The spinal roots and the proximal and distal portions of the peripheral nerves can be stimulated by a rapidly changing magnetic field, which induces an electrical field in the tissues through which it passes. Cerebral responses are elicited by this means and can be recorded over the scalp. In patients with radiculopathy, initial study suggests that the response is delayed,[121] but this needs to be established more clearly.

Marsden et al.[117] showed that percutaneous electrical stimulation over the cervical or lumbar vertebral column can elicit responses from muscles of the upper and lower limbs, and this relates primarily to excitation of the proximal portion of the motor roots.[73] Tabaraud et al.[122] have evaluated the role of recording these motor evoked responses in the diagnosis of radiculopathy. They recorded bilaterally from the tibialis anterior and soleus muscles after lumbar spinal stimulation in 25 control subjects and in 45 patients with unilateral L-5 or S-1 root pain from disc protrusions that were radiologically demonstrated. The motor evoked response latency was prolonged on the symptomatic side by more than 3 standard deviations of the normal mean interside latency difference in 72% of patients with an L-5 lesion and 66% of those with an S-1 lesion, regardless of whether objective neurologic deficits were present on clinical examination.[122] Chokroverty et al.[123,124] used magnetic lumbar stimulation to evaluate patients with lumbosacral or cervical root lesions. Thus they studied five patients with an L-5 or S-1 root lesion confirmed by imaging studies or surgery. A magnetic coil placed over the central sacral region produced pulsed magnetic fields that generated electric currents, activating nerve impulses. They reported prolonged latencies and decreased amplitudes of the evoked motor responses recorded from the soleus and tibialis anterior muscles supplied by the affected roots.[123,124] It remains to be established whether this approach will permit the diagnosis of root lesions when other electrophysiologic techniques fail to reveal any abnormalities.

It is not clear whether magnetic stimulation of nerve roots has any advantage over electrical stimulation by means of a monopolar needle electrode placed on the spinal lamina. In fact, preliminary studies suggest that electrical stimulation may be the superior approach. In another study, Evans et al.[72] showed that magnetic stimulation of C-5–C-6 spinal nerves elicited motor responses with amplitudes and areas of the CMAPs generally comparable to those obtained with electrical stimulation, whereas for the deeper C-8–T-1 spinal nerves, the responses to magnetic stimulations were often submaximal. Moreover, stimulation with the needle electrodes resulted in depolarization of the spinal nerves close to the cord, whereas with magnetic stimulation, some authors have found that the site of excitation yielding maximum motor responses is somewhat more distal.[72,125] In addition, responses elicited in lower limb muscles by paravertebral magnetic stimulation may include components derived from proximally generated F waves and H waves,[126] further complicating the use of this technique to evaluate the functional integrity of nerve roots. Finally, although magnetic stimulation is less uncomfortable for patients, it nevertheless requires the delivery of repeated stimuli, while a search is conducted to determine the optimal site at which to place the coil.

THERMOGRAPHY

Thermography provides a means of determining the functional integrity of the autonomic nervous system. It is thus the only procedure described in this chapter that assesses nerve fibers other than large myelinated ones. Because it is noninvasive, poses no particular risks to patients, is relatively easy to perform, and can be used to follow changes over time, some authors contend that thermography is a useful means of evaluating patients with radiculopathies.

At the present time, however, thermography should not be accepted as a valid diagnostic procedure for neuromuscular disorders in general, or radiculopathies in particular, because of the paucity of properly performed studies to determine its efficacy. Nevertheless, it is being used by certain physicians for this purpose and therefore merits some comment.

An accurate, visual representation of the temperature over the surface of the body can be obtained by liquid crystal thermography or by telethermography. The preferred technique is *infrared imaging* or *telethermography* because temperature measurements can be made with great sensitivity and speed, large regions of the body can be studied, contact of the body with temperature-sensitive material is not required, and dynamic studies can be performed when desired. An infrared camera scans the body, and the information obtained is relayed electronically to a video display unit where different colors representing areas of different temperature, or heat emisison, are used to produce an image of the body. Depending on the equipment, it may also be possible to measure the mean temperature in selected regions using a direct digital readout. The image may be stored digitally for subsequent use, printed on paper, or photographed. Thermal discrimination in the order of 0.1°C generally can be obtained with modern instruments.

Studies are performed in a draft-free environment, with an ambient stable temperature between 68°F and 72°F. The undressed patient is allowed to equilibrate with the environment for 15 to 20 minutes before being imaged. Three sets of images are obtained, with 15 to 20 minutes elapsing between the acquisition of each set, and the images are then compared to ensure that the patient is in equilibrium and that any abnormalities are consistent. The area that is imaged depends on the clinical or diagnostic problem necessitating the study. The temperature of a specific region of the body can be compared with adjacent regions and to corresponding regions on the opposite side of the body. Regional temperature changes may reflect a change in the cutaneous blood supply as a consequence of neurologic or vascular pathology or of local inflammatory processes. Regional thermographic abnormalities are therefore nonspecific—they may relate to peripheral vascular disease, trauma, hematoma, local inflammatory responses, muscle activity, peripheral sensory stimulation, changes in sympathetic or parasympathetic activity, and somatosympathetic reflexes.[127–129]

Findings in normal subjects

The body temperature normally is bilaterally symmetric,[128–130] but it is lower in distal than proximal segments. Normative data must be obtained under specified conditions before thermography is undertaken for clinical purposes because the bounds of normality are influenced by recording conditions, such as the ambient temperature. Arbitrary definitions of abnormality that neglect the extent of any normal variation are clearly inappropriate. The optimal approach is to divide the body and extremities into discrete regions based on the distribution of nerves and nerve roots and then measure the average temperature of each region. The normal interside temperature differences for these areas should be expressed as the mean and standard deviation, determined on healthy volunteers. Only temperature differences that exceed the normal mean by 2.5 or 3 standard deviations should be regarded as abnormal, the latter criterion being preferred when numerous regional comparisons are made.[128,129]

A thermographic abnormality consists of an excessive difference in temperature between a specific region and either the corresponding region on the other side or other (often adjacent) regions in the same limb. Because the temperature may be either increased or decreased in the affected area, it is difficult to determine the abnormal side or region by the thermographic findings alone.

Findings with nerve root compression

In 1964, Albert et al.[131] described the thermographic findings associated with a herniated disc, reporting a *hot spot* overlying the area of pathology. Ching and Wexler[132] subsequently imaged the lower extremities as well as the back in suspected lumbar radiculopathy and reported hot spots in the lumbar region, combined with temperature changes in the buttocks and legs. These findings and subsequent studies led Wexler to conclude that thermography was a useful complimentary technique for evaluating patients with suspected root lesions.[133] Since that time, there have been numerous reports concerning the detection of radiculopathies with thermography, but most have depended on visual reading of a color-coded thermogram and have failed to include a control group studied under identical conditions to determine the bounds of normality. In many of these studies, an interside difference in skin temperature of more than 1°C was regarded as abnormal, but the actual temperature was measured only rarely, and the 1°C criterion was applied arbitrarily to different regions of the body, without taking into account the greater variability of distal skin temperature.[129,134]

Only two attempts to compare patients' data quantitatively to a group of healthy control subjects have been reported. The first showed an abnormality rate of 85% in patients with myelographic abnormalities, but the thermographic abnormality was defined as an interside temperature difference exceeding the normal mean by only 1 standard deviation.[134] This definition of abnormality is inappropriate clinically because of the high false-positive rate, especially when multiple test parameters are considered in the same patient.

So et al.[128] studied 27 normal patients and 30 patients with low back pain to determine the utility and accuracy of thermography in the diagnosis in lumbosacral radiculopathy. They defined thermographic abnormality as the presence of either an interside temperature difference that exceeded the normal mean by more than 3 standard deviations or an abnormal heat pattern overlying the lower back. Thermography was found to be abnormal as often as electrophysiologic studies in patients with clinically unequivocal radiculopathy, and the results of these two investigative techniques showed concordance in 71% of cases. The electrophysiologic findings, however, were of localizing and prognostic im-

portance, whereas the thermographic findings were of much lesser value. In themselves, they failed to identify the side of the lesion, and they did not follow a dermatomal distribution. Thus they did not identify the clinical or electrophysiologic level of the radiculopathy in most cases. So et al. therefore concluded that the thermographic findings were nonspecific and of little clinical utility.

In the correspondence that followed the publication of the paper of So et al. it was pointed out that more favorable results probably would have been obtained if stress tests had been used.[135] Stress testing, however, generally is not performed routinely, the optimal stress procedure to adopt is unclear, and the utility of such testing in the evaluation of radiculopathies is uncertain.[127]

The reason that thermographic abnormalities sometimes occur in lumbosacral radiculopathy is not known. Sympathetic fibers cannot be directly compressed in most patients because preganglionic sympathetic fibers do not exit through the neural foramina below the L-2 level. Ochoa[136] has suggested that unmyelinated sensory fibers may antidromically produce vasodilatation in some pathologic circumstances, perhaps by secretion of vasoactive substances at the nerve endings, but this fails to account for the limb cooling that occurs with some radiculopathies. Stimulation of peripheral somatic afferent fibers may produce peripheral vasoconstriction by a somatosympathetic spinal reflex,[137] but whether this accounts for the thermographic findings is unknown. In any event, the application for clinical purposes of thermography to the investigation of patients with suspected lumbosacral radiculopathy seems unjustified at the present time.

CONCLUSIONS AND RECOMMENDATIONS

The specific approach used by electromyographers when evaluating patients with suspected radiculopathies is not standardized. Regardless of the particular methods used, the study should be comprehensive enough that the risk of both false-positive and false-negative studies is minimized. To achieve these results, we recommend the following guidelines:

1. Do not perform the study until an appropriate time after onset of symptoms or after the onset of new symptoms; this means that at least 3 weeks should elapse before the NEE is undertaken.

2. Always perform motor and sensory NCS on the affected limb and, if necessary, on the asymptomatic limb for comparative purposes. Not only can mononeuropathies be mistaken for radiculopathies, but both disorders may coexist, and the mononeuropathy actually may be responsible for the patient's current symptoms.[43]

3. Obtain H responses on all patients with lower extremity symptoms, particularly with suspected S-1 radiculopathy or possible lumbar canal stenosis. Bilateral H wave studies are indicated if the first is abnormal or if symptoms are bilateral. These may prove to be the only abnormal component of the entire electrodiagnostic evaluation.

4. Perform an adequate NEE. One method of accomplishing this is to perform a general survey or *root search* on the affected limb by assessing at least two muscles from each myotome as well as examining the appropriate paraspinal muscles. At least one *marker* muscle of each myotome should be assessed. If a specific root is suspected clinically, additional muscles within its myotome should be sampled. When the myotome extends throughout the limb, that is, L-5 and S-1, always examine both proximal and distal myotomal muscles. With chronic, static radiculopathies, the focus should be on the more distal muscles of the myotome because they are much more likely to contain abnormalities than proximal muscles.

5. Sample muscles in the contralateral limb whenever necessary, for example, when definite evidence of a radiculopathy is found in the ipsilateral limb; when abnormalities are found in only one or two muscles of the symptomatic limb; when an H wave is unelicitable in the contralateral limb (in these situations, at least one or two S-1-innervated muscles should be assessed, such as the medial gastrocnemius and the abductor hallucis); and in patients with suspected lumbar canal stenosis.

6. Be cognizant of abnormalities that are seen so frequently on lower extremity NEE that they are best regarded as variants of normal, without clinical significance. These include fibrillation potentials limited to one or both extensor digitorum brevis muscles; fasciculation potentials in the abductor hallucis muscles; complex repetitive discharges in the iliacus muscles; difficulty in obtaining full interference patterns in the gastrocnemius, abductor hallucis, and the abductor digiti quinti pedis muscles; many serrated MUPs potentials in the extensor hallucis and adductor longus muscles; and chronic neurogenic MUP changes in the intrinsic foot muscles of elderly patients.

7. Consider only fibrillation potentials and chronic neurogenic MUP changes in a myotomal distribution of diagnostic significance, because employing less stringent, more controversial NEE abnormalities for diagnosis invariably results in high numbers of false-positive studies.

8. Appreciate that with chronic, static lumbosacral radiculopathies, fibrillation potentials or sometimes just chronic neurogenic MUP changes may be limited to only some of the myotomal muscles, particularly the more distal ones.

9. Always sample the appropriate paraspinal muscles unless there has been a prior laminectomy performed through the midline posterior approach. It is often helpful to assess the paraspinal muscles below (as well as at) the level of the suspected root; because of the cascade innervation of the paraspinal muscles, fibrillation potentials often are found caudal to the level of root involvement.

10. Follow the electrodiagnostic criteria rigorously in regard to both recognition and localization of a radiculopathy. Avoid the temptation to liberalize them whenever the clinical history or examination is suggestive. Patients are referred to the EMG laboratory for an *independent* confirmation of their clinical diagnosis. If the electrodiagnostic impression is based primarily on the clinical, rather than the electrophysiologic, findings, this independence is lost.

11. Acknowledge that many electrodiagnostic evaluations with suspected radiculopathies will be inconclusive, and label them as such.

12. Appreciate that some false-negative studies inevitably result when patients with suspected root compression undergo electrodiagnostic examinations, particularly when the symptoms are solely sensory in nature and of long duration. Accordingly, never regard a radiculopathy as excluded by a normal electrodiagnostic examination.

13. Finally, evaluate critically any new electrodiagnostic procedure before using it to investigate patients with suspected radiculopathy, espe-

cially at this time of escalating medical costs. SEPs elicited by nerve trunk stimulation are of no value in detecting isolated root lesions, whereas SEPs elicited by cutaneous nerve or dermatomal stimulation are generally too insensitive or time-consuming for general use. Magnetic stimulation is a new technique, and its value in the diagnosis of root lesions is currently being assessed. Thermography is widely used by certain practitioners, but its utility is unproved, and it does not permit the accurate localization of a radiculopathy or its distinction from more peripheral neuropathic processes.

REFERENCES

1. Ehni G. Historical writings on spondylotic caudal radiculopathy and its effects on the nervous system. In: Weinstein PR, Ehni G, Wilson CB, eds. Lumbar spondylosis. Chicago: Year Book, 1979: 1–12.
2. Latchlaw JP. A historical note on sciatica. In: Hardy RW, ed. Lumbar disc disease. New York: Raven Press, 1982: 1–4.
3. Wilkinson M. Historical introduction. In: Wilkinson M, ed. Cervical spondylosis. Philadelphia: WB Saunders, 1971: 1–9.
4. Mixter W, Barr J. Rupture of the intervertebral disc with involvement of the spinal canal. N Engl J Med 1934; 211:210–214.
5. Wilbourn AJ. Radiculopathies: History and pathophysiology. In Syllabus: AAEE Course D: Radiculopathies. Rochester, MN: American Association of Electromyography and Electrodiagnosis, 1989: 7–10.
6. Knutsson B. Comparative value of electromyographic, myelographic, and clinical-neurological examinations in the diagnosis of lumbar root compression syndromes. Acta Orthop Scand 1961; 49 (suppl): 1–135.
7. Semmes RE, Murphey F. The syndrome of unilateral rupture of the sixth cervical vertebral disc with compression of the seventh cervical nerve root: A report of four cases with symptoms simulating coronary disease. JAMA 1943; 121:1209–1214.
8. Verbiest H. Neurogenic intermittent claudication. New York: American Elsevier, 1976.
9. Brain WR, Northfield DWC, Wilkinson M. Neurological manifestations of cervical spondylosis. Brain 1952; 75:187–225.
10. Epstein NE, Epstein JA. Individual and coexistent lumbar and cervical canal stenosis. Spine: State of the Art Reviews 1987; 1:401–420.
11. Laureno R. Radiculopathies: Clinical and anatomic aspects, in syllabus: AAEE Course D: Radiculopathies. Rochester, MN: American Association of Electromyography and Electrodiagnosis, 1989: 11–22.
12. MacNab I. The pathogenesis of spinal stenosis. Spine: State of the Art Reviews 1987; 1:369–381.
13. Weinstein PR. Lumbar canal stenosis. In: Hardy RW, ed. Lumbar disc disease. New York: Raven Press, 1982: 257–276.
14. Weinstein PR. Pathology of lumbar stenosis and spondylosis. In: Weinstein PR, Ehni G, Wilson CB, eds. Lumbar spondylosis. Chicago: Year Book, 1979: 43–91.
15. Love JC, Keefer EJ. Root pain and paraplegia due to protrusions of thoracic intervertebral disks. J Neurosurg 1950; 7:62–69.
16. Weddell G, Feinstein B, Pattle RE. The electrical activity of voluntary muscle in man under normal and pathological conditions. Brain 1944; 67:178–257.
17. Jasper HH, Ballem G. Unipolar electromyograms of normal and denervated human muscle. J Neurophysiol 1949; 12:231–244.
18. Kugelberg E, Petersen I. "Insertion activity" in electromyography with notes on denervated muscle response to constant current. J Neurol Neurosurg Psychiatry 1949; 12:268–273.
19. Brazier MA, Watkins AL, Michelsen JJ. Electromyography in differential diagnosis of ruptured cervical disc. Arch Neurol Psych 1946; 56:651–658.
20. Shea PA, Woods WW, Werden DR. Electromyography in diagnosis of nerve root compression syndrome. Arch Neurol Psych 1950; 64:93–104.
21. Woods WW, Shea PA. The value of electromyography in neurology and neurosurgery. J Neurosurg 1951; 8:595–607.
22. Marinacci AA. Clinical electromyography. Los Angeles: San Lucas Press, 1955.
23. Kambin P, Smith JM, Hoerner EF. Myelography and myography in diagnosis of herniated intervertebral disk. JAMA 1962; 181:472–475.
24. Knutsson B. Aspects of the neurogenic electromyographic records of voluntary contraction in cases of nerve root compression. Electromyography 1962; 238–242.
25. Mendelsohn RA, Sola A. Electromyography in herniated lumbar disks. Arch Neurol Psych 1958; 79:142–145.
26. Wise CS, Ardizzone J. Electromyography in intervertebral disc protrusions. Arch Phy Med Rehabil 1954; 35:442–446.
27. Goss CM, ed. Gray's anatomy of the human body, ed 29 (American). Philadelphia: Lea & Febiger, 1973.
28. Wilbourn AJ, Aminoff MJ. AAEE Minimonograph #32: The electrophysiologic examination in patients

with radiculopathy. Muscle Nerve 1988; 11:1099–1114.

29. Cohen MS, Wall EV, Brown RA, et al. Cauda equina anatomy II: Extrathecal nerve roots and dorsal root ganglia. Spine 1990; 15:1248–1251.

30. Wall EJ, Cohen MS, Massie JB, et al. Cauda equina anatomy I: Intrathecal nerve root organization. Spine 1990; 15:1244–1247.

31. Goodgold J, Eberstein A. Electrodiagnosis of neuromuscular diseases, ed 3. Baltimore: WIlliams & Wilkins, 1983: 349.

32. van der Most van Spijk D, Vingerhoets HM. Disorders of lumbosacral roots and nerves. In: Notermans SLH, ed. Current practice of clinical electromyography. Amsterdam: Elsevier Scientific, 1984: 255–278.

33. Liveson J, Spielholz N. Peripheral neurology: Case studies in electrodiagnosis. Philadelphia: FA Davis, 1979.

34. Thage O. The myotomes L2-S2 in man. Acta Neurol Scand 1965; 13: (suppl 41): 241–243.

35. Gilliatt RW. Acute conduction block. In: Sumner AJ, ed. The physiology of peripheral nerve disease. Philadelphia: WB Saunders, 1980: 287–315.

36. Gilliatt RW. Physical injury to peripheral nerves. Mayo Clin Proc 1981; 56:361–370.

37. McDonald WI. Physiological consequences of demyelination. In: Sumner AJ, ed. The physiology of peripheral nerve disease. Philadelphia: WB Saunders, 1980:265–286.

38. McDonald WI. Pathophysiology of nerve and tract conduction. In: Cobb WA, Duijn H, eds. Contemporary clinical neurophysiology (EEG Suppl No. 34). Amsterdam: Elsevier, 1978: 386–392.

39. McDonald WI. Structural and functional changes in human and experimental neuropathy. In: Williams D, ed. Modern trends in neurology—4. London: Butterworth, 1967: 145–164.

40. Benecke R, Conrad B. The distal sensory nerve action potential as a diagnostic tool for the differentiation of lesions in dorsal roots and peripheral nerves. J Neurol 1980; 223:231–239.

41. Branstader ME, Fullerton M. Sensory nerve conduction studies in cervical root lesions. Can J Neurol Sci 1983; 10:152.

42. Kuchera M, Wilbourn A. Cutaneous sensory responses with cervical radiculopathies. EEG Clin Neurophysiol 1983; 56:S119.

43. Daube JR. Electrodiagnostic studies in radiculopathies. In syllabus: Course A: Basic electrophysiological testing in mononeuropathy. Rochester, MN: American Association of Electromyography and Electrodiagnosis, 1985: 37–44.

44. Spaans F. Lesions of the brachial plexus and upper limb nerves. In: Notermans SLH, ed. Current practice of clinical electromyography. Amsterdam: Elsevier Scientific, 1984: 213–253.

45. Wilbourn AJ. The value and limitations of electro-

myographic examination in the diagnosis of lumbosacral radiculopathy. In: Hardy RW, ed. Lumbar disc disease. New York: Raven Press, 1982: 65–109.

46. Carpenter DE, Subramony SH. Electromyography. In: Youmans J, ed. Neurological surgery, ed 3. Vol 1. Philadelphia: WB Saunders, 1990: 470–499.

47. Wilbourn AJ. AAEE Case Report #12: Common peroneal mononeuropathy at the fibular head. Muscle Nerve 1986; 9:825–836.

48. Burke D. Value and limitations of nerve conduction studies. In: Delwaide PJ, Gorio A, eds. Clinical neurophysiology in peripheral neuropathies. Amsterdam: Elsevier, 1985: 91–102.

49. Johnson EW, Stocklin R, LaBan MM. Use of electrodiagnostic examination in a university hospital. Arch Phys Med Rehabil 1965; 46:575–578.

50. Eisen A. Electrodiagnosis of radiculopathies. Neurol Clin 1985; 3:495–510.

51. Eisen A, Schomer D, Melmed C. An electrophysiological method for examining lumbosacral root compression. Can J Neurol Sci 1977; 4:117–123.

52. Eisen A, Schomer D, Melmed C. The application of F wave measurements in the differentiation of proximal and distal upper limb entrapments. Neurology (Minneap) 1977; 27:662–668.

53. Fisher MA. F responses latency determination. Muscle Nerve 1982; 5:730–734.

54. Fisher MA, Shidve AJ, Teixera C, et al. The F response—a clinically useful physiological parameter for the evaluation of radicular injury. Electromyogr Clin Neurophysiol 1979; 19:65–75.

55. Kimura J. Clinical value and limitations of F wave determination: A reply. Muscle Nerve 1979; 1:250–251.

56. Panayiotopoulos CP. F chronodispersion: A new electrophysiological method. Muscle Nerve 1979; 2:68–72.

57. Tonzola RF, Ackil AA, Shahani BT, et al. Usefulness of electrophysiological studies in the diagnosis of lumbosacral root disease. Ann Neurol 1981; 9:305–308.

58. Young RR, Shahani BT. Clinical value and limitations of F wave determination. Muscle Nerve 1978; 1:248–249.

59. Aminoff MJ, Goodin DS, Parry GJ, et al. Electrophysiological evaluation of lumbosacral radiculopathies; electromyography, late responses and somatosensory evoked potentials. Neurology (NY) 1985; 35:1514–1518.

60. Ludin H-P. Electromyography in practice. New York: Thieme-Stratton, 1980.

61. Tackman W, Rader EW. Observations on the application of electrophysiological methods in the diagnosis of cervical root compressions. Eur Neurol 1983; 22:397–404.

62. Weintraub JR, Madalin K, Wong M, et al. Achilles tendon reflex and the H response. Their correlation in 400 limbs. Muscle Nerve 1988; 11:972.

63. Braddom RL, Johnson EW. H-reflex: Review and classification with suggested clinical uses. Arch Phys Med Rehabil 1974; 55:412–417.

64. Braddom R, Johnson E. Standardization of the "H" reflex and diagnostic use in S1 radiculopathy. Arch Phys Med Rehabil 1974; 55:161–166.

65. Johnson EW. Electrodiagnosis of radiculopathy. In: Johnson EW, ed. Practical electromyography, ed 2. Baltimore: Williams & Wilkins, 1988: 229–245.

66. Schuchmann J. H reflex latency in radiculopathy. Arch Phys Med Rehabil 1978; 59:185–187.

67. Shahani BT. Late responses and the "silent period." In: Aminoff M, ed. Electrodiagnosis in clinical neurology, ed 2. New York: Churchill-Livingstone, 1986: 333–345.

68. Shahani B, Young R. Studies on reflex activity from a clinical viewpoint. In: Aminoff M, ed. Electrodiagnosis in clinical neurology. New York: Churchill-Livingstone, 1980: 290–304.

69. Berger AR, Busis MD, Logigian MD, et al. Cervical root stimulation in the diagnosis of cervical radiculopathy. Neurology (NY) 1987; 37:329–332.

70. MacLean IC. Nerve root stimulation to evaluate conduction across the lumbrosacral plexus. Acta Neurol Scand 1979; 60(suppl 73):270.

71. Periris OA. Conduction in the fourth and fifth lumbar and first sacral nerve roots; preliminary communication. NZ Med J 1974; 80:502–503.

72. Evans BA, Daube JR, Litchy WJ. A comparison of magnetic and electrical stimulation of spinal nerves. Muscle Nerve 1990; 13:414–420.

73. Mills KR, Murray NMF. Electrical stimulation over the human vertebral column; which neural elements are excited? EEG Clin Neurophysiol 1986; 63:582–589.

74. Eisen A, Aminoff MJ. Somatosensory evoked potentials. In: Aminoff MJ, ed. Electrodiagnosis in clinical neurology, ed 2. New York: Churchill Livingstone, 1986: 535–573.

75. American Electroencephalographic Society. Guidelines for clinical evoked potential studies. J Clin Neurophysiol 1984; 1:3–53.

76. Seyal M, Gabor AJ. The human posterior tibial somatosensory evoked potential: Synapse dependent and synapse independent spinal components. Electroencephalogr Clin Neurophysiol 1985; 63:323–331.

77. Aminoff MJ, Goodin DS, Barbaro NM, et al. Dermatomal somatosensory evoked potentials in unilateral lumbosacral radiculopathy. Ann Neurol 1985; 17:171–176.

78. Feinsod M, Blau D, Findler G, et al. Somatosensory evoked potentials to peroneal nerve stimulation in patients with herniated lumbar discs. Neurosurgery 1982; 11:506–511.

79. El Negamy E, Sedgwick EM. Delayed cervical somatosensory potentials in cervical spondylosis. J Neurol Neurosurg Psychiatry 1979; 42:238–241.

80. Ganes T. Somatosensory conduction times and peripheral, cervical and cortical evoked potentials in patients with cervical spondylosis. J Neurol Neurosurg Psychiatry 1980; 43:683–689.

81. Yiannikas C, Shahani BT, Young RR. Short-latency somatosensory evoked potentials from radial, median, ulnar, and peroneal nerve stimulation in the assessment of cervical spondylosis. Comparison with conventional electromyography. Arch Neurol 1986; 43:1264–1271.

82. Eisen A, Hoirch M, Moll A. Evaluation of radiculopathies by segmental stimulation and somatosensory evoked potentials. Can J Neurol Sci 1983; 10:178–182.

83. Perlik S, Fisher MA, Patel DV, et al. On the usefulness of somatosensory evoked responses for the evaluation of lower back pain. Arch Neurol 1986; 43:907–913.

84. Seyal M, Sandhu LS, Mack YP. Spinal segmental somatosensory evoked potentials in lumbosacral radiculopathies. Neurology 1989; 39:801–805.

85. Green J, Gildenmeister R, Hazelwood C. Dermatomically stimulated somatosensory cerebral evoked potentials in the clinical diagnosis of lumbar disc disease. Clin Electroencephalogr 1983; 14:160.

86. Machida M, Asai T, Sato K, et al. New approach for diagnosis in herniated lumbar discs: Dermatomal somatosensory evoked potentials (DSSEPs). Spine 1986; 11:380–384.

87. Scarff TB, Dallman DE, Toleikis JR, et al. Dermatomal somatosensory evoked potentials in the diagnosis of lumbar root entrapment. Surg Forum 1981; 32:489–491.

88. Katifi HA, Sedgwick EM. Evaluation of the dermatomal somatosensory evoked potential in the diagnosis of lumbosacral root compression. J Neurol Neurosurg Psychiatry 1987; 50:1204–1210.

89. Seyal M, Palma GA, Sandhu LS, et al. Spinal somatosensory evoked potentials following segmental sensory stimulation: A direct measure of dorsal root function. Electroencephalogr Clin Neurophysiol 1988; 69:390–393.

90. Seyal M, Emerson RG, Pedley TA. Spinal and early scalp-recorded components of the somatosensory evoked potential following stimulation of the posterior tibial nerve. Electroencephalogr Clin Neurophysiol 1983; 55:320–330.

91. Leblhuber F, Reisecker F, Boehm-Jurkovic H, et al. Diagnostic value of different electrophysiologic tests in cervical disc prolapse. Neurology 1988; 38:1879–1881.

92. Leyshon A, Kirwan EG, Wynn Parry CB. Electrical studies in the diagnosis of compression of the lumbar root. J Bone Joint Surg 1981; 63B:71–75.

93. Swash M, Schwartz MS. Neuromuscular diseases, ed 2. New York: Springer-Verlag, 1989.

94. Lambert E. Electromyography and electrical stimulation of peripheral nerves and muscle. In: Mayo

Clinic: Clinical examinations in neurology, ed 3. Philadelphia: WB Saunders, 1971: 271–299.

95. Lambert E. Electromyography. In: Youmans J, ed: Neurological surgery. Vol 1. Philadelphia: WB Saunders, 1973: 358–367.

96. Aminoff MJ. Clinical electromyography. In: Aminoff MJ, ed. Electrodiagnosis in clinical neurology, ed 2. New York: Churchill Livingstone, 1986:231–263.

97. Johnson EW, Melvin JL. Value of electromyography in lumbar radiculopathy. Arch Phys Med Rehabil 1971; 52:239–243.

98. See D, Kraft G. Electromyography in paraspinal muscles following surgery for root compression. Arch Phys Med Rehabil 1975; 56:80–83.

99. Weingarden HP, Mikolich LM, Johnson EW. Radiculopathies. In: Johnson EW, ed. Practical electromyography. Baltimore: Williams & Wilkins, 1980:91–109.

100. Van Harreveld A. Reinnervation of denervated muscle fibers by adjacent functioning motor units. Am J Physiol 1945; 144:477–493.

101. Nutter P, Collins K. Diffuse positive waves: Case report. Arch Phys Med Rehabil 1988; 69:295–296.

102. Weichers DO, Johnson EW. Diffuse abnormal electromyographic insertional activity: A preliminary report. Arch Phys Med Rehabil 1979; 60:419–422.

103. Wright KC, Ramsey-Goldman R, Nielsen VK. Syndrome of diffuse abnormal insertional activity: Case report and family study. Arch Phys Med Rehabil 1988; 69:534–536.

104. Wilbourn AJ. An unreported distinctive type of increased insertional activity. Muscle Nerve 1982; 5:S101–S105.

105. Johnson EW. Electromyography. Arch Phys Med Rehabil 1974; 55:96.

106. Kimura J. Electrodiagnosis in diseases of nerve and muscle: Principles and practice. Philadelphia: FA Davis, 1983:672.

107. Johnson EW, Pease WS, Cannell C. Polyphasic motor unit potentials in early radiculopathy. Arch Phys Med Rehabil 1986; 67:639.

108. LaJoie WJ. Introduction to clinical electromyography. Instructional Course, American Association of Orthopedic Surgery. 1972; 21:23–41.

109. Crane CR, Krusen EM. Significance of polyphasic potentials in the diagnosis of cervical root involvement. Arch Phys Med Rehabil 1968; 49:403–406.

110. Hoover BB, Caldwell JW, Krusen EM, Muckelroy RN. Value of polyphasic potentials in diagnosis of lumbar root lesions. Arch Phys Med Rehabil 1970; 51:546–548.

111. LaJoie WV. Nerve root compression: Correlation of electromyographic, myelographic and surgical findings. Arch Phys Med Rehabil 1972; 53:390–392.

112. Waylonis GW. Electromyographic findings in chronic cervical radicular syndromes. Arch Phys Med Rehabil 1968; 49:407–412.

113. Merritt HH. A textbook of neurology, ed 5. Philadelphia: Lea & Febiger, 1973.

114. Simeone FA. Cervical disc disease with radiculopathy. In: Rothman RH, Simeone FA eds. The spine, ed 3. Philadelphia: WB Saunders 1992 (vol. 1):553–560.

115. Kramer J. Intervertebral disc disease: Causes, diagnosis, treatment and prophylaxis. London: Yearbook Medical Publishers, 1981.

116. Marinacci AA. A correlation between operative findings in cervical herniated disc with the electromyograms and opaque myelograms. Electromyography 1966; 6:5–20.

117. Marsden CD, Merton PA, Morton HB. Percutaneous stimulation of spinal cord and brain: Pyramidal tract conduction velocities in man. J Physiol (Lond) 1982; 328:6p.

118. Yoss RE, Corbin KB, MacCarthy CS, Love JG. Significance of signs and symptoms in localization of involved roots in cervical disc protrusion. Neurology (Minneap) 1957; 7:673–683.

119. Wilbourn AJ. Electrodiagnosis of plexopathies. Neurol Clin 1985; 3:511–529.

120. Chu J. Lumbosacral radicular symptoms: Importance of bilateral electrodiagnostic studies. Arch Phys Med Rehabil 1981; 62:522.

121. Tsuji S, Murai Y, Yarita M. Somatosensory potentials evoked by magnetic stimulation of lumbar roots, cauda equina, and leg nerves. Ann Neurol 1988; 24:568–573.

122. Tabaraud F, Hugon J, Chazot F, et al. Motor evoked responses after lumbar spinal stimulation in patients with L5 or S1 radicular involvement. Electroencephalogr Clin Neurophysiol 1989; 72:334–339.

123. Chokroverty S, Sachdeo R, DiLullo J, Duvoisin RC. Magnetic stimulation in the diagnosis of lumbosacral radiculopathy. J Neurol Neurosurg Psych 1989; 52:767–772.

124. Chokroverty S, DiLullo J. Magnetic stimulation of the human cervical vertebral column. Neurology 1989; 39(suppl 1):394.

125. Conway RR, Hof J, Buckelew S. Lower cervical magnetic stimulation: Comparison with C8 needle root stimulation and supraclavicular stimulation. Muscle Nerve 1988; 11:997.

126. Britton TC, Meyer B-U, Herdmann J, Benecke R. Clinical use of the magnetic stimulator in the investigation of peripheral conduction time. Muscle Nerve 1990; 13:396–406.

127. Aminoff MJ, So YT, Olney RK. Thermography. Neurology 1990; 40:561–562.

128. So YT, Aminoff MJ, Olney RK. The role of thermography in the evaluation of lumbosacral radiculopathy. Neurology 1989; 39:1154–1158.

129. So YT, Olney RK, Aminoff MJ. Evaluation of thermography in the diagnosis of selected entrapment neuropathies. Neurology 1989; 39:1–5.

130. Uematsu S, Jankel WR, Edwin DH, et al. Quantification of thermal asymmetry. Part 2: Application in
low-back pain and sciatica. J Neurosurg 1988;
69:556–561.
131. Albert SM, Glickman M, Kallish M. Thermography
in orthopedics. Ann NY Acad Sci 1964; 121:157–
170.
132. Ching C, Wexler CE. Peripheral thermographic
manifestations of lumbar-disc disease. Appl Radiol
1978; 7:53–110.
133. Wexler CE. Thermographic evaluation of trauma
(spine). Acta Thermogr 1980; 5:3–11.
134. Uematsu S, Edwin DH, Jankel WR, et al. Quantification of thermal asymmetry. Part 1: Normal values
and reproducibility. J Neurosurg 1988; 69:552–555.
135. Hubbard JE. Thermography. Neurology 1990;
40:560.
136. Ochoa J. The newly recognized painful ABC syndrome: Thermographic aspects. Thermology 1986;
2:65–107.
137. Sato A, Schmidt RF. Somatosympathetic reflexes:
Afferent fibers, central pathways, discharge characteristics. Physiol Rev 1973; 53:916–947.

8

The Electrodiagnosis
of Plexopathies

Andrew A. Eisen

CONTENTS

LIST OF ACRONYMS

CMAP	compound muscle action potential
EMG	electromyography
MU	motor unit
SEP	somatosensory evoked potential
SNAP	sensory compound nerve action potential

Evaluating lesions involving the plexuses is frequently challenging. Physicians are often daunted because of the relatively complex anatomy. The physician-electromyographer however often has more opportunities to become familiar with such lesions than other physicians. It is mandatory to work with good anatomical charts of the affected regions as an aid to the best selection, application and interpretation of any electrophysiological tests applied for the purposes of better localizing and characterizing lesions involving the plexuses.

Electrophysiologic assessment of plexopathies aims to localize the site and extent of the lesion as accurately as possible while determining its severity and prognosis. When it comes to plexopathies, there are few other investigative procedures that can compete with the importance of electrophysiologic studies. Like the spinal roots, however, the proximal position of the plexuses, especially those of the leg, render them relatively inaccessible to conventional conduction studies. Needle electromyography (EMG) remains the best method for plotting the anatomic distribution of lesions, especially in the presence of axonopathy.

Plexopathies must be differentiated from radiculopathies and more distal peripheral nerve lesions. The clinical deficit produced by a plexopathy may closely mimic either. Clinically neck or back pain, partial muscle weakness and wasting in a myotomal distribution, and sensory deficit in a dermatomal distribution are all helpful in suggesting a root lesion.

The single most useful electrophysiologic marker of a radiculopathy is paraspinal denervation (fibrillation potentials or positive sharp waves) associated with normal compound sensory nerve action potentials (SNAPs). On the other hand, peripheral nerve lesions, although more restricted in terms of their anatomic distribution, often produce a more severe neurologic deficit than does a plexopathy but like them are associated with abnormalities of motor and sensory conduction.

BRACHIAL PLEXUS: ANATOMIC AND CLINICAL CONSIDERATIONS

The brachial plexus[1] (Figures 8.1 and 8.2; Table 8.1) is derived from the anterior rami of C-5 through T-1 spinal roots. The nerve to rhomboids (C-5), the dorsal scapular nerve (C-5, C-6) innervating the subscapularis, and the long thoracic nerve (C-5, C-6, C-7) supplying serratus anterior arise directly from the spinal roots proximal to the formation of the trunks.

① the subscapular nerve

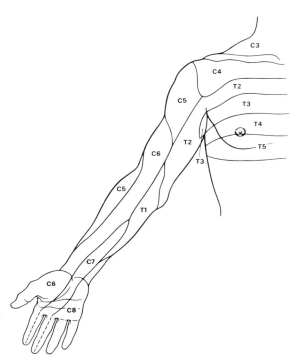

FIGURE 8.1. *The dermatomes of the upper limb. (From Foerster. Brain 1933; 56:1. With permission from Oxford University Press.)*

Paralysis or paresis of these muscles is therefore evidence of radicular involvement, which may be confirmed by finding fibrillation potentials and positive sharp waves in the cervical paraspinal muscles.

Trunks

The *upper trunk* is formed from the junction of C-5 and C-6 spinal roots. The suprascapular nerve innervating the supraspinatus and infraspinatus muscles and the nerve to subclavius arise from the upper trunk. Lesions of the upper trunk result in weakness of shoulder abduction, external rotation, and elbow flexion. The sensory deficit is usually mild and limited to a small patch of skin overlying the deltoid. Upper trunk lesions need to be differentiated from C-5 and C-6 radiculopathies and anterior horn cell disease involving these myotomes. Root lesions are usually accompanied by neck pain, and because of segmental overlap, muscle weakness is often less complete than that occurring with a plexopathy.

The conduction time across the brachial plexus and the amplitude of the motor responses obtained

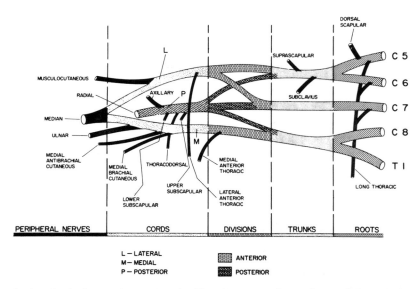

FIGURE 8.2.   *The brachial plexus. (From Goodgold J. Anatomical correlates of clinical electromyography. Baltimore: Williams & Wilkins, 1974:56. Copyright © 1974 The Williams & Wilkins Co. With permission.)*

by stimulating the cervical roots. Erb's point stimulation is less helpful in documenting which part(s) of the plexus are involved. Cervical root stimulation is best achieved through a monopolar needle electrode inserted 2 to 3 cm lateral to the midlnie through the paraspinal muscles until its tip lies against the lamina of the appropriate vertebral body. Compound muscle action potentials (CMAPs) may then be recorded,

TABLE 8.1.   Selected muscles (root values) and sensory nerves useful for delineating brachial plexopathies

	Electromyography/Compound Muscle Action Potentials	*Compound Sensory Nerve Action Potentials*
Roots	Rhomboids (C-5)	None
	Serratus anterior (C-5–C-7)	
Upper trunk	Supraspinatus (C-5,C-6)	None
	Infraspinatus (C-5,C-6)	
Middle trunk	Triceps (C-7,C-8)	Median and
	Pronator teres (C-6,C-7)	radial
	Flexor carpi radialis (C-7,C-8)	
Lower trunk	Thenar (C-8,T-1)	Median and
	Hypothenar (C-8,T-1)	ulnar
	Extensor carpi ulnaris (C-7,C-8)	
Lateral cord	Biceps (C-5,C-6)	Musculocutaneous
	Pronator teres (C-6,C-7)	
Medial cord	Thenar (C-8,T-1)	Median and
	Hypothenar (C-8,T-1)	ulnar
Posterior cord	Deltoid (C-5,C-6)	Musculocutaneous
	Triceps (C-7,C-8)	and radial
	Wrist extensors (C-7,C-8)	

using surface electrodes. The latencies of M potentials representative of various components of the brachial plexus are shown in Table 8.2. Stimulation at Erb's point may also be used to measure conduction across the brachial plexus. This, however, has the disadvantage of often being at, or distal to, the site of the primary pathology. The amplitude of the CMAP is a good reflection of the number of motor axons stiumulated, and side to side comparison is a useful measure of the extent of axonal loss.

When assessing the upper trunk of the brachial plexus, it is desirable to record CMAPs from the supraspinatus or infraspinatus muscles. The deltoid muscle is not optimal because its innervation, through the axillary nerve, arises distally from the posterior cord. Similarly, the innervation of the biceps muscle (musculocutaneous) also arises distally from the lateral cord.

The C-7 root continues as the *middle trunk*, and lesions of the latter may be difficult to distinguish from C-7 radiculopathy. Prominent triceps weakness, loss of triceps deep tendon reflex, and sensory deficit over the dorsum of the hand and adjoining surfaces of the second and third fingers are characteristic of both. Radial motor and sensory conductions are abnormal, and with axon loss, fibrillation potentials are recordable in muscles innervated, by the C-7 root, through the radial nerve. Isolated lesions of the middle trunk of the brachial plexus are rare and must also be distinguished from lesions of the posterior cord. The middle trunk and posterior cord both contain axons derived from the C-7 root. The middle trunk, however, also contains fibers destined for the median nerve, and lesions of it can therefore be recognized by recording an abnormal median compound SNAP and fibrillation potential in the pronator teres and the flexor carpi radialis.

The lower trunk is formed from the C-8 and T-1 spinal roots. The lesions effecting the lower trunk produce a combined median and ulnar "hand" although the ulnar component is often the more severely involved. A lesion of the lower trunk is one of the many causes of the "wasted, weak hand" and must be differentiated from other diseases resulting in this pattern of neurological deficit. The latter pattern includes combined median and ulnar neuropathies, C-8 radiculopathy, diseases affecting the root entry zone as in the case of multiple sclerosis and disorders affecting the motor neurons themselves such as amyotrophic lateral sclerosis, monomelic amyotrophy and syringomyelia. Rarely a similar picture may be produced by lesions affecting the parietal lobe. Any sensory deficit in the hand or forearm excludes amyotrophic lateral sclerosis and monomelic amyotrophy whereas extension of the sensory loss to the medial forearm excludes an ulnar neuropathy at the elbow. Usually by the time either multiple sclerosis or syringomyelia cause significant hand wasting, long-track signs are also obvious.

The chief differential diagnosis is a C-8 radiculopathy. If the T-1 root is involved, Horner's syndrome usually develops. Clues favoring radiculopathy include neck pain induced by neck movement; pain with coughing, sneezing, or Valsalva's maneuver; a normal ulnar compound SNAP; and lower cervical paraspinal denervation.

Key electrophysiologic features confirming a lower trunk plexopathy include (1) slowed motor conduction across the lower trunk (see Table 8.1), (2) prolonged ulnar F wave latencies, (3) absent or reduced size of ulnar compound SNAPs, (4) delayed early latency components of the ulnar somatosensory evoked potential (SEP), and (5) active denervation (fibrillation potentials and positive sharp waves) or

TABLE 8.2.   Motor conduction across the brachial plexus stimulating cervical spinal roots*

Part of Plexus Evaluated	Vertebral Level	Recording Site	Mean Value (ms)	Upper Limit (ms)
Upper trunk	C-5 C-5	Supraspinatus/ infraspinatus	5.1	6.5
Lateral cord	C-5	Biceps	5.1	6.5
Middle trunk	C-6	Triceps	5.7	6.7
Posterior cord	C-6	Deltoid	5.3	6.5
Lower trunk Medial cord	C-7	Hypothenar	12.5	15.5

* Stimulation is through a monopolar needle electrode introduced through the paraspinal muscles 2 cm lateral to the spinous process of the appropriate vertebral body.

chronic partial denervation (complex motor units (MUs) of increased duration and amplitude) in median-supplied and ulnar-supplied hand muscles as well as the radial-supplied extensor and abductor pollicis longus and extensor carpi ulnaris muscles. CMAPs may also be reduced in size in these muscles compared with the noninvolved side.

Cords

The *lateral cord* is formed from the anterior divisions of the upper and middle trunks. Proximally it gives rise to the medial and lateral pectoral nerves supplying the pectoral muscles. It continues as the musculocutaneous nerve to supply the coracobrachialis, biceps, and brachialis muscles. The terminal part of the lateral cord forms the lateral half of the median nerve from which the motor nerve to the pronator teres arises. (The motor supply to all other median-supplied forearm muscles arises from both the medial and the lateral parts of the median nerve. The motor nerves to the intrinsic hand musculature supplied by the median nerve arise only from its medial half.)

Lateral cord lesions are usually easily differentiated from upper trunk lesions by the absence of the *droopy shoulder*, which typifies the latter. Lesions of both, however, may reduce the sizes of the musculocutaneous (biceps) CMAP and median and musculocutaneous compound SNAPs. In lesions affecting the lateral cord, denervation is restricted to the biceps, brachialis, pronator teres, and flexor carpi radialis. Fibrillation potentials or positive sharp waves are not seen in the deltoid, brachioradialis, or spinatae as with upper trunk lesions.

The *medial cord* is formed from the anterior division of the lower trunk. It gives rise to the ulnar nerve and the medial half of the median nerve. The medial brachial and antebrachial cutaneous nerves also arise from the medial cord. Lesions of the medial cord result in a paretic or paralyzed hand and a combined median/ulnar sensory deficit. Differentiating a lower trunk lesion is difficult because abnormalities of nerve conduction are identical in both. Because only the lower trunk contains C-8 motor fibers supplying forearm extensor muscles such as the abductor and extensor policis longus, extensor indicis proprius and extensor pollicis brevis muscles, the finding of fibrillation potentials in these muscles rules out a pure medial cord lesion.

The *posterior cord* is formed from the posterior divisions of all three trunks and continues as the radial nerve. Proximally branches arise to supply the teres major and subscapularis (subscapular nerve, C-5, C-6), latissimus dorsi (thoracodorsal nerve C-6, C-7, C-8), and deltoid and teres minor (axillary nerve, C-5, C-6) muscles. Weakness and wasting of the deltoid, a reduced deltoid CMAP, and fibrillation potential activity in the deltoid and latissimus dorsi muscles are important features differentiating a posterior cord from a radial nerve lesion.

Traumatic Plexopathies

The superficial location, close relationship to many bone structures, and mobility of the shoulder and neck render the brachial plexus particularly vulnerable to injury. Closed traction and stretch injuries of the shoulder commonly injure the trunks of the brachial plexus, whereas open injuries, such as stab and gunshot wounds, usually injure the cords. The chief role of electrophysiologic studies of traumatic brachial plexopathies is to determine whether root avulsion has occurred. Avulsion of the roots is usually a contraindication to surgical repair. Other goals of electrophysiologic testing include determining the anatomic extent of the lesion, the severity of the lesion(s), and the prognosis for recovery. Most traumatic plexopathies result from motor vehicle accidents, and impending litigation makes careful documentation of such lesions important.

Root Avulsion

Avulsion of a cervical root is often apparent myelographically as a small meningocele.[2] Such distentions of the root sleeve, however, may be present in the absence of root avulsion or vice versa. The presence of a flail arm, typical of a severe brachial plexopathy usually with multiple root avulsion, may also be accompanied by evidence of other injuries of the cervical cord. For this reason, myelography or a computed tomographic scan should be considered shortly after the time of the accident even when the clinical evidence strongly suggests root avulsions.

Characteristic electrophysiologic features of root avulsion include the following:

1. Normal compound SNAPs in involved segments. This indicates that even though the central limb of the dorsal root ganglion cell has been severed, the cell body and its peripheral connections remain intact. Such cases are also characterized by skin flare responses of the skin induced by intradermal histamine.[3,4] Absence of a SEP in the face of preserved peripheral sensory conduction is a

useful adjunct to confirming loss of continuity with the central process of the sensory axon.

2. Failure to record a CMAP from paralyzed muscles.

3. Active denervation (fibrillation potentials and positive sharp waves) recorded from the involved muscles and especially the cervical paraspinal muscles. These changes require time to develop. Indirect CMAPs may be elicited for up to 2 to 3 days following severence of a nerve, although size of the potentials fall rapidly within 24 hours postinjury. Fibrillation potentials and positive sharp waves are usually not recordable in the cervical paraspinal muscles for 7 to 10 days and may take up to 21 days to develop in distal muscles and upper limb muscles.

Use of Somatosensory Evoked Potentials in Traumatic Plexopathies

SEPs both have localizing value and add information about the severity of a brachial plexopathy, especially the degree of axonal continuity in sensory fibers (Table 8.3). An absent SEP in the presence of a normal peripheral compound SNAP is good evidence of root avulsion. On the other hand, the presence of a cortical SEP, even in the absence of a peripheral compound SNAP, indicates preservation of continuity in at least some axons.[5] Comparison of the amplitude of the N13 and N9 components is a useful guide of the extent of root avulsion when this is incomplete. Reduction in the size of the median N13 by 40% or more compared with the intact arm indicates injury to the C-6 or C-7 roots, and reduction of the ulnar N13 by 40% or more compared with the intact arm indicates probable injury to the C-8

or T-1 roots.[6] Stimulation of various nerves (median, ulnar, radial, or musculocutaneous) to elicit SEPs may also give information regarding the segmental involvement of the plexus injury.[7–9]

Brachial Neuritis

Paralytic brachial neuritis (also referred to as *neuralgic amyotrophy* and *Parsonage-Turner syndrome*) may closely mimic acute cervical radiculopathy.[10,11] Characteristically the syndrome has an acute onset, often with severe pain, accompanied, or more usually followed in several days, by weakness and subsequent muscle wasting. Patients with mild cases develop pain and weakness but do not go on to develop muscle wasting. The distribution of the pain and weakness is variable and characteristically poorly localized. Careful clinical analysis suggests that the lesion, in many cases of paralytic brachial neuritis, be localized to branching points of the brachial plexus or its major peripheral nerve trunks.[12]

The cause of this disorder is unknown. Approximately 50% of cases are associated with some antecedent event, such as immunization, viral infections, surgery, trauma, pregnancy, drug abuse, or collagen vascular diseases. There is a rare familial form,[13] some cases of which have proved to have tomacular neuropathy,[14] and occasionally the condition is recurrent.[15] The majority of patients make a satisfactory but slow recovery over the next 1 to 2 years. About 10% of patients fail to regain useful function of the involved muscles.

Pathologic observations in brachial neuritis are rare.[16] A report of two patients with recurrent symptoms, who because of developing a tender supraclavicular mass underwent surgery, showed macro-

TABLE 8.3. Nerves stimulated to elicit somatosensory evoked potentials for evaluating brachial plexopathies

Part of Plexus Evaluated	Stimulating Site	Mean Value to N20 (ms)	Upper Limit (ms)
Upper trunk	Musculocutaneous (elbow)	17.4	21
Lateral cord	Radial (wrist)	18.6	22
Middle trunk Posterior cord	Radial (wrist)	18.6	22
Lower trunk	Ulnar (wrist)	20.2	24
Medial cord	Median (wrist)	19.7	23.3

Stimulation should be sufficient to induce slight muscle contraction. Recording is scalp bipolar C-3/C-4 Fcz.

scopic fusiform segmental swelling of the trunks of the brachial plexus. Microscopically the lesions were characterized by edema, onion bulb formation, and marked focal chronic inflammatory infiltrates with lymphoid follicle formation, limited to the endoneurial compartment.[17]

The severity of electrophysiologic abnormalities varies. Nerve conduction studies are usually normal in brachial neuritis. In severe cases, however, the amplitude of the CMAP is reduced, and compound SNAPs may be small or unrecordable in the distribution of the lesion. Needle EMG is the most relevant aspect of the electrophysiologic examination. Even in mild cases, there is abnormal MU recruitment coinciding with the onset of the disease. Onset firing frequencies of individual MUs are increased (>10 c/s), and the ratio of the firing rate of a MU to the number of units already discharging is elevated (normal <5). Depending on the severity, fibrillation potentials and positive sharp waves may be sparse or profuse. Absence of cervical paraspinal denervation is a useful negative feature when cervical radiculopathy is a consideration. With axonal regeneration and muscle reinnervation, fibrillation potentials cease and MUs become enlarged and complex. Unstable units are suggestive of newly formed neuromuscular functions.

Thoracic Outlet Syndromes

The concept of thoracic outlet has evolved over the past century, although controversy surrounds virtually every aspect of the disorder.[18] In the context of this chapter, however, the critical issue lies in the differential diagnosis of root lesions, especially involving C-8, T-1 cervical roots. Pragmatically it may be argued that most if not all thoracic outlet syndromes are of two types: the rare *true neurogenic thoracic outlet syndrome* and the common *droopy shoulder syndrome*.

Neurogenic thoracic outlet syndrome has been well delineated by Gilliatt et al.[19,20] It is rare; the author has seen fewer than 20 cases in 25 years of neurologic and electromyographic practice. Typically it affects young women and presents with painless, partial, thenar wasting. In contradistinction to carpal tunnel syndrome, however, sensory complaints, when they occur, involve the medial aspect of the forearm and ulnar side of the hand. The symptoms are directly due to pressure or stretching of the lower trunk or C-8, T-1 spinal roots from a fibrous band attached to a supernumerary rib or elongated

C-7 transverse process. Where extra ribs are present, they often occur bilaterally, but usually it is the less prominent rib (with the longer fibrous band) that is responsible for symptoms. Radiographs or computed tomographic scans do not always show an extra rib or elongated C-7 transverse process. Hence normal radiologic studies do not rule out neurogenic thoracic outlet syndrome.

Electrophysiologic studies are helpful in the diagnosis and localization of the lesion.[21,22] A constellation of characteristic abnormalities have evolved. These include (1) a much reduced median maximum CMAP in the face of normal median compound SNAPs, (2) a reduced or absent ulnar compound SNAP in the face of a normal or only modestly reduced ulnar maximum CMAP, (3) absent or prolonged latency hypothenar F wave, (4) SEPs that may reveal a small or absent median or ulnar N13 with a relatively normal N9 component (sometimes the N9 peak is delayed and reduced in size with a prolonged N9-N13 interpeak conduction time),[23] and (5) needle electromyographic evidence for chronic partial denervation in the C-8 and T-1 supplied muscles.

In contrast, the droopy shoulder syndrome, a term coined by Swift et al.,[24] is common and accounts for many other cases of thoracic outlet syndrome. This syndrome is most common in women. Criteria for droopy shoulder syndrome include (1) pain or paresthesia occurring in the shoulder, arm, forearm, or hand; (2) long, graceful, and swan-like neck, low set shoulders, and horizontal or downsloping clavicles; (3) exacerbation of symptoms on palpation of brachial plexus or passive downward traction of the arms; (4) immediate relief of symptoms by passive shoulder elevation; (5) absence of vascular phenomena, muscle atrophy, sensory loss, or reflex changes; (6) T-2 or lower vertebrae visible above the shoulders on lateral cervical spine radiographs; and (7) normal electrophysiologic studies.

Radiation Plexopathy

The brachial plexus is vulnerable to physical radiation injury directed toward treatment for carcinoma of the breast, lung, mediastinum, and axillary nodes. Plexopathy complicating radiation results from fibrosis and is dose dependent. If 6000 cGy are administered, about 75% of patients develop radiation plexopathy. Lower doses administered over longer periods of time are much safer.[25] Typically there is progressive, painless wasting of upper trunk muscles with accompanying lymphedema and skin changes.[26] Associated paresthesias and sensory loss occur. In contrast, tumor infiltration involving the brachial plexus usually induces severe pain, and the neurologic deficit predominantly involves the lower trunk. Associated Horner's syndrome is common.

The earliest electrophysiologic abnormality in radiation plexopathy is a reduced amplitude or absent compound SNAP. The median nerve, which contains upper trunk fibers, is involved more than the ulnar nerve.[27,28] Myokymia and low-frequency complex repetitive discharges are often prominent in addition to fibrillation potentials or positive sharp waves. Low-frequency and high-frequency complex repetitive discharges probably reflect ephaptic transmission in demyelinated axons.[29,30]

muscle fibers.

Perioperative Brachial Plexopathy

Perioperative nerve lesions are not infrequent.[31,32] The potential for litigation is high, and it is important to recognize lesions that are clearly the result of the surgery and those that are incidental. For example, an acute wristdrop following abdominal surgery is most probably due to radial nerve compression during the procedure. On the other hand, the development of a femoral neuropathy in a diabetic occurring shortly after surgery is more likely coincidental.

A multifactorial pathogenesis seems likely, and different sites may be simultaneously involved.[31] The mechanism of these lesions is poorly understood.[33] Compression, traction, angulation, and ischemia may all play a role. Whether ischemia is relevant in patients who do not have associated disease such as diabetes is a moot point. In baboons, compression of a nerve that has been rendered ischemic does not cause additional damage.[34]

The brachial plexus is the most susceptible of all nerves to damage from poor positioning during anesthesia. Two mechanisms have been identified. The plexus may be stretched when the arm is abducted and the head flexed laterally in the opposite direction. This usually results in an upper trunk plexopathy. Damage can also follow positioning of a shoulder rest position too far laterally in a patient in the Trendelenburg position. This forces the humeral head down into the axilla causing acute angulation of the plexus. In this situation, the lower trunk is more vulnerable. Most patients recover completely in a few weeks, suggesting that conduction block without significant axonal degeneration underlies the

lesion. Few electrophysiologic studies, however, have been reported for these lesions.[35]

Between 5% and 15% of patients undergoing open heart surgery by a median sternotomy develop a lower trunk brachial plexopathy.[36,37] The side affected does not always correlate with the side of the jugular cannulation; thus although needle trauma may at times be relevant, this is not invariable. Traction may play a role especially in cases requiring left internal mammary artery resection because this procedure necessitates greater chest wall retraction. Electrophysiologic localization of the lesion is often uncertain.[5,33] Most patients recover without going through a phase of axonal degeneration, and the most common mechanism would appear to be one of conduction block.

Brachial plexopathy is now a recognized complication of surgical treatment for thoracic outlet syndrome.[38,39] Its incidence is not known, but when it occurs, it is a serious, difficult to treat, problem. Most cases have been associated with first rib resections performed via the transaxillary approach. The most common clinical features are those of a painful lower trunk/medial cord plexopathy with hand and medial forearm weakness and paresthesias and sensory loss along the medial forearm, hand, and ulnar fingers. Severe, causalgic pain involving the hand is common. Ulnar sensory and ulnar and median CMAPs are usually reduced. Needle EMG characteristically reveals fibrillation potentials in a lower trunk distribution but may be more widespread. These changes of axonal degeneration suggest that the mechanism responsible is due to contusion or traction and not simply conduction block.

Sports-Related Upper Trunk Brachial Plexopathy

Burner or stinger of the football player is a common but controversial disorder of unknown cause. Most evidence, however, points to an upper trunk plexopathy.[40,41] It is commonly induced in football players, who report a sudden jolt, burning, or stinging sensation, for example, throughout the outstretched arm when trying to fend off a tackle. This may be associated with weakness lasting several minutes. The weakness, however, may sometimes persist for many hours and even weeks. EMG has shown the presence of fibrillation potentials and positive sharp waves of upper trunk muscles but not the paraspinal muscles.[40] Others have recorded paraspinal fibrillation potentials, indicating a radiculopathy rather than a plexopathy.[42]

LUMBOSACRAL PLEXUS: ANATOMIC CONSIDERATIONS

The lumbosacral plexus is formed from anterior rami of the five lumbar and four sacral spinal roots[43] (Figure 8.3). The ventral and dorsal divisions are equivalent to the anterior and posterior divisions of the spinal roots forming the brachial plexus. The different terminology is required because of the 90 degree rotation of the leg in relation to the arm. The ventral roots supply the flexor and the dorsal roots the extensor muscles of the leg. The ventral divisions form the iliohypogastric and ilioinguinal; the genitofemoral; the obturator and the tibial portion of the sciatic nerve; and the dorsal divisions form the

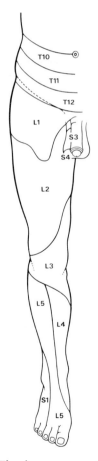

FIGURE 8.3.   *The dermatomes of the lower limb. (From Foerster. Brain 1933; 56:1. With permission from Oxford University Press.)*

lateral femoral cutaneous, the femoral, gluteal nerves, and the common peroneal nerve (Figures 8.2 and 8.3; Table 8.4).

The term *lumbosacral plexus* is used in this section. Simultaneous involvement, however, of both the lumbar and the sacral plexuses is less frequent than their individual involvement.[28] As a group, lumbosacral plexopathies occur less frequently and are more difficult to evaluate than lesions of the brachial plexus. The motor nerves arising from the lumbar plexus (obturator and femoral) innervate proximal muscles, making motor conduction more difficult to assess. Compound SNAPs are also difficult if not impossible to elicit from the cutaneous nerves arising from the lumbar plexus (the iliohypogastric, illoinguinal, genitofemoral, lateral femoral cutaneous, and saphenous). Eliciting SEPs may be a helpful way around this dilemma (Table 8.5). Generally, however, reliance must be largely placed on abnormalities found by needle EMG, which precludes early assessment (Table 8.4). Once fibrillation potentials develop, which takes from 10 to 14 days in proximal muscles, a lumbar plexopathy may be distinguished from a femoral neuropathy by finding fibrillation potentials in obturator innervated muscles, for example, the adductor magnus. Absence of fibrillation potential in the L-1–L-3 paraspinal mucles is important in differentiating a plexopathy from a radioculopathy.

Sacral plexopathies occur more commonly and are easier to evaluate given that the sacral plexus gives rise to the sciatic nerve and its terminal branches the tibial and common peroneal nerves as well as the superficial peroneal and sural cutaneous nerves from which compound SNAPs may be easily recorded.

Lumbosacral plexopathies must be differentiated from radiculopathies, lesions of the cauda equina, and proximal mononeuropathies. Abnormal compound SNAPs (absent or reduced in amplitude) are valuable in ruling out most radiculopathies.[5] It is relatively easy to measure motor conduction across both the lumbar and the sacral plexuses using a monopolar needle electrode to stimulate the lumbosacral roots in a manner similar to that described for the brachial plexus (Table 8.6). Unilateral, proximal muscle denervation (fibrillation potentials or positive sharp waves), in the face of normal paraspinal needle EMG, in more than one myotome, innervated by more than one leg nerve, is, however, the most convincing electrophysiologic means of determining that a lesion involves the plexus.

TABLE 8.4.   Selected muscles (root values) and sensory nerves useful for delineating lumbosacral plexopathies

Electromyography/Compound Muscle Action Potential	Compound Sensory Nerve Action Potential
Lumbar Plexus	
Quadriceps (L-2,L-3,L-4)	Lateral femoral cutaneous and saphenous
Adductor longus (L-2,L-3,L-4)	
Adductor brevis (L-2,L-3,L-4)	
Sacral Plexus	
Gluteus medius (L-4,L-5,S-1)	Sural and
Gluteus maximus (L-5,S-1,S-2)	superficial peroneal
Gastrocnemius (L-5,S-1,S-2)	
Tibialis anterior (L-4,L-5)	

Lumbosacral Plexitis

This is the counterpart of paralytic brachial neuritis affecting the upper limb, but for unknown reasons it occurs much less frequently.[44] For example, at the Mayo Clinic, only 10 cases were collected over a 15-year period.[45] Similar to brachial neuritis, it is associated with an antecedent event (infection, trauma, surgery) in about 50% of cases. Thigh and leg pain, which is initially often severe, is followed by muscle weakness and atrophy in the distribution of the lumbosacral plexus. Despite the inital severity of symptoms, the majority of patients recover without permanent neurologic deficit. In the few cases that have been investigated electrophysiologically, motor conductions were normal, but needle EMG was consistent with an axonal process sparing the paraspinal muscles. Cerebrospinal fluid protein was normal.[44,45]

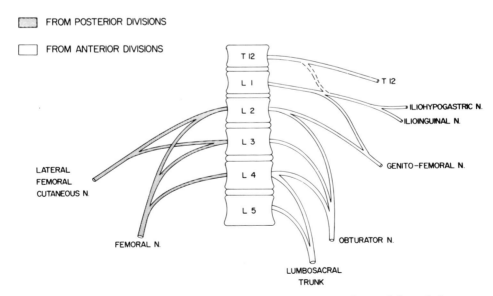

FIGURE 8.4.   *The lumbar plexus. (From Goodgold J. Anatomical correlates of clinical electromyography. Baltimore: Williams & Wilkins, 1974:126. Copyright © 1974 The Williams & Wilkins Co. With permission.)*

TABLE 8.5.   Nerves stimulated to elicit somatosensory evoked potentials for evaluating lumbosacral plexopathies*

Plexus Evaluated	Stimulation Site	Mean Value (ms) to P40	Upper Limit (ms)
Lumbar	Tibial at ankle	38.6	44
Sacral	Peroneal at knee	32.4	38.5

* Stimulation should be sufficient to induce slight muscle contraction. Recording is scalp bipolar Cz-Fpz.

Perioperative Lumbosacral Plexopathies

Genitofemoral or ilioinguinal neuralgia owing to nerve entrapment is a recognized complication of surgery in the inguinal region. Starling and Harms[46] described 36 cases over an 8-year period. Nineteen patients, having had previous inguinal herniorraphy, developed ilioinguinal neuralgia.

Acute lumbosacral plexopathy is a complication of renal transplantation, the treatment of choice for patients with end-stage renal disease from insulin-dependent diabetes. In this situation, the internal iliac artery is used for revascularization of the renal allograft. Symptoms developing usually within 24 hours of surgery are typified by ipsilateral buttock pain, numbness in the leg, and weakness below the knee.[47]

Diabetic Radicular-Plexopathies

Radicular-plexopathies (polyradiculopathy) frequently complicate diabetes. Elderly men with type

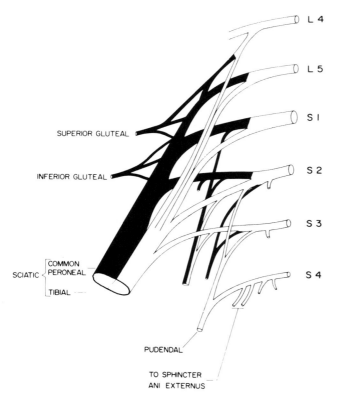

FIGURE 8.5.   *The sacral and coccygeal plexuses. Posterior divisions are in black, anterior divisions in white. (From Good-gold J. Anatomical correlates of clinical electromyography. Baltimore: Williams & Wilkins, 1974:126. Copyright © 1974 The Williams & Wilkins Co. With permission.)*

TABLE 8.6. Motor conduction across the lumbosacral plexus stimulating lumbosacral roots*

Part of Plexus Evaluated	Stimulating Site	Recording Site	Mean Value (ms)	Upper Limit (ms)
Lumbar plexus	L-2–L-4	Vastus medialis	8.8	12.4
Sacral plexus	S-1,S-2	Gastrocnemius	10.4	13.5

* Stimulation is through a monopolar needle passed through the paraspinal muscles to the lamina of the appropriate vertebral body.

II diabetes are particularly prone. Most frequently, the myotomes of the anterior thigh (L-2, L-3, L-4) are involved.[48] Although usually unilateral at onset, many cases go on to involve the contralateral side, not necessarily in a symmetric fashion. Pain, typically acute in onset, is followed by muscle wasting and weakness, depression or loss of reflexes, and sensory loss. Diabetic amyotrophy, described originally by Garland,[49] can be reasonably regarded as a specific variant of diabetic radicular-plexopathy. Garland[49] was impressed by the severe muscle wasting that so frequently occurs.

Clinical and electrophysiologic localization indicate that there may be involvement of root, plexus, or nerve, or more usually a combination of all three. Proximal diabetic radicular-plexopathies often occur on a background of the much more common diabetic symmetric polyneuropathy.[50–52] The sacral plexus and lower lumbar and sacral roots and cervical roots and brachial plexus are affected rarely compared with the upper lumbar roots and the lumbar plexus. Severe involvement of, for example, the C-5 and C-6 roots should prompt one to seek an alternative cause for the radiculopathy.

The chronic complications of diabetes result from the interaction of hyperglycemia and other metabolic consequences of insulin deficiency as well as poorly understood but independent genetic and environmental factors. Rises in tissue sorbitol secondary to glucose concentration–dependent activation of polyol pathway activity and an accompanying fall in tissue myo-inositol and sodium-potassium-adenosinetriphosphatose activity have been linked to a self-reinforcing cyclic metabolic defect to account for rapidly reversible slowing of conduction in peripheral nerve.[53] Treatment aimed at neutralizing this series of events is the obvious approach for the future. Pancreatic transplantation has been shown to prevent development of neuropathy in inbred diabetic rats[54,55] and ameliorate complicating neuropathy in humans.[56]

Miscellaneous Lumbosacral Plexopathies

There are other causes of lumbosacral plexopathy, often reported as single cases. They include compression from a hematoma, usually complicating anticoagulant therapy or hemophilia[57,58]; amyloidosis, sarcoidosis, and leprosy[59–61]; and spinal cord infarction.[62]

REFERENCES

1. Goodgold J. Anatomical correlates of clinical electromyography. Baltimore: Williams & Wilkins, 1974:56.
2. Yeoman PM. Cervical myelography in traction injuries of the brachial plexus. J Bone Joint Surg 1968; 50B:253–260.
3. Bonney G, Gilliatt RW. Sensory nerve conduction after traction lesion of the brachial plexus. Proc R Soc Med 1958; 51:365–367.
4. Warren J, Guttmann L, Figueroa AJ, et al. Electromyographic changes of brachial plexus root avulsions. J Neurosurg 1969; 31:137–140.
5. Eisen A. Radiculopathies and plexopathies. In: Brown WF, Bolton CF, eds. Clinical electromyography, ed 1. Boston: Butterworths, 1987:51–73.
6. Jones SJ, Wynn Parry CB, Landi A. Diagnosis of brachial plexus traction lesions by sensory nerve action potentials and somatosensory evoked potentials. Injury 1981; 12:376–382.
7. Synek VM. Somatosensory evoked potentials from musculocutaneous nerve in the diagnosis of brachial plexus injury. J Neurol Sci 1983; 61:443–452.
8. Yiannikas C, Shahani BT, Young RR. The investigation of traumatic lesions of the brachial plexus by electromyography and short latency somatosensory potentials evoked by stimulation of multiple nerves. J Neurol Neurosurg Psychiatry 1983; 46:1014–1022.
9. Eisen A. Use of somatosensory evoked potentials for

the evaluation of the peripheral nervous system. Neurol Clin 1988; 6:825–838.

10. Parsonage MJ, Turner JWA. Neurologic amyotrophy: The shoulder-girdle syndrome. Lancet 1948; 1:973–978.

11. Turner JWA, Parsonage MJ. Neurologic amyotrophy (paralytic brachial neuritis). Lancet 1957; 2:209–212.

12. England JD, Sumner AJ. Neurologic amyotrophy: An increasingly diverse entity. Muscle Nerve 1987; 10:60–68.

13. Dunn HG, Daube JR, Gomez MR. Heredofamilial brachial plexus neuropathy (hereditary neuralgic amyotrophy with brachial predilection) in childhood. Dev Med Child Neurol 1978; 20:28–46.

14. Madrid R, Bradley WG. 1975. The pathology of neuropathies with focal thickening of the myelin sheath (tomaculous neuropathy). J Neurol Sci 25:415–448.

15. Bradley WG, Madrid R, Thrush DC. Recurrent brachial plexus neuropathy. Brain 1975; 98:381–398.

16. Tsairis P, Dyck P, Mulder DW. Natural history of brachial plexus neuropathy. Arch Neurol 1972; 27:109–117.

17. Cusimano MD, Bilbao JM, Cohen SM. Hypertrophic brachial plexus neuritis: A pathological study of two cases. Ann Neurol 1988; 24:615–622.

18. Cuetter AC, Bartoszek DM. The thoracic outlet syndrome: Controversies, overdiagnosis, overtreatment and recommendations for management. Muscle Nerve 1989; 12:410–419.

19. Gilliatt RW. Thoracic outlet compression syndrome. Br Med J 1976; 1:1274–1275.

20. Gilliatt RW, Willison RG, Dietz V, Williams IR. Peripheral nerve conduction in patients with cervical rib and band. Ann Neurol 1978; 4:124–129.

21. Wilbourn AJ. True neurogenic thoracic outlet syndrome. Rochester, MN: American Association of Electromyography and Electrodiagnosis, 1982.

22. Wilbourn AJ, Aminoff MJ. The electrophysiological examination in patients with radiculopathies. Rochester, MN: American Association of Electromyography and Electrodiagnosis Minimonography #32, 1988.

23. Yiannikas C, Walsh JC. Somatosensory evoked responses in the diagnosis of thoracic outlet syndrome. J Neurol Neurosurg Psychiatry 1983; 46:234.

24. Swift TR, Nichols FT. The droopy shoulder syndrome. Neurology 1984; 34:212–215.

25. Stewart JD. Focal peripheral neuropathies. New York: Elsevier, 1987:93–118.

26. Kori SH, Foley KM, Posner JB. Brachial plexus lesions in patients with cancer: 100 cases. Neurology 1981; 31:45–50.

27. Lederman RJ, Wilbourn AJ. Brachial plexopathy: Recurrent cancer or radiation? Neurology 1984; 34:1331–1335.

28. Wilbourn AJ. Electrodiagnosis of plexopathies. Neurol Clin 1985; 3:511–529.

29. Stohr M. Special types of spontaneous electrical activity in radiogenic nerve injuries. Muscle Nerve 1982; 5:S78–S83.

30. Jablecki C, Schultz P. Single muscle fiber recordings in the Schwartz-Jampel syndrome. Muscle Nerve 1982; 5:S64–S69.

31. Dawson DM, Krarup C. Perioperative nerve lesions. Arch Neurol 1989; 46:1335–1360.

32. Dawson M, Hallett Millender LH. Entrapment neuropathies, ed 2. Boston: Little, Brown, 1990:375–386.

33. Morin JE, Long R, Elleker MG, et al. Upper extremity neuropathies following median sternotomy. Ann Thorac Surg 1982; 34:181–185.

34. Williams IR, Jefferson D, Gilliatt RW. Acute nerve compression during limb ischemia: An experimental study. J Neurol Sci 1980; 46:199–207.

35. Trojaborg W. Electrophysiological findings in pressure palsy of the brachial plexus. Neurol Neurosurg Psychiatry 1977; 40:1160–1165.

36. Hanson MR, Breuer AC, Furlan AJ, et al. Mechanism and frequency of brachial plexus injury in open heart surgery: A prospective analysis. Ann Thorac Surg 1983; 36:675–682.

37. Lederman RJ, Breuer AC, Hanson MR, et al. Peripheral nervous system complications of coronary artery bypass graft surgery. Ann Neurol 1982; 12:297–301.

38. Cherington M, Happer I, Mechanic B, Parry L. Surgery for thoracic outlet syndrome may be hazardous to your health. Muscle Nerve 1986; 9:632–634.

39. Wilbourn AJ. Thoracic outlet syndrome surgery causing severe brachial plexopathy. Muscle Nerve 1988; 11:66–74.

40. Robertson WC, Eichman PL, Clancy WG. Upper trunk brachial plexopathy in football players. JAMA 1979; 241:1480.

41. Cofield RH, Simonet WT. The shoulder in sports. Mayo Clin Proc 1984; 59:157.

42. Poindexter DP, Johnson EW. Football shoulder and neck injury: A study of the "stinger." Arch Phys Med Rehabil 1984; 65:601.

43. Goodgold J. Anatomical correlates of clinical electromyography. Baltimore: Williams & Wilkins, 1975:126.

44. Sander JE, Sharp FR. Lumbosacral plexus neuritis. Neurology 1981; 31:470–473.

45. Evans BA, Stevens C. Lumbosacral plexus neuropathy. Neurology 1981; 31:1327–1330.

46. Starling JR, Harms BA. Diagnosis and treatment of genitofemoral and ilioinguinal neuralgia. World J Surg 1989; 13:586–591.

47. Hefty TR, Nelson KA, Hatch TR, Barry JM. Acute lumbosacral plexopathy in diabetic women after renal transplantation. J Urol 1990; 143:107–109.

48. Wilbourn AJ. The diabetic neuropathies. In: Brown WF, Bolton CF, eds. Clinical electromyography ed 1. Boston: Butterworths, 1987:329–364.

49. Garland H. Diabetic amyotrophy. Br Med J 1955; 2:1287–1290.

50. Asbury AK. Proximal diabetic neuropathy. Ann Neurol 1977; 2:179–180.
51. Bastron JA, Thomas JE. Diabetic polyradiculopathy. Mayo Clin Proc 1981; 56:725–732.
52. Brown MJ, Asbury AK. Diabetic neuropathy. Ann Neurol 1984; 15:2–12.
53. Greene D. The pathogenesis and prevention of diabetic neuropathy and nephropathy. Metabolism 1988; 37:25–29.
54. Orloff MJ, Macedo A, Greenleaf GE. Effect of pancreas transplantation on diabetic somatic neuropathy. Surgery 1988; 104:437–444.
55. Sima AA, Zhang WX, Tze WJ, et al. Diabetic neuropathy in STZ-induced diabetic rat and effect of allogenic islet cell transplantation. Morphometric analysis. Diabetes 1988; 37:1129–1136.
56. Sutherland DE, Kendall DM, Moudry KC, et al. Pancreas transplantation in nonuremic, type I diabetic recipients. Surgery 1988; 104:453–464.
57. Chiu WS. The syndrome of retroperitoneal hemorrhage and lumbar plexus neuropathy during anticoagulant therapy. South Med J 1976; 69:595–599.
58. Emery S, Ochoa J. Lumbar plexus neuropathy resulting from retroperitoneal hemorrhage. Muscle Nerve 1978; 1:330–334.
59. Munsat TL, Poussaint AF. Clinical manifestations and diagnosis of amyloid polyneuropathy. Neurology 1965; 15:1147–1154.
60. Weiderholt WC, Siekert RG. Neurological manifestations of sarcoidosis. Neurology 1965; 15:1147–1154.
61. Rosenberg RN, Lovelace RE. Mononeuritis multiplex in lepromatous leprosy. Arch Neurol 1968; 19:310–314.
62. Lerin KH, Daube JR. Spinal cord infarction: Another cause of "lumbosacral polyradiculopathy." Neurology 1984; 34:389–390.

9

Median Nerve

Jun Kimura

CONTENTS

ANATOMIC CONSIDERATIONS

Sensory Innervation

The median nerve is derived from C-6, C-7, C-8, and T-1 roots and arises from the lateral and median cords of the brachial plexus. It supplies the skin over the lateral aspect of the palm and the dorsal surfaces of the terminal phalanges along with the volar surfaces of the first three digits and the lateral half of the fourth digit. The skin of the third digit is subserved by the C-7 root through the middle trunk and lateral cord, whereas the sensory fibers of the first two digits enter the C-6 and C-7 root through the upper or middle trunk and the lateral cord.

Motor Innervation

The median nerve supplies no muscles in the upper arm, but it innervates most flexors in the forearm and the muscles of the thenar eminence. As it enters the forearm, it passes between the two heads of the pronator teres, which it supplies. It then innervates flexor carpi radialis, palmaris longus, and flexor digitorum superficialis before giving rise to the anterior interosseous nerve. This pure motor branch innervates the flexor pollicis longus, pronator quadratus, and flexor digitorum profundus I and II. The main branch descends the forearm and enters the hand by passing through the carpal tunnel between the wrist and palm. It gives rise to the recurrent thenar nerve at the distal edge of the carpal ligaments, which innervates the abductor pollicis brevis, the lateral half of the flexor pollicis brevis, and the opponens pollicis. After giving off the motor branch to the thenar eminence, the terminal branches of the median nerve supplies lumbricals I and II.

CLINICAL ENTITIES

The entrapment neuropathy or injury of the median nerve occurs at several common sites along its course. Selective lesions of the median nerve are rare in the shoulder girdle. Further distally the median nerve is compressed at three common sites along its course. Entrapment at the elbow involves either the nerve trunk between the two heads of the pronator teres or more distally the anterior interosseous branch. In the carpal tunnel syndrome, the lesions primarily lie at the distal edge of the transverse carpal ligament and less commonly within the intermetacarpal tunnel.

Injury in the Shoulder Girdle

Spontaneous entrapment of the median nerve in the region of the shoulder is rare.[1] Trauma or external compression accounts for the majority of these lesions, which usually result in multiple nerve injuries rather than isolated median neuropathy. Traumatic conditions that could cause median nerve palsies include fracture of the humerus, more commonly associated with radial nerve paralysis,[2] and anterior dislocation of the shoulder, which typically gives rise to axillary nerve paralysis.[3] External compression of the median nerve may result from improper use of axillary crutches or sleeping with arms hanging over chairs or benches, as in *Saturday night palsy*[4] or over the partner's head as in *honeymoon palsy.*[5] Many of these conditions accompany radial and ulnar nerve injuries.

A complete injury to the median nerve in the region of the shoulder gives rise to weakness in pronation and wrist flexion and loss of hand function. With paralysis of pronator teres and pronator quadratus, brachioradialis may provide some pronation. Weak wrist flexion is typically associated with ulnar deviation, indicating sparing of the flexor carpi ulnaris despite the loss of the flexor carpi radialis. Extrinsic flexors of the digits affected by median nerve injury include flexor pollicis longus, flexor digitorum superficialis of all digits, and flexor digitorum profundus of the second and third digits. The patient is unable to flex interphalangeal joints of the first to third digits and the proximal interphalangeal joints of the fourth and fifth digits. The latter is best tested with the distal interphalangeal joints held straight to minimize the action of the flexor digitorum profundus. Median nerve injury spares the flexion of the metacarpophalangeal joints, which is maintained by ulnar-innervated muscles. Paralysis of median-innervated thenar muscles results in absent or weak abduction and opposition of the first digit.

Entrapments at the Elbow

Pronator teres syndrome

The median nerve traverses between the two heads of the pronator teres before passing under it in 83% of dissections.[6] Compression results from trauma, fracture, muscle hypertrophy, or an anomalous fibrous band connecting the pronator teres to the tendinous arch of the flexor digitorum sublimis. Regardless of the responsible lesion, injury of the nerve at this point gives rise to the pronator teres syndrome.[7,8] The patient complains of pain and tenderness over the pronator teres and weakness of flexor pollicis and abductor pollicis brevis with preservation of forearm pronation. In contrast to the carpal tunnel syndrome, sensory changes spare the thenar eminence innervated by the branch that passes superficially to the flexor retinaculum. Conduction studies show mild slowing across the lesion in the proximal forearm, whereas the distal latency and compound sensory nerve action potentials recorded at the wrist are normal.[8] Surgical decompression may be indicated, although injection of corticosteroids into the pronator teres may relieve the pain, aiding the diagnosis.[9]

A similar entrapment may involve the median nerve as it crosses the ligament of Struthers, a fibrous band attached to an anomalous spur on the anteromedial aspect of the lower humerus.[10] This ligament may also compress the brachial artery above the elbow, obliterating the radial pulse with full extension of the forearm. The site of the lesion usually lies proximal to the innervation to the pronator teres, which therefore shows weakness and electromyographic abnormalities. This finding thus serves to differentiate the condition from the pronator teres syndrome, which usually spares the muscle.[11,12]

Anterior interosseous nerve syndrome

Selective injury of the anterior interosseous nerve results in the syndrome of Kiloh and Nevin.[13] In this entity, the nerve is trapped distal to the pronator passage, unilaterally or bilaterally, as it branches off the median nerve trunk.[14] Although the patient commonly complains of pain in the forearm or elbow, careful sensory examination reveals no distinct abnormalities.[15–17] Because of the selective weakness, the patient is unable to form a circle with the first two digits. Formation of a triangle instead results in the so-called pinch sign. The symptom usually abates in 6 weeks to 18 months. Neuralgic amyotrophy with lesions in the brachial plexus may mimic an anterior interosseous nerve palsy.[18] This finding indicates that the spinal root fibers already form groupings for terminal nerve branches at the level of the brachial plexus.[19] For the same reason, compression at an antecubital level can also cause selective injury of the bundles that are destined to form the anterior interosseous nerve.[20]

Nerve conduction studies reveal no abnormalities of the median nerve per se,[21] but the compound muscle action potential recorded from the pronator quadratus may show a delay in latency after stimulation of the anterior interosseous nerve at the el-

bow.[14] Electromyographic studies confirm the diagnosis with the evidence of selective denervation in the flexor pollicis longus, flexor digitorum profundus I and II, and pronator quadratus.

Carpal Tunnel Syndrome

Anatomic characteristics

This syndrome is by far the most common entrapment neuropathy. The tunnel is bounded by the carpal bones and contains the median nerve and nine extrinsic digital flexors. The transverse ligament, attached to the scaphoid, trapezoid, and hamate, forms the roof. Anatomic studies show the most narrow cross-section at 2 to 2.5 cm distal to the entrance. Here the tunnel is rigidly bound on three sides by bone structures and roofed by a thickened transverse carpal ligament.[22] Pathologically myelinated fiber size is strikingly reduced under the retinaculum at this point.[23]

Careful studies in healthy subjects reveal the slowest nerve conduction at a point corresponding to the origin of the ligament, that is, 2 to 4 cm distal to the distal crease of the wrist.[24] Thus there seems to be a mild compression of the median nerve at this particular level even in clinically unaffected hands. A histologic study also documented focal abnormalities at this site in five of 12 median nerves at routine autopsy.[25] None of the subjects had any symptoms suggestive of the carpal tunnel syndrome in life.[26] Some individuals have certain anatomic peculiarities, such as a smaller cross-sectional area of the tunnel, with the tendency to the entrapment neuropathy.[27,28] Any expanding lesions in the closed space of the carpal tunnel may also predispose the subject to this compression.

Incidence and associated disorders

Carpal tunnel syndrome is more common in women. Symptoms appear most commonly in the fifth or sixth decades, usually involving the dominant hand[29] or contralateral to amputation.[30] The carpal tunnel syndrome often affects people with jobs that require heavy and repeated use of the hands.[31] Symptoms with onset during pregnancy may resolve after delivery. The majority of patients suffer from carpal tunnel syndrome alone,[32] although the syndrome may rarely be familial[33] or accompany a variety of polyneuropathies and systemic illnesses.[34–38]

Patients with acromegaly have a higher incidence of carpal tunnel syndrome, one study reporting 35 of 100 patients with this neuropathy.[39,40] Amyloidosis, especially that associated with multiple myeloma, may also give rise to diffuse neuropathy.[39,41] Approximately 23% of patients with rheumatoid arthritis develop carpal tunnel syndrome as the initial manifestation of the tenosynovitis affecting the wrist flexor. In rheumatoid patients, however, thenar atrophy may also result from disuse, cervical spine disease, or compression of the ulnar nerve at the elbow. Carpal tunnel syndrome may develop in eosinophilic fasciitis,[42] myxedema,[43,44] lupus erythematosus,[45] hyperparathyroidism,[46] and toxic shock syndrome.[47–49]

In cases in which a nonspecific tenosynovitis is associated with carpal tunnel symptoms, other signs of degenerative arthritis, such as trigger finger, bursitis, tendinitis, and tennis elbow may be present. In addition to the chronic intracanal entrapment, acute compression of the median nerve at the wrist may result from trauma including Colles' fracture,[50] isolated fracture of capitatum[51] or hamate,[52] acute soft tissue swelling following crush injury of the hand, and acute intraneural hemorrhage.[53] Emergency decompression of the median nerve is necessary in most of these cases.

Symptoms and signs

Paresthesias in the hand frequently awaken these patients at night. The pain may extend to the elbow and sometimes the shoulder, mimicking a cervical spine disease or high median nerve compression.[54] Manipulation of the neck or shoulder girdle exacerbates the symptoms of proximal lesions. In contrast, moving the hand alleviates the pain in the carpal tunnel syndrome. Involvement of peripheral autonomic fibers causes defective vasomotor reflex.[55] Patients with systemic diseases such as rheumatoid arthritis often develop Raynaud's phenomenon.[56]

Sensory changes involve the first three digits and the radial half of the fourth digit or, not uncommonly, only the second or third digit. Patients may complain of a hypesthesia outside the median nerve distribution. In one series, sensory disturbance was confined to the tip of the third digit in 83% of 384 patients.[57] Sensory changes vary greatly in the early stages but typically spare the skin of the thenar eminence innervated by the palmar cutaneous branch that arises proximal to the carpal tunnel. Characteristic sensory splitting of the fourth digit into median and ulnar halves is rarely seen in radiculopathies.

Major wasting of thenar muscles, considered a distinctive feature of the syndrome in advanced cases, does not occur in early carpal tunnel syndrome. Patients may, however, develop slight weakness of the affected hand compared with the normal side. The abductor pollicis brevis is best tested in relative isolation, with the patient pressing the thumb upward perpendicular to the plane of the palm. To test the opponens, the patient is asked to press the tip of the thumb against the tip of the little finger. The deep and superficial heads of the flexor pollicis brevis receive variable median and ulnar innervation.

Symptoms may worsen following passive flexion or hyperextension of the affected hand at the wrist for more than 1 minute.[58] This maneuver may also enhance a delay of motor or sensory conduction across the wrist.[59,60] Tinel's sign, or paresthesia of the digits induced by percussion of the median nerve at the wrist, has no diagnostic value specific to the carpal tunnel syndrome.[61] In fact, based on electrophysiologic data, the compressed segment usually lies about 2 to 3 cm distal to the traditional percussion site on the volar aspect of the wrist.[24] The phenomenon was originally described to localize the proximal stump of an injured nerve by tapping.[62] Paresthesia induced by this maneuver serves as an indication for axonal regeneration and not for entrapment neuropathy.[63,64]

Cause and differential diagnosis

Ischemia of the arm worsens symptoms of the carpal tunnel syndrome.[65] Such susceptibility correlates well with the severity of the pain and paresthesia but not the extent of muscle wasting or duration of symptoms.[66] These findings suggest rapidly reversible changes in the nerve fibers induced by ischemic attacks. Sharply focal structural changes, however, prevail in compression neuropathy, indicating that mechanical factors play an important role in the pathogenesis.[67,68]

The disorder must be differentiated from a polyneuropathy with distally prominent symptoms, high median nerve compression at the elbow, a C-6 radiculopathy, and traumatic injury at the wrist such as a handcuff neuropathy.[69] Degenerative cervical spine diseases may accompany the carpal tunnel syndrome. Despite the popular designation, the *double-crush syndrome*,[70] the combination may represent a chance occurrence of two common entities. This possibility nonetheless should alert the examiner to conduct adequate electrophysiologic assessments in the presence of one condition to rule out the other. The median nerve may be compressed by the lateral border of the flexor digitorum sublimis muscle against the forearm fascia and other flexor tendons. In this rare entity, symptoms are similar to the carpal tunnel syndrome, although the patient also complains of local tenderness and firmness in the forearm.[71]

Digital Nerve Entrapment

Median sensory fibers supply the skin of the index and middle fingers and half of the ring finger by the digital nerve. Entrapment of these small sensory branches against the edge of the deep transverse metacarpal ligament appears in association with trauma, tumor, phalangeal fracture, or inflammation of the metacarpophalangeal joint or tendon.[9] The patient complains of pain in one or two fingers, especially when hyperextending the affected digits laterally, together with tenderness and dysesthesia over the palmar surfaces between the metacarpals. The symptoms may abate after local infiltration of the steroid that assists in diagnosis.[72] Abnormal median sensory potentials may be attributable to unsuspected digital nerve lesions rather than disease of the nerve trunk.[73]

ELECTROPHYSIOLOGIC ASPECTS

Principles of Conduction Studies

Motor fibers

The median nerve takes a relatively superficial course in its entire length from the axilla to the palm. Thus the nerve is accessible to percutaneous stimulation in the Erb's point, axilla, elbow, wrist, and palm.[74,75] In our laboratory, the cathode is placed over the brachial pulse near the volar crease at the elbow and 3 cm proximal to the distal crease at the wrist with the anode 2 cm proximal to the cathode. The ground electrode is located around the forearm usually between the stimulating and recording electrodes (Figure 9.1).

For recording, an active electrode (G1) is over the belly of the abductor pollicis brevis and an indifferent electrode (G2) just distal to the metacarpophalangeal joint (Figure 9.2). With this electrode positioning, all median nerve–innervated intrinsic hand muscles contribute to the evoked response. Distal and proximal stimulation elicits dissimilar compound muscle action potentials if there is an anomalous crossover between the median and ulnar nerve in the forearm. Their latencies, representing two different nerves, cannot be used for calculation of the nerve conduction velocity.

Stimulation at Erb's point or the axilla tends to

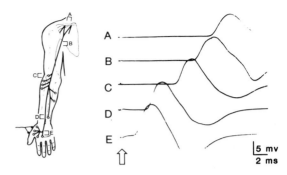

FIGURE 9.1. *Motor nerve conduction study of the median nerve. The sites of stimulation include Erb's point (A), axilla (B), elbow (C), wrist (D), and palm (E). Compound muscle action potentials are recorded with surface electrodes placed on the thenar eminence.*

coactivate other nerves in close proximity,[76] requiring a collision technique to circumvent the problem. In the palm, the motor axons take a recurrent course along the thenar nerve off the median nerve trunk. Thus unless dealing with the exposed nerve for intraoperative monitoring,[77] surface stimulation at the palm may inadvertently activate unintended portions of the thenar nerve.

If stimulation aimed at the origin of the thenar nerve in the palm depolarizes the distal branch near the motor point, measured latency is erroneously short. The latency difference between the wrist and palm then is unreasonably large, presenting a fallacious impression of the carpal tunnel syndrome. One must avoid this error by carefully selecting the most distal point of the palm at which stimulation elicits an appropriate twitch of the abductor pollicis brevis. The recurrent branch may take an anomalous course in rare instances, further compounding the problem.[78] Tables 9.1 and 9.2 summarize normal values in our laboratory.

Sensory fibers

Stimulation is delivered at the same sites as the motor fibers, and antidromic compound sensory nerve action potentials are recorded from the second digit[79] with ring electrodes placed around the proximal (G1) and distal (G2) interphalangeal joints (Figure 9.2). We place the cathode at the wrist 3 cm proximal to the distal crease of the wrist[24] and 5 cm distally at the palm (Figure 9.3). Some investigators use a fixed distance from the recording electrode, most com-

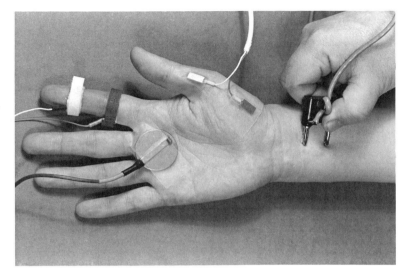

FIGURE 9.2. *Motor and sensory conduction studies of the median nerve. Stimulation at the wrist, 3 cm proximal to the distal crease, and recording over the belly (G1) and tendon (G2) of the abductor pollicis brevis for motor conduction and around the proximal (G1) and distal (G2) interphalangeal joints of the second digit for antidromic sensory conduction. The ground electrode is located in the palm.*

monly 12 to 14 cm.[80] Tables 9.1 and 9.2 summarize normal values for the digital potentials recorded.

The compound sensory nerve action potentials may also be recorded from the first or third digit (Figure 9.4) or lateral half of the fourth digit, sometimes identifying abnormalities not otherwise detectable. Because of mixed sensory innervation, potential is also elicited over the first or fourth digit, after stimulation of the radial or ulnar nerve. Thus one must avoid inadvertent spread of stimulating current to the other nerves. Responses recorded from the third digit are affected by lesions of C-7 root, middle trunk, or lateral cord. Similarly, the potentials from the first digit are a measure of C-6 or C-7 roots,

TABLE 9.1. Median nerve*

	Site of Stimulation	Amplitude† (mV for Motor; μV for Sensory)	Latency‡ to Recording Site (ms)	Difference between Right and Left (ms)	Conduction Time between Two Points (ms)	Conduction Velocity (m/s)
Motor Fibers	Palm	6.9 ± 3.2 (3.5)§	1.86 ± 0.28 (2.4)¶	0.19 ± 0.17 (0.5)¶		
	Wrist	7 ± 3 (3.5)	3.49 ± 0.34 (4.2)	0.24 ± 0.22 (0.7)	1.65 ± 0.25 (2.2)**	48.8 ± 5.3 (38)**
	Elbow	7 ± 2.7 (3.5)	7.39 ± 0.69 (8.8)	0.31 ± 0.24 (0.8)	3.92 ± 0.49 (4.9)	57.7 ± 4.9 (48)
	Axilla	7.2 ± 2.9 (3.5)	9.81 ± 0.89 (11.6)	0.42 ± 0.33 (1.1)	2.42 ± 0.39 (3.2)	63.5 ± 6.2 (51)
Sensory Fibers	Digit					
	Palm	39 ± 16.8 (20)	1.37 ± 0.24 (1.9)	0.15 ± 0.11 (0.4)	1.37 ± 0.24 (1.9)	58.8 ± 5.8 (47)
	Wrist	38.5 ± 15.6 (19)	2.84 ± 0.34 (3.5)	0.18 ± 0.14 (0.5)	1.48 ± 0.18 (1.8)	56.2 ± 5.8 (44)
	Elbow	32 ± 15.5 (16)	6.46 ± 0.71 (7.9)	0.29 ± 0.21 (0.7)	3.61 ± 0.48 (4.6)	61.9 ± 4.2 (53)

* Mean ± standard deviation (SD) in 122 nerves from 61 patients, 11 to 74 years of age (average 40), with no apparent disease of the peripheral nerves.

+ Amplitude of the evoked response measured from the baseline to negative peak.

‡ Latency measured to the onset of the evoked response.

§ Lower limits of normal based on the distribution of the normative data.

¶ Upper limits of normal calculated as mean +2 SD.

** Lower limits of normal calculated as mean −2 SD.

TABLE 9.2.   Latency comparison between two nerves in the same limb*

	Site of Stimulation	Median Nerve (ms)	Ulnar Nerve (ms)	Difference (ms)
Motor Fibers	Wrist	3.34 ± 0.32 (4)[+]	2.56 ± 0.37 (3.3)[+]	0.79 ± 0.31 (1.4)[+]
	Elbow	7.39 + 0.72 (8.8)	7.06 ± 0.79 (8.6)	0.59 ± 0.60 (1.8)
Sensory Fibers	Palm	1.33 ± 0.21 (1.8)	1.19 ± 0.22 (1.6)	0.22 ± 0.17 (0.6)
	Wrist	2.80 ± 0.32 (3.4)	2.55 ± 0.30 (3.2)	0.29 ± 0.21 (0.7)

* Mean ± standard deviation (SD) in 70 nerves from 35 patients 14 to 74 years of age (average 37), with no apparent disease of the peripheral nerve.
[+] Upper limits of normal calculated as mean + 2 SD.

upper or middle trunk, and lateral cord. Postganglionic lesions cause degeneration of the sensory axons, whereas preganglionic root avulsion spares the sensory potential of the anesthestic digits.

Compound muscle action potentials maintain nearly the same amplitude regardless of stimulus sites. In contrast, the antidromically activated digital potentials diminish substantially with increasing distance between the stimulating and recording sites. Indeed, stimulation at Erb's point or the axilla often fails to elicit unequivocal digital potentials because temporal dispersion between fast and slow conducting fibers results in duration-dependent phase cancellation.[81,82] Naturally recurring orthodromic sensory impulses may also partially extinguish the antidromic impulse by collision in proportion to the distance between the stimulating and recording electrodes.

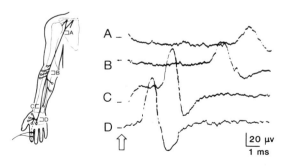

FIGURE 9.3.   *Sensory nerve conduction study of the median nerve. The sites of stimulation include axilla (A), elbow (B), wrist (C), and palm (D). Antidromic compound sensory nerve action potentials are recorded with a pair of ring electrodes placed around the second digit.*

Motor axons and large myelinated sensory axons have a similar threshold. Thus coactivated action potentials from distal muscles obscure the antidromically recorded sensory potential. Stimulation in the palm distal to the origin of the recurrent motor fibers, however, circumvents this problem. Comparison to the pure compound sensory nerve action potential thus recorded helps detect compound muscle action potentials, if elicited with more proximal stimulation, by a change in wave form.[24] In contrast to the antidromic sensory potentials, digital[83–86] or palmar stimulation elicits[87,88] the orthodromic compound sensory nerve action potential recordable at the palm, wrist, or elbow with either surface or needle electrodes. Electronic averaging makes it much easier to detect smaller sized orthodromic compound nerve action potentials, especially in abnormal nerves.

Stimulation of the palmar cutaneous branch of the median nerve about 5.5 cm proximal to the radial styloid elicits antidromic compound sensory nerve action potentials over the midthenar eminence. Reported normal values over 10 cm segments include the onset latency of 2.6 ± 0.2 ms (mean ± SD) and amplitude of 12 ± 4.6 μV.[89] The carpal tunnel syndrome spares the palmar cutaneous branch, which arises proximal to the compression site.

Assessments of Carpal Tunnel Syndrome

Sensitivity of various methods

Simpson[90] originally demonstrated focal slowing of the median nerve at the wrist in the carpal tunnel syndrome. Since then, a number of investigators have published conduction studies in this common entity.[58,91–96] Electrophysiologic procedure can confirm

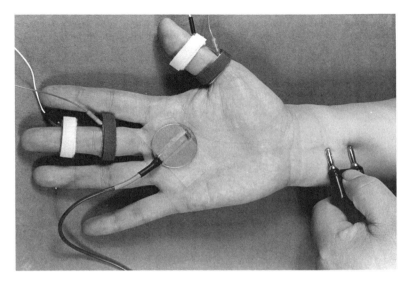

FIGURE 9.4. *Alternative recording sites for sensory conduction study of the median nerve, with the ring electrodes placed around the proximal (G1) and distal (G2) interphalangeal joints of the third digit or the base (G1) and the interphalangeal joint (G2) of the first digit.*

the clinical diagnosis in the majority of patients. It also detects an incidental finding in some asymptomatic subjects. One must therefore carefully weigh the test results and the clinical findings before resorting to surgical intervention.

In previous work, sensory conduction testing was said to have revealed a higher incidence of abnormality than studies of the motor axons.[85,95,96] Our series,[24] however, showed a comparable incidence of abnormalities in the sensory and motor conduction. Further, involvements of motor fibers do not necessarily accompany similar abnormalities of sensory conductions or vice versa.

In advanced stages, axons may degenerate not only distal to the entrapment, but also in the forearm as a result of a severe compression at the wrist.[97,98] Slowed conduction velocity proximal to the site of lesion may simply reflect the loss of fast conducting fibers distal to the compression site.

The sensitivity of the motor and sensory conduction studies may be improved by a number of methods. These include measuring the difference between the right and left sides, which, although useful in unilateral lesions, is of limited help in assessing bilateral cases. Median sensory latencies may also be compared with radial or ulnar sensory latencies especially if the distances are the same.[99] For example, comparison of median and ulnar compound sensory nerve action potentials recorded from the fourth digit or median and radial sensory potentials from the first digit may be made.[100,101] In addition, the motor terminal latencies in the median and ulnar nerves, if

adjusted to the same distance, may also be compared. Prolongation of the motor terminal latency in patients with the carpal tunnel syndrome increases the residual latency[102] and decreases the terminal latency index ratio.[103,104]

In cases with involvement of motor fibers, electromyographic abnormalities include fibrillation potentials and positive sharp waves in the median-innervated intrinsic hand muscles. Spontaneous rhythmic discharges of motor unit potential are seen in occasional patients, presumably originating distally in the nerve near the area of compression.[105] Despite complete denervation of the thenar muscles, the first and second lumbricals may survive, reflecting a deeper location of their motor funiculi.[106] In some patients, the carpal tunnel syndrome may be accompanied by ulnar nerve lesion at the wrist,[107,108] although other studies have failed to show this association.[32,85]

Clinical value of palmar stimulation

Conduction abnormalities often selectively involve the wrist to palm segment of the median nerve for both sensory[74,83,85–87,109,110] and motor fibers.[24,75] In one series,[24] complete studies including palmar stimulation confirmed sensory or motor conduction abnormality or both in all but 13 (8%) of 172 clinically affected hands. Without palmar stimulation, an additional 32 (19%) hands would have escaped detection. In another study, the conventional criteria revealed abnormalities of the orthodromic sensory conduction in only 53% of 72 suspected hands, but addition of palmar stimulation increased the detection percentage of 67%.[111]

Using palmar stimulation, it is also possible to differentiate compression by the transverse carpal ligament from diseases of the most terminal segment in a distal neuropathy.[112] Palmar stimulation also provides a means to record compound nerve action potential simultaneously from the digit and the median nerve trunk at the wrist. This method allows instantaneous comparison of the two segments based

on the antidromic compound sensory nerve action potential distally and mixed orthodromic sensory and antidromic motor compound nerve action potential proximally.[113]

Multiple stimulation across the carpal ligament

Palmar stimulation helps identify conduction abnormalities of sensory or motor fibers under the transverse carpal ligament[114] and differentiate the carpal tunnel syndrome from a distal neuropathy.[112] The median nerve may be stimulated at 1-cm increments (Figure 9.5) to localize further the point of maximal conduction delay within the distal segment across the wrist.[24,74] Sensory latencies normally change 0.16 to 0.20 ms per cm with stimulation between the midpalm and distal forearm (Figure 9.6). In about one-half of the affected hands with focal abnormalities of the median nerve, the latency increases sharply across a 1-cm segment (Figures 9.7 and 9.8), most commonly 2 to 4 cm distal to the origin of the transverse carpal ligament.[24] In these hands, the average focal latency change across the affected 1-cm segment exceeds four times that of the adjoining

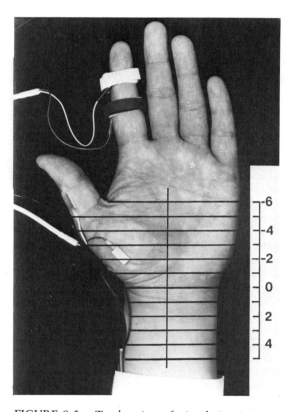

FIGURE 9.5.   *Twelve sites of stimulation in 1-cm increments along the length of the median nerve. The 0 level at the distal crease of the wrist corresponds to the origin of the transverse carpal ligament. Recording arrangement for compound sensory nerve action potentials from the second digit and compound muscle action potentials from the abductor pollicis brevis. (Reprinted with permission from Kimura J. The carpal tunnel syndrome. Localization of conduction abnormalities within the distal segment of the median nerve. Brain 1979; 102:619–635.)*

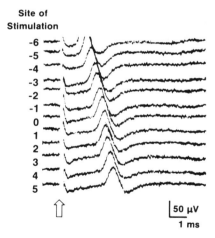

FIGURE 9.6.   *Compound sensory nerve action potentials in a normal subject recorded after stimulation of the median nerve at multiple points across the wrist. The numbers on the left indicate the site of each stimulus (compare with Figure 9.5). The latency increased linearly with stepwise shifts of stimulus site proximally in 1-cm increments. (Reprinted with permission from Kimura J. The carpal tunnel syndrome. Localization of conduction abnormalities within the distal segment of the median nerve. Brain 1979; 102:619–635.)*

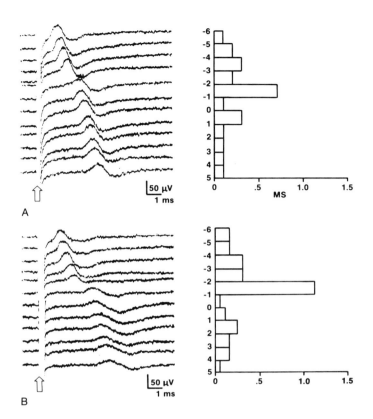

FIGURE 9.7. *Compound sensory nerve action potentials in a patient with the carpal tunnel syndrome. Both hands showed a sharply localized slowing from −2 to −1, with the calculated segmental conduction velocity of 14 m/s on the left (A) and 9 m/s on the right (B). Note a distinct change in wave form of the compound sensory nerve action potential at the point of localized conduction delay. Double-humped appearance at −2 on the left suggests sparing of some sensory axons at this level. (Reprinted with permission from Kimura J. The carpal tunnel syndrome. Localization of conduction abnormalities within the distal segment of the median nerve. Brain 1979; 102:619–635.)*

distal or proximal 1-cm segments. In the remaining hands, conduction delay, although maximal at the site described here, involves more than one 1-cm segment across the carpal tunnel. Incremental stimulation of the motor axons in short segment is technically more difficult because of the recurrent course of the thenar nerve, which varies anatomically from one subject to another.[115]

Spread of the Stimulus Current

Shocks of an inappropriately high intensity may spread to a nerve or muscle not being tested. This leads to fallacious determination of latencies because of volume conducted potentials from distant muscles.[116,117] The problem may be identified by visual inspection of the contracting muscle. More selective recording of the signal may be helped by employing the collision technique to block the unwanted responses to stimulation of other nerves.[118] Recording from limited areas by the use of needle electrodes also helps identify innervation by individual motor branches and recognize patterns of anomaly. The electrical activity registered from a restricted area in the muscle, however, fails to provide any information on the size of compound muscle action potentials.

Axillary stimulation and collision technique

Stimulation intended for the median nerve at the wrist or elbow may simultaneously activate the ulnar nerve only if the shock intensity is unusually high.[117] At the axilla, however, ordinary stimulation usually excites both the median and ulnar nerves, which lie in close proximity.[119] If the current spreads to the ulnar nerve, not only median-innervated muscles, but also ulnar-innervated muscles contribute to the potential recorded by the electrodes placed on the thenar eminence. The measured latency will then be normal in the carpal tunnel syndrome, reflecting ulnar conduction despite slowing of the median nerve (Figure 9.9). In the same case, a stimulus at the elbow, which activates only the median nerve, shows a prolonged latency. The calculated latency difference between the axilla and elbow would then be erroneously small, leading to an unreasonably fast conduction velocity along this segment. In extreme cases, the latency of the ulnar response after stimu-

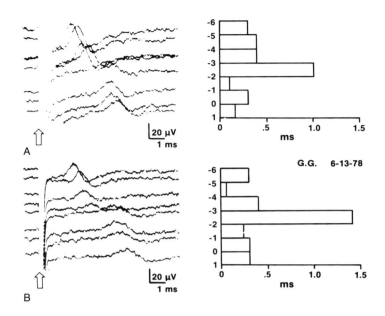

FIGURE 9.8.   *Compound sensory nerve action potential in a patient with the carpal tunnel syndrome. Both hands show a sharply localized slowing from −3 to −2, with a segmental conduction velocity of 10 m/s on the left (A) and 7 m/s on the right (B). An abrupt change in wave form of the compound sensory nerve action potential also indicates the point of localized conduction delay. (Reprinted with permission from Kimura J. The carpal tunnel syndrome. Localization of conduction abnormalities within the distal segment of the median nerve. Brain 1979; 102:619–635.)*

lation at the axilla falls short of that of the median component elicited with shocks at the elbow.

A physiologic nerve block with collision allows selective recording of the median component despite coactivation of the ulnar nerve proximally.[118] If one delivers a distal stimulus to the ulnar nerve (Figure 9.10), the antidromic impulse from the wrist collides with the orthodromic impulse from the axilla, allowing only the median impulse to reach the muscle. The much earlier ulnar response induced by the distal stimulus usually does not obscure the median compound muscle action potential under study. If nec-

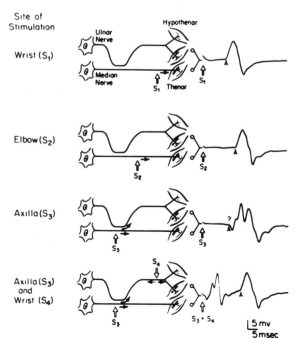

FIGURE 9.9.   *A 39-year-old man with carpal tunnel syndrome. The stimulation of the median nerve at the wrist (S1) or elbow (S2) elicited a compound muscle action potential with increased latency in the thenar eminence. Spread of axillary stimulation (S3) to the ulnar nerve (third tracing from top) activated ulnar-innervated thenar muscles with shorter latency. Another stimulus (S4) applied to the ulnar nerve at the wrist (bottom tracing) blocked the proximal impulses by collision. The compound muscle action potential elicited by S4 occurred much earlier. The diagnosis on the left shows collision between the orthodromic (solid arrows) and antidromic (dotted arrows) impulses. (Reprinted with permission from Kimura J. Collision technique. Physiologic block of nerve impulses in studies of motor nerve conduction velocity. Neurology (Minneap) 1976; 26:680–682.)*

essary, one may deliver the distal stimulus a few milliseconds before the proximal stimulation to separate these two responses further. Should this time interval exceed the conduction time between the two points of stimulation, however, the antidromic impulse from the distal point passes the proximal site of stimulus without collision.

The collision technique may help resolve confusing results of motor nerve conduction studies in pa-

tients with the carpal tunnel syndrome. With spread of stimulus, distal and proximal stimuli may give rise to markedly different wave forms of the evoked potentials, as shown in the illustrated cases. With a less apparent discrepancy, blocking unwanted nerve stimulation may be necessary to uncover the true response. The collision technique, similar to a procaine nerve block previously employed,[116,120] improves the accuracy of latency determination when one fails to stimulate the median nerve selectively at a proximal point. The use of needle electrodes, recording from a restricted area, also allows reliable assessment of latency but not amplitude of a compound muscle action potential, as stated before.

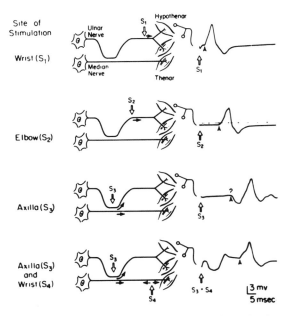

FIGURE 9.10.   *A 29-year-old man with tardy ulnar palsy. Stimulation at the wrist (S1) or elbow (S2) selectively activated the ulnar nerve, giving rise to an abnormally delayed compound muscle action potential over the hypothenar eminence. Spread of axillary stimulation (S3) to the median nerve (third tracing from top) elicited an additional short latency median response with initial positivity. This potential, registered through volume conduction, obscured the onset (arrowhead) of the muscle response under study. Another stimulus (S4) applied to the median nerve at the wrist (bottom tracing) blocked the proximal impulses by collision. The positive median potential elicited by S4 did not interfere because it clearly preceded the ulnar component under study. (Reprinted with permission from Kimura J. Collision technique. Physiologic block of nerve impulses in studies of motor nerve conduction velocity. Neurology (Minneap) 1976; 26:680–682.)*

Segmental stimulation across the palm

Palmar stimulation contributes importantly in evaluation of the distal segment of the median nerve despite some technical problems.[24,75,83,86,87] Serial stimulation in 1-cm increments increases the sensory latency linearly from palm to wrist. Studies of the motor conduction in this region, however, sometimes show unexpected latency changes because the motor fibers take a recurrent course. Thus spread of a stimulus directed to the origin of the thenar nerve may excite the terminal portion near the motor point. Another stimulus, delivered 1 cm proximally, activates only the median nerve trunk. The unreasonably large latency difference between the two stimulus points fallaciously suggests a focal slowing (Figure 9.11). A disproportionate latency increase does indicate a localized pathology if serial stimulation in the segment proximal and distal to the site of lesion shows a linear latency change (Figure 9.12).

Accurate calculation of motor latency over the wrist-to-palm segment requires activating the median nerve precisely at the origin of the recurrent thenar branch. If the site of stimulation is moved from the wrist toward the digit with the cathode distal to the anode, the recurrent branch may be activated at the anode (which acts as floating cathode), even when the actual cathode is positioned distal to the origin of the recurrent branch. Surface distances, if measured to the cathode, would overestimate the nerve length and result in an erroneously rapid conduction velocity. To avoid this error, the stimulus should be moved from the distal palm toward the wrist with the cathode positioned proximal to the anode. With this approach, palmar stimulation of the deep ulnar branch initially causes thumb adduction. With the cathode just over the origin of the thenar nerve, thumb abduction occurs. This point usually lies 3 to

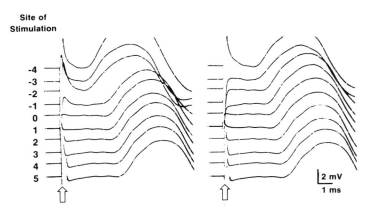

Site of Stimulation

FIGURE 9.11.   *Compound muscle action potentials in a normal subject recorded after stimulation of the median nerve at multiple points across the wrist. On the initial trial (left), the latency decreased, with the cathode inching proximally from −4 to −2, indicating inadvertent spread of stimulating current to a distal portion of the thenar nerve. An apparent steep latency change from −2 to −1 gave an erroneous impression of a focal slowing at this level. A more careful placement of the cathode (right) eliminated unintended activation of the thenar nerve. The 0 level at the distal crease of the wrist corresponds to the origin of the transverse ligament. (Compare with Figure 9.5.)*

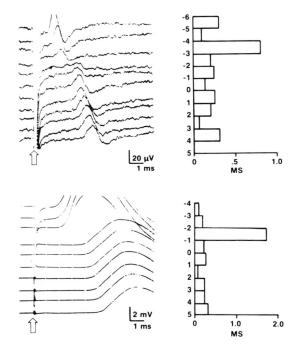

FIGURE 9.12.   *Compound sensory nerve action potentials (top) and compound muscle action potentials (bottom) in a symptomatic hand with the carpal tunnel syndrome. Serial stimulation showed a linear motor latency increase from −4 to −2 and from −1 to 5, with a localized slowing between −2 and −1. A temporally dispersed, double-peaked sensory nerve potential indicates the point of localized conduction delay from −4 to −3. (Reprinted with permission from Kimura J. The carpal tunnel syndrome. Localization of conduction abnormalities within the distal segment of the median nerve. Brain 1979; 102:619–635.)*

4 cm from the distal crease of the wrist, which approximately corresponds to the edge of the transverse carpal ligament.[115]

Anomalies as Sources of Error

Martin-Gruber anastomosis

Martin[121] and Gruber[122] first described anomalous communication from the median to the ulnar nerve at the level of the forearm. This anastomosis, predominantly consisting of motor axons with rare sensory contributions, often originates from the anterior interosseous nerve. The communicating branch usually innervates ulnar intrinsic hand muscles, for example, the first dorsal interosseous, adductor pollicis, and abductor digiti minimi.[123–125] The number of axons taking the anomalous course varies widely. The nerve fibers forming the anastomosis run in a separate bundle, rather than scattered randomly. Thus by properly adjusting electrical stimulus delivered at the elbow, one may activate the anomalous fibers maximally and selectively, without exciting the median nerve proper or vice versa[126] (Figure 9.13).

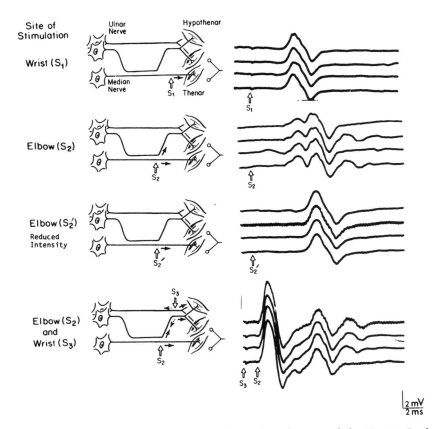

FIGURE 9.13. *A 46-year-old woman with the carpal tunnel syndrome and the Martin-Gruber anomaly. Stimulation at the elbow (S2) activated not only the median nerve, but also communicating fibers, giving rise to a complex compound muscle action potential. With proper adjustment of electrode position and shock intensity, another stimulus at the elbow (S2) excited the median nerve selectively without activating the anastomosis. Another stimulus (S3) applied to the ulnar nerve at the wrist (bottom tracing) achieved the same effect by blocking the unwanted impulse transmitted through the communicating fibers. (Reprinted with permission from Kimura J. Electrodiagnosis in diseases of nerve and muscle. Principles and practice, 2nd Ed, 1989; F.A. Davis.)*

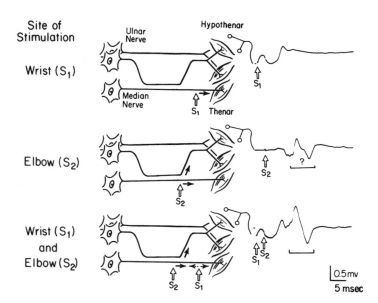

FIGURE 9.14. *Compound muscle action potentials recorded from the hypothenar eminence after stimulation of the median nerve at the wrist (S1) or elbow (S2). The top tracing shows a volume conducted potential from thenar muscles (U-shaped wave of positive polarity). The middle tracing reveals a small negative potential superimposed on the thenar component. In the bottom tracing, collision technique clearly separated the anomalous response (bracket), with S1 preceding S2 by 4 ms. (Reprinted with permission from Kimura J. Electrodiagnosis in diseases of nerve and muscle. Principles and practice, 2nd Ed, 1989; F.A. Davis.)*

This anomaly, occurring in 15% to 31% of an unselected population, tends to involve the arms bilaterally.[126] The incidence of this anastomosis is high among the congenitally abnormal fetus in general and those with trisomy 21 in particular.[124,127] The communicating fibers usually cross from the median to the ulnar nerve in the forearm and only rarely to the opposite direction.[128]

Careful analysis of the compound muscle action potentials readily reveals the presence of a Martin-Gruber anomaly during the routine nerve conduction studies. Stimulation of the median nerve at the elbow evokes not only median-innervated thenar muscles, but also ulnar muscles anomalously innervated by the crossing fibers. In contrast, stimulation of the median nerve at the wrist elicits a smaller response without the ulnar component. In the studies of the ulnar nerve, proximal and distal stimulation shows a reverse discrepancy in the amplitude of thenar or hypothenar compound muscle action potentials. In

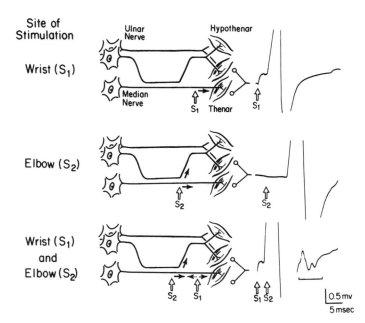

FIGURE 9.15. *Compound muscle action potentials recorded from the thenar eminence after stimulation of the median nerve at the wrist (S1) or elbow (S2) as in Figure 9.13. In the middle tracing, a large compound muscle action potential buried a small anomalous response mediated by the anastomosis. In the bottom tracing, a collision technique separated the anomalous response (bracket), with S1 preceding S2 by 4 ms. (Reprinted with permission from Kimura J. Electrodiagnosis in diseases of nerve and muscle. Principles and practice, 2nd Ed, 1989; F.A. Davis.)*

this case, stimulation at the elbow spares the communicating branch still attached to the median nerve, whereas stimulation at the wrist activates all the axons, including the additional anomalous fibers, giving rise to a full response.

In equivocal cases, the evidence of anastomosis depends on selective recording action potentials from the ulnar-innervated muscles after stimulation of the median nerve at the elbow. When recording from the ulnar side, median-innervated muscles may also give rise to a distant potential, usually with initial positivity.[85,94,116,118,129] Such volume conducted potentials appear regardless of the site of stimulus, whereas an anomalous response is elicited only by proximal stimulation. Restricted recording by a needle electrode also localizes the origin of the recorded response, although with intramuscular recording, distant activities are not entirely eliminated.

Alternatively, the collision technique may be employed to block selectively the unwanted impulses transmitted via the communicating fibers (Figure 9.14). Antidromically directed impulses from distal stimulation normally block the orthodromic impulses derived by proximal stimulation in the same nerve.[130,131] Orthodromic impulses traveling through an anastomotic branch to the ulnar nerve, however, bypass the antidromic impulses.[118] The technique helps characterize the anomalous response, allowing

one to calculate conduction velocity accurately. In the collision technique, a small response elicited by proximal stimulation through anastomosis tends to overlap with a large median potential evoked by distal stimulation (Figure 9.15). Satisfactory separation of the two responses results if one delivers the distal stimulus a few milliseconds before the proximal stimulation. With the interval exceeding the conduction time between the two stimulus sites, however, the orthodromic impulse escapes antidromic collision even in a normal subject without an anomalous route of transmission.

If the carpal tunnel syndrome accompanies this anastomosis, stimulation of the median nerve at the elbow evokes a normal ulnar and a delayed, temporally dispersed, median component. The initial ulnar response has a short latency, erroneously suggesting the presence of normally conducting median fibers. The response evoked by stimulation of the median nerve at the wrist is delayed without an ulnar component.[94,118,132] The latency difference between proximal and distal stimulation would result in an unreasonably rapid conduction velocity from the elbow to the wrist.[85,94,118] The ulnar muscles lie at some distance from the recording electrodes placed on the thenar eminence. Thus the anomalous ulnar component often displays an initial positive deflection.[133,134] As mentioned earlier, one may resort to a

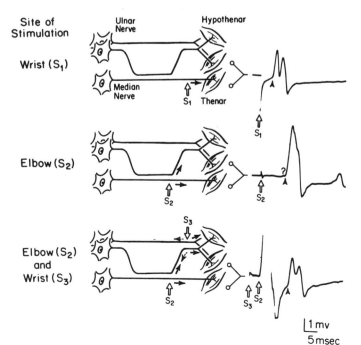

FIGURE 9.16. *A 55-year-old man with the carpal tunnel syndrome and the Martin-Gruber anastomosis. Stimulation at the elbow (S2) spread to the ulnar nerve through the anomalous communication (middle tracing). Another stimulus (S3) applied to the ulnar nerve at the wrist (bottom tracing) blocked the impulses transmitted through the communicating fibers. In the bottom tracing, S3 preceded S2 by 4 ms to avoid the overlap of the muscle responses elicited by S1 and S2. (Reprinted with permission from Kimura J. Electrodiagnosis in diseases of nerve and muscle. Principles and practice, 2nd Ed, 1989; F.A. Davis.)*

collision technique to block impulses in the anomalous fibers for selective transmission along the median nerve proper (Figure 9.16).

Severance or severe injury of the median nerve at the elbow may result in wallerian degeneration of communicating fibers. In extreme cases, separation of the median nerve at the elbow may affect all the intrinsic hand muscles. This rare condition is called the *all median hand* because all ulnar muscles in the hand receive innervation via the communicating fibers.[135] Electromyography may reveal abnormalities in the ulnar-innervated muscles after an injury to the median nerve at the elbow. An anomaly of this type therefore leads to considerable confusion in the interpretation of electrophysiologic findings.

Anomalies of the hand

Anomalies of the peripheral nerves may give rise to variations in the innervation of the intrinsic hand muscles. Although less commonly recognized than the median to ulnar communication, these are nonetheless important sources of error in the evaluation of nerve conduction and electromyography. Electrophysiologic studies may suggest the presence of such anastomoses, although anatomic analysis is necessary to characterize and delineate precisely the extent of anomaly.[136] Such anomalies include communications between motor branches of the median and ulnar nerves in the lateral portion of the hand[137,138] and ulnar or dual ulnar and median innervation of the flexor pollicis brevis [139] and the thenar muscles, which may derive their supply exclusively from either the median or ulnar nerve. Other anomalies include congenital absence of thenar muscles, which may give rise to a false impression of the carpal tunnel syndrome.[140]

REFERENCES

1. Spinner M. Injuries to the major branches of peripheral nerves of the forearm. Philadelphia: WB Saunders, 1972.
2. Sunderland S. Nerves and nerve injuries. Edinburgh: Churchill Livingstone, 1978.
3. Blom S, Dahlback LO. Nerve injuries in dislocations of the shoulder joint and fractures of the neck of the humerus. A clinical and electromyographical study. Acta Chir Scand 1970; 136:461.
4. Marinacci A. The value of electromyogram in the diagnosis of pressure neuropathy from "handing arm." Electromyogr Clin Neurophysiol 1967; 7:5.
5. Roth G, Ludy JP, Engloff-Baer S. Isolated proximal median neuropathy. Muscle Nerve 1982; 5:247.
6. Anson BJ. An atlas of human anatomy, ed 2. Philadelphia: WB Saunders, 1963.
7. Esposito GM. Peripheral entrapment neuropathies of upper extremity. NY State J Med 1972; 72:717–724.
8. Morris HH, Peters BH. Pronator syndrome: Clinical and electrophysiological features in seven cases. J Neurol Neurosurg Psychiatry 1976; 39:461–464.
9. Kopell HP, Thompson WAL. Peripheral entrapment neuropathies, ed 2. Huntington, NY: Robert E. Krieger, 1976.
10. Marquis JW, Bruwer AJ, Keith HM: Supracondyloid process of the humerus. Proc Staff Meet Mayo Clin 1957; 32:691–697.
11. Aiken BM, Moritz MJ. Atypical electromyographic findings in pronator teres syndrome. Arch Phys Med Rehabil 1987; 68:173–175.
12. Suranyi L. Median nerve compression by Struthers ligament. J Neurol Neurosurg Psychiatry 1983; 46:1047–1049.
13. Kiloh LG, Nevin S. Isolated neuritis of the anterior interosseous nerve. Br Med J 1952; 1:850–851.
14. Nakano KK, Lundergan C, Okihiro MM. Anterior interosseous nerve syndromes. Diagnostic methods and alternative treatments. Arch Neurol 1977; 34:477–480.
15. Gardner-Thorpe C. Anterior interosseous nerve palsy: Spontaneous recovery in two patients. J Neurol Neurosurg Psychiatry 1974; 37:1146–1150.
16. Lake PA. Anterior interosseous nerve syndrome. J Neurosurg 1974; 41:306–309.
17. Neundorfer B, Kroger M. The anterior interosseous nerve syndrome. J Neurol 1976; 213:347–352.
18. Rennels GD, Ochoa J. Neuralgic amyotrophy manifesting as anterior interosseous nerve palsy. Muscle Nerve 1980; 3:160–164.
19. Schady W, Ochoa JL, Torebjork HE, Chen LS. Peripheral projections of fascicles in the human median nerve. Brain 1983; 106:745–760.
20. Wertsch JJ, Sanger JR, Matloub HS. Pseudo-anterior interosseous nerve syndrome. Muscle Nerve 1985; 8:68–70.
21. O'Brien MD, Upton ARM. Anterior interosseous nerve syndrome. A case report with neurophysiological investigation. J Neurol Neurosurg Psychiatry 1972; 35:531–536.
22. Robbins H. Anatomical study of the median nerve in the carpal tunnel and etiologies of the carpal-tunnel syndrome. J Bone Joint Surg 1963; 45A:953–966.
23. Thomas PK, Fullerton PM. Nerve fibre size in the carpal tunnel syndrome. J Neurol Neurosurg Psychiatry 1963; 26:520–527.

24. Kimura J. The carpal tunnel syndrome. Localization of conduction abnormalities within the distal segment of the median nerve. Brain 1979; 102:619–635.

25. Neary D, Ochoa J, Gilliatt RW. Sub-clinical entrapment neuropathy in man. J Neurol Sci 1975; 24:283–298.

26. Gilliatt RW. Sensory conduction studies in the early recognition of nerve disorders. Muscle Nerve 1978; 1:352–359.

27. Bleecker ML, Bohlman M, Moreland R, Tipton A. Carpal tunnel syndrome: Role of carpal canal size. Neurology 1985; 35:1599–1604.

28. Dekel S, Coates R. Primary carpal stenosis as a cause of "idiopathic" carpal tunnel syndrome. Lancet 1979; 2:1024.

29. Reinstein L. Hand dominance in carpal tunnel syndrome. Arch Phys Med Rehabil 1981; 62:202–203.

30. Reddy MP. Nerve entrapment syndromes in the upper extremity contralateral to amputation. Arch Phys Med Rehabil 1984; 65:24–26.

31. Gainer JV Jr, Nugent GR. Carpal tunnel syndrome. Report of 430 operations. South Med J 1977; 70:325–328.

32. Harrison MJG. Lack of evidence of generalized sensory neuropathy in patients with carpal tunnel syndrome. J Neurol Neurosurg Psychiatry 1978; 41:957–959.

33. Braddom RL. Familial carpal tunnel syndrome in three generations of a black family. Am J Phys Med 1985; 64:227–234.

34. Bastian FO. Amyloidosis and the carpal tunnel syndrome. Am J Clin Pathol 1974; 61:711–717.

35. Halter SK, Delisa JA, Stolov WC, et al. Carpal tunnel syndrome in chronic renal dialysis patients. Arch Phys Med Rehabil 1981; 6:197–201.

36. Klofkorn RW, Steigerwald JC. Carpal tunnel syndrome as the initial manifestation of tuberculosis. Am J Med 1976; 60:583–586.

37. Vallat JM, Dunoyer J. Familial occurrence of entrapment neuropathies. Arch Neurol 1979; 36:323.

38. Yu J, Bendler EM, Mentari A. Neurological disorders associated with carpal tunnel syndrome. Electromyogr Clin Neurophysiol 1979; 19:27–32.

39. O'Duffy JD, Randall RV, MacCarty CS. Median neuropathy (carpal-tunnel syndrome) in acromegaly. A sign of endocrine overactivity. Ann Intern Med 1973; 78:379–383.

40. Kyle RA, Bayrd ED. Amyloidosis: Review of 236 cases. Medicine 1975; 54:271–299.

41. Khaleeli AA, Levy RD, Edwards RHT, et al. The neuromuscular features of acromegaly: A clinical and pathological study. J Neurol Neurosurg Psychiatry 1984; 47:1009–1015.

42. Jones HR Jr, Beetham WP Jr, Silverman ML, Margles SW. Eosinophilic fasciitis and the carpal tunnel syndrome. J Neurol Neurosurg Psychiatry 1986; 49:324–327.

43. Murray IPC, Simpson JA. Acroparesthesias in myxedema: A clinical and electromyographic study. Lancet 1958; 1:1360.

44. Scarpalezos S, Lygidakis C, Papageorgiou C, et al. Neural and muscular manifestations of hypothyroidism. Arch Neurol 1973; 29:140–144.

45. Sidiq M, Kirsner AB, Sheon RP. Carpal tunnel syndrome. First manifestation of systemic lupus erythematosus. JAMA 1972; 222:1416–1417.

46. Valenta LJ. Hyperparathyroidism due to parathyroid adenoma and carpal tunnel syndrome. Ann Intern Med 1975; 82:541–542.

47. Sahs AL, Helms CM, Dubois C. Carpal tunnel syndrome. Complication of toxic shock syndrome. Arch Neurol 1983; 40:414–415.

48. Nakano KK. The entrapment neuropathies of rheumatoid arthritis. Orthop Clin North Am 1975; 6:837–860.

49. Vemireddi NK, Redford JB, Pombejara CN. Serial nerve conduction studies in carpal tunnel syndrome secondary to rheumatoid arthritis: Preliminary study. Arch Phys Med Rehabil 1979; 60:393–396.

50. Lewis MH. Median nerve decompression after Colles' fracture. J Bone Joint Surg 1969; 60B:195–196.

51. Schmitt O, Temme CH. Carpal tunnel syndrome bei pseudarthrosebildung nach isolierter fraktur des os capitatum. Arch Orthop Tramat Surg 1978; 93:25–28.

52. Manske PR. Fracture of the hook of the hamate presenting as carpal tunnel. Hand 1978; 10:191.

53. Hayden JW. Median neuropathy in the carpal tunnel caused by spontaneous intraneural hemorrhage. J Bone Joint Surg 1964; 46A:1242–1244.

54. Cherington M. Proximal pain in carpal tunnel syndrome. Arch Surg 1974; 108:69.

55. Aminoff MJ. Involvement of peripheral vasomotor fibres in carpal tunnel syndrome. J Neurol Neurosurg Psychiatry 1979; 42:649–655.

56. Lindscheid RL, Peterson LFA, Juergens JL. Carpal tunnel syndrome associated with vasospasm. J Bone Joint Surg 1967; 49A:1141–1146.

57. Phalen GS. Reflections of 21 years experience with the carpal tunnel syndrome. JAMA 1970; 212:1365–1367.

58. Phalen GS. The carpal-tunnel syndrome. Seventeen years' experience in diagnosis and treatment of six hundred fifty-four hands. J Bone Joint Surg 1966; 48A:211–228.

59. Marin EL, Vernick S, Friedmann LW. Carpal tunnel syndrome: Median nerve stress test. Arch Phys Med Rehabil 1983; 64:206–208.

60. Schwartz MS, Gordon JA, Swash M. Slowed nerve conduction with wrist flexion in carpal tunnel syndrome. Ann Neurol 1980; 8:69–71.

61. Stewart JD, Eisen A. Tinel's sign and the carpal tunnel syndrome. Br Med J 1978; 2:1125–1126.

62. Tinel J. Le Signe du "Fourmillement" dans les Le-

sions des Nerfs Peripheriques. Press Med 1915; 47:388. [Transl by Kaplan EB. In: Spinner M, ed. Injuries to the major branches of peripheral nerves of the forearm, ed 2. Philadelphia: WB Saunders, 1978.]

63. Spinner M. Injuries to the major branches of peripheral nerves of the forearm, ed 2. Philadelphia: WB Saunders, 1978.

64. Wilkins RH, Brody IA. Tinel's sign. Arch Neurol 1971; 24:573.

65. Gilliatt RW, Wilson TG. Ischaemic sensory loss in patients with peripheral nerve lesions. J Neurol Neurosurg Psychiatry 1954; 17:104–114.

66. Fullerton PM. The effect of ischaemia on nerve conduction in the carpal tunnel syndrome. J Neurol Neurosurg Psychiatry 1963; 26:385–397.

67. Fullerton PM, Gilliatt RW. Median and ulnar neuropathy in the guinea-pig. J Neurol Neurosurg Psychiatry 1967; 30:393–402.

68. Ochoa J, Marotte L. The nature of the nerve lesion caused by chronic entrapment in the guinea-pig. J Neurol Sci 1973; 19:491–495.

69. Levin RA, Felsenthal G. Handcuff neuropathy: Two unusual cases. Arch Phys Med Rehabil 1984; 65:41–43.

70. Upton ARM, McComas AJ. The double crush in nerve-entrapment syndromes. Lancet 1973; 2:359–362.

71. Gardner RC. Confirmed case and diagnosis of pseudocarpal-tunnel (sublimis) syndrome. N Engl J Med 1970; 282:858.

72. Nakano KK. Entrapment neuropathy from Baker's cyst. JAMA 1978; 239:135.

73. Jablecki C, Nazemi R. Unsuspected digital nerve lesions responsible for abnormal median sensory responses. Arch Phys Med Rehabil 1982; 63:135–138.

74. Kimura J. A method for determining median nerve conduction velocity across the carpal tunnel. J Neurol Sci 1978; 38:1–10.

75. Roth G. Vitesse de conduction motrice du nerf median dans le canal carpien. Ann Med Phys 1970; 13:117–132.

76. Ginzburg M, Lee M, Ginzburg J, Alba A. Median and ulnar nerve conduction determinations in the Erb's point-axilla segment in normal subjects. J Neurol Neurosurg Psychiatry 1978; 41:444–448.

77. Brown WF, Ferguson GG, Jones MW, Yates SK. The location of conduction abnormalities in human entrapment neuropathies. Can J Neurol Sci 1976; 3:111–122.

78. Werschkul JD. Anomalous course of the recurrent motor branch of the median nerve in a patient with carpal tunnel syndrome. Case report. J Neurosurg 1977; 47:113–114.

79. Mavor H, Shiozawa R. Antidromic digital and palmar nerve action potentials. Electroencephalogr Clin Neurophysiol 1971; 30:210–211.

80. DiBenedetto M, Mitz M, Klingbeil G, Davidoff DD. New criteria for sensory nerve conduction especially useful in diagnosing carpal tunnel syndrome. Arch Phys Med Rehabil 1986; 67:586–589.

81. Buchthal F, Rosenfalck A. Evoked action potentials and conduction velocity in human sensory nerves. Brain Res 1966; 3:1–122.

82. Kimura J, Machida M, Ishida T, et al. Relationship between size of compound sensory or muscle action potentials, and length of nerve segment. Neurology 1986; 36:647–652.

83. Buchthal F, Rosenfalck A. Sensry conduction from digit to palm and from palm to wrist in the carpal tunnel syndrome. J Neurol Neurosurg Psychiatry 1971; 34:243–252.

84. Buchthal F, Rosenfalck A. Sensory potentials in polyneuropathy. Brain 1971; 94:241–262.

85. Buchthal F, Rosenfalck A, Trojaborg W. Electrophysiological findings in entrapment of the median nerve at wrist and elbow. J Neurol Neurosurg Psychiatry 1974; 37:340–360.

86. Wiederholt WC. Median nerve conduction velocity in sensory fibers through carpal tunnel. Arch Phys Med Rehabil 1970; 51:328–330.

87. Daube JR. Percutaneous palmar median nerve stimulation for carpal tunnel syndrome. Electroencephalogr Clin Neurophysiol 1977; 43:139–140.

88. Eklund G. A new electrodiagnostic procedure for measuring sensory nerve conduction across the carpal tunnel. Upsala J Med Sci 1975; 80:63–64.

89. Lum PB, Kanakamedala RV. Conduction of the palmar cutaneous branch of the median nerve. Arch Phys Med Rehabil 1986; 67:805–806.

90. Simpson JA. Electrical signs in the diagnosis of carpal tunnel and related syndromes. J Neurol Neurosurg Psychiatry 1956; 19:275–280.

91. Duensing F, Lowitzsch K, Thorwirth V, Vogel P. Neurophysiologische Befunde beim Karpaltunnelsyndrom. Korrelationen zum klinischen Befund. Z Neurol 1974; 206:267–284.

92. Gilliatt RW, Sears TA. Sensory nerve action potentials in patients with peripheral nerve lesions. J Neurol Neurosurg Psychiatry 1958; 21:109–118.

93. Kaesar HE. Diagnostische Probleme beim Karpaltunnelsyndrom. Deutsche Zeitschrift Fur Nervenheilkunde 1963; 185:453–470.

94. Lambert EH. Diagnostic value of electrical stimulation of motor nerves. Electroencephalogr Clin Neurophysiol 1962; (suppl 22):9–16.

95. Melvin JL, Schuchmann JA, Lanese RR. Diagnostic specificity of motor and sensory nerve conduction variables in the carpal tunnel syndrome. Arch Phys Med Rehabil 1973; 54:69–74.

96. Thomas JE, Lambert EH, Cseuz KA. Electrodiagnostic aspects of the carpal tunnel syndrome. Arch Neurol 1967; 16:635–641.

97. Anderson MH, Fullerton PM, Gilliatt RW, Hern

JEC. Changes in the forearm associated with median nerve compression at the wrist in the guinea-pig. J Neurol Neurosurg Psychiatry 1970; 33:70–79.

98. Stohr M, Petruch F, Shceglmann K, Schilling K. Retrograde changes of nerve fibers with the carpal tunnel syndrome. An electroneurographic investigation. J Neurol 1978; 218:287–292.

99. Carroll GJ. Comparison of median and radial nerve sensory latencies in the electrophysiological diagnosis of carpal tunnel syndrome. Electroencephalogr Clin Neurophysiol 1987; 68:101–106.

100. Johnson EW, Kukla RD, Wongsam RE, Piedmont A. Sensory latencies to the ring finger: Normal values and relation to carpal tunnel syndrome. Arch Phys Med Rehabil 1981; 62:206–208.

101. Johnson EW, Sipski M, Lammertse T. Median and radial sensory latencies to digit I: Normal values and usefulness in carpal tunnel syndrome. Arch Phys Med Rehabil 1987; 68:140–141.

102. Kraft GH, Halvorson GA. Median nerve residual latency: Normal value and use in diagnosis of carpal tunnel syndrome. Arch Phys Med Rehabil 1983; 64:221–226.

103. Kimura I, Ayyar DR. The carpal tunnel syndrome: Electrophysiological aspects of 639 symptomatic extremities. Electromyogr Clin Neurophysiol 1985; 25:151–164.

104. Shahani BT, Young RR, Potts F, Maccabee P. Terminal latency index (TLI) and late response studies in motor neuron disease (MND), peripheral neuropathies and entrapment syndromes. Acta Neurol Scand 1979; 73 (suppl):60.

105. Spaans F. Spontaneous rhythmic motor unit potentials in the carpal tunnel syndrome. J Neurol Neurosurg Psychiatry 1982; 45:19–28.

106. Desjacques P, Egloff-Baer S, Roth G. Lumbrical muscles and the carpal tunnel syndrome. Electromyogr Clin Neurophysiol 1980; 20:443–450.

107. Cassvan A, Rosenberg A, Rivera L. Ulnar nerve involvement in carpal tunnel syndrome. Arch Phys Med Rehabil 1986; 67:290–292.

108. Sedal L, McLeod JG, Walsh JC. Ulnar nerve lesions associated with the carpal tunnel syndrome. J Neurol Neurosurg Psychiatry 1973; 36:118–123.

109. Brown WF, Yates SK. Percutaneous localization of conduction abnormalities in human entrapment neuropathies. J Can Neurol Sci 1982; 9:391–400.

110. Monga TN, Shanks GL, Poole BJ. Sensory palmar stimulation in the diagnosis of carpal tunnel syndrome. Arch Phys Med Rehabil 1985; 66:598–600.

111. Mills KR. Orthodromic sensory action potentials from palmar stimulation in the diagnosis of carpal tunnel syndrome. J Neurol Neurosurg Psychiatry 1985; 48:250–255.

112. Casey EB, Le Quesne PM. Digital nerve action potentials in healthy subjects, and in carpal tunnel and diabetic patients. J Neurol Neurosurg Psychiatry 1972; 35:612–623.

113. Maccabee PJ, Shahani BT, Young RR. Usefulness of double simultaneous recording (DSR) and F response studies in the diagnosis of carpal tunnel syndrome (CTS). Neurology 1980; 30:18P.

114. Stevens JC. AAEE Minimonograph #26: The electrodiagnosis of carpal tunnel syndrome. Muscle Nerve 1987; 2:99–113.

115. Johnson RK, Shrewsbury MM. Anatomical course of the thenar branch of the median nerve—usually in a separate tunnel through the transverse carpal ligament. J Bone Joint Surg 1970; 52A:269–273.

116. Gassel MM. Sources of error in motor nerve conduction studies. Neurology (Minneap) 1964; 14:825–835.

117. Kaeser HE. Nerve conduction velocity measurements. In: Vinken PJ, Bruyn BW, eds. Handbook of clinical neurology. Vol 7. Amsterdam: North Holland, 1970:116–196.

118. Kimura J. Collision technique. Physiologic block of nerve impulses in studies of motor nerve conduction velocity. Neurology (Minneap) 1976; 26:680–682.

119. Kimura J. F-wave velocity in the central segment of the median and ulnar nerves. A study in normal subjects and in patients with Charcot-Marie-Tooth disease. Neurology (Minneap) 1974; 24:539–546.

120. Hopf HC, Hense W. Anomalien der motorischen Innervation an der Hand. Z EEG-EMG 1974; 5:220–224.

121. Martin R. Tal om Nervers allmanna egenskaper i manniskans kropp. Stockholm: L Salvius, 1963.

122. Gruber W. Ueber die Verbindung des Nervus medianus mit dem Nervus ulnaris am Unterarme des Menschen und der Saugethiere. Arch Anat Physiol Med, Leipzig, 1870:501–522.

123. Mannerfelt L. Studies on the hand in ulnar nerve paralysis. A clinical-experimental investigation in normal and anomalous innervation. Acta Orthop Scand 1966; (suppl 87):23–176.

124. Srinivasan R, Rhodes J. The median-ulnar anastomosis (Martin-Gruber) in normal and congenitally abnormal fetuses. Arch Neurol 1981; 38:418–419.

125. Wilbourn AJ, Lambert EH. The forearm median-to-ulnar nerve communication: Electrodiagnostic aspects. Neurology (Minneap) 1976; 26:368.

126. Kimura J, Murphy JM, Varda DJ. Electrophysiological study of anomalous innervation of intrinsic hand muscles. Arch Neurol 1976; 33:842–844.

127. Bunnels S. Surgery of the hand, ed 4. Philadelphia: JB Lippincott, 1964.

128. Streib EW. Ulnar-to-median nerve anastomosis in the forearm: Electromyographic studies. Neurology (New York) 1979; 29:1534–1537.

129. Simpson JA. Fact and fallacy in measurement of conduction velocity in motor nerves. J Neurol Neurosurg Psychiatry 1964; 27:381–385.

130. Hopf HC. Untersuchungen uber die Unterschiede in der leitgeschwindigkeit motorischer Nervenfasern beim Menschen. Deutsche Zeitschrift Fur Nervenheilkunde 1962; 183:579–588.

131. Thomas PK, Sears TA, Gilliatt RW. The range of conduction velocity in normal motor nerve fibres to the small muscles of the hand and foot. J Neurol Neurosurg Psychiatry 1959; 22:175–181.

132. Iyer V, Fenichel GM. Normal median nerve proximal latency in carpal tunnel syndrome: A clue to coexisting Martin-Gruber anastomosis. J Neurol Neurosurg Psychiatry 1976; 39:449–452.

133. Gutmann L. Important anomalous innervations of the extremities. American Association of Electromyography and Electrodiagnosis Meeting, Rochester, MN, 1977.

134. Gutmann L. Median-ulnar nerve communications and carpal tunnel syndrome. J Neurol Neurosurg Psychiatry 1977; 40:982–986.

135. Marinacci AA. Diagnosis of "all median hand." Bull LA Neurol Soc 1964; 29:191–197.

136. Sunderland S. Nerves and nerve injuries, ed 2. Edinburgh: Churchill Livingstone, 1978.

137. Cannieu JMA. Note sur une anastomose entre la branche profonde du cubital et le median. Bull Soc D'Anat Physiol Bordeaux 1897; 18:339–340.

138. Richie P. Le nerf cubital et les muscles de l'eminence thenar. Bull Mem Soc Anat Paris 1897; 72:251–252 (Series 5).

139. Seddon H. Surgical disorders of the peripheral nerves, ed 2. Edinburgh: Churchill Livingstone, 1975:203–211.

140. Cavanagh NPC, Yates DAH, Sutcliffe J. Thenar hypoplasia with associated radiologic abnormalities. Muscle Nerve 1979; 2:431–436.

10

Ulnar Nerve Lesions

Robert G. Miller

LIST OF ACRONYMS

ADM	abductor digiti minimi
CMAP	compound muscle action potential
CT	cubital tunnel
EMG	electromyography
FCU	flexor carpi ulnaris
FDI	first dorsal interosseous
FDP	flexor digitorum profundus
ME	medial epicondyle
NAP	nerve action potential
NCV	nerve conduction velocity
NP	not provided
SD	standard deviation

Precise localization of an ulnar nerve lesion on the basis of clinical information is sometimes impossible. In the majority of cases, however, the clinical electromyographer can precisely and confidently localize the lesion even if sometimes more sophisticated approaches than those employed in routine practice may have to be used. All of these techniques can and should be employed in standard clinical neurophysiologic practice. In this chapter, the most common lesions at the elbow are considered separately in their acute and chronic forms. Both clinical and electrophysiologic findings are discussed. Information of both diagnostic and prognostic value from the electrophysiologic studies is emphasized.

ANATOMY

The ulnar nerve is derived from C-8 and T-1 roots and continues as the major extension of the medial cord of the brachial plexus. In the axilla, it is somewhat posterior along with the axillary artery, and in the arm, it travels near the median nerve and brachial artery. It traverses the medial aspect of the medial head of triceps and remains very superficial as it descends to the ulnar groove between the olecranon and the medial epicondyle. There are usually two branches to the flexor carpi ulnaris (FCU), one to each head of the muscle. The first branch arises at or just distal to the entrance of the cubital tunnel, a dense aponeurosis that connects the two heads of FCU, usually located between 3 and 20 mm distal to the medial epicondyle.[1,2] A further branch, to the flexor digitorum profundus (FDP) of the fourth and fifth fingers, arises in this same area, and the nerve descends under the belly of the FCU through the forearm. The nerve exits from the FCU after an intramuscular course of several centimeters, where a tough intramuscular septum between FCU and FDP may entrap the nerve.[3] At the wrist, the nerve is again superficial and lies between the tendon of flexor digitorum sublimis laterally and FCU medially. The nerve enters the canal of Guyon at the level of the proximal wrist crease and divides into the superficial and deep branches. Distal to the branch to the abductor digiti minimi (ADM), the deep branch leaves the canal through the rigid space between the hamate and pisiform bones. The deep branch traverses the palm and supplies the motor fibers to the ulnar intrinsic hand muscles, including the first dorsal interosseous (FDI). Between the pisiform and the hook of the hamate, the superficial cutaneous branch of the ulnar nerve leaves the main trunk to provide sensation for the palmar aspect of the fifth and the medial half of the fourth digits. The dorsal sensory branch leaves the main trunk of the ulnar nerve 5 to 8 cm proximal to the ulnar styloid and innervates the dorsal aspect of the same digits.

CLASSIFICATION OF ULNAR NEUROPATHIES

By far, the most common site of entrapment of the ulnar nerve is in the region of the elbow. Much less commonly, entrapment occurs at the wrist or in the palm. Compressive neuropathy may also occur in the upper arm or forearm, although these are probably rare causes of ulnar neuropathy. The following brief discussion of a working classification of ulnar neuropathies starts with the most common condition and ends with less frequently encountered focal lesions.

Tardy ulnar palsy was first described in 1878 in connection with the late development of ulnar neuropathy at the elbow in patients with a residual bone deformity from an earlier fracture in the region of the elbow.[4] It subsequently became widely recognized that ulnar neuropathy may be a late complication of a traumatic deformity of the elbow region. Of course, other causes of joint deformity such as rheumatoid arthritis may also be associated with ulnar neuropathy at the elbow. The concept of the cubital tunnel was introduced by Feindel and Stratford[5] to describe the course of the ulnar nerve as it runs beneath the aponeurosis of the FCU muscle just distal to the medial epicondyle. They reported three patients with entrapment of the nerve within this tunnel, two of whom also had obvious posttraumatic joint deformity, suggesting that two separate pathologic processes might be important.[6] Subsequently, it has become clear that patients without trauma or joint deformity may also develop ulnar neuropathy at the elbow.[7] Many of these patients have focal abnormalities in the ulnar nerve at the level of the cubital tunnel, and the findings are often bilateral. Such patients often give a history of repeated elbow flexion and engaging in activities that result in repeated contraction of FCU, which narrows the cubital tunnel.[6] Not all ulnar neuropathies at the elbow originate in the cubital tunnel, as compression and injury to the nerve may occur in the ulnar groove at or just proximal to the medial epicondyle.[8] Patients with an underlying polyneuropathy are particularly susceptible to develop ulnar neuropathy at the elbow superimposed on the underlying polyneuropathy. Thus ulnar neuropathy at the elbow constitutes a heterogeneous group of conditions with varying causes; taken together, however, it is the second most common site of entrapment of peripheral nerves in the upper extremity second only to carpal tunnel syndrome.

Ulnar neuropathy at or distal to the wrist is perhaps more common than generally recognized. Such neuropathies may be confused with ulnar neuropathies at the elbow or with the focal onset of anterior horn cell disease in patients without sensory symptoms. Varying patterns of weakness of intrinsic hand muscles with or without sensory loss have been observed.[9–11] Ulnar neuropathy in the forearm, at the point of exit from the cubital tunnel, has also been documented as the nerve passes through the dense fascia that separate FCU and FDP.[3] More detailed discussion of these distal ulnar neuropathies is provided later in the chapter.

Entrapment of the ulnar nerve proximal to the elbow is distinctly unusual. The arcade of Struthers is formed by superficial fibers of the medial head of the triceps muscle, by attachments of the internal brachial ligament, and anteriorly by the medial intermuscular septum. Compression of the ulnar nerve under the arcade may occur up to 7 cm proximal to the medial epicondyle.[12] Similarly, compression may occur under the anconeus epitrochlearis, an anomalous muscle arising from the medial border of the olecranon and the adjacent triceps tendon and inserting into the medial epicondyle.[1,12] Either of these anomalies may contribute to compression of the ulnar nerve proximal to the elbow.

An important point in classification derives from the temporal development of the neuropathy. Acute compressive neuropathy resulting from a single episode of compression during general anesthesia or a drunken stupor presents a different clinical, electrophysiologic, and prognostic picture when compared with chronic entrapment.[13] Most importantly, the management may be entirely different for these two different conditions.[14] This point is highlighted in further detail in the section dealing with specific types of ulnar neuropathies.

PATHOLOGY AND PATHOPHYSIOLOGY OF ULNAR NEUROPATHY

There is little information available about the pathology of ulnar neuropathy in humans. It has been demonstrated, however, that neuromatous thickening primarily on the basis of increased endoneurial area is present at the level of the lesion. Demyelination and small clusters of regenerating fibers at the

level of the cubital tunnel have been documented along with fascicular enlargement, numerous Renaut bodies, and reductions in nerve fiber density. Selective loss of the larger myelinated nerve fibers together with marked increases in the numbers of small-diameter (2 to 4 μ) fibers indicating nerve regeneration, have been observed at the site of the primary pathologic change.[15]

Abnormalities in the ulnar nerve at the elbow may be extremely common in the general population, as suggested by the study of Neary et al.,[16] wherein mild but definite pathologic changes of compressive neuropathy in the ulnar nerve at the cubital tunnel were observed in five of 12 ulnar nerves from autopsy patients without signs or symptoms of neuropathy. Increased Renaut bodies and abnormalities observed in teased fibers indicating previous demyelination were also present. The appearance of internodes was altered, with bulbous swelling at one end and thinning and retraction of myelin at the other; in some nerves, intercolated segments were also found.[16] These findings were similar to those observed in experimental compression neuropathy in both the guinea pig and the baboon with recurrent trauma or recurrent compression.[17,18] Moreover, Neary and Eames[15] found similar but less severe pathologic changes in the asymptomatic ulnar nerves of two autopsy patients with idiopathic contralateral ulnar neuropathy. Similarly, abnormal motor and sensory nerve conduction has been reported in the clinically normal arms of patients with unilateral ulnar neuropathy.[19–21] Further, the finding of abnormal slowing across the elbow in a normal series of ulnar nerve conduction studies suggests that many individuals have subclinical entrapment of the ulnar nerve at the elbow.[22–24] The difficult question of determining normal values and the precise site of entrapment are discussed in more detail subsequently.

The gross appearance of the nerve was described in a series of patients with cubital tunnel syndrome.[7] Eleven of 15 ulnar nerves were explored surgically. There was a dense aponeurosis at the cubital tunnel, where the nerve was swollen, edematous, and hyperemic proximal to the tunnel. After the aponeurosis was sectioned, the segment underlying the tight band was seen to be narrowed and pale. Before section, the tunnel was examined with the elbow in extension and in 90 degrees flexion, and in each case the nerve was tightly compressed by the aponeurosis in 90 degrees flexion. Nerve conduction studies were performed at operation in seven patients and confirmed localization of the abnormal conduction to the cubital tunnel.

Important observations on experimental compression neuropathy in the baboon using the sphyg-momanometer cuff have yielded information that bears directly on the problems encountered in the clinical laboratory (reviewed in references 17 and 25). In this animal model, the conduction block was found to be localized to both the proximal and the distal ends of the cuff. A dramatic reduction in the amplitude of the evoked muscle response was found when comparing stimulation just proximal with that just distal to the edge of the cuff. It is of great practical interest that in the region of the peripheral nerve beneath the cuff, the threshold for stimulation was higher for damaged fibers. Thus an increase in stimulus intensity was required to ensure supramaximal stimulation of fibers conducting in this segment of nerve, as compared with the segment distal to the blood pressure cuff. Teased fiber studies by Ochoa et al.[18] revealed displacement of the nodes of Ranvier under the edges of the cuff. Serial studies revealed subsequent development of paranodal demyelination and subsequent remyelination.

In the model of acute compression neuropathy in the baboon already described, the degree of conduction block (e.g., the percentage of fibers that were electrically inexcitable proximal to the lesion) was directly proportional to both the amount and the duration of the pressure exerted through the cuff.[25] When the block was incomplete, the amplitude of the proximal response was reduced compared with the response to distal stimulation. In addition, the latency of the proximal response was initially increased, indicating slowing of conduction across the lesion. When there was a complete block, subsequent resolution was characterized by an initially prolonged latency. It is worth pointing out that simple comparison of the amplitudes of the compound muscle action potential (CMAP) evoked by proximal and distal stimulation is insufficient to determine the presence or absence of conduction block. Only by comparing the area of the response with proximal and distal stimulation can one be certain about the presence or absence of conduction block.[26,27] Where the area of the motor responses is similar but the amplitude is markedly diminished in response to proximal stimulation compared with distal stimulation, conduction slowing and increased temporal dispersion are more likely causes of the reduction in amplitude than conduction block. The area is diminished as well in response to proximal compared with distal stimulation; however, conduction block, at least in some fibers, is probably present.

Data from this baboon model also provided evidence about the differential susceptibility of axons to compression according to their external diameter.

Structural damage was greater in larger myelinated fibers with relative sparing of smaller myelinated fibers with an external diameter less than 5 μm.[25] Unmyelinated fibers were affected only when compression was so severe that substantial axonal degeneration occurred in the larger fibers. It appears that fiber size is more important in determining susceptibility to compression than whether the fibers are efferent or afferent because these two types of axons have shown a similar susceptibility to compression in this experimental model.

A further point that emerged from the study of experimental compression neuropathy is the difference between the acute and the chronic compressive lesion. The histology is different, inasmuch as the chronic lesion generally covers a wider area of the nerve with a different histologic appearance compared with the acute lesion.[18] The initial stage is retraction of the myelin sheath from one end of the internode leading to paranodal demyelination. Complete internodal demyelination then occurs, with a tendency to more marked distortion of the internodes on the proximal as opposed to the distal side of the compressive lesion. With increasing amount and duration of compression, wallerian degeneration appears distal to the site of compression. Although the data from the experimental neuropathy does not permit precise comparison between the physiologic implications of acute as opposed to chronic compression, the data do suggest that in the chronic compressive neuropathy, conduction block is less common than in the acute compressive neuropathy. These findings are supported by the report of Brown et al.,[8] who found conduction block in only one-third of entrapped ulnar nerves and one-quarter of entrapped median nerves studied at surgery for treatment of chronic compressive neuropathy. Our own experience with the acute compressive neuropathy occurring during compression of the ulnar nerve in patients undergoing major surgery indicated a significant conduction block in three of eight patients.[28] These small studies do not provide clear evidence of a difference in the degree of conduction block in acute as opposed to chronic neuropathy. This point deserves further study.

ELECTROPHYSIOLOGIC TECHNIQUES

Motor Nerve Conduction Studies

The hallmark of nerve compression is abnormally slowed nerve conduction velocity. One might reasonably ask, however, what constitutes slowing in the ulnar nerve across the elbow. Should one set an arbitrary lower limit, or should there be a comparison between the distal or proximal segment of the same nerve or perhaps the contralateral side? Should we consider motor or sensory conduction or both? Several technical questions need to be considered. First, the position of the limb is important in determining conduction velocity in various segments. Checkles et al.[24] showed that motor nerve conduction velocities are substantially slower when the elbow is extended compared with the elbow flexed[29,30] (Table 10.1). Presumably the measurement of nerve length is more accurate in the elbow-flexed position compared with the extended position, where the nerve may be kinked.[31] Thus the elbow-flexed position (135 degrees; full extension = 0 degrees) is probably superior, markedly reducing the variation between different segments of the nerve.[32] The second point concerns the selection of a nerve segment in the elbow region. One can evaluate focal slowing of motor nerve conduction velocity at the elbow only when stimulation is performed both above and below the elbow, in addition to the wrist and axilla. The major advantage of determining the conduction in the smallest affected segment is to increase the yield of abnormal findings. This point has been dem-

onstrated for carpal tunnel syndrome,[33] wherein stimulation in the palm and recording at the wrist increase the sensitivity of the method, compared with stimulating at the digit and recording at the wrist.[33] Presumably the length of normal nerve distal to the carpal tunnel may disguise the abnormally slowed segment under the carpal ligament. Carrying the point one step further, Brown et al.[8] have demonstrated the same phenomenon at the cubital tunnel in a patient with normal motor nerve conduction velocity in the 10-cm across-elbow segment but with prolonged conduction time in two 1-cm segments studied intraoperatively. The disadvantage of trying to study the across-elbow segment, as pointed out by Odusote and Eisen,[20] is the occasional difficulty of obtaining a good motor response when stimulating over the belly of FCU. There are two ways of minimizing the error introduced by either insufficient stimulus intensity or abnormal stimulus spread owing to very high stimulus intensity. Either near-nerve stimulation with needle electrodes can be performed, or above-elbow stimulation can be performed 5 cm above the medial epicondyle and below-elbow stimulation at 5 cm below the medial epicondyle, thus providing interstimulus electrode distance of 10 cm and remaining over the relatively thin proximal por-

TABLE 10.1.   Reported values for ulnar nerve conduction velocity*

| | | Motor Nerve Conduction | | |
Reference	Elbow Position	Upper Arm	Across Elbow	Below Elbow
34	Flexed	52	50	49
24	Flexed	NP	52	53
8	Flexed	58	47	50
35	Flexed	46	45	45
29	Flexed	50	49	49
19	Extended	60	44	56
24	Extended	NP	34	52
22	Extended	43	38	41
29	Extended	50	38	53

| | | Sensory Nerve Conduction | | |
Reference	Elbow Position	Across Elbow	Wrist to Below Elbow	Digit 5 to Wrist
19	Extended	50	63	49
23	Extended	44	59	44
29	Flexed	51	54	NP

* The lower limit of normal (95% confidence level) is taken from each study.

NP, Not provided.

tion of the FCU muscle. This stimulus point will, in almost all cases, still be located distal to the cubital tunnel roof.[2,7] Finally, the importance of temperature requires either heating the limb or measuring temperature and using a correction factor.

The lower limits of normal for conduction in the upper arm, across-elbow, and below elbow segments of the ulnar nerve recorded by various investigators are shown in Table 10.1. In general, slower values for motor nerve conduction velocity across the elbow were recorded in each study in which the elbow was extended. On the basis of these studies, a lower limit of normal for ulnar nerve motor conduction in the across-elbow segment of 49 meters per second with the elbow flexed 135 degrees appears reasonable.[30] In the elbow-extended position, Eisen[22] suggested a lower limit of 38 m per second on the basis of findings from 48 normal control subjects. The conduction velocity across the elbow, however, was below 42 m per second in six subjects and below 32 m per second in two. In the study by Checkles et al.,[24] a value of 34 m per second was the lower limit of normal found from 31 ulnar nerve studies; however, a relatively short mean interstimulus distance of 8.1 cm was used. In Payan's study,[19] no subject with less than 44 m per second in the across-elbow segment was seen, although only 20 control subjects were included. In a study by Kincaid et al.,[29] the lowest value observed in 50 subjects was 38 m per second in the across-elbow segment, with an interstimulus electrode distance of 10 cm. I am now persuaded that the elbow-flexed (135 degrees) position should be used to assess conduction across the elbow.

With regard to the question of comparing the across-elbow velocity with adjacent segments, there is no difference between the mean velocities across the elbow and in the forearm with the elbow flexed.[24,29] Kincaid[30] accepted 11.4 m per second as the maximum difference in conduction velocity between the across-elbow segment and the forearm with flexed elbow, a criterion that also appears sound based on another recent study.[35] With the subject's elbow extended, Eisen[22] found that seven of 48 normal subjects exceeded 10 m per second difference between the across-elbow and adjacent segments of the ulnar nerve. It is probably safe to conclude that because 15% of normal subjects in Eisen's study demonstrated a drop of greater than 10 m per second in the across-elbow segment compared with adjacent segments, this criterion would provide too many false-positive results. In a group of patients with mild ulnar neuropathy at the elbow, the incidence of slowing across the elbow in excess of 10 m per second

increased to only 20%, thus providing evidence of the limited utility of this criterion in the elbow-extended position. Studies comparing magnetic and electrical stimulation have failed to demonstrate any superiority of magnetic stimulation in localizing focal disturbances of nerve conduction.[36]

M Wave Analysis

Although focal slowing of conduction velocity is helpful in localizing a compressive ulnar nerve lesion, valuable information may be obtained by comparing the amplitude and configuration of the CMAP in response to stimulation at different points along the nerve. It is worth pointing out that if even a few large and fast axons are still conducting normally through a site of compression, there will be no slowing of maximum motor nerve conduction velocity. When a significant number of axons are slowed, the CMAP may become dispersed, indicating differential slowing at the site of compression. Conduction distal to the point of compression will, however, be normal. When compression is more severe, conduction block may occur in individual axons. In that situation, both the amplitude and the area of the response to stimulation proximal to the site of compression will be reduced as compared with responses elicited with distal stimulation. With temporal dispersion, increased duration occurs along with reduced amplitude of the proximally elicited CMAP, but the area under the curve of the proximal CMAP may be preserved. On the other hand, conduction block is associated with a reduced amplitude and area of the proximally elicited CMAP potential and is usually associated with clinical evidence of weakness.

These observations constitute the basis for analysis of the M wave in localizing the ulnar nerve lesion. Standard procedures for ulnar nerve stimulation and recording are used.[7] A median to ulnar nerve anastomosis in the forearm must be carefully evaluated in each instance. This is easily accomplished by stimulating the median nerve at the elbow and recording the response in the ulnar-innervated hand muscle. If the evoked CMAP is predominantly initially positive (downgoing) and the evoked responses from ulnar stimulation at the wrist and elbow are predominantly initially negative (upgoing), the presence of a Martin-Gruber anastomosis is excluded.

We have reported our normal data using recordings of the CMAP from 37 control nerves.[26,27] Amplitude was measured from baseline to negative peak, and duration was measured along the baseline as that of the initial negative M response. The area measured using a digital image analyzer (MPO-3, Carl Zeiss, Inc., West Germany) was that of the negative component of each M response. In addition, the M index was calculated from the amplitude and duration of each potential (M index = ½ amplitude × duration) as a convenient estimate of the area, using only the initial negative component as the M response.[37] Each of the four variables (amplitude, duration, M index, and M area) was statistically analyzed as the percent change in the proximal CMAP value in comparison with the distal one. A positive value indicates that the change was in the predicted direction. For amplitude, M index, and area, a positive value indicates a reduction in the variable with proximal stimulation, whereas for duration, a positive sign indicates proximal prolongation. The results are listed in Table 10.2.

Relative frequency histograms and descriptive statistics revealed a normal distribution for duration, amplitude, M index, and area from each stimulation site and for the percent change in duration, M index, and area. Using the arbitrary upper limit of normal as the mean plus 2.5 standard deviations for the 37 control nerves, the amplitude of the proximal CMAP was reduced up to 19% of the CMAP obtained by wrist stimulation. With elbow flexed, Kincaid et al.[29] found a maximum amplitude drop of 10% across the elbow. Comparing stimulation at elbow and wrist, the M index was reduced up to 20%, integrated area was reduced up to 16%, and the duration of the proximal CMAP was increased up to 15% (Table 10.2). We found in analyzing the upper limit of change from above elbow to below elbow in 32 ulnar nerves that the integrated area was reduced less than 7%, the amplitude was reduced less than 14%, and the duration was prolonged up to 8%.[27]

When changes in the M wave, comparing proximal and distal stimulation, are significant, using the inching technique with the nerve stimulator may permit more precise localization of the lesion.[7] By stimulating the nerve at the level of the medial epicondyle and in 2-cm increments both below and above that point, an abrupt change in the amplitude and configuration of the CMAP may be localized. Careful attention to stimulus intensity must be used such that the stimulation is only 10% above that necessary to elicit the maximum amplitude CMAP. Stimulus spread from excessive stimulus intensity will distort the results. The application of this technique is described in more detail under acute ulnar neuropathy at the elbow, later. Methods for evaluating short segments of motor nerve conduction intraoperatively

have been described using 1-cm segments from well above to well below the elbow.[8,38]

Changes in amplitude and duration seen in normal ulnar nerves are primarily as a result of dispersion on the basis of the wide range of conduction velocities of normal motor axons and increased desynchronization in the activation of motor units with stimulation at more proximal sites. The observation of longer duration and lower amplitude as well as reduced area of CMAPs obtained with proximal compared with distal stimulation is due to the desynchronization of the CMAP.[27]

Compound Sensory and Mixed Nerve Action Potentials

Sensory nerve conduction studies have considerable potential for localizing a nerve lesion. In one large series of patients with carpal tunnel syndrome, it was possible to localize the lesion from abnormal sensory conduction in 25% of patients in whom motor conduction and electromyography (EMG) were normal.[39] The same principle applies in ulnar neuropathy at the elbow. In 48 ulnar nerves with lesions at the elbow, abnormal sensory conduction was found in 34, whereas slowing of motor conduction velocity was present in only 25.[19] In another study, the duration of the compound sensory nerve action potential recorded above the elbow in response to stimulation of the fifth finger was prolonged in 84.6% of symptomatic limbs.[20] These reports constitute good evidence for the increased sensitivity of sensory nerve conduction studies in localizing the lesion; however, near-nerve needle electrode recording was used in both reports, a technique that is described in detail later. Two studies have demonstrated the utility of antidromic stimulation of ulnar sensory fibers recording with ring electrdes over the fifth finger.[30,40] Occasionally it is difficult to separate the antidromic compound sensory nerve action potential from the volume conducted CMAP. The lower limit of normal sensory conduction velocity in the elbow segment was 50 m per second and the lower limit of amplitude was 4 μV.[30] The difference between sensory conduction velocity in the forearm and in the elbow segment did not exceed 9% in normal subjects. The change in amplitude of the evoked compound sensory nerve action potential, comparing stimulation above the elbow with that below the elbow, did not exceed 43% in normal subjects.[30,39,41]

It goes without saying that routine sensory nerve studies between finger and wrist have no localizing value when considering the ulnar nerve lesion at the

TABLE 10.2. M response data

Group	Stimulation Site	Variable: Mean (Range)							
		Duration (ms)		Amplitude (mV)		M index (mVms)		Area (mVms)	
Compression neuropathy									
Conduction block* (N=7)	Wrist	6.2	(4.5–9)	8	(5.2–9.8)	25.4	(16.5–32.8)	22.3	(14.8–32.7)
	Above-elbow	6.2	(4.6–7.8)	4.3	(2–7)	12.8	(7.7–23.5)	14	(3.7–26.6)
	% change‡	0.8%	(−16.4–13.3)	46.8%	(23–72.6)*	47.1%	(25.2–76.4)*	36.8%	(18.2–75.2)*
Conduction block and temporal dispersion (N=4)⁺	Wrist	7.5	(7–9.8)	3.6	(0.7–7)	13	(3.4–24.5)	13.6	(2.7–27)
	Above-elbow	13.8	(8.8–17.7)	1.1	(0.3–2.8)	5.7	(2.7–12.3)	6.5	(1.8–16.2)
	% change‡	84.2%	(25.7–120)	68.7%	(57.1–89)	44.6%	(20.6–75.9)	44.2%	(26.1–77.5)
Temporal dispersion (N=3)⁺	Wrist	6.5	(4.8–7.3)	5.6	(3.8–8)	19	(9.1–29.2)	22	(10.2–32.6)
	Above-elbow	9.4	(7.1–11.6)	3.7	(2.3–5.2)	18	(8.2–24.9)	19.8	(9.4–29.4)
	% change‡	45.6%	(30.1–58.9)	34.4%	(29.4–39.5)	4.1%	(−12.4–14.7)	9.6%	(7.2–11.9)
Control Group N=37	Wrist	6.1	(4.2–8.6)	9.1	(4.1–15)	28.2	(9.6–51)	31.7	(17.3–57.1)
	Above-elbow	6.3	(4.4–9)	8.4	(3.8–14.2)	26.9	(10.3–49.5)	29.9	(16–53.8)
	% change‡	3.5%	(−6.7–14.9)	7%	(−3.3–17.7)	3.8	(−8.3–20.9)	5.6%	(−5.6–15.3)

* Different from control group; P <0.001 for all comparisons where significant difference exists.

⁺ Subgroup was not included in analysis of variance.

‡ Percent change for each M response variable was calculated comparing the M response obtained with stimulation above the elbow to that obtained with stimulation at the wrist, using the following formula: Percent change $= \dfrac{M_W - M_{AE}}{M_W} \times 100\%$

elbow. A slightly prolonged latency may be seen when the largest and fastest fibers are no longer conducting, and a reduced amplitude reflects the amount of axonal degeneration from the proximal lesion. Thus the conduction study between finger and wrist provides important data about the amount of axonal degeneration but gives virtually no information about localization of the lesion.

At least three different investigators have established the efficacy of sensory nerve conduction studies across the elbow using near-nerve recording.[10,20,23] In these studies, the recording electrodes were (1) a macroelectrode (bared tip, 3 mm) positioned 0.5 to 1 mm from the nerve and (2) a remote electrode (bared tip, 5 mm) placed at a transverse distance of 3 to 4 cm from the nerve. The noise from the tissue-metal junction of the electrode pair was 0.5 to 1 μV peak to peak (20 to 4000 c/s).[23] the potentials were amplified by a low-noise amplifier with a short blocking time. A high gain sensory amplifier (amplification capability of 0.4 μV per division) has been used in some laboratories. The responses were electronically averaged, and consecutively averaged traces following 32, 64, 128, and sometimes 256 sweeps were compared. In this way, it was possible to recognize which of the smallest peaks had grown and were therefore representative of a true nerve potential. Peaks that progressively declined in amplitude were interpreted as reflecting electronic noise. The temperature of the limb surface in these studies was kept within 36 to 38°C corresponding to 35 to 37°C near the nerve.[23]

A large needle electrode placed at a distance from the nerve was chosen so fibers from the total cross-section of the nerve would then contribute to the potential approximately equally. A microelectrode inserted into the nerve would reflect only the single fibers closest to it, and information about remaining fibers could not be obtained. On the other hand, the advantage of the gross needle electrode over percutaneous electrodes is twofold: First, the amplitude of the potential is two to three times larger, and second, the noise from the electrode-tissue surface is two to three times lower. Thus a signal to noise ratio five times higher than that achieved with percutaneous electrodes reduced the averaging time by a factor of 25 times. In this recording situation, the surface of the electrode is larger than the nerve diameter; therefore the amplitude does not change with small movements of the electrode. Nonetheless, the distance between nerve and electrode is critical in obtaining maximal amplitude responses. This is a clear-cut limitation of the method because the electrode cannot always be placed at a well-defined distance from the nerve. Administering stimuli through the needle and adjusting the electrode until the motor threshold is 0.5 to 1 mA is the best way to ensure optimal electrode placement. Using this method with repeated investigations of the same nerve in the same normal subject, the variation in observed amplitude was 20% to 30%, a variation that was attributed primarily to differing distances between electrode and nerve.[23] The variation in amplitude between subjects was two times greater because of individual anatomic differences as well as the possibility that some control subjects have subclinical nerve damage.

This method was used to study maximum sensory conduction velocity in the ulnar nerves of normal control subjects as a function of age (Figure 10.1). The amplitude and the maximum conduction velocity of the compound sensory nerve action potentials decreased with increasing age, and early recognition of nerve disorders required that findings in patients be compared with normal subjects of similar age.[23] The tendency toward reduced velocity and amplitude in normal controls over 50 years of age probably reflects both aging and subclinical ulnar neuropathy. The suggestion of subclinical ulnar neuropathy is reinforced by a comparison of the normal control data from the ulnar nerve with similar data from the median nerve, where changes in amplitude and conduction velocity with age are less marked.[23]

Electromyography

Needle EMG may be used to establish both the severity and the localization of the lesion. Even when conduction studies disclose unequivocal evidence of a localized neuropathy, the information obtained from needle EMG is valuable. The presence or absence of abnormal spontaneous activity provides some indication of the tempo of partial denervation and reinnervation. Similarly, the configuration of motor units and the numbers of motor units under voluntary control provide needed information about voluntary contraction. At the very least, the abductor pollicis brevis is usually sampled to exclude the possibility of a radiculopathy or brachial plexus lesion. In addition, ADM, FDI, FDP, and FCU are sampled in every patient.

Nerve Conduction Studies Across the Wrist and Palm

Ulnar neuropathy at the wrist or in the palm is relatively uncommon. Usually the interosseous muscles are more severely involved than the hypothenar

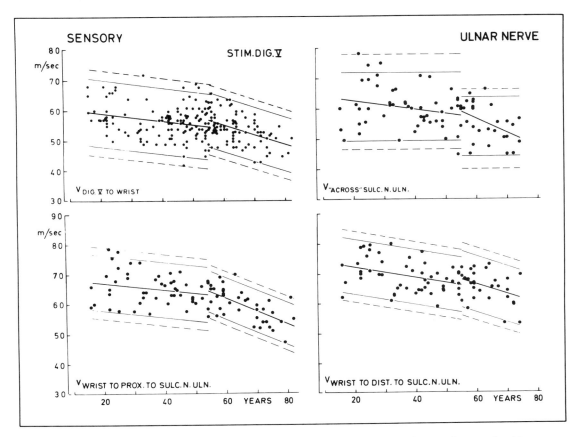

FIGURE 10.1. *Maximum sensory conduction velocity in the ulnar nerves of normal control subjects as a function of age. Above left: from the fifth finger to the wrist (202 nerves). Above right: "across" sulcus nervi ulnaris—that is, from 5 cm distal to sulcus nervi ulnaris to 5 cm proximal to sulcus nervi ulnaris (80 nerves). Below left: from wrist to 5 cm proximal to sulcus nervi ulnaris (88 nerves). Below right: from wrist to 5 cm distal to sulcus nervi ulnaris (80 nerves). Stimulus to fifth finger. The thick lines are the regression lines calculated by the method of least squares; thin lines represent 95%, and broken lines 99%, upper and lower confidence limits. The confidence limits for the velocities "across" the sulcus nervi ulnaris were determined from the cumulated distribution of velocities. (Reprinted with permission from Rosenfalck A. Early recognition of nerve disorders by near-nerve recording of sensory action potentials. Muscle Nerve 1978; 1:360–367. Copyright © 1978 John Wiley & Sons, Inc.)*

muscles. It is therefore necessary to study a muscle innervated by the deep branch of the ulnar nerve as well as the hypothenar muscles.

In a study of 373 ulnar nerves, the active recording electrode was placed over the maximum convex bulge of the FDI muscle approximately at the midpoint between the first and second metacarpophalangeal joints with the reference electrode over the second metacarpophalangeal joint.[42] In this location, the amplitude of the CMAP is maximized, but there is usually a small initial positive deflection. The ac-

tive recording electrode over ADM was placed at the motor point as located at the site where submaximal percutaneous stimulation over the muscle produced the maximum visible twitch, and the reference was placed over the fifth metacarpophalangeal joint. Distal motor latency was measured to the first deflection from baseline, which was always negative for the ADM and usually a small brief positive deflection for the FDI. Amplitude measurements were made from baseline to negative peak. The mean and range for distal motor latency to ADM and FDI are shown in Table 10.3. With advancing age, there was an increase in the distal motor latency for each muscle: approximately 0.05 ms per decade. The side to side difference in latency to each muscle and the ipsilateral difference in distal latencies between the two muscles did not significantly change with advancing age. Greater variability was found with amplitude measurements, as shown in Table 10.4. There was a tendency toward decreased amplitude with increasing age of approximately ½ mV per decade. The amplitude of the CMAP over ADM was never less than 5 mV, nor was it ever less than 6 mV for FDI. The amplitude of FDI was greater than ADM by an average of 3 mV, but occasionally the difference was more than 11 mV. In 20% of the nerves studied, the amplitude of ADM was larger than FDI but never by more than 5 mV. Frequently a bifid contour was observed in the negative component of the CMAP recorded over ADM, whereas the negative component of the CMAP over FDI always had a smooth contour. In summary, amplitudes less than 6 mV for FDI and 5 mV for ADM may be considered abnormal.

A comparison of distal latencies is most helpful in this situation. Maximum observed distal motor latencies of 3.4 ms and 4.5 ms for ADM and FDI were not exceeded in a large control series.[42] The maximum difference between the latency to FDI and the latency to ADM was 2 ms (mean 0.9 ± 0.3 ms SD). This is slightly less than the value of 2.4 ms reported in an earlier, smaller series.[40] The difference

TABLE 10.3. Mean and range for distal motor latency by decade

		Latency (ms)	
Age (years)	No.	Abductor Digiti Minimi*	First Dorsal Interosseous*
<20	14	2.5 (2.2–2.9)	3.3 (2.7–4.2)
20–29	48	2.5 (2–3)	3.4 (2.6–4.1)
30–39	103	2.4 (1.8–3.2)	3.3 (2.5–4.4)
40–49	82	2.5 (2–3)	3.2 (2.3–4.2)
50–59	84	2.6 (2–3.4)	3.4 (2.6–4.4)
60–69	34	2.7 (2.2–3.1)	3.6 (3–4.5)
>70	8	2.7 (2.3–3.1)	3.6 (3–4.2)
Side to side difference			
ADM*	0.2 ms (0–1)		
FDI*	0.2 ms (0–1.3)		
Ipsilateral difference			
FDI – ADM*	0.9 ms (0.2–2)		

*Mean (range).

TABLE 10.4. Mean and range for amplitude by decade

		Amplitude (mV)	
Age (years)	No.	Abductor Digiti Minimi*	First Dorsal Interosseous*
<20	14	13 (11–16)	15 (8–23)
20–29	48	12 (5–20)	14 (8–22)
30–39	103	12 (6–21)	15 (6–24)
40–49	82	12 (6–19)	13 (6–22)
50–59	84	11 (7–17)	13 (6–20)
60–69	34	12 (6–15)	12 (7–20)
>70	8	10 (8–13)	12 (8–15)

* Mean (range).

between distal motor latencies when comparing the same nerve in opposite hands did not exceed 1 ms for ADM or 1.3 ms for FDI.[42]

Sensory nerve conduction studies are often completely normal in subjects with wrist or palm lesions. We ordinarily use orthodromic sensory conduction with ring electrodes around the fifth digit, with the cathode around the proximal interphalangeal joint and the anode around the distal joint. Surface recording electrodes are positioned at the wrist, with the cathode at the proximal wrist crease and the anode placed 2 cm proximal to that. In our laboratory, the upper limit of normal distal sensory latency is 3.4 ms, and the lower limit of amplitude is 8 μV. This response is generally decreased in amplitude with lesions of the ulnar nerve proximal to the wrist as well as in lesions involving the medial cord of the brachial plexus. The effect of varying interelectrode distance, age, temperature, and longitudinal versus transverse electrode placement on amplitude, duration, and latency of compound sensory nerve action potentials is considerable,[43] so these variables must be controlled and carefully considered.

When the ulnar nerve is compressed at the wrist and there is sensory loss, evaluation of the dorsal sensory branch of the ulnar nerve may be most helpful. Because this nerve leaves the main trunk of the ulnar nerve 5 to 8 cm proximal to the ulnar styloid, it is never involved in wrist or palm lesions. On the other hand, with an elbow lesion, both sensory studies should be equally abnormal.

To evaluate the dorsal sensory branch, the active recording electrode is placed over the junction between the fourth and the fifth metacarpals with the reference electrode at the base of the fifth digit. Stimulation of the dorsal sensory branch is accomplished at a distance of 8 cm from the active electrode with the stimulator placed in the space between the ulna and the FCU tendon or placed in such a way that it straddles the ulna bone.[44] The patient is supine with the arm alongside the body and the hand pronated. This study is especially useful in patients with severe ulnar lesions at the wrist and very little interfering CMAP responses. In such cases, proximal stimulation of the ulnar nerve above the elbow can also be performed, whereas in normal individuals the CMAP provides substantial interference. Normal values from one study of 50 normal limbs included a mean distal sensory latency of 2 ± 0.3 ms (mean $\pm$ SD), with a conduction velocity between elbow and forearm that was greater than 52 meters per second (2 SD below the mean).[44] The lower limit of normal amplitude was 8 μV with distal stimulation. Thus the presence of a normal dorsal sensory branch potential and an abnormal potential recorded from the palmar branch is strong evidence of a lesion at the wrist.

FINDINGS IN ULNAR NEUROPATHIES

Acute Ulnar Neuropathy at the Elbow

Examples of acute compressive neuropathy in humans include the classic Saturday night palsy, which affects the radial nerve, is commonly associated with an episode of alcohol intoxication, and is generally associated with a rapid recovery in 3 to 6 weeks.[45] Another example of a human compressive neuropathy is the pneumatic tourniquet lesion occurring intraoperatively during an attempt to obtain a bloodless field distal to the cuff. Patients with reported cases of this kind of compressive neuropathy recover more slowly (50% recovery at 4 months).[46,47] Obviously when there is axonal degeneration as well as conduction block, recovery is substantially slower and incomplete. An estimate of the amount of axonal degeneration can be obtained by comparing the amplitude of the CMAP in response to distal stimulation of the nerve below the lesion with that obtained on the opposite side. The test must be performed at least 7 to 10 days following the compression to allow fibers that are undergoing axonal degeneration to become electrically inexcitable.[48]

Postoperative ulnar neuropathy, resulting from compression of the ulnar nerve at the elbow during operations involving general anesthesia, is another example of an acute compressive neuropathy in humans. We saw eight patients with this neuropathy during a three-year period. In every patient, the initial symptom was numbness in the ulnar distribution of the affected hand, which was noted immediately on wakening from general anesthesia in five patients and within 24 to 48 hours after surgery in three patients who had severe postoperative pain.[28] Only three of these patients experienced pain in the arm, and this was usually located in the forearm. By contrast, in our experience with chronic compression at the cubital tunnel, seven of nine patients complained of pain.[7] Tinel's sign was present, with tenderness over the cubital tunnel in only one patient with postoperative ulnar neuropathy. Atrophy and moderate to severe weakness of ulnar-innervated hand muscles and weakness of the FDP of the fourth and fifth digits were present in every patient. FCU was normally strong in every case. All patients had hypesthesia and hypalgesia in the distribution of the ulnar nerve. The presence of ulnar distribution sensory loss with weakness of ulnar-innervated hand muscles and FDP of the fourth and fifth fingers documents the presence of an ulnar neuropathy at the elbow. The presence of diminished sensation is strong evidence against motor neuron disease, and the absence of weakness in median-innervated hand muscles provides evidence against a cervical radiculopathy or a medial cord lesion in the brachial plexus. The latter must be thoroughly evaluated in patients who have had cardiac surgery.[49]

Motor nerve conduction velocities were determined for three segments of the ulnar nerve: from axilla to above elbow, across elbow, and from below elbow to wrist.[28] The subject was supine with the arm at 5 degrees to the trunk, the elbow extended, and forearm supinated. Standard distances across the elbow (10 cm) and from axilla to above elbow (12 cm) were used. The CMAP was recorded with surface electrodes over the ADM muscle. In patients in whom a dispersed low-amplitude response was obtained by stimulating above the elbow, the inching technique in which the stimulator was moved along the nerve in several steps was used to detect the site at which abrupt change occurred in the amplitude of the CMAP. Abnormal nerve conduction was localized to the cubital tunnel between 1.5 and 4 cm distal to the median epicondyle. The same procedure was repeated intraoperatively in one patient, during surgical exploration, and the findings confirmed the results in the clinical laboratory. In most cases, the motor nerve conduction velocity was normal in the above-elbow segment and in the forearm. Motor nerve conduction velocity in the 10 cm across the elbow, which included the cubital tunnel, was reduced below 42 m per second in all but one patient and below 34 m per second in three patients. Distal motor latency was prolonged in only one patient, probably reflecting loss of the fastest fibers.

The amplitude of the CMAP following both proximal and distal stimulation was normal in only two cases. In three cases, the CMAP amplitude was smaller and desynchronized when stimulating above the elbow than when stimulating below the elbow. Precise localization of the conduction block was possible in only one patient and depended on an abrupt amplitude change at the cubital tunnel using the inching technique, such that the CMAP amplitude was smaller when stimulating just proximal to the cubital tunnel compared with the larger response to distal stimulation (Figure 10.2). In every patient, stimulation of the median nerve at the elbow and at the wrist was also performed to exclude the possibility of anomalous innervation. A median to ulnar communication was not found in any patient in this series.

Needle EMG gave similar results in the FDI and ADM muscles in any given patient. Signs of partial denervation were seen in every case, and fibrillation potentials and positive sharp waves were evident in six. In all patients, there was a moderate to substantial reduction in the number of motor unit potentials under voluntary control at maximum effort. In the FCU, there was no abnormality in three patients, and a few potentials with increased duration and polyphasia were observed at maximum effort in two patients. In the median-innervated abductor pollicis brevis, there was no abnormality in five patients, and in three patients with mild polyneuropathy, there was a slight reduction in the number of motor unit potentials under voluntary control at maximum effort.

The compound sensory nerve action potential, recording at the wrist and stimulating the fifth finger, could not be obtained in six of eight ulnar nerves; in two cases in which it was present, it was normal in latency but dispersed in form and reduced in amplitude. Intraoperative findings in three patients in this series who subsequently underwent exploration included substantial narrowing of the ulnar nerve under the FCU aponeurosis with proximal swelling and hyperemia of the nerve.

Evidence for localization of the compressive lesion in postoperative ulnar neuropathy comes from clinical, electrophysiologic, and intraoperative observations (Table 10.5). The clinical finding of normal median nerve function, normal strength in FCU, and weakness of FDP suggest that the lesion occurs

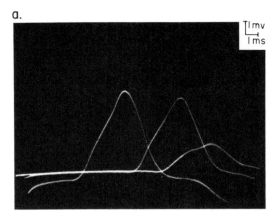

a.

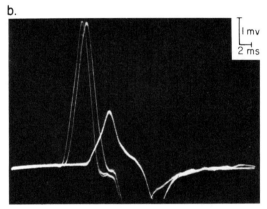

b.

FIGURE 10.2. *These responses were obtained from a 56-year-old woman with a moderately severe ulnar neuropathy at the elbow. The CMAP recorded over ADM, following stimulation at the wrist, below elbow and above elbow, was dispersed and smaller with above-elbow stimulation (top). Precise localization of abnormal conduction was found between the medial epicondyle (ME) and a point 4 cm distal to the ME, since the response to stimulation 2 cm distal to the ME was much smaller and delayed compared to those elicited from stimulation at 4 cm and 6 cm distal to the ME (bottom).*

distal to the point where the branch for FCU exits the main nerve trunk, and proximal to the branch for FDP. Thus the clinical information localizes the problem at the elbow. Even in severe ulnar neuropathy at the elbow, FCU is usually clinically normal. In mild ulnar neuropathy, where FDP may be normally strong, localization is more difficult because

TABLE 10.5. Electrophysiologic criteria for localizing a nerve lesion

Motor nerve conduction
    Reduced amplitude (or area) of the CMAP with proximal stimulation
        Ensure supramaximal stimulation
        Search for anomalous innervation
    Desynchronization of CMAP with proximal stimulation
    Focal slowing of maximum motor nerve conduction
CNAP
    Focal slowing of nerve conduction (prolonged latency)
    Focal amplitude reduction or desynchronization of CNAP
Electromyography—location of most proximal abnormal finding (e.g., forearm muscles in ulnar
    neuropathy at the elbow)

CMAP, compound muscle action potential; CNAP, compound nerve action potential.

the lesion might be anywhere between the wrist and the elbow.

In this series of postoperative ulnar neuropathy, slowing of motor nerve conduction velocity at the ulnar nerve across the elbow was present in four patients, and a significant reduction in amplitude of the CMAP comparing proximal and distal stimulation was found in three patients. Thus on the basis of the motor nerve conduction velocities and the CMAP amplitude reduction, abnormal conduction could be localized to the elbow in five of eight patients. The abnormal compound sensory nerve action potential in every patient provided no evidence for localization. The distal sensory latency was normal when it could be recorded, whereas the sensory action potential was diminished in amplitude or there was no detectable response. Thus a diminished number of axons were present, and the lesion responsible for this finding could have occurred anywhere from the dorsal root ganglion to the wrist.

The EMG findings indicated partial denervation in the intrinsic hand muscle supplied by the ulnar nerve. When abnormalities were detected in FCU, localization could be accomplished on the basis of electromyography. The presence of mild abnormalities in FCU with much more marked abnormalities in the hand suggests a lesion at the elbow (Table 10.5). Muscle sampling in FDP is more often abnormal than in FCU, but this was not performed in these patients.

One report described slowing of motor nerve conduction across the elbow in the contralateral (asymptomatic) arm in 12 of 14 patients with postoperative ulnar neuropathy at 6 month follow-up.[21] The authors suggested that some patients have subclinical entrapment that may predispose to the development of compressive neuropathy during anesthesia. Fur-

ther study is needed to determine the precise factors that produce postoperative ulnar neuropathy.

Chronic Ulnar Neuropathies at the Elbow

We reported nine patients with entrapment of the ulnar nerve in the cubital tunnel, six of whom had the syndrome bilaterally[7] (Table 10.6). There was no history of trauma and no evidence of joint deformity at the elbow in any patient; thus precise localization of the lesion was difficult on the basis of clinical

TABLE 10.6. Cubital tunnel syndrome

No history of trauma or arthritis
No joint deformity
Clinical signs of ulnar neuropathy
    Usually involves FDI, ADM, FDP 3, 4 equally
    Usually spares flexor carpi ulnaris
    Usually splits ring finger (sensory loss)
Often bilateral
Palpation of ulnar nerve
    Swollen usually
    Taut, immobile in elbow flexion
Electrophysiologic findings
    Partial denervation FDI, ADM, FDP (EMG)
    Slowed NCV across elbow
    Reduced CMAP with proximal stimulation
    Abnormal compound sensory nerve action potential
    Look for underlying polyneuropathy
Operative findings
    Swollen engorged nerve
    Tight tunnel in flexion
Decompression may be better than transposition

FDI, First dorsal interosseous; ADM, abductor digiti minimi; FDP, flexor digitorum profundus; EMG, electromyography; NCV, nerve conduction velocity; CMAP, compound muscle action potential.

information alone. In this series of nine patients, seven complained of pain. Localization of pain, however, was often misleading. Pain was primarily localized at the elbow in only two patients, in the forearm in four, the hand in four, and shoulder in three.

Paresthesias were noted in all patients and were primarily experienced as numbness of the fourth and fifth fingers on both the palmar and the dorsal surfaces. Thus the location of the sensory symptoms in the presence of objective sensory loss was helpful in delineating an ulnar nerve lesion but not in determining precise localization. Clearly the elbow is the most common site of nerve entrapment producing ulnar sensory loss; however, a lesion at the wrist may also produce palmar sensory symptoms. Palpation of the nerve in the ulnar groove revealed entrapment of seven nerves with substantially diminished mobility in the groove in 12 of the 15 ulnar nerves. In each case, the nerve was especially taut at 90 degrees flexion of the elbow. There was atrophy and moderate to severe weakness of the ulnar-innervated hand muscles in every case. The FDP muscle of the fourth and fifth digits was weak in 13 of the 15 arms, whereas FCU was weak in only two. All patients had hypesthesia and hypalgesia in the distribution of the ulnar nerve. Thus on the basis of clinical information, the most helpful localizing sign was the presence of weakness in the FDP with sparing of FCU (Table 10.5). The pattern of sensory loss confirmed that the lesion involved the ulnar nerve. Abnormalities on palpation of the ulnar nerve at the elbow were confirmatory, although there is a considerable margin of uncertainty in this determination.

Electrophysiologic studies were performed according to methods previously described.[7] CMAP was recorded with surface electrodes over the ADM muscle. A local demyelinative lesion was diagnosed when the following three criteria were present: (1) an abrupt amplitude change at the cubital tunnel, such that with stimulation just proximal to the tunnel, the CMAP amplitude was reduced by more than 40% compared with stimulation distal to the tunnel; (2) slowing of motor nerve conduction velocity to less than 35 m per second in the across-elbow segment, which included the cubital tunnel; and (3) a change in form of the CMAP toward a desynchronized response with stimulation above the elbow compared with the wrist. These criteria have subsequently been revised as already described and now include (1) an amplitude change exceeding 10% in the across-elbow segment and (2) motor conduction

velocity below 50 m per second with elbow flexed to 135 degrees (0 degrees = extended). Nonetheless, the findings in these patients with classic cubital tunnel syndrome are instructive.

Motor nerve conduction velocity was normal in the above-elbow segments and normal or slightly diminished in the forearm, with a normal or slightly prolonged distal motor latency to the ADM. Motor nerve conduction velocity in a 10-cm segment across the elbow, which included the cubital tunnel, was reduced below 35 m per second in 13 of the 15 ulnar nerves (Table 10.7). Neither of the two patients with an across-elbow velocity exceeding 35 m per second worsened within a year, and the patients were not operated on. In both cases, however, the across-elbow velocity was substantially less than the forearm velocity, a difference of 16 m per second in one case and 26 m per second in the other.

When the amplitude of the CMAP with stimulation above the elbow was less than that produced by stimulation below the elbow or at the wrist, the percentage amplitude reduction was determined (Table 10.7). Precise localization of the conduction

TABLE 10.7. Abnormal ulnar motor nerve conduction across the cubital tunnel

Amplitude of Compound Muscle Action Potential (above CT/below CT)*	Amplitude Reduction (%)	Motor Nerve Conduction Velocity (m/s)
Definite		
6/1	83	30
2.5/0.5	80	23
4.5/1	78	23
12/5	58	19
4/2	50	19
4/2	50	29
3.4/1.8	47	32
0.7/0.4	43	19
1.4/0.8	43	32
4.2/2.9	31	26
4.5/3	33	31
5/3	40	47
0.8/0.8	0	26
12/10	17	22
Indefinite		
6/5	17	40

* Definite—abrupt amplitude change at the CT or slowing of motor nerve conduction across the elbow; indefinite—insufficient amplitude change or slowing for localization. CT, Cubital tunnel.

block depended on an abrupt amplitude change at the cubital tunnel using the inching technique, such that the CMAP amplitude was reduced when stimulation was compared just proximal and just distal to the cubital tunnel (see Table 10.5). Precise localization at the cubital tunnel was possible in 12 nerves, with an amplitude reduction exceeding 40% in nine nerves and 30% in three (see Table 10.7). In one case in which there was long-standing partial denervation, an identical low amplitude response was elicited by stimulation at all sites. In addition to the diminished amplitude obtained from proximal stimulation, marked desynchronization of the response was often seen. The marked dispersion of the action potential indicates the variable amount of slowing in different axons, whereas the diminished area of the action potential is evidence that some fibers are completely blocked.

In every patient, stimulation of the median nerve at the elbow and at the wrist was also performed to exclude the possibility of anomalous innervation. A Martin-Gruber anastomosis was found in only one case, and in this patient, the amplitude reduction was still greater than 50%, even after the contribution of the median nerve was subtracted.

Muscle sampling with a needle electrode gave similar results in the FDI and ADM muscles in any given patient. Fibrillation potentials and positive sharp waves were seen in seven hands. In all cases, there were motor unit potentials of increased duration and polyphasia, with a reduction in the number of motor unit potentials under voluntary control at maximum effort. The latter finding was also observed in the FCU in two cases.

The compound sensory nerve action potential recorded at the wrist with surface electrodes when stimulating the fifth finger was normal in only one of the ulnar nerves. It was not obtainable with 32 superimposed sweeps in nine cases and was diminished in amplitude and desynchronized in five patients.

Another series of 14 patients with compressive ulnar neuropathy at the elbow is summarized in Table 10.2.[26] In three patients with amplitude reductions of 29% to 40% and duration prolongation of 30% to 59%, the integrated area was reduced by less than 16%, which is within normal limits. Thus in these patients, there was evidence for marked temporal dispersion without significant conduction block; these three subjects are classified in Table 10.2 under temporal dispersion. The remaining 11 patients with compressive ulnar neuropathy had evi-

dence for conduction block based on a greater than 16% reduction in the integrated area of the proximal CMAP in comparison with the distal CMAP. There was conduction block as well as temporal dispersion in four of the 11; these four are classified under conduction block and temporal dispersion. The CMAP duration from proximal stimulation was prolonged by 26% to 120% above the normal limit. The remaining seven patients with compression neuropathy showed no evidence of temporal dispersion. These seven patients are classified under conduction block in Table 10.2.

Thus a comparison of the proximal and distal CMAP may be extremely useful in localizing a compressive lesion of the ulnar nerve. A change in the amplitude of the evoked potential, when it clearly exceeds normal limits, may be associated with conduction block or temporal dispersion. When there is prolonged duration in the proximal CMAP, there is some temporal dispersion. More precise quantification of the presence of conduction block, a potentially reversible cause of weakness, is possible using area measurements of the M wave. In temporal dispersion, weakness is not necessarily present, as seen in patients recovering from the Guillain-Barré syndrome, when full recovery of strength may be seen despite persistence of slow motor nerve conduction velocity with dispersed M waves.[50]

Using near-nerve recordings in a study of 13 patients with mild cubital tunnel syndrome, dispersion in the compound sensory nerve action potential recorded above the elbow was found in 84% of symptomatic limbs and in 50% of contralateral, asymptomatic limbs.[20] Thus study of the above-elbow compound sensory nerve action potential substantially improved the diagnostic yield. The dispersion or extent of desynchronization of the above-elbow compound sensory nerve action potential was the most useful characteristic in this study. Increased dispersion, a reflection of segmental demyelination, could be localized to the elbow using this technique in the majority of patients.[20] The findings from a patient with mild cubital tunnel syndrome, in whom other physiologic studies were completely normal, are shown in Figure 10.3. The extraordinary sensitivity of this technique makes it worth considering in spite of the technical difficulties.

Ulnar Neuropathies at the Wrist or Palm

We studied 16 patients with ulnar neuropathy at or distal to the wrist.[51] The mean age was 46, with a

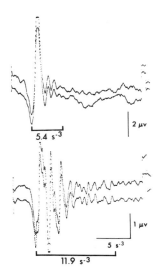

FIGURE 10.3. *Sensory action potentials recorded above the cubital sulcus in a normal subject (top pair) and a patient (bottom pair). The labeled bars mark the total dispersion of the responses, which are an average of 128 sweeps. The procedure was carried out twice in each patient. Normal dispersion was <6.9 s⁻³. The patient had a mild sensory deficit; other physiologic studies were normal. (Reprinted with permission from Odusote K, Eisen A: An electrophysiological quantitation of the cubital tunnel syndrome. Can J Neurol Sci 1979; 6:403–410.)*

range from 8 to 74. The chief complaint was painless weakness in half of the patients. In patients with pain, fractures or coexistent carpal tunnel syndrome were responsible for pain in six of nine. Examination of the wrist near the canal of Guyon provided supportive evidence for a lesion in this region in 40% of the patients. A palpable mass or a positive Tinel's sign at the canal of Guyon was found in one-third of the patients. All patients had weakness of the FDI, whereas weakness of ADM was either less severe or absent in the majority of patients. Fewer than 25% had numbness of the fifth finger. All five reported patterns of involvement were represented as follows: (1) weakness only, limited to interossei (four cases); (2) weakness only, including interosseous and hypothenar muscles (eight cases); (3) interosseous and hypothenar weakness associated with sensory involvement and with normal dorsal cutaneous function (two cases); (4) pure sensory loss with normal dorsal cutaneous and motor responses (one case); and (5) interosseous weakness associated with sensory involvement but hypothenar and dorsal cutaneous functions normal (one case). Causes included ganglionic cysts (four), tumors (four), blunt injuries (four), injuries with fracture (two), aberrant artery (one), and idiopathic (one).

The nerve conduction study of the FDI was the most helpful single test in most patients. The greater severity of interosseous involvement is clearly illustrated by diminished evoked potential amplitude over FDI. In 13 of 16 patients with weakness in FDI, the amplitude over this muscle was reduced below 1.5 mV. In contrast, an evoked CMAP below 1.5 mV over ADM was seen in only one of 12 patients with weakness in the hypothenar muscles. Prolonged distal motor latencies were most commonly seen to FDI, and fibrillation potential and positive sharp wave activity was most commonly found on EMG in that muscle. Normal findings were obtained on EMG and nerve conduction studies of ADM in one-third of patients in this study. Myokymia associated with tremor was described in the third and fourth dorsal interosseous muscles in a patient with distal ulnar neuropathy,[52] a finding that is rare in our experience and not specific for distal ulnar nerve lesions. The digital compound sensory nerve action potential (palmar branch) was abnormal in only four of 18 patients, and the dorsal cutaneous action potential was normal in all patients. The latter is particularly helpful in evaluating distal ulnar neuropathies because it is unaffected by a distal lesion but usually abnormal with an elbow lesion.[11]

Recognition of distal ulnar neuropathies is important for proper management. Only two of 18 patients improved without surgical exploration. Both of these had obvious history of recurrent blunt trauma to the hand that could be easily avoided. Imaging studies may be useful in identifying structural causes of distal ulnar neuropathy, especially with a tumor or ganglion cyst.[53] In 14 of 16 patients in this series, surgical exploration was performed and usually was followed by improvement. In one patient, surgical exploration was negative.

In 1960, Ebeling et al.[9] proposed that distal ulnar neuropathies at the wrist could be divided into three types. Seven of their nine patients had weakness in the interossei with normal hypothenar strength and normal sensation. The other two patients had severe interosseous weakness with mild hypothenar weakness and no sensory loss. A third group with both sensory and motor involvement was described based on other reported cases. Shea and McClain[10] described patients with pure distal ulnar sensory loss without weakness, a group that constituted 18% of reported cases. Dorsal cutaneous action potentials were not performed to confirm the distal localization of the ulnar neuropathy. The development of a deep branch lesion of the ulnar nerve with prolonged bicycle or motorcycle riding has become well recognized also.[54] The deep branch is compressed in the palm and frequently follows unaccustomed, prolonged bicycling. This lesion usually has an excellent prognosis for spontaneous recovery and is preventable with patient education, padding of the hand grip, and improved position.

Thus in the majority of reported cases, careful study of the FDI was most likely to reveal abnormalities. Most patients have no or minimal abnormalities in ADM and normal sensory function clinically and electrophysiologically. When there is clinical evidence of abnormal sensation in the fifth digit, the presence of a normal dorsal cutaneous action potential and an abnormal palmar sensory study is strong evidence for a wrist lesion.

AN OVERVIEW OF ELECTROPHYSIOLOGIC TESTING IN ULNAR NEUROPATHIES

In mild ulnar neuropathy, the electrodiagnostic study may well be completely normal. Eisen[22] found that 42% of patients with mild ulnar neuropathy at the elbow had a proximal motor latency in excess of 8.8 ms. He proposed that this might be a useful criterion. Unfortunately, this measurement includes a very long segment of normal nerve distal to the compressive lesion, as mentioned previously, thus limiting the sensitivity of this indicator as well. In the study of Payan,[19] 85% of patients with ulnar neuropathy at the elbow had slowing in the across-elbow segment. This figure was obtained when studies were performed to both the FDI and the ADM; the figure was 75% when only one hand muscle was studied. A higher yield of conduction abnormalities was found in a study that compared abnormalities to the FDI and the ADM; the difference was attributed to differential susceptibility to compression in different nerve fascicles.[55] Another obvious advantage to studying both muscles is to look for excessive slowing in the deep branch of the ulnar nerve to the FDI. As mentioned previously, the distal motor latency to the ADM is sometimes abnormal in patients with ulnar neuropathy at the elbow but provides no lo-

calizing value and probably simply reflects loss of the fastest and largest fibers. Increased diagnostic yield may be obtained by wave form analysis, comparing the proximal and distal CMAP, in terms of amplitude, duration, and area.[26]

Careful attention to electromyographic findings may add substantial information about localization as well as severity of the neuropathy. In one study of 34 ulnar nerves from patients with clear-cut clinical evidence of ulnar nerve compression at the elbow, there was evidence of active denervation (fibrillation potentials or positive sharp waves outside the end plate zone) in the FDI (50%), ADM (36.8%), and FCU (5.9%).[19] Reduced recruitment of motor unit potentials with increased numbers of large polyphasic potentials were noted in the ADM of every patient and in the FDI of all patients but one. These abnormalities were noted in the FCU in 26.5% of patients.[19] When abnormalities are found in the FCU, the lesion clearly must be as high as the elbow. Unfortunately, many patients with ulnar neuropathy at the elbow exhibit no abnormality in the FCU because the branch for that muscle is less susceptible to compression as it travels alongside the larger main nerve trunk passing through the ulnar groove and cubital tunnel.[7] The FDP of the fourth and fifth fingers is often clinically weak in patients with ulnar neuropathy at the elbow, and although it is sometimes difficult to sample these muscles reliably, when they are abnormal it is very helpful in localizing the neuropathy.

Finally, important prognostic information may be obtained from analysis of the CMAP. Focal disturbances in conduction that produce conduction block, slowed conduction velocity, or temporal dispersion are usually associated with normal responses to distal stimulation. When there is axonal degeneration, a diminished amplitude and area of the CMAP is observed in response to distal stimulation. Thus the amplitude of the CMAP in response to distal stimulation is proportional to the number and size of muscle fibers that remain viable within the muscle. An approximation of the degree of axonal degeneration can be obtained by comparing the amplitude of the distal CMAP with the contralateral side in an individual subject. In a large number of patients with facial nerve lesions, the amplitude of the CMAP in response to stimulation distal to the nerve lesion was the best indicator of prognosis.[56] When the amplitude of the CMAP was less than 10% of the contralateral (unaffected) side, there was a high risk of unsatisfactory outcome. This measurement was more reliable than an attempt to quantify the numbers of fibrillation potentials or positive waves, threshold for nerve excitability, or distal motor latency.

Thus analysis of the evoked CMAP in response to both proximal and distal stimulation yields substantial information about focal disturbances in conduction and the extent of axonal degeneration. Taken together, the electrophysiologic results provide considerable data that constitute a basis for prognosis as well as precise diagnosis.

REFERENCES

1. Campbell WW, Pridgeon RM, Riaz G, et al. Variations in anatomy of the ulnar nerve at the cubital tunnel: Pitfalls in the diagnosis of ulnar neuropathy at the elbow. Proc Congr Neurol Surg 1986; 36:152–154.
2. Campbell WW, Pridgeon RM, Riaz G, et al. Sparing of the flexor carpi ulnaris in ulnar neuropathy at the elbow. Muscle Nerve 1989; 12:965–967.
3. Campbell WW, Pridgeon RM, Sahni SK. Entrapment neuropathy of the ulnar nerve at its point of exit from the flexor carpi ulnaris muscle. Muscle Nerve 1988; 11:467–470.
4. Panas P. Sur une cause peu connue de paralysie du nerf cubital. Arch Gen Med 1878; 2:5–7.
5. Feindel W, Stratford J. Cubital tunnel compression in tardy ulnar palsy (short communication). Can Med Assoc J 1958; 78:351–353.
6. Feindel W, Stratford J. The role of the cubital tunnel in tardy ulnar palsy. Can J Surg 1958; 1:287–300.
7. Miller RG. The cubital tunnel syndrome. Diagnosis and precise localization. Ann Neurol 1979; 6:56–59.
8. Brown WF, Ferguson GG, Jones MW, et al. The location of conduction abnormalities in human entrapment neuropathies. Can J Neurol Sci 1979; 3:111–122.
9. Ebeling P, Gilliatt RW, Thomas PK. A clinical and electrical study of ulnar nerve lesions in the hand. J Neurol Neurosurg Psychiatry 1960; 23:1–9.
10. Shea JD, McClain EJ. Ulnar nerve compression syndromes at and below the wrist. J Bone Joint Surg (Br) 1969; 51A:1095–1103.
11. Olney RK, Hanson M. AAEE Case Report #15. Ulnar neuropathy at or distal to the wrist. Muscle Nerve 1988; 11:828–832.
12. Spinner M. Injuries to the major branches of peripheral nerves of the forearm. Philadelphia: WB Saunders, 1978:230–266.
13. Dawson DM, Krarup C. Perioperative nerve lesions. Arch Neurol 1989; 46:1355–1360.
14. Miller RG. Acute vs. chronic compressive neuropathy. Muscle Nerve 1984; 7:427–430.
15. Neary D, Eames RA. The pathology of ulnar nerve compression in man. Neuropathol Appl Neurobiol 1975; 1:69–88.
16. Neary D, Ochoa J, Gilliatt RW. Subclinical entrapment neuropathy in man. J Neurol Sci 1975; 24:283–298.
17. Gilliatt RW. Chronic nerve compression and entrapment. In: Sumner AJ, ed. The physiology of peripheral nerve disease. Philadelphia: WB Saunders, 1980:316–339.
18. Ochoa J, Fowler TJ, Gilliatt RW. Anatomical changes in peripheral nerves compressed by pneumatic tourniquet. J Anat 1972; 113:433–455.
19. Payan J. Electrophysiological localization of ulnar nerve lesions. J Neurol Neurosurg Psychiatry 1969; 32:208–220.
20. Odusote K, Eisen A. An electrophysiological quantitation of the cubital tunnel syndrome. J Can Sci Neurol 1979; 6:403–410.
21. Alvine FG, Schurrer ME. Postoperative ulnar nerve palsy. Are there predisposing factors? J Bone Joint Surg (Br) 1987; 69A:255–259.
22. Eisen A. Early diagnosis of ulnar nerve palsy. Neurology 1974; 24:256–262.
23. Rosenfalck A. Early recognition of nerve disorders by near-nerve recording of sensory action potentials. Muscle Nerve 1978; 1:360–367.
24. Checkles NS, Russakov AD, Piero DL. Ulnar nerve conduction velocity—effect of elbow position on measurement. Arch Phys Med Rehab 1971; 52:362–365.
25. Gilliatt RW. Acute compression block. In: Sumner AJ, ed. The physiology of peripheral nerve disease. Philadelphia: WB Saunders, 1980:287–315.
26. Olney RK, Miller RG. Conduction block in compression neuropathy: Recognition and quantification. Muscle Nerve 1984; 7:662–667.
27. Olney RK, Budingen HJ, Miller RG. The effect of temporal dispersion on compound action potential area in human peripheral nerve. Muscle Nerve 1987; 10:728–733.
28. Miller RG, Camp PE. Postoperative ulnar neuropathy. JAMA 1979; 242:1636–1639.
29. Kincaid JC, Phillips LH, Daube JR. The evaluation of suspected ulnar neuropathy at the elbow: Normal conduction study values. Arch Neurol 1986; 43:44–47.
30. Kincaid JC. The electrodiagnosis of ulnar neuropathy at the elbow. Muscle Nerve 1988; 11:1005–1015.
31. Harding C, Halar E. Motor and sensory ulnar conduction velocities: Effect of elbow position. Arch Phys Med Rehab 1983; 64:227–232.
32. Miller RG. Ulnar neuropathy at the elbow. Muscle Nerve 1991; 14:97–101.
33. Kimura J. The carpal tunnel syndrome: Localization

of conduction abnormalities within the distal segment of the median nerve. Brain 1979; 102:619–635.

34. Kaeser HE. Nerve cnduction velocity measurements. In: Vinken PJ, Bruyn GW, eds. Handbook of clinical neurology. Vol 7. New York: Elsevier, 1970:116.

35. Bielawski M, Hallett M. Position of the elbow in determination of abnormal motor conduction of the ulnar nerve across the elbow. Muscle Nerve 1989; 12:803–809.

36. Olney RK, So YT, Goodin DS, Aminoff MJ. A comparison of magnetic and electrical stimulation of peripheral nerves. Muscle Nerve 1990; 13:957–963.

37. Gans BM, Kraft GH. M-response quantification: A technique. Arch Phys Med Rehab 1981; 62:376–380.

38. Campbell WW, Sahni SK, Pridgeon RM, et al. Intraoperative electroneurography: Management of ulnar neuropathy at the elbow. Muscle Nerve 1988; 11:75–81.

39. Buchthal F, Rosenfalck A, Trojaborg W. Electrophysiological findings in entrapment of the median nerve at wrist and elbow. J Neurol Neurosurg Psychiatry 1974; 37:340–360.

40. Felsenthal G, Freed MJ, Kalafut R, Hilton B. Across-elbow ulnar nerve sensory conduction technique. Arch Phys Med Rehab 1989; 70:668–672.

41. Tackman W, Vogel P, Kaeser HE, Ettlin TH. Sensitivity and localizing significance of motor and sensory electroneurographic parameters in the diagnosis of ulnar nerve lesions at the elbow. J Neurol 1984; 231:204–211.

42. Olney RK, Wilbourn AJ. Ulnar nerve conduction study of the first dorsal interosseous muscle. Arch Phys Med Rehab 1985; 66:16–18.

43. Anderson K. Surface recording of orthodromic sensory nerve action potentials in median and ulnar nerves in normal subjects. Muscle Nerve 1985; 8:402–408.

44. Jabre JF. Ulnar nerve lesions at the wrist: New technique for recording from the sensory dorsal branch of the ulnar nerve. Neurology 1980; 30:873–876.

45. Trojaborg W. Rate of recovery in motor and sensory fibres of the radial nerve: Clinical and electrophysiological aspects. J Neurol Neurosurg Psychiatry 1970; 33:625–638.

46. Rudge P. Tourniquet paralysis with prolonged conduction block: An electrophysiological study. J Bone Joint Surg (Br) 1974; 56B:716–720.

47. Bolton CF, McFarlane RM. Human pneumatic tourniquet paralysis. Neurology 1978; 28:787–796.

48. Miller RG. Injury to a peripheral motor nerve. Muscle Nerve 1987; 10:698–710.

49. Seyfer AE, Grammer NJ, Bogumil GP, et al. Upper extremity neuropathies after cardiac surgery. J Hand Surg 1985; 10A:16–19.

50. Sumner AJ. The physiological basis for symptoms in Guillain-Barré syndrome. Ann Neurol 1981; 9(suppl 9):28–30.

51. Olney RK, Wilbourn AJ, Miller RG: Ulnar neuropathy at or distal to the wrist (abstr.). Neurology 1983; 33(suppl 2):185.

52. Streib EW. Distal ulnar neuropathy as a cause of finger tremor: A case report. Neurology 1990; 40:153–154.

53. Giuliani G, Poppi M, Pozzati E, Forti A. Ulnar neuropathy due to a carpal ganglion: The diagnostic contribution of CT. Neurology 1990; 40:1001–1002.

54. Hankey GJ, Gubbay SS. Compressive mononeuropathy of the deep palmar branch of the ulnar nerve in cyclists. J Neurol Neurosurg Psychiatry 1988; 51:1588–1590.

55. Stewart JD. The variable clinical manifestations of ulnar neuropathies at the elbow. J Neurol Neurosurg Psychiatry 1987; 50:252–258.

56. Olsen PZ. Prediction of recovery in Bell's palsy. Acta Neurol Scand 1975; 61(suppl):1–121.

11

Other Mononeuropathies of the Upper Extremities
Morris A. Fisher

CONTENTS

This chapter concentrates on mononeuropathies other than of the median and ulnar nerves affecting the upper limbs. These remaining neuropathies may present special problems for the clinical neurophysiologist. Conduction directly across a site of injury may not be possible. Comparison between normal and abnormal sides may therefore be more important than in some other areas of electrophysiologic analysis. It is often impossible to stimulate these nerves in their more proximal courses without stimulating other neural components in the region of the shoulder girdle or brachial plexus. The unwanted stimulation of these other neural components can sometimes cause interpretive problems because of volume pickup at the recording site from muscles activated by the unwanted spread of the stimulus current. Moreover, because of the wide distribution of the innervation zones in some of the proximal muscles, needle electromyographic rather than surface recordings are at times required for accurate definition of the onset of electrical responses in the muscles.

Despite these and other limitations, techniques have been developed for helping to define the location, severity, and probable duration of the nerve lesion as well as contributing to our knowledge of the likely underlying changes in the peripheral nerve in a manner akin to more readily accessible nerves such as the median and ulnar nerves.

RADIAL NERVE

Anatomy

The radial nerve, the major terminal branch of the posterior cord of the brachial plexus, contains fibers derived from the C-5 through C-8 roots and frequently from the T-1 root. It descends behind the axillary artery to reach the angle between the medial aspect of the arm and the posterior border of the axilla (brachioaxillary angle) (Figure 11.1) then inclines obliquely before entering the spinal groove, passing between the origins of the medial and lateral heads of the triceps. At the latter level, it traverses a fibrous arch formed by the tendon of the lateral head of the triceps.[1] Within the spinal groove, the nerve lies next to the humerus; turning forward, it then pierces the lateral intermuscular septum below the deltoid insertion to reach the anterior compartment of the arm. Where it descends, it is covered by the brachioradialis and extensor carpi radialis longus and brevis muscles before crossing the lateral capsule of the elbow joint to reach the supinator. Here the

nerve divides into its two major terminal branches: the posterior interosseous and superficial radial nerves.

The posterior cutaneous nerve of the arm arises in the axilla, whereas the posterior cutaneous nerve of the forearm originates either in the axilla or spinal groove. The lower lateral cutaneous nerve of the arm originates either with the posterior cutaneous nerve of the forearm or separately within the spinal groove.

Motor branches supplying the triceps originate in the axilla, brachioaxillary angle, and spiral groove.[2] The medial head of the triceps receives its supply from the ulnar collateral branch, which arises predominantly within the brachioaxillary angle and accompanies the ulnar nerve. A branch from this radial branch to the medial head goes on to supply the anconeus muscle; this branch as well as collateral fibers from the ulnar nerve supplies articular twigs to the elbow joint. The brachioradialis and extensor carpi radialis receive their motor supply from the radial nerve proximal to the lateral nerve at the level of the epicondyle, whereas the extensor carpi radialis longus may receive its innervation from the radial nerve distal to the elbow. The extensor carpi radialis brevis is innervated largely distal to the elbow. The supinator may also receive radial nerve branches below the epicondyle. In this region, articular branches pass to the lateral elbow.

The region where the radial nerve passes just before entering the supinator muscle has been called the *radial tunnel*. Proximally this tunnel is made up by the space between the brachialis muscle medially; the brachioradialis and extensor carpi radialis successively, anteriorly, and laterally; and the capitulum of the humerus posteriorly. Within this tunnel, the radial nerve divides into the terminal posterior interosseous and superficial radial nerves. The site of this division is variable but in most individuals occurs within 3 to 4 cm distal to the lateral epicondyle.[2]

The point at which the posterior interosseous nerve pierces the superficial head of the supinator muscle has been called the *arcade of Frohse*.[3] This is a fibrous arch in the origin of the muscle between the lateral and medial aspect of the lateral epicondyle. The lateral half is tendinous, whereas the medial half under which the posterior interosseous nerve passes is membranous in 70% of individuals and tendinous in 30%.[4] Proximally in its course within the supinator, the nerve is contiguous to the bicipitoradial and interosseous bursae of the elbow. Within the supinator, the posterior interosseous nerve lies between the superficial and deep heads. In

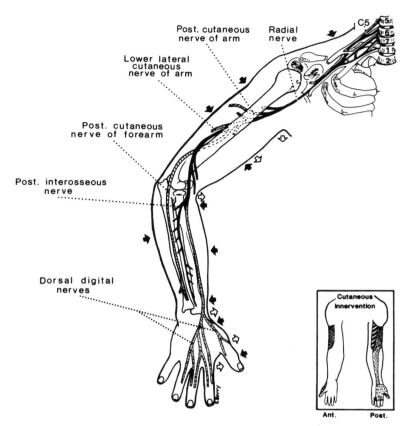

FIGURE 11.1.   *Course and cutaneous distribution of the radial nerve. Stimulus sites (solid arrows) for evoked motor responses are shown on the outer aspect of the figure, whereas on the inner aspect, stimulus (solid arrows) and recording sites (open arrows) for sensory potentials are indicated.*

this location, the nerve may be in direct contact with the radius as the nerve passes laterally along the upper portion of the shaft. The nerve then emerges posteriorly from the supinator to descend along the posterior aspect of the forearm to end in terminal filaments, which innervate the wrist and carpal joints.

The main innervation of the supinator is from the posterior interosseous nerve. Constant branches arise before the nerve entering the supinator, while additional branches commonly arise within the substance of the muscle itself. At the lower border of the supinator, the nerve may divide into two branches. One innervates the medial extensors (extensor carpi ulnaris, extensor digitorum communis, and extensor digiti minimi), whereas the other supplies the remaining forearm extensor muscles. The usual order of posterior interosseous innervation is extensor dig-

itorum communis, extensor carpi ulnaris, abductor pollicis longus, extensor pollicis brevis, and extensor indicis propius. Deviations from this order are, however, common.

In contrast to the motor posterior interosseous nerve, the superficial radial nerve is strictly sensory. The nerve passes distally, becoming cutaneous at the level of the lower one-third of the forearm and then descending across the extensor retinaculum to divide into medial and lateral branches. The lateral branch crosses the tendon of the extensor polics longus superficially at the *anatomic snuff box.*

Function

Radial supplied muscles are responsible for extension of the elbow, wrist, and metacarpophalangeal joints as well as extension of the carpometacarpal and interphalangeal joints of the thumb. The long head of the triceps can aid in extension (as well as adduction) of the shoulder. Supinator contraction produces supination of the forearm (radial-ulnar joints). The extensors digitorum communis, indicis propius, and digiti minimi assist in extension of the interphalangeal joints of the second through fifth fingers, whereas the abductor pollicis longus assists in wrist flexion. Clinically, however, it is important to appreciate that every movement produced through the action of muscles supplied by the radial nerve can be carried out to a limited extent by other muscles or *trick* movements even when the radial nerve injury is complete.[5]

The usual cutaneous innervation of the posterior and lower lateral cutaneous nerves of the arm, the posterior cutaneous nerve of the forearm, and the superficial radial nerve are shown in Figure 11.1. As always with cutaneous innervation patterns, however, variations are common. The skin area normally supplied by the superficial radial nerve may be reduced or even completely supplied by fibers from the ulnar, median, and lateral or posterior cutaneous nerves of the forearm. Less commonly, the terminals of the superficial radial nerve may supply a larger than expected cutaneous area.

The radial nerve also supplies bones and joints. This type of innervation is important clinically but often forgotten. Portions of the upper humerus and posterior aspect of the radius and ulna are innervated by twigs that penetrate through from adjacent radially supplied muscles. The lateral elbow and dorsal wrist and carpal bones receive branches from nerve trunks. The dorsum of the phalanges of the thumb and adjacent one and one-half fingers are supplied by filaments from the superficial radial nerve.

Mode of Injury

Compression

Compression is a well-recognized cause of injury to the radial nerve. The nerve may be compressed at the axillary outlet[6] against the fibrotendinous tissue junction of the long head of the triceps with the tendons of the latissimus dorsi and teres major. Such compression may be caused by misuse of an axillary crutch or the pressure on a dependent arm from a chair edge. Injuries to the radial nerve in the axilla may cause paralysis of all radially supplied muscles, including the triceps, and a sensory loss that includes the distribution of the posterior cutaneous nerve of the forearm.

The radial nerve may also be compressed in the arm inferior to the lowest point of the deltoid insertion[6] where it pierces the lateral intermuscular septum. At this level, the nerve is exposed because although it lies closely applied to the humerus, it is no longer covered by the triceps and has not yet reached its more protected position between the brachioradialis and brachialis muscles. In such a pressure palsy, all radially supplied muscles beyond the triceps may be affected. Associated damage to the posterior cutaneous nerve with hypesthesia over the dorsum of the forearm varies somewhat from patient to patient because of variations in the origin and course of this nerve and perhaps to a lesser degree because of liability to compression injury of sensory compared with motor fibers.

The most common compressive injury affecting the radial nerve is the so-called Saturday night palsy, in which because of deep sleep, or ingestion of drugs or alcohol, or simply fatigue, the nerve is compressed in its course behind the spiral groove between the underlying unyielding humerus and external compressive force.

Compression of the radial nerve in the arm has been reported from a number of other causes, including rifle-slings,[7] wheelchairs,[8] and tourniquets. Even frequent blood pressure measurements may pose a risk in infants.[9] Pressure injury during surgical anesthesia occurs,[10,11] for example, secondary to compression of the arm against a table edge or an armboard.

The superficial radial nerve may be injured by compression at the wrist, causing numbness and at times hyperpathia in the cutaneous distribution of the nerve. Such an injury may be produced by wearing tight watch bands[12,13] as well as handcuffs.[14,15] The latter may be associated with fracture of the radial styloid.[16] The mononeuropathy affecting the superficial radial nerve has been called *cheiralgia paresthetica*[17] (hand pain) because of its similarity to meralgia paresthetica (thigh pain).

The radial nerve may also be compressed by a hematoma, and radial nerve palsy may rarely be a complication of anticoagulant therapy.[18] Computed tomography may be helpful in such cases as a way of visualizing the hematoma.

Entrapment

The radial nerve may also be *entrapped* by fibrous bands or in a fibrous or fibro-osseous tunnel. As with other entrapment neuropathies, the damage may be induced through compression, angulation, or stretch or various combinations of these factors.

Radial nerve injury has been reported to follow strenuous muscular effort involving the triceps. This neuropathy may be acute and cause paresis of all radially innervated muscles and beyond the triceps as well as sensory loss in the distribution of both the posterior cutaneous nerve of the forearm and the superficial radial nerve. This neuropathy has been attributed to compression of the nerve as it passes through the distal portion of the spinal groove by a fibrous arch in the lateral head to the triceps.[1] The effect of angulation of the nerve at the lateral intermuscular septum has also been thought to be an important factor causing injury to the nerve at this level.[19] A progressive palsy as a result of compression of the radial nerve by the lateral head of the triceps in the absence of any defined fibrous arch has been reported.[20]

Injury to the posterior interosseous nerve in the region of the elbow may be caused by repeated contraction of the supinator muscle.[21–25] Injury to the posterior interosseous nerve as it passes through the supinator muscle has been called the *supinator channel syndrome*.[26,27]

The actual site of entrapment, however, may lie at the most proximal part of the superficial head of the supinator muscle,[28–30] where a fibrous band, the arcade of Frohse, may be present. Pressures on the radial nerve caused by contraction of the supinator muscle may be as much as three or four times greater where this band is fibrous rather than simply membranous.[25] The fibrous edge of the origin of the extensor carpi radialis brevis muscle may also be a potential entrapment site.[30–33]

The radial tunnel syndrome[23,29,34] is an inclusive concept that includes potential sites of injury to the radial nerve from the region of the lateral epicondyle to the supinator muscle. This course embraces all those potential sites of entrapments discussed here as well as other possible sites, such as the tethering of the radial nerve to radiohumeral joint.[29] The term *radial tunnel syndrome,* however, is unfortunate because the tunnel itself is not a well-defined entity but rather a potential space; therefore localization of neuropathies to this level should imply no specific causative mechanism as being the cause of the radial neuropathy. Simply localizing the level of the injury to the elbow is sufficient and carries no implications as to the presumed cause.

Radial neuropathies at the level of the elbow primarily involve the posterior interosseous nerve, producing a motor syndrome that may be gradually progressive without sensory loss. Pain may be present, perhaps as a result of the involvement of skeletal afferents carried by the recurrent branch to the lateral epicondyle.[32] Entrapment of the radial nerve at the elbow must be included within the differential diagnosis of lateral epicondylitis (*tennis elbow*), that is, tendinitis of the common origin of the forearm extensor muscles. With lateral epicondylitis, there is tenderness over the lateral epicondyle and pain in the same region produced by flexion of the wrist and fingers with the elbow extended. Radial nerve injuries at the elbow, by contrast, are accompanied by local tenderness, which is maximal about 5 cm distal to the lateral epicondyle, as well as by pain produced through resisted extension of the middle finger or from resisted supination of the forearm.[23] In practice, the clinical distinction between radial nerve injury at the elbow and lateral epicondylitis may be difficult and the two conditions may coexist. Refractory tennis elbow by itself should not be considered an indication for surgery.[35]

Entrapment of the posterior cutaneous nerve of the arm has been reported in a drummer most likely owing to stress on the nerve in the region of the long head of the triceps.[36]

Musculoskeletal inflammation

Other inflammatory processes have been associated with elbow pain and dysfunction of the posterior interosseous nerve. These include bursitis, synovitis and synovial rupture, and tenosynovitis of the thumb (De Quervain's disease).[37–44]

Tumors and cysts

The radial nerve may also be damaged by noninflammatory masses in the arm. Lipomas almost always involve the posterior interosseous nerve in the proximal forearm[45–51] but may also cause a radial neuropathy in the arm between the medial and lateral heads of the triceps.[52] These syndromes present as painless masses with weakness in the radial nerve distribution. The lipomas may often be seen on x-ray examination, and surgery has produced good results.

Radial neuropathies have been caused by other tumors. Fibromas and neuromas of the nerve in the region of the elbow cause progressive paresis in the radial nerve distribution, sometimes unassociated with any palpable swelling of the nerve.[53–56] Radial nerve paresis has also been reported with benign extraneural tumors (cavernous hemangioma),[57] benign neural tumors (schwannoma,[58] lipofibromatous hamartoma[59]), and malignant tumors (malignant granular cell,[60] angiosarcoma[61]). Malignant tumors affecting the radial nerve were much more commonly associated with pain compared with benign tumors. The posterior interosseous nerve or radial sensory fibers may be compressed by ganglion cysts in the region of elbow.[62,63]

Trauma

Because of its course, the radial nerve is readily injured by fractures of the humerus. This can occur at the time of the accident but also in the course of closed or open reduction of the fracture.[64] Treatment has been controversial. Laceration of the radial nerve can occur,[65] and early exploration has been advocated.[66] At the same time, owing to the high rate of (70%[67]–95%[68]) spontaneous recovery, a more conservative approach is generally favored.[19,68,69] Spiral fractures in the distal third of the humerus are associated with proximal and radialward deviation of the distal fragment. With the latter fractures, the radial nerve is particularly vulnerable to injury[70] between bone fragments because of the nerve's relative fixation where it leaves the spinal groove. The argument for early exploration seems stronger for these fractures, but even here the chance of spontaneous recovery is high.[68] Other indications for early exploration include open fractures (or closed fractures requiring open reduction), paralysis following closed manipulation, or progressive paresis following the fracture.[19,64] Even where delayed exploration may be indicated, questions remain as to the appropriate waiting period following the injury when exploration may be justified. Although spontaneous recovery may occur as much as a year following the injury, 2 to 3 months seems a reasonable period to wait before making any decision about exploration. The critical issue governing the need and timing for exploration is whether evidence for recovery of radial nerve function is present after an appropriate interval given the site of the injury as well as the severity and type of injury present. Reconstructive tendon repairs should be performed only when it is clear the nerve injury is irreparable, that is, when there is no meaningful recovery after a year has elapsed following the original injury or any attempts at repair.

Because the posterior interosseous nerve within the supinator channel is relatively fixed and closed related to bone, the nerve may be damaged by fractures of the proximal one-third of the radius. The nerve is also vulnerable to injury in fractures of the shaft of the ulna with associated anterior dislocation of the radial head (Monteggia fractures). The radial nerve may be lacerated or compressed at the arcade of Frohse or stretched over the radial head.[71,72] Spontaneous recovery of the radial injury is the rule.[73–75] Paresis in the territory of the posterior interosseous nerve has been reported up to 47 years after a fracture of the elbow[76–78] (tardy radial palsy).

The radial nerve may be injured directly. During the two World Wars, the radial nerve was damaged more often than any other nerve, primarily through gunshot wounds.[19] The nerve may also be injured by venipuncture,[79] elbow arthroscopy,[80] injections of local anesthetics and steroids about the elbow,[81] and in surgical procedures on the head of the radius.[82]

Systemic illnesses

Radial neuropathies may occur in diabetes mellitus, disorders associated with arteritis, and connective tissue diseases. Focal constrictive fibrosis of the radial nerve has been described in polyarteritis nodosa.[83] The radial nerve may also be involved in leprosy even when the nerve appears clinically normal.[84] Finger and wrist extensor weakness is common in the neuropathy of lead intoxication.[85] Because the weakness may be assymmetric and characteristically spares the brachioradialis, lead poisoning enters into the differential diagnosis of posterior interosseous injury.

Radial injury in the newborn

Radial palsies have been well described in the newborn, causes for which include hematoma, pressure owing to uterine contractions, and traction of the posterior interosseous nerve owing to prolonged intrauterine palmar flexion.[86–89] Radial nerve palsy has also been reported with localized sclerema (hardening of the subcutaneous fat) neonatorum.[90] The prognosis for recovery appears uniformly good.

Electrophysiologic Diagnosis of Radial Neuropathies

Electrical responses to stimulation of nerve and muscle have long been used for the diagnosis of radial nerve injury[91] (see Figure 11.1). Our present techniques for electrophysiologically studying the radial nerve as well as other nerves developed largely during World War II as ways to evaluate traumatic nerve lesions more accurately.[92] Hodes et al.[93] in 1948 were the first to measure motor conduction velocities by stimulating proximally and distally along the course of a nerve. The identification of radial nerve injury following surgical procedures using needle electromyography (EMG) was reported in 1958,[94] and a radial nerve lesion secondary to a humeral fracture was localized using electrophysiologic techniques including conduction velocities in 1961.[95]

In 1964, Gassel[96] measured the latencies to a number of muscles of the shoulder girdle. Recordings were made with concentric needle electrodes and with stimulation at Erb's point with bifocal surface electrodes. The distance from the stimulating electrodes to the *active* or G1 recording electrode was measured with obstetric calipers and control values for the latencies obtained (Table 11.1). In muscles where the innervation zone is longitudinally distributed throughout the muscle, as it is in the triceps, the latency increases as the recording electrode is positioned more distally within the innervation zone. The technique was used to show abnormally prolonged latencies in cases of acute and recurrent polyneuritis.

At about the same time, Gassel and Diamantopoulos[97] reported conduction studies of the radial nerve. The nerve was stimulated with surface electrodes at Erb's point, the junction of the upper and mid one-third of a line drawn between the deltoid insertion and lateral epicondyle of the humerus and 5 cm superior and slightly posterior to the lateral epicondyle. Recordings were made with concentric needle electrodes from the anconeus, brachioradialis, and extensor digitorum communis muscles, that is, muscles receiving their innervation by branches taking their origin from the radial nerve in the upper arm, the region of the lateral epicondyle, and forearm. Distances were measured using obstetric calipers from the point midway between the cathode and anode of the stimulating electrodes. The motor distal latency and conduction velocities between proximal and distal stimulation sites for recording from the anconeus, brachioradialis, and extensor digitorum communis are shown in Table 11.1. Three cases of radial nerve injury associated with fractures of the humerus as well as six patients with pressure palsies were described. Using their techniques, the authors were able to localize the nerve injury and by serial studies define progression or healing of the lesions.

Trojaborg and Sindrup[98] studied motor conduction of the radial nerve by recording with concentric needle electrodes in the triceps, brachioradialis, extensor digitorum communis, extensor policis longus, and extensor indicis muscles. Needle electrode stimulation was used. The stimulus cathode was positioned as close to the nerve as possible by adjusting the position of the electrode to a point where the maximum compound muscle action potential could be elicited with the least stimulus activity. The radial nerve was stimulated in the forearm 8 cm proximal to the ulnar styloid, 6 cm proximal to the lateral epicondyle of the humerus, and between the coracobrachialis and medial edge of the triceps 18 cm proximal to the medial epicondyle of the humerus. The limbs were heated to maintain an even temperature. The conduction velocity between the elbow and forearm was about 10% lower than that across the upper arm. Specific values reported for conduction velocities, latencies, and amplitudes are shown in Table 11.1.

In 1969, Jebsen[99] described a useful method for assessing conduction in the distal radial nerve. Recordings were made with an intramuscular needle electrode inserted into the extensor indicis muscle 4 cm proximal to the ulnar styloid. The posterior interosseous nerve was electrically stimulated 3 to 4 cm proximally and in its superficial course 6 to 7 cm proximal to the lateral epicondyle. Normal condition velocities were reported as 59.7 ± 6.7 m per second. With this technique, Jebsen found conduction slowing in four patients with polyneuropathies.

Shortly afterward, Jebsen[100] extended his observations to include conduction in the more proximal radial nerve by adding a stimulation site at Erb's point. Based on cadaver studies, measurements were made with calipers with the arm closely abducted to the side. Distance measurements between the stimulation sites in the upper arm and forearm were made with a steel tape with the elbow slightly flexed and forearm pronated. The normal values (see Table 11.1) for the proximal conduction were slightly faster than the conduction velocities for the distal segment. Jebsen considered that a proximal conduction velocity of less than 60 m per second or distal conduction velocity exceeding the proximal conduction velocity by 6 m per second or more constituted probable evidence for abnormal conduction slowing in the radial nerve between Erb's point and the distal upper arm stimulation site. Proximal slowing of conduction velocity and dispersion of the evoked compound muscle action potential were described in one case of crutch paralysis, whereas in a second patient, normal radial conduction velocities helped differentiate a radial neuropathy from a cervical radiculopathy.

Normal conduction for the radial nerve between the axilla and elbow recording from the extensor indicis has been reported as 72.5 ± 4.7 m per second. Based on measurements in cadavers, distances for this segment were most accurate using tape rather than caliper measurements.[101]

TABLE 11.1. Conduction in motor fibers of the radial nerve and amplitude of compound muscle action potentials

Muscle	Conduction Between	Conduction Velocity* (m/s) or Motor Distal Latencies (ms)	Amplitude* (mV)	Distance* (cm)
Conduction Velocity				
Anconeus[99]	Erb's point–arm	66 ± 9.2		
Brachioradialis[99]	Erb's point–arm	74 ± 6.7		
Extensor indicis[98]	Erb's point–elbow	72 + 6.3		
Brachioradialis[98]	Axilla–elbow	70 ± 4.9	14 ± 5.7	16.2 ± 2.7
Extensor digitorum communis[98]	Axilla–elbow	60 ± 5	13 ± 4.7	18.2 ± 2.3
Extensor pollicis longus[98]	Axilla–elbow	67 ± 8.7	15 ± 5.4	16.3 ± 2.5
Extensor digitorum communis[98]	Arm–elbow	72 ± 6.1	13 ± 8.2	18.1 ± 1.5
Extensor indicis[98]	Elbow–forearm	62 ± 5.1		
Motor Distal Latencies				
Triceps brachii[96]	Erb's point–arm	4.5 ± 0.4		20–23
		4.9 ± 0.45		25–28
		5.3 ± 0.5		30–33
Triceps brachii[98]	Axilla–muscle	2.7 ± 0.5	23 ± 8.1	11.3 ± 1.6
Anconeus[99]	Arm–muscle	3.8 ± 0.5		7–12
Brachioradialis[99]	Elbow–muscle	3.4 ± 0.65		8–12
Brachioradialis[98]	Elbow–muscle	2.5 ± 0.3	17 ± 6.1	9.5 ± 1.1
Extensor digitorum communis[98]	Elbow–muscle	2.9 ± 0.3	16 ± 6.5	9.9 ± 1.3
Extensor digitorum communis[99]	Elbow–muscle	3.7 ± 0.4		9–14
Extensor pollicis longus[98]	Elbow–muscle	4.4 ± 0.6	14 ± 6.1	19.0 ± 2.0
Extensor indicis[98]	Forearm–muscle	2.4 ± 0.5	14 ± 6.1	6.2 ± 0.9

* Mean ± standard deviation or range.

Ample conduction techniques and control data are therefore available for defining injury to radial motor fibers. Some of these techniques examine a restricted portion of the radial nerve or require multiple needle recordings. Despite these disadvantages, acquaintance with these techniques can at times be important for defining localization or type of nerve injury. The standard clinical method for evaluating motor conduction in the radial nerve is essentially that described by Jebsen,[99,100] that is, recording from the extensor indicis with stimulation more proximally in the forearm, in the region of the elbow, and at Erb's point. Stimulation in the forearm 8 to 12 cm proximal to the recording electrode is feasible and less technically demanding than the 4 cm used by Jebsen. For meaningful results, attention to detail is important. The forearm should be pronated and

the elbow extended. Stimulation at the elbow should be between the biceps and triceps and the stimulating electrodes moved proximally to the medial groove as needed. Recordings can be made with surface (active on the muscle belly, indifferent 5 cm distal on the ulnar styloid) or needle electrodes. What is important is that identical responses are obtained from all stimulation sites. Needle electrodes have the advantage of decreasing the effects of volume conduction but the disadvantage of increased movement with stimulation. The extensor indicis is the preferred recording muscle because it is the most distal innervated radial muscle. Any forearm extensor muscle, however, may be used. At times, it is preferable to record from the extensor digitorum communis when evaluating more proximal conductions. This muscle's larger bulk provides a more stable recording site as well as further limiting the effects of pickup from other muscles.

The first reports of sensory conduction studies of the radial nerve were presented by Downie and Scott in 1964.[102] They recorded from the nerve where it lies superficial in the spiral groove. Downie and Scott themselves appreciated the need for improvements in their technique. In 1967,[103] they advocated placing the active recording electrode directly over the radial nerve where it is palpable as it crosses the tendon of the extensor pollicis longus. This remains recognized as the best site for surface recordings of superficial radial sensory potentials. The authors studied patients with pressure or traumatic neuropathies. In some, the compound sensory nerve action potentials were delayed or absent, and the authors concluded that the outlook for recovery was good where the potential was preserved.

Buchthal and Rosenfalck[104] included studies of the radial nerve in their extensive evaluation of sensory conductions. The authors used near-nerve monopolar needle recording techniques with the indifferent electrodes placed at transverse distances of 5 cm and 3 cm. Conduction times were measured to the first positive peak. Amplitude was measured peak to peak. Orthodromic potentials were elicited by stimulating the fingers with the cathode placed on the middle phalanx of the thumb for the radial nerve. The total error in measurement of distal conduction times was thought to be 6% to 9%. This included errors in distance measurements as well as the possibility of stimulus lead displacement whereby the nerve trunk is progressively excited ahead of the cathode as the stimulus strength is increased. Errors in measurement of amplitude of the potentials in the same subject from study to study were approximately 20% to 30% and were probably mainly due to differences in position of the recording electrode in relation to the nerve. Potential durations were 1.84 ± 0.05 ms measured between the initial positive peak to the intersection of the following negative to positive going component of the spike with the baseline. The lower limit of normal (98% confidence limits) for radial orthodromic sensory conduction between the finger and wrist was 45.5 m per second; between the wrist and elbow, 55.5 m per second; and between the elbow and axilla, 54.4 m per second. The comparable lower confidence limit for radial compound sensory nerve action potential amplitudes recorded at the wrist was 6 μV. Other normal values for radial sensory latencies, conduction velocities, and amplitudes for this study (as well

as for studies discussed subsequently) are shown in Table 11.2.

Trojaborg and Sindrup[98] recorded compound sensory nerve action potentials using methods similar to those of Buchthal and Rosenfalck[104] discussed previously (Figure 11.2). The conduction velocities across the forearm and upper arm following radial nerve stimulation at the wrist were about 3 to 4 m per second below the comparable velocities obtained by stimulating the thumb. This was true even though the amplitude of the compound sensory nerve action potentials was two and one-half to six times greater with wrist stimulation presumably because of the greater number of nerve fibers. The authors also emphasized the inevitability of at least some volume conduction from the median nerve when the radial nerve was stimulated at the thumb.

Antidromic methods for assessing radial sensory conduction have been reported since 1967.[105–110] The results of these studies indicate that antidromic studies are preferable to orthodromic for routine clinical use. The response should be recorded using surface electrodes from the superficial radial nerve where it crosses the extensor pollicis tendon. In comparison to ring electrode recording of digital fibers of the thumb, recordings from the *anatomic snuffbox* are two to four times larger in amplitude and are not contaminated by discharges in median sensory fibers. The nerve should be stimulated in the lateral forearm, where it becomes superficial. Recordings have been made with distances between stimulation and recording sites of 11 to 18 cm. The maximum distance possible is preferable to minimize errors in the calculation of conduction owing to errors in distance measurements. The subjects' hands should be warmed if the temperature is less than 31°C.[109]

Normative values for radial compound sensory nerve action potentials are shown in Table 11.2. These observations were taken from studies in which the latencies were measured to the onset of the initial negative potential, that is, the peak of the initial positive phase. Conductions in the superficial radial nerve have been reported abnormal if they are less than 7 m per second in comparison to conductions in the lateral antebrachial nerve.[111]

Several studies have shown slowed sensory conduction velocities and reductions in superficial radial compound sensory nerve action potential amplitude with age.[107,108,112] Regression equations relating conduction velocity and amplitude to age are available.[113–115] The declines are of the order of 1 m per second and 0.05 μV per year of age.

TABLE 11.2. Conduction in sensory fibers of the radial nerve and amplitude of compound sensory nerve action potentials

Recording	Stimulation	Distance (cm) or Segment	Latency (ms)* or Velocity (m/s)	Amplitude (μV)
Axilla (n)[104]	Thumb	Elbow–axilla	68.7 ± 8 m/s	3 ± 1
Axilla (n)[104]	Thumb	Wrist–axilla	67.7 ± 5.2 m/s	
Axilla (n)[100]	Thumb	Elbow–axilla	71 ± 5.2 m/s	4 ± 1.4
Elbow (n)[104]	Thumb	Wrist–elbow	69.5 ± 6.9 m/s	4 ± 2
Elbow (n)[100]	Thumb	Wrist–elbow	69 ± 5.7 m/s	5 ± 2.6
Forearm[107]	Thumb	11	1.98 ± 0.41 ms	
		Thumb–forearm	54.4 ± 5.3 ms	
Forearm[107]	Thumb	14	2.5 ± 0.02 ms	6.6 ± 1
		Thumb–forearm	56 ± 1.3 m/s	
Wrist (n)[104]	Thumb	14 ± 0.4	2.5 ± 0.1 m/s	12 ± 6
		Thumb–wrist	56.3 ± 5.3 m/s	
Wrist (n)	Thumb	Thumb–wrist	58 ± 6 m/s	13 ± 7.5
Web space	Spiral groove	Spiral groove–elbow	77 ± 8.8 m/s (61.5–97) m/s	
	Elbow	Elbow–mid-forearm	61.5 ± 5 m/s (52–75)	
	Midforearm	Midforearm–wrist	65 ± 7.1 m/s (53–76)	
	Wrist	Distance not specified	1.33 ± 0.23 ms (1.0–1.9)	54.3 ± 25.9 (20–150)
Web space[108]	Forearm	10	2.11 ± 0.15 ms	35.4 ± 11
Web space[109]	Forearm	14	2.4 ± 0.15 ms	31 ± 20
Web space[110]	Forearm	10	1.6 ± 0.1 ms (1.4–1.9)	42.2 ± 14.9 (16–80)
	Forearm–web space	62.1 ± 4.9 m/s	(52.6–71.4)	
Thumb[105]	Forearm	11–18	2.6 ± 0.3 ms (20–3.3)	21.4 ± 4.8 (15–35)
	Forearm–thumb		58.1 ± 4.7 m/s (50–68)	
Thumb[109]	Forearm	14	2.8 ± 0.25 ms	12 ± 8
Thumb[110]	Forearm	15–17	2.8 ± 0.2 ms (2.5 ± 3.3)	12.3 ± 4.9 (5–23)
	Forearm–thumb		57.1 ± 5.3 m/s (48.5–66)	

* Mean ± standard deviation (range).
n, Needle recording.

Ma and Liveson[116] have described an antidromic method for studying the posterior cutaneous nerve of the forearm. Surface stimulation was performed at the elbow just above the lateral epicondyle, with surface recording approximately 12 cm (10 to 14 cm) distally along a line extending from the stimulation point to the middorsum of the wrist. Normal latencies measured to onset were 1.9 ± 0.3 ms (range 1.5 to 2.4 ms), amplitudes measured peak to peak were 8.6 ± 3.9 μV (range 5 to 20 μV), and conduction velocities were 64 + 7.4 m per second (range 51.3 to 73.7 m/s).

Using methods similar to that described previously,[100] Trojaborg[117] reported his electrophysiologic observations on radial neuropathies in 58 patients. Stimulation and recording sites were in the proximal

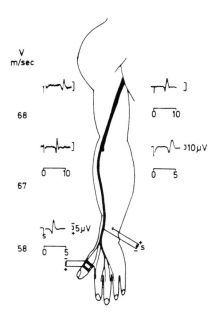

FIGURE 11.2. *Radial sensory potentials recorded at the wrist, elbow, and axilla by stimulating the thumb (left) and those recorded at the elbow and axilla following wrist stimulation (right). Time scale in milliseconds. (Reprinted with permission from Trojaborg W, Sindrup EH. Motor and sensory conduction in different segments of the radial nerve in normal subjects. J Neurol Neurosurg Psychiatry 1969; 32:354–359.)*

and distal upper arm as well as in the forearm 8 cm proximal to the ulnar styloid. Because of contamination of the radial compound sensory nerve action potentials by activation of median nerve fibers with thumb stimulation, the radial nerve was also stimulated at the wrist. Five hundred to 1000 responses were averaged in which the compound sensory nerve action potential was less than 2 μV in size. Electromyographic examinations of the triceps, brachioradialis, and extensor digitorum communis muscles were carried out using concentric needle electrodes; the pattern and amplitudes of the motor unit (MU) potentials at full effort, signs of denervation (i.e., fibrillation potentials, positive sharp waves), the mean duration of at least 20 different potentials, and the numbers of polyphasic MU potentials were evaluated.

In 29 patients, the radial neuropathy was caused by compression at the spiral groove during sleep. In five of these individuals, weakness was limited to the wrist and finger extensors, with sensory loss being

apparent in only one. In the remaining 24 patients, the brachioradialis was also involved, and in 17 of these, there was sensory loss in the hand alone (10) or hand and forearm (seven). Of the 29 other patients (15 with fractures of the humerus), 21 had clinical evidence of involvement of the brachioradialis as well as more distally radially innervated muscles, and 18 of this group had sensory loss in the forearm or hand. In eight patients, weakness was limited to wrist and finger extensors and was associated with sensory changes in the hand in only three. The variability of the pattern of sensory changes in the hand was noted; nearly half of these disturbances were confined to the thumb. Patients were examined 1 day to 12 months after injury. In 21 of the patients, repeat examinations were carried out one or more times.

Regardless of cause, needle examinations of paretic muscles at least 2 weeks after onset of the injury revealed reduced MU recruitment in about 90% of patients and complete paralysis of the muscles in 30%. Fibrillation potentials or positive sharp waves were seen in 60% to 70% of those patients with compressive neuropathies and 85% to 95% of patients with other radial neuropathies. Increased durations of MU potentials and increased numbers of polyphasic MU potentials were seen, however, only in patients with noncompressive radial neuropathies, and these findings were present even when patients were reinvestigated 4 months to 2 years after onset.

In two of the patients with compressive neuropathies, no compound muscle action potential or compound sensory nerve action potential could be elicited distally (or proximally) to the elbow. In the remainder of the patients with compressive radial neuropathies, the latencies and size of the compound muscle action potentials were within normal limits as were the sensory conduction velocities between the wrist and elbow and the size of the compound sensory nerve action potentials as recorded at the elbow. Proximal to the elbow, motor and sensory conduction velocities were reduced as were evoked response amplitudes. The latter abnormalities tended to recover by about 7 weeks after onset (Figure 11.3). There was a good correlation between recovery of sensory conduction velocities and the sizes of the recorded evoked compound sensory nerve action potentials. Even in two of the patients in whom stimulation of the radial nerve proximal to the elbow failed to elicit any compound muscle action potentials or compound nerve action potentials distal to the elbow, complete clinical recovery followed in 1 to 1.5 years. Electrophysiologic evidence of injury to

EVOKED ACTION POTENTIALS FROM M. BRACHIO-RADIALIS

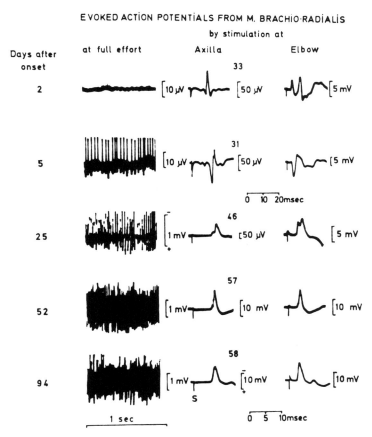

FIGURE 11.3.   *Recovery after radial nerve palsy caused by compression shown from recordings in the brachioradialis. The interference patterns at full effort as well as the evoked responses after stimulation at the axilla and elbow are presented in a sequential fashion from the days since onset. The numbers above the potentials in the middle series indicate the maximum motor conduction velocity between the axilla and elbow. (Reprinted with permission from Trojaborg W. Rate of recovery in motor and sensory fibers of the radial nerve: Clinical and electrophysiological aspects. J Neurol Neurosurg Psychiatry 1970; 33:625–638.)*

sensory nerve fibers was common where there was no clinically apparent sensory loss. Overall, Saturday night palsy was considered to be primarily due to transient block (neurapraxia) with local demyelination as the main underlying pathologic change.

In six of the patients with noncompressive injuries of the radial nerve, motor and sensory conduction velocities were normal. The electromyographic study of affected muscles provided the only evidence for the radial neuropathy. In other patients, in whom compound muscle action potentials and compound nerve action potentials were initially absent in the distribution of the radial nerve but in whom recovery occurred, conduction in motor fibers apparently re-

turned before sensory conduction. In those patients with fractures of the humerus, there was a good correlation between the clinical and electrophysiologic findings as to the site of the lesion.

Trojaborg[117] pointed out the frequent occurrence of electromyographic evidence of denervation in radial-innervated muscles with conduction block injury of the radial nerve and that indeed denervation could be the only evidence of such injury after clinical recovery. Negrin and Fardin[118] found evidence of denervation in electromyographic studies in six of 10 patients as much as 4 months to 2 years following the acute onset of a radial neuropathy even when the clinical recovery was apparently complete.

Focal conduction block has been reported in two patients who experienced the sudden onset of paresis of wrist and finger extensors following muscular effort.[19] This was attributed to compression of the radial nerve in its passage through the triceps. When studied 2 to 4 days after the onset of the neuropathy, no voluntary MU activity was present in the extensor indicis, and no motor potentials could be elicited in the latter by supramaximal stimulation of the radial nerve at the axilla or at Erb's point. Spontaneous and rapid recovery ensued.

Electrodiagnosis can help to establish the degree of radial nerve injury following fractures of the humerus as well as provide evidence for recovery. The data would suggest caution in the need for early tendon transfer.[69]

Studies of conduction of the posterior interosseous nerve have been reported.[119,120] Recordings were made with surface electrodes from the extensor indicis proprius muscle and stimulating the radial nerve in the spiral groove as well as *5 cm distally to the site of maximal nerve tenderness* in the region of the supinator muscles. Conduction velocities in control subjects were 65.8 ± 5.9 m per second[119] and 71.4 ± 2.9 m per second.[120] Although conduction slowing has been reported in entrapment of the posterior interosseous nerve,[120] conduction slowing is not a sensitive test in this condition. Asymmetric prolongation of latencies stimulating at the spiral groove with the forearm supinated may be a more sensitive test.[119] Abnormalities of MU amplitudes, durations, and phases have been observed with needle electromyographic examination in muscles innervated by the posterior interosseous nerve in patients with entrapment of this nerve.

Electrodiagnostic studies of the radial nerve have been helpful as a way of showing radial nerve injury in rheumatoid arthritis,[40–43] where it is sometimes difficult to recognize the neuropathy because of pain or tendon ruptures. Radial nerve studies can localize the radial neuropathies, which sometimes complicate injections in the arm[79,81] or develop in patients with arteritis[83] as well as for testing the function of radial nerve grafts.[121] Abnormal superficial radial compound sensory nerve action potentials—absent potentials or prolonged latencies and diminished amplitudes—have also been shown in cheiralgia paresthesia resulting from the use of handcuffs.[14,15]

Studies in patients with carpal tunnel syndromes in which the median compound sensory nerve action potentials were either delayed or absent have been used to demonstrate volume conduction of superficial radial compound sensory nerve action potentials to median recording sites.[122]

Antidromic sensory nerve conduction velocities in the radial nerve may be measured by surface electrode recordings from the branch of the radial nerve to the index finger while stimulating the radial nerve 14 cm proximally.[84] Latencies to onset were 2.2 ± 0.4 m per second, and peak to peak amplitudes were 19 ± 12 μV. Because biopsy specimens of the radial index branch can be readily obtained, such studies may be useful as one way of revealing early pathologic and physiologic abnormalities in as yet clinically uninvolved nerves in patients with leprosy as well as in close contacts of lepers.[84,123]

Electrodiagnostic techniques have also been applied to the study of radial nerve injuries in the newborn. For example, the presence of fibrillation potentials in muscles innervated by the radial nerve as early as 7 days after birth has been put forward as evidence of prenatal injury to the radial nerve.[124]

Electrodiagnostic techniques for examining the radial nerve have become a useful tool for defining radial neuropathies and providing some indication as to the localization, nature, and severity of the neuropathy. In addition, the techniques are helpful indicators of recovery or lack of recovery in these neuropathies. C-7 radiculopathies may mimic radial neuropathies; electrodiagnostic studies can provide definitive information about this differential diagnosis. The clinical problem presented by hysterical paralysis affecting what seems to be primarily radially supplied muscles and the sometimes confusing compensatory actions of muscles not supplied by the radial nerve are additional reasons for performing electrodiagnostic studies of the radial nerve.

Methods for studying conduction in the posterior cutaneous nerve of the arm have not been described, and those for the posterior cutaneous nerve of the forearm have not received wide clinical application. The latter could be helpful for localizing radial neuropathies, especially because the posterior cutaneous nerve of the forearm may provide the radial cutaneous innervation of the hand. Because of volume conduction of electrical activity from the median nerve to radial nerve recording sites at the wrist, it may be difficult to show whether conduction in the distal portion of the superficial radial nerve has been completely lost.

In addition to electrodiagnostic examinations, other techniques such as plain films, computed tomography, and magnetic resonance imaging are sometimes helpful in revealing the probable site of the injury to the radial nerve. This is especially true in patients in whom the neuropathy is caused by a tumor (benign or otherwise). The clinical examination remains an important tool for examining the radial nerve but is limited by anatomic variations in the sensory innervation pattern of the forearm and hand and limitations of movement imposed by pain.

Controversies remain as to the role of the radial nerve in tennis elbow[29,38] or the need for and timing of surgical explorations of the radial neuropathies associated with fractures. These issues could perhaps be clarified by closer clinical and electrodiagnostic studies, supplemented whenever possible by further careful clinical electrodiagnostic correlations. Intraoperative electrophysiologic studies of the radial nerve have not been reported. Such studies might help in better defining the localization and physiologic character of radial neuropathies.

MUSCULOCUTANEOUS NERVE

Anatomy

The musculocutaneous nerve (Figure 11.4) originates from the lateral cord of the brachial plexus and contains fibers from the C-5, C-6, and, to a lesser extent, C-7 roots. Arising near the inferior border of the pectoralis minor, the nerve passes inferiorly and laterally and pierces the coracobrachialis to lie between the brachialis and biceps brachii before emerging 2 to 5 cm above the elbow crease as the lateral cutaneous nerve of the forearm. The nerve then divides into its terminal anterior and posterior divisions.

The coracobrachialis receives innervation from branches of the musculocutaneous nerve both proximally and as the nerve passes through the muscle, whereas biceps and brachialis receive their innervations as the nerve descends between these muscles. The elbow may receive a filament from the branch to the biceps and brachialis. The anterior division of the lateral cutaneous nerve of the forearm runs subcutaneously along the anterolateral aspect of the forearm and supplies terminal filaments to the thenar eminence. The posterior division traverses the posterolateral aspect of the forearm to terminate over the dorsum of the wrist and the base of the first two metacarpals. Both terminal divisions send articular twigs to the wrist and carpal bones.

The musculocutaneous nerve is relatively fixed at the coracobrachialis as it passes between the biceps

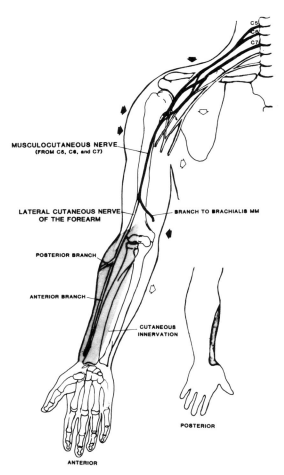

FIGURE 11.4.   *Course and cutaneous distribution of the musculocutaneous nerve. Arrows as indicated in Figure 11.1.*

and brachialis and at the point where it exits through the deep fascia at the elbow. Anatomic variations are common.[125] Musculocutaneous nerve fibers, including their motor or sensory fibers, may run for a variable distance with the median nerve. The brachialis may be supplied by the median nerve, the pronator teres by the musculocutaneous, the lateral cutaneous nerve of the forearm distribution by the median nerve, and the superficial radial cutaneous area by the musculocutaneous.

Function

The coracobrachialis flexes and adducts the shoulder as well as stabilizing the head of the humerus in the glenoid fossa. The brachialis and biceps brachii are flexors of the elbow. The biceps brachii also acts to supinate the forearm.

Even where there is complete paralysis of the biceps brachii and brachialis, supination of the forearm is still possible through the supinator and brachioradialis muscles and elbow flexion by the brachioradialis and pronator teres muscles. Even with paralysis of the biceps, brachialis, and pronator teres muscles, full flexion against mild resistance can be performed by the brachioradialis alone.[5]

Because of extensive overlap in cutaneous innervation from territories of adjacent cutaneous nerve, lesions of the musculocutaneous nerve may result in anesthesia only in a narrow band along the radial margin of the forearm. None of 19 patients who had a musculocutaneous neurotomy for treatment of spastic elbow flexion complained of impaired sensation in the distribution of the lateral cutaneous nerve of the forearm.[126]

Mode of Injury

Musculocutaneous nerve injuries are uncommon.[127] In its short course before entering the coracobrachialis, the nerve is deeply placed and closely related to the lateral cord of the brachial plexus. As a result, it is unusual for isolated musculocutaneous lesions to occur in this region. More distally, the nerve is relatively fixed at several points and is therefore more subject to traction injury as in traumatic injuries of the shoulder.[127,128] The nerve may be particularly vulnerable to downward traction and external rotation.[129] Injuries to the nerve when combined with vascular insufficiency appear to have a poor prognosis.[130] Stretch injury has been reported with violent forearm extension.[131] Painless neuropathies affecting the musculocutaneous nerve have been reported to follow heavy exercise[132] and have been attributed to compression by the coracobrachialis muscle or stretch of the nerve. Similar mechanisms have been proposed for postoperative musculocutaneous paresis.[133–135]

The lateral cutaneous nerve of the forearm may be damaged by the pressure in the antecubital fossa, such as from the strap of a handbag.[136] Entrapment neuropathy affecting the lateral cutaneous nerve of the forearm has been described by Bassett and Nunley[137] and attributed to compression by the lateral edge of the biceps aponeurosis with the elbow in full extension and the forearm in maximal pronation. The neuropathy is accompanied by anterolateral elbow pain and sometimes acutely by dysesthes-

ias along the radial aspect of the forearm as well as limitation of elbow extension when the forearm is pronated. Surgical release produced relief in those who failed to recover spontaneously. The musculocutaneous nerve may be absent in Edwards' syndrome (trisomy 18).[138]

Electrodiagnosis

In 1958, Redford[139] described a method for studying conduction in the musculocutaneous nerve. Stimuli were given just posterior to the distal border of the pectoralis major near its insertion on the humerus, while recordings were made from the biceps brachii belly, preferably at its midpoint because this corresponded to the end plate region of the muscle.[140] Prolonged motor distal latencies were seen in patients with peripheral neuropathies. Gassel,[96] Vacek and Drugova,[141] and Kraft[142] have all reported motor latencies for the musculocutaneous nerve using the now standard technique of stimulating at Erb's point and recording from the biceps muscle. These values are shown in Table 11.3.

Measurements of the maximum motor conduction velocity in the musculocutaneous nerve were first reported by Nelson and Currier in 1969.[143] Surface stimulation was carried out at Erb's point and in the axilla and surface recordings made from the mid biceps. Measurements were made with a flexible steel ruler, and conduction velocities of 75 ± 11 m per second (range 61 to 89 m/s) were reported. Conduction velocity slowing was seen in patients with musculocutaneous nerve injury.

Trojaborg[131] measured sensory as well as motor conduction velocities in the musculocutaneous nerve (Figure 11.5). The biceps compound muscle action potentials were recorded with concentric needle electrodes in the *end plate zone*, while near-nerve stimulation was carried out at Erb's point and the axilla (in the latter instance between the axillary artery and median nerve medially and the coracobrachialis laterally). Compound sensory nerve action potentials were recorded with the same near-nerve electrodes (with electronic averaging as needed) following stimulation of the lateral cutaneous nerve of the forearm at the elbow. Conduction times were measured to the onset of the action potential, amplitudes were measured peak to peak, and distances were measured with an obstetric caliper. The values from these studies are shown in Table 11.3.

Trojaborg[131] presented three cases illustrating the usefulness of these studies. In two, an electrodiagnostic pattern consistent with C-5 root avulsion was

TABLE 11.3.   Musculocutaneous motor and sensory conductions and amplitudes*

Stimulus or Nerve Segment	Distance (cm)	Age (years)	Latency (ms), Velocity (m/s), Amplitude (μV)	Comments
Motor (Recording biceps brachii)				
Axilla	7		2(1.3–2.6)[+] ms	Latency increases
	13		2.9(2.3–3.6)ms	0.16 ms/cm
Erb's point	25		4.8(4.1–5.5)ms	
	33		6(5.4–6.7)ms	
	19–21[96]		4.6 ± 0.6[‡] ms	
	23–25[96]		4.7 ± 0.6 ms	
	27–29[96]		5 ± 0.5 ms	
	23–30[141]		4–5.1[§] ms	
	30–36[141]		4.1–5.7 ms	
	23.5–29[142]		4.5 ± 0.6 ms	
Erb's point–axilla		15–24	70(63–78) m/s	Velocity
		65–74	58(50–66) m/s	decreases
				2 m/s 10 years
Axilla		15–24	17(9–32) mV	Amplitude
		65–74	12(6–22) mV	decreases with
Erb's point		15–24	14(7–27) mV	age and proximal
		65–74	9(5–19) mV	stimulation
Sensory				
Elbow–axilla		15–24	68(61–75) m/s	Velocity decreases
(19 ± 2.2 cm)		65–74	58(51–65) m/s	2 m/s 10 years
Axilla–Erb's point		15–24	68(59–76) m/s	
(19 ± 1.8 cm)		65–74	55(47–64) m/s	
Elbow–axilla		15–24	36(17–75) μV	Amplitude decreases
		65–74	28(13–59) μV	about 2 μV/10 years;
Axilla–Erb's point		15–24	11(3.5–30) μV	75% decrease from
		65–74	4(1.5–12) μV	axilla to Erb's point

* Data from reference 123 except as indicated.
[+] Mean (95% limits).
[‡] Mean ± standard deviation.
[§] Range.

seen: *complete denervation* in C-5 supplied muscles, including the biceps brachii, and abolition of motor responses but well-preserved sensory conductions in the musculocutaneous nerves. The third case involved an injury to the musculocutaneous nerve following violent extension of the forearm. At the time of the initial examination, the evidence pointed to complete disruption of motor and sensory functions in the musculocutaneous nerve, but 21 months later, there was electrodiagnostic (as well as clinical) evidence of recovery, including reinnervation of the biceps and return of both compound muscle action potentials and compound sensory nerve action potentials in the territory of the nerve.

Spindler and Felsenthal[144] have described a more convenient technique for assessing antidromic con-duction in the lateral cutaneous nerve of the forearm. The nerve was stimulated at the elbow just lateral to the biceps tendon, and surface recordings were made 12 cm distally along a straight line extending between the stimulus cathode and the radial artery at the wrist. The mean latency to the onset of the compound nerve action potential was 1.8 ± 0.1 ms (range 1.6 to 2.1 ms) and the conduction velocities 65 ± 3.6 m per second (range 57 to 75 m/s). The mean amplitude (peak to peak) was 24 ± 7.2 μV (range 12 to 50 μV). The authors noted that such potentials could be obtained in patients with polyneuropathies even where more distal potentials were absent. The finding of a normal lateral cutaneous compound nerve action potential is to be expected in preganglionic C-5 and C-6 root avulsions. In addition, study of

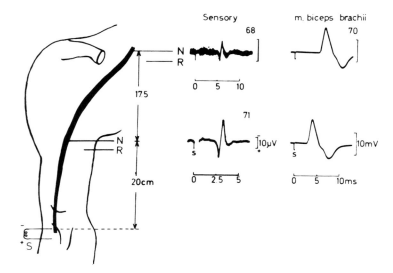

FIGURE 11.5.   *Evoked motor responses recorded from biceps brachii (right) after stimulation at Erb's point and the axilla as well as sensory potentials recorded at these sites after stimulation at the elbow. The numbers above the traces indicate the maximum conductions distal to the stimulation sites. N, Near-nerve electrode; R, remote (indifferent) electrode. (Reprinted with permission from Trojaborg W. Motor and sensory conduction in the musculocutaneous nerve. J Neurol Neurosurg Psychiatry 1976; 39:890–899.)*

conduction in the lateral cutaneous nerve of the forearm may be helpful in localizing and assessing the severity of brachial plexus injuries.

Izzo et al.[145] reported data recording from the lateral cutaneous nerve of the forearm in 155 normal subjects ranging in age from 17 to 80 years. Mean amplitudes decreased steadily with age, whereas conduction velocities showed a less consistent decrease.

Needle electromyographic abnormalities in the biceps brachii and brachialis muscles as well as prolonged conduction times from Erb's point to the biceps may be helpful in diagnosing musculocutaneous nerve palsies as well as for following recovery.[132,134] Techniques are therefore available for measuring conduction in both motor and sensory fibers belonging to the musculocutaneous nerves. Accurate measurements of distance, however, and orthodromic sensory recording studies are listed by the low amplitudes of the potentials. Isolated injuries of the musculocutaneous nerve are rare, but studies of the musculocutaneous nerve can also be helpful for defining brachial plexus dysfunction as well as separating nerve from root injury.

AXILLARY NERVE

Anatomy

The axillary (circumflex) (Figure 11.6) nerve is the smaller of the two terminal divisions of the posterior cord of the brachial plexus. The nerve is derived from

the C-5 and C-6 nerve roots and descends on the subscapularis, to pass posteriorly through the quadrilateral (or quadrangular) space. This space is bounded by the teres minor and capsule of the shoulder joint above, the surgical neck of the humerus laterally, the long head of the triceps medially, and the teres major posteriorly. In this space, the nerve is accompanied by the posterior circumflex humeral artery. After traversing the quadrilateral space, the nerve lies deep to the deltoid and divides into its terminal divisions.

The posterior terminal division sends twigs to the teres minor and supplies the posterior part of the deltoid before piercing the deep fascia to become the upper lateral cutaneous nerve of the arm and supplying the skin of the upper lateral aspect of the arm. The anterior terminal division turns laterally around the surgical neck of the humerus accompanied by the posterior circumflex humeral artery. This division innervates the anterior and central portions of the deltoid as well as supplying a few cutaneous twigs.

The axillary nerve may be derived entirely from the C-5 root and at times contains fibers from the C-7 root. The nerve may partially innervate the subscapularis, the long head of the triceps, and the infraspinatus muscles.

Function

The deltoid is the prime shoulder abductor at the glenohumeral joint. This is achieved chiefly by the middle fibers, with stabilization being carried out by

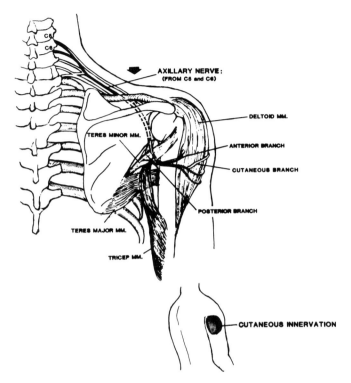

FIGURE 11.6.   *Course of the axillary nerve showing its passage through the quadrilateral space. The potential stimulation site at Erb's point is indicated by the arrow.*

anterior and posterior fibers. The anterior fibers also flex and medially rotate the shoulder, whereas the posterior fibers extend and laterally rotate.

The flexor, extensor, and rotary functions of the deltoid may be carried out by other muscles. Deltoid paralysis can seriously impair shoulder abduction, but varying degrees of abduction, even full abduction, are still possible with time and training without the deltoid.[146–149] Electromyographic recordings can help define the pattern of the compensatory actions in other muscles. Paralysis of the teres minor is not easily demonstrated clinically because compensation readily occurs.

Injury to the upper lateral cutaneous nerve of the arm produces loss of sensation that is most consistently seen and most pronounced in the central area of the nerve's cutaneous distribution. Sensation may be normal even when motor dysfunction is severe.

Mode of Injury

Although isolated injury of the axillary nerve is uncommon,[150] the nerve is vulnerable in shoulder trauma. The axillary nerve is free for only a short distance in the axilla before becoming relatively fixed by its deltoid branches. The nerve may be stretched under the head of the humerus during hyperabduction sufficient to dislocate the shoulder or during the downward traction accompanying inferior dislocation of the shoulder. Axillary nerve injuries may occur with blunt trauma,[151] fractures of the neck of the humerus[128] and acromion,[152] and shoulder dislocation.[128,153] Axillary neuropathy is one of the most common complications of shoulder dislocation, and the axillary nerve is said to be the most frequently injured infraclavicular branch of the brachial plexus.[154] As a complication of shoulder dislocations and fractures about the shoulder, axillary nerve injury is more common in those aged over 50 years and is commonly associated with reduced shoulder mobility.[128] Infraclavicular brachial plexus injuries have a generally good prognosis but this may be less true where there is isolated injury to the axillary nerve.[155] Axillary nerve injury may also be associated with traumatic hematoma in the quadrilateral space.[127]

The axillary nerve may also be damaged by penetrating wounds such as those caused by bullets or upward pressure in the axilla such as from a misused crutch. This is usually associated with radial nerve injury. Entrapment of the anterior branch of the axillary nerve owing to hypertrophied muscles in the quadrilateral space has also been described.[156] A syndrome characterized by anterior shoulder pain has been attributed to entrapment of the axillary nerve and compression of the posterior humeral circumflex artery in the quadrilateral space.[157] Axillary paresis may, of course, occur with brachial plexopathies.

Electrodiagnosis

Conduction studies for the axillary nerve have been limited to the measurement of the latency to muscle response recorded from the deltoid in response to stimulation at Erb's point. Recording with concentric needle electrodes, Gassel[96] reported mean latencies of 4.3 ± 0.5 ms at caliper-measured distances of 15 to 16 cm and 4.4 ± 0.35 ms at distances of 18 to 19 cm. Vacek and Drugova[141] found latencies of 3.4 to 4.6 ms at distances of 16 to 22 cm and 3.8 to 5 ms at distances of 22 to 25 cm. Kraft[142] noted latencies of 3.9 ± 0.5 ms (range 2.8 to 5 ms) at distances of 14.8 to 21 cm.

Needle electromyographic examination of axillary-supplied muscles, the deltoid primarily, is a useful way to recognize axillary nerve injuries. These studies also provide a guide to recovery[128,151] as well as help select those patients who might benefit from neurolysis.[158]

SUPRASCAPULAR NERVE

Anatomy

The suprascapular nerve (Figure 11.7) is the only branch of the upper trunk of the brachial plexus. The fibers derive primarily from C-5 with contributions usually from C-6 and occasionally C-4. The nerve arises in the posterior triangle of the neck and passes beneath the trapezius to reach the upper border of the scapula. The nerve then traverses the suprascapular notch to reach the supraspinous fossa. The notch is bridged by the transverse scapular ligament to form a fibro-osseous foramen. Within the supraspinous fossa, the nerve supplies branches and acromioclavicular joints. The nerve then continues around the lateral border of the spine of the scapula to enter the infraspinatus fossa to supply the infraspinatus muscle as well as more twigs to the shoulder. In passing into the infraspinatus fossa, the nerve traverses the spinoglenoid notch, which is frequently covered by the spinoglenoid (or inferior transverse scapular) ligament. Although the suprascapular nerve is generally considered a purely motor nerve, a cutaneous branch overlapping in distribution that of the axillary nerve has been described.[159]

Function

The supraspinatus muscle is a shoulder abductor, although full abduction is still possible following

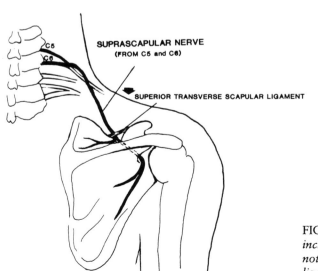

FIGURE 11.7. *Course of the suprascapular nerve, including its passage through the suprascapular notch (bounded by the superior transverse scapular ligament) as well as the spinoglenoid notch. Potential stimulation site at Erb's point (arrow).*

paralysis of this muscle. The infraspinatus muscle is the prime external rotator of the arm at the shoulder. With paralysis, there is only poor compensation by the teres minor and anterior fibers of the deltoid. Paresis of the infrascapular muscle is therefore readily recognized by weakness of external rotation of the shoulder. The supraspinatus and infraspinatus, along with the teres minor and suprascapularis, form the rotator cuff, which stabilizes the humeral head in the glenoid fossa and provides a fulcrum for the deltoid.

Mode of Injury

Trauma is a frequent cause of suprascapular injury. The nerve is the highest branch of the brachial plexus and therefore subject to traction injury in falls where there is an increase in the acromiomastoid angle. In addition, the suprascapular nerve may be compressed in fractures of the scapular notch,[160] and the nerve may be injured in shoulder dislocations[161] or other trauma involving the shoulder.[162]

The suprascapular nerve is susceptible to injury because it is relatively fixed at its origin from the brachial plexus as well as at its muscular and joint attachments. As such, the nerve can be tightened at the foraminal edges by forward motion of the shoulder girdle. The resulting entrapment neuropathy has been well described[163–169] and may be bilateral.[170] This syndrome is characterized by shoulder pain aggravated by movement that is accompanied by weakness, especially of external rotation of the shoulder. Clear precipitating factors are not always present. A shallow suprascapular notch may be a predisposing factor in suprascapular neuropathy.[171] The differential diagnosis in patients with suprascapular nerve entrapment includes subacromial bursitis, tenosynovitis, and particularly rotator cuff injury.[172] With rotator cuff injury, the supraspinatus and infraspinatus muscles may appear weak because of unstable insertions and pain, and the muscles may become atrophied from disuse.

Entrapment of the nerve at the spinoglenoid notch with selective involvement of the infraspinatus muscle has been described.[173,174] The resultant shoulder pain and weakness of shoulder external rotation has been relieved by section of the inferior transverse scapular ligament. Selective injury to the inferior division of the suprascapular nerve has also been described from compression by ganglion cysts.[175,176] The suprascapular nerve may occasionally be injured in radical neck dissection.[177]

Studies of suprascapular neuropathy in baseball pitchers have indicated that the nerve injury is not always due to entrapment at the suprascapular or spinoglenoid notches. Other proposed mechanisms include stretch or ischemic injury to the suprascapular nerve.[178]

Electrodiagnosis

Motor latencies for the suprascapular nerve have been determined[97,142,179] by stimulating percutaneously at Erb's point and recording with concentric needle electrodes from both the supraspinatus and the infraspinatus muscles. Calipers should be used to measure the distance between the sites of stimulation and recording. Normal values are shown in Table 11.4. A method for evaluating conduction in the articular branch of the suprascapular nerve has been described.[180]

Despite the fact that motor conduction velocities cannot be measured, needle electromyographic studies of the supraspinatus and infraspinatus muscles is still a valuable way of assessing patients in whom movement of the shoulder is restricted and painful. Prolonged motor latencies are also valuable indicators of neuropathy.[170,171] Electrodiagnostic studies

TABLE 11.4. Normal motor latencies for the suprascapular nerve*

Muscle Recorded	Distance (cm)	Latency+ (ms)	Range (ms)
Supraspinatus	8–9[97]	2.6 ± 0.32	
	10–11[97]	2.7 ± 0.27	
	7.4–12[142]	2.7 ± 0.5	1.7–3.7
		2.7[179]	1.7–3.7
Infraspinatus	13–15[97]	3.4 ± 0.4	
	16–18[97]	3.4 ± 0.4	
	10.6–15[142]	3.3 ± 0.5	2.4–4.2

* Stimulation site: Erb's point
+ Mean ± standard deviation.

may also help to delineate selective involvement of the inferior branch of the suprascapular nerve[173–177] (Figure 11.8). Arthrography and magnetic resonance imaging studies may also help in the assessment of the painful shoulder.

LONG THORACIC NERVE

Anatomy

The long thoracic nerve (Figure 11.9) is formed from the C-5, C-6, and C-7 nerves. In about 8% of subjects, the branch from the C-7 root is absent, and in another 8% of subjects, there may be contributions from the C-8 root.[181] The contributions from the C-5 and C-6 roots traverse the scalenus medius muscle, unite, and then are joined by branches from more caudal roots to form the long thoracic nerve. The nerve passes behind the clavicle at the junction of its medial two-thirds and lateral one-third. The nerve is angulated as it enters the axilla, passing over the first and second ribs before descending along the thoracic wall on the surface of the serratus anterior muscle. The long thoracic nerve in its course also lies close to the subcoracoid and subscapular bursae.

Function

Winging of scapula owing to paralysis of the serratus anterior was described as early as 1825.[182] The serratus anterior arises from the outer and superior surfaces of the first eight to 10 ribs and inserts into the costal margin of the scapula. During elevation of the arm, the middle fibers assist the lower fibers in bringing the scapula forward, and the lower fibers rotate the inferior angle of the scapula upward and laterally. With the scapula fixed by the rhomboids in adduction, the serratus anterior can also act as an accessory muscle of respiration.

Paralysis of the serratus limits and may appear to weaken abduction of the shoulder, particularly abduction exceeding 90 degrees, which primarily de-

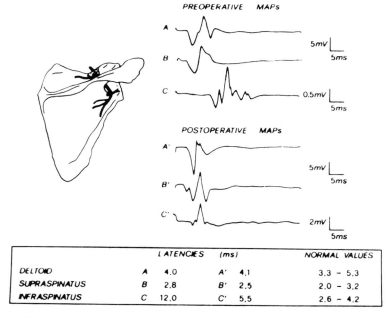

FIGURE 11.8.   *Needle recordings from the deltoid (A), supraspinatus (B), and infraspinatus (C) muscles after stimulation at Erb's point. The data are consistent with entrapment of the suprascapular nerve at the spinoglenoid notch, with improvement after surgical excision of the inferior transverse scapular ligament (C'). Note the decrease in latency, increase in amplitude, and decrease in dispersion of the infraspinatus evoked motor response postoperatively. (Reprinted with permission from Aiello I, Serra G, Traina GC, et al. Entrapment of the suprascapular nerve of the spinoglenoid notch. Ann Neurol 1982; 12:314–316.)*

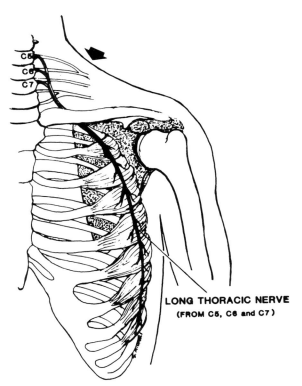

FIGURE 11.9. *Course of the long thoracic nerve with site of stimulation at Erb's point (arrow).*

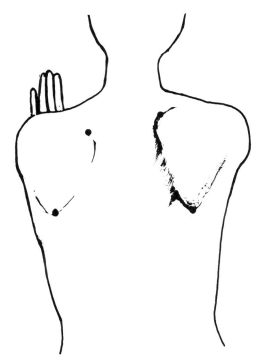

FIGURE 11.10. *Winging of the right scapula with forward flexion of the extended arms owing to long thoracic nerve injury. Dots indicate the positions of the superior and inferior angles of the scapula. On the right, note the upward and medial displacement of the scapula as well as external rotation (inferior angle more lateral) owing to unopposed normal actions of the levator scapulae and rhomboids.*

pends on scapulothoracic motion. When the arm is flexed, the poor fixation of the scapula to the thorax and difficulties stabilizing the inferior angle of the scapula seen in paralysis of the serratus anterior account for the well-recognized and often prominent scapular winging owing to poor fixation of the scapula to the thorax (Figure 11.10). When the individual is at rest, there is usually little if any displacement of the scapula. The trapezius and rhomboids compensate in part for weakness of the serratus anterior.

Mode of Injury

Because of the fixation of the long thoracic nerve at the scalenus medius and serratus anterior as well as the angulation of the nerve as it enters the axilla, the long thoracic nerve is prone to traction injury. This can be caused by acute trauma or may be due to recurrent stressful movements of the shoulder.[183–188] Skillern's[183] case, for example, occurred in a machine operator who reached forward 800 times a night.

Similar paresis, however, may occur in those engaged in what are usually considered benign activities, such as playing tennis[189] or carrying a knapsack.[190] Even a particular arm position during sleep has been causally related to long thoracic paresis.[184,191,192] The nerve may be injured by direct blows to the shoulder or lateral thoracic wall such as in falls or in sports (e.g., football). Stretch injury of the long thoracic nerve during surgery has long been recognized,[183,192,193] and this type of injury as well as direct trauma has been reported as a complication of resection of the first rib.[194]

Long thoracic neuropathy may occur in diphtheria and infectious mononucleosis[195] as well as an isolated manifestation of brachial neuritis.

The prognosis for recovery of long thoracic neuropathies may be relatively good following, for example, minor trauma or brachial neuritis but may be less satisfactory with severe injury to the nerve. Surgical attachment of the sternal portion of the pectoralis major to the lower pole of the scapula has been recommended for functional improvement if recovery has not occurred by 6 months following traumatic winging of the scapula.[187]

Electrodiagnosis

Reports have emphasized the importance of needle electromyographic study of the serratus anterior muscle for confirmation of lesions affecting the long thoracic nerve and following any subsequent recovery as a guide to management.[187,189,196,197] Needle electromyographic studies must be done carefully to avoid penetration of the pleura and are performed most safely by examining the muscle at the inferior angle of the scapula.

Conduction in the long thoracic nerve is most easily measured by stimulating at Erb's point and recording with surface electrodes parallel to the fifth or sixth ribs.[116] The active electrode is placed at the midaxillary line with the reference electrode parallel but more medial. The active electrode should not be placed more posteriorly to avoid recording from the latissimus dorsi. The mean latency is 3 ± 0.2 ms (range 2.8 to 3.4).

Conduction studies have been performed recording with monopolar[197] or concentric[198] needle electrodes from digitations of the serratus anterior in the region of the anterior to midaxillary lines at the level of the fifth or sixth ribs. These studies have been used to follow recovery in patients with serratus anterior palsy. Complete lesions have been characterized by failure to elicit a motor response following Erb's point stimulation, whereas incomplete lesions were marked by prolonged latencies, polyphasic responses of prolonged duration, and reduced amplitudes.[198]

Despite the well-recognized clinical picture of long thoracic paresis, the value of electrodiagnosis for evaluating such lesions has become accepted. At the least, these studies can help evaluate patients whose scapulothoracic motion is abnormal but in whom it cannot be clearly established clinically whether the cause lies in weakness of the serratus anterior muscle alone or in the action of other muscles acting on the scapula.

Long thoracic palsy may enter into the differential diagnosis of Sprengel's deformity.[199]

SPINAL ACCESSORY NERVE

Anatomy

The spinal accessory nerve (XI cranial nerve) arises from motoneurons of the first four cervical segments. The root fibers unite to form a common trunk, which ascends to enter the intracranial cavity through the foramen magnum. This trunk then exits with the vagus through the jugular foramen to pierce the sternocleidomastoid muscle subsequently and descend obliquely across the floor of the posterior triangle of the neck to the trapezius muscle. In the posterior triangle, the nerve lies superficially covered only by fascia and skin. The spinal accessory forms a plexus with fibers from the C-3, C-4, and, to a lesser degree, C-2 nerves. There is debate as to the extent, if any, of the motor innervation of the trapezius by the cervical nerves.[200–202]

Function

The spinal accessory nerve innervates the sternocleidomastoid and trapezius muscles, but the trapezius is the only muscle that affects arm movements. This large, broad muscle adducts the scapula (chiefly middle fibers), rotates the glenoid cavity upward (chiefly upper and lower fibers), and elevates and depresses the scapula.

Weakness of the trapezius causes shoulder droop.[203] This drooping is thought capable of stretching the nerves and roots of the brachial plexus and may cause pain that is sometimes severe and localized in the shoulder. Because of the relatively unopposed pull of the arm on the shoulder, the inferior angle of the scapula may be rotated nearer to the midline than is the case on the normal side. Winging of the scapula is accentuated by abduction at the shoulder—not by forward flexion of the humerus as in serratus anterior palsies (Figure 11.11). Atrophy of the trapezius results in loss of shoulder contour and accentuation of the supraclavicular fossa.

Trapezius paralysis weakens elevation of the shoulders and may severely impair abduction of the shoulder as well. The rhomboids, levator scapulae, and serratus anterior muscles may all help to compensate for the trapezius weakness, and shoulder abduction remains full.[5,203] Combined trapezius and serratus paralysis, however, produces a serious disability with abduction limited to less than 90 degrees because of poor shoulder fixation and the abnormal scapulothoracic motion.

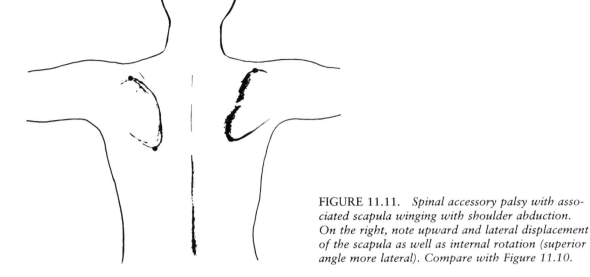

FIGURE 11.11. *Spinal accessory palsy with associated scapula winging with shoulder abduction. On the right, note upward and lateral displacement of the scapula as well as internal rotation (superior angle more lateral). Compare with Figure 11.10.*

Mode of Injury

There are many reports of injury to the spinal accessory nerve from surgery in the posterior triangle of the neck, where the nerve lies superficially.[204–215] These lesions are characterized by sparing of the sternocleidomastoid because the injury is distal to the innervation of the latter muscle. Lesions may complicate such minor surgical procedures as lymph node biopsies or the removal of cysts in the region. Damage to the accessory may also follow surgery in the anterior cervical triangle.[215] Although adequate spontaneous functional recovery can occur, this is not always true, and there may be residual disability owing to pain, limitation of motion, and shoulder and scapula dislocation.[216] Conservative therapy has included support slings, whereas operative therapy has included nerve suture[205,207,217] and facial slings.[214] In the past, the spinal accessory nerve has been routinely sacrificed in radical neck dissections. The importance of accessory nerve function is indicated by the number of articles indicating such sacrifice is neither desirable nor necessary.[218–222]

Iatrogenic injury is the most common cause of spinal accessory paresis. Other causes, however, are not infrequent. Because of its superficial location, the nerve is subject to injury in shoulder trauma[128,223] as well as from direct pressure, such as from a sling,[224] hanging (unsuccessful),[225] or neck biting during lovemaking.[226] The nerve may be stretched during thoracotomy as well as with quick head turning with

the arm pulled down by heavy objects.[227] Isolated, idiopathic spinal accessory paresis characterized by shoulder or neck pain and shoulder weakness has been described.[228–231] The sternocleidomastoid as well as trapezius may be paretic.

The spinal accessory nerve may be involved by pathologic processes that affect cranial nerves. Trapezius (as well as sternocleidomastoid) involvement is said to be a feature of the jugular foramen syndrome.[232]

Electrodiagnosis

In 1963, Skorpil and Zverina[233] reported motor conduction velocities in the accessory nerve of 71 ± 11 m per second (range 40 to 75 m/s). The nerve was stimulated percutaneously both at the upper and at the lower portions of the posterior triangle of the neck, while making recordings with needle electrodes in the upper trapezius.

In 1968, Cherrington[234] described a now standard technique involving percutaneous stimulation of the accessory nerve in the middle of the posterior triangle of the neck and recording with surface electrodes from the upper trapezius with the active electrode about 5 cm lateral from the C-7 spinous process. The range of normal latencies was 1.8 to 3 ms. Delay was reported in a patient with accessory nerve injury caused by posterior fossa meningioma.

Eisen and Bertrand,[235] using a similar technique, reported prolonged latencies and reduced muscle potential amplitudes in patients with idiopathic accessory palsies (Figure 11.12); electrophysiologic improvement accompanied clinical recovery in these patients.

Krongness[236] stimulated in front of the mastoid and recorded with needle electrodes in the ipsilateral upper trapezius and sternocleidomastoid. With trapezius recording, the latency was 3.5 ± 0.5 ms at a distance of 12.5 ± 1.4 cm. Comparable values for the sternocleidomastoid were 2.3 ± 0.5 ms at a distance of 9.6 ± 0.14 cm. These studies were used to follow recovery in a patient with accessory paresis following a lymph node biopsy.

Latencies can be recorded from the upper as well as the lower and middle trapezius.[237] Such studies can be used to define differential effects of spinal accessory nerve injury.[238] Needle electromyographic studies of the trapezius are also helpful as an aid in diagnosis and prognosis.[212,213,216,229]

Whether because of the growing recognition of accessory paresis or the ready availability of electrodiagnostic techniques to study these neuropathies, it is clear that there has been an increased awareness of accessory nerve injuries. Given the complexity of shoulder motion, it may simply be that electrodiagnostic analysis has provided a readily available tool for defining and following isolated accessory palsies, whereas this was previously difficult based on clinical examination alone.

DORSAL SCAPULAR NERVE

The dorsal scapular nerve (Figure 11.13) arises within the scalenus medius from fibers of the C-5 root. After emerging from the muscle, the nerve passes obliquely backward deep to the levator scapulae, which it innervates before descending to supply the major and minor rhomboids.

The levator scapulae elevates the scapula. Its clinical importance lies primarily in its ability to compensate for paresis of the upper trapezius.

The rhomboids retract the scapula, elevate its vertebral border, and rotate the scapula such that its inferior angle moves medially. With paralysis of the rhomboids, there may be slight scapula winging at rest and lateral displacement of the inferior angle of the scapula during activity. Paralysis of the rhomboids alone (or levator scapulae muscle) does not usually produce much functional impairment because of the compensatory actions of other muscles.

Conduction studies have not been reported. Techniques for the needle electromyographic examination of the levator scapulae and rhomboids are well described.[239,240] Although examination of the rhomboids or levator scapulae is not routinely carried out, the absence of clinical or electrophysiologic reports of isolated dorsal scapula neuropathies argues against *entrapment* of this nerve, as described by Kopell and Thompson,[241] occurring with any degree of frequency.

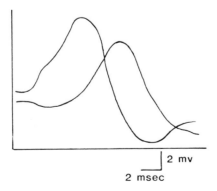

2 mv
2 msec

FIGURE 11.12.   *Surface-recorded evoked motor responses from the trapezius muscles after spinal accessory stimulation with lower tracing, indicating latency delay associated with nerve dysfunction. (Reprinted with permission from Eisen A, Bertrand G. Isolated accessory nerve palsy of spontaneous origin. Arch Neurol 1972; 27:496–502.)*

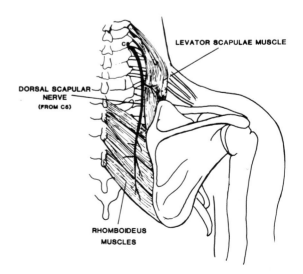

LEVATOR SCAPULAE MUSCLE

DORSAL SCAPULAR NERVE (FROM C5)

RHOMBOIDEUS MUSCLES

FIGURE 11.13.   *Course of dorsal scapular nerve.*

SUBSCAPULAR NERVE

The subscapular nerves arise from the posterior cord of the brachial plexus. They contain fibers from the C-5 and C-6 spinal roots. The upper subscapular nerve passes downward to supply the subscapularis, whereas the lower passes more laterally, sending a branch to the subscapularis and terminating in the teres major.

The subscapularis and teres major act primarily to rotate the shoulder medially. Paralysis of these muscles may be accompanied by some external rotation of the shoulders at rest, but the resulting functional disability as a consequence of paralysis of the muscles is minimized by the compensatory actions of the pectoralis major, anterior fibers of the deltoid, and latissimus dorsi muscle.

Subscapular nerve palsies have been found in brachial plexus injuries. Isolated nerve injuries have not been reported.

Needle examination of the teres major is possible.[240] The usefulness of this procedure would seem limited to the evaluation of brachial plexus injury. Conduction studies have not been reported.

THORACODORSAL NERVE

As with the subscapular nerve, the thoracodorsal is a branch of the posterior cord of the brachial plexus (C-6, C-7, C-8). The nerve runs a long, exposed course along the posterior axilla to reach the deep surface of the latissimus dorsi. The latissimus dorsi acts primarily to rotate, adduct, and extend the shoulder medially.

Thr thoracodorsal may be injured by lesions of the brachial plexus as well as surgical procedures in the axilla. Strong shoulder adduction may as a consequence be impaired. Conduction studies have not been described for the thoracodorsal nerve.

MEDIAL AND LATERAL PECTORAL NERVES

The medial and lateral pectoral (anterior thoracic) nerves (Figure 11.14) are so named because they arise from the most proximal portion of the medial cord (C-8, T-1) and lateral cords (C-5, C-6, C-7) of the brachial plexus. The lateral pectoral nerve passes superficial to the axillary artery before terminating deep to the clavicular and upper sternocostal portions of the pectoralis major. The medial pectoral nerve descends between the axillary artery and vein before supplying the pectoralis minor and inferior portion of the sternocostal portion of the pectoralis major.

The pectoral nerves may be injured as part of a brachial plexopathy as well as in surgery.[242] With paralysis of the pectoralis minor, there may be weakness of the arm extension owing to poor scapula

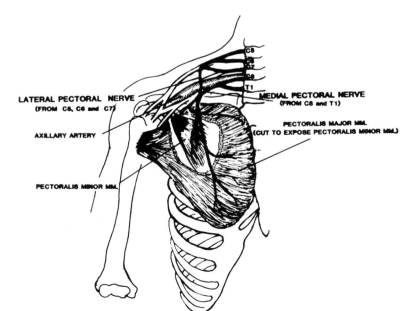

FIGURE 11.14. *Course of the medial and lateral pectoral nerves, indicating their relation to the axillary artery and innervation of the pectoral muscles.*

fixation; with paralysis of the pectoralis major, there may be weakness of arm adduction.

Electromyographic examination of the pectoral muscles can be helpful for evaluating brachial plexus injuries. Avoiding injury to the pectoral nerves in mastectomy procedures is important for cosmetic reasons.[242] Conduction studies of the pectoral nerves have not been reported.

MEDIAL CUTANEOUS NERVES OF THE ARM AND FOREARM

The medial cutaneous nerves of the arm (T-1) and forearm (C-8, T-1) (Figure 11.15) arise from the medial cord of the brachial plexus. They travel with the ulnar nerve as far as the level of the attachment of the coracobrachialis to the humerus. The medial cutaneous arm (upper) then becomes superficial to pass down the inner aspect of the arm to the elbow. The medial cutaneous nerve of the forearm becomes superficial above the elbow and then descends subcutaneously in the forearm anteromedially (anterior division) and posteromedially (posterior division) to the hand. The medial cutaneous nerves of the arm and forearm supply cutaneous fibers to the inner aspect of the arm and forearm.

Given their superficial location, injury to the medial cutaneous nerves might be expected frequently, yet this has not been reported. This may be because, owing to overlap with other cutaneous nerves, the area of involvement is small or the loss is transient.

Antidromic conduction studies of the medial cutaneous nerve of the forearm have been reported.[145,243,244] Izzo et al.[145] stimulated about 5 cm proximal to the medial epicondyle and recorded from the anteromedial surface of the forearm 14 cm distally. Based on a series of 155 nerves, the mean amplitude (peak to peak) was 11.4 ± 5.2 μV, the mean conduction velocity (measured to onset) was 62.7 ± 4.9 m per second, and the mean latency (mea-

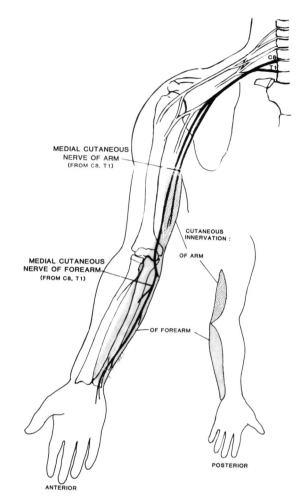

FIGURE 11.15. *Course of the medial cutaneous nerves of the arm and forearm.*

sured to peak) was 2.7 ± 0.2 ms. Reports of conduction studies of the medial cutaneous nerve of the arm are not available.

REFERENCES

1. Lotem M, Fried A, Solzii P, et al. Radial nerve palsy following muscular effort. J Bone Joint Surg 1971; 53-B:500–506.
2. Sunderland S. Nerves and nerve injuries. New York: Churchill Livingstone, 1978:802–819.
3. Frohse LF, Frankel M. Die Muskein des menschlichen Armes. Jena: G Fischer, 1908.
4. Spinner S. The arcade of Froshe and its relationship to posterior interosseous nerve paralysis. J Bone Joint Surg (Br) 1968; 50:809–812.
5. Sunderland S. Voluntary movements and the deceptive action of muscles in peripheral nerve lesions. Aust NZ J Surg 1944; 13:160–183.
6. Sunderland S. Traumatic injuries of peripheral nerves. I. Simple compression injuries of the radial nerve. Brain 1945; 68:58–72.
7. Muntz HH, Coonrad RW, Murchison RA. Rifle-sling palsy. US Armed Forces Med J 1955; 6:353–358.

8. Hortigan JD. The dangerous wheelchair. J Am Geriatr Soc 1981; 30:572–573.

9. Tollner U, Bechinger D, Pohlandt R. Radial nerve palsy in a premature infant following long-term measurement of blood pressure. J Pediatr 1980; 95:921–922.

10. Dhuner KG. Nerve injuries following operations: A survey of cases occurring during a six-year period. Anesthesiology 1950; 11:289–293.

11. Parks BJ. Postoperative peripheral neuropathies. Surgery 1974; 74:348–357.

12. Matzdorff F. Zwei seltene Falle nonperipherer sensibler Lahmung. Klin Wochenschr 1926; 5:1187.

13. Rask MR. Watchband superficial facial neurapraxia. JAMA 1979; 241:2702.

14. Massey EW, Pleet BA. Handcuffs and cheiralgia paresthetica. Neurology 1978; 28:1312–1313.

15. Dorfman LJ, Jayaram LA. Handcuff neuropathy. JAMA 1978; 239:957.

16. Richmond PW, Fligelstone LJ, Lewis E. Injuries caused by handcuffs. Br Med J 1988; 297:111–112.

17. Wartenberg R. Cheiralgia paresthetica (isolierte Neuritis der Ramus superficlis Nervi radialis). Z Ges Neurol Psychiatr 1932; 141:145–155.

18. Hoyt TE, Tiwari R, Kusske JA. Compressive neuropathy as a complication of anticoagulant therapy. Neurosurgery 1983; 12:268–271.

19. Sunderland S. Nerves and nerve injuries. New York: Churchill Livingstone, 1978:820–842.

20. Manske PR. Compression of the radial nerve by the triceps muscles. J Bone Joint Surg 1977; 59-A:835–836.

21. Guillain G, Courtellemont. L'action du muscle court supinateur dans la paralysie du nerf radial. Presse Med 1905; 25:50–52.

22. Woltman HW, Learmonth JR. Progressive paralysis of the nervous interosseous dorsalis. Brain 1934; 57:25–31.

23. Lister GD, Belsole RB, Kleinert HE. The radial tunnel syndrome. J Hand Surg 1979; 4:52–59.

24. Framm CJ, Peters BH. Unusual cause of nerve entrapment. JAMA 1979; 242:2557–2558.

25. Werner CO, Haeffner F, Rosen I. Direct recording of local pressure in the radial tunnel during passive stretch and active contraction of the supinator muscle. Arch Orthop Traumat Surg 1980; 96:299–301.

26. Mumenthaler M, Schiack H. Lasionen peripherer Nerven. Stuttgart: Georg Thieme Verlag, 1965:220.

27. Blom LS, Hele P, Porkman L. The supinator channel syndrome. Scand J Plast Reconstr Surg 1971; 5:71–73.

28. Spinner M. The arcade of Frohse and its relationship to posterior interosseous nerve paralysis. J Bone Joint Surg (Br) 1968; 50:809–812.

29. Roles NC, Maudsley RH. Radial tunnel syndrome. J Bone Joint Surg (Br) 1972; 54:499–508.

30. DeZanche L, Negrin P, Fardin P, et al. Paralysis of the deep branch of the radial nerve due to an entrapment neuropathy. Eur Neurol 1978; 17:56–59.

31. Kopell HP, Thompson WAL. Peripheral entrapment neuropathies. Baltimore: Williams & Wilkins. 1963:121–128.

32. Inove Y, Suzuki N, Saito T, et al. Entrapment neuropathy of radial nerve: A review of 4 cases. Nagoya Med 1971; 17:15–24.

33. Goldman S, Honet JC, Sobel R, et al. Posterior interosseous palsy in the absence of trauma. Arch Neurol 1969; 21:435–441.

34. Narakis AD, Crawford GP. Les aspects etipathoogeniques, cliniques, anatopathologiques, ainsi que le traitement chirugical dans l'epicondylite chronique. Ther Umscau 1977; 34:70–80.

35. Van Rossum J, Buruma OJS, Komphuisen HAC, et al. Tennis elbow—a radial tunnel syndrome? J Bone Joint Surg (Br) 1978; 60:197–198.

36. Makin GJV, Brown WF. Entrapment of the posterior cutaneous nerve of the arm. Neurology 1985; 35:1677–1678.

37. Agnew. Bursal tumour producing loss of power of forearm. Am J Med Soc 1863; 46:404–405.

38. Weinberger LM. Non-traumatic paralysis of the dorsal interosseous nerve. Surg Gynecol Obstet 1939; 69:358–363.

39. Kruse F. Paralysis to the dorsal interosseous nerve not due to direct trauma. Neurology 1958; 8:307–308.

40. Marmor L, Lawrence JF, Dubois EL. Posterior interosseous nerve palsy due to rheumatoid arthritis. J Bone Joint Surg 1967; 49-A:381–383.

41. Chang LW, Gowens JDC, Granger CU, et al. Entrapment neuropathy of the posterior interosseous nerve. Arthritis Rheum 1972; 15:350–352.

42. Milender LH, Naleboff EA, Holdsworth DE. Posterior interosseous nerve syndrome secondary to rheumatoid arthritis. J Bone Joint Surg (Am) 1973; 55:753–757.

43. Fernandes L, Goodwin CH, Srivatsa SR. Synovial rupture of rheumatoid elbow causing radial nerve compression. Br Med J 1979; 2:17–18.

44. Rask MR. Superficial radial neuritis and DeQuervain's disease. Clin Orthop 1978; 131:176–178.

45. Campbell CS, Wulf RF. Lipoma producing a lesion of the deep branch of the radial nerve. J Neurosurg 1954; 11:310–311.

46. Richmond DA. Lipoma causing a posterior interosseous nerve lesion. J Bone Joint Surg (Br) 1953; 35:83.

47. Hustead AP, Mulder DW, MacCarty CS. Non-traumatic, progressive paralysis of the deep radial (posterior interosseous) nerve. Arch Neurol Psychiatry 1958; 79:269–274.

48. White WL, Hanna DC. Troublesome lipomata of the upper extremity. J Bone Joint Surg (Am) 1962; 44:1353–1359.

49. Moon N, Marmer L. Parosteal lipoma of the proximal part of the radius. J Bone Joint Surg (Am) 1964; 46:608–614.

50. Capener N. The vulnerability of the posterior interosseous nerve of the forearm. J Bone Joint Surg 1966; 48-B:770–773.

51. Kwang-Tzen W, Jordan FR, Eckert C. Lipoma, a cause of paralysis of deep radical (posterior interosseous) nerve: Report of a case and review of the literature. Surgery 1974; 75:790–795.

52. Phalen GS, Kendrick JI, Rodriguez JM. Lipomas of the upper extremity. Am J Surg 1971; 121:298–306.

53. Ostenasek FJ. Progressive paralysis of the nervus interosseous dorsalis: Pathological findings in one case. John Hopkins Hosp Bull 1947; 81:163–167.

54. Whiteley WH, Alpers BJ. Posterior interosseous nerve palsy with spontaneous neuroma formation. Arch Neurol 1959; 1:226–229.

55. Mulholland RC. Non-traumatic progressive paralysis of the posterior interosseous nerve. J Bone Joint Surg (Br) 1966; 48:781–785.

56. Sharrard WJW. Posterior interosseous acuratis. J Bone Joint Surg 1966; 4:777–780.

57. Barber KW, Bianco AJ, Soule EH, Maclarty CS. Benign extraneural soft-tissue tumors of the extremities causing compression of nerves. J Bone Joint Surg (Am) 1962; 44:98–104.

58. Hecht OA, Hass A. Regional multiplicity of a neurilemoma. Hand 1982; 1:97–99.

59. Herrick RT, Godsil RD Jr, Widener JH. Lipomatous hamartoma of the radial nerve: A case report. J Hand Surg 1980; 5:211–213.

60. Usui M, Ishii S, Yamawaki S, et al. Malignant granular cell tumor of the radial nerve. Cancer 1977; 39:1547–1555.

61. Bricklin AS, Rushton HW. Angiosarcoma of venous origin arising in radial nerve. Cancer 1977; 39:1556–1558.

62. Bowen T, Stone KH. Posterior interosseous nerve paralysis caused by a ganglion at the elbow. J Bone Joint Surg 1966; 48B:774.

63. Hermansdorfer JD, Greider JL, Dell PC. A case report of a compressive neuropathy of the radial sensory nerve caused by a ganglion cyst at the elbow. Orthopedics 1986; 9:1005–1006.

64. Shaw JL, Sakellarides H. Radial nerve paralysis associated with fractures of the humerus. J Bone Joint Surg (Am) 1967; 49:899–902.

65. Martin DF, Tolo VT, Sellers DS, et al. Radial nerve laceration and retraction associated with a supracondylar fracture of the humerus. J Hand Surg 1989; 14A:542–545.

66. Parker JW, Foster RR, Garcia A, et al. The humeral fracture with radial nerve palsy: Is exploration warranted? Clin Orthop 1972; 88:34–38.

67. Kettelkamp DB, Alexander H. Clinical review of radial nerve injury. J Trauma 1967; 7:424–432.

68. Shah JJ, Bhatti NA. Radial nerve paralysis associated with fractures of the humerus. Clin Orthop 1983; 172:171–176.

69. Seddon JH. Surgical disorders of peripheral nerves. Edinburgh: Churchill Livingstone, 1975.

70. Holstein A, Lewis G. Fractures of the humerus with radial nerve paralysis. J Bone Joint Surg (Am) 1963; 45:1382–1388.

71. Stein F, Grabias LSL, Deffer PA. Nerve injuries complicating Monteggia lesions. J Bone Joint Surg (Am) 1971; 53:1432–1436.

72. Spar I. Neurological complications following Monteggia fracture. Clin Orthop 1977; 122:207–209.

73. Smith FM. Monteggia fractures. Surg Gynecol Obstet 1947; 85:630–640.

74. Spinner M, Freundlich BD, Teicher J. Posterior interosseous nerve palsy as a complication of Monteggia fractures in children. Clin Orthop 1968; 58:141–145.

75. Boyd HB, Boals JC. The Monteggia lesion. Clin Orthop 1969; 66:94–100.

76. Adams JP, Rizzoli HV. Tardy radial and ulnar nerve palsy. J Neurosurg 1959; 16:342–344.

77. Sharrard WJW. Posterior interosseous neuritis. J Bone Joint Surg (Br) 1966; 48:777–780.

78. Lichter RL, Jacobsen T. Tardy palsy of the posterior interosseous nerve with a Monteggia fracture. J Bone Joint Surg (Am) 1975; 57:124–125.

79. Edwards LWC, Lamar LF. Radial nerve palsy following venipuncture. J Hand Surg 1981; 5:468–469.

80. Thomas MA, Fast A, Shapiro D. Radial nerve damage as a complication of elbow arthroscopy. Clin Orthop 1987; 215:130–131.

81. Hirasawa Y, Inove A, Ban S, et al. Radial nerve paralysis caused by drug injection. Arch Jap Chir 1980; 49:129–134.

82. Strachen JCH, Ellis BW. Vulnerability of the posterior interosseous nerve during radial head resection. J Bone Joint Surg (Br) 1971; 53:320–323.

83. Belsole RJ, Lister GD, Kleinert HE. Polyarteritis: A cause of nerve palsy in the extremity. J Hand Surg 1978; 3:320–325.

84. Anita MH, Mehta L, Shetty V, et al. Clinical, electrophysiological, quantitative, histological and ultrastructural studies of the index branch of the radial cutaneous nerve in leprosy. Int J Lepr 1975 43:106–113.

85. Goldstein NP, McCall JT, Dyck PJ. Metal neuropathy. In: Dyck PJ, Thomas PK, Lambert EH, eds. Peripheral neuropathy. Philadelphia: WB Saunders, 1975:1227–1262.

86. Smith HL. Two cases of obstetrical paralysis involving only the musculospinal nerve. Am J Dis Child 1916; 11:333–341.

87. Morgan L. Radial nerve palsies in the newborn. Arch Dis Child 1948; 23:137–139.

88. Feldman GV. Radial nerve palsies in the newborn. Arch Dis Child 1957; 32:469–471.

89. Craig WS, Clark JMP. Of peripheral nerve palsies in

the newly born. J Obstet Gynecol Br Emp 1958; 65:229–237.

90. Coppotelli BA, Lonsdale JD, Kass E. Sclerna neonatorum complicated by radial nerve palsy following nontraumatic delivery. Mt Sinai J Med 1979; 46:143–144.

91. Dejerine MM, Bernheim. Sur un cas de paralysie radiale par compression, suivi d'autopsie. Rev Neurol 1989; 7:785–788.

92. Harvey AM, Kuffler LSW. Motor nerve function with lesions of the peripheral nerves. Arch Neurol Psychiatry 1944; 52:317–322.

93. Hodes R, Larrabee MG, German W. The human electromyogram in response to nerve stimulation and the conduction velocity of motor axons. Arch Neurol Psychiatry 1948; 60:340–365.

94. Marinacci AA, Rand CW. Electromyogram in peripheral nerve complications following general surgical procedures. West J Surg Obstet Gynecol 1959; 67:199–204.

95. Bouwens P. Electrodiagnosis revisited. Tenth John Stanley Coulter Memorial Lecture. Arch Phys Med Rehab 1961; 42:6–18.

96. Gassel MM. A test of nerve conduction to muscles to the shoulder girdle as an aid in the diagnosis of proximal neurogenic and muscular disease. J Neurol Neurosurg Psychiatry 1964; 27:200–205.

97. Gassel MM, Diamantopoulos IE. Patterns of conduction times in the distribution of the radial nerve. Neurology 1964; 14:222–231.

98. Trojaborg W, Sindrup EH. Motor and sensory conduction in different segments of the radial nerve in normal subjects. J Neurol Neurosurg Psychiatry 1969; 32:354–359.

99. Jebsen RH. Motor conduction velocity in proximal and distal segments of the radial nerve in normal subjects. Arch Phys Med Rehab 1966; 47:12–16.

100. Jebsen RH. Motor conduction velocity in proximal and distal segments of the radial nerve. Arch Phys Med Rehab 1966; 47:597–602.

101. Kalantri A, Visser BD, Dumitru D, et al. Axilla to elbow radial nerve conduction. Muscle Nerve 1988; 11:133–135.

102. Downie NW, Scott TR. Radial nerve conduction studies. Neurology 1964; 14:839–843.

103. Downie AW, Scott TR. An improved technique for radial nerve conduction studies. J Neurol Neurosurg Psychiatry 1967; 30:332–336.

104. Buchthal F, Rosenfalck A. Evoked action potentials and conduction velocity in human sensory nerves. Brain Res 1966; 3:1–119.

105. Shahani B, Goodgold J, Spielholz JI. Sensory nerve action potentials in the radial nerve. Arch Phys Med Rehab 1967; 48:602–605.

106. Shirali CS, Sandler B. Radial nerve sensory conduction velocity: Measurement by antidromic technique. Arch Phys Med Rehab 1972; 53:457–460.

107. Feibel A, Foca FJ. Sensory conduction of radial nerve. Arch Phys Med Rehab 1974; 55:314–316.

108. Critchlow JF, Seybold ME, Jablecki CJ. The superficial radial nerve: Techniques for evaluation. J Neurol Neurosurg Psychiatry 1980; 43:929–933.

109. MacKenzie K, DeLisa JA. Distal sensory latency measurement of the superficial radial nerve in normal subjects. Arch Phys Med Rehab 1981; 62:31–34.

110. Ma CM, Kim SH, Spielholtz M, et al. Sensory conduction study of distal radial nerve. Arch Phys Med Rehab 1981; 62:562–564.

111. Spindler HA, Dellon AL. Nerve conduction studies in the superficial radial nerve entrapment syndrome. Muscle Nerve 1990; 13:1–5.

112. Dylewska D. Conduction in sensory nerve fibers of the radial nerve in healthy subjects. Neurol Neurochem (Pol) 1972; 8:513–519.

113. Vandenriessche G, Vonhecke J, Roselle N. Normal sensory conduction in the distal segments of the median and radial nerve: Relation to age. Electromyogr Clin Neurophysiol 1981; 21:511–519.

114. Buchthal F, Rosenfalck A, Behse F. Sensory potentials of normal and diseased nerves. In: Dyck PJ, Thomas PK, Lambert ED, eds. Peripheral neuropathy. Philadelphia: WB Saunders, 1975:442–464.

115. Tackmann W, Spalke G, Oginszus HJ. Quantitative histometric studies and relation of number and diameter of myelinated fibers to electrophysiological parameters in normal sensory nerves of man. J Neurol 1976; 212:71–84.

116. Ma DM, Liveson JA. Nerve conduction handbook. Philadelphia: FA Davis, 1983.

117. Trojaborg W. Rate of recovery in motor and sensory fibers of the radial nerve: Clinical and electrophysiological aspects. J Neurol Neurosurg Psychiatry 1970; 33:625–638.

118. Negrin P, Fardin P. "Sleep paralysis" of the radial nerve: Clinical and electromyographic evaluation of 10 cases. Electromyogr Clin Neurophysiol 1979; 19:435–441.

119. Rosen I, Werner CO. Neurophysiological investigation of posterior interosseous nerve entrapment causing lateral elbow pain. Electromyogr Clin Neurophysiol 1980; 50:125–133.

120. Falck B, Hurme M. Conduction velocity of the posterior interosseous nerve across the arcade of Frohse. Electromyogr Clin Neurophysiol 1983; 23:567–576.

121. Dolene V, Trontelj JV, Tonko M. Neurophysiological evaluation of microsurgically implanted nerves bridging peripheral nerve defaults. Acta Neurochir 1979; 28(suppl):608–612.

122. Smith J. Radial nerve conduction in patients with carpal tunnel syndrome. Appl Neurophysiol 1981; 44:363–367.

123. Shetty VP, Mehta LN, Irani PF, et al. Study of evo-

lution of nerve damage in leprosy. Lepr India 1980; 52:19–25.

124. Ross D, Jones R Jr, Fisher J, et al. Isolated radial nerve lesion in the newborn. Neurology (Cleve) 1983; 33:1354–1356.

125. Sunderland S. Nerves and nerve injuries. New York: Churchill Livingstone, 1978:769–801.

126. Garland DE, Thompson R, Waters RL. Musculocutaneous neurotomy for spastic elbow flexion in nonfunctional upper extremities in adults. J Bone Joint Surg (Am) 1980; 62:108–112.

127. Bateman JE. Nerve injuries about the shoulder in sports. J Bone Joint Surg (Am) 1967; 47:785–792.

128. Blom S, Dahlback LO. Nerve injuries in dislocations of the shoulder joint and fractures of the neck of the humerus. Acta Chir Scand 1970; 136:461–466.

129. Milton GW. The mechanism of circumflex and other nerve injuries in dislocation of the shoulder, and the possible mechanism of nerve injuries during reduction of dislocation. Aust J Surg 1953; 23:25–30.

130. Batey MR, Makin GS. Neurovascular traction injuries of the upper limb roof. Br J Surg 1982; 69:35–37.

131. Trojaborg W. Motor and sensory conduction in the musculocutaneous nerve. J Neurol Neurosurg Psychiatry 1976; 39:890–899.

132. Braddom RL, Wolfe C. Musculocutaneous nerve injury after heavy exercise. Arch Phys Med Rehab 1978; 59:290.

133. Ewing MR. Postoperative paralysis in the upper extremity. Lancet 1959; 1:99–103.

134. Zeuk VW, Heidrich R. Pathogenese der isolilerten, post-operative Lahmung des Nerves musculocutaneous. Schweiz Arch Neurol Neurochir Psychiatry 1974; 114:289–294.

135. Dundore DE, DeLisa JA. Musculocutaneous nerve palsy: An isolated complication of surgery. Arch Phys Med Rehab 1979; 60:130–133.

136. Hale BR. Handbag paresthesia. Lancet 1976; 2:470.

137. Bassett III FH, Nunley JA. Compression of the musculocutaneous nerve at the elbow. J Bone Joint Surg (Am) 1982; 62:1050–1052.

138. Aziz MA. Muscular and other abnormalities in a case of Edward's syndrome (18-Trisomy). Teratology 1979; 20:303–312.

139. Redford WJB. Conduction time in motor fibers of nerves which innervate proximal muscles of extremities in normal persons and in patients with neuromuscular disease. University of Minnesota: Thesis, 1958.

140. Coers C, Woolf AL. The innervation of muscle. Oxford: Blackwell, 1959.

141. Vacek J, Drugova B. Proximal amyotrophy EMG stimulation of Erb's point. Cesk Neurol 1967; 30:183–190.

142. Kraft GH. Axillary, musculocutaneous, and suprascapular nerve latency studies. Arch Phys Med Rehab 1972; 53:383–387.

143. Nelson RM, Curier DP. Motor conduction velocity

144. Spindler HA, Felsenthal G. Sensory conduction in the musculocutaneous nerve. Arch Phys Med Rehab 1978; 59:20–23.

145. Izzo KL, Aravabhumi S, Jafri A, et al. Medial and lateral antebrachial cutaneous nerves: Standardization of technique, reliability and age effect on healthy subjects. Arch Phys Med Rehab 1985; 66:592–597.

146. Staples OS, Watkins AL. Full active abduction with traumatic paralysis of the deltoid. J Bone Joint Surg (Am) 1943; 25:85–89.

147. Wynn Parry CB. Shoulder abduction with deltoid paralysis. Ann Phys Med 1953; 2:178–179.

148. Dehne E, Hall RM. Active shoulder motion in complete deltoid paralysis. J Bone Joint Surg (Am) 1959; 41:745–748.

149. Babcock JL, Wray JB. Analysis of abduction in a shoulder with deltoid paralysis due to axillary nerve injury. Clin Orthop 1970; 68:116–120.

150. Sunderland S. Nerves and nerve injuries. New York: Churchill Livingstone, 1978:843–848.

151. Berry H, Bril V. Axillary nerve palsy following blunt trauma to the shoulder region: A clinical and electrophysiological review. J Neurol Neurosurg Psychiatry 1982; 45:1027–1032.

152. McGahan JP, Rab GT. Fracture of the acromion associated with an axillary nerve deficit. Clin Orthop 1980; 147:216–218.

153. Pasila M, Jaroma H, Kiviluoto O, et al. Early complications of primary shoulder dislocations. Acta Orthop Scand 1978; 49:260–263.

154. Bateman JE. Nerve lesions about the shoulder. Orthop Clin North Am 1980; 11:307–326.

155. Leffert RD, Seddon H. Infraclavicular brachial plexus injuries. J Bone Joint Surg (Br) 1956; 47:9–22.

156. Kirby JF, Kraft GH. Entrapment neuropathy of anterior branch of axillary nerve: Report of case. Arch Phys Med Rehab 1972; 53:383–387.

157. Chill BR, Palmer RE. Quadrilateral space syndrome. J Hand Surg 1983; 8:65–69.

158. Petrucci FS, Morelli A, Raimondi PL. Axillary nerve injuries—21 cases treated by nerve graft and neurolysis. J Hand Surg 1982; 7:271–287.

159. Horiguchi M. The cutaneous branch of some human suprascapular nerves. J Anat 1980; 130:191–195.

160. Solheim LF, Roaas A. Compression of the suprascapular nerve after fracture of the scapular notch. Acta Orthop Scand 1978; 49:338–340.

161. Zoltan JD. Injury to the suprascapular nerve associated with anterior dislocation of the shoulder: Case report and review of the literature. J Trauma 1979; 19:203–206.

162. Toon TN, Bravois M, Guillen M. Suprascapular nerve injury following trauma to the shoulder. J Trauma 1981; 21:652–655.

of the musculocutaneous nerve. Phys Ther 1969; 49:586–589.

163. Kopell HP, Thompson WAL. Pain and the frozen shoulder. Surg Gynecol Obstet 1959; 109:92–96.

164. Kopell HP, Thompson WAL. Peripheral entrapment neuropathies. Baltimore: Williams & Wilkins, 1963:130–142.

165. Clein LJ. Suprascapular entrapment neuropathy. J Neurosurg 1975; 43:337–342.

166. Rask MR. Suprascapular nerve entrapment: A report of two cases treated with suprascapular notch resection. Clin Orthop 1977; 123:73–75.

167. Reid AC, Hazelton RA. Suprascapular nerve entrapment in the differential diagnosis of shoulder pain. Lancet 1979; 2:477.

168. Gelmers HJ, Guys DA. Suprascapular entrapment neuropathy. Acta Neurochir 1977; 38:121–124.

169. Swafford AR, Lichtman DH. Suprascapular nerve entrapment—case report. J Hand Surg 1982; 7:57–60.

170. Garcia G, McQueen D. Bilateral suprascapular nerve entrapment syndrome. J Bone Joint Surg (Am) 1981; 63:491–492.

171. Rengachary SS, Bur D, Lucas S, et al. Suprascapular entrapment neuropathy: A clinical, anatomical, and comparative study. Neurosurgery 1979; 5:447–451.

172. Donovan WH, Kraft GH. Rotator cuff tear versus suprascapular nerve injury—a problem in differential diagnosis. Arch Phys Med Rehab 1974; 55:424–428.

173. Ailello I, Serra G, Traina GC, et al. Entrapment of the suprascapular nerve injury—a problem in differential diagnosis. Arch Phys Med Rehab 1974; 55:424–428.

174. Kiss G, Komar J. Suprascapular nerve compression at the spinoglenoid notch. Muscle Nerve 1990; 13:556–557.

175. Ganzhorn RW, Hacker JT, Horowitz M, et al. Suprascapular nerve entrapment. J Bone Joint Surg (Am) 1981; 63:492–494.

176. Thompson RC, Schneider W, Kennedy T. Entrapment neurology of the inferior branch of the suprascapular nerve by ganglia. Clin Orthop 1982; 166:185–187.

177. Swift TR. Involvement of peripheral nerves in radical neck dissection. Am J Surg 1970; 119:694–698.

178. Ringel SP, Treihaft M, Carry M, et al. Suprascapular neuropathy in pitchers. Am J Sports Med 1990; 18:80–86.

179. Khalili AA. Neuromuscular electrodiagnostic studies in entrapment neuropathy of the suprascapular nerve. Orthop Rev 1974; 3:27–28.

180. Inouye Y. Conduction along the articular branch of the suprascapular nerve. Acta Neurol Scand 1978; 58:230–240.

181. Horowitz MT, Tocantins LM. An anatomical study of the role of the long thoracic nerve and the related scapular bursae in the pathogenesis of local paralysis of the serratus anterior muscle. Anat Rec 1938; 71:375–385.

182. Velpeau AALM. Traite d'anatomie chirugicale, ou anatomie des regions, consideree dans ses rapports avec la chirugie. Paris: Crevot, 1825.

183. Skillern PG. Serratus magnus palsy with proposal of a new operation for intractable cases. Ann Surg 1913; 57:909–915.

184. Overpeck DO, Ghormley RK. Paralysis of the serratus magnus muscle. JAMA 1940; 1994–1996.

185. Ellis JD. Delayed traumatic serratus paralysis. Arch Neurol Psychiatry 1929; 22:1233–1236.

186. Goodman CE, Kenrick MM, Blum MV. Long thoracic nerve palsy: A follow-up study. Arch Phys Med Rehab 1975; 56:352–355.

187. Gonza ER, Harris WR. Traumatic winging of the scapula. J Bone Joint Surg (Am) 1979; 61:1230–1233.

188. Shah K, Stefaniwesky L. Long thoracic nerve palsy: Case report. Arch Phys Med Rehab 1982; 62:585–586.

189. Gregg JR, Labosky D, Harty M, et al. Serratus anterior paralysis in the young athlete. J Bone Joint Surg (Am) 1979; 61:825–832.

190. Ilfeld FW, Holder HG. Winged scapula: Case occurring in shoulder from a knapsack. JAMA 1942; 120:448–449.

191. Potts CS. Isolated paralysis of the serratus magnus. Arch Neurol Psychiatry 1928; 20:184–186.

192. Thorek M. Compression paralysis of the long thoracic nerve following an abdominal operation. Ann J Surg 1926; 40:26–27.

193. Lorhan PH. Isolated paralysis at the serratus magnus following surgical procedures. Arch Surg 1957; 54:656–659.

194. Wood VE, Frykman GK. Winging of the scapula as a complication of first rib resection. Clin Orthop 1980; 149:160–163.

195. Radin EL. Peripheral neuritis as a complication of infectious mononucleosis. J Bone Joint Surg (Am) 1967; 49:533–538.

196. Hammond SR, Danta G. A clinical and electrophysiological study of neurogenically induced winging of the scapula. Clin Exp Neurol 1981; 17:153–166.

197. Kaplan PE. Electrodiagnosis confirming of long thoracic nerve palsy. J Neurol Neurosurg Psychiatry 1980; 43:50–52.

198. Petera JE, Trojaborg W. Conduction studies of the long thoracic nerve in serratus anterior palsy of different etiology. Neurology (Cleve) 1984; 34:1033–1037.

199. Nobel W. Serratus anterior palsy stimulating Sprengel's deformity. Bull Hosp Joint Dis 1946; 7:51–58.

200. Fahrer H, Ludin HP, Mumenthaler M, et al. The innervation of the trapezius muscle. J Neurol 1974; 207:183–188.

201. Logigian EL, McInnes JM, Berger AR, et al. Stretch-induced spinal accessory nerve palsy. Muscle Nerve 1988; 11:146–150.

202. Seddon H. Surgical disorders of the peripheral nerves. New York: Churchill Livingstone, 1975.

203. Brunnstrom S. Muscle testing around the shoulder girdle. J Bone Joint Surg (Am) 1941; 23:263–272.
204. Wulff HB. The treatment of tuberculous cervical lymphoma: Late results in 230 cases treated partly surgically, partly radiographically. Acta Chir Scand 1941; 84:343–366.
205. Norden A. Peripheral injuries to the spinal accessory nerve. Acta Chir Scand 1946; 94:512–532.
206. Mead S. Posterior triangle operations and trapezius paralysis. Arch Surg 1952; 64:752–756.
207. Woodhall B. Operative injury to the accessory nerve in the posterior cervical triangle. Ann Surg 1952; 136:375–380.
208. Woodhall B. Operative injury to the accessory nerve in the posterior cervical triangle. AMA Arch Surg 1957; 74:122–127.
209. Schneck SA. Peripheral and cranial nerve injuries resulting from general surgical procedures. AMA Arch Surg 1960; 81:855–859.
210. Gordon SL, Graham WP, Black JT, et al. Accessory nerve function after surgical procedures in the posterior triangle. Arch Surg 1977; 112:264–268.
211. Olarte M, Adams D. Accessory nerve palsy. J Neurol Neurosurg Psychiatry 1977; 40:1113–1116.
212. Saeed MA, Gatens PF. Winging of the scapula. Am Fam Phys 1981; 24:139–143.
213. Saeed MA, Gatens PF. Accessory nerve palsy—a hazard of lymph node biopsy: Case reports. Milit Med 1982; 147:586–588.
214. King RJ, Motta G. Iatrogenic spinal accessory nerve palsy. Ann R Coll Surg 1983; 65:35–37.
215. Sarala PK. Accessory nerve palsy: An uncommon etiology. Arch Phys Med Rehab 1982; 63:445–446.
216. Valtonen EJ, Lilius HG. Late sequelae of iatrogenic spinal accessory nerve injury. Acta Chir Scand 1974; 140:453–455.
217. Cherrington M, Hendee R, Roland R. Accessory nerve palsy—a painful cranial neuropathy: Surgical cure. Headache 1978; 18:274–275.
218. Roy PH, Beahrs OH. Spinal accessory nerve in radial nerve dissections. Am J Surg 1969; 116:800–804.
219. Carenfelt C, Eliasson K. Occurrence, duration and prognosis of unexpected accessory nerve paresis in radical neck dissection. Acta Otolaryngol 1980; 90:470–473.
220. Carenfelt C, Eliasson K. Cervical metastases following radical neck dissection that preserved the spinal accessory nerve. Head Neck Surg 1980; 2:181–184.
221. Brandenburg JH, Lee CYS. The eleventh nerve in radial neck surgery. Laryngoscope 1981; 91:1851–1859.
222. Pearlman NW, Meyers AD, Sullivan WG. Modified radical neck dissection for squamous carcinoma of the head and neck. Surg Gynecol Obstet 1982; 154:214–216.
223. Patterson WR. Inferior dislocation of the distal end of the clavicle. J Bone Joint Surg (Am) 1967; 49:1184–1186.
224. Woodruff AW. Unilateral spinal accessory nerve palsy caused by an arm sling. Br Med J 1959; 2:821–822.
225. Singh S, Schlagenhauff RE. Pressure palsy of accessory nerve. Neurol India 1971; 19:122–125.
226. Pajarvi L, Partenen J. Biting palsy of the accessory nerve. J Neurol Neurosurg Psychiatry 1980; 43:744–746.
227. Morrell S, Roberson JR, Rooks MD. Accessory nerve palsy following thoracotomy. Clin Orthop 1989; 103:237–240.
228. Spillane JD. Isolated unilateral spinal accessory nerve palsy of obscure origin. Br Med J 1949; 2:365–366.
229. Eisen A, Bertrand G. Isolated accessory nerve palsy of spontaneous origin. Arch Neurol 1972; 27:496–502.
230. Laha RK, Panchal P. Isolated accessory nerve palsy. South Med J 1979; 72:1005–1007.
231. Doriguzzi C, Palmucci L, Troni W. Isolated accessory nerve palsy: Case report. Ital J Neurol Sci 1982; 2:135–138.
232. Robbins TK, Fenton RS. Jugular foramen syndrome. J Otolaryngol 1980; 9:505–516.
233. Skorpil V, Zverina E. The speed of conduction in the cranial nerves in man (in Czech). Cesk Neurol 1963; 26:152–157.
234. Cherrington M. Accessory nerve conduction studies. Arch Neurol 1968; 18:708–709.
235. Eisen A, Bertrand G. Isolated accessory nerve palsy of spontaneous origin. Arch Neurol 1972; 27:496–502.
236. Krongness K. Serial conduction studies of the spinal accessory nerve used as a prognostic tool in a lesion caused by a lymph node biopsy. Acta Chir Scand 1974; 140:7–11.
237. Green RF, Brien M. Accessory nerve latency to the middle and lower trapezius. Arch Phys Med Rehabil 1985; 66:23–24.
238. Shankar K, Means KM. Accessory nerve conduction in neck dissection subjects. Arch Phys Med Rehab 1990; 71:403–405.
239. Goodgold J. Anatomical correlates of clinical electromyography. Baltimore: Williams & Wilkins, 1974.
240. Delagi EF, Perotto A. Anatomical guide for the electromyographer. Springfield, IL: Charles C. Thomas, 1975.
241. Kopell HP, Thompson WAL. Peripheral entrapment neuropathies. Baltimore: Williams & Wilkins, 1974.
242. Scanlon EF. The importance of the anterior thoracic nerves in modified radical mastectomy. Surg Gynecol Obstet 1981; 152:789–791.
243. Pribyl R, You SB, Jantra P. Sensory nerve conduction velocity of the medial antebrachial cutaneous nerve. Electromyogr Clin Neurophysiol 1979; 19:41–46.
244. Reddy MP. Conduction studies of medial cutaneous nerve of forearm. Arch Phys Med Rehab 1983; 64:209–211.

12

Mononeuropathies of the Lower Extremities

John D. Stewart

CONTENTS

ACRONYMS

CT   computed tomography
MRI   magnetic resonance imaging
EMG   electromyography
ALS   amyotrophic lateral sclerosis
EDB   extensor digitorum brevis

The nerves to the legs arise from the spinal nerve roots L-1–S-3. Those from L-2, L-3, L-4 form the lumbar plexus from which are derived the femoral and obturator nerves and the lateral cutaneous nerve of the thigh (see Fig. 12.6). Some of the L-4 nerve fibers join those from L-5 to form the lumbosacral trunk. This crosses into the pelvis to form with spinal nerves S-1–S-3, the sacral plexus (see Fig. 8.5). The principal nerve from the sacral plexus is the sciatic nerve, which divides into the common peroneal and the tibial nerves. Other nerves arising from the sacral plexus are the two gluteal nerves, the posterior cutaneous nerve of the thigh, and the pudendal nerve.

In the evaluation of patients with a possible peripheral nerve lesion in the leg, it is important to keep in mind the differential diagnosis of *radiculopathy* (see Chapter 7) versus *plexopathy* (see Chapter 8) versus *individual mononeuropathy,* versus *mononeuropathy multiplex*—involvement of more than one individual peripheral nerve. In addition, disorders of the anterior horn cells such as amyotrophic lateral sclerosis and polio may present as focal weakness in one or both legs. Occasionally central nervous system disorders such as a unilateral lesion of the corticospinal tracts or a focal dystonia may masquerade as a peripheral neurologic lesion.

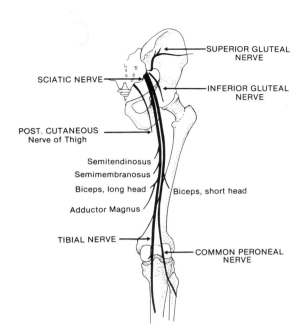

FIGURE 12.1. *Posterior view of the course and branches of the sciatic nerve. (Reprinted with permission from Stewart JD. Focal peripheral neuropathies. New York: Elsevier Science Publishing, 1987:273.)*

SCIATIC NERVE

Anatomy

The sciatic nerve is formed from the sacral plexus and contains nerve fibers from L-4, L-5, S-1, and S-2 spinal nerve roots. It leaves the pelvis through the sciatic notch along with the superior and inferior gluteal nerves and the posterior cutaneous nerve of the thigh (Figure 12.1). The sciatic nerve usually passes below the piriformis muscle, but the whole nerve, or more commonly one of its trunks, may pass over or through this muscle. It courses behind the hip joint and then deep in the thigh. The sciatic nerve is made up of two *trunks,* the medial and the lateral. The medial becomes the tibial nerve, whereas the lateral forms the common peroneal nerve. The two trunks normally diverge in the upper popliteal fossa.

All of the hamstring muscles are supplied by branches from the medial trunk of the sciatic nerve with one exception, the short head of the biceps femoris; this is supplied by the only branch arising from the lateral trunk. This branch is very important

to the electromyographer, as is discussed later. Neither trunk gives off sensory branches.

Disorders

Most sciatic nerve lesions result from trauma such as fracture-dislocations of the hip joint and as complications of hip replacement procedures[1–10] (Table 12.1). Misplaced injections can also damage the nerve. *External compression* occurs mainly during coma, anesthesia, protracted periods of confinement in bed, and prolonged sitting on a hard edge.[9,10] Constriction of the nerve can result from muscle fibrosis following injections and scarring in the region of the ischial tuberosity.[11,12] Several deep masses can involve or compress the nerve. Endometriosis can damage the sciatic nerve within the pelvis, at the sciatic notch, or more distally in the thigh.[13,14] Other masses that can compress the nerve in the gluteal region include hematomas that may follow hip surgery, the use of anticoagulants, or both; lipomas; schwannomas; and gluteal artery aneurysms.[15–19]

The *piriformis syndrome* is a controversial entity.

TABLE 12.1.   Causes of sciatic neuropathy

In the sciatic notch/gluteal region
  Trauma
    Pelvic and hip joint fractures
    Missile wounds
  Hip surgery
  External compression
  Injection injury
  Compression from deeply situated lesions
    Endometriosis
    Hematoma
    Fibrosis
    Lipoma
    Aneurysms
  Schwannoma, neurofibroma
  Piriformis syndrome (?)
In the thigh
  Missile wounds
  Soft tissue injury
  Fractures of the femur
  External compression
  Hematoma
  Schwannoma, neurofibroma
  Myositis ossificans

The close and variable relationship between the sciatic nerve and the piriformis muscle in the sciatic notch has led to the suggestion that *sciatica* could result from nerve compression by this muscle.[20–24] Some of these reports antedate the use of myelography and computed tomography (CT) scanning, or these investigations were not done; these patients may well have had radiculopathy. Few patients alleged to have this syndrome have had significant neurologic deficits; indeed some authors have insisted that lack of neurologic deficit is an essential criterion for this diagnosis. Only two patients with electromyographic abnormalities in muscles innervated by the sciatic nerve have been described.[25,26] A number of patients have been explored surgically, and the findings, when described, have been unimpressive; no patients had an anatomic abnormality of the sciatic nerve and piriformis muscle. The symptoms, however, were allegedly relieved by division of the piriformis muscle in most of these patients.

Clinical Evaluation

In many patients, the site of the sciatic neuropathy is obvious from the history or examinations or both. An example is a patient with a fracture-dislocation of the hip. In other patients, it may not be at all obvious that the lesion is in the sciatic nerve or, even if it is, exactly where it lies.

A severe lesion of the sciatic nerve produces paralysis of the hamstring muscles and of all the muscles below the knee, with sensory loss in the distribution of the tibial and common peroneal nerves (see Figure 12.3). A very common occurrence is preferential involvement of the lateral rather than the medial trunk of the sciatic nerve.[17] One study of 68 sciatic neuropathies showed predominantly lateral trunk involvement in 57%, predominantly medial trunk in 9%, and both trunks equally affected in 34%.[27] The reason for this preferential involvement of the lateral trunk is not known with certainty. Sunderland[28] suggests two possibilities: Because this trunk contains larger fascicles and less connective tissue than the medial trunk, it has less tensile strength; the lateral trunk is more firmly fixed and angulated in the sciatic notch, and the common peroneal nerve is also quite firmly fixed at the fibular neck, so it may be less resistant to stretch than the medial trunk. The greater vulnerability of the lateral trunk has been noted in many different causes of sciatic neuropathies. This unequal and partial involvement has major clinical importance: A lesion exclusively of the lateral trunk of the sciatic nerve produces exactly the same clinical picture as a common peroneal neuropathy.

Examination of the leg should be aimed at determining first if the gluteal muscles are involved because weakness here indicates a lesion in L-5 or S-1 roots, sacral plexus, or very proximal sciatic nerve as it exits through the sciatic notch. Such a lesion of the nerve at the notch may be difficult to distinguish from a sacral plexopathy. Radiologic investigations, particularly CT scanning, are required to differentiate between these two entities.

A sciatic neuropathy in which the lateral trunk is chiefly or exclusively involved has to be distinguished from a common peroneal neuropathy. An example of such a situation is a patient with footdrop following hip surgery: Is the footdrop due to partial sciatic nerve damage during the surgery or to intraoperative pressure on the common peroneal nerve at the neck of the fibula? In examining such a patient, it is important to look for even minor motor, sensory, and reflex signs in the distribution of the tibial nerve; these would imply medial trunk involvement. In a common peroneal neuropathy, there may also be tenderness of the nerve at the fibular neck. The one muscle supplied by the lateral trunk above the knee, the short head of the biceps femoris, cannot be examined clinically, and electromyographic evaluation of this muscle is particularly helpful.

Some sciatic neuropathies, particularly those caused by misplaced injections, produce a lot of neuropathic pain in the leg and foot. The motor and sensory deficits may be very subtle and found only by careful examination.

Pelvic or rectal examinations sometimes reveal the cause of proximal sciatic neuropathies, or a mass may be palpable through the gluteus maximus muscle. Tenderness of the sciatic nerve in this area is not a useful sign because this may be found in patients with lumbar and sacral radiculopathies.

Investigations

Nerve conduction studies of the sciatic nerve are difficult to perform because the nerve lies so deeply that long needle electrodes are required to stimulate it proximally. Motor conduction studies of the peroneal and tibial nerves may show reduced amplitudes with minor conduction velocity changes, but these are of little localizing value. F wave latencies may be prolonged, although this may also be found in all other proximal lesions, including radiculopathies and plexopathies. Abnormal peroneal or sural compound sensory nerve action potentials show the lesion *not* to be a radiculopathy because in these the sensory nerves are damaged proximal to the dorsal root ganglia; therefore the distal segment of the sensory nerves remains intact.

Needle electromyographic studies are much more useful than nerve conductions in diagnosing and localizing sciatic neuropathies. Electromyography (EMG) of the paraspinal and gluteal muscles helps to distinguish a sciatic neuropathy from a radiculopathy and plexopathy. In distinguishing a lesion of the lateral trunk of the sciatic nerve from a common peroneal neuropathy, electromyographic abnormalities in the short head of the biceps femoris shows the lesion to be in the lateral trunk. Further evidence for sciatic neuropathy, even when predominantly affecting the lateral trunk, is the presence of electromyographic abnormalities in the muscles innervated by the medial trunk and tibial nerve as well as abnormal compound sensory nerve action potentials in the sural nerve.

CT scanning is useful for showing tumors and other masses in the pelvis and sciatic notch. CT scanning also shows a hematoma in some patients with sciatic neuropathy following hip replacement.

Magnetic resonance imaging (MRI) may be even more sensitive in detecting small nerve tumors.[29]

SUPERIOR AND INFERIOR GLUTEAL NERVES

Anatomy

The superior gluteal nerve (L-4, L-5, S-1) exits the pelvis through the sciatic notch deep to the gluteal muscles (see Figure 12.1). It turns rostrally to supply the gluteus medius and minimus and the tensor fascia lata muscles. The inferior gluteal nerve (L-5, S-1, S-2) also leaves the pelvis through the sciatic notch along with the superior gluteal and sciatic nerves, and supplies the gluteus maximus muscle.

Disorders

Because the superior gluteal nerve is the only nerve to pass through the sciatic notch above the piriformis muscle, it may be damaged when the other nerves of the sciatic notch are spared. This rare neuropathy usually results from misplaced injections. A single patient with entrapment of this nerve between the upper edge of the piriformis and the ilium has been reported; a previous fall on the buttock and a hip fracture may have caused muscle fibrosis. Surgical division of the muscle relieved the pain.[30]

The inferior gluteal nerve is almost always damaged in association with the sciatic and pudendal nerves or the posterior cutaneous nerve of the thigh. Mass lesions in the sciatic notch described earlier as damaging the sciatic nerve often also involve the inferior gluteal nerve. There is a report of patients with recurrent colorectal carcinoma compressing both the inferior gluteal nerve and the posterior cutaneous nerve of the thigh but not the sciatic nerve.[31]

Evaluation

Patients with superior gluteal neuropathies have wasting and weakness of the gluteus medius and minimus and tensor fascia lata muscles and no sensory abnormalities. An inferior gluteal nerve lesion produces wasting and weakness of the gluteus maximus muscle and no sensory loss. Electromyographic studies help to confirm that the lesion is restricted to an individual gluteal nerve or if there is coexisting damage to other nerves of the sciatic notch or of the sacral plexus. Imaging, particularly CT scanning of the pelvis, is useful in identifying mass lesions affecting these nerves.

POSTERIOR CUTANEOUS NERVE OF THE THIGH AND PUDENDAL NERVE

Anatomy

The posterior cutaneous nerve of the thigh (S-1–S-3) leaves the sciatic notch to supply the skin of the lower buttock and posterior thigh. The pudendal nerve (S-2–S-4) passes through the lower part of the sciatic notch and medially to the perineum. Motor fibers innervate the external anal sphincter, muscles of the perineum, erectile tissue of the penis, and the external urethral sphincter. Sensory fibers supply the skin of the perineum and genitalia.

Disorders

Posterior cutaneous nerve of the thigh lesions are rare and are caused by injections, pressure from prolonged cycling, and presacral tumors.[17] Injuries to the pudendal nerve are also rare. It can be damaged together with other nerves in this area by buttock injections and pelvic fractures. Both pudendal nerves may be damaged during operations for hip fractures. This has been attributed to pressure from the perineal post, a device that fits into the groin and allows traction to be applied to the leg during the operation.[32] Prolonged cycling can also compress these nerves.[33] The syndrome of idiopathic fecal continence has been attributed to stretch of the pudendal nerves resulting from the descent of the pelvic floor during childbirth or repeated straining during defecation.[34]

Evaluation

The symptom of a posterior cutaneous nerve of the thigh lesion is sensory disturbance in the posterior thigh. Pudendal neuropathy results in numbness of half or all of the penis (or the labia majora) and perineum, depending on the site of the nerve damage and whether one or both nerves are affected. Male patients may also have erectile impotence, although this may be due to additional damage to autonomic nerves or blood vessels rather than to the pudendal nerve itself.[35] Bulbocavernosus reflex testing and EMG of the external anal sphincter are methods that can be used to evaluate the pudendal nerves.[34,36]

COMMON PERONEAL NERVE

Anatomy

This nerve descends obliquely through the popliteal fossa to wind around the neck of the fibula (Figure 12.2). It then passes through the attachment of the superficial head of the peroneus longus muscle, the *fibular tunnel*, and divides into the superficial and deep peroneal nerves. The former innervates the per-

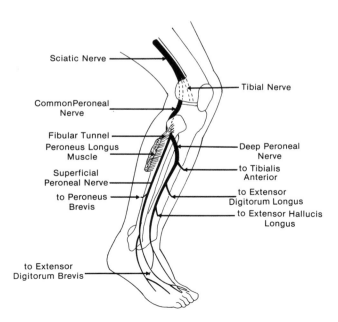

FIGURE 12.2. *Anterolateral view of the right leg showing the course, clinically relevant anatomic relations, and major branches of the common peroneal nerve. (Reprinted with permission from Stewart JD, Aguayo AJ. Compression and entrapment neuropathies. In: Dyck PJ, Thomas PK, Lambert EH, Bunge R, eds. Peripheral neuropathy, ed 2. Philadelphia, WB Saunders, 1984:1448.)*

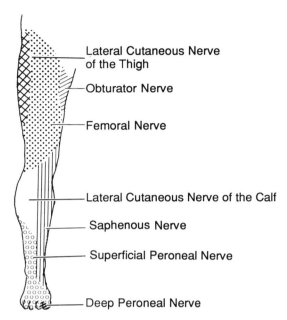

Lateral Cutaneous Nerve of the Thigh

Obturator Nerve

Femoral Nerve

Lateral Cutaneous Nerve of the Calf

Saphenous Nerve

Superficial Peroneal Nerve

Deep Peroneal Nerve

FIGURE 12.3. *Anterior view of the right leg to show the distribution of the major sensory nerves. (Reprinted with permission from Stewart JD, Aguayo AJ. Compression and entrapment neuropathies. In: Dyck PJ, Thomas PK, Lambert EH, Bunge R, eds. Peripheral neuropathy, ed 2. Philadelphia, WB Saunders, 1984:1448.)*

TABLE 12.2.   Causes of common peroneal neuropathy

External compression
During anesthesia, coma, sleep, bed rest
Plaster casts, braces
Habitual leg crossing
Sitting cross-legged
Prolonged squatting
Direct trauma
Blunt injuries, lacerations, gunshot wounds
Fractures of the fibula
Adduction injuries, dislocations of the knee
Surgical procedures in popliteal fossa and knee
Traction injuries
Acute plantar flexion-inversion injuries at the ankle, sprains, torn ligaments, fractures of lower tibia and fibula
Masses
Ganglia, Baker's cysts, fabella, hematomas, callus, fibular tumors, lipomas, osteomas, nerve sheath ganglia
Entrapment
In the fibular tunnel
Vascular conditions
Vasculitis, local vascular disease
Diabetes mellitus
Leprosy
Idiopathic

oneus longus, brevis, and tertius muscles and then continues as the superficial peroneal (sensory) nerve to supply the skin of the distal lateral leg and dorsum of the foot (Figure 12.3). The deep peroneal nerve runs in the anterior compartment of the leg then across the ankle into the dorsum of the foot. It supplies the dorsiflexors of the foot and toes: the tibialis anterior, extensor hallucis longus, extensor digitorum longus, and brevis muscles. Its terminal branch supplies the skin between the first and second toes (Figure 12.3). An additional sensory branch is the lateral cutaneous nerve of the calf, which arises from the peroneal nerve in the popliteal fossa.

Disorders

The common peroneal nerve is vulnerable to external compression in its course around the head and neck of the fibula (Table 12.2). This can occur during sleep, coma, anesthesia, and prolonged bed rest or from plaster casts, leg braces, and tight bandages around the knee.[17] Quite frequently there is no obvious cause. When symptoms of peroneal neuropathy are noticed on awakening from a night's sleep, the neuropathy is probably the result of sleeping in a position causing nerve compression. Habitual crossing of the legs may be another frequent cause, although this is such a common habit its role is hard to assess.[37] This is probably the cause in obese patients who have recently lost weight because obese persons cannot cross their legs and take pleasure in doing so when they have become slimmer.[38] Prolonged squatting, as in some gardening jobs, can also kink and compress the nerve.[39] The nerve may also be compressed by ganglia and cysts arising from the knee joint, lipomas, popliteal aneurysms, tumors of the fibular, or callus from old fibula fractures.[17]

Cadaver dissection studies have shown that sometimes the fibrous arch of the peroneus longus muscle that roofs the fibular tunnel is thick and tight.[40] True entrapment of the common peroneal nerve within this tunnel is probably rare,[41] although several such cases have been confirmed surgically, with improvement following division of the fibrous arch.

Common peroneal neuropathy may be noncompressive in etiology, as in diabetes,[42,43] vasculitis,[44,45] or leprosy. Most common peroneal neuropathies are benign disorders with no clear cause. Many probably result from pressure on the nerve during sleep or from habitual leg crossing.

The *deep peroneal nerve* is compressed by muscle swelling within the anterior compartment in the anterior tibial syndrome. This results from excessive exercise, trauma, occlusion of the anterior tibial artery or its parent trunk, or restoration of blood flow after acute arterial insufficiency of the leg.[46] The deep peroneal nerve may also be compressed by ganglia.[70]

Entrapment of the terminal branches of the *superficial peroneal nerve* where they pierce the deep fascia of the lower leg above the ankle has been described following minor trauma. These nerves may also be compressed by tight shoes.

Clinical Evaluation

A complete lesion of the common peroneal nerve leads to paralysis of dorsiflexion of the foot and toes and of eversion of the foot. A characteristic footdrop and slapping gait result. The sensory loss extends over the anterolateral surface of the lower leg and dorsum of the foot.

The motor and sensory deficits that occur in common peroneal neuropathies are often quite variable.[39,48] The muscles supplied by the deep branch are more frequently and more severely affected than those innervated by the superficial branch. The sensory loss varies from involving skin innervated by all three sensory branches of the nerve to no loss of sensation. The most likely explanation for these findings is differing degrees of damage to individual fascicles within the nerve.[48]

A common peroneal neuropathy must be distinguished from an L-5 radiculopathy, a lesion of the lumbosacral plexus, partial sciatic neuropathy, and amyotrophic lateral sclerosis. In an L-5 radiculopathy, there is weakness of the foot and toe dorsiflexor muscles and sensory abnormalities over the dorsum of the foot, but muscles supplied by L-5 through nerves other than the common peroneal, such as the gluteal muscles (superior and inferior gluteal nerves), and the invertor of the foot, tibialis posterior (tibial nerve), are also involved; the ankle reflex is often depressed owing to the frequent mild concomitant involvement of the S-1 root.

The lumbosacral trunk is the continuation of the L-5 spinal nerve root, joined by some of the fibers from L-4, that passes over the ala of the sacrum to join the sacral plexus. Damage to this trunk results from trauma to the posterior pelvis, pressure during prolonged childbirth, and from mass lesions in the pelvis.[17] Muscles innervated by L-5 via nerves other than the common peroneal (e.g., the tibialis posterior muscle) are involved in lumbosacral trunk lesions.

A proximal sciatic neuropathy principally affecting the lateral trunk may be almost indistinguishable from a common peroneal palsy, as discussed earlier. Amyotrophic lateral sclerosis can present with footdrop, but there is usually more extensive muscle weakness, hyperreflexia, and no sensory abnormalities. The anterior compartment syndrome is recognized by pain, swelling, and redness in the anterior lower leg, with motor and sensory dysfunction of the deep peroneal nerve.

It is important to examine the popliteal fossa carefully for mass lesions. Tenderness of the peroneal nerve, with or without Tinel's sign, is a useful sign of local damage to the nerve.

Investigations

The usual method of assessing motor nerve conduction is to record from the extensor digitorum brevis muscle while stimulating the nerve first at the ankle and then above and below the head of the fibula. Slowing or blocking of conduction is detected in up to two-thirds of patients with peroneal neuropathies.[49–51] This can be increased by stimulating the common peroneal nerve at more proximal sites within the popliteal fossa and recording from other muscles such as tibialis anterior and peroneus brevis.[48,52] Sensory nerve conduction studies of the superficial peroneal nerve may show reduced amplitudes; careful studies with needle electrodes may localize slowing of conduction to the fibular neck. Sensory studies of the terminal branch of the deep peroneal nerve are technically difficult.

EMG is an essential adjunct to nerve conduction studies and often provides more information. Muscles supplied by the deep and superficial branches of the common peroneal nerve should be examined. Two other key muscles should also be examined: the short head of the biceps femoris (supplied by the lateral trunk of the sciatic nerve above the knee) and the tibialis posterior (supplied by the tibial nerve from L-4, L-5, i.e., the same root innervation as the tibialis anterior muscle). It may also be necessary to include electromyographic studies of paraspinal and gluteal muscles.

Radiographs of the fibula, arthrograms, and CT scans of the popliteal fossa may all be of value to diagnose mass lesions causing the peroneal neuropathy.

Treatment

If no structural cause is found for the common peroneal neuropathy, the patient should be advised to avoid pressure on the nerve at the knee, and the clinical course should be followed carefully. Most patients with a clear history of external pressure or those who developed the neuropathy during sleep will improve. The very few who do not may have a true compressive neuropathy that requires surgical exploration. Because some of the soft tissue masses that can compress the common peroneal nerve are not identifiable radiologically and also because there is no way to diagnose entrapment in the fibular tunnel preoperatively, surgical exploration should be carried out in patients with progressive peroneal neuropathies. The anterior compartment syndrome is a surgical emergency; prompt fasciotomy is important for good recovery of both the muscle and the nerve.

TIBIAL NERVE

Anatomy

The tibial nerve is the continuation of the medial trunk of the sciatic nerve. It passes through the popliteal fossa and then deep to the gastrocnemius mus-

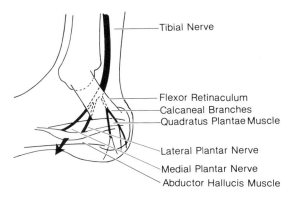

Tibial Nerve

Flexor Retinaculum
Calcaneal Branches
Quadratus Plantae Muscle

Lateral Plantar Nerve
Medial Plantar Nerve
Abductor Hallucis Muscle

FIGURE 12.4. *Medial aspect of the right ankle, showing the course of the distal tibial nerve and its terminal branches. The abductor hallucis muscle has been displaced downward (arrow), showing the course of the plantar nerves. (Reprinted with permission from Stewart JD, Aguayo AJ. Compression and entrapment neuropathies. In: Dyck PJ, Thomas PK, Lambert EH, Bunge R, eds. Peripheral neuropathy, ed 2. Philadelphia, WB Saunders, 1984:1448.)*

cle. At the ankle, the nerve passes under the flexor retinaculum into the foot (Figure 12.4). This retinaculum consists of thin fascia (quite unlike the thick transverse carpal ligament of the wrist)[53] and forms the roof of the tarsal tunnel. Within or just distal to the tarsal tunnel, the tibial nerve divides into the calcaneal sensory branches and the two plantar nerves. The calcaneal branches supply cutaneous sensation to the sole of the heel (Figure 12.5). The plantar nerves pass deep to the abductor hallucis muscle then take separate courses between the intrinsic foot muscles. They innervate these muscles and the skin of the anterior two-thirds of the sole (Figure 12.5) and end by forming the interdigital nerves. The branch of the medial plantar nerve that courses along the medial side of the big toe is called the *medial plantar proper digital nerve.*

The sural nerve divides from the tibial nerve in the popliteal fossa and descends to pass behind the lateral malleolus to supply the skin over the lateral aspect of the ankle and border of the foot as far as the little toe.

Disorders

Proximal tibial nerve lesions

Damage in the popliteal fossa is uncommon, by contrast with lesions here affecting the common peroneal nerve. Baker's cysts, popliteal artery aneurysms, and nerve sheath ganglia can compress and damage the tibial nerve alone or in association with the common peroneal nerve.[54]

Tarsal tunnel syndrome and plantar neuropathies

The tibial nerve and its terminal branches, the plantar and calcaneal nerves, can be compressed within the tarsal tunnel. External compression from ill-fitting footwear or tight plaster casts is probably the most common cause. Posttraumatic fibrosis occurring years after injury may constrict the nerve.[55–60] Tendon sheath cysts, tenosynovitis, ganglia, rheumatoid arthritis, hypothyroidism, and acromegaly are less frequent causes or associations.[55,61–63] A true entrapment neuropathy from a thickened or tight flexor retinaculum is rare.[55,56,64,65] In some patients, surgical exploration has shown fibrosis or dilated veins within the tunnel, the significance of which is uncertain.[56,65] In other patients, no specific abnormality was found, yet most improved postoperatively.[65]

The *plantar nerves* may be damaged within the tarsal tunnel or more distally in their course through

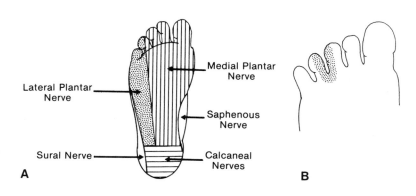

FIGURE 12.5.   *(A) Plantar aspect of the right foot showing the cutaneous distributions of the nerves that supply the sole. (B) The distribution of a digital nerve. (Reprinted with permission from Stewart JD. Focal peripheral neuropathies. New York: Elsevier Science Publishing, 1987:311.)*

the arch and sole of the foot. Thus depending on the site of the injury, a plantar neuropathy may or may not be considered as a type of tarsal tunnel syndrome. The causes of plantar nerve injuries within the tunnel are the same as those already listed. Distal to the tunnel, causes of *medial plantar* neuropathy include compression by tendon sheath cysts and hypertrophy or fibrosis of the abductor hallucis muscle.[57,58] Compression of the *lateral plantar nerve* is less well documented. Scarring following injury to the foot may be one cause. Spontaneous entrapment has been reported, but no details of the surgical findings have been provided.[56,66]

Digital neuropathies (Morton's Neuroma)

The interdigital nerves may be compressed between adjacent metatarsal heads or stretched where they cross the deep metatarsal ligaments.[67,68] The nerve in the third metatarsal interspace is most frequently involved. The digital nerve on the medial side of the big toe may be compressed by ill-fitting shoes or by scars following bunion surgery (Joplin's neuroma).[69]

Sural neuropathy

Compression of this nerve can occur in the popliteal fossa from a Baker's cyst,[54] but damage more distally is common. Resting the calf against hard objects or the upper edge of a ski boot can compress the nerve. Damage can occur during vein stripping. At the ankle, the sural nerve can be compressed by tendon sheath cysts, ganglia, and scar tissue.[17] More distally in the foot itself, the nerve can be entrapped following a fracture of the base of the fifth metatarsal bone.[70]

Clinical Evaluation

A tibial nerve lesion at the knee produces weakness of the calf and intrinsic foot muscles and sensory loss in the distribution of the sural and plantar nerves. This is unlikely to be confused with an S-1 radiculopathy, which would involve the gluteal and hamstring muscles also. A partial sciatic neuropathy mainly involving the medial trunk could be confused with a tibial neuropathy, but the former will also affect the hamstring muscles. When a proximal tibial neuropathy is diagnosed, the popliteal fossa must be examined carefully for mass lesions.

Tarsal tunnel syndrome and plantar neuropathies are uncommon disorders that present with pain in the foot and ankle and numbness in the sole of the foot. Accurate mapping of the sensory abnormalities is essential. When the sensory loss involves the heel, the calcaneal sensory branches are involved, localizing the lesion to within or proximal to the tarsal tunnel. Clinical evaluation of the intrinsic foot muscles is difficult, but wasting and weakness may be detected by comparing the affected foot with the other, if the signs are unilateral. It is useful to assess muscle bulk by palpation and strength by testing toe clawing. Weakness of the intrinsic foot muscles, when the gastrocnemius muscle and ankle reflex are normal, localizes the neuropathy to the distal tibial or plantar nerves. Swellings may be present on the medial side of the ankle, and local tenderness there on palpation or percussion is a valuable diagnostic sign.

Investigations

In a tibial neuropathy, nerve conductions show reduced amplitudes of the motor response from the abductor hallucis muscle. Unless deep needle electrodes are used to stimulate the sciatic nerve in the thigh (see earlier), it it usually impossible to stimulate the nerve above a popliteal fossa lesion. The sural sensory amplitude is usually reduced in amplitude. Electromyographic studies are more accurately localizing: Abnormalities in the gastrocnemius and intrinsic foot muscles, when the hamstring muscles are normal, are strong evidence for a tibial nerve lesion. Imaging of the popliteal fossa with CT scanning is useful for detecting masses that may be compressing the nerve.

For diagnosing tarsal tunnel syndrome and plantar neuropathies, motor nerve conduction studies can be performed along the medial and lateral plantar nerves by recording from the abductor hallucis and abductor digiti minimi muscles following stimulation of the tibial nerve at the ankle. These conductions, however, are often only abnormal when the nerve lesion is severe. Sensory conduction studies of the plantar nerves, best performed with needle recording electrodes and averaging techniques, are more likely to show abnormalities of the distal tibial or plantar nerves.[66,71,72] Normal values vary considerably, so it is best to compare the results with the other foot if it is unaffected. EMG of the intrinsic foot muscles is a valuable adjunct to the physical examination because these muscles are so difficult to examine clinically. A few denervation potentials and some neurogenic changes, however, may be found in these muscles in normal persons, so it is best, when possible, to compare the muscles of the affected foot with those of the other foot.[73] In an individual plantar neuropathy, EMG of the abductor hallucis can be compared with that of the abductor digiti minimi muscle.

Morton's neuroma is usually easily diagnosed by the characteristic symptoms of pain and numbness in the forefoot on walking and standing, tenderness on palpation of the interdigital space, and sensory loss on the adjacent surfaces of two toes (Figure 12.5). A technique for doing nerve conduction studies to confirm this neuropathy has been described and should be used if there is doubt about the diagnosis.[74,75] A sural neuropathy produces sensory loss in the distribution of this nerve and can be confirmed by nerve conduction tests.

Treatment

A mass in the popliteal fossa causing tibial neuropathy usually requires surgical excision. If a tarsal tunnel syndrome is clearly attributable to tight footwear, simply changing this may be effective. For persistent and progressive tarsal tunnel syndrome or medial plantar neuropathy, however, surgical exploration is indicated. This involves exposing the nerves in the tarsal tunnel and following the medial plantar nerve into the abductor hallucis muscle; if the nerve is constricted at that site, this should be corrected.

For mild symptoms of Morton's syndrome,

changing from high-heeled to flat shoes is often all that is required. Pads under the appropriate metatarsal heads to separate these bones when the patient stands may relieve symptoms.[76] Local injections of corticosteroids and anesthetics have also been used. If these measures fail, surgical treatment is indicated. Both excision of the thickened plantar digital nerve and incising the transverse deep intermetacarpal ligament are effective.[67,68,77]

FEMORAL NERVE

Anatomy

The femoral nerve arises from the lumbar plexus within the psoas muscle (L-2–L-4). It emerges from the psoas, passes under the iliacus fascia in the iliacus compartment, then courses deep to the inguinal ligament (Figure 12.6). It then divides into branches to the quadriceps muscles and cutaneous branches to the anterior thigh (see Figure 12.3). It ends as the *saphenous nerve*, which descends on the medial side of the knee and leg to the ankle, supplying sensation along its length (see Figure 12.3).

Disorders

Direct trauma such as stab wounds and injuries causing hip and pelvic fractures can damage the nerve. It can be compressed by hematomas and abscesses within the iliacus compartment.[78–80] Pelvic operations such as hysterectomy and renal transplantation may be complicated by compression of the femoral nerve from self-retaining retractors or hematomas.[81–83] Hip arthroplasty operations may also result in femoral nerve damage alone or in association with sciatic neuropathy.[2] Prolonged procedures in the lithotomy position such as vaginal hysterectomy have resulted in bilateral femoral neuropathies, perhaps owing to kinking and compression of the nerve beneath the inguinal ligament.[82,84] Femoral neuropathy following coma or drunken sleep may also be due to this mechanism.[10] Direct damage to the nerve can occur during inguinal lymph node biopsies, femoral herniorrhaphies, and femoral artery cannulations.

Diabetes mellitus can cause quadriceps weakness, and this has been attributed to femoral neuropathy.[85,86] Most of these patients, however, have evidence of more extensive damage involving the nerve roots and lumbar plexus (diabetic amyotrophy, diabetic lumbar plexopathy, polyradiculoplexopathy), although often with the greatest damage to the femoral nerve. The cause is thought to be multiple infarcts in the lumbosacral plexus, spinal nerve roots,

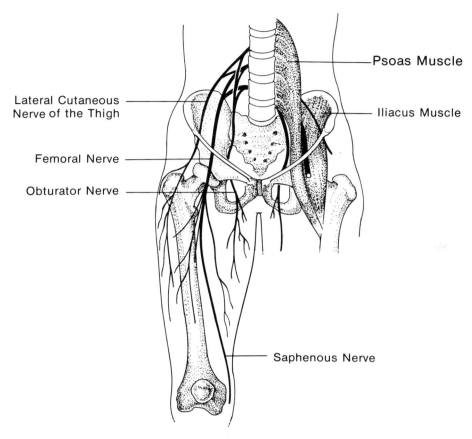

FIGURE 12.6. *Anterior view of the lower trunk and upper right leg to show the origin, course, and distribution of the femoral and obturator nerves and the lateral cutaneous nerve of the thigh. (Reprinted with permission from Stewart JD. Focal peripheral neuropathies. New York: Elsevier Science Publishing, 1987:323.)*

and proximal segments of the femoral and obturator nerves.[87,88] Idiopathic femoral neuropathy has also been described, although it is likely that many of these patients had diabetic radiculoplexopathy.[89]

Clinical Evaluation

A severe femoral neuropathy produces wasting and weakness of the quadriceps muscle, an absent knee reflex, and sensory impairment over the anteromedial aspect of the thigh and the medial aspect of the lower leg. Partial nerve lesions often produce little or no sensory deficit. Important muscles to test, in addition to the quadriceps, are the iliopsoas and the hip adductors. Weakness of the iliopsoas shows that

either the upper lumbar plexus or the L-2 or L-3 spinal nerve roots are involved. The hip adductors are supplied by the obturator nerve. This has the same root (L-2–L-4) and plexus origins as the femoral nerve (see Figure 12.6), so concomitant weakness of the hip adductors shows that the patient either has a lumbar plexopathy or a lesion of one or more of these roots but not an isolated femoral neuropathy.

The onset of symptoms in diabetic amyotrophy may be gradual or sudden. There is often severe back, hip, and thigh pain, which can mimic radiculopathy, although sometimes pain is entirely absent. There is usually wasting and weakness in the thighs and hip girdle mainly involving the quadriceps.

Investigations

The electrophysiologic evaluation should be directed at establishing whether the motor and sensory signs are restricted to the femoral nerve distribution. Femoral nerve motor conduction studies, in which the nerve is stimulated proximal to the inguinal ligament with recording from the quadriceps muscle, provide little specific information. Saphenous nerve sensory studies may or may not be abnormal. EMG is much more useful; the important muscles to evaluate are the quadriceps, hip adductors, iliopsoas, and paraspinal muscles. It is important to stress that in the syndrome of diabetic amyotrophy, denervative changes are often found in the paraspinal muscles,[88] presumably because the spinal nerve roots as well as the plexus are involved. Unfortunately, therefore the presence or absence of paraspinal electromyographic abnormalities do not distinguish this syndrome from radiculopathy with certainty. Radiographs of the lumbar and sacral spine, myelography, CT scanning, or MRI may be needed to distinguish between lumbosacral radiculopathy, retroperitoneal, and intrapelvic lesions affecting the plexus or proximal femoral nerve.

Treatment

The neuropathies caused by iliacus compartment hematomas have been treated both conservatively and by evacuation of the clot, with equally good results. Femoral neuropathies occurring after surgical procedures usually recover in time except in the rare situation in which the nerve is totally transected.

SAPHENOUS NERVE

Despite its long and superficial course, the saphenous nerve is infrequently injured except by lacerations. It is in particular danger during operations on varicose veins and when the saphenous vein is removed for use as an arterial graft.[90,91] Attempts to cannulate the saphenous vein at the ankle may injure the nerve and produce permanent painful paresthesias. The nerve can be compressed during anesthesia if the leg is improperly supported by stirrups or braces.

Entrapment of the saphenous nerve at the site where it pierces the fascia to emerge from the distal end of the subsartorial canal just above the knee has been alleged, but the evidence is not convincing.[92,93]

The *infrapatellar branch* of the saphenous nerve may be damaged during knee operations and by direct blunt trauma and accidental lacerations to the anteromedial surface of the knee.[94] These injuries usually produce minor sensory symptoms that are seldom reported by the patient, but sometimes painful neuromas occur. The spontaneous onset of paresthesias in the distribution of this nerve has been described (*gonyalgia paresthetica*). It is possibly the result of entrapment of the nerve where it pierces the sartorius tendon. Alternatively, it could be due to compression of one knee against the other because in some persons the nerve crosses the medial epicondyle of the femur.[94]

LATERAL CUTANEOUS NERVE OF THE THIGH

Anatomy

This nerve arises from the lumbar plexus and contains fibers from L-2 and L-3 spinal nerve roots. It emerges from the lateral border of the psoas muscle, crosses the iliacus muscle, then usually passes through a tunnel formed by a small split in the lateral end of the inguinal ligament (see Figure 12.6). Anatomic variations in this course through the inguinal ligament are common. The nerve is purely sensory and supplies the anterolateral and the lateral aspects of the thigh (see Figure 12.3).

Disorders

The most common cause of damage to this nerve is entrapment or kinking of the nerve as it passes through or under the inguinal ligament.[95] This usually occurs for no identifiable reason, and perhaps minor anatomic variations of the course predispose certain persons to the neuropathy. It is more frequent in obese or pregnant patients, and the symptoms disappear with weight loss or delivery; possibly the nerve is kinked and compressed by the protuberant abdomen. Meralgia paresthetica following general anesthesia may be due to prolonged kinking of the nerve as it passes through the inguinal ligament or from external pressure during the operation. Repeated external pressure on the nerve, for example, by leaning against a workbench or wearing tight corsets or braces, is another cause. Direct damage can occur during operations for removal of iliac crest bone for grafting.[96] More proximal damage to the nerve is rare. Causes include psoas hematomas, retroperitoneal tumors, masses in the iliac fossa, and postoperative scarring of the iliacus fascia.[97,98]

Clinical Evaluation

Damage to this nerve causes the syndrome of *meralgia paresthetica*. Numbness and paresthesias are present on the lateral aspect of the thigh, and the skin may be sensitive to touch. Symptoms often are worsened by prolonged standing or walking. On examination, the sensory abnormalities are usually confined to a much smaller area than the total distribution of the nerve. Sensation may be reduced, and yet the skin may be exquisitely sensitive. Pain may be present on deep palpation of the lateral aspect of the inguinal ligament, but this is an unreliable sign. Meralgia paresthetica is occasionally bilateral.

The differential diagnosis includes a femoral neuropathy and a L-3 radiculopathy. In these conditions, the sensory changes usually extend more anteriorly; the iliopsoas or quadriceps muscles, or both, are often weak, and the knee reflex is depressed.

Investigations

The clinical picture is usually so characteristic that the diagnosis can be made confidently on clinical grounds only. Nerve conduction studies of the lateral cutaneous nerve of the thigh are difficult to perform reliably. This is probably due to difficulty in knowing where best to stimulate the variable branches of the nerve in the thigh and also where best to place the recording electrodes given the variable course of the nerve. Normal electromyographic studies of paraspinal, iliopsoas, and quadriceps muscles are of value in excluding femoral neuropathy and radiculopathy.

Treatment

Meralgia paresthetica usually improves spontaneously. Analgesics can be helpful. In obese patients, weight loss and exercises of the abdominal muscles may help. Hydrocortisone and local anesthetic injections at the lateral end of the inguinal ligament can provide temporary relief. Recurrences are quite common. Surgery is indicated for intractable or recurrent cases. The usual procedure is to release the lateral end of the inguinal ligament. Sectioning the nerve is also usually effective, and complications such as recurrence of symptoms owing to neuroma formation are surprisingly few.

OBTURATOR NERVE

Anatomy

The obturator nerve is formed within the psoas muscle from the anterior divisions of the ventral rami of the L-2–L-4 spinal nerve roots (see Figure 12.6). It thus contains fibers from the same roots as the femoral nerve, which arises from the posterior divisions of these ventral rami. It descends through the psoas muscle into the pelvis and curves laterally around the wall of the pelvic cavity to leave it through the obturator foramen. In the thigh, it innervates the hip adductor muscles and supplies a small area of skin (Figure 12.7).

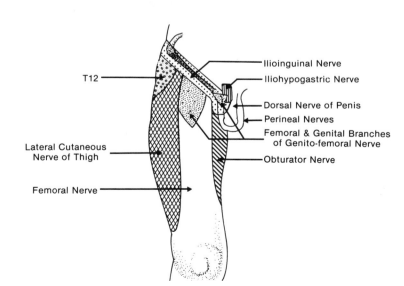

T12

Ilioinguinal Nerve
Iliohypogastric Nerve
Dorsal Nerve of Penis
Perineal Nerves
Femoral & Genital Branches of Genito-femoral Nerve
Obturator Nerve

Lateral Cutaneous Nerve of Thigh

Femoral Nerve

FIGURE 12.7.   *View of the inguinal region and right thigh to show the cutaneous innervation in this area. (Reprinted with permission from Stewart JD. Focal peripheral neuropathies. New York: Elsevier Science Publishing, 1987:345.)*

Disorders

Injuries to this nerve are uncommon. In prolonged or difficult labor, it can be compressed between the fetal head and pelvic wall.[99] Pelvic malignancies may invade the nerve.[98] It can also be damaged in pelvic fractures and occasionally during hip replacement, although this is much less frequent than damage to the sciatic nerve.[2] Obturator hernias can compress the nerve within the obturator canal.[93]

Clinical Evaluation

The usual complaint is of weakness in the leg and sometimes also paresthesias in the upper inner thigh. On examination, weakness is confined to the hip adductor muscles with a small area of sensory loss in the medial thigh. The quadriceps muscle and knee reflex should be examined carefully because of the shared root and plexus derivation of the femoral and obturator nerves. The diagnosis of obturator neuropathy can be made with confidence only when femoral nerve function is absolutely normal.

Investigations

The diagnosis of obturator neuropathy is best confirmed by demonstrating electromyographic abnormalities in the hip adductors but not in the quadriceps muscles. If no cause for the neuropathy is apparent, an intrapelvic tumor must be suspected, so a careful vaginal or rectal examination should be done and imaging studies undertaken. If these are all entirely negative, compression by a hernia within the obturator canal should be suspected.

Treatment

Postpartum obturator neuropathies usually resolve spontaneously. If no cause is apparent from the history and investigations, exploration of the obturator canal is warranted.

ILIOHYPOGASTRIC, ILIOINGUINAL, AND GENITOFEMORAL NERVES

Anatomy

The iliohypogastric, ilioinguinal, and genitofemoral nerves arise from the upper lumbar plexus and contain fibers from T-12–L-1, L-2 spinal nerve roots. These nerves supply the skin in the inguinal region, the upper and medial thigh, and part of the genitalia (see Figure 12.7). An important anatomic point is that the ilioinguinal and genitofemoral nerves both pass through the inguinal canal and are therefore susceptible to injury during herniorrhaphies.

Disorders

The iliohypogastric nerve can be damaged by surgical incisions in the lower quadrant of the abdomen[100]; the sensory deficit is in the suprapubic region and is usually trivial. Damage to the ilioinguinal nerve usually occurs during herniorrhaphies and appendectomies, but considering the frequency of these operations, such damage occurs surprisingly seldom.[100–103] Entrapment of the nerve as it passes through the muscles of the abdominal wall medial to the anterior superior iliac spine has also been described.[104,105] Genitofemoral nerve damage is usually the result of an appendectomy with subsequent scarring and adhesions.[106,107]

Clinical Evaluation

The symptoms are numbness and paresthesias, or both, and sometimes pain in the inguinal area. To make the diagnosis with absolute certainty, an area of sensory abnormality must be found. Very careful testing with a pin is required. Another helpful finding is a Tinel's sign producing painful electrical sensations, reproducing the patient's symptoms. Because of the motor fibers present in the ilioinguinal and iliohypogastric nerves, there may be some bulging of the abdominal wall muscles above the inguinal ligament, but this is probably uncommon and difficult to detect. The genitofemoral nerve supplies the cremaster muscles, but surprisingly abnormalities of the cremaster reflex have not been described in patients with this neuropathy.

Investigations

These nerves cannot be evaluated by conduction studies. Nerve blocks are helpful in that if pain and particularly the paresthesias are improved, this is suggestive that the symptoms are due to a damaged nerve. Because nerve blocks may alleviate pain arising from nonneural structures, however, and also because these three nerves run so closely together, it is often difficult to draw specific conclusions as to the cause of pain and which nerve is involved. The principal differential diagnosis is a L-1 or L-2 radiculopathy. These are rare and should be suspected when there has been no previous surgery of the kind associated with damage to these three nerves and also when back pain is present. Electromyographic studies of the paraspinal muscles and imaging help to diagnose radiculopathy.

Treatment

In some patients, repeated local anesthetic injections have been curative.[104] If this is ineffective or when symptoms are severe, surgical exploration of the nerve is indicated. It is thought that resecting the nerve proximal to the site of damage is the most effective procedure.

REFERENCES

1. Huittinen VM, Slatis P. Nerve injury in double vertical pelvic fractures. Acta Chir Scand 1972; 138:571–575.
2. Weber ER, Daube JR, Coventry MB. Peripheral neuropathies associated with total hip arthroplasty. J Bone Joint Surg 1976; 58A:66–69.
3. Evarts CM, DeHaven KE, Nelson CL et al. Interim results of Charnley-Muller total hip arthroplasty. Clin Orthop 1973; 95:193–200.
4. Coventry MB, Nolan DR, Beckenbaugh RD. "Delayed" prophylactic anticoagulation: A study of results and complications in 2,012 total hip arthroplasties. J Bone Joint Surg 1973; 55A:1487–1492.
5. Casagrande PA, Danahy PR. Delayed sciatic-nerve entrapment following the use of self-curing acrylic: A case report. J Bone Joint Surg 1971; 53A:167–169.
6. Edwards MS, Barbaro NM, Asher SW, et al. Delayed sciatic palsy after total hip replacement: Case report. Neurosurgery 1981; 9:61–63.
7. Rodriguez MJ, Austin E, McBride EJ. Peroneal nerve damage following insertion of Austin-Moore prosthesis. Arch Phys Med Rehabil 1964; 45:283–285.
8. Campbell RD, Mason JB, Wilson PD Jr., et al. The use of intramedullary prosthetic replacement in fractures of the femoral neck. Am J Surg 1960; 99:745–755.
9. Stewart JD, Angus E, Gendron D. Sciatic neuropathies. Br Med J 1983; 287:1108–1109.
10. Shields RW, Root KE, Wilbourne AJ. Compartment syndromes and compression neuropathies in coma. Neurology 1986; 36:1370–1374.
11. Pearce JMS. Peripheral nerve lesions in the muscle compartment syndrome. Br Med J 1980; 280:109–110.
12. Parks BJ. Postoperative peripheral neuropathies. Surgery 1973; 74:348–357.
13. Denton RO, Sherrill JD. Sciatic syndrome due to endometriosis of sciatic nerve. South Med J 1955; 48:1027–1031.
14. Baker GS, Parsons WR, Welch JS. Endometriosis within the sheath of the sciatic nerve: Report of two patients with progressive paralysis. J Neurosurg 1966; 25:652–655.
15. Fleming RE, Michelsen CB, Stinchfield FE. Sciatic paralysis: A complication of bleeding following hip surgery. J Bone Joint Surg 1979; 61A:37–39.
16. Leonard MA. Sciatic nerve paralysis following anticoagulant therapy. J Bone Joint Surg 1972; 54B:152–153.
17. Stewart JD. Focal peripheral neuropathies. New York: Elsevier Science Publishing, 1987.
18. Vanneste JAL, Butzelaar RMJM, Dicke HW. Ischiadic nerve entrapment by an extra- and intrapelvic lipoma: A rare cause of sciatica. Neurology 1980; 30:532–534.
19. Meek GN, Hill RL. Surgical treatment of gluteal artery aneurysms. Am J Surg 1968; 116:731–734.
20. Freiberg AH. Sciatic pain and its relief by operations on muscle and fascia. Arch Surg 1937; 34:337–350.
21. Robinson DR. Pyriformis syndrome in relation to sciatic pain. Am J Surg 1947; 73:355–358.
22. Adams JA. The pyriformis syndrome—report of four cases and review of the literature. South Afr J Surg 1980; 18:13–18.
23. Solheim LF, Siewers P, Paus B. The piriformis muscle syndrome: Sciatic nerve entrapment treated with section of the piriformis muscle. Acta Orthop Scand 1981; 52:73–75.
24. Pace JB, Nagle D. Piriform syndrome. West J Med 1976; 124:435–439.
25. Nakano KK. Sciatic nerve entrapment: The piriformis syndrome. J Musculoskel Med 1987; 4(2):33–37.
26. Synek VM. The pyriformis syndrome: Review and case presentation. Clin Exp Neurol 1987; 23:31–37.
27. Johnston W, Stewart JD. Sciatic neuropathies: A 10 year experience. Can J Neurol Sci 1990; 17:249.
28. Sunderland S. The relative susceptibility to injury of the medial and lateral popliteal divisions of the sciatic nerve. Br J Surg 1953; 41:2–4.
29. Pillay PK, Russell WH, Wilbourn AJ, et al. Solitary primary lymphoma of the sciatic nerve: Case report. Neurosurgery 1988; 23:370–371.
30. Rask MR. Superior gluteal nerve entrapment syndrome. Muscle Nerve 1980; 3:304–307.
31. LaBan MM, Meerschaert JR, Taylor RS. Electromyographic evidence of inferior gluteal nerve compromise: An early representation of recurrent colorectal carcinoma. Arch Phys Med Rehabil 1982; 63:33–35.

32. Hofmann A, Jones RE, Schoenvogel R. Pudendal-nerve neurapraxia as a result of traction on the fracture table: A report of four cases. J Bone Joint Surg 1982; 64A:136–138.

33. Desai KM, Gingell JC. Hazards of long distance cycling. Br Med J 1989; 298:1072–1073.

34. Snooks SJ, Barnes PRH, Swash M. Damage to the innervation of the voluntary anal and periurethral sphincter musculature in incontinence: An electrophysiological study. J Neurol Neurosurg Psychiatry 1984; 47:1269–1273.

35. Schulak DJ, Bear TF, Summers JL. Transient impotence from positioning on the fracture table. J Trauma 1980; 20:420–421.

36. Mehta AJ, Viosca SP, Korenman SG, Davis SS. Peripheral nerve conduction studies and bulbocavernosus reflex in the investigation of impotence. Arch Phys Med Rehabil 1986; 67:332–335.

37. Nagler SH, Rangell L. Peroneal palsy caused by crossing the legs. JAMA 1947; 133:755–761.

38. Sprofkin BE. Peroneal paralysis—a hazard of weight reduction. Arch Intern Med 1958; 102:82–87.

39. Garland H, Moorhouse D. Compressive lesions of the external popliteal (common peroneal) nerve. Br Med J 1952; 2:1373–1378.

40. Sandhu HS, Sandhey BS. Occupational compression of the common peroneal nerve at the neck of the fibula. Aust N Z J Surg 1976; 46:160–163.

41. Sidey JD. Weak ankles. A study of common peroneal entrapment neuropathy. Br Med J 1969; 3:623–626.

42. Mulder DW, Lambert EH, Bastron J, Sprague RG. The neuropathies associated with diabetes mellitus. A clinical and electromyographic study of 103 unselected diabetic patients. Neurology 1961; 11:275–284.

43. Fraser DM, Campbell IW, Ewing DJ, et al. Mononeuropathy in diabetes mellitus. Diabetes 1979; 28:96–101.

44. Bleehen SS, Lovelace RE, Cotton RE. Mononeuritis multiplex in polyarteritis nodosa. Q J Med 1963; 32:193–209.

45. Moore PM, Fauci AS. Neurologic manifestations of systemic vasculitis. Am J Med 1981; 71:517–524.

46. Lunceford EM. The peroneal compartment syndrome. South Med J 1965; 58:621–623.

47. Brooks DM. Nerve compression by simple ganglia. J Bone Joint Surg 1952; 34:391–400.

48. Sourkes M, Stewart JD. Common peroneal neuropathy: A study of selective motor and sensory involvement. Neurology 1991; 41:1029–1033.

49. Singh N, Behse F, Buchthal F. Electrophysiological study of peroneal palsy. J Neurol Neurosurg Psychiatry 1974; 37:1202–1213.

50. Pickett JB. Localizing peroneal nerve lesions to the knee by motor conduction studies. Arch Neurol 1984; 41:192–195.

51. Katirji MB, Wilbourn AJ. Common peroneal mononeuropathy: A clinical and electrophysiologic study of 116 lesions. Neurology 1988; 38:1723–1728.

52. Kanakamedala RV, Hong CZ. Peroneal nerve entrapment at the knee localized by short segment stimulation. Am J Phys Med Rehabil 1989; 68:116–122.

53. Irani KD, Grabois M, Harvey SC. Standardized technique for diagnosis of tarsal tunnel syndrome. Am J Phys Med 1982; 61:26–31.

54. Nakano KK. Entrapment neuropathy from Baker's cyst. JAMA 1978; 239:135.

55. Edwards WG, Lincoln CR, Bassett FH, Goldner JL. The tarsal tunnel syndrome: Diagnosis and treatment. JAMA 1969; 207:716–720.

56. Linscheid RL, Burton RC, Fredericks EJ. Tarsal tunnel syndrome. South Med J 1970; 63:1313–1323.

57. Mann RA. Tarsal tunnel syndrome. Orthop Clin North Am 1974; 5:109–115.

58. Goodgold J, Kopell HP, Spielholz NI. The tarsal tunnel syndrome. N Engl J Med 1965; 273:742–745.

59. Wilemon WK. Tarsal tunnel syndrome: A 50 year survey of the world literature and a report of two cases. Orthop Rev 1979; 8:111–117.

60. Bourrel P, Rey A, Blanc JF, et al. Syndrome du canal tarsien: à propos de 15 cas "purs" et do 100 cas "associés" à la lèpre ou au diabète. Rev Rhum Mal Osteoartic 1976; 43:723–728.

61. DiStefano V, Sack JT, Whittaker R, et al. Tarsal-tunnel syndrome: Review of the literature and two case reports. Clin Orthop 1972; 88:76–79.

62. Baylan SP, Paik SW, Barnert AL, et al. Prevalence of the tarsal tunnel syndrome in rheumatoid arthritis. Rheumatol Rehabil 1981; 20:148–150.

63. Schwartz MS, Mackworth-Young CG, McKeran RO. Short report: The tarsal tunnel syndrome in hypothyroidism. J Neurol Neurosurg Psychiatry 1983; 46:440–442.

64. Keck C. The tarsal tunnel syndrome. J Bone Joint Surg 1962; 44:180–182.

65. Lam SJS. Tarsal tunnel syndrome. J Bone Joint Surg 1967; 49B:87–92.

66. Oh SJ, Sarala PK, Kuba T, et al. Tarsal tunnel syndrome: Electrophysiological study. Ann Neurol 1979; 5:327–330.

67. Kite JH. Morton's toe neuroma. South Med J 1966; 59:20–25.

68. Betts LO. Morton's metatarsalgia: Neuritis of the fourth digital nerve. Med J Aust 1940; 1:514–515.

69. Joplin RJ. The proper digital nerve, vitallium stem arthroplasty, and some thoughts about foot surgery in general. Clin Orthop 1971; 76:199–212.

70. Gould N, Trevino S. Sural nerve entrapment by avulsion fracture of the base of the fifth metatarsal bone. Foot Ankle 1981; 2:153–155.

71. Behse F, Buchthal F. Normal sensory conduction in

the nerves of the leg in man. J Neurol Neurosurg Psychiatry 1971; 34:404–414.

72. Guiloff RJ, Sherratt RM. Sensory conduction in medial plantar nerve: Normal values, clinical applications, and a comparison with the sural and upper limb sensory nerve action potentials in peripheral neuropathy. J Neurol Neurosurg Psychiatry 1977; 40:1168–1181.

73. Falck B, Alaranta H. Short report: Fibrillation potentials, positive sharp waves and fasciculation in the intrinsic muscles of the foot in healthy subjects. J Neurol Neurosurg Psychiatry 1983; 46:681–683.

74. Oh SJ, Kim HS, Ahmad BK. Electrophysiological diagnosis of interdigital neuropathy of the foot. Muscle Nerve 1984; 7:218–225.

75. Falck B, Hurme M, Hakkarainen S, et al. Sensory conduction velocity of plantar digital nerves in Morton's metatarsalgia. Neurology 1984; 34:698–801.

76. Milgram JE. Morton's neuritis and management of post-neurectomy pain. In: Omer GE, Spinner M, eds. Management of Peripheral Nerve Problems. Philadelphia: WB Saunders, 1980: 203–215.

77. Gauthier G. Thomas Morton's disease: A nerve entrapment syndrome: A new surgical technique. Clin Orthop 1979; 142:90–92.

78. Chiu WS. The syndrome of retroperitoneal hemorrhage and lumbar plexus neuropathy during anticoagulant therapy. South Med J 1976; 69:595–599.

79. Aichroth P, Rowe-Jones DC. Iliacus compartment compression syndrome. Br J Surg 1971; 58:833–834.

80. Goodfellow J, Fearn CBd'A, Matthews JM. Iliacus haematoma: A common complication of haemophilia. J Bone Joint Surg 1967; 49B:748–755.

81. Rosenblum J, Schwarz GA, Bendler E. Femoral neuropathy—a neurological complication of hysterectomy. JAMA 1966; 195:409–414.

82. Hopper CL, Baker JB. Bilateral femoral neuropathy complicating vaginal hysterectomy: Analysis of contributing factors in 3 patients. Obstet Gynecol 1968; 32:543–547.

83. Vaziri ND, Barton CH, Ravikumar GR, et al. Femoral neuropathy: A complication of renal transplantation. Nephron 1981; 28:30–31.

84. Sinclair RH, Pratt JH. Femoral neuropathy after pelvic operation. Am J Obstet Gynecol 1972; 112:404–407.

85. Goodman JI. Femoral neuropathy in relation to diabetes mellitus. Diabetes 1954; 3:266–273.

86. Calverley JR, Mulder DW. Femoral neuropathy. Neurology 1960; 10:963–967.

87. Raff MC, Sangalang V, Asbury AK. Ischemic mononeuropathy multiplex associated with diabetes mellitus. Arch Neurol 1968; 18:487–499.

88. Bastron JA, Thomas JE. Diabetic polyradiculopathy: Clinical and electromyographic findings in 105 patients. Mayo Clin Proc 1981; 56:725–732.

89. Biemond A. Femoral neuropathy. In: Vinken PJ, Bruyn GW, eds. Handbook of clinical neurology. New York, American Elsevier, 1970: 303–310.

90. Garnjobst W. Injuries to the saphenous nerve following operations for varicose veins. Surg Gynecol Obstet 1964; 119:359–361.

91. Lederman RJ, Breuer AC, Hanson MR, et al. Peripheral nervous system complications of coronary artery bypass graft surgery. Ann Neurol 1982; 12:297–301.

92. Mozes M, Ouaknine G, Nathan H. Saphenous nerve entrapment simulating vascular disorder. Surgery 1975; 77:299–303.

93. Mumenthaler M. Some clinical aspects of peripheral nerve lesions. Eur Neurol 1969; 2:257–268.

94. Wartenberg R. Digitalgia paresthetica and gonyalgia paresthetica. Neurology 1954; 4:106–115.

95. Ghent WR. Meralgia paraesthetica. Can Med Assoc J 1959; 81:631–633.

96. Weikel AM, Habal MB. Meralgia paresthetica: A complication of iliac bone procurement. Plast Reconstr Surg 1977; 60:572–574.

97. Flowers RS. Meralgia paresthetica: A clue to retroperitoneal malignant tumor. Am J Surg 1968; 116:89–92.

98. Sunderland S. Nerves and nerve injuries, ed 2. Edinburgh: Churchill Livingstone, 1978.

99. Donaldson JO. Neurology of pregnancy. Philadelphia: WB Saunders, 1978:49.

100. Stulz P, Pfeiffer KM. Peripheral nerve injuries resulting from common surgical procedures in the lower portion of the abdomen. Arch Surg 1982; 117:324–327.

101. Winer JB, Harrison MJG. Iatrogenic nerve injuries. Postgrad Med J 1982; 58:142–145.

102. Bohm E, Fiorillo A, Pellettieri L. Ilio-inguinal neuralgia: A forgotten disease. Acta Neurol Scand 1979; 34:33–38.

103. Sterling JR, Harus BA, Schroder ME, Eichman PL. Diagnosis and treatment of genitofemoral and ilioinguinal entrapment neuropathy. Surgery 1987; 102:581–586.

104. Mumenthaler A, Mumenthaler M, Luciani G, et al. Das Ilioinguinalis-Syndrom: Beschreibung von sieben eigenen Beobachtungen. Dtsch Med Wochenschr 1965; 90:1073–1078.

105. Kopell HP, Thompson WAL, Postel AH. Entrapment neuropathy of the ilioinguinal nerve. N Engl J Med 1962; 266:16–19.

106. Magee RK. Genitofemoral causalgia (a new syndrome). Can Med Assoc J 1942; 46:326–329.

107. Lyon EK. Genitofemoral causalgia. Can Med Assoc J 1945; 53:213–216.

13

Traumatic Peripheral Nerve Lesions

Henry Berry

CONTENTS

ACRONYMS

EMG   Electromyography
MRC   Medical Research Council
MU   Motor unit

ELECTROPHYSIOLOGIC ASSESSMENT OF PERIPHERAL NERVE INJURIES

Categories of Injury

There are different degrees of injury to the peripheral nerves, and these vary from the mildest stretch or pressure injury; to those that involve loss of axonal continuity with preservation of endoneural and perineural continuity; to the most extreme form, in which there is complete mechanical disruption of the peripheral nerve and its fascicles. Seddon[1] has coined the terms *neurapraxia, axonotmesis,* and *neurotmesis* to indicate the clinical counterparts of these increasing degrees of severity, and Sunderland[2] has enlarged on these concepts and has described the degrees of nerve injury in greater detail.

The mildest form of injury appears to disturb the axoplasmic flow and blood-nerve barrier,[3] as in intermittent compression, impingement, and stretching, by a constriction of the axis cylinder and an obstruction of the distal flow of axoplasm. The normal transient sensations of numbness of an extremity after lying or sitting in a certain position or after a blow to the ulnar nerve at the elbow occur, at least in part, on this basis.

The next degree of injury causes a distortion of the myelin in the area between the nodes of Ranvier. Experimental studies have revealed that the myelin lamellae appear to slide away from the point of compression and to telescope through the node of Ranvier. Localized pressure or stretch that causes structural distortion results in detachment of the inner myelin lamella, and the histologic appearance is that of paranodal and segmental demyelination.[4] Axonal function cannot be restored to normal until there is regeneration of the myelin sheath in the affected segment, and as the axon and its associated Schwann cells are intact proximal and distal to the site of injury, remyelination can occur rapidly.

If local injury has been severe enough to damage the axon irreversibly, the distal part of the axon becomes separated from its cell body and it disintegrates. The chain of Schwann cells distal to the point of injury digests their myelin as in wallerian degeneration,[5] leaving behind a band of Schwann cells enclosed in the basement membrane system of the original fibres, without myelin or axons. In order that regeneration may occur, the proximal intact axon must provide axon sprouts that traverse the chain of Schwann cells until they reinnervate motor fibers and regenerate nerve endings.[6,7] The Schwann cells then remyelinate the larger axons, and there is

a return of function when the fibers achieve their normal caliber.

In the final category of injury, there is gross disruption and severance of large numbers of nerve fibers, and this may include fascicles or the entire nerve such that the endoneurium and perineurium are not preserved. There is no guiding channel for axonal regrowth and reinnervation, and regrowth results in a tangled mass of Schwann cells, axons, and fibroblasts, which form a neuroma. Mechanical disruption or severance of a larger nerve with disruption of the perineurium that surrounds each fascicle or of the epineurium, that is, the fibrous fatty covering of multiple fascicles, often results in a gap between opposing ends that cannot possibly be bridged by the process of growth. Further, local fibrosis, either intrafascicular or on a larger scale, can constitute a mechanical barrier to reinnervation. At a microscopic level, it is recognized that the severity of involvement is not necessarily uniform; some fibers are minimally damaged and recover function within a few weeks, whereas adjacent fibers may have suffered axonal disruption such that recovery can occur only through regeneration, over a matter of months, and the time of recovery will be determined by the length of the nerve distal to the site of injury. It is the aim of clinical and electrophysiologic examination to determine the predominant category of involvement and severity and to express this in terms such as partial, be it mild, moderate, severe, or as complete.

It is well established that conduction velocity increases with the increasing diameter of the nerve fiber, and this is largely due to the presence of myelin. Normal nerve conduction depends on a wave of depolarization along the nerve (saltatory conduction), which does not travel at a uniform rate but which "jumps" from node to node.[8,9] When a segment of myelin is damaged such that saltatory conduction is interfered with, nerve conduction is considerably slowed, and it approaches those values seen in unmyelinated fibers. Unmyelinated fibers conduct at rates as slow as 1 to 2 m per second. Every nerve contains fibers of different diameters, and measurement of sensory and motor conduction, expressed as a latency or as a calculated velocity, is based on the maximal velocity, that is, the velocity of the most rapidly conducting fibers as evoked by appropriate electrical stimuli.

The larger diameter fibers appear to be more sensitive to pressure and mechanical injury, presumably because of the effect on myelin. When myelin is damaged over a segment of these larger fibers or when the axis cylinder is damaged, the nerve conducts at a slower rate because of the loss of saltatory conduction, or it ceases to conduct, as in complete severance. Conduction now occurs through the slower fibers, which serve to reduce the maximum conduction velocity. It is now established that there are two main pathologic types of peripheral neuropathy: demyelinative neuropathy (segmental demyelination), in which there is marked slowing of conduction down to a value of less than 70% of normal owing to an interference with saltatory conduction, and primary axonal neuropathy, in which axonal and wallerian degeneration have usually affected the larger diameter fibers, with a resultant mild slowing such that nerve conduction is lowered slightly and remains above about 70% of normal. Peripheral nerve trauma largely mimics the findings of axonal neuropathy in that there is mild slowing of motor nerve conduction despite a wide spectrum of partial involvement from mild to severe, with a complete absence of conduction in conditions of conduction block or complete severance. Berry and Richardson,[10] in a review of the clinical and electrophysiologic features of common peroneal nerve palsy, noted the relationship between the severity of the palsy and the amount of slowing of conduction; this relationship is similar to the prolongation of the motor latency, which parallels the duration and severity of symptoms in patients with carpal tunnel syndrome. In the nerve regeneration that follows complete severance or transection, the compound nerve action potential is at first severely diminished in amplitude, and there is considerable slowing. Regeneration is known to proceed at a faster rate than remyelination, and, from animal experiments, it is known that regeneration nerve fibers may achieve 80% of normal conduction, although they have a more slender axon and a thinner myelin sheath with shorter internodal distances.[11,12]

Historical Considerations

Erb[13] introduced the use of galvanic (on-off) and faradic (repetitive) stimulation of muscles at their point of innervation as tests of *the electrical reactions of muscles* in 1883. These proved to be of little value to the clinician. It was time-consuming to plot the intensity/duration curves. The results were inconsistent, and they did not prove to be useful in the detection of partial denervation. In 1929, Adrian and Bronk[14] used a bipolar (concentric) needle electrode to record muscle activity and advances in electronics; the development of the amplifier and the cathode ray

oscilloscope provided the technical basis for the investigation of motor unit (MU) activity. In 1938, Denny-Brown and Pennybacker[15] described the spontaneous electrical activity of a denervated muscle. Buchthal and Clemmesen in 1941[16] and Weddell et al. in 1944[17] applied these techniques to the investigation of peripheral nerve injury and neurogenic muscular atrophy. Kugelberg in 1947[18] recognized the differing wave forms of MU potentials in different types of muscle wasting, and electromyography (EMG) thereby became useful in the distinction between myogenic and neurogenic weakness.

The electrical examination of nerve function was limited to nerve stimulation and the detection of a corresponding muscle response until the development of techniques for measuring motor nerve conduction velocity by Simpson[19] and sensory nerve conduction by Gilliat and Sears.[20] These methods reflected an important advance in the diagnosis of peripheral neuropathy, the detection of entrapment and pressure palsy, and in some conditions, it allowed the identification of the actual site of the lesion. Further refinement became possible with the development of quantitative evaluation of electromyographic recordings.[21,22] The invention of the digital computer and its use as a signal averager have created the ability to detect action potentials of very low amplitude; this has permitted the measurement and analysis of compound nerve action potentials as well as their evoked cortical counterparts.

These advances in electrical testing have helped to clarify the nature and clinical features of various forms of peripheral nerve disorders. They have made it possible to demonstrate objectively slowing of nerve conduction in those portions of the nerve that have been subjected to pressure or entrapment. Their use has laid the groundwork for a better understanding of previously known conditons, such as palsy of the ulnar, radial, common peroneal, and other nerves. Measurement of motor nerve conduction has led to the recognition of carpal tunnel syndrome, a common condition that until then had been diagnosed as a form of scalenus anticus or thoracic outlet syndrome or as acroparesthesia of unknown origin.

Nerve conduction studies and EMG have led to the development of more rational methods of management of nerve palsies of spontaneous as well as traumatic origin. For example, examination of the facial nerve and muscles, in facial nerve trauma and Bell's palsy, has allowed a determination of the severity of the lesion and has provided indications for surgical or other management. When there has been peripheral nerve trauma, pressure palsy, or entrapment, the combined investigations of motor and at times sensory nerve conduction and the electromyographic detection of surviving MUs have permitted a more accurate assessment of severity and prognosis. The preservation of motor conduction, as evidenced by MUs under voluntary control or on electrical stimulation of the nerve, indicates a degree of physical continuity, and this has important implications for management and prognosis.

Nerve conduction and electromyographic examinations are most useful when they are performed by a clinician who possesses neurologic expertise. Although routine measurements of sensory and motor conduction velocity, distal latency, evoked compound nerve action potentials by the signal averaging method and the recording of elecromyographic potentials can be accurately done by a suitably trained technician, the assessment of more complex diagnostic problems requires a different approach, and the details of the clinical picture must be kept clearly in mind. A knowledge of the symptoms and signs—the presence of absence of wasting, weakness, and sensory loss—and the territory of suspected nerve involvement; the identification and electromyographic sampling of individual muscles in the case of a localized peripheral nerve injury; and an awareness of the anatomic arrangements of nerves and of the differential diagnoses are required to perform a precise and useful examination.

Electromyography

A normal muscle does not show any spontaneous activity in the relaxed state, and after a brief discharge of short-duration, low-amplitude potentials that transiently follows needle electrode insertion, and except for high-frequency, low-amplitude end plate noise and spike potentials, which can be mistaken for fibrillation potentials, it is electrically silent. With voluntary contraction, MU discharges or action potentials are seen, and they increase in number and in firing rate as the strength of contraction increases. These MU action potentials are biphasic or triphasic, and their amplitude and duration vary with the muscle under contraction. Values of 2 to 10 ms in duration and 500 μV to 2 mV are common for limb muscles. The number of phases and the duration and amplitude of the action potential are altered by neurogenic changes as well as by other nontraumatic conditions. A slight contraction allows individual MUs to be inspected on the oscilloscope screen and permits an assessment of wave form, am-

plitude, and duration. As the strength of contraction increases, there is a parallel increase in the discharge of MUs, and these summate into an interference pattern. The interference pattern is incomplete when the strength of contraction is limited either voluntarily, in which MUs discharge at a slow rate, or by partial paralysis, owing to conduction block or denervation in which the rate is unusually rapid.

After 10 to 14 days of denervation, spontaneous electrical activity appears in the muscle at rest in the form of fibrillation positive sharp waves and occasionally as fasciculation. Fasciculation consists of discharge of individual MUs, and these are more characteristic of disease of the anterior horn cell than of traumatic injury. Fibrillation potentials represent the electrical activity of a discharging individual muscle fiber, and this produces a brief low-amplitude biphasic or triphasic potential, 1 to 5 ms in duration and 20 to 200 μV in amplitude. Positive sharp waves are similar in amplitude but are of longer duration (10 ms or more) than fibrillation potentials; they consist of an initial positive spike followed by a slow negative deflection that resembles a sawtooth. Fasciculation potentials are identical in appearance to MU discharges, and they represent the spontaneous discharge of a MU. It is important that the muscle be at rest and that the patient not be cold or shivering because MU discharges under such circumstances can be misinterpreted as fasciculation potentials. If the needle is in the end plate region, end plate activity consisting of low-voltage undulations, 10 to 50 μV in amplitude and 1 to ms in duration, or of higher voltage spikes, 100 to 200 μV and 3 to 4 ms in duration, may be seen and be mistaken for positive sharp waves or fibrillation potentials.

The wave form of MU acton potential is altered by disease, as for exmaple in the appearance of the short-duration polyphasic potentials of polymyositis and muscular dystrophy. Similar low-voltage polyphasic potentials are also recorded as paralyzed muscle is reinnervated (nascent potentials), and they increase in amplitude and number with further recovery. The wave form has more phases than the normal MU action potential, that is, four or more, and the amplitude, although low in the early stages of recovery, gradually increases to larger values of up to 10 mV or greater. In longstanding neurogenic atrophy, as for example in a chronic pressure palsy; in spinal cord trauma in which anterior horn cells have been involved; and in motor neuron disease, large-amplitude or giant potentials owing to collateral innervation and of long duration (15 to 30 ms) are seen. Electromyographic examination performed under proper conditions with the patient relaxed and cooperating with willed movements and with sampling of the appropriate muscles provides data as to the preservation of MUs under voluntary control, evidence of denervation, the degree of paralysis, and evidence of recovery through reinnervation.

In neurogenic paralysis, evidence of denervation occurs after about 10 to 14 days and persists for a number of months and as long as there is viable muscle tissue. The greater degrees of weakness and associated muscle wasting are readily detected on clinical examination. In the patient without any clinical findings, but in whom mild injury is suspected, electromyographic examination can reveal subclinical changes; in such conditions as a mild brachial plexus stretch injury, in our experience, it is more common to find polyphasic MUs in the recovery phase rather than fibrillation potentials in the acute stage of subclinical injury.

In severe pressure or stretch injuries, paralysis is obvious, and recovery is usually delayed. In such patients, EMG often provides the first evidence of recovery in the form of low-voltage polyphasic nascent potentials appearing first at rest, increasing in number, and then appearing on volition as early evidence of reinnervation.

At rest, apart from low-voltage brief duration end plate potentials, normal muscle is electrically silent. MU action potentials appear during slight contraction and increase with the strength of contraction. A finding of incomplete paralysis of recent onset, with denervation, indicates a lesion in continuity and usually indicates a good prognosis. Fibrillation and positive sharp waves at rest with MU potentials during voluntary contraction indicate that some denervation has occurred but that there is continuity. There are the usual findings in patients who have suffered peripheral nerve trauma, such as a common peroneal nerve palsy owing to pressure or local trauma or a brachial plexus stretch injury.

Complete paralysis in conjunction with denervation is of special concern to the neurosurgeon, and although it may indicate a lesion in continuity, it may also indicate that the nerve has been severed and that nerve suture or grafting is required (Figure 13.1). The clinical and electrophysiologic features of lesions in continuity and in discontinuity are summarized in Figures 13.2 and 13.3. If a complete lesion is confirmed electromyographically, serial examinations are required to assess the pace of recovery. The earliest sign of recovery is the appearance of low-voltage nascent potentials, spontaneously and then on attempted contraction, and a gradual in-

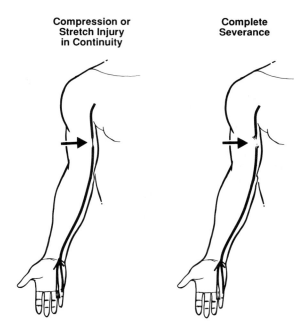

Compression or Stretch Injury in Continuity   **Complete Severance**

FIGURE 13.1.   *The fundamental distinction in diagnosis is that between a lesion in continuity and that of complete severance and discontinuity.*

crease in their number with further axonal regrowth. This is the earliest evidence of recovery, and it is seen a few weeks before there is visible contraction and often long before motor nerve conduction can be demonstrated by electrical stimulation.

An important concept in the assessment of traumatic palsies is that of what we have termed *the pace of recovery*, as illustrated in Figures 13.2 and 13.3. When a nerve lesion has been judged to be complete but in continuity, the time and distance relationships of reinnervation must be carefully considered. Reinnervation occurs at a rate of approximately 1 mm per day or 1 inch per month. A motor nerve that supplies branches to individual muscles along its linear course should show the first evidence of recovery in the muscle most proximal to the lesion after the appropriate time for reinnervation has elapsed. A muscle supplied at a distance about 3 inches from a site of injury as in axillary nerve palsy following blunt injury should show evidence of regeneration after 3 to 4 months have elapsed. If this does not occur, the pace of recovery is unduly slow, and the likelihood of a complete severance of the nerve or a mechanical obstruction to reinnervation must be considered. In our experience, serial electromyographic examinations have been a useful indicator

1. Usually blunt non-penetrating trauma
2. Clinically incomplete
3. Clinically complete but preserved
   motor units on EMG

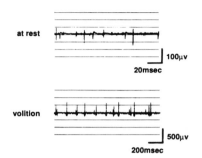

4. Satisfactory pace of recovery
   (time vs re-innervation distance relationship)

DELTOID EMG ON VOLITION IN AXILLARY NERVE PALSY
(estimated re-innervation distance 5 - 7 cm)

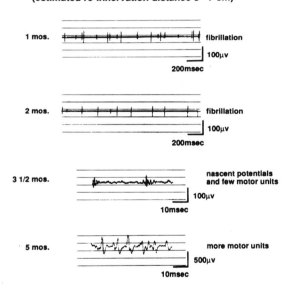

FIGURE 13.2. *Features of a traumatic lesion in continuity and the relevant electromyographic findings. The estimated reinervation distance defines the* pace of recovery *and indicates the time at which nascent potentials should appear. Serial electromyographic examinations are required to monitor the pace of recovery, and these are shown in a patient with circumflex nerve palsy after a shoulder dislocation. The reinervation distance is approximately 5 to 7 cm, and the appearance of nascent potentials between 3 and 4 months indicated a satisfactory pace of recovery.*

of the pace of recovery in patients with nerve lesions in continuity in the presence of a complete loss of function, and the *pace of recovery rule* has been of considerable help in the management of such patients. An excessively slow pace of recovery can indicate an unsuspected section of the nerve or an impediment to reinnervation by neuroma formation or fibrosis, and surgical exploration may therefore be required.

A denervated muscle eventually undergoes complete atrophy, and this progressive loss of viable muscle occurs over a matter of months. If denervated muscle can be reinnervated within a matter of a few months, some function can be restored. If, however, the muscle has undergone complete atrophy or if there has been an ischemic complication and the muscle has atrophied owing to an associated arterial injury, nerve regrowth is to no avail. As a general guide, it can be said that denervated muscle usually must be reinnervated within about 6 to 8 months in order that useful function can be restored. The verification of the nature of the lesion and the timing of an operative exploration of a nerve are contingent on an assessment of the pace of recovery and an awareness of the limited lifespan of denervated muscle.

Nerve Conduction

Motor nerve conduction, expressed as a latency or as a calculated motor conduction velocity, refers to the speed of transmission of the most rapidly conducting fibers, the large myelinated motor fibers. Gradual compression of motor nerve fibers, as in carpal tunnel syndrome or ulnar nerve pressure palsy, tends to effect the larger, myelinated, rapidly conducting fibers selectively. We do find, however, that the conduction velocity can be normal in patients with common peroneal nerve palsy and dropfoot, although the compound action potential (the amplitude of a motor response evoked by stimulation above the lesion and consisting of numerous MUs) is considerably diminished. Slowing of motor conduction is greatest over the region of entrapment or pressure; when the nerve has a long course and is superficial and accessible, it is possible, by stimulation at successive points, to demonstrate localized slowing, as for example at the elbow in ulnar pressure palsy. There are limitations to this technique, however, and our reliance on it has been a cautious one because errors in measurement are greater when dealing with short nerve segments.

When a mixed nerve is subject to pressure or entrapment, the earliest change involves sensory con-

1. More severe or penetrating injury
2. Complete paralysis (clinical and electrical)
3. Estimated pace of recovery not fulfilled
   (time vs re-innervation distance)

DELTOID EMG ON VOLITION IN AXILLARY NERVE PALSY
(estimated re-innervation distance 5 - 7 cm)

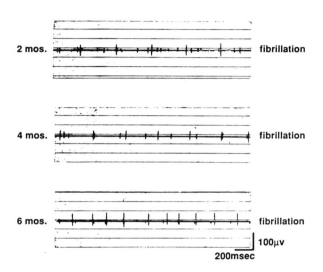

2 mos.   fibrillation

4 mos.   fibrillation

6 mos.   fibrillation

                                           100μv
           200msec

FIGURE 13.3.   *Features of a traumatic lesion in discontinuity and the electromyographic findings. Serial electromyographic examinations do not show any recovery at the expected time, and the estimated pace of recovery is therefore not fulfilled.*

duction, and motor conduction may remain normal. This is often seen in mild ulnar pressure palsy and in the milder cases of carpal tunnel syndrome. Electromyographic examination is usually within normal limits at this stage. When the lesion is more severe, conduction of the most rapidly conducting fibers is impaired, and there is a mild slowing of motor conduction. The disturbance of sensory conduction is usually greater at this stage, with a prolonged latency and conduction velocity and a considerably reduced or an absent sensory evoked response. Changes in the wave form and the duration of the sensory evoked response are of value in the detection of early involvement, and there is also dispersion of the compound motor action potential evoked by nerve stimulation.

The compound action potential, that is to say the action potential wave form that is made up or compounded of the multiple MUs evoked by stimulation of a motor nerve, is of some value in the assessment of the severity of peripheral nerve involvement and of the amount of residual muscle that is capable of contraction. A significant reduction of the compound action potential on maximal stimulation proximal to a localized nerve lesion indicates a conduction block, that is, a loss of conduction of some fibers across the lesion. Compound action potentials are properly recorded by the use of surface electrodes; modified compound action potentials of lower voltage with amplitudes up to several millivolts can be recorded by the concentric needle electrode at the time of electromyographic examination and are of less value for assessing conduction block. The amplitude of the compound action potential as recorded with surface electrodes is valuable for the assessment of the small muscles of the hands, feet, and facial muscles but is not so readily applicable to examination of the more proximal muscles.

Motor Conduction Latency Values to a Proximal Muscle

For practical purposes, the nerves that innervate proximal muscles, such as the deltoid, supraspinatus, and biceps, are not accessible to stimulation at two points, and therefore a conduction velocity cannot be calculated. Nerve stimulation at one point, however, provides a latency value, and this is a measure of motor conduction of that nerve. These latency determinations are easy to obtain and are prolonged in incomplete nerve injuries. We have found them of value, however. We rely on electromyographic sampling of the involved muscles for the detection of denervation, surviving MUs under voluntary control, and motor nascent potentials of reinnervation. Normal range of latencies for the accessory and musculocutaneous nerves and for the deltoid, triceps, supraspinatus, and infraspinatus muscles as well as other nerves have been published by Ludin[23] and by Gassel.[24]

When a motor or mixed nerve is completely severed at some distance from the muscle, the nerve distal to the lesion remains excitable for some time, and electrical stimulation of the nerve results in muscle contraction. Gilliatt and Taylor[25] demonstrated that the distal facial nerve fibers remain excitable and conduct at a normal velocity for about 4 to 5 days after intracranial section of the VII cranial nerve at the time of operation for acoustic neuroma. The amplitude of the evoked motor potential gradually declined over this time without any change in latency, and conduction was completely lost after about the fifth day. Interference with axoplasmic flow and the early changes of wallerian degeneration are responsible for this loss of conduction. We have observed preservation of a motor response to electrical stimulation of the distal portion of a severed sciatic nerve for about 2 weeks after injury. Gilliatt and Hjorth[26] found no motor response in monkeys on stimulation of the distal stump after about 6 days, but precise information as to the duration of preserved nerve conduction following severance of the longer nerves in humans is not available. This preservation of nerve conduction in response to electrical stimulation distal to the lesion can be misleading when the patient is examined in the early days after injury.

If electrical studies confirm that the paralysis is complete, serial examinations are required to determine whether there is recovery and, if so, whether it is occurring at a satisfactory pace. Electromyographic examination of the muscle closest to the site of the presumed lesion must be done because recovery will be first detected there. For example, in a radial nerve palsy at the level of the spiral groove and with a rate of recovery of approximately 1 inch per month, evidence of reinnervation should be first detectable in the proximal portion of the brachioradialis muscle after about 3 to 4 months. The next site of recovery is that of the upper fibers of the extensor digitorum communis muscle, and if recov-

ery is not detected within about 4 to 5 months at these sites, it is reasonable to conclude that the nerve has been transected or that there is a mechanical impediment to reinnervation and that surgical exploration should be undertaken.

Intraoperative Recording

The majority of nerve injuries do not result in complete interruption or severence, and a neuroma often develops during the process of recovery. Kline and Nulsen[27] described the incidence of neuromas in continuity, made up of sworls of disorganized axonal and connective tissue, to be 60%. Recovery of function under such circumstances can be minimal, and the question does arise as to whether this can be improved by a resection of the neuroma with reanastomosis of the nerve ends or by a nerve graft procedure. Kline and Nulsen have assessed continuity by the technique of bipolar electrical stimulation proximal to the neuroma and an attempted recording of a compound nerve action potential distal to the neuroma along with an electromyographic response in the appropriate muscle. In their experience, the presence of a compound nerve action potential is regarded as an indication for external neurolysis, whereas the absence of a potential should lead to resection and suture of the lesion.

Williams and Terzis[28] described the results of bipolar stimulation and recording from single fascicles that had been dissected out of the neuroma to detect continuity and to provide a rational basis for a more selective resection and suture. The authors believed, on comparison with the more radical resection of an entire neuroma, that the outcome had been improved by this single fascicle recording technique.

Electrical stimulation has also been used to identify fascicles, as an adjunct to nerve repair. The introduction of the operating room microscope in the early 1970s made it possible to suture individual fascicles, and considerable effort has been directed to obtaining correct fascicular orientation at the time of suture. Discrete stimulation of individual fascicles by a needle electrode has been used to identify the motor fasciculi in the distal segment and the sensory fasciculi in the proximal segment.[29,30] In this procedure, it is assumed that fasciculi in the proximal segment that are not sensory are therefore motor. The identification of motor fasciculi in the proximal and distal segments probably does permit a more accurate suture technique.

Hakstian[31] gave an earlier report of this method by the use of a unipolar needle stimulating electrode in the awake patient. The patient must be awake, able to cooperate, and indicate the region of the hand in which sensation is felt when the proximal segment is stimulated, whereas a motor response can be observed on stimulation of the distal stump. The fascicles are then labeled with a dye or a stitch, and the proximal and distal stumps are matched in such a way that the labeled proximal funicular ends are joined to the appropriate distal ones. Gaul[30] has reported good results obtained by this method.

Mackinnon and Dellon[32] have commented on these techniques. Under appropriate anesthesia, the nerve is explored and the nerve ends are prepared for electrical evaluation. The patient is then wakened, and the fascicles of the proximal stump are stimulated electrically to identify the sensory fascicles and those that are silent and therefore assumed to be motor fascicles. Stimulation of the sensory fascicles results in pain or sensation in a distinct cutaneous region. Stimulation of the motor fascicles does elicit a slight aching sensation in a deeper, less well-defined location, corresponding to the approximate location of the muscle. Stimulation of the distal stump elicits a motor contraction only in the early days after a complete transection.

Clinical Examination

In every case of peripheral nerve injury, a neurologic examination of sensory motor function by the referring physician or surgeon is a necessary prelude to an informed request for electrophysiologic investigation. The electrophysiologic examination is best regarded as an extension of the clinical examination, and to provide precise and authoritative results, the electromyographer must perform an examination that is appropriate to the nature and complexity of the diagnostic problem. The examiner must possess a thorough knowledge of peripheral nerve anatomy, including a knowledge of the segments of origin of the major peripheral nerves, their course, branches, muscles supplied by those nerves, and their sensory supply as well as the anatomy of the brachial and lumbosacral plexuses. To facilitate this, we have made up poster-sized charts of the major nerves—the ulnar, radial, median, sciatic, medial, and lateral popliteal nerves—and of the brachial and lumbosacral plexuses, all of which are mounted on the walls of the EMG/Nerve Conduction laboratory, in full view of the examining area. The individual drawings have been adapted from the MRC Handbook on peripheral nerve examination, a publication that has now been revised as *Aids to the Examination of*

the Peripheral Nervous System (1986).[33] In addition, we have devised a brachial plexus assessment chart and a lumbosacral plexus chart, each of which contains a drawing of the respective plexus and a list of the major muscles and their segmental origin, with columns to contain the clinical findings appropriate to such plexus injuries, as shown in Figures 13.4 and 13.5. These devices have proved of considerable teaching value, have permitted a more rapid and accurate evaluation of individual patients, and have been especially useful in the documentation and analysis of the more complex problems of brachial and lumbosacral plexus injury.

An important finding in patients with obvious or suspected nerve injury is that of *functional overlay*: findings of a sensory or a motor involvement that are nonanatomic and out of proportion to any possible physical cause. For example, a patient with an isolated ulnar nerve palsy or with a mild residual sensory motor median nerve defect following an occupational injury at the level of the wrist may show a diffuse loss to pinprick and vibration extending up to the shoulder along with a generalized weakness of the entire extremity. Similarly, functional sensory motor abnormalities may be found in patients in whom there is no demonstrable nerve lesion. Such findings provide the basis for a diagnosis of a conversion (hysterical) reaction. The detection of a functional disorder or overlay is important; its presence is an indication of the patient's illness behavior and response to bodily symptoms, and it has implications for prognosis. In our experience, patients with functional overlay often do not respond well to treatment and may remain troubled and disabled by minor residual symptoms that would be ignored by another subject. Their continuing complaints may lead to unnecessary investigations and treatments that may serve to ingrain further the illness behavior. An awareness of the presence of a functional disorder assists the clinician and the electrophysiologist in interpreting the significance of minor clinical and electrical changes that might otherwise be given undue emphasis. We regard the presence of a functional disorder or overlay as a poor prognostic indicator, and it may represent a contraindication to an elective surgical procedure for pain or other discomfort when objective clinical or electrophysiologic findings are minimal or absent.

We also believe it is important to recognize that the electrophysiologic investigation is an extension of the clinical neurologic examination and that the application of the specific techniques and methods of electrical examination and the interpretation of

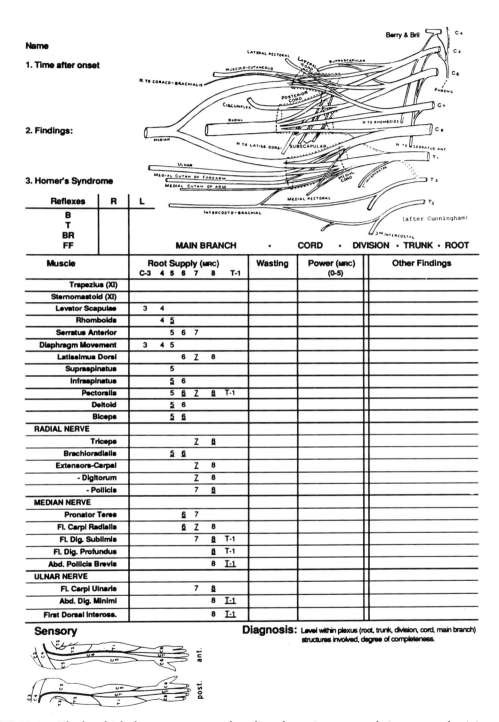

Muscle	Root Supply (MRC) C-3 4 5 6 7 8 T-1	Wasting	Power (MRC) (0-5)	Other Findings
Trapezius (XI)				
Sternomastoid (XI)				
Levator Scapulae	3 4			
Rhomboids	4 5			
Serratus Anterior	5 6 7			
Diaphragm Movement	3 4 5			
Latissimus Dorsi	6 7 8			
Supraspinatus	5			
Infraspinatus	5 6			
Pectoralis	5 6 7 8 T-1			
Deltoid	5 6			
Biceps	5 6			
RADIAL NERVE				
Triceps	7 8			
Brachioradialis	5 6			
Extensors-Carpal	7 8			
- Digitorum	7 8			
- Pollicis	7 8			
MEDIAN NERVE				
Pronator Teres	6 7			
Fl. Carpi Radialis	6 7 8			
Fl. Dig. Sublimis	7 8 T-1			
Fl. Dig. Profundus	8 T-1			
Abd. Pollicis Brevis	8 T-1			
ULNAR NERVE				
Fl. Carpi Ulnaris	7 8			
Abd. Dig. Minimi	8 T-1			
First Dorsal Inteross.	8 T-1			

Diagnosis: Level within plexus (root, trunk, division, cord, main branch) structures involved, degree of completeness.

FIGURE 13.4.   *The brachial plexus assessment chart lists the major nerves, their segmental origins, the muscles that they supply, and the dermatomes and contains headings for the clinical information that is essential to diagnosis. The diagnosis should attempt to indicate the site of the lesion, be it the root, spinal nerve, trunk, division, or cord, and it should also indicate any involvement of single or multiple branches and of any of the long nerves.*

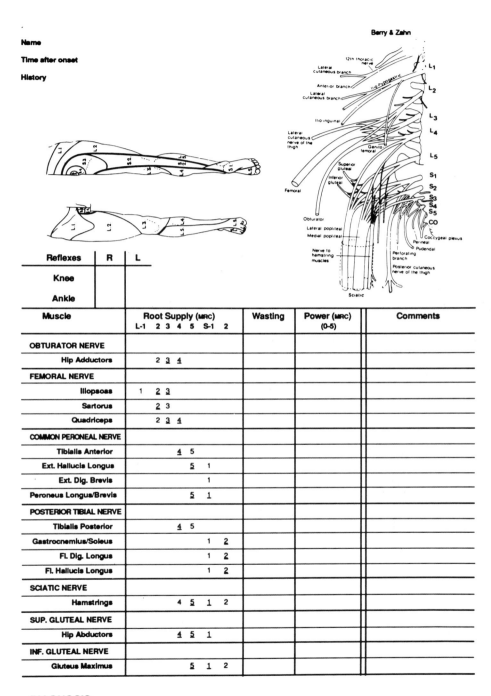

Name

Time after onset

History

Berry & Zahn

Reflexes	R	L
Knee		
Ankle		

Muscle	Root Supply (MRC) L-1 2 3 4 5 S-1 2	Wasting	Power (MRC) (0-5)	Comments
OBTURATOR NERVE				
Hip Adductors	2 3 4			
FEMORAL NERVE				
Iliopsoas	1 2 3			
Sartorus	2 3			
Quadriceps	2 3 4			
COMMON PERONEAL NERVE				
Tibialis Anterior	4 5			
Ext. Hallucis Longus	5 1			
Ext. Dig. Brevis	1			
Peroneus Longus/Brevis	5 1			
POSTERIOR TIBIAL NERVE				
Tibialis Posterior	4 5			
Gastrocnemius/Soleus	1 2			
Fl. Dig. Longus	1 2			
Fl. Hallucis Longus	1 2			
SCIATIC NERVE				
Hamstrings	4 5 1 2			
SUP. GLUTEAL NERVE				
Hip Abductors	4 5 1			
INF. GLUTEAL NERVE				
Gluteus Maximus	5 1 2			

DIAGNOSIS:

FIGURE 13.5.　*The lumbosacral plexus assessment chart lists the major nerves, their segmental origins, the muscles that they supply, and the dermatomes, and it contains the headings for the clinical information that is essential to diagnosis. The diagnosis should attempt to indicate the site of the lesion, be it the root, spinal nerve, trunk, or division, and it should indicate any involvement of single or multiple branches and of the long nerves.*

the findings are based on a proper clinical understanding of the nature of the diagnostic problem. For example, electrophysiologic studies in an older patient may reveal mild sensory motor changes of an ulnar pressure palsy at the elbow when the patient is entirely asymptomatic; when there is no muscle wasting, weakness, or definite sensory loss; and when treatment, other than the advice to avoid excessive elbow pressure, is not required. Similar electrical values may be obtained in a patient with wasting and weakness of the ulnar-supplied muscles who has been unresponsive to conservative treatment and in whom surgical treatment is required. This important distinction and its implications for treatment can be made only on clinical grounds.

ULNAR NERVE INJURIES AT THE ELBOW

The ulnar nerve arises from the medial cord of the brachial plexus, containing fibers from the C-8 and T-1 nerve and, in the majority of patients, from the C-7 root. It lies alongside of the axillary and then the brachial artery, and it pierces the medial intermuscular septum and descends in front of the medial head of the triceps to reach the space between the olecranon and the medial epicondyle of the humerus. An aponeurotic arch between the epicondyle and the olecranon covers the ulnar nerve, and it then enters the forearm between the humeral and ulnar origins of the flexor carpi ulnaris and descends between the flexor carpi ulnaris and flexor digitorum profundis muscles. It becomes more superficial in the distal half of the forearm, lying on the medial side of the ulnar artery and overlapped by the tendon of the flexor carpi ulnaris muscle. Just proximal to the flexor retinaculum, it pierces the deep fascia in company with the artery and passes to the front of the retinaculum at the lateral side of the pisiform bone, where it divides into its two terminal branches, the superficial and deep. The ulnar nerve gives off no branches until it reaches the forearm. The ulnar nerve can be involved in acute injuries that involve laceration or penetration, but it is most commonly involved in pressure or compressive injuries as a result of a single compression or of multiple minor pressure injuries, as in the common tardy ulnar nerve palsy or ulnar sensorimotor neuritis at the elbow.

The ulnar nerve is in its most vulnerable position at the elbow, behind the medial epicondyle of the humerus as it lies in the cubital tunnel. The floor of this tunnel consists of the ulnar collateral ligament of the elbow, and the roof consists of the aponeu-

rosis, which bridges the two heads of the flexor carpi ulnaris muscle. Anatomic variations in this region appear to determine the vulnerability of the nerve to pressure palsy. The depth of the postcondylar groove; the mobility of the nerve; the degree to which the proximal portion of the aponeurosis (the arcuate ligament) tightens on elbow flexion with associated compression of the nerve; the presence of overlying subcutaneous fat as a protective layer and any local pathologic condition of the joint such as degenerative change, deformity, or thickening of the joint capsule all determine the vulnerability of the nerve to local pressure and trauma. Systemic conditions such as diabetes mellitus, alcoholism, or other diseases that can cause generalized peripheral neuropathy also influence vulnerability; the combination of these along with the mechanical factors and the effect of local pressure or trauma results in the palsy.

A history of repeated pressure on the elbow as in leaning on a desk or during telephone work is obtained in some patients. Postoperative ulnar nerve palsy represents a distinct etiologic group, and the condition is also seen after fractures around the elbow. In the majority of patients, in our experience, there is either a history of repeated pressure or of elbow trauma.

Ulnar nerve palsies occur following penetrating injuries and lacerations or local contusions, following a surgical procedure as a postanesthetic palsy,[34,35] as a sleep or *Saturday night palsy*, after coma,[36] following fractures around the elbow with or without dislocation,[36] and as a result of recurrent dislocation of the ulnar nerve.[37] They have also been described as a type of occupational palsy.

In our experience of 1245 patients with ulnar nerve palsy verified by electrical study, the majority were men between the ages of 40 and 60. Symptoms had usually been present for a few months to a year, and the condition was usually unilateral. Patients most frequently complained of numbness involving the fourth and fifth fingers in a characteristic distribution, and weakness was noted in about one-third. The condition can be asymptomatic, and it was detected as an incidental finding by electrical studies alone in about 20% of cases at the time of electrophysiologic examination for a suspected carpal tunnel syndrome, peripheral neuritis, or entrapment elsewhere.

On clinical examination, minimal wasting is best detected by examining the first dorsal interosseous muscle and comparing it with the opposite side. Hypothenar muscle bulk can be assessed by palpation of the muscle between the examiner's thumb and index fingers. It is important to compare long finger flexor strength of the fourth and fifth fingers with the adjacent third and fourth fingers because this helps to distinguish ulnar nerve palsy at the elbow from the much rarer condition of ulnar nerve palsy at the wrist. Sensation is readily assessed, and minor sensory changes can often be confirmed by the loss of two-point discrimination over the fifth and adjacent half of the fourth finger when two-point discrimination is used as a test of peripheral nerve function and not of parietal lobe sensory function.

The most common consideration in differential diagnosis is that of cervical disc disease and C-7 or C-8 nerve root involvement. A history of neck pain along with loss of triceps reflex, at times accompanied by wasting and weakness, is diagnostic of C-7 nerve root involvement. The rarer condition of C-8 nerve root compression closely mimics the motor involvement of ulnar nerve palsy, but there is also weakness of thumb and finger extension and thinning and weakness of abductor pollicis brevis muscle action because these functions are subserved by the C-8 root. Wasting of the small muscles of the hand can occur in syringomyelia, and the accompanying dissociated sensory loss should serve to indicate this diagnosis. Motor neuron disease of the amyotrophic lateral sclerosis or progressive muscular atrophy type can produce wasting of the small muscles of the hand sometimes with fasciculation, evident progression, and evidence of more widespread muscle involvement together with signs of upper motor neuron involvement in the case of amyotrophic lateral sclerosis and no accompanying sensory loss.

In more advanced cases, there is well-defined muscle atrophy and weakness as well as sensory loss, and the diagnosis can be confidently made without the use of electrical tests. The technique of electrical assessment involves stimulation of the ulnar nerve just above the elbow as well as below it and at the wrist with a recording of a compound action potential by surface or concentric needle electrodes from the abductor digiti minimi muscle. Sensory conduction is determined by stimulation of the fifth or fourth fingers with ring electrodes and detection of a sensory evoked response at the wrist by the single sweep or signal averaging method. The sensory response can also be detected at the elbow in a similar manner. We record the sensory response at the wrist as a distal latency and amplitude measurement. We do not routinely record the sensory evoked responses at the elbow, although a recording of these potentials does allow calculation of a trans elbow and forearm maximum conduction velocity for ulnar sensory fibers. Motor conduction may be expressed as a distal

latency between a stimulus site above the elbow and hypothenar, first dorsal interosseus, or flexor carpi ulnaris motor points, as a calculated maximum forearm conduction velocity, a trans sulcal velocity and the size of the surface recorded compound muscle action potential can also be recorded. The calculation of the trans-sulcal velocity, expressed as meters per second, may reveal a localized slowing corresponding to the site of the lesion and sometimes to a recognition of a conduction block but may also be misleading. The elbow segment is short and extends over a curved pathway. Exact measurement of this distance is difficult, with small discrepancies in the measurement of the nerve length easily leading to erroneous calculations of conduction velocity.

In mild cases of ulnar neuropathy, motor conduction may be normal between the proximal elbow and wrist stimulus sites, whereas sensory conduction is usually impaired; the sensory evoked response at the wrist, on stimulation of the fifth finger, is reduced in amplitude, usually with a normal latency, or it may be absent. In more advanced cases, slowing of motor conduction between the proximal elbow to wrist segment is usually demonstrable. Electromyographic examination may reveal some denervation with loss of MUs in ulnar intrinsic muscles and, later in the recovery stage, evidence of reinnervation with polyphasic action potentials. Finally, in the later stages, larger amplitude MU action potentials may be found.

The common site of the lesion in ulnar neuritis is at the elbow, and although earlier reports have emphasized prior fracture of the humerus, arthritis, or other abnormalities around the elbow as possible contributing factors in tardy ulnar nerve palsy, we have not found any predisposing abnormality in the majority of our patients. Gilliatt and Sears[38] have demonstrated the recording of compound nerve action potentials in patients with ulnar nerve lesions at the elbow, and Gilliatt and Thomas[39] described nerve conduction studies in 14 patients with chronic lesions at the elbow. Payan[40] described detailed studies of sensory and motor conduction as they could be applied to the localization of the lesion in ulnar nerve palsy and found that three-quarters of the lesions were due to unknown causes. Sensory fibers were the first to be affected, and the majority of lesions could be localized by electrophysiologic means to the elbow.[41] Investigation of a small number of patients before and after operative transposition of the nerve and after conservative management alone did not reveal any difference in outcome. The earliest electrophysiologic sign of recovery was an increase in conduction velocity across the sulcus, in both sensory and motor fibers. Adequate controlled observations of conservative versus operative management are required, but it does appear that operations are being performed unnecessarily.

In our experience, the common pattern of electrophysiologic abnormalities is that of a below normal, borderline, or slightly slowed forearm conduction velocity with a diminished to absent sensory evoked response. The sensory abnormality may be the only finding in patients with a minimal sensory ulnar neuritis.

Ulnar nerve palsy is not always a progressive condition. The majority of mild cases can be treated conservatively. We recommend conservative treatment alone, the advice to avoid elbow pressure, in the patient with a minimal sensory motor or a pure ulnar sensory neuritis. The presence of muscle wasting and weakness requires a consideration of the surgical treatment of decompression, with or without anterior transposition. An ulnar sensory motor neuritis attributable to a single accident or incident of ulnar nerve pressure can be followed as to gradual improvement, and surgical treatment can be avoided in most instances. In the more severe cases, recovery can be detected by clinical examination as well as by electrical tests. With recovery, motor conduction velocity improves, a larger number of MUs are detected during voluntary contraction, and the compound action potential of the abductor digiti minimi muscle as measured by surface electrodes also increases. When the paralysis is moderate in degree, closer follow-up assessment is required. If there is no improvement in the electrical parameters over the next months, if there is any suggestion of worsening, or if there is reason to believe that additional nerve pressure will occur because of abnormal angulation or other abnormality at the elbow, operative treatment is usually advisable. The decision as to surgical management has to be made after a consideration of the causation, the duration and severity, the likelihood of recurrent compression of the nerve, the anatomic features of the cubital tunnel, and the presence of any progression of the palsy, as balanced against the possibility of disruption of the blood supply to the ulnar nerve at the elbow and of other possible complications.

Improvement after surgical treatment may occur over a matter of months. The prognosis is poorer if atrophy has been longstanding, that is, for more than 8 months or so, or if the patient is suffering from a generalized peripheral neuropathy, as in alcoholism or diabetes.

The ulnar nerve is occasionally injured at a higher level, in the upper arm or close to the brachial plexus.

Because the ulnar nerve does not give off any branches in the upper arm and apart from evidence of local trauma and slowing of ulnar nerve conduction at a higher level, the clinical and electrophysiologic picture is identical to that of ulnar nerve palsy at the elbow. High ulnar nerve lesions can occur as part of brachial plexus injuries, and they may be combined with injury to the adjacent median and radial nerves and to the medial or other cords of the plexus.

ULNAR NERVE INJURY IN THE ARM AND FOREARM

The common ulnar nerve palsy occurs behind the elbow, and a traumatic incident cannot usually be identified. We have seen a number of ulnar nerve palsies following trauma to the forearm or around the elbow and upper arm, such as after a fall on the elbow, fracture and fracture dislocation around the elbow, crush and penetrating injury, stab wounds, or lacerations, and the palsies have usually been incomplete. The median nerve in the forearm may provide motor fibers to the hypothenar muscles via the ulnar nerve; this anomalous innervation (the Martin-Gruber anastomosis) and the preservation of function of this muscle, in the presence of a complete ulnar lesion at or above the elbow, can lead to the mistaken conclusion that the lesion is a partial one. The examination of ulnar nerve forearm motor conduction velocity by stimulation above and below the elbow, examination of sensory conduction, and electromyographic examination of individual ulnar-supplied muscles, along with clinical assessment, usually leads to accurate diagnosis and localization.

ULNAR NERVE PALSY AT THE WRIST

The ulnar nerve crosses superficial to the transverse carpal ligament, runs lateral to the pisiform bone, and enters Guyon's canal. This canal is formed by an extension of the tendon of the flexor carpi ulnaris muscle, which forms the roof, and its only contents are the ulnar nerve and artery. The nerve divides into superficial and deep branches inside the canal, and the superficial branch supplies the cutaneous distribution of the ulnar nerve in the hand. The deep branch passes between the heads of the flexor and abductor digiti minimi, winding around the hook of the hamate and deep into the palm. It runs laterally within the concavity of the palmar arch. The deep branch supplies the hypothenar muscles: the flexor and abductor digiti minimi, the interossei, the third and fourth lumbricals, and the adductor pollicis. In one-third of patients, the flexor pollicis muscle is also supplied.

Ulnar nerve palsies at the wrist have been described and classified by Wu et al.[42] The condition has been described following fractures at the wrist,[43] after fractures of the distal radius,[44] and after prolonged bicycle riding.[45] Several authors have reviewed the anatomy of Guyon's canal and its variants.[46,47] Dodds et al.[47] performed 58 wrist dissections and found a 22% incidence of anomalous muscles that pass through the canal. Aberrant branching of the ulnar nerve in the canal is rare and was seen only in 2% of the 58 wrist dissections. Still and Kleinert[48] described ulnar nerve entrapment at the wrist by anomalous muscles, and Swanson et al.[49] described ulnar nerve compression owing to an anomalous muscle in the Guyon's canal. Ulnar neuropathy at the wrist has also been reported with aberrant flexor carpi ulnaris insertion.[50] Zook et al.[51]

described palmar wrist pain owing to ulnar nerve entrapment within the flexor carpi ulnaris tendon. Ulnar nerve involvement at the wrist can also be due to lipoma[52] and rheumatoid arthritis,[53] to compression secondary to a rheumatoid synovial cyst,[54] and to mutilating injuries of the wrist.[55]

Ulnar nerve lesions around the wrist can be divided into three groups according to the clinical signs and the apparent site of the lesion[56]: pure motor lesions of the deep palmar branch, pure motor lesions of the proximal palmar motor branch, and sensory/motor ulnar palsy at the wrist, as in Figure 13.6. In our series of 32 palsies at the wrist, 20 involved the deep palmar motor branch, eight involved the proximal motor palmar branch, and four had sensorimotor involvement.

Deep Palmar Motor Branch Palsy

Involvement of the deep palmar branch of the ulnar nerve is the most common form of ulnar palsy in

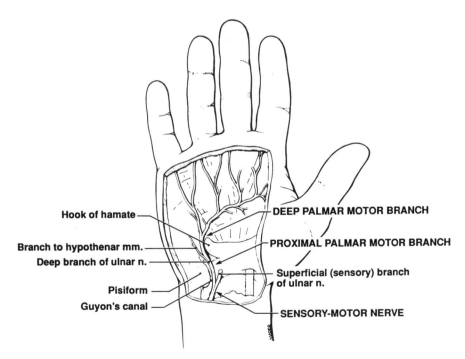

FIGURE 13.6.   *Ulnar nerve palsy at the wrist can be conveniently divided into three groups. The most distal lesion is that of the deep branch (deep or distal palmar motor branch) of the ulnar nerve in the palm, and this is a purely motor lesion that involves the interosseous muscles. A slightly more proximal lesion (proximal palmar motor branch) within Guyon's canal involves the nerve to the hypothenar muscle, and it is also a purely motor lesion. An even more proximal lesion (sensory motor branch), at the level of the pisiform bone, transverse ligament, or proximal to it, involves the sensory as well as the motor branch.*

this region. In this condition, the deep palmar branch is involved after the hypothenar muscles have been supplied; the hypothenar muscles are therefore normal in bulk and strength, and sensation is not affected. The condition is seen over a wide age range, and there is usually a history of hand trauma or unusual and excessive usage of the hand in work that involves pressure on the palm. Weakness develops over weeks to a few months, and some patients have improved with conservative treatment alone, with the advice to avoid pressure on that portion of the palm. We recommend surgical exploration if the wasting and weakness are unusually severe or if there has not been improvement over a follow-up interval of about 2 to 4 months. At exploration, a carpal synovioma is a common finding. Thickening of the pisohamate ligament with an overhanging hook of the hamate has also been described.[57]

In our series, we have seen 20 patients with deep palmar branch involvement, six with a more proximal but purely motor lesion that also involves the abductor digiti minimi muscle, and eight with an even more proximal lesion around the wrist with involvement of the sensory supply in addition to the aforementioned motor involvement. Sixteen out of 20 patients gave a history of trauma, and the most common cause was that of the repeated use of hand tools such as an awl, screwdriver, pliers, staple gun, or vibrating tool, in seven patients. Three were associated with other forms of manual labor, and in two patients, the onset occurred after unusual activity, such as shoveling snow or breaking ice. Two patients had suffered lacerations, and one had suffered a crush injury. One patient was an amputee who used crutches.

The clinical picture is that of wasting and weakness of the first dorsal interosseous as well as the other interosseous muscles, with sparing of the abductor digiti minimi. There is no sensory abnormality. Some patients have a callus over the region of the pisiform and hook of the hamate (Guyon's canal). The differential diagnosis must include other causes of wasting of the small muscles of the hand with sparing of sensation such as motor neuron disease (progressive muscular atrophy). Syringomyelia can cause wasting of the small hand muscles, but the wasting is usually more diffuse, and there is a dissociated sensory loss with preservation of light touch and with loss of pain and temperature sensation. Cervical disc disease with involvement of the C-8 root can result in wasting of the small muscles of the hand, but involvement goes beyond the ulnar nerve territory and usually includes the thenar eminence,

with weakness of the abductor pollicis brevis muscle and the forearm thumb extensors.

Electrical studies confirm the site of the lesion. On stimulation of the ulnar nerve at the wrist, the distal motor latency to the abductor digiti minimi muscle is normal, but the latency to the first dorsal interosseous muscle is usually but not invariably prolonged. The electromyogram of the first dorsal interosseous muscle reveals denervation with a diminished interference pattern. We usually do not examine the other interossei. Electromyographic examination of the abductor digiti minimi muscle is within normal limits. The ulnar nerve sensory evoked response at the wrist is normal, and the wrist to above elbow motor conduction velocity is also normal. This combination of findings is diagnostic of a lesion of the deep palmar branch of the ulnar nerve.

The latency to the first dorsal interosseous muscle, on stimulation of the ulnar nerve at the wrist, was prolonged in 13 of our patients (the upper limit of normal in our laboratory is 5.1 ms), and the increase in latency varied from 5.3 to 13.5 ms, with an average of 7.3 ms. The latency was normal in the remaining seven patients. The compound action potential was not recorded in our earlier patients, but it was abnormal in at least one of the patients in the normal latency group. The latency to the abductor digiti minimi muscle was within normal limits, with an average value of 3.2 ms. The sensory branch is spared in this condition, and ulnar nerve sensory responses are therefore entirely normal. The usual findings on electromyographic examination of the first dorsal interosseous muscle were those of fibrillation potentials and reduced recruitment. Nine patients underwent surgical exploration, and this revealed fibrous bands in four, a ganglion in Guyon's canal in two and ligamentous thickening in two, and the nerve was found to be unusually tight around the hook of the hamate in one. Seddon[58] reported four cases caused by a ganglion arising from the palmar aspect of one of the carpal joints, which compressed the deep palmar branch of the nerve, and additional cases were described by Ebeling et al.[57]

Proximal Palmar Motor Branch Palsy

We have had eight patients with the more proximal variant of palsy, in which there is involvement of the deep palmar branch along with the branch to the abductor digiti minimi muscle. There is purely motor involvement, and the sensory branch is spared. There was a history of trauma in two patients (wrist fracture and severe blow to the elbow); one patient had used a cane for many years, and another was a laborer. The onset appeared to be spontaneous in two patients. The clinical picture of wasting of the ulnar-supplied small muscles of the hand but without sensory involvement or involvement of the long finger flexors of the fourth and fifth fingers was distinctive. Motor latency values to both the first dorsal interosseous and the abductor digiti minimi muscle were prolonged in three patients and were prolonged only to the first dorsal interosseous muscle in two patients. Latency values were entirely normal in one patient. Electromyographic examination of the first dorsal interosseous and abductor digiti minimi muscles revealed fibrillation potentials and positive sharp waves. All patients came to surgical exploration, with the findings of a ganglion in the region of Guyon's canal in two, fibrous tissue bands in two, and scarring or ligamentous thickening in two. Mallett and Zilkha[59] reported two cases, both men over the age of 40 with a history of chronic occupational trauma in one and of an acute wrist strain in another; a ganglion was found on operation in both.

The site of the lesion can be confirmed by electrical studies, and the changes are identical to those described for the deep palmar branch lesion except for the additional finding of involvement of the hypothenar muscles characterized by denervation, diminished MUs, and a reduction in the interference pattern. The distal latency to the abductor digiti minimi muscle is often prolonged, and it has ranged from 2.8 to 6.7 ms. The latency to the first dorsal interosseous muscle is also prolonged and in our experience has ranged from 6.7 to 9.2 ms. The sensory evoked response over the ulnar nerve at the wrist is normal, and the ulnar nerve forearm conduction velocity is also normal.

Lesions of the Ulnar Nerve at the Wrist Involving the Sensory and Motor Branch

In this condition, the lesion is a little more proximal to the previous ones, and it involves the motor as well as the sensory supply. The clinical picture is one of both motor and sensory involvement: weakness and wasting of the ulnar-supplied small muscles of the hand and a sensory loss of the fifth and adjacent half of the fourth fingers and palm. This condition can be distinguished from ulnar nerve palsy at the elbow by the preservation of long flexor action of the fourth and fifth fingers and of the flexor carpi ulnaris muscle. The dorsal cutaneous branch of the ulnar nerve is not involved, and normal sensation may therefore be demonstrated on the dorsum of the

ulnar-supplied fingers, as a clue to the site of the ulnar nerve involvement.

In our experience, electrical studies, in combination with careful clinical examination, allow localization of the lesion. Denervation is present in the abductor digiti minimi and the first dorsal interosseous muscles exhibit reduced recruitment of MUs and prolonged distal motor latencies to the abductor digiti minimi and first dorsal interosseous muscles. There is little or no slowing of motor conduction of the elbow to the wrist nor directly over the transsulcal portion of the ulnar nerve. Compound sensory nerve action potentials are reduced or absent at the wrist and elbow.

In our series of eight patients, three followed fractures about the wrist; four patients had suffered lacerations, and two of these had associated median nerve and tendon injuries. The other two patients had experienced a blow to the wrist and a pressure type injury. Motor latency values to the first dorsal interosseous and abductor digiti minimi muscles were delayed to both muscles in three patients, were not obtainable in two, and were delayed to one muscle and normal to the other in three patients. Both motor latency values were normal in one patient. The sensory response at the wrist was absent in eight patients, and there was diminished amplitude in one patient; that patient also had normal motor latency values. The latency to the abductor digiti minimi muscle was prolonged to an average of 5.3 ms, and, to the first dorsal interosseous, to an average of 10.6 ms. The sensory response was absent in our four patients, and the ulnar forearm motor conduction velocity was normal. Electromyographic examination revealed findings of denervation and diminished MUs in those patients with incomplete lesions, and there was no detectable MU activity in the two patients in whom the lesion was complete. Two patients improved without surgical treatment, and one remained unchanged.

RADIAL NERVE

The radial nerve is the continuation into the upper limb of the posterior cord of the brachial plexus. It usually contains fibers from all of the segments that form the posterior cord: C-5, C-6, C-7, and C-8 segments. As a variation, the C-5 segment may not make any contribution,[60] and the first thoracic nerve may also not contribute. The radial nerve passes through the axilla, and then it lies to the medial side of the humerus, passing between the long and medial heads of the triceps to reach the spiral groove; it passes laterally and downward in the groove around the back of the humerus and under cover of the lateral head of the triceps, piercing the intermuscular septum at the lateral border of the triceps and passing to the front of the lateral epicondyle of the humerus, where it lies deeply between the brachioradialis and the brachialis muscles, after which it becomes the posterior interosseous nerve. It gives off four sets of branches. The posterior cutaneous nerve of the arm arises at the level of the axilla and supplies the skin of the posterior surface of the upper arm. Muscular branches arise medially to the humerus and supply the long, medial, and lateral heads of the humerus above the level of the spiral groove, and a branch descends along the humrus and behind the lateral epicondyle to terminate in the anconeus muscle. This latter branch is of some practical significance because the anconeus muscle is usually spared in the common radial nerve palsy that occurs at the level of the spiral groove. The lower lateral cutaneous nerve of the arm rises from the upper portion of the radial nerve, as does the posterior cutaneous nerve of the forearm before its entry into the spiral groove. The former nerve supplies the lower lateral and adjacent aspects of the upper arm, below the territory of supply of the axillary nerve, and the posterior cutaneous nerve of the forearm supplies a band of sensation down the posterior part of the forearm as a continuation of the area of supply of the lower lateral cutaneous nerve. The posterior cutaneous nerve of the forearm territory extends to the level of the wrist and at times over the dorsum of the hand. High lesions of the radial nerve therefore result in a loss of sensation over the posterior aspect of the upper arm, below the area supplied by the circumflex nerve, extending over and beyond the elbow, and in a band-like area of loss over the extensor surface of the forearm, which extends down into the dorsum of the hand. Some sensory branches arise in the forearm and extend down to the level of the wrist, the dorsum of the hand, and occasionally the dorsum of the thumb. At the lateral side of the humerus are found muscular branches to the brachioradialis and extensor carpi radialis longus and brevus muscles.

Radial nerve palsy is a common complication of fractures of the humerus,[61,62] and it has been described with neurilemoma,[63] as a complication of elbow arthroscopy,[64] and following fracture-dislocations around the elbow.[65] It is a common form of pressure palsy, as in *Saturday night* paralysis.

A high radial nerve lesion, at the level of the axilla or upper portion of the brachium, therefore results in an extensive sensory loss involving the brachium, forearm, and dorsum of the hand in addition to weakness, wasting, and denervation of all of the muscles within the radial nerve territory, the triceps, anconeus, brachioradialis, and extensor carpi radialis longus muscles as well as the forearm muscles within the posterior interosseous nerve territory. A complete lesion is occasionally seen following penetrating injury, but in our experience it is most common as part of a brachial plexus injury with posterior cord involvement.

The usual radial nerve palsy occurs at the level of the spiral groove following midhumerus fracture and other forms of trauma and in *Saturday night* paralysis. In such patients, the triceps muscle is spared, with a preserved triceps tendon jerk, and either no sensory loss or loss within the territory of the dorsal cutaneous nerve of the forearm. The anconeus muscle can be palpated just behind the head of the radius, in front of the posterior border of the ulna, and it can be seen to be spared and to contract on elbow extension. The brachioradialis muscle is paralyzed, and the wrist, finger, and thumb extensor muscles are involved. The paralysis, on clinical examination, is usually incomplete and the wrist-drop is symmetric; that is to say, in those patients with incomplete lesions who have preserved wrist extension, the wrist extends without drift to either side. This is in contradistinction to posterior interosseous nerve palsy, in which wrist extension results in a radial drift owing to preservation of extensor carpi radialis longus action in the presence of involvement of the extensor carpi radialis brevis and extensor carpi ulnaris muscles. The sensory disturbance is usually minimal and involves a small patch over the dorsal aspect of the base of the thumb; this is absent in some patients, and the radial nerve sensory evoked response is preserved. The prognosis in these cases is usually good, with gradual improvement over weeks to a few months and with ultimate full recovery.

The diagnosis of a radial nerve lesion at the level of the spiral groove can be confidently made on the basis of clinical examination alone. There is a dropped wrist as well as dropping of the fingers and thumb and loss of brachioradialis contraction. Radial nerve involvement at the spiral groove level can be readily distinguished from the considerably less common condition of posterior interosseous nerve involvement in that wrist extension as well as brachioradialis action is spared in the latter. A spiral groove radial nerve palsy results in a dropped wrist, fingers, and thumb; a posterior interosseous palsy results in a dropped fingers and thumb with radial deviation of the extended wrist. A lesion of the C-8 root or spinal nerve in cervical disc disease results in triceps muscle weakness along with some weakness of the forearm, wrist, and thumb extensors, and careful examination may reveal some weakness of the finger flexors supplied by the median and ulnar nerves. The brachioradialis muscle is not involved, and these features, along with a history of neck and upper limb pain, readily distinguished this segmental lesion from radial nerve palsy.

The diagnosis of radial nerve palsy in the upper arm, at the spiral groove or at a higher level, can be made on clinical examination alone, and electrophysiologic investigations are not strictly necessary. When the palsy appears to be complete on clinical examination, electromyographic examination is useful because it can detect surviving MUs as evidence of continuity. The typical electromyographic findings in a patient with a radial nerve palsy, examined about 14 days after onset, reveal denervation with fibrillation potentials and positive sharp waves, with or without surviving MUs. With an electromyographic needle in place in the forearm extensor muscles and on stimulation of the radial nerve at the level of the elbow, spiral groove, and high in the axilla, conduction latency values can be obtained when there is continuity. These are used by some laboratories in the assessment of radial nerve palsy,[66] although we have not found these to be necessary and we do not use them.

If the paralysis is complete by clinical and electrical examination and the injury a penetrating one or of a type suggestive of severance of the nerve, early surgical exploration should be considered. If, however, there has been a blunt or stretch injury, serial examinations can be done to monitor recovery. An incomplete radial nerve palsy on initial examination usually does not require electrical testing and can be followed by clinical examination alone. A complete radial nerve palsy, at the level of the spiral groove, if in continuity, should show the earliest electromyographic evidence of reinnervation by about 3 to 4 months, in the upper fibers of the brachioradialis muscle, a reinnervation distance of a few inches only. If this does not occur, surgical exploration becomes advisable.

Techniques of radial nerve motor conduction measurement have been described by numerous authors.[66] Stimulation at Erb's point, the lateral mid-humerus, and at a point 5 cm superior to the lateral epicondyle, with recordings in the brachioradialis and forearm muscles, can provide nerve conduction latency measurements such that motor conduction values can be calculated.

In our personal series of 114 patients, 76 were on a traumatic basis and 38 occurred spontaneously and mainly on awakening as a form of *Saturday night* palsy. The involvement was incomplete in virtually all of the spontaneous cases. Of the 76 traumatic radial nerve palsies, 36 occurred in association with fracture of the humerus, and half of these were incomplete. In 10 patients, the palsy followed blunt trauma to the upper arm; in eight, a hypodermic injection; and in four, a compressive upper arm injury. In a few patients, the cause was that of a laceration, a gunshot wound, and the removal of fixation plates used to stabilize a fracture of the humerus. The degree of paralysis in the patients who had received injections was usually complete, but the other forms of trauma were equally divided between complete and incomplete involvement.

High Radial Nerve Palsy

In high radial nerve palsy, the lesion is above the level of the spiral groove and yet distal to the posterior cord such that the anconeus, all or part of the triceps, and the more distal muscles supplied by the radial nerve, are involved. We have examined nine patients with this condition. Two of these were nontraumatic, owing to a mass in the axilla and a posterior cord neuroma. Of the seven traumatic cases, four followed a fractured humerus, and the others were seen after a fall down the stairs, the use of crutches, and as a postoperative complication of excision of a neuroma of the posterior cord. With the exception of that which followed excision of the neuroma, all of the traumatic cases were incomplete.

POSTERIOR INTEROSSEOUS NERVE

The radial nerve, as it passes under the upper fibers of the brachioradialis muscle, becomes the posterior interosseous nerve, which then passes around the lateral side of the head and neck of the radius to pierce the supinator muscle. It passes down the dorsal surface of the forearm deep to the superficial extensor muscles, superficial to the abductor pollicis longus, and then passes deep to the extensor pollicis longus and lies on the interosseous membrane, where it terminates at the wrist. Apart from small articular branches to the intercarpal joints, it is a purely motor nerve, and as it passes across the elbow and down the forearm, it supplies in turn the extensor carpi radialis brevis, supinator, extensor digitorum, extensor digiti minimi, and extensor carpi ulnaris muscles. More distally, it supplies the abductor pollicis longus, extensor pollicis longus and brevis muscles, and the extensor indicis. It supplies the extensor carpi radialis brevis and the supinator muscles before it enters the supinator.

Posterior interosseous nerve palsy can be looked on as a partial form of radial nerve palsy; radial nerve palsy results in a drop wrist as well as dropped fingers and thumb, whereas a posterior interosseous nerve palsy results in dropped fingers and thumb only; in posterior interosseous nerve palsy, the lesion is below the branch to the extensor carpi radialis longus muscle. The extensor carpi radialis brevis muscle has a dual supply, from the radial as well as the posterior interosseous nerve, and wrist extension is therefore preserved and at or near full strength albeit with radial deviation. The supinator muscle can be tested by an attempt to pronate the hand when the elbow is fully extended and the forearm is fully supinated. In our experience, on clinical examination, the supinator muscle is often spared in this condition. When the arm is held outstretched, the fingers and thumb are dropped (the *dropped fingers and thumb sign*), and when the palsy is complete, there is no demonstrable extensor strength of the fingers or the thumb. Because the lumbrical muscles have an extensor action at the proximal interphalangeal joints and because they are supplied by the median and ulnar nerves, extensor strength can be demonstrated there when the metacarpophalangeal joints are held in a flexed position. Thumb abduction is weakened, and unless it is recalled that the abductor pollicis longus muscle is supplied by the posterior interosseous nerve, a diagnosis of median nerve involvement will be incorrectly made. Finger abductor strength (ulnar nerve supplied) also appears weak when testing is done with the arm in the usual outstretched position, and this can lead to the wrongful conclusion that there is ulnar nerve or C-8 root involvement. The hand must be placed on a flat, relatively friction-free surface with the wrist either in a neutral or extended position to test the finger abductors and adductors (interossei muscles) properly. Otherwise, the abducted fingers, when tested, slip into a flexed position, which gives the false impression of an abductor (ulnar-supplied) weakness. The brachioradialis muscle can be readily observed to be intact because it derives its supply from the radial nerve and is therefore spared.

The differential diagnosis of posterior interosseous nerve palsy includes radial nerve palsy at a higher level, C-8 nerve or root involvement as in cervical disc disease or brachial plexus trauma, and forearm muscle involvement in amyotrophic lateral sclerosis. A careful examination of the muscles supplied by the posterior interosseous nerve should exclude all of these conditions. C-8 segmental involvement results in dropped fingers, thumb, and wrist, and there is demonstrable weakness of finger abductors and adductors (ulnar nerve territory) as well as of the abductor pollicis brevis muscle (median nerve territory). The triceps reflex may also be diminished, and the history is that of neck and radicular pain and numbness as in cervical disc disease or that of trauma to the brachial plexus. The onset, in amyotrophic lateral sclerosis, is gradual without pain or history of injury, and a careful examination should reveal muscle involvement, which is usually outside of the territory of the posterior interosseous nerve. Electromyographic sampling of the forearm and adjacent muscles usually reveals evidence of chronic denervation with giant potentials, and there is often evidence of chronic denervation in muscles of the other extremities. In our experience, posterior interosseous nerve palsy is considerably less frequent than radial nerve palsy, and we have seen 25 cases of the former as opposed to 114 of the latter.

Carfi and Dong[67] reviewed retrospectively 12 patients, seven of whom had a history of elbow trauma with a blunt injury, fracture-dislocation, or a laceration. Five patients gave no history of injury, and the symptoms were those of weakness of the finger or wrist extensors, elbow pain, and, surprisingly, numbness of the forearm and hand in four patients. The authors point out that several normally present anatomic structures may compress the posterior interosseous nerve: fibrous bands anterior to the radial head, the recurrent radial fan of vessels, the tendinous margin of the extensor carpi radialis brevis, the arcade of Frohse, and the distal edge of the supinator muscle. Nontraumatic palsy has been attributed to tumors, rheumatoid disease, cysts, and repeated extension of the elbow along with extreme pronation and supination, which draws the edge of the extensor carpi radialis brevis muscle and arcade of Frohse into the nerve. Kaplan[68] described 15 patients with posterior interosseous neuropathy, 12 of whom were followed for 5 years. Seven patients had suffered closed injuries to the elbow, and eight had experienced the spontaneous onset of the condition association with heavy racquetball or tennis activity. All patients had tenderness over the lateral humeral epicondyle with the usual distribution of weakness of the thumb and fingers without any wrist weakness or sensory abnormality. The onset was gradual in the spontaneous cases, whereas it was sudden following elbow trauma. Electrodiagnostic testing was consistent with posterior interosseous neuropathy in all patients, and they were all treated conservatively. A few of the patients were treated with finger and wrist splinting to prevent overstretching of the extensor muscles, and gentle range-of-motion exercises were prescribed, followed by strengthening exercises as improvement occurred. Residual stiffness or weakness was not described, and those patients in whom the onset corresponded with heavy tennis and racquetball play had reduced their playing or had stopped playing. None of the patients were treated surgically. All recovered within 5 years, and it was suggested that this satisfactory natural course was the probable explanation for the good results of surgical decompression.

Holst-Nielsen and Jensen[69] described four patients who developed posterior interosseous nerve palsy during adulthood, with an average interval of 37 years after an unreduced dislocation of the radial head accompanying a Monteggia fracture in childhood. Surgical treatment by division of the ligament of Frohse was recommended. Jones et al.[70] reported an instance of an elderly patient with synovial chondromatosis at the elbow with posterior interosseous nerve compression, and El-Hadidi and Burke[71] described a palsy owing to a cystic bursa in the region of the supinator muscle that was attached to the distal biceps tendon. A case report of the sudden onset of wrist and finger extension weakness on the basis of posterior interosseous nerve palsy was reported after deep palpation near the right elbow.[72] The condition has also been described owing to lipoma,[73] rheumatoid arthritis,[74] and amyloid neuropathy.[75] Cravens and Kline[76] noted that, over a 15-year period, only 32 out of 170 patients with radial nerve disorders had posterior interosseous nerve involvement. The causes were entrapment at the arcade of Frohse in 14 patients, laceration in six, fracture in six, compression or contusion in three, and tumor in three. The ratio of men of women was 2:1, and the right arm was involved twice as frequently. Two patients had bilateral lesions, and 26 underwent surgical treatment.[76]

In our series of 25 patients, the most common cause was that of fracture of the head or proximal radius in eight patients, at times associated with fracture of the ulna or distal humerus. The condition came on postoperatively in five patients, after a local exploration for tennis elbow, resection of the head of the radius for a nonunited fracture, removal of fixation pins, and excision of a subcutaneous lump.

The palsy followed blunt trauma to the upper forearm in one patient and occurred after a traction injury of the upper extremity in another. In three patients, there was no definite trauma, although the palsy came on after a prolonged sleep, after hanging some heavy object, and after an insect bite to the forearm; in two patients of the spontaneous-onset group, there was an underlying peripheral neuropathy. Posterior interosseous palsy is usually incomplete, and this was so in 19 of our 23 patients. Complete paralysis was found in four patients, after a lacerating injury or a surgical exploration.

EMG is the investigation of choice in patients with posterior interosseous nerve palsy. A knowledge of the muscles supplied by the nerve readily permits its distinction, on clinical examination, from radial nerve palsy and from a rare C-8 nerve radiculopathy. Electromyographic studies are not mandatory for diagnosis but do provide prognostic information. Examination is best done after the fourteenth day following onset because fibrillation potentials are then usually present. Denervation can readily be confirmed in the extensor digitorum communis or the extensor pollicis longus muscles, and the electromyographic examination will identify whether the lesion is a partial or complete one by the presence or absence of surviving MU action potentials under voluntary control. Examination before 14 days reveals diminished to absent MUs without evidence of denervation.

Management is largely determined by the clinical picture. If there is a laceration in the region of the posterior interosseous nerve or a possibility that the nerve has been sectioned and the electrical findings are those of denervation without any MUs under voluntary control or in response to electrical stimulation of the radial nerve at a higher level, a severed nerve should be suspected and surgical exploration is advisable. If there has been blunt elbow trauma or if the palsy is of spontaneous onset, surviving MUs are usually demonstrable, and this indicates continuity and a good prognosis; a follow-up electromyographic examination can therefore be done after a few weeks to assess the pace of recovery. If there are no surviving MUs, the lesion may be in continuity, and follow-up examination may reveal the appearance of MUs under voluntary control. In our experience with blunt injuries around the elbow or cases of spontaneous onset, the lesions are usually incomplete as evidenced by surviving MUs under voluntary control. In patients with posterior interosseous nerve palsy, the site of the nerve lesion and the most proximal point of muscle innervation are only a few centimeters apart, and the *pace of recovery* rule dictates that in a complete lesion, the short reinnervation distance of about 3 to 5 cm should be traversed in about 2 months' time; reinnervation, as evidenced by motor nascent potentials and MUs, should appear in the uppermost fibers of the extensor digitorum communis muscle after about 2 months if there is no obstruction to reinnervataion. If there has been no recovery after 2 months, we recommend surgical exploration.

In addition to electromyographic examination of muscles within the posterior interosseous nerve territory, it is useful to perform sensory motor nerve conduction on the median and ulnar nerves of the upper extremity to exclude an underlying generalized neuropathy; the presence of generalized neuropathy indicates an increased vulnerability to pressure palsy and in our experience can also reduce the prognosis for a full recovery.

The technique of nerve conduction latency measurement and of stimulation of the radial nerve at multiple points to obtain a conduction velocity value has been applied to the assessment of posterior interosseous nerve function by Falck and Hurme[77] they give a detailed description of stimulation a few centimeters above the lateral epicondyle and several centimeters below it with the recording of a compound action potential from the extensor indicus proprius muscle such that a conduction velocity across the arcade of Frohse could be calculated. These elegant techniques are of considerable technical interest and are suitable for special study and research. For practical purposes, a thorough and satisfactory assessment can be obtained by the combination of a careful clinical examination and electromyographic sampling as we have described it.

ANTERIOR INTEROSSEOUS NERVE (MEDIAN NERVE AT THE ELBOW)

The anterior interosseous nerve is the large, purely motor branch of the median nerve that arises in the cubital fossa, passing between the two heads of the pronator teres muscle and then anterior to the interosseous membrane and posterior to the pronator quadratus muscle. It supplies the flexor pollicis longus, the lateral half of the flexor digitorum profundus, and the pronator quadratus muscle. Lesions of the anterior interosseous nerve are rare, and they have been described in isolated case reports and in small series.[78–80]

The nerve can be injured as a complication of a supracondylar fracture of the humerus in children, after penetrating injuries, blunt trauma, and compression injuries of the upper forearm. The clinical picture is characteristic and consists of pain at the onset in some patients, with weakness of the index finger and thumb flexion. When the patient attempts to make a fist, the index and thumb remain extended. When the ability to make a pinching movement with the thumb and index finger (the pinch test) is tested, the thumb and index finger extend rather than flex at their distal joints. The pronator quadratus muscle is also involved, and when the elbow is flexed to minimize action of the intact pronator teres muscle, a loss of forearm pronation strength can be demonstrated. There is no accompanying sensory disturbance, and if the weakness is severe and of sudden onset, an incorrect diagnosis of tendon rupture may be made. When the weakness of the flexor pollicis longus and flexor digitorum profundus to the index finger is mild in degree, recovery can occur over a matter of weeks.

If the paralysis is incomplete at the onset or improvement has occurred over a matter of weeks, follow-up is appropriate, and a satisfactory outcome can usually be expected.[81] If paralysis is complete on clinical examination or there is reason to suspect a section of the nerve because of fracture or penetrating injury, electromyographic studies may reveal surviving MUs in the involved muscles as evidence of continuity. In those patients in whom paralysis is found to be complete, by clinical and electrical examination, follow-up should reveal evidence of recovery within 3 to 4 months, and serial electromyographic examination should be attempted to detect this. If significant disability and paralysis persist for more than 3 months without improvement, the nerve should probably be explored. O'Brien and Upton[78] reviewed 23 cases drawn from the literature and noted that 13 patients underwent operative exploration. Constricting fibrous bands were found in seven patients and a neuroma in one.

Anterior interosseous nerve palsy has been reported as a result of arcuate ligament entrapment,[82] after the use of a sling for acromioclavicular joint dislocation,[83] and as a complication of irreducible supracondylar fracture of the humerus.[84] The condition has been referred to by several authors as the Kiloh-Nevin syndrome.[82,85,86] Hill et al.[87] described 33 cases of an incomplete anterior interosseous nerve syndrome in which there was isolated involvement of the flexor pollicis longus or of the flexor digitorum profundus of the index finger and stressed that this partial syndrome must be distinguished from flexor tendon rupture, adhesion, or stenosing tenosynovitis. They recommended surgical exploration in patients with complete paralysis who show no improvement clinically or electromyographically after 12 weeks of observation, and they note that the finding at operation is usually that of compression of the nerve by fibrous bands originating from the deep head of the pronator teres and extending to the brachialis fascia. Less common causes are fibrous bands from the superficial head of the pronator teres, bands from the superficialis arcade, the anomalous passage of the nerve deep to both heads of the pronator teres, or compression by a double lacertus fibrosis. In their series, most patients recovered spontaneously and did not require surgical exploration.

Electrical studies in these patients demonstrate a normal motor conduction velocity to the abductor pollicis brevis muscle, and the median nerve sensory responses at the wrist and elbow are also entirely normal. Electromyographic examination involves the accurate placement of needle electrodes into the deeper forearm muscles. O'Brien and Upton[79] published the electrical studies in a single patient, and there was normal sensory and motor conduction of the median nerve distally as well as in the forearm and upper arm; electromyographic examination revealed a diminished interference pattern of the pronator quadratus, the median-supplied portion of the flexor digitorum profundus, and of the flexor pollicis longus muscles. The variations of this rare nerve palsy are discussed in detail by Lake[87] and Spinner.[88]

Our series consists of 11 patients, and the majority of these cases occurred after trauma of diverse types, including knife injury with laceration, localized blunt injury, venipuncture, arthroscopy of the elbow, stretch injury of the forearm, localized pressure injury, and upper forearm fractures that required débridement and plate fixation. In one patient, the palsy occurred many years after a childhood forearm fracture. In three patients, it developed after carrying or pulling a heavy object with that upper limb.

Electromyographic examination requires careful needle placement into the appropriate forearm muscles. If denervation can be demonstrated in the suspected muscles, this confirms that the needle electrode has been accurately placed, and the presence of surviving MUs can be ascertained. In deeply placed muscles that cannot be identified by palpation or by surface anatomy, surviving MUs are easily missed on serial examinations, and in our experience, serial examinations are therefore not very reliable. We prefer to confirm the diagnosis by careful clinical examination of the thumb and index flexors, and we have not placed much reliance on the assessment of pronator quadratus strength. We perform a routine examination of the median nerve motor conduction to the abductor pollicis brevis muscle as well as assessment of the median nerve sensory responses at the wrist along with ulnar nerve sensory motor conduction to rule out an associated peripheral neuropathy, and we do not rely on EMG to confirm the specific muscle involvement. We take care to assess whether there is any residual long flexor action, that is, whether the paralysis is partial rather than complete, because this is important for prognosis. Because recovery is the rule and because it can be more confidently predicted in those with partial weakness, we restrict our attempts at sampling the involved muscles to those patients judged to have remained complete for about 3 months after onset and in whom the question of surgical exploration is being considered. Findings of polyphasic nascent potentials at the same insertion site in which there is denervation constitute strong evidence of continuity and reinnervation and are therefore an indication for further conservative management.

PRONATOR TERES SYNDROME

The pronator teres syndrome can be regarded as a slightly more proximal form of median nerve involvement in which the anterior interosseous nerve as well as the main trunk of the median nerve from which it has taken its origin are involved. In addition to features of anterior interosseous nerve palsy, there is altered sensation in the distribution of the median nerve, and innervation to pronator teres, flexor carpi radialis, and flexor digitorum sublimis is interfered with. There are three syndromes of compression of the median nerve in the proximal forearm or about the elbow: the pronator teres syndrome, anterior interosseous nerve syndrome, and the supracondylar process syndrome.[85] The pronator teres and supracondylar process syndromes are identical in that they involve all of the median nerve functions in the forearm and hand. The signs and symptoms of pronator teres syndrome are similar to those of carpal tunnel syndrome, with the addition of weakness of the long flexors of the thumb, index, and middle finger and of pronator quadratus action. It becomes apparent therefore that a patient with a good history of carpal tunnel syndrome, without any electrical abnormalities, may in fact have a pronator teres or supracondylar syndrome. The finding of weakness of the three long flexors and of pronation would confirm the diagnosis. It may be therefore that the diagnosis of this condition is being missed in those patients who appear to have the symptoms of carpal tunnel syndrome but who have normal electrical findings.

Entrapment of the median nerve in the proximal forearm takes two forms: the pronator teres and the anterior interosseous nerve syndrome. Both syndromes are rare and according to Nigst and Dick,[85] they constitute about 1% of the upper limb compression syndromes that come to surgical treatment. These authors describe nine cases of pronator teres syndrome, eight of which improved following surgical treatment. Both syndromes are noted to have a favorable prognosis, and the authors recommended operative treatment only in those patients who did not improve after about 8 weeks.

Entrapment of the median nerve by the upper portion of the pronator teres muscle has also been described by Seyffarth.[89] Kopell and Thompson[90] published a case report with operative confirmation of an anomalous fibrous band between the two heads of the pronator teres muscle that indented the median nerve. Morris and Peters[91] described the clinical and electrophysiologic features in seven cases. The majority responded to steroid injection in the upper portion of the pronator teres muscle, and the patients were advised to alter their activities. There was a history of considerable forearm and hand activity including forceful pronation, and the presenting symptoms were pain; tenderness of the proximal forearm; and numbness of the forearm, thumb, and index finger. Weakness of the flexor pollicis longus and abductor pollicis brevis muscles was almost always present, and the flexor digitorum profundus and opponens pollicis muscles were also described as weak. It was remarked that weakness could be missed if the strength was not compared with that of the opposite side. Sensory loss in a median nerve distribution was described in several patients, and there was tenderness over the pronator teres muscle and a positive Tinel's sign over the median nerve at that point. Motor conduction of the median nerve in the elbow to wrist segment was usually slowed, and distal motor latency was normal.

Despite a large laboratory experience, we have encountered only four patients in whom the diagnosis of pronator teres syndrome could be confidently made. The median nerve involvement was incomplete in all, and median nerve sensory motor conduction over the forearm and distal segments as well as electromyographic sampling of the abductor digiti minimi was within normal limits in three pa-

tients. In the remaining patient, forearm motor conduction was slowed with a diminished compound action potential and occasional fibrillation potential, of the abductor pollicis brevis muscle. In the three patients with normal electrophysiologic studies, the diagnosis was based on findings of weakness and wasting in one and on the operative findings of a tendinous band and of compression by the deep head of the pronator teres in the other two patients.

In our experience, the diagnosis of pronator teres syndrome is suggested by the referring clinician in patients who have pain around the elbow without demonstrable neurologic signs, and we have usually not been able to confirm the existence of any median nerve lesion in such patients. The diagnosis appears to be speculatively applied at times as an explanation for pain around the elbow and upper anterior forearm when there is no obvious basis for the pain.

The median nerve can be injured in the forearm by laceration and penetrating injuries. Assessment involves the recognition of the sites of branching of the median nerve as it traverses the forearm as well as an attempt to define whether the lesion is complete or incomplete. Lacerations can involve the smaller branches to individual muscles. Follow-up examination involves an application of the principle of the time/reinnervation distance relationship and an awareness of the appropriate pace of recovery.

MEDIAN NERVE AT THE WRIST (CARPAL TUNNEL SYNDROME)

The median nerve arises from the lateral and medial cords of the brachial plexus. The lateral root contains contributions from the C-5, C-6, C-7 nerves and is joined by components of the C-8 and T-1 roots in the proximal part of the upper arm, before descending alongside the brachial artery. In the hollow of the elbow, it lies behind the bicipital aponeurosis and passes into the forearm between the two heads of the pronator teres muscle. The median nerve does not give off any branches in the upper arm nor does it have any cutaneous distribution in the upper arm or forearm. It extends downward along the middle of the forearm, between the more superficial flexor digitorum sublimis and the deeper flexor digitorum profundis muscles. The median nerve becomes more superficial as it approaches the wrist and enters the palm by passing deep to the flexor retinaculum and in front of the tendons of the flexor digitorum sublimis. In the hand, it spreads out at the distal border of the flexor retinaculum under cover of the palmar aponeurosis and arch and separates into its six terminal branches. In the forearm, it supplies the pronator teres, flexor carpi radialis, palmaris longus, flexor digitorum sublimis, and the index and middle finger portions of the flexor digitorum profundus muscle. The nerve to the pronator teres is the first branch in the forearm, and it often arises in the hollow of the elbow. The anterior interosseous nerve arises in the cubital fossa, extending downward in front of the interosseous membrane and behind the pronator teres and pronator quadratus muscles; it supplies the flexor pollicis longus and the lateral half of the flexor digitorum profundus as well as the pronator quadratus muscles. The sensory fibers of the median nerve are given off in the hand and supply the palmar aspects of the thumb, index, middle, and medial half of the ring fingers; the adjacent palm up to the wrist; and the terminal portions of the dorsum of the thumb, index, and middle fingers.

Median nerve injuries do occur in the region of the carpal tunnel syndrome following crush injury, Colles' fracture, cast immobilization, and penetrating injuries. The clinical picture is that of sensory motor involvement at or around the wrist, and the electrophysiologic examination is identical to that used in the diagnosis of carpal tunnel syndrome except that stimulation of the nerve well above the level of the wrist may be appropriate. A carpal tunnel syndrome can develop as a complication of Colles' fractures, and we have seen numerous examples of this.

The most common median nerve lesion is that of entrapment at the wrist as in the carpal tunnel syndrome. This is the single most identifiable cause of numbness in the upper limbs. Patients with carpal tunnel syndrome are predominantly women usually between the ages of 40 and 60. Symptoms are bilateral in 20% to 30% of cases and usually of 6 to 12 months' duration. Numbness, tingling, and pain are often described and frequently involve the entire hand as well as the forearm. The thumb, index, and middle fingers are the areas of greatest numbness, and a characteristic feature is that the symptoms are worse at night (nocturnal precipitation or aggravation) and often troublesome during manual activity such as driving an automobile (the *steering wheel sign*). Repetitive hand and wrist movements have been implicated in the cause of carpal tunnel syndrome,[92] but in our experience, an occupational association has not been common. The condition is more common during pregnancy and often improves or subsides after delivery. Although the early reports included the clinical features of wasting of the thenar

muscle, we now see patients in the earlier stages, when there is usually no demonstrable wasting, although slight weakness of the abductor pollicis brevis muscle may be demonstrable in about 20% of patients. Clinical sensory examination is normal except in the more advanced cases.

In about half of the patients, the clinical symptoms are typical, and the diagnosis can be made with a high degree of certainty on clinical grounds alone. In the remainder, the clinical picture is atypical and can lead to a mistaken diagnosis. Pain may be prominent and may extend up to involve the forearm and entire upper limb such as to suggest cervical nerve root compression. Degenerative cervical changes and nerve root compression may coexist, and this combination has been termed the double *crush syndrome*.[93] In about 10% of patients, despite suggestive symptoms, nerve conduction studies are within normal limits in our experience. Symptoms suggestive of carpal tunnel syndrome are seen in patients who have cold, sweaty hands or other symptoms suggestive of Raynaud's phenomenon and also in patients who have generalized sensory motor neuropathy.

The diagnosis maybe confirmed by nerve conduction studies. On stimulation of the median nerve at the wrist with recording from the abductor pollicis brevis muscle by surface or a concentric needle electrode, the motor conduction latency is prolonged. The electromyographic examination is usually normal, although enlarged MU action potentials are seen when the condition has been longstanding and with associated muscle atrophy. On stimulation of the thumb, index, and middle fingers by ring electrodes with recording at the wrist, sensory latencies are delayed and compound sensory nerve action potential amplitudes are diminished. In our experience, the earliest changes in carpal tunnel syndrome involve prolongation of the distal sensory values, with a corresponding reduction of the compound sensory nerve action potential amplitude in one or more digits. The distal motor latency may as yet be within normal limits or fall within the upper limit of the range of normal. As the condition progresses, sensory and motor latencies become more prolonged, and the compound sensory nerve action potentials may eventually disappear. At this stage, the distal motor latency exceeds the upper limit of the range of normal by 1 or 2 ms. In advanced cases, the distal motor latency may be prolonged to two to three times normal; the compound sensory nerve action potentials are absent and sensory loss and mild wasting of the abductor pollicis brevis muscle present.

We occasionally encounter patients in whom one

sensory latency value is abnormal and everything else is within normal limits. These changes may represent the earliest manifestations of a carpal tunnel syndrome, but we do not regard them as definite enough to establish the diagnosis. Other techniques have been reported, such as palmar stimulation of sensory fibers,[94,95] and this appears to offer a more sensitive method. We have not had any experience with this technique; however, the value of very early diagnosis of carpal tunnel syndrome is questionable. We advise a follow-up examination of those patients in whom the only finding is that of a mildly abnormal sensory value in one or two fingers, and if a carpal tunnel syndrome is confirmed by reexamination, it can be readily dealt with. There is a low but definite incidence of complications with surgical treatment, and the advisability of surgical release at a very early stage has not been proven.

Although carpal tunnel syndrome usually develops spontaneously and without any local trauma, it is a recognized complication of Colles' fracture, of fracture of the carpal bones, and of local trauma. In our experience with these conditions, clinical and electrical sensory motor abnormalities are usually well developed. We have seen examples of a complete loss of median sensory motor function in patients who have had penetrating injuries and lacerations at the wrist level.

When there has been a severe localized injury of the median nerve at the wrist or a laceration treated by reanastomosis, clinical and electrical follow-up examination may be carried out at intervals according to the *reinnervation distance formula* as previously described. The reinnervation distances are short, measuring 50 to 80 mm, and in the presence of continuity, electrical studies at 2 to 3 months after onset should reveal evidence of reinnervation. When the lesion is at the level of the wrist and MU action potentials cannot be demonstrated in the abductor pollicis brevis muscle by about the third month, loss of continuity may be presumed and surgical exploration may be appropriate.

MEDIAN NERVE TRAUMA IN THE FOREARM AND UPPER ARM

We have seen a few patients with forearm lacerations that have involved the median and ulnar nerve. These have usually been complete. We have also seen a few examples of complete median nerve lesions after a gunshot injury of the forearm. Our few cases of median nerve palsy following crush injuries of the forearm, with or without fractures of the radius and ulna, have usually been incomplete.

MUSCULOCUTANEOUS NERVE

The musculocutaneous nerve of the arm arises from the lateral cord of the plexus and includes contributions from the C-5 and C-6 roots and from the C-4 root in over half of patients. The musculocutaneous nerve separates from the lateral cord to lie between the coracobrachialis muscle and the axillary artery. It passes between the two parts of the coracobrachialis and runs between the biceps and brachialis muscles to the elbow, where it pierces the deep fascia over the front of the elbow and terminates as the lateral cutaneous nerve of the forearm. It supplies the two heads of the biceps and the brachialis while it lies between these muscles and supplies the coracobrachialis as well. The nerve to the coracobrachialis is usually incorporated with the trunk of the musculocutaneous nerve, although it has an independent origin from the sixth or seventh spinal nerves. The lateral cutaneous nerve of the forearm divides into anterior and posterior branches, and these supply a strip-like area over the anterior and posterior aspects of the lateral portion of the forearm from the level of the elbow down to the wrist.

Isolated paralysis of the musculocutaneous nerve is rare, but it has been reported as a complication of surgical procedure for shoulder dislocation,[96] after coracoid process transfer for clavicle instability,[97] and as an isolated complication of positioning during an abdominal surgical procedure that involved abduction and external rotation of the shoulder joint.[98] Ewing,[99] in his study of cadavers with the arm abducted and externally rotated, noted that the brachial plexus was stretched as it passed over the head of the humerus and that in most cases, the musculocutaneous nerve was at the prominence of the curve, accounting for its particular susceptibility to injury. The Trendelenburg position, which depresses the shoulder girdle with respect to the rib cage, may cause the plexus to stretch over the acromial process and contribute to nerve injury in this manner. Zeuke and Heidrich[100] reported three cases in the German literature and postulated that the nerve is injured as it travels through the tunnel in the coracobrachialis muscle.

The clinical picture of musculocutaneous nerve palsy is that of weakness and wasting of the biceps muscle with loss of the reflex. This may be associated with a sensory loss over the lateral and posterior aspects of the forearm down to the level of the wrist. The biceps muscle can be easily sampled electromyographically, and the presence of denervation, surviving MU action potentials, the completeness of the interference pattern, and the appearance of nascent potentials during the recovery phase can be looked for. A conduction latency value can also be determined by stimulation of the nerve in the region of Erb's point,[24] although we do not usually perform this measurement.

In our experience with four patients with isolated musculocutaneous nerve palsy, the causes were recurrent shoulder dislocation in two, a fall of about 10 feet in which the axilla was caught on a crossbar in one, and a heavy lifting strain in one. The lesions were all incomplete, and a sensory loss over the forearm was present in two patients. It is more common for the musculocutaneous nerve to be injured in combination with other nerves, and this occurred with circumflex nerve injury in 10 patients, with the radial nerve in two, and with C-5–C-6 nerve root or spinal nerve injury in another two patients. These combined lesions occurred after a fall, fracture-dislocation, an automobile and motorcycle accident, a gunshot wound, and a conveyor belt injury in which the arm was subject to severe traction.

AXILLARY (CIRCUMFLEX) NERVE

The circumflex nerve arises from the posterior cord, and it contains fibers of the C-5 and C-6 segments. It passes through the axilla, and it divides into an anterior and a posterior branch. The longer anterior branch winds laterally around the back of the surgical neck of the humerus and enters the deep surface of the deltoid muscle as a number of branches. A few of these nerves pass through the muscle and become cutaneous. The posterior branch supplies the teres minor, provides a few twigs to the posterior part of the deltoid muscle, and then curves around the posterior border of the deltoid muscle to become the upper lateral cutaneous nerve of the arm and to supply the skin overlying the deltoid muscle and adjacent upper arm in a wide area. The anatomic features are such that the nerve is free only for a short distance in the axilla and for the remainder of its length is attached to the deltoid muscle by numerous branches. This renders it susceptible to stretch injury as in dislocation and blunt trauma. The injury is most commonly seen with fracture of the neck of the humerous or shoulder dislocation, and in many patients, the nerve complication is prob-

ably undetected because it is mild in degree or because the joint or bone injuries dominated the clinical picture. Its occurrence after blunt shoulder trauma suggests that the extreme scapular thoracic movement and shoulder displacement, with relative fixation of the proximal portion of the axillary nerve, posterior cord, and brachial plexus, also can be a mechanism of injury.

Although axillary nerve palsy is commonly due to trauma, it represents less than 1% of nerve injuries.[101,102] It is usually caused by fracture-dislocation of the surgical neck of the humerus. The posterior branch, which is almost entirely motor, is responsible for almost the entire motor supply of the deltoid muscle, and it takes a course that renders it vulnerable in this injury. Blom and Dahlback[103] found clinical or electromyographic evidence of axillary nerve palsy, usually mild in degree, in 26 out of 73 patients with fracture-dislocation of the humerus.

In our experience of 55 patients with axillary nerve palsy, the causes were shoulder dislocation with or without fracture in 26 cases and blunt trauma to the shoulder associated with fracture of the clavicle, scapula, or distal humerus in 20 patients; a few examples of palsy were seen following fracture of the neck of the humerus, shoulder strain, and axillary and breast surgery. Of the 26 cases that followed shoulder dislocation, 16 were incomplete. Of the 20 cases that followed blunt trauma, 13 were complete. We had previously reported a series of 13 patients with axillary nerve palsy following blunt trauma to the shoulder[206] that were not associated with fracture, dislocation, or evidence of penetrating injury, and the mechanism appeared to be that of a stretch injury. Of these 13 patients, seven showed minimal or no recovery of deltoid muscle function, and six went on the complete or near complete recovery.

Those cases that follow shoulder dislocation or humeral fracture usually go on to a full recovery. The palsy is often missed initially after fracture-dislocation because the shoulder is painful and immobilized; the paralysis is noticed when shoulder movements become possible and when wasting of the deltoid muscle becomes conspicuous. This delay in diagnosis occurred in about one-quarter of the patients referred to us. The development of a frozen shoulder (capsulitis) also often serves to delay the recognition of axillary nerve palsy.

The clinical picture is that of weakness and wasting of the deltoid muscle, at times accompanied by sensory loss over the deltoid and adjacent regions. The posterior branch supplies virtually all of the deltoid muscle, and the anterior sensory branch is frequently spared; in our series of patients following blunt trauma, just over half (eight out of 13) had sensory involvement.

The diagnosis is readily made because there is usually a clear relationship to trauma. Paralysis is localized to the deltoid muscle without involvement of other muscles of C-5 segmental origin. A sudden onset of painful paralysis of the deltoid and adjacent muscles is a feature of neuralgic amyotrophy (brachial plexus neuritis), and although other proximal muscles are frequently involved, the paralysis can, in rare instances, be isolated to the deltoid muscle.

The degree of involvement of nerve function must be carefully assessed by clinical examination, and it is important to detect any flicker of preserved muscle action. When the palsy is incomplete on clinical examination, electrical tests are not essential; the nerve can be said to be in continuity, and some recovery can therefore be expected. When the clinical paralysis appears to be complete, however, electromyographic examination should be undertaken. It has been our general experience in the assessment of different nerve palsies that about 15% of those judged to be complete by clinical examination will, in fact, be incomplete as evidenced by the finding of MUs under voluntary control on electromyographic examination. When MU action potentials are present on volition, the lesion is in continuity and gradual improvement can usually be expected over a matter of a few months and up to about 12 months. A daily routine of shoulder exercises should be prescribed because this prevents the troublesome and painful complication of glenohumeral joint fixation (frozen shoulder).

When the palsy appears to be complete by clinical and electromyographic criteria, follow-up examinations should be done at intervals of about 1 month. The innervation distance of the axillary nerve is a short one, and the pace of recovery is therefore such that there should be some recovery between the third and fourth month after onset. Nascent potentials, as evidence of reinnervation, should be looked for. If there is no sign of reinnervation by about the fourth month, the lesion may be in discontinuity, and surgical exploration and reanastomosis of a nerve graft may therefore be appropriate.

SUPRASCAPULAR NERVE

The suprascapular nerve arises from the back of the upper trunk of the brachial plexus. Its fibers derive from the C-4, C-5, and C-6 nerves. It lies about the cords of the plexus and courses downward and lat-erally toward the superior border of the scapula, where it passes through the suprascapular notch to the dorsum of the scapula. It supplies the supraspinatus muscle and then passes through the spinal glenoid notch and terminates in the infraspinatus muscle.

The nerve is relatively fixed at the suprascapular foramen and possibly subject to traction there. Kopell and Thompson,[104] Ford,[105] and Clein[106] have described entrapment syndromes apparently on this basis, and Bateman[107] has described injury to the nerve after blows to the suprascapular region in sporting accidents. The nerve is the only branch of the lateral cord and is involved along with injuries to the brachial plexus. Suprascapular nerve palsy has been reported after intensive exercises such as weight-lifting[108] and following repair work on a ceiling.[109] Isolated nerve palsies have been described after trauma[110] and in association with a rotator cuff tear.[111] Weaver[112] has reviewed the anatomic features and the published literature on isolated suprascapular nerve lesions.

Trauma to the suprascapular nerve usually involves other nerves such as the circumflex, musculocutaneous, long thoracic, and the posterior cord of the brachial plexus. The clinical picture of isolated suprascapular palsy is that of wasting and weakness of the supraspinatus and infraspinatus muscles. The first 30 degrees of abduction of the shoulder is effected by the supraspinatus muscle, and the milder degrees of weakness can be detected by comparison with the strength of the opposite side. Infraspinatus involvement results in weakness of shoulder external rotation. These muscles along with other adjacent muscles can also be involved in brachial plexus neuritis and in polymyositis, conditions that are of spontaneous onset and that are readily distinguished from traumatic palsy.

The supraspinatus and infraspinatus muscles are readily accessible for electromyographic sampling, and the distinction of a complete from an incomplete lesion can easily be made. Motor latency values to these muscles can be obtained, as described by Gassell[24] and Ludin,[23] but we do not use these techniques usually. We sample the supraspinatus and infraspinatus muscles looking for denervation, numbers of surviving MUs, completeness of the interference pattern, and, during the recovery phase, the presence of any polyphasic nascent potentials as evidence of reinnervation. If the lesion is electrically complete, the usual principles of follow-up, with respect to the estimated reinnervation distance, the pace of recovery, and the timing of any relevant surgical exploration, do apply.

In our eight patients with isolated involvement of the suprascapular nerve, the paralysis was incomplete, and MUs were always demonstrable in the supraspinatus muscle but were frequently absent in the infraspinatus. The condition followed blunt trauma to the shoulder in three patients and was associated with a fracture of the scapula in one. It occurred after lifting weights or wrestling in three patients, and in one patient, it followed excision of a schwannoma in the region of the brachial plexus.

NERVE TO SERRATUS ANTERIOR (LONG THORACIC NERVE)

This nerve is formed from the backs of the fifth, sixth, and seventh spinal nerves as they emerge from the intervertebral foramina. The upper two roots unite into one after they pierce the scalenus medius muscle and are then joined by the root from the C-7 nerve. In the neck, the nerve extends behind the cords of the brachial plexus and enters the axilla between the upper edge of the serratus anterior muscle and the axillary artery. The nerve descends down the thoracic wall on the surface of the serratus anterior and is attached to it by the filaments that pass to and supply the several digitations of that muscle. The upper part of the serratus muscle is innervated by the fifth nerve alone, the middle by the fifth and sixth, and the lower part by the sixth and seventh nerves.

The nerve is angulated as it enters the axilla, and it lies 1.5 to 2 cm behind the clavicle.[113,114] It is also angulated over the first rib, where it turns downward to follow the thoracic wall in an almost vertical downward course. It is therefore likely to be stretched when the shoulder is depressed or when the neck is flexed to the opposite side.

The clinical picture is that of dull, aching pain around the shoulder and weakness of the shoulder on raising the arm. The function of the muscle is to fix and stabilize the shoulder girdle by pulling the scapula forward during pushing movements with the arm. Its lower fibers, acting at the inferior angle, assist the trapezius in rotating the scapula outward when the arm is elevated in forward flexion or abduction. With serratus anterior palsy, there is usually no deformity when the arm is at rest. The inferior angle of the scapula, however, rotates backward and medially when the extended arm is flexed, and it protrudes posteriorly when the extended arm is used to push against resistance, such as a push against a wall. Abduction of the arm is usually limited to about 90 degrees because the scapula is not prevented from rotating inward.

It is important to distinguish serratus anterior from trapezius muscle palsy. The posterior border of the scapula does become more prominent with spinal accessory nerve palsy because of wasting of the overlying fibers of the trapezius. The inferior angle of the scapula rotates inwardly on abduction of the arm with both trapezius and serratus anterior palsies, but the posterior protrusion of the scapula when the outstretched arm is pushed against a wall is diagnostic of serratus anterior palsy. Palpation of the upper fibers of the trapezius muscles and their comparison with the intact opposite side reveal wasting of that muscle, indicative of trapezius muscle involvement.

The condition has been described as a result of repeated reaching movements,[115] and it is common in patients who perform heavy labor.[116] It has been described after the limb has been overstretched.[117] Gregg et al.[118] described 10 cases of isolated complete paralysis of the serratus anterior muscle in young athletes on the basis of a traction injury to the long thoracic nerve of Bell; full recovery occurred in an average of 9 months. Isolated paralysis of the serratus anterior muscle has been reported as a weight-training injury,[119] following axillary node dissection,[120] as an occupational palsy in slaughterhouse workers,[121] and in association with a cervical rib.[122] Foo and Swann[123] reported 20 cases, the majority of which were of spontaneous onset, and noted that a full recovery of function could take up to 2 years.

In our experience with 20 cases of isolated paralysis of the long thoracic nerve, seven occurred after a heavy lifting or carrying strain, three followed a fall, and another three occurred after a stretch injury. The onset was spontaneous in three patients. We encountered single cases after a laceration and blunt trauma, and two followed local surgical procedures. The paralysis, as determined by electromyographic examination of the serratus anterior muscle, was incomplete in 16 patients, and this was so in the majority of those that followed carrying, lifting, stretch, or similar injuries.

Although a diagnosis of serratus anterior muscle weakness can usually be made with confidence on the basis of clinical examination alone, it is extremely difficult to detect a mild to moderate contraction of surviving muscle by clinical examination. We routinely sample two or three digitations of the serratus anterior muscle in the midaxillary line. The individual ribs are identified, and the needle is carefully inserted at an angle into the muscle as it overlies the rib. Care is taken to avoid insertion into the intercostal space. Denervation, surviving MU action potentials, and, in the recovery stage, nascent potentials, are looked for as indicators of severity and continuity as the patient pushes the outstretched, extended limb against resistance. Intercostal muscle activity may be mistaken for residual serratus anterior activity. Any contribution from the intercostal muscles can be assessed by a comparison of the level of electromyographic activity when the patient takes a deep breath with that obtained during attempted contraction of the serratus muscle. Because the reinnervation distance is a long one, it may take up to 6 months for the appearance of nascent potentials in a complete lesion that is in continuity.

ACCESSORY NERVE PALSY

The spinal portion of the accessory nerve descends from the jugular foramen into the neck, and it lies along with other nerves between the internal jugular vein and the internal carotid artery. It then passes downward and laterally, under cover of the posterior portion of the digastric muscle, and it pierces the deep surface of the sternomastoid muscle and supplies it. It enters the posterior triangle at the posterior border of the sternomastoid muscle, at or below the junction of the middle thirds, and it runs obliquely downward and backward in the fascial roof of the posterior triangle to reach the anterior border of the trapezius muscle. It then passes under the muscle, and it helps to supply it along with the branches of the cervical plexus. The accessory nerve communicates with the C-2, C-3, and C-4 nerves as part of the cervical plexus in the region of the sternomastoid, the posterior triangle, and the trapezius muscle. It is intimately associated with lymph nodes in its course beneath the sternomastoid and in the posterior triangle.

The posterior triangle is formed by the middle third of the clavicle, the posterior border of the sternomastoid, and the anterior border of the trapezius. It has a muscular floor formed by the scalenus capitus, the levator scapuli, and the scalenus medius and posterior muscles, all of which run obliquely downward and backward. The muscular floor is covered with a layer of fascia and with the motor nerves to four muscles: the levator scapuli (C-3, C-4), rhomboids (C-5), serratus anterior (C-5, C-6, C-7), and the diaphragm (C-3, C-4, C-5). The nerves to the first three muscles are found in the area below the

accessory nerve and above the upper border of the brachial plexus and are therefore vulnerable to injury along with the accessory nerve. Several sensory nerves—the lesser occipital (C-2, C-3), the greater auricular (C-2, C-3), the anterior cutaneous colli (C-2, C-3), and the supraclavicular nerves (C-3, C-4)—are also found in the posterior triangle, and they can be involved along with the accessory nerve.

Accessory nerve palsy commonly occurs as a result of surgical trauma within the posterior triangle,[36,124–127] usually at the time of lymph node excision.[128–131] It has also been described following accidental laceration,[128] carotid endarterectomy,[132,133] irradiation,[134] blunt trauma,[135] and as a spontaneous event.[136]

The clinical picture is that of wasting and weakness of the trapezius muscle. The bulk of the upper fibers of the trapezius can be assessed by grasping them between the thumb and index finger and by a comparison with that of the opposite side. Atrophy of the middle and lower portions of the muscle results in an increased prominence of the scapula, and in some patients, the underlying rhomboid muscle becomes more visible. Scapular position at rest is altered, and the unsupported scapula and shoulder sag downward and laterally. Under normal conditions, the upper portion of the muscle is most active during scapular elevation and the mid and lower parts during abduction and flexion of the limb. With trapezius weakness, the scapula is already displaced downward and laterally at rest, and it rotates inwardly during abduction such that arm abduction is lmited to about 90 degrees. The increased prominence of the medial border of the scapula is sometimes confused with serratus anterior palsy. Careful examination, with the outstretched arm held horizontal, in flexion at the shoulder, reveals that the scapula does not displace posteriorly as it does in serratus anterior palsy. At rest, the medial border of the scapula is more prominent, but this prominence virtually disappears when the *push test* for serratus anterior palsy is done. The latter creates a useful point of distinction in that axial pressure on the outstretched arm in the forward flexed position results in scapular prominence with serratus anterior palsy, whereas the scapular prominence disappears with trapezius muscle palsy. Sternomastoid bulk may be assessed by inspection and palpation of that muscle with the head and neck rotated in the opposite direction and also by forward flexion of the neck and head against resistance. Evidence for injury to adjacent nerves should also be looked for, that is, sensory loss around the angle of the mandible and the pinna of the ear owing to greater auricular nerve involvement, the back of the pinna and adjacent occipit to a lesion of the lesser occipital nerve, sensory loss around the clavicle owing to supraclavicular nerve lesions, and loss below the angle of the jaw and in front of the mastoid owing to involvement of the anterior cutaneous colli nerve. The diagnosis of accessory nerve palsy is usually evident on clinical examination alone.

Electromyographic examination reveals evidence of denervation; loss of MU action potentials, with preservation of some MUs in an incomplete lesion; and the appearance of nascent potentials when there is reinnervation. We usually examine the upper trapezius muscle fibers and in some instances the mid and lower fibers. The mid and lower portions are said to receive a greater contribution from the cervical plexus[137]; although this would suggest that surviving MUs of cervical origin could interfere with the assessment of a complete accessory nerve palsy, we have not found this to be of any practical significance.

In our review of 23 patients with accessory nerve palsy, the single most common cause was injury to the nerve at the time of surgical removal of an enlarged lymph node or similar mass in the posterior triangle. Other nonsurgical traumatic causes included blunt injuries in automobile accidents in two patients, a fall and head blow in one, and a beating with a baseball bat in another. Accidental laceration as a form of penetrating injury was seen in three patients and a stretch injury, in which the upper limb was caught in machinery or in which there was sudden angulation or traction, was encountered in three patients. In two patients, the condition occurred spontaneously, without any definable cause.

In our patients, about half had isolated accessory nerve involvement and about half of these in turn had involvement of the trapezius muscle only; this indicated that the lesion was below the level of supply to the sternomastoid muscle. In our reported series of 23 patients, approximately half had additional nerve and muscle involvement: the greater auricular and lesser occipital, supraclavicular, and the recurrent laryngeal nerves and the serratus anterior, rhomboid, suprascapular, and levator scapuli muscles. Multiple nerve involvement is more common after node excision and penetrating injury; under such circumstances and when electromyographic sampling reveals a complete lesion with denervation, surgical exploration is usually appropriate, and neurolysis, reanastomosis, or sural nerve grafting can lead to a degree of recovery. Overall, the outcome is poorest when the palsy has followed lymph node excision or accidental penetrating injury and is best when it has been caused by blunt trauma and in those rare cases of spontaneous onset.

FEMORAL NERVE

The femoral nerve arises within the psoas major muscle from the L-2, L-3, and L-4 nerves and posterior to the obturator nerve. It passes obliquely through the psoas major muscle and emerges from its lateral border just below the iliac crest. It then runs inferiorly to enter the thigh behind the inguinal ligament, lateral to the femoral sheath and femoral vessels. It breaks up into a large number of branches, which supply the pectineus, sartorius, and quadriceps muscles. The vastus lateralis and rectus femoris are supplied on their deep surfaces by separate branches, and the vastus intermedius muscle is supplied superficially. The vastus medialis is supplied by two branches. The cutaneous branches are the intermediate and medial cutaneous nerves as well as the saphenous nerve. The intermediate and medial cutaneous nerves of the thigh supply the anterior portion of the thigh. The saphenous nerve may be regarded as a terminal branch of the femoral nerve. It descends from its origin in the femoral triangle down to the medial side of the knee joint, where it becomes cutaneous; it supplies the medial portion of the knee and lower leg down to the level of the ankle, and it lies adjacent to the long saphenous vein.

The femoral nerve is vulnerable to injury because of its anatomic relationship to the lower abdomen, pelvis, hip joint, and inguinal region and its passage through the iliopsoas muscle and sheath. Femoral nerve paralysis has been described following laparoscopy,[138] tubal microsurgery,[139] vaginal hysterectomy,[140] renal transplantation,[141,142] abdominal hysterectomy,[143] and appendectomy[144]; it is a well-recognized complication of total hip arthroplasty.[145–147] Hudson et al.[146] described 18 cases of iatrogenic femoral nerve trauma, the majority of which were complete and which followed hip joint surgery; only one patient made a full recovery. Femoral nerve palsy has also occurred as a complication of aortic surgery,[148] accidental femoral nerve block during local anesthesia for inguinal hernia,[149] ruptured abdominal aortic aneurysm,[150] radiotherapy for malignancy,[151] and a variety of gynecolgic operations.[152] Because the nerve passes through the psoas major muscle, it is therefore vulnerable to hematoma of a traumatic type,[153] and it is an often reported complication of retroperitoneal[154] and iliopsoas compartment hematomas in hemophilia[155] and during anticoagulant therapy.[156–158] The nerve does not appear to be involved in entrapment.

In our personal series of 70 patients with femoral nerve palsy, 29 were traumatic and 41 were spontaneous in onset. Of these 41 patients, 33 were diabetics, usually of long standing, and were in the older age group. The spontaneous cases were almost invariably incomplete. Of the 29 traumatic palsies, seven followed hip replacement, and the paralysis was usually complete or very severe in degree. In four patients, the paralysis occurred as a complication of kidney transplantation, and in three patients, it occurred after a heavy lifting strain. In three patients, the paralysis was a result of pelvic fracture, and other regional nerves were involved. A few cases and isolated cases were seen following a femoral arteriogram, arterial surgery and sympathectomy, pelvic surgery, laminectomy, gunshot, lacerating and penetrating injuries, pressure palsy, and retroperitoneal hemorrhage. With the exception of the usual complete involvement following hip replacement, there was an equal likelihood of complete or incomplete involvement in the other examples of trauma.

The clinical picture of unilateral wasting and weakness of a quadriceps muscle with associated pain can occur in high lumbar disc lesions (L-4); in such patients, the history of low back pain, a positive femoral stretch test (pain on hip hyperextension), numbness in an L-4 distribution, and mild weakness of adjacent muscles innervated by the L-4 segment (tibialis anterior and posterior) allow this diagnosis to be made. Bilateral quadriceps wasting and weakness are seen in quadriceps myopathy on the basis of polymyositis, sarcoidosis, and muscular dystrophy, and involvement of adjacent muscles is usually demonstrable in such patients.

The femoral nerve is an exception to the general rule that conduction velocities cannot be calculated for the proximally supplied muscles. This is possible because the fibers of the rectus femoris muscle originate from a thin, central tendon such that the end plate zone forms a largely vertical band along the muscle,[22,159,160] whereas in other muscles, the zone of innervation usually runs transversely, across the belly of the muscle and at right angles to the length of the muscle. Femoral nerve conduction latencies and velocities can therefore be measured by stimulation of the femoral nerve at the inguinal ligament and recording of evoked muscle potentials at successive distances along the rectus femoris muscle.[159]

We have used the femoral nerve conduction technique described by Gassel,[159] which provides latency values to the femoral muscle. Concentric needle electrodes are inserted at three equidistant points and a supramaximal stimulus applied at the femoral ligament. In our series, we have found motor conduction, as determined by latency values, to be slowed in about 50% of patients with femoral neuropathy (mononeuritis) and also with femoral nerve palsy following hip surgery. EMG provides evidence of the completeness of the lesion, of denervation, and of reinnervation; the *pace of recovery rule* may be used to guide serial examinations and any decision as to surgical exploration.

SCIATIC NERVE

The sciatic nerve is the thickest nerve in the body, and it consists of two nerves, the medial and lateral popliteal, bound together by a sheath. The lateral popliteal nerve arises from the posterior trunks of the L-4 and L-5 and the first and second sacral nerves; the anterior trunks of these nerves along with part of the third sacral nerve unite to form the medial popliteal nerve. In the thigh, branches from the medial and lateral popliteal nerves supply the hamstring and biceps femoris muscles. The sciatic nerve leaves the pelvis, enters the gluteal region through the greater sciatic foramen, and runs laterally and downward between the greater trochanter of the femur and the ischial tuberosity, where it is covered by the gluteus maximus posteriorly. It runs down the back of the thigh on the posterior surface of the adductor magnus and is covered by the long head of the biceps femoris muscle. The sciatic nerve terminates at the proximal angle of the popliteal fossa by dividing into the medial and lateral popliteal nerves. The nerves to the hamstring muscles arise from all roots of the medial popliteal nerve, that is, the L-4 and L-5 and the first three sacral nerves. The nerve to the short head of the biceps arises from the lateral popliteal trunk in the proximal part of the thigh and is usually of L-5 and first and second sacral origin. The nerve to the adductor magnus muscle arises in common with the nerve to the semimembranosus component of the hamstring muscle, in the upper posterior thigh.

The clinical picture of a sciatic nerve lesion in its most proximal portion includes involvement of the hamstring and biceps femoris muscles as well as of medial and lateral popliteal function, and the degree of involvement is determined by the severity of the lesion. Proximal injuries and injuries to the plexus may involve the superior and inferior gluteal nerves. The superior gluteal nerve innervates the gluteus medius muscle and the inferior gluteal nerve, the gluteus maximus muscle. These muscles can be tested by assessing hip abduction and extension. The muscles can also be palpated during contraction and assessed by electromyographic sampling. Proximal lesions may also involve the nerve to the adductor magnus, and we have encountered this in pelvic injuries.

Sciatic nerve palsy is a recognized complication of total hip replacement, along with femoral nerve palsy. Roblin et al.[161] described 48 cases of paralysis of the femoral or sciatic nerves complicating hip surgery, mostly commonly after total hip arthroplasty. The prognosis was better for cases of paralysis of the femoral than of the sciatic nerve. Sciatic neuropathy has been reported in childhood[162] as an example of a nerve compression syndrome. The pyriformis syndrome has been described by Symek[163] as a rare type of entrapment neuropathy, although we have not encountered any examples of this condition.

The sciatic nerve is not readily accessible to direct stimulation and measurement of motor conduction because it lies deeply within the posterior thigh. Gassel and Trojaborg[164] have described a technique of sciatic nerve examination by the use of simulating needle electrodes inserted close to the sciatic nerve, although we have not had any experience with this. The hamstring muscles and biceps femoris can be easily sampled by electromyographic examination, and the medial and lateral popliteal nerve functions can be readily accessed for measurement of motor conduction and for electromyographic studies of their muscle supply. Our laboratory clinically and electromyographically assesses the hamstring and biceps femoris muscles, measures medial and conduction in the lateral popliteal nerves, and electromyographically studies their muscles.

Of our 34 patients with sciatic nerve palsy, 32 were secondary to trauma. Of these, 16 followed fractures of the pelvis, including the upper femur and hip joint. The paralysis was complete in 12 patients and incomplete in four, and several of these complete injuries followed motorbike accidents. Total hip replacement, blunt injury, and penetrating injury were each complicated by paralysis in three patients. Other isolated causes were those of hip dislocation, pressure palsy following drug overdose, posterior abdominal surgery, and an injection into the buttock region.

COMMON PERONEAL (LATERAL POPLITEAL) NERVE

The common peroneal nerve arises from the posterior portion of the sacral plexus and is derived from the L-4 and L-5 and first two sacral nerves. The nerve is incorporated along with the medial popliteal nerve into the sciatic nerve in the gluteal region. It descends as a component of the sciatic nerve through the thigh, down to the bifurcation of the nerve at the upper border of the popliteal fossa then downward and inferolaterally under the cover of the biceps tendon, and it is separated from the lateral femoral condyle by the upper portion of the gastrocnemius and plantaris muscles. The nerve continues posterior to the tendon of the popliteus muscle and to the tendinous attachment of the soleus to the fibular head. The common peroneal nerve now curves around the neck of the fibula, and it is applied to the periosteum of the fibula for a total of about 10 cm.[10] The nerve passes through a fibro-osseous tunnel, the roof of which is formed by the origin of the peroneus longus muscle and the intermuscular septum. The upper portion of the arch of the tunnel is attached to the head of the fibula and the lower portion of the arch, to the lateral aspect of the upper portion of the shaft of the fibula. Kopell and Thompson[104] note that the fibromuscular opening of the tunnel may have a J-shaped outline and that the curved portion of the J forms the inferior margin of the opening.

The common peroneal nerve divides into the deep peroneal (anterior tibial nerve), which passes through a second fibro-osseous canal formed by the origin of the extensor digitorum longus muscle about 4 cm below the first tunnel and supplies the muscles of the anterior compartment. The superficial peroneal (musculocutaneous) nerve runs deep to and between the peroneal muscles and supplies the peroneus longus and brevis muscles and the skin.

There are several peculiarities of the common peroneal nerve that make it vulnerable to injury. It is exposed over the bony prominence of the upper fibula for about 4 cm, covered only by skin and superficial fascia, and is susceptible to direct blows and lacerations. It is readily compressed at the latter site when the legs are crossed or when consciousness is diminished or where there has been a nearby fracture. Nobel[165] noted the limited longitudinal mobility of the nerve, and our dissection studies show that the passage of the common and deep peroneal nerves through the two tunnels limits its mobility in a longitudinal direction to about 0.5 cm.[10] The branching of the nerve immediately below the knee contributes to this fixation. The epineurium is not usually adherent to the superficial fascia or periosteum, but adhesions may occur following injury, and this was encountered at the time of surgical exploration in several of our patients. Longitudinal stretch applied to the nerve, as in forced ankle inversion, or in proximal injuries such as posterior hip dislocation can injure the common peroneal nerve in the region of the knee. Haftek[166] has noted that the relative thickness of the epineurium to the fascicular area on cross-section does influence the susceptibility to stretch injury. A thicker epineurium protects the nerve; the epineurium is thickest over the sciatic nerve in the gluteal region and is thinnest around the common peroneal nerve.[167]

Passage through the fibro-osseous tunnel can contribute to injury if any of the structures should be involved in swelling or hemorrhage. This may be the basis of the delayed type of palsy that we have seen following blunt trauma around the knee. Nobel[165] found hematomas within the nerve sheath at the level of the popliteal fossa in two patients who developed painful common peroneal nerve palsy after a twisting injury of the knee.

The clinical picture, when paralysis is severe or complete, is that of a footdrop, and with walking, there is a characteristic elevation of the entire leg in order that the drooping toes may clear the ground. There is weakness of the tibialis anterior muscle on attempted dorsiflexion and of the peronei on ankle eversion. In the mildest cases, the gait may be normal, and there may be only mild weakness on extension of the toes and ankle. Muscle wasting results in a flattening of the normal surface convexity of the anterior tibial compartment, an increased prominence of the anterior border of the tibia, and *sharpening* of the tibial border on palpation with the flat of the hand. It is important to compare carefully the bulk of the contracted extensor digitorum brevis muscle on the involved side with that of the opposite side because this may be the only definite site of wasting in the patient with a mild nerve palsy.

The usual cause of unilateral footdrop is common peroneal nerve palsy of a spontaneous, traumatic, or pressure type. In rare instances, the palsy can be progressive. The diagnosis is usually obvious on careful clinical examination. Footdrop may also be caused by a herniated intravertebral disc with compression of the L-5 root or spinal nerve. The pattern of muscle involvement within the territory of the common peroneal nerve is identical, although the muscle paralysis is always incomplete. The sensory disturbance is also similar, but an important distinguishing point is demonstrable weakness of the tibialis posterior muscle on ankle inversion. Although this muscle has L-5 segmental supply, it is innervated through the medial popliteal nerve and is therefore spared in common

peroneal nerve palsy. Back pain, sciatica, and limitation of straight leg raising are evident, and the two conditions are readily distinguished. In rare instances, intervertebral disc disease with multiple root involvement (L-5, S-1) may result in a footdrop with additional muscle involvement: wasting and weakness of the calf muscles and of the small muscles of the foot. Motor neuron disease of the progressive muscular atrophy type can occasionally present with weakness around the ankle, and bilateral footdrop is seen in generalized neuropathy, Charcot-Marie-Tooth disease, and lumbosacral arachnoiditis.

Sorell et al.[168] described 26 cases of traumatic common peroneal nerve palsy, of which 15 were complete. Peroneal nerve palsy has also been described following minor athletic trauma[169] and following ankle inversion injury.[170] The condition has also been described as a complication of fractures of the femur,[168] tibia, and fibula,[169] after exercise,[171] and in runners[172]; as a result of knee dislocation,[173] inversion ankle injury[170]; laceration by a skate blade in hockey players,[174] as a tennis footdrop,[175] and after general anesthesia for a variety of surgical procedures.[176,177] It has also been reported as a complication of blood pressure measurements in the infant[178] and as an undetected and possibly preventable pressure neuropathy in head-injured adults.[179]

In our review of 145 patients with common peroneal nerve palsy, 77 were due to identifiable trauma. Thirty-seven of these occurred postoperatively, following hip replacement or arthroplasty, arterial bypass surgery, meniscectomy, osteotomy, knee replacement, or other procedures. Of the 40 nonsurgical trauma patients, the more common causes were sudden ankle inversion; lacerations; fractures around the knee involving the tibia, fibula, or femur; ligamentous injury; and crush and blunt injuries around the knee. Palsies caused by lacerations or trauma tended to be severe or complete, and complete lesions were likely after hip surgery and replacement. In the remaining nonsurgical trauma patients, the involvement was usually incomplete.

Electrical studies are not always required in the diagnosis of footdrop, but they are of value in assessing prognosis and in detecting early signs of recovery. Slowed motor conduction of other nerves may reveal an underlying generalized neuropathy. We find it helpful to sample the tibialis anterior muscle and occasionally the peroneal compartment as well as to obtain motor conduction velocities across the fibular head for both the tibialis anterior and extensor digitorum brevis muscles. Sometimes the extensor digitorum brevis muscle is totally denervated or inaccessible owing to local swelling, and the conduction velocities for this muscle cannot be measured, but latencies to other muscles can be determined.[180] Our experiences with the latter technique have been too limited to allow any useful comment. In the presence of a lesion at the neck of the fibula, stimulation of the nerve above and below it may demonstrate a reduction in the size of the compound action potential of the tibialis anterior and the extensor digitorum muscles, suggesting conduction block.[181] Stimulation of the nerve at consecutive points, in the popliteal fossa and above and below the neck of the fibula, while recording from the tibialis anterior muscle[181] allows calculation of motor conduction velocity over this short nerve segment to define the site of the lesion, and the technique of sciatic nerve conduction can be used to detect lesions within the thigh.[164] In patients with complete paralysis, we have found the earliest evidence of recovery to occur within the upper portion of the tibialis anterior muscle; nascent MU potentials should be looked for; in our experience and with a lesion at the neck of the fibula, these were usually detected within 2 to 3 months after onset.

The lateral half of the extensor digitorum brevis muscle may be innervated by a branch of the superificial peroneal (musculocutaneous) nerve. Lambert,[182] by means of nerve stimulation, found this to be so in 22% of limbs. The practical importance of this *accessory deep peroneal nerve* is not great because the site of most lesions is at or proximal to the neck of the fibula and is therefore above the origin of the accessory branch. We have not encountered any misleading observations that could be attributed to this anatomic variant.

When the palsy is incomplete and there is slight to moderate weakness, the prognosis is uniformly good, and the patient can be reassured of this. If the footdrop develops after local trauma and is mild in degree, there is usually no clear indication for any further medical or electrophysiologic investigation, and these patients usually recover over the next weeks. When the condition develops spontaneously or after diminished consciousness following head injury, anesthesia, or other cause, an inquiry as to general health, diabetes, or alcoholism is relevant. In such patients, nerve conduction studies may show sensorimotor abnormalities in other nerves indicative of a generalized neuropathy as a factor that predisposes to pressure palsy. Progressive cases require investigation, and an underlying neuropathy should be looked for. Electrical testing can serve to confirm the progression, and if the cause is not apparent, it is reasonable to recommend surgical exploration.

A complete common peroneal palsy, apart from the occasional patient with severe generalized neuropathy or a progressive palsy, is almost always caused by trauma. In blunt injuries around the knee, severance of the nerve is unlikely and is also unlikely in most patients with dislocation of the hip or knee or fractures of the femur, tibia, fibula, or following ankle injuries. If the lesion is incomplete clinically, there may be no need for electrical testing, and recovery can be followed by clinical observation alone. In those patients in whom the lesion appears to be complete, electrical testing and more careful follow-up are required. Electromyographic evidence of recovery should be looked for, and in our experience, this usually occurs within 2 to 3 months. If continuity of the nerve is in doubt, it is probably unreasonable to wait for evidence of recovery beyond 6 months, and surgical exploration can be advised. This was performed in three of our patients, 3 months, 6 months, and 1 year after injury, and continuity was found in all. Some patients will have already undergone exploration at the time of a surgical repair of the knee and observations made at the time of surgical exposure, as to the appearance of the nerve, bruising, attenuation, and the length of an injured segment, will reveal the severity of the injury and help to indicate whether recovery will be delayed or incomplete.

Although published reports have given a poor prognosis for stretch injuries following hip dislocation, our experience justifies a more optimistic outlook, and four out of five of our patients experienced a return of useful function. We would therefore wait for evidence of recovery and would postpone surgical exploration of the common peroneal nerve for about 6 months unless there should be an additional reason to suspect discontinuity of the nerve.

MEDIAL POPLITEAL (TIBIAL) NERVE

The medial popliteal nerve arises from the anterior surface of the lumbosacral plexus, usually from the L-4 and L-5 and first three sacral nerves and like the common peroneal nerve, is incorporated into the sciatic trunk in the gluteal region and extends down the thigh to the point of bifurcation just above the popliteal fossa. There it separates from the trunk of the sciatic nerve, passing through the popliteal fossa, where it is concealed by the semimembranosis and other hamstring muscles. It passes behind the popliteal vessels and extends downward behind the popliteal muscle and under cover of the gastrocnemius and plantaris muscles. In the popliteal fossa, it provides branches to the two heads of the gastrocnemius and to the plantaris muscles. Branches are also supplied to the soleus and popliteus muscles and the tibialis posterior. The cutaneous branch is the sural nerve. It passes between the two heads of the gastrocnemius muscle and lies on the lateral border of the Achilles' tendon. The posterior tibial nerve is the direct continuation of the medial popliteal nerve, beginning at the distal border of the popliteus muscle and passing downward as it lies on the tibialis posterior muscle and tibia along with the posterior tibial vessels. It supplies branches to the tibialis posterior, the flexor digitorum longus, and flexor hallucis longus muscles, and its terminal branches are the medial and lateral plantar nerves. The cutaneous branch is the sural nerve; it arises in the popliteal fossa, extends down the back of the leg piercing the deep fascia in the middle third of the back of the leg and reaching the foot by winding around the back of the lateral malleolus. It supplies the lateral side and back of the distal third of the leg, the ankle and heel, and the lateral border of the foot.

The medial popliteal nerve, in its course, is well protected by muscle, and it is not subject to pressure palsy. It can, however, be involved in penetrating injuries, and it has been reported as a complication of closed tibial fracture[183] and other forms of penetrating and nonpenetrating injuries.[184]

The clinical picture is that of weakness and wasting of the calf muscles, a diminished to absent ankle reflex and loss of sensation over the lower posterior leg and lateral border of the ankle and foot. The medial popliteal nerve conduction velocity from the popliteal fossa to the abductor hallucis muscle can be determined, and electromyographic examination of the calf muscles and small muscles of the foot provides evidence of denervation, surviving MUs, and recovery.

We have seen isolated involvement of the nerve in six patients, as a complication of total knee replacement; of mid and upper tibial fracture, which required open reduction; and of penetrating and gunshot injuries of the thigh and lower leg. In one patient with a Baker's cyst, it appeared to have been precipitated by a fall while skiing. The involvement was complete in four patients and this included those with penetrating injuries and fractures. It was incomplete but dense following total knee replacement and

in the patient with a Baker's cyst. The motor nerve conduction velocity was normal in this patient albeit with a reduced compound action potential. The sural nerve sensory responses were absent in all of our patients.

OBTURATOR NERVE

The obturator nerve, in a manner similar to the femoral nerve, arises within the substance of the psoas major muscle from the L-2, L-3, and L-4 nerves and in front of the femoral nerve. The nerve passes downward; emerges from the psoas major muscle at its medial border behind the common iliac vessels; and passes anteriorly below the pelvic brim, behind the os pubis, through the obturator foramen, and into the thigh. In the thigh, it supplies the adductor longus, gracilis, and adductor brevis muscles, and there is a variable cutaneous branch that supplies sensation to the upper medial portion of the thigh.

Isolated obturator nerve paralysis appears to be extremely rare, and a review of the literature has revealed it as a complication of labor during pregnancy.[185] Siliski and Scott[186] have described four instances of palsy resulting from intrapelvic extrusion of cement during total hip replacement. We encountered one patient with an isolated complete obturator nerve palsy following avulsion fracture of the pubic and ischial rami. In our experience with two other patients, the paralysis was incomplete, and it was accompanied by femoral and sciatic nerve palsy following severe trauma and pelvic fracture.

Adductor muscle bulk can be assessed during contraction by palpation and can be compared with the opposite side. Strength can also be readily assessed. The nerve is easily sampled for evidence of denervation, MU activity, and reinnervation.

TARSAL TUNNEL SYNDROME

The posterior tibial nerve terminates in the medial and lateral plantar nerves. The medial plantar nerve is analogous to the median nerve in the hand. It courses forward in the sole of the foot under cover of the flexor retinaculum and abductor hallucis muscle, supplying branches to the abductor hallucis and flexor digitorum brevis; cutaneous branches to the medial part of the sole of the foot; and terminal branches to the intrinsic muscles of the foot and to the skin of the sides of the first, second, third, and fourth toes. The lateral plantar nerve is analogous to the ulnar nerve in the hand. From its origin under cover of the flexor retinaculum, it passes forward and laterally in the sole to supply the abductor digiti minimi, the accessory flexor digitorum, and the intrinsic muscles, and it provides a cutaneous supply to the lateral border of the foot and the fifth and the lateral half of the fourth toes. The clinical picture of tarsal tunnel syndrome is described as pain and burning in the foot along with numbness and sensory loss in the medial and lateral plantar nerve territories. Wasting of the abductor hallucis muscle has been noted.[187,188]

Takakura et al.[189] described the operative findings in 50 feet of 45 patients with a diagnosis of tarsal tunnel syndrome. The most common causes were ganglia and a bony prominence from the talocalcaneal junction, with a few cases being attributable to injury and tumor; there was no obvious cause in nine patients. Grumbine et al.[190] described 87 cases and noted multiple causes, with no definite cause in some patients. Taguchi et al.[191] described two cases owing to neurilemoma and subperiosteal ganglion, and tarsal tunnel syndrome has been implicated in the burning feet syndrome.[192] The condition has been reported in rheumatoid arthritis[193] and in association with varus heel deformity[194] Kaplan[195] has stressed that a reduction in amplitude and an increased duration of the evoked motor potentials are more sensitive indicators of this condition than the distal motor latencies and that the lateral plantar branch of the posterior tibial nerve is probably affected earlier than the medial plantar branch.

Although tarsal tunnel syndrome has been described as a common condition by some of these authors, we have encountered only 10 patients in whom the diagnosis appeared to be tenable by clinical, electrical, or combined criteria. There were six posttraumatic cases; three cases followed fractures around the ankle. There were single examples after an inversion injury, a blow to the inside of the sole by a falling object, and a tibial fracture complicated by Volkmann's ischemic contracture. Those cases that followed fractures around the ankle all had considerable prolongation of distal motor latency to the abductor hallucis and abductor digiti quinti muscles with diminished MUs on electromyographic examination and with evident thinning of those muscles on inspection and palpation. Plantar sensation was diminished in two patients. Although a diagnosis of tarsal tunnel syndrome was made in the remaining four nontraumatic cases, one of whom had not experienced any relief following a tarsal tunnel de-

compression several months previously, we were not able to confirm any electrical abnormalities except in a single surgically treated patient, and we therefore did not feel confident about the diagnosis. It is evident from the literature that this condition is often diagnosed in patients with painful feet and burning soles, but the evidence for the diagnosis is not convincing in our view.

BRACHIAL PLEXUS INJURY

Brachial plexus trauma is common in comparison with lumbosacral plexus injuries, and we have seen 424 cases of brachial plexus trauma, usually as a form of stretch injury after motorcycle accidents, falls, shoulder dislocations, occasionally automobile accidents, and occasionally gunshot wounds. There are three general patterns of involvement: segmental owing to root, spinal nerve, or trunk injury; lesions of the various branches of the brachial plexus or trunk; and lesions of the cords of the brachial plexus, often combined with branch and major long nerve injuries. The most common group is that of segmental injuries, and of these, the most common subgroup is that of involvement of the C-5–C-6 segment involvement. This results in weakness of the supraspinatus and infraspinatus muscles, the deltoid, the biceps, and the brachioradialis; this combination of involvement within the suprascapular, circumflex, musculocutaneous, and radial nerve territories is diagnostic of a more proximal lesion involving C-5–C-6 segmental innervation. The addition of triceps involvement to this pattern of motor weakness indicates that there is also C-7 segment involvement. The lower roots, spinal nerves, and trunks are also frequently involved, and this results in weakness and wasting of the small muscles of the hand, the triceps, and forearm extensors on the basis of C-8 and T-1 involvement.

The next common pattern of injury is that of lesions of the nerve branches of the cords or trunks, often without involvement of the cords or trunks. The common combinations are circumflex and suprascapular nerve; circumflex, suprascapular, and musculocutaneous; musculocutaneous and radial; circumflex with high radial nerve involvement; circumflex and musculocutaneous; and suprascapular and radial. In some instances, the nerve to the rhomboids and the accessory nerve are involved along with the aforementioned combinations. A degree of cord involvement can also be combined with these individual nerve injuries.

The third pattern of involvement is that of a predominantly cord lesion; the posterior cord is most commonly affected, and this results in a loss of function within the territories of the radial and circumflex nerves and of the latissimus dorsi muscle. The medial cord is less commonly involved, and this results in a loss of ulnar nerve function and a loss of function of that portion of the median nerve that is derived from the medial cord. Lateral cord involvement is the least common type of cord injury in our experience.

The electrophysiologic assessment of these injuries is discussed along with the assessment of lumbosacral plexus lesions. In some patients with complete plexus lesions, surgical repair by primary suture, by grafting, and by intercostal-musculocutaneous nerve anastomosis has resulted in the return of function around the shoulder and of elbow flexion; this has avoided limb amputation, but the expectation of recovery of forearm or hand reinnervation has not been fulfilled.

LUMBOSACRAL PLEXUS INJURY

In contrast to the incidence of brachial plexus involvement, lumbosacral plexus injuries are very rare, and we have seen 12 cases, following osteotomy, fracture of the acetabulum, hip replacement, and extensive laminectomy procedures. The clinical picture is of a loss of function within the major nerve territories of the plexus: the superior and inferior gluteal, the femoral, and sciatic nerves. Injury to the branches of the plexus are also seen, as, for example, in isolated involvement of the nerves to the gluteus maximus and medius muscles following an acetabulum fracture and hip surgery.

Diagnosis is based on a careful clinical examination with an awareness of the complex anatomy of these regions, and in our work, we frequently refer to our brachial and lumbosacral plexus assessment charts. We do not perform motor conduction latency measurements of the proximal muscles, but we do rely on electromyographic sampling for evidence of denervation, surviving MUs, and reinnervation, combined with a careful clinical examination, to reach an accurate diagnosis. It is important to recall that in the acute stage of a complete lesion, conduction is preserved for up to a week or so in the portion of a long nerve such as the median, ulnar, radial, or sciatic distal to the lesion. The motor conduction velocity of these long nerves is frequently diminished when there has been a severe proximal lesion and

the compound motor action potential is diminished. When the lesion is complete, there is complete loss of motor conduction. The compound sensory nerve action potentials, however, can be preserved in complete lesions, when the lesion is preganglionic as in brachial plexus root avulsions,[196] and findings at operation have confirmed this in several of our patients. In other words, the assessment of plexus injuries is largely based on a careful clinical examination in combination with electromyographic sampling of appropriate muscles as to completeness or incompleteness of the lesion, the presence or absence of a sensory response, and a follow-up examination at appropriate intervals to assess the pace of recovery.

FACIAL NERVE

The facial nerve leaves the lateral aspect of the brain stem at the lower border of the pons, and together with the intermedius and the VIII cranial nerves, it enters the internal auditory meatus and passes through it. It then enters the facial canal, which, in its first part, is directed laterally. At the geniculate ganglion, it makes a sharp bend in a posterolateral direction, proceeds caudally, and leaves the skull through the stylomastoid foramen. The facial canal lies close to the tympanic cavity and in its dorsolateral and caudal course is separated from it only by a thin bone lamella. On leaving the stylomastoid foramen, the facial nerve pierces the parotid gland and splits into several branches, which spread out in a fan-like manner to reach the facial muscles. It also gives off motor fibers to the stapedius muscle in the middle ear and to the stylohyoid and posterior belly of the digastric muscles and to the platysma.

The facial nerve is vulnerable to injury in its intracranial portion during the excision of an acoustic neuroma or other local tumor, and it is also injured in fractures of the base of the skull. The degree of paralysis can range from a slight to a total involvement. Clinical examination involves the assessment of eye closure, forehead wrinkling, symmetry of the face at rest and during movements, and ability to retract the angles of the mouth. The strength of orbicularis oculi and oris muscles in their sphincter action can be tested by an attempt to overcome their action with the examining fingers. The mildest degree of facial paresis appears as a slight flattening of the lower face at rest and of the arch of the upper lip on that side when the mouth is opened widely. The ability to bury the eyelashes, on orbicularis oculi contraction, as compared with the intact side, is a useful indicator of mild to moderate weakness. With total paralysis, the eyelids cannot be apposed, whereas with mild residual strength, apposition is possible. The mild to moderate degrees of palsy are easy to detect because residual facial movement is demonstrable. In those patients in whom the palsy appears to be complete on clinical examination, we have found that the ability to appose the lids fully indicates that the lesion is, in fact, incomplete and that this can be confirmed by nerve conduction studies and electromyographic examination. That is to say, the ability to appose the lids, in an otherwise immobile face, indicates an incomplete lesion with continuity, and it indicates a good prognosis.

The most common cause of facial paralysis is Bell's palsy of spontaneous onset. Facial palsy is also seen with geniculate herpes, and bilateral facial palsy occurs as part of a more widespread involvement of cranial nerve function in the Guillain-Barré syndrome. Facial palsy is also seen with infarction of the lateral brain stem. Involvement of the nuclear or infranuclear portion of the facial nerve simulates the lower motor neuron lesion of Bell's palsy or of traumatic facial palsies. Facial paralysis of an upper motor neuron type occurs as a part of the common hemiplegic stroke, and the upper face is spared in this type of paralysis because of its bilateral innervation. Lower motor neuron facial paralysis results in an equal involvement of the upper and lower portions of the face.

Facial nerve function can be further assessed by the testing of lacrimation and of taste of the anterior two-thirds of the tongue (chorda tympani function), and the latter can be evaluated by electrogustometry.[197,198] We have found electrogustometry to be a difficult examination. Many patients are not able to perceive the stimulus (a metallic taste) clearly; because the threshold is often not reproducible, we do not routinely use the test.

Traumatic facial nerve palsy is commonly due to longitudinal and transverse fractures of the temporal bone[199,200] and can be associated with disruption of the auditory ossicle chain.[201] Ghorayeb and Rafie[202] have described the findings on high-resolution CT of temporal bone fractures in 110 patients, in whom there was immediate onset of facial paralysis in 64 and a delayed onset in 13. Silverstein[203] described injury to the facial nerve as a result of temporal bone fractures, blunt trauma, and penetrating wounds and occasionally after iatrogenic injury during ear surgery. Yamamoto et al.[204] described 23 cases of facial palsy out of 781 patients with head injury, and com-

plete recovery occurred in 16 patients. The mechanism of the delayed onset of facial paralysis following head injury remains unclear.[205]

A review of our experience of 41 cases of traumatic facial nerve palsy revealed that 13 occurred after head injury. The head injury was usually of a severe type with unconsciousness and skull fracture, the paralysis was incomplete in 10 of the 13 patients. The paralysis was postoperative in 25 patients, 12 cases of which followed the removal of an acoustic neuroma (schwannoma); about half of these cases were incomplete. Facial paralysis followed parotid tumor surgery in four patients, and it was complete in two of these. The remaining postoperative group was composed of single cases following a variety of procedures such as cosmetic and temporomandibular joint surgery, removal of a cholesteatoma, and other surgical procedures on the ear. In two patients, the paralysis followed blunt trauma to the side of the face.

Facial nerve conduction can be assessed by the insertion of concentric needle electrodes into the various facial muscles; we routinely sample the frontalis/orbicularis oculi junction above the midpoint of the orbital rim, the orbicularis oculi about 1 cm lateral to the lateral orbital margin, the levator anguli oris about 2 cm lateral to the angle of the mouth. On stimulation of the facial nerve in the preauricular region, conduction latency values can be determined, and the compound action potential amplitude can be seen and measured. The normal latency values for our laboratory, on supramaximal stimulation, are 2.1 to 3.8 ms to the frontalis orbicularis oculi junction and 2.3 to 4.1 ms to the levator anguli oris and the orbicularis oris. When the nerve has been completely severed in its intracranial portion, as for example, during a surgical procedure for acoustic neuroma, conduction is preserved in the more distal portion of the nerve by the aforementioned technique until about the fourth or fifth day[25] without any change in the latency values but with a progressive decline of the compound action potential until it disappears at about the fourth or fifth day.

We measure the motor latency value to the three facial muscles as well as the compound action potential amplitude, and we look for evidence of denervation, the completeness of the interference pattern, and the appearance of nascent potentials in the recovery phase. In patients with traumatic facial palsies and in patients who have suffered basal skull fracture and an associated facial palsy, examination before 5 to 6 days after injury can be misleading because there may be a response to nerve stimulation in the presence of a complete lesion without any surviving MUs. An examination at this stage can be useful if it detects surviving MU activity, but in the absence of that activity, it can be misleading because nerve conduction is temporarily preserved.

The severity of the lesion can be assessed in a manner that is similar to that in Bell's palsy. Normal or near-normal latency values with normal to near-normal compound action potential amplitude are seen in the milder degrees of involvement. Prolonged latency values of 6 to 7 ms to the frontalis with a considerably diminished compound action potential down to the microvolt range indicate a more severe lesion. Although in Bell's palsy the severity of involvement tends to be uniform with equal involvement of all divisions of the facial nerve, traumatic facial palsies may result in a dense or complete involvement in one facial area with milder involvement in another. For example, the frontalis or orbicularis oculi involvement may be complete or near complete, whereas orbicularis oris and levator anguli oris action may be well preserved.

In an examination of the patient following hypoglossal-facial anastomosis, the usual technique of facial nerve stimulation cannot be applied. The various facial muscles are sampled with concentric needle electrodes, and the patient is instructed to move the tongue to bring out any volitional MU activity as evidence of recovery and of reinnervation.

ACKNOWLEDGMENT

The author wishes to acknowledge the technical and clinical assistance of Annette Mrazek, R.N., Chief Technologist, Department of Neurophysiology, St. Michael's Hospital, Toronto, and to acknowledge the numerous patient referrals by Dr. Alan Hudson and by other colleagues, without whose collaboration this clinical and electrophysiologic experience would not have been possible.

REFERENCES

1. Seddon H. Degeneration and regeneration. In: Seddon H. Surgical disorders of the peripheral nerves. Edinburgh: E & S Livingstone, 1972:9–31.
2. Sunderland S. A classification of peripheral nerve injuries producing loss of function. Brain 1951; 74:491.
3. Ochsner A, Gage M, DeBakey M. Scalenus anticus (Naffziger) syndrome. Am J Surg 1935; 28:669–695.
4. Ochoa J, Fowler TJ, Gilliat RW. Anatomical changes in peripheral nerves compressed by a pneumatic tourniquet. J Anat 1972; 113:433–455.
5. Waller A. Experiments on the section of the glossopharyngeal and hypoglossal nerves of the frog. Phil Trans Roy Soc (Lond) 1850; 140:423–429.
6. Morris JH, Hudson AR, Weddell G. A study of degeneration and regeneration in the divided rat sciatic nerve based on electron microscopy. Z Zellforsch 1972; 124:76–203.
7. Denny-Brown D, Brenner C. Paralysis of nerve induced by direct pressure and by tourniquet. Arch Neurol Psychiat 1944; 51:1.
8. Boyd IA, Davey MR. Composition of peripheral nerves. Edinburgh: E & S Livingstone, 1968.
9. Gasser HS, Erlanger J. The role played by the sizes of the constituent fibers of a nerve trunk in determining the form of its action potential wave. Am J Physiol 1927; 80:522–547.
10. Berry H, Richardson PM. Common peroneal nerve palsy: A clinical and electrophysiological review. J Neurol Neurosurg Psychiatry 1976; 39:1162–1171.
11. Cragg BG, Thomas PK. The conduction velocity of regenerated peripheral nerve fibres. J Physiol (Lond) 1964; 171:164–175.
12. Trojaborg W. Rate of recovery in motor and sensory fibres of the radial nerve: Clinical and electrophysiological aspects. J Neurol Neurosurg Psychiatry 1970; 33:625–628.
13. Erb W. Handbook of electrotherapy. New York, 1883.
14. Adrian E, Bronk D. The discharge of pulses in motor nerve fibres. J Physiol (Lond) 1929; 67:119–251.
15. Denny-Brown D, Pennybacker J. Fibrillation and fasciculation in voluntary muscle. Brain 1938; 61:311–344.
16. Buchthal F, Clemmesen S. Differentiation of muscle atrophy by electromyography. Acta Psychiat (KbH) 1941; 16:143–181.
17. Weddell G, Fernstein B, Pattie R. The electrical activity of voluntary muscle in man under normal and pathological conditions. Brain 1944; 67:178–256.
18. Kugelberg E. Electromyograms in muscular disorders. J Neurol Neurosurg Psychiatry 1947; 10:122–133.
19. Simpson JA. Electrical signs in the diagnosis of carpal tunnel and related syndromes. J Neurol Neurosurg Psychiatry 1956; 19:275–280.
20. Gilliat RW, Sears TA. Sensory nerve action potentials in patients with peripheral nerve lesions. J Neurol Neurosurg Psychiatry 1958; 21:109–118.
21. Buchthal F, Pinelli P, Rosenfalck, P. Action potential parameters in normal human muscle and their physiological determinants. Acta Physiol Scand 1954; 32:219–229.

22. Lenman JA, Ritchie AE. Clinical electromyography. Philadelphia: JB Lippincott, 1970.
23. Ludin H-P. Electromyography in practice. New York: Georg Thieme Verlag, 1980.
24. Gassel MM. A test of nerve conduction to muscles of the shoulder girdle as an aid in the diagnosis of proximal neurogenic and muscular disease. J Neurol Neurosurg Psychiatry 1964; 27:200–205.
25. Gilliatt RW, Taylor JC. Electrical changes following section of the facial nerve. Proc Roy Soc Med 1959; 52:1080–1083.
26. Gilliatt RW, Hjorth RJ. Nerve conduction during wallerian degeneration in the baboon. J Neurol Neurosurg Psychiatry 1972; 35:335–341.
27. Kline DG, Nulsen FE. The neuroma in continuity: Its preoperative and operative managment. Surg Clin North Am 1972; 52(5):1189–1209.
28. Williams HB, Terzis JK. Single fascicular recordings: An intraoperative diagnostic tool for the management of peripheral nerve lesions. Plast Reconstr Surg 1976; 57(5):562–569.
29. Nakatsuchi Y, Matsui T, Handa Y. Funicular orientation by electrical stimulation and internal neurolysis in peripheral nerve suture. Hand 1980; 12(1):65–74.
30. Gaul JS Jr. Electrical fascicle identification as an adjunct to nerve repair. Hand Clin 1986; 2(4):709–722.
31. Hakstian RW. Funicular orientation by direct stimulation. J Bone Joint Surg 1968; 50A(6):1178–1186.
32. Mackinnon SE, Dellon AL. Surgery of the peripheral nerve. New York: Thieme Medical Publishers, 1988.
33. Aids to the examination of the peripheral nervous system. MRC Nerve Injuries Committee. London: Bailliere Tindall, 1986.
34. Wadsworth TG. The cubital tunnel and the external compression syndrome. Anesth Analg 1974; 53:303.
35. Wadsworth TG. The external compression syndrome of the ulnar nerve at the cubital tunnel. A clinical study of external compression ulnar neuropathy at elbow level and a classification of the cubital tunnel syndrome. Clin Orthop 1977; 124:189.
36. Sunderland S. Nerves and nerve injuries, ed 2. Edinburg: Churchill/Livingstone, 1978:822.
37. Osborne G. Compression neuritis of the ulnar nerve at the elbow. Hand 1970; 2:10.
38. Gilliatt RW, Sears TA. Sensory nerve action potentials in patients with peripheral nerve lesions. J Neurol Neurosurg Psychiatry 1972; 35:335–341.
39. Gilliatt RW, Thomas PK. Changes in nerve conduction with ulnar lesions at the elbow. J Neurol Neurosurg Psychiatry 1960; 23:312–320.
40. Payan J. Anterior transposition of the ulnar nerve. An electrophysiological study. J Neurol Neurosurg Psychiatry 1970; 33:157–165.
41. Brown WF, Ferguson GG, Jones MW, et al. The location of conduction abnormalities in human entrapment neuropathies. Can J Neurol Sci 1976; 3:111–122.
42. Wu JS, Morris JD, Hogan GR. Ulnar neuropathy at the wrist: Case report and review of literature. Arch Phys Med Rehabil 1985; 66(11):785–788.
43. Vance RM, Gelberman RH. Acute ulnar neuropathy with fractures at the wrist. J Bone Joint Surg (Am) 1978; 60(7):962–965.
44. Poppi M, Padovani R, Martinelli P, Pozzati E. Fracture of the distal radius with ulnar nerve palsy. J Trauma 1978; 18(4):278–279.
45. Eckman PB, Perlstein G, Altrocchi PH. Ulnar neuropathy in bicycle riders. Arch Neurol 1975; 32(2):130–132.
46. Gross MS, Gelberman RH. The anatomy of the distal ulnar tunnel. Clin Orthop 1985; (196):238–247.
47. Dodds GA III, Hale D, Jackson WT. Incidence of anatomic variants in Guyon's canal. J Hand Surg (Am) 1990; 15(2):352–355.
48. Still JM Jr, Kleinert HE. Anomalous muscles and nerve entrapment in the wrist and hand. J Plast Reconstr Surg 1973; 52(4):394–400.
49. Swanson AB, Biddulph SL, Baughman FA Jr, De Groot G. Ulnar nerve compression due to an anomalous muscle in the canal of Guyon. Clin Orthop 1972; 83:64–69.
50. O'Hara JJ, Stone JH. Ulnar neuropathy at the wrist associated with aberrant flexor carpi ulnaris insertion. J Hand Surg (Am) 1988; 13(3):370–372.
51. Zook EG, Kucan JO, Guy RJ. Palmar wrist pain caused by ulnar nerve entrapment in the flexor carpi ulnaris tendon. J Hand Surg (Am) 1988; 13(5):732–735.
52. McFarland GB Jr, Hoffer MM. Paralysis of the intrinsic muscles of the hand secondary to lipoma in Guyon's tunnel. J Bone Joint Surg (Am) 1971; 53(2):375–376.
53. Taylor AR. Ulnar nerve compression at the wrist in rheumatoid arthritis. Report of a case. J Bone Joint Surg (Br) 1974; 56(1):142–143.
54. Dell PC. Compression of the ulnar nerve at the wrist secondary to a rheumatoid synovial cyst: Case report and review of the literature. J Hand Surg (Am) 1979; 4(5):468–473.
55. Bennett JE, Hayes JE, Robb C. Mutilating injuries of the wrist. J Trauma 1971; 11(12):1008–1020.
56. Hudson A, Berry H, Mayfield F. Chronic injuries of peripheral nerves by entrapment. In: Youmans JR, ed. Neurological surgery, ed 2. Vol 4. Philadelphia: WB Saunders, 1982:2454–2456.
57. Ebeling P, Gilliatt RW, Thomas PK. A clinical and electrical study of ulnar nerve lesions in the hand J Neurol Neurosurg Psychiatry 1960; 23:1–9.
58. Seddon H. Carpal ganglion as a cause of paralysis of the deep branch of the ulnar nerve. J Bone Joint Surg 1952; 34–B:386.
59. Mallett B, Zilkha K. Compression of the ulnar nerve at the wrist by a ganglion. Lancet 1955; 1:890–891.

60. Brosh JC, Jamieson EB, eds. Cunningham's text-book of anatomy, ed 8. London: Oxford University Press, 1947:1041.

61. Shah JJ, Bhatti NA. Radial nerve paralysis associated with fractures of the humerus. A review of 62 cases. Clin Orthop 1983; (172):171–176.

62. Shaw JL, Sakellarides H. Radial nerve paralysis associated with fractures of the humerus. A review of forty-five cases. J Bone Joint Surg (Am) 1967; 49(5):899–902.

63. Dinakar I, Rao SB. Neurilemomas of peripheral nerves. Int Surg 1971; 55(1):15–19.

64. Papilion JD, Neff RS, Shall LM. Compression neuropathy of the radial nerve as a complication of elbow arthroscopy: A case report and review of the literature. Arthroscopy 1988; 4(4):284–286.

65. Olney BW, Menelaus MB. Monteggia and equivalent lesions in childhood. J Pediatr Orthop 1989; 9(2):219–223.

66. Young AW, Redmond MD, Hemler DE, Belandres PV. Radial motor nerve conduction studies. Arch Phys Rehabil 1990; 71:399–402.

67. Carfi J, Dong M. Posterior interosseous syndrome revisited. Muscle Nerve 1985; 8:499–502.

68. Kaplan PE. Posterior interosseous neuropathies: Natural history. Arch Phys Med Rehabil 1984; 65:399–400.

69. Holst-Nielsen F, Jensen V. Tardy posterior interosseous nerve palsy as a result of an unreduced radial head dislocation in Monteggia fractures: A report of two cases. J Hand Surg 1984; 9A(4):572–575.

70. Jones JR, Evans DM, Kaushik A. Synovial chondromatosis presenting with peripheral nerve compression—a report of two cases. J Hand Surg 1987; 12B(1):25–27.

71. El-Hadidi S, Burke FD. Posterior nerve syndrome caused by a bursa in the vicinity of the elbow. J Hand Surg 1987; 12B(1):23–24.

72. Geiringer SR, Leonard JA Jr. Posterior interosseous palsy after dental treatment: Case report. Arch Phys Med Rehabil 1985; 66:711–712.

73. Pidgeon KJ, Abadee P, Kanakamedala R, Uchizono M. Posterior interosseous nerve syndrome caused by an intermuscular lipoma. Arch Phys Med Rehabil 1985; 66(7):468–471.

74. Ishikawa H, Hirohata K. Posterior interosseous nerve syndrome associated with rheumatoid synovial cysts of the elbow joint. Clin Orthop 1990; (254):134–139.

75. Rayan GM, Conner S. Posterior interosseous nerve paralysis and amyloid neuropathy of multiple myeloma. Clin Orthop 1982; (171):202–205.

76. Cravens G, Kline DG. Posterior interosseous nerve palsies. Neurosurgery 1990; 27(3):397–402.

77. Falck B, Hurme M. Conduction velocity of the posterior interosseus nerve across the arcade of Frohse. Electromyogr Clin Neurophysiol 1983; 23:567–576.

78. Lake PA. Anterior interosseous nerve syndrome. J Neurosurg 1974; 41:306–309.

79. O'Brien MD, Upton ARM. Anterior interosseous nerve syndrome. Neurol Neurosurg Psychiatry 1972; 35:531–536.

80. Smith BH, Herbst BA. Anterior interosseus nerve palsy. Arch Neurol (Chicago) 1974; 30:330–331.

81. Gardner-Thorpe C. Anterior interosseous nerve palsy: Spontaneous recovery in two patients. J Neurol Neurosurg Psychiatry 1974; 37:1146–1150.

82. Rask MR. Anterior interosseous nerve entrapment (Kiloh-Nevin syndrome): Report of seven cases. Clin Orthop 1979; (142):176–181.

83. O'Neill DB, Zarins B, Gelberman RH, et al. Compression of the anterior interosseous nerve after use of a sling for dislocation of the acromioclavicular joint. A report of two cases. J Bone Joint Surg (Am) 1990; 72(7):1100–1102.

84. Moehring HD. Irreducible supracondylar fracture of the humerus complicated by anterior interosseous nerve palsy. Clin Orthop 1986; (206):228–232.

85. Nigst H, Dick W. Syndromes of compression of the median nerve in the proximal forearm (pronator teres syndrome; anterior interosseous nerve syndrome). Arch Orthop Trauma Surg 1979; 93(4):307–312.

86. Stern MB. The anterior interosseous nerve syndrome (the Kiloh-Nevin syndrome). Report and follow-up study of three cases. Clin Orthop 1984; (187):223–227.

87. Hill NA, Howard FM, Huffer BR. The incomplete anterior interosseous nerve syndrome. J Hand Surg (Am) 1985; 10(1):4–16.

88. Spinner M. Injuries to the major branches of peripheral nerves of the forearm. Philadelphia: WB Saunders, 1972.

89. Seyffarth H. Primary myoses in the m. pronator teres as cause of lesion of the n. medianus (pronator syndrome). Acta Psychiat Neurol Scand 1951; 74(suppl):251–254.

90. Kopell HP, Thompson WAL. Pronator syndrome. N Engl J Med 1958; 259:713–715.

91. Morris HH, Peters BH. Pronator syndrome: Clinical and electrophysiological features in seven cases. J Neurol Neurosurg Psychiatry 1976; 39:566–570.

92. Feldman RG, Travers PH, Chirico-Post J, Keyserling WM. Risk assessment in electronic assembly workers: Carpal tunnel syndrome. J Hand Surg 1987; 12A(5 Pt.2):849–855.

93. Upton ARM, McComas AJ. Double crush in nerve-entrapment syndromes. Lancet 1973; 2:359–361.

94. Wongsam PE, Johnson EW, Weinerman JD. Carpal tunnel syndrome: Use of palmar stimulation of sensory fibers. Arch Phys Med Rehabil 1983; 64:16–19.

95. Buchthal F, Rosenfalck A. Sensory conduction from digit to palm and from palm to wrist in the carpal

tunnel syndrome. J Neurol Neurosurg Psychiatry 1971; 34:243–252.

96. Bach BR Jr, O'Brien SJ, Warren RF, Leighton M. An unusual neurological complication of the Bristow procedure. A case report. J Bone Joint Surg (Am) 1988; 70(3):458–460.

97. Caspi I, Ezra E, Nerubay J, Horoszovski H. Musculocutaneous nerve injury after coracoid process transfer for clavicle instability. Report of three cases. Acta Orthop Scand 1987; 58(3):294–295.

98. Dundore DE, DeLisa JA. Musculocutaneous nerve palsy: An isolated complication of surgery. Arch Phys Med Rehabil 1979; 60(3):130–133.

99. Ewing MR. Postoperative paralysis in upper extremity: Report of five cases. Lancet 1950; 1:99–103.

100. Zeuke VW, Heidrich R. Pathogenese der isolierten, post-operative Lähmung des Nerves musculocutaneus. Schweiz Arch Neurol Neurochir Psychiatr 1974; 114:289–294.

101. Pollock LJ, Davis L. Peripheral nerve injuries. Incidence. Am J Surg 1932; 15:179–181.

102. Pollock LJ, Davis L. Peripheral nerve injuries. The axillary nerve. Am J Surg 1932; 17:462–471.

103. Blom S, Dahlback LD. Nerve injuries in dislocations of the shoulder joint and fractures of the neck of the humerus. Acta Chir Scand 1970; 136:461–466.

104. Kopell HP, Thompson WAL. Peripheral entrapment neuropathies. Baltimore: Williams & Wilkins, 1963.

105. Ford FR. Diseases of the nervous system in infancy, childhood and adolescence, ed 6. Springfield, IL: Charles C. Thomas, 1973:1313.

106. Clein JJ. Suprascapula entrapment neuropathy. J Neurosurg 1975; 43:337.

107. Bateman JE. Nerve injuries about the shoulder in sports. J Bone Joint Surg 1967; 49–A:785.

108. Agre JC, Ash N, Cameron MC, House J. Suprascapular neuropathy after intensive progressive resistive exercise: Case report. Arch Phys Med Rehabil 1987; 68:236–238.

109. Montagna P. Suprascapular neuropathy after muscular effort. Electromyogr Clin Neurophysiol 1983; 23:553–557.

110. Foerster O. Die Symptomatologie der Schussverletzungen der peripheren Nerven. In: Lewandowsky M, ed. Handbuch der Neurologie. Ergänzungsband, Part 2. Berlin: Springer, 1929.

111. Kaplan PE, Kernahan WT Jr. Rotator cuff rupture: Management with suprascapular neuropathy. Arch Phys Med Rehabil 1984; 65:273–275.

112. Weaver HL. Isolated suprascapular nerve lesions. Injury 1983; 15(2):117–126.

113. Horwitz MT, Tocantins LM. An anatomical study of the role of the long thoracic nerve and the related scapular bursae in the pathogenesis of local paralysis of the serratus anterior muscle. Anat Rec 1938; 71:375.

114. Horwitz MT, Tocantins LM. Isolated paralysis of the serratus anterior (magnus) muscle. J Bone Joint Surg 1938; 20:720.

115. Skillern PG. Serratus magnus palsy with proposal of a new operation for intractable cases. Ann Surg 1913; 57:909.

116. Overpeck DO, Ghormley RK. Paralysis of the serratus magnus muscle caused by lesions of the long thoracic nerve. JAMA 1940; 14:1994.

117. Prescott MU, Zollinger RW. Alar scapula. An unusual surgical complication. Am J Surg 1944; 65:98.

118. Gregg JR, Labosky D, Harty M, et al. Serratus anterior paralysis in the young athlete. J Bone Joint Surg (Am) 1979; 61(6A):825–832.

119. Stanish WD, Lamb H. Isolated paralysis of the serratus anterior muscle: A weight training injury. Case report. Am J Sports Med 1978; 6(6):385–386.

120. Duncan MA, Lotze MT, Gerber LH, Rosenberg SA. Incidence, recovery, and management of serratus anterior muscle palsy after axillary node dissection. Phys Ther 1983; 63(8):1243–1247.

121. Porsman O. Serratus anterior paresis as an occupational disease in slaughterhouse workers. An occupational medicine analysis. Ugeskr Laeger 1977; 139(5):291–292.

122. del Sasso L, Mondini A, Brambilla S. A case of isolated paralysis of serratus anterior. Ital J Orthop Traumatol 1988; 14(4):533–537.

123. Foo CL, Swann M. Isolated paralysis of the serratus anterior. A report of 20 cases. J Bone Joint Surg (Br) 1983; 65(5):552–556.

124. King RJ, Motta G. Iatrogenic spinal accessory nerve palsy. Ann R Coll Surg Eng 1983; 65(1):35–37.

125. Becker GP, Parell GT. Technique of preserving the spinal accessory nerve dissection. Laryngoscope 1979; 89:827–831.

126. Petrera JE, Trojaborg W. Conduction studies along the accessory nerve and follow-up of patients with trapezius palsy. J Neurol Neurosurg Psychiatry 1984; 47(6):630–636.

127. Woodall B. Trapezius paralysis following minor surgical procedures in the posterior cervical triangle: Results following cranial nerve suture. Ann Surg 1952; 136:375–380.

128. Gordon SL, Graham WP, Black JT, Miller SH. Accessory nerve function after surgical procedures in the posterior triangle. Arch Surg 1977; 112:264–268.

129. Norden A. Peripheral injuries to the spinal accessory nerve. Acta Chir Scand 1946; 94:515–532.

130. Olarte M, Adams D. Accessory nerve palsy. J Neurol Neurosurg Psychiatry 1977; 40:1113–1116.

131. Wright TA. Accessory spinal nerve injury. Clin Orthop Related Surg 1975; 108:16–18.

132. Swann KW, Heros RC. Accessory nerve palsy following carotid artery endarterectomy. Report of two cases. J Neurosurg 1985; 63(4):630–632.

133. Sarala PK. Accessory nerve palsy, an uncommon etiology. Arch Phys Med Rehabil 1982; 63(9):445–446.

134. Berger PS, Bataini JP. Radiation-induced cranial nerve palsy. Cancer 1977; 40(1):152–155.

135. Berry H, MacDonald EA, Mrazek AC. Accessory nerve palsy: A review of 23 cases. Can J Neurol Sci 1991; 18:337–341.

136. Eisen A, Bertrand G. Isolated accessory nerve palsy of spontaneous origin. A clinical and electromyographic study. Arch Neurol 1972; 27(6):496–502.

137. Haymaker W, Woodhall B. Peripheral nerve injuries. Principles of diagnosis. Philadelphia: WB Saunders, 1953:201–208.

138. Hershlag A, Loy RA, Lavy G, DeCherney AH. Femoral neuropathy after laparoscopy. A case report. J Reprod Med 1990; 35(5):575–576.

139. Hassan AA, Reiff RH, Fayez JA. Femoral neuropathy following tubal microsurgery. Fertil Steril 1986; 45(6):742–889.

140. Jurgens R, Haupt WF. Femoral nerve paralysis after vaginal hysterectomy. Its causes and forensic significance. Dtsch Med Wochenschr 1984; 109(48):1848–1850.

141. Vaziri ND, Barton CH, Ravikumar GR, et al. Femoral neuropathy: A complication of renal transplantation. Nephron 1981; 28(1):30–31.

142. Pontin AR, Donaldson RA, Jacobson JE. Femoral neuropathy after renal transplantation. S Afr Med J 1978; 53(10):376–378.

143. Georgy FM. Femoral neuropathy following abdominal hysterectomy. Am J Obstet Gynecol 1975; 123(8):819–822.

144. Kourtopoulos H. Femoral nerve injury following appendectomy. Case report. J Neurosurg 1982; 57(5):714–715.

145. Solheim LF, Hagen R. Femoral and sciatic neuropathies after total hip arthroplasty. Acta Orthop Scand 1980; 51(3):531–534.

146. Hudson AR, Hunter GA, Waddell JP. Iatrogenic femoral nerve injuries. Can J Surg 1979; 22(1):62–66.

147. Muller ME. Total hip prostheses. Clin Orthop 1970; 72:46–68.

148. Boontje AH, Haaxma R. Femoral neuropathy as a complication of aortic surgery. J Cardiovasc Surg (Torino) 1987; 28(3):286–289.

149. Berliner SD. Accidental femoral nerve block during local anaesthesia for inguinal hernia repair (letter). Anaesthesia 1989; 44(3):261.

150. Razzuk MA, Linton RR, Darling RC. Femoral neuropathy secondary to ruptured abdominal aortic aneurysms with false aneurysms. JAMA 1967; 201(11):817–820.

151. Laurent LE. Femoral nerve compression syndrome with paresis of the quadriceps muscle caused by radiotherapy of malignant tumours. A report of four cases. Acta Orthop Scand 1975; 46(5):804–808.

152. Buchthal A. Femoral nerve paresis as a complication of gynaecological operations. Dtsch Med Wochenschr 1973; 98(43):2024–2027.

153. Ginanneschi U, Capus L, Smrekar V, et al. Partial paralysis of the right lumbar plexus caused by a traumatic hematoma of the ileo-psoas muscle. Chir Ital 1985; 37(2):165–173.

154. Tittel K. CT scanning in the diagnosis of a retroperitoneal haematoma. Aktuel Traumatol 1979; 9(1):11–13.

155. Goodfellow J, Fearn CB, Matthews JM. Iliacus haematoma. A common complication of haemophila. J Bone Joint Surg (Br) 1967; 49(4):748–756.

156. Stern MB, Spiegel P. Femoral neuropathy as a complication of Heparin anticoagulation therapy. Clin Orthop Related Res 1975; 106:140–142.

157. Spiegel PG, Meltzer JL. Femoral-nerve neuropathy secondary to anticoagulation. Report of a case. J Bone Joint Surg 1974; 56A(2):425–427.

158. Dhaliwal GS, Schlagenhauff FE, Megahed SM. Acute femoral neuropathy induced by oral anticoagulation. Dis Nerv Syst 1976; 37(9):539–541.

159. Gassel MM. A study of femoral nerve conduction time. Arch Neurol (Chicago) 1963; 9:607–614.

160. Chopra JS, Hurwitz LJ. Femoral nerve conduction in diabetes and chronic occlusive vascular disease. J Neurol Neurosurg Psychiat 1968; 31:28.

161. Roblin L, Tea S, Le Saout J, et al. Nerve paralysis after surgery of the hip. Apropos of 48 cases. Rev Chir Orthop 1989; 75(2):104–111.

162. Jones HR Jr, Gianturco LE, Gross PT, Buchhalter J. Sciatic neuropathies in childhood: A report of ten cases and review of literature. J Child Neurol 1988; 3(3):193–199.

163. Synek VM. The pyriformis syndrome: Review and case presentation. Clin Exp Neurol 1987; 23:31–37.

164. Gassel MM, Trojaborg W. Clinical and electrophysiological study of the pattern of conduction times in the distribution of the sciatic nerve. J Neurol Neurosurg Psychiatry 1964; 27:351–357.

165. Nobel W. Peroneal palsy due to hematoma in the common peroneal nerve sheath after distal torsional fractures and inversion ankle sprains. J Bone Joint Surg 1966; 48A:1484–1495.

166. Haftek J. Stretch injury of peripheral nerve. J Bone Joint Surg 1970; 52B:354–365.

167. Sunderland S. Nerves and nerve injuries. Baltimore: Williams & Wilkins, 1968.

168. Sorell DA, Hinterbuchner C, Green RF, Kalisky I. Traumatic common peroneal nerve palsy: A retrospective study. Arch Phys Med Rehabil 1976; 57(8):361–365.

169. Streib EW. Traction injury of peroneal nerve caused by minor athletic trauma: Electromyographic studies. Arch Neurol 1983; 40(1):62–63.

170. Stoff MD, Greene AF. Common peroneal nerve palsy following inversion ankle injury: A report of two cases. Phys Ther 1982; 62(10):1463–1464.
171. Braune HJ, Huffmann G. Exercise-induced partial damage of the n. peroneus profundus. Dtsch Med Wochenschr 1990; 115(25):974–976.
172. Leach RE, Purnell MB, Saito A. Peroneal nerve entrapment in runners. Am J Sports Med 1989; 17(2):287–291.
173. Sisto DJ, Warren RF. Complete knee dislocation. A follow-up study of operative treatment. Clin Orthop 1985; (198):94–101.
174. Shevell MI, Stewart JD. Laceration of the common peroneal nerve by a skate blade. Can Med Assoc J 1988; 139(4):311–312.
175. Barbour PJ, Levitt LP. Tennis foot drop. J Sports Med Phys Fitness 1983; 23(4):427–428.
176. Herrera-Ornelas L, Tolls RM, Petrelli NJ, et al. Common peroneal nerve palsy associated with pelvic surgery for cancer. An analysis of 11 cases. Dis Colon Rectum 1986; 29(6):392–397.
177. Hatano Y, Arai T, Iida H, Soneda J. Common peroneal nerve palsy. A complication of coronary artery bypass grafting surgery. Anaesthesia 1988; 43(7):568–569.
178. Giacoia GP. Peroneal nerve palsy in a premature: Complication of multiple blood pressure measurements. Clin Pediatr (Phila) 1981; 20(9):591.
179. Garland DE, Bailey S. Undetected injuries in head-injured adults. Clin Orthop 1981; (155):162–165.
180. Redford JB. Nerve conduction in motor fibers to the anterior tibial muscle in peroneal palsy. Arch Phys Med Rehabil 1964; 45:500–504.
181. Katirji MB, Wilbourn AJ. Common peroneal mononeuropathy: A clinical and electrophysiologic study of 116 lesions. Neurology 1988; 38:1723–1728.
182. Lambert EH. The accessory deep peroneal nerve. Neurology (Minneap) 1969; 19:1169–1176.
183. Brunner WG, Spencer RF. Posterior tibial nerve neurotmesis complicating a closed tibial fracture. A case report. S Afr Med J 1990; 78(10):607–608.
184. Peck JJ, Eastman AB, Bergan JJ, et al. Popliteal vascular trauma. A community experience. Arch Surg 1990; 125(10):1339–1343.
185. Hopf HC. Obturator nerve paralysis during parturition (author's trans.). J Neurol 1974; 207(2):165–166.
186. Siliski JM, Scott RD. Obturator-nerve palsy resulting from intrapelvic extrusion of cement during total hip replacement. Report of four cases. J Bone Joint Surg (Am) 1985; 67(8):1225–1228.
187. Oh SJ, Sarala PK, Kuba T, Elmore RS. Tarsal tunnel syndrome: Electrophysiological study. Ann Neurol 1979; 5:327–330.
188. Edward WG, Lincoln GR, Bassett III FH, Goldman JL. The tarsal tunnel syndrome: Diagnosis and treatment. JAMA 1969; 207(4):716–720.
189. Takakura T, Kitada C, Sugimoto K, et al. Tarsal tunnel syndrome. Causes and results of operative treatment. J Bone Joint Surg (Br) 1991; 73(1):125–128.
190. Grumbine NA, Radovic PA, Parsons R, Scheinin GS. Tarsal tunnel syndrome. Comprehensive review of 87 cases. J Am Podiatr Med Assoc 1990; 80(9):457–461.
191. Taguchi Y, Nosaka K, Yasuda K, et al. The tarsal tunnel syndrome. Report of two cases of unusual cause. Clin Orthop 1987; (217):247–252.
192. Babbage NF. "Burning feet" syndrome (letter). Med J Aust 1987; 146(12):657.
193. Grabois M, Puentes J, Lidsky M. Tarsal tunnel syndrome in rheumatoid arthritis. Arch Phys Med Rehabil 1981; 62(8):401–403.
194. Radin EL. Tarsel tunnel syndrome. Clin Orthop 1983; (181):167–770.
195. Kaplan PE, Kernahan WT Jr. Tarsal tunnel syndrome: An electrodiagnostic and surgical correlation. J Bone Joint Surg 1981; 63(1):96–99.
196. Warren J, Gutmann L, Figueroa AF, Bloor BM. Electromyographic changes of brachial plexus root avulsions. J Neurosurg 1969; 31:137–140.
197. Krarup B. Electrogustometry: A method for clinical taste examinations. Acta Otolaryngol 1958; 49:294.
198. Harbert FS, Wagner S, Young IM. The quantitative measurement of taste function. Arch Otolaryngol 1962; 75:138.
199. Lindeman RC. Temporal bone trauma and facial paralysis. Otolaryngol Clin North Am 1979; 12(2):403–413.
200. Adour KK, Boyajian JA, Kahn ZM, Schneider GS. Surgical and nonsurgical management of facial paralysis following closed head injury. Laryngoscope 1977; 87(3):380–390.
201. Gunnel F. Surgical findings and results following traumatic destruction of the auditory ossicle chain and facial nerve injury. Z Arztl Fortbild (Jena) 1966; 60(5):250–251.
202. Ghorayeb BV, Rafie JJ. Fracture of the temporal bone. Evaluation of 123 cases. J Radiol 1989; 70(12):703–710.
203. Silverstein H. Surgery of the facial nerve. J Otolaryngol 1981; 10(6):449–458.
204. Yamamoto T, Sato S, Nakao S, et al. Facial palsy following head injury: Topognosis, prognosis and indications for surgical decompression. No Shinkei Geka 1984; 12(7):807–813.
205. Puvanendran K, Vitharana M, Wong PK. Delayed facial palsy after head injury. J Neurol Neurosurg Psychiatry 1977; 40(4):342–350.
206. Berry H, Bril V. Axillary nerve palsy following blunt trauma to the shoulder region: A clinical and electrophysiological review. J Neurol Neurosurg Psychiatry 1982; 45:1027–1032.

14

Ischemic Neuropathy

Asa J. Wilbourn
Kerry H. Levin

CONTENTS

ACRONYMS

AH	abductor hallucis
CMAP	compound muscle action potential
CTS	carpal tunnel syndrome
DRG	dorsal root ganglion
EDB	extensor digitorum brevis
IMN	ischemic monomelic neuropathy
MNM	mononeuropathy multiplex
MUP	motor unit potential
NCS	nerve conduction studies
NEE	needle electrode examination
SNAP	sensory nerve action potential
TA	tibialis anterior

To maintain their physical and functional integrity, nerve fibers must receive an adequate blood supply.[1] When this requirement is not met, they become ischemic. Short-lived ischemia produces primarily physiologic changes along the affected portions of the nerve fibers, temporarily impairing their ability to conduct impulses. With more severe ischemia, however, the nerve fibers themselves sustain structural damage to varying degrees, and an *ischemic neuropathy* has occurred. The term is a general one, encompassing all types of nerve fiber injury caused by decreased blood flow.[2–4] Nonetheless, it is often restricted to situations in which the circulatory compromise is physically obvious, and other limb structures, primarily soft tissues, also have been injured. Considered in the broad sense, an ischemic neuropathy can be produced by lesions affecting vascular structures of virtually all dimensions, ranging from the aorta to the microvasculature. The primary causes for ischemic neuropathy are exceptionally diverse, ranging from immunologic disease to violent trauma; many are iatrogenic in nature.

Although it seems obvious that adequate blood flow is a prerequisite for normal functioning of nerve, historically the first articles attributing *neuritis* to ischemia apparently did not appear in the medical literature until the latter half of the 19th century.[3] Moreover, many of the modern concepts regarding impaired circulation and subsequent neuromuscular injury are of surprisingly recent vintage, having been formulated over the past two decades. Thus the fact that, in humans, diffuse limb ischemia can produce significant nerve injury without preceding or coexisting muscle damage, the characteristic presentation of ischemic monomelic neuropathy, was not appreciated until the 1970s.[5] Serving as even more striking examples are the compartment syndromes, which become symptomatic when the microvasculature of nerve and muscle is compromised. Although some types were first recorded by Volkmann and Lesser in the 1880s,[6] almost all the unifying concepts regarding their underlying pathophysiology, which serve as the basis for current diagnosis and management, were formulated over the past 25 years.[6–8]

ANATOMIC AND PHYSIOLOGIC PRINCIPLES

Peripheral nerve trunks are supplied by a succession of nutrient arteries along their extent, which enter at irregular intervals and vary in both number and size. Most are direct branches derived from major arteries supplying the limb, but some are subsidiary branches, arising from passing arteries that primarily supply muscles. On the surface of the nerves, the nutrient arteries typically divide into descending and ascending branches, which, after following a tortuous course, anastomose with similar branches derived from adjacent nutrient arteries. Branches arising from this superficial arterial system enter the nerve and then, in turn, divide into descending and ascending branches. In this manner, superficial and deep longitudinal arterial chains result, linked by anastomoses and extending the full length of the nerve. Whenever a branch arises from a nerve, or the latter divides, vascular networks continuous with those in the parent nerve accompany each branch or division. Thus although a nerve receives its blood supply in essentially a segmental fashion, there is considerable overlap in the distribution of the nutrient arteries supplying it at successive levels. Consequently, its circulation is not dominated by a single vessel over its entire length. Nonetheless, there are gaps in the system, some fairly constant for a given nerve trunk, in which a considerable segment of nerve receives only a single nutrient artery, for example, the median nerve in the forearm and the sciatic nerve in the thigh. For this reason, the nerve fibers in these regions are more susceptible to injury under ischemic conditions.[1,3]

Peripheral nerve has energy requirements for the maintenance of structural integrity, for the upkeep of energy-dependent ion channels in its excitable membrane, and for the propagation of nerve action potentials. Aerobic metabolism is responsible for most of its energy production. The oxygen requirements of mammalian nerve are relatively low and less than for many other tissues, for example, about $\frac{1}{20}$ of that of the cerebral cortex. Peripheral nerve, however, lacks autoregulation of blood flow.[9–12] Muscle also has a highly developed collateral vascular network. Moreover, its resting oxygen consumption is even lower than that of peripheral nerve and muscle has autoregulatory capacity.[12,13] For these reasons, nerve and muscle are relatively resistant to ischemic injury. There is general agreement, however, that the threshold for ischemic dysfunction is lower for peripheral nerve than for muscle; that is, limb nerves cease to conduct impulses under ischemic conditions before limb muscles become inexcitable.[14,15] If the ischemia is short-lived, the structural integrity of the nerve is maintained even though its ability to propagate nerve action potentials is temporarily lost. In contrast to the consensus regarding their relative ischemic dysfunction threshold, the relative infarction threshold of muscle and nerve is controversial. Most animal research suggests that muscle is structurally injured by ischemia before nerve.[4,16] The opposite, however, is characteristic of one type of human ischemic neuropathy, ischemic monomelic neuropathy, in which distal nerve fibers degenerate without any associated muscle fiber injury being evident.[13] Presumably this divergence between the experimental and the clinical and electrophysiologic studies results from differences in limb vascular supply in various species.

PATHOPHYSIOLOGY OF ISCHEMIC LESIONS

Limb ischemia can damage both nerve and muscle fibers. Usually injuries of one of these structures can be separated from those of the other in the electromyography (EMG) laboratory because their electrodiagnostic features differ for the most part.

With few exceptions (which are discussed subsequently), ischemic injuries of nerve fibers present as axon loss. These lesions do not materially differ from any other type of axon loss lesion. Although obviously dependent on such factors as the location, severity, duration of the process, and on the degree of collateral circulation, ischemic injury of nerve fibers produces alterations of the nerve conduction studies (NCS) and needle electrode examination (NEE) in a characteristic manner. When very mild axon loss lesions involve mixed nerves, the only detectable change is seen on the NEE, some 3 or more weeks after onset: a minimal to modest number of fibrillation potentials. If the axon loss is more severe, the amplitudes of the sensory nerve action potentials (SNAPs) decrease appreciably (below laboratory normal limits for age, or less than 50% of the amplitude of the corresponding response in the contralateral limb). Whenever substantial axon loss occurs, additional changes are noted, on both the NCS and the NEE, as the affected muscles are assessed: The compound muscle action potential (CMAP) amplitudes drop, and decreased recruitment, or a neurogenic motor unit potential (MUP) firing pattern (decreased numbers of MUPs, firing at rapid rates) are seen on attempted maximal activation (Table 14.1). If the muscle is reinnervated, highly polyphasic MUPs are found in it as this process occurs. Conversely, if the muscle is severely denervated and not reinnervated within 18 to 24 months, its fibers undergo irreversible degenerative changes, and it becomes electrically silent; that is, the insertional activity is markedly decreased or absent, no spontaneous activity is seen, and no MUPs can be activated.

In contrast to the aforementioned, direct ischemic injury of muscle, when incomplete, often initially produces a mixture of fibrillating and electrically silent fibers, at least in certain areas of the muscle, because some of the fibers actually undergo degeneration, whereas others, although they survive, are denervated, owing to degeneration of the intramuscular nerve fibers supplying them.[17,18] If some of the muscle fibers of an ischemic muscle remain viable and under voluntary control, polyphasic MUPs can be seen on activation immediately after onset because the muscle fiber loss has occurred in a random fash-

TABLE 14.1. Electrodiagnostic findings*

| Lesion Severity | Nerve Conduction Studies | | Needle Electrode Examination | |
	SNAP Amplitudes	CMAP Amplitudes	Fibrillation Potentials—Amount	MUPs Firing— Maximal Effort
Mild	Normal	Normal	Minimal/modest	Normal
Moderate	Low	Normal	Modest/moderate	Normal
Modestly severe	Very low/ no response	Low	Moderate/moderately abundant	Normal/mild decrease
Severe	No response	Very low	Moderately abundant	Moderate decrease
Very severe	No response	No response	Abundant	Severe decrease
Total	No response	No response	Abundant	None fire

* The electrodiagnostic changes typically seen with relatively recent onset (of greater than 3 weeks duration) focal axon-loss lesions. In the last column, the MUPs, when they fire in reduced numbers, do so at a rapid rate, thereby permitting maximal effort to be distinguished from incomplete voluntary effort.

SNAP, Sensory nerve action potential; CMAP, compound muscle action potential; MUP, motor unit potential.

ion, depleting many of the intact MUPs of some of their constituent muscle fibers. With more severe ischemia, however, all the individual muscle fibers may undergo ischemic degeneration, and the muscle then is essentially electrically silent from onset. Shortly thereafter, if circulation is not restored, the muscle fibers become necrotic. If some circulation returns, however, fibrosis develops in the degenerating muscle,[17,18] yielding a characteristic finding on NEE: a muscle that is electrically silent or nearly silent (containing only a few, tiny, scattered fibrillation potentials) along with the so-called *gritty* feel on needle insertion, caused by abrupt, *substantial* changes in mechanical resistance to needle advancement through the fibrotic muscle. Motor NCS using the ischemic muscle as the recording site yield low-amplitude or unelicitable CMAPs, depending on the degree of muscle fiber and intramuscular nerve fiber involvement. Conversely, the responses obtained on sensory NCS, the SNAPs, are not affected by ischemic muscle injuries per se.

There are two situations in which distinguishing ischemic lesions of nerve from those of muscle proves difficult. First, within a few weeks after onset, if highly polyphasic MUPs are found in a muscle near the lesion site. These could equally be due to nerve fiber injury with subsequent reinnervation and to primary muscle fiber injury with resultant disintegration of the motor units. Second, a year or more after a severe lesion, a completely atrophic muscle may be found that contains no insertional activity, no appreciable spontaneous activity (i.e., fibrillation potentials), and no voluntary MUPs. Typically the mechanical resistance to needle insertion is markedly increased in an irregular fashion (gritty feel). With such *end stage* muscle, it is impossible to determine, by NEE, whether the injurious process was severe primary denervation with absence of reinnervation and subsequent secondary muscle fiber degeneration or whether it was primary muscle degeneration owing to direct muscle fiber damage.

VARIOUS TYPES OF ISCHEMIC NEUROPATHIES

In the remainder of this chapter, a number of conditions in which symptomatic nerve or muscle ischemia occurs are reviewed. Omitted from discussion are certain disorders, for example, various types of diabetic neuropathy, in which ischemic nerve damage may be the primary cause but which are not customarily considered *ischemic neuropathies*.[19]

Brief Physician-Induced Limb Ischemia

The effect of short-lived ischemia—usually of less than 40 minutes duration and induced by a pneumatic cuff placed around the arm or thigh—on human limb nerves has been the subject of a number of investigations this century. The report by Lewis et al.,[20] although one of the earliest, probably has been the most influential. Their experiments suggested that ischemia caused loss of motor and sensory function in the limb, that always began distally and progressed proximally, with the function of large fibers compromised before that of small fibers. They attributed these changes to ischemia of the nerve segment beneath the cuff rather than of more distal segments (this concept has been challenged in some later reports[21,22]). Subsequent investigators dealt with various motor and sensory phenomena associated with the ischemic and postischemic states and with their modifications by different types of peripheral nervous system (PNS) and central nervous (CNS) system disorders affecting the limb.[21-32] Most of these studies were devoted to clinical research and had little practical application. Nonetheless, it is pertinent to note that one of the very first articles to describe carpel tunnel syndrome (CTS) as it is known today, authored by Kremer et al. and published in *Lancet* in 1953,[33] was immediately followed by an article by Gilliatt and Wilson,[34] in which they advocated using upper extremity limb ischemia as a diagnostic test for that entity because it could provoke the patient's CTS symptoms or cause early sensory loss in a median finger distribution. Obviously that provocative test for CTS was rendered obsolete a few years later when NCS (specifically, median motor and sensory NCS) became a clinical tool. Consequently, at present, induced limb ischemia apparently plays only a minor role in clinical research and practice.

Regarding clinical research, induced limb ischemia is used to demonstrate a curious fact about patients with diabetes mellitus: Their peripheral nerves function longer under ischemic conditions than do the nerves of persons who are not diabetic. This paradoxical phenomenon was first reported in regard to vibratory perception in 1959.[35] Subsequently, various investigators have shown that under ischemic conditions, the various components (amplitudes, latencies, conduction velocities) of the sensory and motor NCS are all less affected in diabetic patients than in normals.[36-39] The ability of diabetic nerves to tolerate ischemia more than normal ones is lost when the patients are brought under rigid diabetic control. Moreover, this resistance to ischemia is not limited to diabetics because it can also be seen in patients with uremia and other disorders (see Chapter 18).

Induced limb ischemia can be used in clinical practice to diagnose myophosphorylase deficiency, myasthenia gravis, and spasmophilia.

The *forearm ischemic exercise test* has been used to diagnose myophosphorylase deficiency since the condition was first described by McArdle in 1951. Following exercise of the forearm muscles under ischemia, neither the venous lactate nor pyruvate level rises, as they do in normals; also, if a needle recording electrode is inserted into one of the exercised muscles, it can be shown that the painful contraction that occurs is actually a contracture, rather than a cramp, because it is an electrically silent event. Of note is that this electromyographic finding is not pathognomonic of myophosphorylase deficiency because it also can be seen with other metabolic blocks along the glycolytic or glycogenolytic pathways, for example, debrancher deficiency and phosphofructokinase deficiency.[40]

Harvey and Masland first described the value of repetitive stimulation studies (RSS) to diagnose myasthenia gravis. They were also the first to note that the safety factor for neuromuscular transmission could be reduced by ischemia, thereby causing RSS to be more sensitive. Subsequently, a testing procedure for myasthenia gravis, combining RSS and ischemia, was devised, although apparently it is seldom employed at present.[41]

Spasmophilia, also known as *cryptotetany* and *latent tetany*, is a disorder that has received far more attention in Europe than in North America.[42,43] It is usually described as being more prevalent in women than in men and as presenting with a number of nonspecific complaints, many psychiatric in nature, including generalized weakness, hand and feet cramping, distal paresthesias, anxiety, and depression.[42,44-46] Some investigators consider the entity synonymous with *chronic hyperventilation syndrome*, although the serum calcium levels typically are normal. Others attribute it to a chronic magnesium deficit, often marginal in degree, although in some of the well-documented cases, the serum magnesium levels have been normal as well. Spasmophilia has also been called *chronic constitutional tetany*, but the link between it and the relatively few well-reported cases of patients having normal serum calcium and magnesium levels who, on an inherited basis, experience repeated attacks of painful carpopedal spasms (and sometimes childhood convulsions as well), is unclear.[47,48]

Limb ischemia has been used to diagnose spasmophilia as well as other disorders causing tetany for almost 50 years[49]; an entire book was devoted to the use of electromyography in this regard in the late 1950s.[43] Judging by the literature, the procedure most often used in the EMG laboratory to diagnose spasmophilia is a modification of von Bonsdorff's clinical test to diagnose subclinical tetany, which combines hyperventilation with ischemia.[46,48] In our EMG laboratory, when confronted with patients having some of the symptoms described here, we employ a more simple protocol. We place a pneumatic cuff around the arm, inflate it above systolic pressure, and maintain it at that level for 3 minutes, while monitoring the first dorsal interosseus muscle with a needle recording electrode. In most patients, no spontaneous activity is seen during the observation period, or, at most, a few random fasciculations appear during the last minute. In some patients, however, spontaneous potentials develop as early to 20 to 30 seconds after cuff inflation. These have the appearance of MUPs, firing either singly or as doublets and triplets, in a rapid, repetitive fashion. Similar firing potentials are progressively recruited, so very soon the screen is filled with this activity. Nonetheless, careful visual and auditory analysis suggests that this *full interference pattern* is not identical to that seen with normal complete voluntary activity. All these repetitive potentials produced by ischemia disappear promptly (within 10 s) after cuff deflation.

The nonspecific nature of this electromyographic activity was noted by Eisinger,[50] who labeled it *spasmorhythmia*. He found it in 21% of normal men and 30% of normal women during 10 minutes of pneumatic cuff-induced ischemia and cautioned that it should not be considered indicative of spasmophilia unless the clinical presentation was appropriate.[50]

Blood Flow Interruption in Large Arteries

Although the term *peripheral arterial occlusion*[51] often is used in lieu of the more unwieldy title of this section, the latter is actually more accurate because arterial blood flow can be compromised by nonoccluding events such as penetrating injuries and shunt placements.[13] Whenever the arterial blood supply to a limb is seriously disrupted, the results can be extremely variable, depending on such factors as the site of interruption; the cause of the lesion; the abruptness and duration of the process; and the status, size, number, and location of the nutrient vessels in regard to the lesion site.[3,13,52] Because of these variables, a broad spectrum of pathologic and pathophysiologic changes can result, ranging from almost no discernible neuromuscular dysfunction to massive limb gangrene, with cases in between in which circulation is barely adequate for limb survival, and the nerves, muscles, or other soft tissues sustain substantial ischemic injury in varying combinations.[3,13] Of these many possible clinical presentations, only some have been labeled with specific names, and more than one can occur simultaneously. These ischemic nerve and muscle lesions have numerous causes, which vary with the circumstances. In wartime, penetrating arterial wounds often are the prime offenders. In civilian populations, they most often are due to emboli, to occlusive vascular disease, to penetrating wounds, and to various iatrogenic causes.[3,4,13,51,52] Some of the more well-described ischemic syndromes associated with the interruption of blood flow in major limb arteries are discussed next.

Severe distal muscle and nerve degeneration: Ischemic Paralysis

This type of abrupt-onset ischemic limb insult was first well described by Tinel,[53] based on his World War I experiences. He saw it exclusively in the upper extremity of a minority of patients who sustained proximal injury of one of the major limb arteries, resulting in its obliteration or ligation.[53] Subsequently, the same syndrome was observed in the lower extremity following injuries to the popliteal and femoral arteries.[1–3] Ischemic paralysis is probably the most severe type of ischemic damage a limb can sustain, "short of early massive gangrene."[2] Two stages are evident. In the first, the distal portion of the limb is edematous, cold, cyanotic, and painful (deep burning or freezing pain). Voluntary movements of the distal muscles are markedly impaired, and even passive movements of the fingers or toes are resisted. Sensory loss is present in a *vaguely segmental* distribution. During the second stage, which soon follows, the edema and pain disappear, but the distal soft tissues undergo *fibrous transformation.* The muscles become very firm and nonfunctional, the overlying skin smooth and shiny with a tendency to ulcerate and to heal slowly, and the fingernails and toenails talon-like. The distal portion of the limb becomes totally anesthetic, and neither active nor passive movements of the fibrotic muscles are possible.[1,2,53]

We have only rarely examined patients with this degree of ischemic limb injury, and it seems likely that the incidence of *ischemic paralysis* has decreased markedly because of treatment advances. Nonetheless, the syndrome is described at length in Sunderland's recently published book on nerve injuries, so apparently it is of more than historical interest.[1]

To our knowledge, no electromyographic examinations have been reported on patients with this type of ischemic lesion. Based on the clinical descriptions, however, most, if not all, of the distal motor disability these patients experience is due to direct muscle ischemia, with resulting muscle fibrosis; nonetheless, the fact that sensation is markedly impaired indicates that permanent nerve injury occurs as well. Consequently, electrodiagnostic studies yield the following: unelicitable motor and sensory NCS responses, recording distally, and essentially electrical silence, with markedly increased mechanical resistance to needle insertion, on NEE of the more distal muscles.

Focal infarction of (proximal) nerve trunks

Relatively few instances of this type of ischemic lesion have been reported, and many of them are dated. Almost all have involved the lower extremity, and most have been attributed to very proximal arterial compromise—either of the aorta, the iliac vessels, or both. Sometimes the neurologic symptoms developed spontaneously, following thromboembolic episodes (and radiation), but more frequently they appeared after surgical procedures, such as abdominal aortic aneurysm repair, endarterectomy, and cannulation for placement of intraaortic balloons. The neural structures reportedly infarcted have included the lumbosacral roots, the lumbosacral plexuses, the brachial plexus, and various peripheral nerves: femoral, sciatic, and especially peroneal. Even some of the authors of these reports, however, concede that precisely locating the exact site of nerve fiber injury in many of these patients was, at best, arbitrary; for example, ischemic spinal cord lesions could not be definitely excluded in some patients considered to have ischemic radiculopathies.[4,10,54–61]

The electrophysiologic data are sparse concerning lesions of this type. In many instances, electromyographic examinations either were not performed or were less than comprehensive. Thus in some reports, the results were limited to the findings on NEE of scattered muscles (which typically consisted of fibrillation potentials and MUP loss) and one or more lower extremity motor conduction velocities (which were either normal or slowed).

We have studied a few patients with lower extremity dysfunction caused by ischemic intraspinal canal lesions sustained during aortic surgical procedures. Severe axon loss was present in the affected extremities. The sural and superficial peroneal sensory SNAPs were normal because the sensory fibers were injured proximal to their dorsal ganglia (DRG). In contrast, the lower extremity CMAPs were low in amplitude or unelicitable; with predominant L-5 segment/root involvement, the peroneal motor NCS responses, recording extensor digitorum brevis and particularly tibialis anterior, were most affected, whereas with predominant S-1 involvement, the posterior tibial motor responses, recording abductor hallucis, and the M-component of the H wave test recorded from the gastrocnemius/soleus muscles, were most involved. The H waves usually were unobtainable. NEE revealed fibrillation potentials and severe MUP loss in the distribution of the involved segments/roots. In the cases we have seen, the process usually has been bilateral, although sometimes asymmetrical, suggesting spinal cord or cauda equina involvement.

Focal infarction of major nerve trunks should produce electrodiagnostic findings identical to those seen with any other type of axon loss lesion at the same location. Thus with rather severe sciatic nerve involvement, the NCS should reveal unelicitable sural and superficial peroneal sensory SNAPs, along with low-amplitude or unelicitable peroneal and posterior tibial CMAPs. In contrast to the findings with ischemic monomelic neuropathy (discussed later), the motor NCS responses recorded from leg muscles (peroneal motor, recording tibialis anterior; posterior tibial motor, recording gastrocnemius/soleus as a component of the H wave test) should be as affected as the peroneal and posterior tibial motor NCS responses, recording intrinsic foot muscles. Similarly, at least with recent-onset lesions, NEE should reveal fibrillation potentials and MUP loss that are equally prominent in all muscles distal to the lesion site.

The intraarterial injection of various drugs, usually inadvertent, can damage nerve and muscle as well as other tissues on an ischemic basis. Many of the reported cases have involved injections into various upper extremity arteries, particularly the brachial, at the elbow. Distal limb ischemia, often requiring amputation, has been the most common complication.[62–64] Judging by the clinical descriptions provided, however, some patients developed forearm compartment syndromes in addition to more distal ischemic damage; the former has resulted in median nerve injury.[63,64] A special situation was encountered in England in the late 1940s, when neonates developed unilateral buttock gangrene and a sciatic neuropathy after analeptics were mistakenly injected into their umbilical arteries (instead of veins) during resuscitation.[65–67] Also, ischemic injuries of the lumbosacral plexus have followed intragluteal drug injections, presumably because the needle tip inadvertently entered the inferior gluteal artery.[68]

To our knowledge, no detailed information is available regarding the electrodiagnostic changes seen with these subgroups of patients; some were infants, and many sustained their injuries before the modern era of electrodiagnosis.

Infarction of distal limb nerve fibers: ischemic monomelic neuropathy

This entity consists of multiple axon loss mononeuropathies that develop acutely and simultaneously in the distal portion of the limb, with a prominent distal to proximal gradient, caused by transient loss of arterial blood flow; the latter results from occlusion of the major proximal limb artery or the shunting of blood away from it. Characteristically no evidence of associated ischemic injury of soft tissues (skin, muscle) is evident.[13,69] Ischemic monomelic neuropathy (IMN) was first reported to occur in the upper extremity of uremic patients who had arteriovenous shunts placed in their arms for renal dialysis, and most reports have focused on that cause.[5,70–72] Nonetheless, lower extremity involvement occurs much more frequently.[13,51]

IMN is probably the most common type of *ischemic neuropathy* seen in the EMG laboratory. In the largest series so far reported (30 patients), men outnumbered women almost 2 to 1.[51] Although IMN affects both upper and lower extremities, there are certain differences between lesions at these two locations.

Patients with lower extremity IMN are more numerous, as noted, and are considerably older overall. This is because the majority have underlying atherosclerotic occlusive disease. The reported causes for lower extremity IMN include aortoiliac emboli, acute superficial femoral or iliofemoral artery thrombosis, and cannulation of the superficial femoral artery for intraaortic balloon pump use and for cardiopulmonary bypass. Thus lower extremity IMN may be due to both noniatrogenic and iatrogenic causes, with the former predominating.[13,51]

In contrast, upper extremity IMN occurs almost exclusively in uremic patients, after they undergo arteriovenous shunt placement in the arm or antecubital fossa region for dialysis purposes. Although specifically stated in only one of the reports, it appears likely that almost all of these patients had diabetic nephropathy as the underlying cause for their renal failure. Thus upper extremity IMN affects younger patients, on average, and is almost always iatrogenic in nature.[5,13,70–72] The only reports describing other causes for upper extremity IMN include that of Matolo et al.[70] (one patient) and Lachance and Daube[51] (eight patients); the latter lists the following causes for the upper extremity IMN; "hypercoagulable states, thoracic outlet obstruction (angiographic confirmation), laceration of the brachial artery, intraarterial injection, and cellulitis." Unfortunately, no further details are provided.

The clinical presentation of IMN is remarkably stereotyped. Persistent deep, burning pain is the most prominent symptom. It is most severe in the palm and fingers in the upper extremity and in the foot and toes in the lower extremity. Sensory and motor deficits are also found, which characteristically are prominent only in the hand and foot; a distal to proximal gradient of change is obvious, with minimal to no abnormalities being present proximal to the midforearm or midleg. Also, the changes are not limited to or distinctly more pronounced in the distribution of a single peripheral nerve; instead, they are fairly uniform circumferentially at a given level, regardless of the nerve supply.

The electrodiagnostic features of IMN have been reported in detail. In fact, the characteristic presentation of IMN was first well defined in the EMG laboratory.[13] To summarize in one sentence: IMN presents electrophysiologically as a rather severe axon loss peripheral polyneuropathy involving a single limb. Thus on NCS the amplitudes are essentially the only component affected, and a distal to proximal gradient of change can be demonstrated if multiple studies are performed. For example, with upper extremity IMN, the median and ulnar SNAPs typically are unelicitable or very low in amplitude, whereas the radial SNAPs sometimes are slightly more preserved, and the lateral antebrachial cutaneous SNAPs usually are normal. These variations reflect the fact that progressively more proximal (and therefore less affected or unaffected) nerve segments are being assessed. For the same reason, the median and ulnar CMAPs, recording from the intrinsic hand muscles, are both very low in amplitude, whereas the ulnar motor NCS, recording forearm muscles, is

usually normal or near normal, as is the radial motor NCS, recording proximal-midextensor forearm.

We have studied a few patients with very mild lower extremity IMN in whom the only findings were fibrillation potentials and MUP loss in the intrinsic foot muscles. In most instances, however, the process extends proximal enough that the sural and superficial peroneal sensory SNAPs are affected (usually being unelicitable), whereas the peroneal and posterior tibial motor CMAPs, recording intrinsic foot muscles, are generally unelicitable or low in amplitude. In contrast, the peroneal motor CMAP, recording tibialis anterior, and the posterior tibial CMAP, recording gastrocnemius/soleus, tend to be normal or only modestly reduced in amplitude. H waves usually are preserved with lower extremity IMN; relatively few, if any, of the fibers that subserve it are damaged because of their more proximal location in the limb.[13]

The distal to proximal shading of axon loss, characteristic of IMN, is most convincingly demonstrated on NEE (Figure 14.1). Fibrillation potentials and MUP loss are usually prominent in the intrinsic hand and foot muscles and equally severe in all muscles, regardless of peripheral nerve supply. They are much less prominent in the muscles immediately proximal to the wrist and ankle, whereas the proximal forearm and leg muscles usually are normal or nearly so.[13]

One of the key features of IMN is that neither clinical nor electromyographic evidence of primary muscle fiber injury is evident when the patients are studied soon after onset. If electromyographic examinations are performed during the period when the distal muscles are reinnervating, however, polyphasic MUPs can be seen on NEE, which can be mistaken for *myopathic* changes. The fact that structural damage occurs to nerve fibers, as opposed to mere temporary loss of function, before any evident ischemic muscle damage develops is at variance with almost all the results of animal research.[16]

If adequate electrodiagnostic studies are performed, IMN of relatively recent onset usually can be confidently diagnosed in the EMG laboratory. A number of confounding factors, however, can render a definite diagnosis much more difficult, if not impossible. These include advanced age, bilateral lower extremity lesions, and the presence of coexisting nerve lesions (either focal or generalized). Moreover, the electrodiagnostic studies are often indeterminate if the lesion is of prolonged duration at the time of the assessment. These confounding factors are briefly discussed here. In many persons over the age of 60, the lower extremity sensory NCS responses are une-

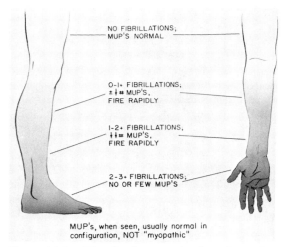

NO FIBRILLATIONS;
MUP'S NORMAL

0-1+ FIBRILLATIONS;
± ↓ # MUP'S,
FIRE RAPIDLY

1-2+ FIBRILLATIONS,
↓↓# MUP'S,
FIRE RAPIDLY

2-3+ FIBRILLATIONS;
NO OR FEW MUP'S

MUP's, when seen, usually normal in
configuration, NOT "myopathic"

Figure 14.1.   *The distal to proximal gradient of needle electrode examination abnormalities characteristically seen with ischemic monomelic neuropathy.*

licitable bilaterally (as are plantar responses and H waves). Because lower extremity IMN occurs almost exclusively in older patients, invariably some patients with suspected IMN have unelicitable sural and superficial peroneal sensory responses bilaterally. Differentiating IMN from chronic, combined L-5, S-1 radiculopathies, in which fibrillation potentials can be limited to the more distal lower extremity muscles, may be difficult in these instances. Bilateral lower extremity IMN, caused by saddle emboli, can have an electrodiagnostic presentation similar to a moderate axon loss polyneuropathy. In our limited experience with such lesions, however, the findings in the two limbs have been asymmetrical enough to suggest bilateral IMN. Also, in many patients, IMN is superimposed on a generalized polyneuropathy, either diabetic or, less often, uremic. (As previously noted, almost all the reported cases of upper extremity IMN have occurred in diabetics with uremia.) If the polyneuropathies are mild or are producing primarily demyelination rather than axon loss, a superimposed IMN is readily demonstrable. If the polyneuropathies are axon loss in type and severe in degree, however, so that the standard sensory and motor NCS response amplitudes are severely affected and fibrillation potentials are abundant in the intrinsic muscles on NEE, the definite diagnosis of a superimposed IMN becomes impossible. Nonetheless, at times IMN still may be suspected if the axon loss is disproportionately worse in one limb than in the

contralateral limb, as judged by the severity of both the SNAP and CMAP amplitude changes and by the NEE findings. As would be expected, IMN becomes more difficult to diagnose if there are coexisting nerve fiber lesions, or the residuals of such lesions, in the affected limb (e.g., CTS, ulnar neuropathy at the elbow, peroneal neuropathy, radiculopathies) because the abnormalities in the distribution of the affected nerves must be discarded when attempting to diagnose IMN. Finally, when studying lesions of long duration, lower extremity IMN can be confused with a focal axon loss sciatic neuropathy of remote onset. These are readily distinguished from one another when both are of recent onset because a distal to proximal shading of abnormalities is found with IMN, on both NCS and NEE, whereas a sharp line of demarcation between normal and abnormal is seen with the focal sciatic neuropathy. Unfortunately, as time passes, these electrodiagnostic distinctions fade. Because of progressive proximal to distal reinnervation with the latter, a shading of abnormalities ultimately can be found that is indistinguishable from that seen with more severe lower extremity IMN. Consequently, if patients with suspected lower extremity ischemic nerve lesions are studied many months after onset, it may be impossible to determine whether their abnormalities are due to IMN or to a focal sciatic nerve lesion. (Saphenous NCS theoretically should be helpful in making this distinction, because they would be affected by IMN but normal with sciatic neuropathies. Unfortunately, in almost all patients with suspected IMN, they are unelicitable bilaterally because of age or an underlying polyneuropathy.)

Electromyographers should be aware that iatrogenic, and sometimes even noniatrogenic, IMN has significant medicolegal implications. We have personal knowledge of lawsuits that have been initiated because upper extremity IMN followed arteriovenous shunt placements and lower extremity IMN followed use of an intraaortic balloon pump. This is decidedly unfair for the physicians involved because in the vast majority of cases, the IMN was both unpredictable and unavoidable. Our experience suggests that the ischemic nerve damage probably can develop within a few hours after limb blood flow is reduced, so the process may be already established before the patient even leaves the recovery room.[13]

Chronic obliterative peripheral vascular disease

Many patients, mostly elderly, have symptomatic ischemia of the lower extremity owing to chronic, progressive obliterative arteriosclerosis. The symptoms typically are restricted to skin and, with limb use, to muscle (intermittent claudication). According to some authorities, the peripheral nerves of the limb in such patients, even the distal segments, are not injured because their blood supply is not substantially compromised.[73] Nonetheless, even before the turn of the century, reports began to appear associating arteriosclerotic vascular disease and neurologic complications.[9] Since then, several clinical articles have described such neurologic involvement. Distal sensory loss has been the most common finding, but loss of deep tendon reflexes and distal limb weakness have been observed.[9,10,74] Moreover, nerves obtained from both biopsy and from amputated limbs (owing to atherosclerotic gangrene) frequently, but not invariably, have shown abnormalities of nerve fibers, primarily the myelinated ones, consisting of axon degeneration and regeneration, demyelination and remyelination, and endoneurial fibrosis.[9,73,74] Thus ischemic injury of nerve fibers appears to be more common than generally appreciated with chronic occlusive vascular disease, although often unrecognized.[73,74]

The electromyographic confirmation of this ischemic nerve damage, however, has been neither extensive nor totally conclusive, although articles were published on the subject at least as early as 1962.[75] Unfortunately, most of them have been restricted in scope (e.g., focused on the NEE findings in a single lower extremity muscle[75,76] or one lower extremity motor NCS[56,77,78]). Moreover, the majority contain no information regarding lower extremity sensory NCS, in large part because they appeared more than a quarter century ago, before sural (and later superficial peroneal sensory) NCS came into widespread use. Even the NCS data provided typically are incomplete, being limited to conduction velocities and sometimes latencies; only rarely are CMAP (or SNAP) amplitudes mentioned, although they are the only component of the NCS consistently affected by axon loss lesions. In one of the more informative studies, reported by Miglietta in 1967[79] and limited to motor NCS and H wave testing, the following results were noted: (1) In 15% to 20% of 50 patients, the peroneal or posterior tibial motor CMAPs, recording intrinsic foot muscles, could not be elicited, whereas in many of the remaining patients, they were very low in amplitude and dispersed. (2) The peroneal and posterior tibial motor conduction velocities, when obtainable, were generally in the 30 to 40 m per second range and, on average, 5 m per second slower than those found in aged-matched

asymptomatic controls. (3) The peroneal and posterior tibial distal latencies were somewhat prolonged. (4) H waves were unelicitable in 50% of the patients, and markedly prolonged in latency in the remainder. Unfortunately, NEEs were not performed. It is very likely that the 50 patients in this series had advanced chronic occlusive vascular disease, not only because all had signs of arterial insufficiency in the examined lower extremity, but also because all previously had undergone amputation of the other lower extremity owing to gangrene.[79] Nonetheless, some confounding factors were present, including the fact that limb temperatures were uncontrolled, and six of the patients with abnormal findings had diabetes mellitus. The former could have had a significant effect because, in our experience, the majority of patients with substantial ipsilateral chronic occlusive vascular disease have obvious temperature differences between their distal lower extremities, with the symptomatic side being noticeably cooler. This alone could have been responsible for at least a portion of the abnormalities described.

Hunter et al.[80] studied 32 limbs in 25 patients with severe lower extremity atherosclerotic disease, before and after operative reconstructive vascular procedures were performed. They reported the peroneal and posterior tibial CMAPs were low, especially the peroneal, and the conduction velocities were modestly slow. The sural peak latencies, however, were normal (amplitudes not mentioned). The major problem with this study is that one-fourth of the patients had diabetes mellitus, and the control group was much younger (30 to 60 years of age, whereas the study group's average age was 64 years). Consequently, at least some of the *abnormalities* seen, for example, peroneal CMAP amplitudes of less than 4 mV, could have been caused by age alone.

In contrast to the aforementioned, Chopra and Hurwitz, in a series of papers,[56,76,81] as well as Kumlin et al.[82] found lower extremity motor conduction slowing in only a distinct minority of patients, if at all. Chopra and Hurwitz noted, for example, that the conductions in their peripheral vascular group were generally within the normal range and better than in their diabetic groups, especially those diabetics with neuropathy. Their study patients, however, may have had less severe limb ischemia than those reported by Miglietta and Hunter et al.

It is pertinent to note that in those reports that detail lower extremity motor NCS abnormalities, the peroneal nerve often has been more affected, although usually just modestly so, than the posterior tibial nerve.

Whether the lower extremity NCS results change appreciably following operative vascular procedures has been considered in two reports, with conflicting results. Kumlin et al.[82] found improvement in both the peroneal and the posterior tibial motor conduction velocity in four of five patients (80%), whereas Hunter et al.[80] found no improvement in these NCS; moreover, the latter noted an increase in the sural distal latency in some patients, which they attributed to *deterioration of function.*

In regard to the NEE findings of patients with occlusive vascular disease, the data are even more sparse. This is despite the fact that this point has been specifically addressed in two papers: by Serra,[75] who studied the gastrocnemius muscle (which one, medial or lateral, not stated), and by Chopra,[76] who assessed the tibialis anterior muscle. Unfortunately, both these reports are seriously flawed, in that only a single muscle in the ischemic limb was studied, and that muscle was located in the mid, rather than the distal, portion of the extremity. Nonetheless, Serra reported finding *neurogenic* MUP changes, although the MUPs were of decreased, rather than increased, duration as well as being of increased amplitude and polyphasic. Chopra's results were somewhat puzzling, in that he found more abnormalities in the limbs of younger patients with peripheral vascular disease than in the older ones. Thus fibrillation potentials were present in almost 50% of those under the age of 50 but in only 25% of those over the age of 50. Similarly, compared with normals, the MUP durations were more prolonged, and the instance of polyphasic MUPs was much greater in the younger compared with the older patients. He found the mean MUP amplitude to be lower, rather than higher, in those with peripheral vascular disease, and, once again, the changes were more pronounced in the younger group. Similar to the NCS changes reported by Chopra and Hurwitz in another paper,[56] with relatively few exceptions the NEE findings seen in patients with peripheral vascular disease tended to be similar to those seen in normals or in diabetics without neuropathy and to be much less pronounced than in the group of diabetic patients with neuropathy.[76]

We have studied many patients referred by peripheral vascular physicians with a question of distal ischemic nerve damage caused by chronic occlusive vascular disease. Although lower extremity abnormalities almost always have been present, their relationship to ischemia generally has been unclear because of the presence of a host of confounding factors. Almost all the patients have been elderly,

most have been diabetic, many have had lumbar canal stenosis (frequently with prior lumbar laminectomies), and some have had multiple prior surgical procedures performed on the limb, particularly those of a vascular and orthopedic nature. Consequently, these processes in various combinations could have been responsible for the typical abnormalities seen, without the necessity of invoking an additional component attributable to ischemia. These findings usually included the following bilaterally: on NCS, unelicitable sural and superficial peroneal SNAPs; low-amplitude or unelicitable peroneal and posterior tibial motor CMAPs, recording intrinsic foot muscles, with borderline to mildly slowed conduction velocities; and unelicitable H waves; on NEE, fibrillation potentials and MUP loss in the more distal muscles.

In the majority of patients having strictly unilateral symptoms, the differences in temperature between the two lower extremities usually could explain many of the relatively slight differences found between them on electrodiagnostic studies.

Such limb cooling can be a vexing problem when studying patients under these circumstances. Not only can it cause slowing of nerve impulse transmission, thereby producing slowed conduction velocities and prolonged distal latencies, but also it can cause an increase in the NCS amplitudes (motor and sensory) along with, on NEE, a decrease or disappearance of fibrillation potentials and an increase in the duration of the MUPs. Thus rather paradoxically, cooling can simultaneously both simulate and conceal evidence of peripheral nerve dysfunction. Because the limbs in these patients have such precarious blood supplies, most electromyographers consider attempts to warm them unwise. Consequently, the only recourse available is the use of various *correction factors* for the NCS results, with their inherent limitations.

Occlusion of Median and Small-Sized Arteries

In clinical practice, compromise of median and small arteries is an important cause of ischemic neuropathy. Included among arteries of these sizes are those with diameters of 50 to 300 μm, "the precise spectrum of the vasa nervorum."[83] Formerly, discussion of PNS lesions caused by occlusion of such vessels was almost limited to a characteristic presentation and a few causes: mononeuropathy multiplex caused by diabetes mellitus, polyarteritis nodosa, or a collagen vascular disease.[83,84] A considerable amount of clinical investigation over the past two decades, however, has revealed that the situation is far more complex and variable than previously thought.[85] The relationship between vasculitis and mononeuropathy multiplex, formerly considered to be almost one to one, is now known to be much more inconstant: Vasculitis has several other PNS presentations, and mononeuropathy multiplex has a number of other causes.[85–87] Moreover, vasculitis is not a prerequisite for sudden symptomatic restriction of blood flow in the vasa nervorum. One report, for example, described a young woman with sickle cell anemia who developed a median neuropathy in the midarm region that consisted almost solely of a persistent (greater than 3 weeks) conduction block. Presumably the mechanism of injury in that patient was sludging of the red blood cells in a critical nutrient vessel.[88]

Necrotizing angiopathy (necrotizing vasculitis) is a pathologic process wherein inflammation and necrosis affect blood vessel walls, producing partial or complete occlusion, often with resulting ischemia of the structure(s) supplied by the damaged vessels.[84] When nerves are the target organ, a characteristic finding frequently is seen on nerve biopsy: a pattern of patchy asymmetrical nerve fiber loss between and within individual fascicles.[86]

The pathogenesis of the vasculitides is unclear, but an autoimmune mechanism is considered to be the major factor, with many of the disorders grouped under this designation. No detailed classification of these various entities has been generally accepted; their clinical presentations not only are remarkably diverse, but also there is considerable overlap among them. Nonetheless, a broad division into *primary* or *secondary* vasculitis is widely used, depending on whether vasculitis is the major, if not the sole, manifestation of the disorder, for example, polyarteritis nodosa, or whether it is a complication, sometimes a relatively minor one, of another disorder, for example, rheumatoid arthritis.[83,84,89]

When the complete spectrum of vasculitis is considered, virtually any type or size of blood vessel is at risk. Small to medium sized muscular arteries, however, probably are the most often injured when PNS involvement occurs.[84,86] Among the various vasculitic syndromes in which PNS involvement is relatively common are the polyarteritis nodosa group, some of the hypersensitivity vasculitis group (particularly those in the collagen vascular subgroup), and Wegener's granulomatosis.[84,86]

Until rather recently, vasculitic involvement of the PNS was considered to be just one component of a systemic disorder. The concept of *nonsystemic* or *isolated* PNS vasculitis has been raised, however, as

studies have shown that an appreciable number of patients with PNS lesions secondary to necrotizing angiopathy do not show evidence of compromise of other organ systems, either at the time of diagnosis or even after years of subsequent observation.[83,85,90] Nonetheless, the fact that in one series evidence of vasculitis was found in muscle biopsy specimens in more than 80% of 32 patients who appeared to have clinically isolated PNS vasculitis suggests that the vasculitis was not organ specific in these cases, as the clinical picture implied, but rather mild in degree. Consequently, the relatively small number of lesions in other organs remained asymptomatic, whereas those in the PNS were manifested.[91]

Probably the majority of patients with vasculitis are women and are over the age of 50. Otherwise, the clinical features seen with ischemic PNS injury caused by compromise of medium and small-size arteries defy simple characterization; they are extremely variable, depending on the underlying cause. When only PNS symptoms are considered, motor, sensory, or motor and sensory deficits in the distribution of the involved nerves are common. These typically are of abrupt onset and often accompanied by burning pain.[86]

The electrodiagnostic features of such lesions are much more stereotyped. Almost invariably the pathophysiology is one of axon loss. Consequently, depending on the nerve fiber(s) affected, the severity of the lesion, and its duration, the following changes can be seen: On NCS, the SNAPs and CMAPs (particularly the former) are low in amplitude or unelicitable, whereas the latencies and conduction velocities are in the normal or near normal range; the H wave is low in amplitude or, more often, unelicitable; F waves are difficult to obtain but usually of normal latency. On NEE, fibrillation potentials and loss of MUPs (decreased number of MUPs, firing at a rapid rate) are prominent, along with at times *reinnervational* or chronic neurogenic MUP changes.

Transient conduction blocks not caused by focal demyelination are seen if patients are studied within the first week or so of lesion onset. This is not a rare scenario because a substantial number of patients with these lesions are hospitalized as soon as they become symptomatic, or they are already in the hospital because of an underlying disorder. Consequently, they are referred to the EMG laboratory early in their illness. These conduction blocks are present, despite the focal ischemic nerve lesion being one of axon loss, because the distal stump remains capable of conducting impulses for several days after lesion onset (6 days for motor fibers, 9 to 10 days for sensory fibers), even though the fibers that compose it are in the process of degenerating. This type of *axon noncontinuity conduction block* is seen with any type of focal axon loss nerve lesion, if NCS are performed so early after nerve fiber injury. When NCS are repeated 11 or more days after onset, the responses on stimulation distal to the lesion are identical in amplitude to those seen on stimulation proximal to the lesion, being either uniformly low or unelicitable. Thus the conduction block has converted to conduction failure (see Chapter 7).

Prolonged conduction block, suggesting the presence of either some focal metabolic disturbance or of demyelination at the lesion site, has been seen experimentally, but almost no convincing instances in humans have been published.[90,92,93] In one study, for example, that reputedly demonstrated such conduction blocks, the amplitudes of the distal motor responses were very low to begin with (four of five being less than 0.5 mV), and the amplitude changes on proximal stimulations were minuscule (four of five being 0.2 mV or less).[93]

Ischemic neuropathy attributable to small and medium-sized artery compromise has a number of clinical and electrophysiologic presentations, including mononeuropathy, mononeuropathy multiplex, asymmetrical and symmetrical sensorimotor polyneuropathy, and pure sensory polyneuropathy.

Mononeuropathy

Single nerve lesions are one of the PNS presentations of vasculitis, comprising 5% to approximately 20% in various series.[91,94,95] Often they are merely the first of what will ultimately be several such lesions, but at times they persist as the only PNS abnormality for prolonged periods of time. Almost any component of the PNS can be affected, including the roots,[97] the plexuses,[94,96] and various peripheral nerves.[83,91,94,95]

Of the peripheral nerves, the common peroneal is the most likely one to be damaged, in isolation, by vasculitis; for example, in the study of Said et al.,[91] 11 of the 13 patients with ischemic mononeuropathies had peroneal nerve involvement. Other nerves commonly involved are the median and ulnar. These mononeuropathies are almost always axon loss in type. They can be extremely variable in degree, ranging from complete and producing a fixed, severe deficit in the distribution of the nerve to so mild that they are asymptomatic and can be detected only (when a motor nerve) by the presence of a modest number of fibrillation potentials in the appropriate muscles. When abnormalities are restricted to all or a portion of the territory of a single cutaneous nerve, some investigators have chosen to define the lesion as a *cutaneous sensory neuropathy* rather than a mononeuropathy.[96] Although an abrupt onset is considered characteristic, some patients experience a more subacute presentation, extending over several hours to several days.

The responsible lesions along nerve trunks tend to be located at other than the usual compressive/entrapment sites. Nonetheless, it is not uncommon for these ischemic mononeuropathies to be mistaken for compression or entrapment nerve lesions, particularly when the median, ulnar, and peroneal nerves are involved, and for the patient to undergo needless decompressive surgical procedures. This confusion can be prevented, at least with median nerve lesions, if an adequate electrodiagnostic examination is performed. Changes in amplitude, rather than latency, dominate the median motor and sensory NCS, whereas on NEE, fibrillation potentials are found in the median-innervated forearm muscles as well as the median-innervated thenar muscles (because typically median nerve ischemic lesions occur in the midarm). The distinction becomes more difficult with ulnar and, particularly, peroneal mononeuropathies, based on the electromyographic findings alone. Many compressive/entrapment ulnar neuropathies at the elbow present as pure axon loss lesions. Consequently, the ulnar motor and sensory NCS results with them can be identical to those seen with an ischemic nerve lesion located in the midarm: low amplitude or unelicitable ulnar SNAPs and CMAPs with fibrillation potentials and MUP dropout in the ulnar-innervated hand muscles. NEE of the forearm ulnar-innervated muscles (flexor carpi ulnaris; flexor digitorum profundus, medial aspect) may be helpful in this differentiation. If abundant fibrillation potentials are found in them, we consider the lesion is more likely proximal to the elbow segment rather than along it; only rarely in our experience is severe denervation seen in those muscles with axon loss ulnar neuropathies at the elbow, even when the ulnar-innervated hand muscles have been totally denervated. In regard to peroneal mononeuropathies, the distinction between lesion types (ischemic versus compression) generally cannot be made by electrodiagnostic studies. This is because many compressive/traction peroneal mononeuropathies at the fibular head present with pure axon loss, just as virtually all focal ischemic peroneal mononeuropathies do. In our experience, the latter almost always affect the peroneal nerve fibers distal to where the motor branch arises to supply the short head of the biceps femoris, that is, in the middistal thigh. Consequently, their electrodiagnostic presentation is that of a common peroneal mononeuropathy, axon loss in type, located at some point between the fibular head and the midthigh. Unfortunately, this is exactly the same electrodiagnostic presentation of axon loss peroneal neuropathies at the fibular head caused by compression or traction.[97]

Mononeuropathy multiplex

The syndrome of mononeuropathy multiplex (MNM) is defined as the involvement of two or more peripheral nerves, usually sequential and in different limbs.[99] (For unclear reasons, many reports define MNM as "involvement of one or more nerves . . ." This obviously is incorrect; if only one nerve is affected, the problem is a mononeuropathy, not MNM.)

For many years, as noted, MNM was considered to be almost the sole PNS presentation of vasculitis. Almost all investigators now view MNM as merely one of several presentations, and some believe it occurs less frequently than others.[83,85,91,94,98–102] In part this is because of changes in definitions. Many physicians now subdivide MNM into nonconfluent (*true*) MNM, in which compromise of several individual peripheral nerves is obvious, and confluent (*overlapping, extensive*) MNM, in which so many nerves in one or more limbs are affected simultaneously that individual nerve involvement is obscured, both on clinical and on electrodiagnostic examination. There is general agreement that the confluent type of MNM is much more common than the nonconfluent type.[83,94,96] Moreover, when the confluent type of MNM involves homologous limbs, particularly both lower extremities, some designate the pattern that results as *asymmetrical* polyneuropathy.[98,102] This semantic shift decreases the incidence of the MNM presentation, while increasing the incidence of the *polyneuropathy* presentation.

As with vasculitic mononeuropathies, the lesions with MNM are axon loss in type, and the nerves most often affected are the peroneal, ulnar, and median. Involvement of homologous nerves in corresponding limbs (e.g., both peroneal nerves) is common.[95] In these situations, the two nerves often, but not always, are affected asymmetrically. Near-simultaneous involvement of multiple bilateral distal lower extremity nerves (peroneal, tibial, sural) is readily confused with an axon loss polyneuropathy. Also, ischemic MNM can be mistaken for multiple

compression/entrapment neuropathies and lead to unnecessary decompressive surgery. In our experience, this is particularly likely to occur when ischemic neuropathies of median and ulnar nerves coexist in the same limb.

Whenever MNM is present or suspected, extensive electrodiagnostic studies are required. Not only must homologous nerves be assessed, but frequently nonroutine NCS (e.g., radial motor NCS) must be performed. Overall, MNM assessments probably are the most time-consuming studies done in the EMG laboratory, excluding those often required on elderly diabetic patients.

It is pertinent to note that axon loss MNM can be seen with several disorders besides those customarily classified as vasculitides, including diabetes mellitus, leprosy, herpes zoster, acquired immunodeficiency syndrome, carcinomas, and trichinosis.[85,87,90] Also, although not pertinent to this discussion because its predominant pathophysiology is that of demyelinating conduction block, the disorder of inherited tendency to compressive palsies classically presents as MNM.

Polyneuropathy

Only relatively recently have investigators appreciated that vasculitis can present as a polyneuropathy.[83,100] Some now consider it the most common single presentation.[100,102] Harati and Niakan,[100] for example, reported that almost 80% of their 33 patients had a symmetrical polyneuropathy. It is important to note that the polyneuropathy pattern often is subdivided into symmetrical and asymmetrical types, and many physicians would consider at least some of the latter as instances of confluent MNM.

Most vasculitic polyneuropathies are sensorimotor in nature, although we and others have encountered a rare *pure* sensory polyneuropathy case.[90]

The electrodiagnostic assessment of vasculitic polyneuropathy often must be more extensive (and more time-consuming) than that of other polyneuropathies because both lower extremities must be studied to determine if the process is symmetrical or asymmetrical. Also, many patients with symmetrical lower extremity involvement have one or more upper extremity mononeuropathies superimposed.[99]

Cauda equina

We have encountered a pattern suggestive of a cauda equina lesion in a few patients with vasculitis. The peroneal and posterior tibial CMAPs, recording intrinsic foot muscles, are low in amplitude, and fibrillation potentials and MUP loss are seen in the more distal lower extremity muscles bilaterally; yet, the sural SNAPs are normal.[99] Characteristically NEE of the proximal L-5, S-1-innervated muscles is unrevealing, as is NCS and NEE of one upper extremity. Whether this pattern reflects actual bilateral ischemic lesions of the L-5 and S-1 roots or whether it merely results from bilateral distal involvement of the peroneal and tibial nerves with sural nerve sparing often is unclear. If the symptoms are of relatively recent onset and the degree of axon loss in the distal lower extremities is severe, the fact that the hamstrings, glutei, and low lumbar and high sacral paraspinal muscles are normal on NEE speaks against a lumbar intraspinal canal lesion. This presentation, however, typically is encountered in patients with quite chronic lesions, sometimes those having only moderate to modestly severe axon loss in the distal lower extremities, and in such instances the lack of NEE changes in L-5, S-1-innervated muscles situated proximal to the knees is not conclusive. Often with chronic cauda equina lesions, the NEE findings are limited to the more distal limb muscles because the more proximal muscles have been reinnervated (if they were ever denervated), via collateral sprouting (see Chapter 7). In any case, this electromyographic presentation can prove quite misleading to the clinician if vasculitis is not yet suspected; that is, there are no abnormalities elsewhere, such as in the upper extremities, to suggest a diffuse disorder.[99] Performing more extensive electrodiagnostic studies may prevent such electromyographic localization errors, particularly studying the superficial peroneal sensory nerves as well as the sural nerves bilaterally. The motor NCS and the NEE, even when performed bilaterally, are much less likely to be of benefit in these situations because asymmetrical findings on the motor side (peroneal and tibial motor NCS amplitude changes, recording intrinsic foot muscles; NEE abnormalities in the more distal lower extremity muscles) are typically found with compressive cauda equina lesions.

Electrodiagnostic studies are indicated with all types of vasculitic neuropathy. They can reveal involvement of clinically unsuspected nerves as well as demonstrate that what was clinically considered a generalized polyneuropathy is actually multifocal neuropathy.[87] Also, they permit some quantification of the degree of axon loss, based on the SNAP and CMAP amplitudes. These results can serve as baselines for future assessments. Finally, they can prove helpful in diagnosis not only by revealing patterns suggestive of a vasculitic process, but also by assisting in the selection of nerves for biopsy. Two studies have shown that if a normal SNAP is obtained on sural NCS, biopsy of that nerve is unlikely to be revealing. Conversely, if the sural SNAP is unelicitable in the presence of a vasculitic process, biopsy of it probably will be of diagnostic benefit.[98,102] Overall, on NCS, the sensory responses are more affected than the motor, and nerves of the lower extremities are involved more often than those of the upper extremity. Also, the electrodiagnostic studies generally must be quite extensive, usually encompassing three limbs (and the appropriate paraspinal muscles on NEE) at least.

Capillary/Venule Compromise: Compartment Syndromes

The initial description of one of the subtypes of compartment syndrome was published as a case report in 1869. In 1881, Volkmann's classic article on the subject, "Ischemic Muscle Paralysis and Contractures," appeared. In 1914, J. B. Murphy recommended treating some of the subgroups of compartment syndromes with fasciotomy. Volt, in 1943, described the most classic lower extremity compartment syndrome, the anterior tibial compartment syndrome, caused by intensive exercise. Nonetheless, it was not until the 1970s, a full century after the first report appeared, that the current, modern concepts of compartment syndromes were formulated, and it was appreciated that a great number of diverse clinical entities were actually different clinical manifestations of the same pathophysiology.[6,103]

Compartment syndromes are entities of very varied cause in which an increase in tissue pressure within a limited space compromises the microcirculation, and thus the function, of the neuromuscular structures within that space. If the pressure is significantly elevated and unrelieved, the muscles and nerves within the compartment degenerate. Established compartment syndromes have four necessary components:

1. A limiting envelope, which may be fascia alone; various combinations of bone, muscle and fascia; epimysium; skin; or external structures such as circumferential casts and bandages.

2. Elevated tissue pressure, which usually is due to an increase in the compartment's contents, caused by fluid accumulation secondary to bleeding, increased capillary permeability, increased capillary pressure, or infiltrated infusions.

3. Reduced perfusion of neuromuscular structures

within the compartment, owing to reduced tissue circulation rather than to a direct mechanical effect of increased pressure (this is usually attributed to either microvascular occlusion, e.g., capillary closure, or to a decrease in the arteriovenous gradient).

4. Neuromuscular abnormalities, owing to the progressive ischemia.

Initially the ability of the nerves and muscles to function is lost, but their structural integrity is maintained. (For nerves, this loss of function would be designated a neurapraxia.) If the elevated tissue pressure is not reduced within a few hours, however, the nerves and muscles within the compartment degenerate. For nerves, the ischemic event typically produces severe injury both to the axons and to their supporting structures throughout the compartment; the results often are irreversible because spontaneous recovery cannot occur, and the lesions are too extensive to be amenable to surgical repair. For muscles, ischemic necrosis occurs, resulting in extensive fibrosis.[7,8,103,104]

The human body has many compartments. A few years ago, it was reported that there were 46 of these when homologous ones are considered separately, 38 being in the upper and lower extremities.[104,105] Since then, at least one other compartment has been described: the medial brachial fascial compartment, in which the infraclavicular brachial plexus can be compromised following injuries to the axillary artery.[106] Many of these compartments have relatively little significance, either because of their location or the structures they contain or because they are seldom the site of a compartment syndrome. Certain compartments, however, such as the ventral and dorsal forearm compartments in the upper extremity and the gluteal, iliacus, psoas, and especially the anterior leg compartment in the lower extremity, are of particular significance because they are traversed by main nerve trunks or they contain major muscle groups or both, and they have a much greater tendency than other compartments to be the locus of compartment syndromes.

The causes of compartment syndromes are numerous and incredibly varied. In general, they can be divided into those that restrict compartment volume—for example, circumferential dressings and casts, the closure of fascial defects, and thermal injuries with eschar formation—and those that increase compartment contents. The causes for the latter are far more numerous. They include (1) primarily edema accumulation related to postischemic swelling, which can result from arterial in-

juries, prolonged tourniquet operative time, and arterial spasm; from prolonged immobilization with limb compression, such as follows drug overdoses and general anesthesia; from exertion; and from venous diseases, and (2) primarily blood accumulation, which can result from anticoagulation therapy, bleeding disorders, infiltrated transfusions, and vessel lacerations.[7,8] Both edema and blood accumulation can follow fractures and soft tissue injuries.[7,8]

The symptoms and signs of a compartment syndrome include the following: (1) pain, localized to the involved compartment—it is generally deep, unrelenting, and out of proportion to what would be anticipated from the clinical situation; (2) a palpably tense, swollen compartment; (3) hypesthesia, which develops distal to the compartment in the distribution of the nerves traversing it as they become progressively more ischemic; (4) paresis, progressing to paralysis, of the muscles within the compartment or of muscles innnervated by nerves that traverse the compartment (muscle weakness is a late sign with compartment syndromes and generally indicates a need for emergency decompression of the compartment); (5) *normal* distal pulses in the involved limb, even though the major limb arteries may also traverse the compartment, because the elevated compartment pressure never exceeds mean arterial pressure.[104,107]

The most important ancillary study for diagnosing compartment syndromes is the direct measurement of tissue pressure, using the wick or slit catheter. Tissue pressure generally is less than 8 mm Hg. When readings of more than 30 mm Hg are found, a compartment syndrome is likely.[103,108]

Treatment of compartment syndromes consists of opening external envelopes (e.g., removing tight bandages and casts); maintaining local arterial pressure (e.g., prompt treatment of systemic hypotension and avoiding limb elevation); and, when significant neuromuscular deficits are developing, opening internal envelopes by surgically decompressing the involved compartments, generally by means of fasciotomies. The result of failing promptly to surgically decompress a compartment can be severe, resulting in permanent neuromuscular disability. Additional complications are encountered if extensive muscle necrosis occurs. These may be life-threatening and include infection (dead muscle is an excellent culture medium), renal failure from myoglobinuria, and hyperkalemia.[7,103,104] The major exceptions regarding surgical decompression are the iliacus and psoas compartment syndromes, in which dysfunction of the femoral nerve and lumbar plexus results from bleeding into the iliacus or psoas muscles respectively. Experience has shown that these compartments are difficult to decompress, and the ultimate clinical results following conservative treatment have been reported to be as satisfactory as those following surgical decompression.[109]

The value of electrodiagnostic studies with compartment syndromes varies, depending on the particular compartment syndrome present and the timing of the examination. In general, they are of limited usefulness in diagnosing an incipient compartment syndrome simply because, similar to most other laboratory diagnostic studies, they are relatively time-consuming, and with compartment syndromes, as with almost no other PNS lesion, time is of the essence. The so-called golden period—the time that can elapse between onset of symptoms and surgical decompression before irreversible changes supervene—was once thought to be 6 to 8 hours; more recently, it has been reduced to 4 hours.[103,110] Consequently, if any electrodiagnostic studies are to be done, they must be limited in scope and rapidly performed. It has been shown experimentally that the initial weakness is due to conduction block along the large myelinated fibers, which are selectively affected.[110] In some situations, specifically those in which muscle weakness could be due to either a developing compartment syndrome or a lesion along a nerve trunk, a single motor NCS may establish the correct diagnosis. For example, if the tibialis anterior muscle is very weak, recording from it while stimulating the common peroneal nerve distal to the fibular head may establish the diagnosis. If a CMAP of normal amplitude results, a conduction block lesion must be present along the nerve proximal to the stimulation point because both distal nerve and muscle are functioning normally. Conversely, if the response is unelicitable, an anterior compartment syndrome is very likely to be present; not enough time has elapsed since onset of symptoms for the CMAP amplitude to be unelicitable because of an axon loss lesion affecting the peroneal nerve, and conduction block lesions located along the peroneal nerve distal to the fibular head stimulation point but prior to where it enters the anterior compartment are virtually unknown. Thus by elimination, an unelicitable CMAP suggests compromise of the deep peroneal nerve fibers supplying the tibialis anterior muscle, or the tibialis anterior muscle itself, within the anterior compartment syndrome of the leg.

More often, electrodiagnostic studies are employed some time after a compartment syndrome is established, both to determine the full extent of the lesion and, if possible, to confirm its nature. Thus following a severe anterior compartment syndrome, the fact that both the tibialis anterior and extensor digitorum brevis muscles are paralyzed but the tibialis anterior muscle is degenerated, whereas the extensor digitorum brevis muscle is denervated,[111] can readily be demonstrated by NEE: Although neither will possess MUPs under voluntary control, the tibialis anterior muscle will be electrically silent, while the extensor digitorum brevis will be teeming with fibrillation potentials. At times, a clinically unsuspected compartment syndrome can be detected in the EMG laboratory. For example, we studied a young girl who had sustained a sciatic neuropathy during a knee operation, performed under a bloodless field (pneumatic cuff about midthigh). Electrodiagnostic examination performed a few weeks after the surgery showed the following in the affected limb: unelicitable sural and superficial peroneal sensory SNAPs; unelicitable posterior tibial and peroneal CMAPs, recording from both the intrinsic foot and the leg muscles; and abundant fibrillation potentials and MUP loss in all the muscles examined distal to the knee except for the tibialis anterior, which was electrically silent (i.e., no insertional activity and no fibrillation potentials as well as no voluntary MUPs). The electrodiagnostic changes thus suggested that not only had a sciatic neuropathy occurred, but also a simultaneous ischemic insult of the tibialis anterior muscle, causing the muscle fibers of the latter to degenerate. The observation provided to the clinician at that time, that function probably would be recovered in the limb except for the tibialis anterior muscle, which was irreversibly injured, was subsequently confirmed by both clinical and electrodiagnostic studies.

CONCLUSION

Under ischemic conditions, nerve function and then nerve structure are compromised. Ischemic neuropathies can result from interruption of blood flow in vessels of any size, ranging from the aorta to capillaries. With rare exceptions, an ischemic neuropathy is an axon loss lesion. In many situations, nerve ischemia coexists with muscle ischemia. Electrodiagnostic studies can be of considerable benefit in assessing patients with definite, or suspected, ischemic neuropathies.

REFERENCES

1. Sunderland S. Nerve injuries and their repair. Edinburgh: Churchill Livingstone, 1991.
2. Richards RL. Neurovascular lesions. In: Seddon HJ, ed. Peripheral nerve injuries. (MRC Special Report 282). London: Her Majesty's Stationary Office, 1954:186–238.
3. Richards RL. Ischemic lesions of peripheral nerves: A review. J Neurol Neurosurg Psychiatry 1951; 14:76–87.
4. Turley JE, Johnston KW. Ischemic neuropathy. Semin Vas Surg 1991; 4:12–19.
5. Bolton CF, Driedger AA, Lyndsay RM. Ischemic neuropathy in uremic patients caused by bovine arteriovenous shunt. J Neurol Neurosurg Psychiatry 1979; 42:810–814.
6. Garfin SR. Historical review. In: Mubarak SJ, Hargens AR, eds. Compartment syndromes and Volkmann's contracture. Philadelphia: WB Saunders, 1981:17–46.
7. Matsen FA. Compartmental syndromes. New York: Grune & Stratton, 1980.
8. Mubarak SJ. Etiologies of compartment syndromes. In: Mubarak SJ, Hargens AR, eds. Compartment syndromes and Volkmann's contracture. Philadelphia: WB Saunders, 1981:71–97.
9. Daube JR, Dyck PJ. Neuropathy due to peripheral vascular diseases. In: Dyck PJ, Thomas PK, Lambert EH, et al, eds. Peripheral neurology ed 2. Philadelphia: WB Saunders, 1984:1458–1478.
10. Johnson KW. Nonvascular complications of vascular surgery. In: Rutherford RB, ed. Vascular surgery. Vol 1. Philadelphia: WB Saunders, 1989:536–541.
11. Low PA, Tuck RR. Effects of changes of blood pressure, respiratory acidosis, and hypoxia on blood flow in the sciatic nerve of the rat. J Physiol 1984: 347:513–524.
12. Ritchie JM. The oxygen consumption of mammalian non-myelinated nerve fibres at rest and during activity. J Physiol 1967; 188:309–329.
13. Wilbourn AJ, Furlan AJ, Hulley W, Ruschaupt W. Ischemic monomelic neuropathy. Neurology 1983; 33:447–451.
14. Chervu A, Moore WA, Homsher E, et al. Differential recovery of skeletal muscle and peripheral nerve function after ischemia and reperfusion. J Surg Res 1989; 47:12–19.
15. Lewis T. Vascular disorders of the limbs. New York: Macmillan, 1936.
16. Korthals JK, Maki T, Gieron MA. Nerve and muscle vulnerability to ischemia. J Neurolog Sci 1985; 71:283–290.
17. Allbrook DB, Aitken JT. Reinnervation of striated muscle after acute ischemia. J Anat 1951; 85:376–389.
18. Sanderson RA, Foley RK, Malvor GWD, et al. His-tological response of skeletal muscle to ischemia. Clin Ortho Rel Res 1975; 113:27–35.
19. Dyck PJ. Hypoxic neuropathy: Does hypoxia play a role in diabetic neuropathy? Neurology 1989; 39:111–118.
20. Lewis T, Pickering GW, Rothschild P. Centripedal paralysis arising out of arrested blood flow to the limb, including notes on a form of tingling. Heart 1931; 16:1–32.
21. Merrington WR, Nathan PW. A study of post-ischemic paraesthesiae. J Neurol Neurosurg Psychiatry 1949; 12:1–18.
22. Weddell G, Sinclair DC. "Pins and needles": Observations on some of the sensations aroused in a limb by the application of pressure. J Neurol Neurosurg Psychiatry 1947; 10:26–46.
23. Bazett HC, McGlone B. Chemical factor in causation of tingling sensations during and after release of stasis. Proc Soc Exp Biol 1931; 29:87–88.
24. Cobb W, Marshall S. Repetitive discharges from human motor nerves after ischemia and their absence after cooling. J Neurol Neurosurg Psychiatry 1954; 17:183–188.
25. Gilliatt RW. Ischemic sensory loss in patients with spinal and cerebral lesions. J Neurol Neurosurg Psychiatry 1955; 18:145–154.
26. Gilliatt RW, Wilson TG. Ischemic sensory loss in patients with peripheral nerve lesions. J Neurol Neurosurg Psychiatry 1954; 17:104–114.
27. Kibler RF, Nathan PW. Relief of pain and paraesthesiae by nerve block distal to a lesion. J Neurol Neurosurg Psychiatry 1960; 23:91–98.
28. Kugelberg E. Activation of human nerves by ischemia. Trousseau's phenomenon in tetany. Arch Neurol Psych 1948; 60:140–152.
29. Nathan PW. Ischemic and post-ischemic numbness and paresthesia. J Neurol Neurosurg Psychiatry 1958; 21:12–23.
30. Poole EW. Ischemic and post-ischemic paraesthesiae. J Neurol Neurosurg Psychiatry 1956; 19:148–154.
31. Reid C. Experimental ischemia; sensory phenomena, fibrillary twitches, and effects on pulse, respiration and blood pressure. Quart J Exp Physiol 1931; 21:243–251.
32. Zotterman Y. Studies in peripheral nerve mechanisms of pain. Acta Med Scand 1933; 80:185–242.
33. Kremer M, Gilliatt RW, Golding JS, et al. Acroparesthesia in the carpal tunnel syndrome. Lancet 1953; 2:590–595.
34. Gilliatt RW, Wilson TG. A pneumatic test in the carpal tunnel syndrome. Lancet 1953; 2:595–597.
35. Steiness I. Vibratory perception in diabetics during arrested blood flow to the limb. Acta Med Scand 1959; 163:195–205.
36. Castaigne P, Cathala HP, Dry J, et al. Les responses des nerfs et des muscles á 'des stimulations, electriques an cours d'une epreuve de garrot ischemique

chez l'homme normal et chez le diabolique. Rev Neurol 1966; 115:61–66.

37. Gregersen G. A study of the peripheral nerves in diabetic subjects during ischemia. J Neurol Neurosurg Psychiatry 1968; 31:175–181.

38. Senenviratne KN, Peiris OA. The effect of ischemia on the excitability of sensory nerves in diabetes mellitus. J Neurol Neurosurg Psychiatry 1968; 31:348–353.

39. Seneviratne KN, Peiris OA. The effect of ischemia on the excitability of human sensory nerve. J Neurol Neurosurg Psychiatry 1968; 31:338–347.

40. Dimauro S, Bresolin N. Phosphorylase deficiency. In: Engel AG, Banker BQ, eds. Myology. New York: McGraw-Hill, 1986:1585–1601.

41. Brown WF. The physiological and technical basis of electromyography. Boston: Butterworth Publishers, 1984.

42. Durlach J. Neurological manifestations of magnesium imbalance. In: Viken PJ, Bruyn GW, eds. Handbook of clinical neurology. Vol 28. Metabolic and deficiency diseases of the nervous system, Part II. Amsterdam: North-Holland, 1976:545–579.

43. Rosselle N. Électromyographic in nervous disease and in cryptotetany. [English edition] Louvain, Belgium: Éditions E. Nouwelaerts 1959.

44. de Romanis F, Feliciani H, Rosati HV, et al. Spasmophilia: A clinical, neurophysiopathological and biochemical study. Funct Neurol 1987; 2:239–246.

45. Feldman RG, Granger CV. Electromyography in latent tetany. N Engl J Med 1963; 269:1064–1067.

46. Seelig MS, Berger AR, Spielholz N. Latent tetany and anxiety, marginal magnesium deficit and normocalcemia. Dis Nerv Syst 1975; 36:461–465.

47. Day JW, Parry GJ. Normocalcemic tetany abolished by calcium infusion. Ann Neurol 1990; 27:438–440.

48. Isgreen WP. Normocalcemic tetany. Neurology 1976; 26:825–834.

49. Turpin R, Lefebvre J, Lerique J. Les modifications de l'électromyogramme élémentaire et les troubles de la transmission neuromusculaire dans la tétanie. Compt Rend Acad d Sci 1943; 216:579.

50. Eisinger J. Repetitive electromyographic activity, spasmorhythmia and spasmophilia. Magnesium 1987; 6:65–73.

51. Lachance DH, Daube JR. Acute peripheral arterial occlusion: Electrophysiologic study of 32 cases. Muscle Nerve 1991; 14:633–639.

52. Schmidt FE, Hewitt RL. Severe upper limb ischemia. Arch Surg 1980; 115:1188–1191.

53. Tinel J. Nerve wounds. New York: William Wood & Company, 1917.

54. Archie JP. Femoral neuropathy due to common iliac artery occlusion. South Med J 1983; 76:1073.

55. Benjamin HZ, Nagler W. Peripheral nerve damage resulting from local hemorrhage and ischemia. Arch Phys Med Rehabil 1973; 54:263–270.

56. Chopra JS, Hurwitz LJ. Femoral nerve conduction in diabetes and chronic occlusive vascular disease. J Neurol Neurosurg Psychiatry 1968; 31:28–33.

57. D'Amour ML, Lebrun LH, Rabbat A, et al. Peripheral neurological complications of aortoiliac vascular disease. Can J Neurol Sci 1987; 14:127–135.

58. Gerard JM, Frank N, Moussa Z, et al. Acute ischemic brachial plexus neuropathy following radiation therapy. Neurology 1989; 39:450–454.

59. Gilliatt RW. Physical injury to peripheral nerves: Physiologic and electrodiagnostic aspects. Mayo Clin Proc 1981; 56:361–370.

60. Honet JC, Wajszczuk WJ, Rubenfire H, et al. Neurological abnormalities in the leg(s) after use of intraaortic balloon pump: Report of six cases. Arch Phys Med Rehabil 1975; 56:346–352.

61. Voulters L, Bolton C. Acute lumbosacral plexus neuropathy following vascular surgery. Can J Neurosci 1983; 10:153.

62. Cohen SH. Accidental intraarterial injection of drugs. Lancet 1948; 2:409–416.

63. Gaspar MR, Harc RR. Gangrene due to intra-arterial injections of drugs by drug addicts. Surgery 1972; 72:573–577.

64. Morgan NR, Waugh TR, Boback MD. Volkmann's ischemic contracture after intra-arterial injection of secobarbital. JAMA 1970; 212:476–478.

65. Hudson FP, McCandless A, O'Malley AG. Sciatic paralysis in newborn infants. Br Med J 1950; 1:223–225.

66. McFarland B. Neonatal sciatic palsy—comment. J Bone Joint Surg 1950; 32B:47–49.

67. Mills WG. A new neonatal syndrome. Br Med J 1949; 2:464–466.

68. Stöhr M, Dichgans J, Dörstelmann D. Ischaemic neuropathy of the lumbosacral plexus following intragluteal injection. J Neurol Neurosurg Psychiatry 1980; 43:489–494.

69. Levin KH. AAEE case report #19: Ischemic monomelic neuropathy. Muscle Nerve 1989; 12:791–795.

70. Matolo N, Kastagir B, Stevens L, et al. Neurovascular complications of brachial arteriovenous fistula. Am J Surg 1971; 121:716–719.

71. Riggs JE, Moss AH, Labosky DA, et al. Upper extremity ischemic monomelic neuropathy: A complication of vascular access procedures in uremic diabetic patients. Neurology 1989; 39:997–998.

72. Wytrzes L, Markley HG, Fisher, et al. Brachial neuropathy after brachial artery-antecubital vein shunts for chronic hemodialysis. Neurology 1987; 37:1398–1400.

73. Schaumburg HH, Spenser PS, Thomas PK. Disorders of peripheral nerves. Philadelphia: FA Davis, 1983.

74. Eames RA, Lange LS. Clinical and pathological study of ischemic neuropathy. J Neurol Neurosurg Psychiatry 1967; 30:215–226.

75. Serra C. Electromyography of arterial occlusive disease. World Neurol 1962; 3:664–678.

76. Chopra JS. Electromyography in diabetes mellitus and chronic occlusive peripheral vascular disease. Brain 1969; 92:97–108.

77. Miglietta O. Nerve motor fiber characteristics in chronic ischemia. Arch Neurol 1966; 14:448–453.

78. Miglietta O, Lowenthal M. Nerve conduction velocity and refractory period in peripheral vascular disease. J Appl Physiol 1962; 17:837–840.

79. Miglietta O. Electrophysiologic studies in chronic occlusive peripheral vascular disease. Arch Phys Med Rehabil 1967; 48:89–96.

80. Hunter GC, Song GW, Nayak NN, et al. Peripheral nerve conduction abnormalities in lower extremity ischemia: The effects of revascularization. J Surg Res 1988; 45:96–103.

81. Chopra JS, Hurwitz LJ. A comparative study of peripheral nerve conduction in diabetes and non-diabetic chronic occlusive peripheral vascular disease. Brain 1969; 92:83–96.

82. Kumlin T, Seppalainen A, Railo J. Electroneurography in intermittent claudication due to obliterative arteriosclerosis. Angiology 1974; 25:373–380.

83. Kissel JT, Slivka AP, Warmolts JR, et al. The clinical spectrum of necrotizing angiopathy of the peripheral nervous system. Ann Neurol 1985; 18:251–257.

84. Fauci AS, Haynes BF, Katz P. The spectrum of vasculitis: Clinical, pathologic, immunologic and therapeutic considerations. Ann Intern Med 1978; 89:660–676.

85. Hellmann DB, Laing TJ, Petri M, et al. Mononeuritis multiplex: The yield of evaluations for occult diseases. Medicine 1988; 67:145–153.

86. Kissel JT. Neurologic manifestations of vasculitis. Neurol 1989; 7:655–673.

87. Parry GJG. Mononeuropathy multiplex (AAEE Case report #11). Muscle Nerve 1985; 8:493–498.

88. Shields RW, Harris JW, Clark M. Mononeuropathy in sickle cell anemia: Anatomical and pathophysiological basis for its rarity. Muscle Nerve 1991; 14:370–374.

89. Hunder GG, Arend WP, Block DA, et al. The American College of Rheumatology 1990 criteria for the classification of vasculitis. Arthritis Rheumatism 1990; 33:1065–1100.

90. Dyck PJ, Benstead TJ, Conn DL, et al. Nonsystemic vasculitic neuropathy. Brain 1987; 110:843–854.

91. Said G, Lacroix-Ciaudo C, Fugimuri H, et al. The peripheral neuropathy of necrotizing arteritis: A clinicopathological study. Ann Neurol 1988; 23:461–465.

92. Jamieson PW, Giuliaini MJ, Martinez AJ. Necrotizing angiopathy presenting with multifocal conduction blocks. Neurology 1991; 41:442–444.

93. Ropert A, Metral S. Conduction block in neuropathies with necrotizing vasculitis. Muscle Nerve 1990; 13:102–105.

94. Bouche P, Léger JM, Travers MA. Peripheral neuropathy in systemic vasculitis: Clinical and electro-physiologic study of 22 patients. Neurology 1986; 36:1598–1602.

95. Chang RW, Bell CL, Hallett M. Clinical characteristics and prognosis of vasculitic mononeuropathy multiplex. Arch Neurol 1984; 41:618–621.

96. Moore PM, Cupps TR. Neurological complications of vasculitis. Ann Neurol 1983; 14:155–167.

97. Wilbourn AJ. AAEE Case Report #12: Common peroneal neuropathy at the fibular head. Muscle Nerve 1986; 9:825–836.

98. Wees SJ, Sunwoo IN, Oh SJ. Sural nerve biopsy in systemic necrotizing vasculitis. Am J Med 1981; 71:525–532.

99. Battaglia M, Mitsumoto H, Wilbourn AJ, et al. Utility of electromyography in the diagnosis of vasculitic neuropathy. Neurology 1990; 40(suppl 1):427.

100. Harati Y, Niakan E. The clinical spectrum of inflammatory-angiopathic peripheral neuropathy. Neurology 1985; 35(suppl 1):77.

101. Moore PM, Fauci AS. Neurologic manifestations of systemic vasculitis. Am J Med 1981; 71:517–524.

102. Oh SJ. The nerve conduction and sural nerve biopsy helpful in rapid diagnosis of vasculitis. Neurology 1985; 35(suppl 1):240–241.

103. Moore RE, Friedman RJ. Current concepts in pathophysiology and diagnosis of compartment syndromes. J Emerg Med 1989; 7:657–662.

104. Gamron RB. Taking the pressure out of compartment syndrome. Am J Nurs 1988; 88:1076–1080.

105. Garfin SR. Anatomy of the extremity compartments. In: Mubarak SJ, Hargens AR, eds. Compartment syndromes and Volkmann's contracture. Philadelphia: WB Saunders, 1981:6–16.

106. Smith DC, Mitchell DA, Peterson GW, et al. Medial brachial fascial compartment syndrome: Anatomical basis of neuropathy after trans-axillary arteriography. Radiology 1989; 173:149–174.

107. Owen CA. Clinical diagnosis of acute compartment syndromes. In: Mubarak SJ, Hargens AR, eds. Compartment syndromes and Volkmann's contracture. Philadelphia: WB Saunders, 1981:98–105.

108. Hargens AR, Mubarak SJ. Laboratory diagnosis of acute compartment syndromes. In: Mubarak SJ, Hargen AR, eds. Compartment syndromes and Volkmann's contracture. Philadelphia: WB Saunders, 1981:106–122.

109. Mumenthaler M, Schliak H. Peripheral nerve lesions: Diagnosis and therapy. Stuttgart: Thieme, 1991.

110. Hargens AR, Romine JS, Sipe JC, et al. Peripheral nerve-conduction block by high muscle-compartment pressure. J Bone Joint Surg 1979; 61-A:192–200.

111. Seddon H. Surgical disorders of the peripheral nerves, ed 2. Edinburgh: Churchill Livingstone, 1975.

112. Dyck PJ, Conn DL, Okazaki H. Necrotizing angio-

pathic neuropathy. Mayo Clin Proc 1972; 47:461–475.

113. Ferguson FR, Liversedge LA. Ischemic lateral popliteal nerve palsy. Br Med J 1954; 2:333–335.

114. Parkes AR. Traumatic ischemia of peripheral nerves with some observations on Volkmann's ischemic contracture. Br J Surg 1944–45; 32:403–414.

115. Peyronnard JM, Charron L, Beaudet F, et al. Vas-culitic neuropathy in rheumatoid disease and Sjögren syndrome. Neurology 1982; 32:839–845.

116. Schaumberg H, Spencer PS, Thomas PK. Disorders of peripheral nerves. Philadelphia: FA Davis, 1983.

117. Usubiaga JE, Kolodny J, Usubiaga LE. Neurologic complications of prevertebral surgery under regional anesthesia. Surgery 1970; 14:127–130.

15

Classification and Electrodiagnosis of Hereditary Neuropathies

P. K. Thomas

CONTENTS

LIST OF ACRONYMS

AD	autosomal dominant
AR	autosomal recessive
CIDP	chronic inflammatory demyelinating polyneuropathy
CMUA	continuous motor unit activity
CNS	central nervous system
HDL	high-density lipoprotein
HMN	hereditary motor neuronopathy
HMSN	hereditary motor and sensory neuropathy
HSAN	hereditary sensory and autonomic neuropathy
LDL	low-density lipoprotein
OPCA	olivopontocerebellar atrophy

Peripheral nerve involvement may either be the predominant manifestation of a number of inherited conditions, or it may occur as part of a more widespread neurologic or multisystem disorder. Since their introduction, electrodiagnostic studies have played an important part in unraveling this complex group of conditions, in combination with more extensive genetic and morphologic studies. Electromyography (EMG) is helpful in differentiating purely motor neuropathies from myopathic disorders. Nerve conduction studies may detect the presence of subclinical neuropathy, which can be valuable both in the electrodiagnosis of individual patients and in case identification in family studies to establish patterns of inheritance. The severity of reduction in nerve conduction velocity may be useful in predicting the underlying pathology and has proved a valuable asset in the subdivision of groups of disorders that display similar clinical features.

A convenient way of classifying the hereditary neuropathies is to subdivide them into those in which there is a known metabolic basis and those in which the underlying pathogenesis is still obscure. The latter can be further subdivided into the hereditary motor neuronopathies (HMN) (spinal muscular atrophies [SMAs]), the hereditary motor and sensory neuropathies (HMSN), the hereditary sensory and autonomic neuropathies (HSAN), and miscellaneous conditions. A provisional classification based on these principles is given in Tables 15.1 and 15.2. This classification will continue to be modified as new information accrues.

TABLE 15.1.   Classification of hereditary neuropathies associated with specific metabolic defects

Disturbances of lipid metabolism
   Metachromatic leukodystrophy
   Globoid cell leukodystrophy (Krabbe's disease)
   Refsum's disease
   Hereditary high-density lipoprotein deficiency (Tangier disease)
   Abetalipoproteinemia (Bassen-Kornzweig disease)
   Fabry's disease
   Cholestanolosis
   Niemann-Pick disease
   Farber's lipogranulomatosis
Peroxisomal disorders
   Adrenoleukodystrophy and adrenomyeloneuropathy
   Infantile Refsum's disease
   Hyperoxaluria type I
   Benign peroxisomal dysgenesis with ataxia and peripheral neuropathy
Hereditary amyloid neuropathies
Hereditary hepatic porphyria
   Acute intermittent porphyria
   Variegate porphyria
   Hereditary coproporphyria
   ALA dehydratase deficiency
Disorders associated with defective DNA repair
   Ataxia telangiectasia
   Xeroderma pigmentosum
   Cockayne's syndrome
Mucopolysaccharidoses and oligosaccharidoses
Hexosaminidase deficiency

NEUROPATHIES ASSOCIATED WITH SPECIFIC METABOLIC DEFECTS

Disturbances of Lipid Metabolism

Metachromatic leukodystrophy (sulfatide lipidosis)

The metachromatic leukodystrophies comprise at least five genetically separate conditions. All are characterized by the occurrence of demyelination in the central nervous system and the peripheral nervous system. This is associated with the accumulation of galactosyl sulfatide in glia, Schwann cells, and macrophages that stains metachromatically. Late infantile, juvenile, and adult onset forms are associated with a deficiency of arylsulfatase A; multiple sulfatase deficiency with lack of arylsulfatase A, B, and C activity (and lack of activity of other sulfa-

tases); and the AB variant of metachromatic leukodystrophy with a lack of activator protein.

The late infantile form is the most common variety. The onset is between 1 and 4 years of age, usually between 15 and 18 months. Hagberg[1] has divided the condition into four stages. After normal early development, the first stage begins with difficulty in walking owing to limb weakness and ataxia. Peripheral nerve involvement is evidenced by diminution or loss of tendon reflexes. This may antedate central nervous system involvement, but at times the disorder begins with a spastic paraparesis and exaggerated tendon reflexes. In the second stage, mental regression becomes obvious, and the child is no longer able to stand, although he or she is able to sit unsupported. Limb ataxia is more evident, and dysarthria develops. The tendon reflexes remain depressed or absent, and limb pain may reflect neuropathy. In the third stage, the child is quadriplegic and

TABLE 15.2.   Classification of hereditary
neuropathies of unknown causation

Hereditary motor neuronopathies (spinal muscular atro-
  phies [SMA])
  Proximal SMA
  Distal SMA
  SMA with complex distributions
Hereditary motor and sensory neuropathies (HMSN)
  Type I HMSN
  Type II HMSN
  X-linked HMSN
  Type III HMSN
  Complex forms of HMSN
Hereditary sensory and autonomic neuropathies (HSAN)
  Autosomal dominant hereditary sensory neuropathy
  Autosomal recessive hereditary sensory neuropathy
  Familial dysautonomia
  Congenital sensory neuropathy with anhidrosis
  Congenital sensory neuropathy with selective loss of
    small myelinated fibers
Neuropathy in spinocerebellar degenerations, hereditary
  spastic paraplegia, and inherited extrapyramidal disor-
  ders
Inherited recurrent brachial plexus neuropathy
Hereditary liability to pressure palsies
Giant axonal neuropathy
Chediak-Higashi syndrome
Familial multiple symmetrical lipomatosis

---

can no longer sit unsupported. There is severe mental
deterioration, and tonic seizures occur. In the final
stage, there is severe dementia, accompanied by optic
atrophy and blindness, deafness, and decerebrate rigidity. Death usually occurs in the sixth year of life.

Abnormalities of nerve conduction in metachromatic leukodystrophy were first shown by Fullerton.[2]
In six of seven children, severely reduced motor nerve
conduction velocity was demonstrated. This was associated with a reduction in the amplitude of evoked
compound muscle action potentials and was confirmed by Yudell et al.[3] It can be related to the
occurrence of extensive segmental demyelination and
remyelination.[4,5] Compound sensory and mixed
nerve action potentials are of reduced amplitude but
are occasionally normal, as may be true for motor
nerve conduction velocity.[2] Nerve conduction studies
may be important diagnostically in suggesting the
diagnosis of leukodystrophy in children in whom
only central nervous system signs are present in the
initial stages. They could also provide an early non-
invasive method for the detection of the disease in
some instances for genetic studies.

The juvenile form is clinically similar to the late
infantile variety but has an onset in later childhood,
usually before the age of 10 years, although it sometimes occurs in adolescence. Manifestations related
to central nervous system involvement tend to appear
earlier. The adult-onset form usually begins early in
the third decade of life but can develop in late adolescence, and the clinical picture is usually dominated
by behavioral changes and dementia. The tendon
reflexes may be depressed or absent. The adult form
tends to pursue a protracted course. Motor nerve
conduction velocity is reduced, and compound sensory nerve action potentials are of reduced amplitude,[6,7] but these changes are not present in all patients, even when they have clinically advanced
disease.[8] On the other hand, the above-mentioned
changes may develop before clinical evidence of the
disease becomes manifest[9] and may be an important
factor suggesting this diagnosis in cases of progressive dementia and behavioral disorder developing in
late adolescence or early adult life. The pathologic
changes in peripheral nerve in the juvenile and adult
forms resemble those of the late infantile variety,
apart from abnormalities that can be related to
chronicity.[6,10]

Multiple sulfatase deficiency gives rise to a disorder with an age of onset and duration similar to
those of the late infantile form, but in addition, affected children may display ichthyosis, hepatosplenomegaly, and flaring of the rib cage. Motor nerve
conduction velocity is reduced,[11] and nerve biopsies
reveal segmental demyelination with metachromatic
material in Schwann cells and macrophages.[12]

A further variant without arylsulfatase deficiency
has been described,[13,14] related to a deficiency of
activator protein. In the case reported by Hahn et
al.,[14] the patient when aged 21 was severly demented
with a bilateral supranuclear bulbar palsy and spasticity in the upper limbs. This was accompanied by
a moderately severe lower limb neuropathy, where
there was hypotonic weakness and tendon areflexia.
There was a history of progressive psychomotor disorder dating back to early life. Motor nerve conduction velocity in the peroneal nerve was severely reduced (10 m/s), compound sensory nerve action
potentials were unrecordable, and electromyographic studies showed evidence of chronic denervation. Nerve biopsy revealed changes typical of
metachromatic leukodystrophy.[14] Despite normal arylsulfatase A activity, hydrolysis of cerebroside sulfate in this disorder by fibroblasts is defective but is
corrected by activator protein.[15]

Globoid cell leukodystrophy (galactosylceramide lipidosis, Krabbe's disease)

As with metachromatic leukodystrophy, globoid cell leukodystrophy or Krabbe's disease predominantly affects the central nervous system, but there is associated peripheral nerve involvement. The disorder is of autosomal recessive inheritance and is related to a deficiency of galactosylceramidase. The pathologic changes in the central nervous system are characterized by widespread cortical demyelination, variable axonal loss, gliosis, and the presence of large multinucleated *globoid* cells. Signs of the disorder usually appear at the age of 3 to 6 months after a normal neonatal period. Hagberg[284] has recognized three stages in the clinical evolution of the condition. In stage 1, the child becomes irritable and shows hypersensitivity to sensory stimuli. Convulsive seizures may occur. This is succeeded by stage 2, in which rapidly advancing motor and intellectual regression occurs with hypertonicity in the limbs and axial musculature, accompanied by exaggerated tendon reflexes. Seizures continue to occur, and optic atrophy may develop. In stage 3, which may be reached after only a few months, the child becomes blind, deaf, and decerebrate. Death usually occurs within 2 years of the onset.

Clinical evidence of peripheral nerve involvement is not as obtrusive as in metachromatic leukodystrophy, but the tendon reflexes usually become depressed within about 6 months of the onset of symptoms[16] and flaccidity of the limbs in the terminal stages. Nerve biopsy shows moderate fiber loss, segmental demyelination, and the presence of prismatic inclusions in Schwann cells associated both with myelinated and unmyelinated axons,[17,18] Abnormalities are consistently found on electron microscopy.

Motor nerve conduction velocity is reduced in approximately 50% of patients.[12] The degree of reduction may be marked: It was 20 to 25 m per second in the median and ulnar nerves and 18 m per second in the peroneal nerve at the age of 22 months in the patient reported by Hogan et al.,[19] in whom conduction velocity in sensory fibers was also reduced. Slowing of nerve conduction may be detectable as early as 7 weeks postnatally.[20]

Cases with a later onset and a slower course also occur. These may begin in later childhood, adolescence, or adult life. Clinically they are usually characterized by progressive dementia, optic atrophy, and pyramidal signs.[21] Peripheral nerve involvement is generally not prominent in such patients. Thomas et al.[22] have recorded a patient with an onset in early childhood and a clinical picture resembling a spinocerebellar degeneration. This was accompanied by a demyelinating neuropathy with severely reduced motor nerve conduction velocity and loss of compound sensory nerve action potentials.

Refsum's disease (phytanic acid storage disease)

This autosomal recessive disorder has been reported most frequently in Norway, Sweden, the British Isles. Ireland, France, and Germany. The onset of symptoms is usually in the second or third decades but may be in childhood. The clinical features have been reviewed by Refsum et al.[23] The course may be slowly progressive or be marked by exacerbations and remissions and is characterized by a combination of a distal sensorimotor neuropathy usually associated with ataxia, this having led to its designation as heredopathia atactica polyneuritiformis. Pigmentary retinal degeneration is a constant associated feature; anosmia, pupillary changes, and deafness are common. Cardiomyopathy may develop, and the condition may be accompanied by ichthyosis and skeletal malformations. Phytanic acid accumulates in the serum and in a variety of tissues, related to a block in its α-oxidation. The phytanic acid is derived from phytol of dietary origin, and it is likely that it is responsible for the neurologic dysfunction.[23]

Autopsy studies have demonstrated diffuse and often irregular enlargement of nerves and particularly of spinal nerves immediately distal to the dorsal root ganglia. Microscopically there is loss of myelinated nerve fibers and evidence of segmental demyelination. Hypertrophic changes are often prominent.[23] Similar changes may be demonstrable in biopsy specimens from distal sensory nerves,[24] but not infrequently the predominant abnormality in such specimens is axonal degeneration with inconspicuous hypertrophic changes.

EMG of distal muscles demonstrates signs of chronic partial denervation. Motor conduction velocity is reduced, but the magnitude of this is variable. Extremely slow values may be recorded, as in the case reported by Eldjarn et al.,[25] in which it was 7 m per second in the ulnar nerve. Other authors have recorded values of 10 to 50 m per second in the upper limb nerves.[26–29] The findings may be discordant between siblings; motor nerve conduction velocity in the median nerves was 45 and 50 m per second in one patient and 23 and 27 m per second in her sister.[29] Presumably these divergences reflect varying degrees of segmental demyelination in distal limbs,[30] as is evident from the results of nerve biopsy studies as discussed already. Because the hypertrophic changes are more prominent proximally, the findings for F wave latencies would be of interest in patients with relatively preserved motor conduction velocity in the limbs. Compound sensory nerve action potentials are usually abolished.

Refsum's disease may be improved by a diet low in phytol and phytanic acid as well as by plasma exchange.[31] Nerve conduction velocity has been found to parallel the reduction in serum phytanic acid concentrations and clinical recovery.[31–35]

Hereditary high-density lipoprotein deficiency (Tangier disease)

Hereditary high-density lipoprotein (HDL) deficiency or Tangier disease derives its name from Tangier Island in Chesapeake Bay. It is a rare autosomal-recessive disorder in which affected individuals have no detectable normal serum HDL. Cholesterol levels are also reduced, but triglycerides are normal or increased. Obligate heterozygotes have reduced serum HDL concentrations.

The disease may become manifest during childhood or be delayed until adult life. Cholesterol esters are deposited in a wide variety of tissues, where they are present in macrophages. This is particularly evident in the tonsils, which become enlarged and orange in color (*the tangerine tonsils of Tangier disease*) and in the thymus.

Peripheral nerve involvement has been encountered in approximately one-half of the patients so far described. Three variants have been recognized, although it is not yet known whether these are genetically distinct. The first consists of a multifocal neuropathy with repeated transient mononeuropathies.[36] The second is the pseudosyringomyelic form,[37–39] which shows an unusual combination of neurologic features comprising weakness of the facial and distal limb muscles, particularly those of the hands; tendon areflexia; and extensive dissociated pain and temperature sensory loss, which tends to spare the distal extremities. The third is a symmetrical distal sensorimotor polyneuropathy.[40] The pathologic changes in the first type are predominantly demyelination and remyelination, with lipid vacuoles confined almost exclusively to Remak cells.[36] In contrast, the pseudosyringomyelic type shows axonal degeneration, particularly affecting

smaller fibers, without demyelination. Numerous lipid droplets (neutral lipid and cholesterol esters) are present in Schwann cells but not in macrophages. It has been suggested[39,41] that the lipid inclusions within Schwann cells are derived from nerve fiber breakdown that, for reasons not yet established, these cells are unable to transfer to macrophages. In the form with a symmetrical distal sensorimotor polyneuropathy, loss of larger myelinated fibers was found, with an increase in small-caliber fibers, probably related to regeneration. Lipid deposits were present within Schwann cells, predominantly those associated with unmyelinated axons.[40]

In the multifocal type, reduced motor unit (MU) recruitment has been found in affected muscles, with occasional increases in MU potential amplitude indicating chronic partial denervation. Nerve conduction studies have demonstrated focal slowing of motor conduction, sometimes at entrapment sites, and prolonged latencies of compound sensory action potentials in distal limb nerves.[36] In the pseudosyringomyelic form, there is evidence of denervation in affected muscles.[38] Motor nerve conduction velocity has been found to be moderately reduced, by about 25%, and compound sensory nerve action potentials are absent.[41] They are thus important in distinguishing this form of Tangier disease from true syringomyelia, in which compound sensory nerve action potentials are preserved, because the sensory loss is related to damage to the sensory pathway proximal to the dorsal root ganglia. In the form with a symmetrical distal sensorimotor polyneuropathy, signs of denervation were observed in distal muscles. Motor nerve conduction velocity was normal in the upper limbs but reduced in lower limb nerves.[40]

Abetalipoproteinemia (Bassen-Kornzweig disease)

Hereditary absence of low-density lipoproteins (LDL) or Bassen-Kornzweig disease is again of autosomal recessive inheritance, although males are affected more than females. The biochemical features also include hypocholesterolemia and reduced levels of circulating phospholipids, free fatty acid, and chylomicrons. The disorder is probably related to defective synthesis of apoprotein B, which is involved in the transport of triglyceride from the intestinal cells into plasma. Heterozygotes have a normal plasma LDL concentration.

The onset of symptoms is usually in infancy, when evidence of fat malabsorption becomes evident. This tends to decline with age. Neurologic deficits usually become apparent during the first decade and almost always before the age of 20 years. Ataxia is commonly the initial feature, but it may be preceded by tendon areflexia. Cases evolve into a clinical picture resembling Friedreich's ataxia with dysarthria, limb ataxia, areflexia, loss of proprioceptive and vibration sense, and later of all modalities. Weakness is present in the limbs, and the plantar responses may become extensor. Pigmentary retinal degeneration is frequent, and acanthocytes are present in peripheral blood smears. There is now good evidence for believing that the neurologic features associated with abetalipoproteinemia are related to vitamin E deficiency.[42] The absorption of fat-soluble vitamins from the gut is impaired, and serum vitamin E is severely reduced or undetectable from birth.

Peripheral nerve pathology and pathophysiology in abetalipoproteinemia have not been extensively investigated. Sural nerve biopsy has shown a loss of myelinated nerve fibers, mainly of larger size, and sparse segmental demyelination.[43,44] Loss of anterior horn cells has been found at autopsy.[45] EMG has demonstrated changes of chronic partial denervation,[44] although some earlier reports had questioned myopathic changes.[46,47] Motor nerve conduction velocity has been found to be normal and compound sensory nerve action potentials to be variably depressed.[44]

Fabry's disease (α-galactosidase A deficiency)

This disorder is of X-linked recessive inheritance. It has been mapped to the proximal part of Xq.[48] α-Galactosidase is a lysosomal hydrolase, and its deficiency leads to impaired breakdown of glycosphingolipids and their deposition in a variety of tissues. The most characteristic systemic manifestation is a scaly telangiectatic skin rash, angiokeratoma corporis diffusum, which is present mainly over the lower trunk and buttocks. Other systemic manifestations include corneal dystrophy, dilatation of conjunctival vessels, multifocal cerebral ischemic lesions, heart murmurs, and renal failure. Female carriers may exhibit signs of the disease of varying severity, but these are inconsistent and usually mild.

The most important neurologic symptom is pain, which commonly begins in childhood or adolescence. This takes the form of persistent aching in the limbs with severe exacerbations of burning pain (Fabry crises) sometimes provoked by emotional factors. Distal hypohidrosis may be demonstrable.[49] There is deposition of glycolipid in perineurial and capillary

endothelial cells[49,50] and dorsal root ganglion cells[51] and loss of small myelinated and unmyelinated fibers in the peripheral nerves and of small dorsal root ganglion cells.[50,52]

Motor nerve conduction was examined in three separate kindreds with Fabry's disease by Sheth and Swick.[52] Reduced conduction velocity and prolonged distal latencies were recorded in hemizygous males and at times in carrier females. The changes were mild in the ulnar nerve, but values of 21.5 m per second and 8.5 m per second for motor conduction velocity in the peroneal nerve were recorded in two affected males. This is somewhat surprising in view of what is known concerning the pathology, with the selective involvement of small fibers. Motor and sensory conduction was normal in the case reported by Kocen and Thomas.[50]

Cholestanolosis

Cholestanolosis or cerebrotendinous xanthomatosis is a rare lipid storage disease characterized by progressive dementia, cerebellar ataxia, spasticity, and peripheral neuropathy, accompanied by tendon and tuberous xanthomas, cataracts, and premature atherosclerosis. The onset is usually in late childhood or adolescence, and death occurs by the age of 30 to 40 years. Inheritance is autosomal recessive. The diagnosis is established by the finding of high plasma cholestanol levels coupled with normal cholesterol levels. The underlying biochemical disturbance involves defective bile acid synthesis with diversion of cholesterol into cholestanol as a result of a lack of mitochondrial 26-hydroxylase.[53] Chenodeoxycholic acid is virtually absent from the bile, and bile acid precursors (as alcohols) conjugated with glucuronic acid are present in bile and urine. The tendon xanthomas, however, predominantly contain cholesterol with lesser amounts of cholestanol.

Neuropathy is not present in all patients. It is relatively mild and predominantly sensory in type.[54–57] Motor nerve conduction velocity shows mild to moderate reduction, and sensory nerve action potentials are reduced in amplitude.[57] Nerve biopsy shows loss of myelinated nerve fibers, particularly those of large diameter.[57] Some investigators have been impressed with the presence of demyelination and hypertrophic changes.[55,56]

A reduction in blood cholestanol levels and some clinical improvement can be produced by the oral administration of chenodeoxycholic acid to supplement the enterohepatic bile acid pool. Improvement in neuropathy has not been documented, but a beneficial effect on nerve conduction has been shown.[57]

Other disorders of lipid metabolism

Peripheral neuropathy may occasionally occur in the acute neuronopathic form (Crocker type A) of Niemann-Pick disease, which constitutes the most common variant of the sphingomyelin lipidoses. Inheritance is autosomal recessive. This form develops in the first year of life and is characterized by progressive intellectual deterioration, retinal cherry red spots, and sometimes seizures, in association with hepatosplenomegaly. Sphingomyelin accumulates in foamy histiocytes in various tissues. The neuropathy is manifested by hypotonic weakness and tendon areflexia. The peripheral nerves show demyelination and remyelination, the presence of dense bodies in Schwann cells, and foamy macrophages in the endoneurium.[58,59] Electromyographic studies have shown evidence of denervation and markedly reduced motor nerve conduction velocity with values in upper and lower limb nerves of 10 m per second or less at 1 year of age[58] and less severe reductions of motor and sensory conduction velocities in a child of 8 months.[59]

Farber's lipogranulomatosis is a rare disorder of probable autosomal recessive inheritance with onset in infancy. The salient manifestations are the occurrence of joint enlargement and contractures, subcutaneous and periarticular nodules, and pulmonary consolidation. Affected tissues show an infiltration with foam cells and an increased ceramide content. A deficiency of an acid ceramidase probably underlies the condition. Mental deterioration may occur. There is usually severe muscle wasting accompanied by hypotonia and tendon areflexia. Cutaneous hyperesthesia may be evident. Electromyographic studies have shown signs of denervation, related either to anterior horn cell or peripheral nerve involvement, although myopathic changes have also been described.[60] In the peripheral nerves, the Schwann cells contain prominent membrane-bound inclusions.[61] No reports on nerve conduction in this condition appear to have been published.

A single report has been made on a multisystem disorder associated with reduced tissue arachidonic acid levels.[62] This comprised the onset in childhood of mental retardation, pigmentary retinopathy, sensorineural hearing loss, and later distal limb weakness and tendon areflexia. There was electromyographic evidence of denervation and reduced motor and sensory conduction velocity.

Peroxisomal Disorders

Peroxisomes are small intracellular organelles bounded by a single membrane. They contain catalase and a variety of oxidases. These include phytanic acid oxidase and enzymes involved in the β-oxidation of very long-chain fatty acids. Peroxisomes are also involved in glyoxylate metabolism. Peroxisomal disorders can be divided into three categories. The first consists of single enzyme defects with normal peroxisome structure, of which the most common instance is X-linked adrenoleukodystrophy; primary hyperoxaluria also falls into this category. The second category consists of multiple enzyme defects with normal or slightly reduced numbers of peroxisomes. The final category comprises multiple enzyme defects with severely reduced numbers of peroxisomes; it includes Zellweger's syndrome, infantile Refsum's disease, and neonatal adrenoleukodystrophy.

Adrenoleukodystrophy and adrenomyeloneuropathy

X-linked adrenoleukodystrophy affects both the adrenal cortex, giving rise to an addisonian syndrome, and the nervous system, usually causing a progressive cerebral degeneration, in young males. The gene has been mapped to the end of the long arm of the X chromosome.[63] A number of different phenotypes have been recognized,[64] and less severe manifestations may occur in female carriers. The disorder is associated with the accumulation of very long-chain fatty acids, particularly with a 25-carbon and 26-carbon chain length. In particular, this involves hexacosanate, a 26-carbon unbranched fatty acid. The increases are demonstrable in plasma and cultured skin fibroblasts.[65]

Clinically evident peripheral nerve involvement is seen in cases of adrenomyeloneuropathy. Such cases may occur in the same families as examples of adrenoleukodystrophy, and the two presentations are therefore likely to represent different phenotypic manifestations of the same abnormal gene. In patients with adrenomyeloneuropathy, in addition to corticospinal tract involvement, there may be lower motor neuron weakness and depression but not loss of the tendon reflexes. Some but not all patients show a mild or moderate reduction in motor and sensory nerve conduction velocity,[66] together with electromyographic evidence of denervation in limb muscles.

Neonatal adrenoleukodystrophy is an autosomal recessive disorder, genetically distinct from X-linked adrenoleukodystrophy. It does not affect the peripheral nervous system.

Infantile Refsum's disease

This autosomal recessive disorder that has been recognized in recent years[67–69] bears resemblances to Zellweger's syndrome. It is characterized by dysmorphic features, mental retardation, pigmentary retinopathy, severe sensorineural deafness, and hepatomegaly. Serum phytanic acid levels are elevated, and phytanic acid oxidase activity is defective in cultured fibroblasts.[69] Hepatic peroxisomes are deficient.[70] Serum pipecolic acid levels are also increased, as is the ratio of C26:C22 very long-chain fatty acids.[71] Some children have an accompanying peripheral neuropathy. In such patients, motor nerve conduction velocity has been found to be moderately reduced and compound sensory nerve action potentials to be absent.[69] Nerve biopsy has shown demyelination and loss of myelinated nerve fibers without hypertrophic changes.[69]

Hyperoxaluria type I

Type I primary hyperoxaluria (glycolic aciduria) is an autosomal recessive disorder in which the urinary excretion of oxalate and glycocolate is elevated. The peroxisomal enzyme alanine:glyoxylate aminotransferase has been shown to be deficient in the liver.[72] The occurrence of neuropathy has been shown in a few instances. It is rapidly progressive, affects both motor and sensory function, and is of interest in that oxylate crystals are not only deposited in the walls of neural arterioles, but also within nerve fibers, probably within axons.[73] Pathologically a combination of axonal loss and segmental demyelination has been described. Motor nerve conduction velocity has been severely reduced and compound nerve action potentials are of reduced amplitude or are absent.[73,74]

Benign peroxisome dysgenesis with ataxia and peripheral neuropathy

A syndrome has been described in a child that combined ataxia, hypotonia, and tendon areflexia. Nerve conduction velocity was mildly reduced.[75] A panel of peroxisomal markers, including very long-chain fatty acids, phytanic acid, and catalase compartmentation, were abnormal. In contradistinction to other panperoxisomal disorders, this condition was relatively benign.

Hereditary Amyloid Neuropathies

Peripheral neuropathy is a prominent feature in a number of inherited amyloidoses. All show autosomal dominant inheritance. Most are related to variant transthyretin (TTR), previously known as prealbumin. The first condition to be recognized was the Portuguese type originally identified by Andrade.[76] It has been shown to be due to a valine to methionine substitution at position 30 (met 30) in the molecule.[77] The gene has been mapped to the long arm of chromosome 18.[78] The disorder has an insidious onset, usually in the third or fourth decades. Initially there is loss of pain and temperature sensation distally in the lower limbs, often accompanied by spontaneous pain. The upper limbs are affected later. Autonomic symptoms are an early feature. Distal motor involvement, tendon areflexia, and sensory loss for all modalities follow. The loss of pain sensibility frequently leads to persistent foot ulceration and neuropathic joint degeneration. There may be associated renal, cardiac, and ocular manifestations (vitreous opacification). The disorder is steadily progressive; death occurs after about 10 years. Apart from the families in Northern Portugal, the met 30 mutation has been identified in patients from Brazil, Japan, Sweden, Italy, Greece, Cyprus,[79] and the UK.

Two large unrelated kindreds from Indiana[80] and Maryland[81] have shown a different clinical picture with a disorder that begins in the fourth decade, frequently with the carpal tunnel syndrome. More diffuse sensory loss distally in all four extremities follows, together with autonomic symptoms, cardiac involvement, and vitreous opacities. Progression of the disease is slow. The Indiana form has been shown to be related to a serine for isoleucine substitution at position 84 in the TTR molecule[82] and the Maryland form to a histidine for leucine substitution at position 58.[83] Other TTR variants are responsible for the Jewish,[84] Irish-Appalachian,[85] and German forms.[86] These are so far less well characterized clinically, as are those related to further more recently described TTR gene mutations.

The Iowa or Van Allen form[87] has clinical similarities to the Portuguese type, with an onset in the third or fourth decades with a distal sensorimotor neuropathy preferentially affecting pain and temperature sensation in the early stages. Autonomic involvement is less obtrusive. Renal involvement and peptic ulceration are common. Cardiomyopathy may also occur. The amyloid in this disorder is not derived from TTR but from a variant apolipoprotein A1 with an arginine for glycine substitution at position 26 in the molecule.[88]

The Finnish or Meretoja form is clinically different. It consists of cranial neuropathy associated with a corneal lattice dystrophy and cutaneous laxity.[89] A mild neuropathy in the limbs may develop later.[90] The onset is usually in the fifth decade, and progression is slow. The amyloid has been shown to be related to serum gelsolin.[91]

Pathologic studies on the peripheral nervous system have been most extensive in the Portuguese type. Amyloid deposits are present in the endoneurium, perineurium, and epineurium and around the neural blood vessels. They are also evident in dorsal root and sympathetic ganglia.[92] In the earlier stages, there is a preferential loss of small myelinated and unmyelinated axons, which correlates well with the early autonomic involvement and pattern of sensory loss.[93,94] Some accompanying demyelination is also present.

In patients with the Portuguese form of amyloid neuropathy, nerve conduction velocity is usually mildly or moderately reduced[95] but can be quite severely reduced with values down to 20 m per second in the upper limbs and 15 m per second in the lower extremities.[92] Compound sensory nerve action potentials recorded by conventional means may be normal, reduced in amplitude, or undetectable,[94,96] depending on the severity of the disease. Focal

abnormalities related to compression of the median nerve are demonstrable in patients with the Indiana form of hereditary amyloidosis.[81]

Lambert and Dyck[97] have documented their findings for the in vitro recording of the compound sural nerve action potential in a case of dominantly inherited amyloidosis, clinically of the Portuguese type (Figure 15.1). No C fiber potential was detectable, and the A δ potential was considerably reduced in amplitude. In contrast, there was only a moderate reduction in the height of the A α potential, which was of normal configuration and conduction velocity (54 m/s). These changes correlated well with the histologic findings: a virtual absence of unmyelinated fibers and a reduction in the myelinated fiber population, particularly those of small diameter.

Sales Luis[96] has provided evidence that suggested that abnormalities of nerve conduction may be present before the disease becomes clinically overt. How far in advance of the clinical onset such changes may be detectable is not established.

Boysen et al.[90] studied five members of a Danish family with the Finnish type of hereditary amyloid neuropathy. All had a late-onset cranial neuropathy

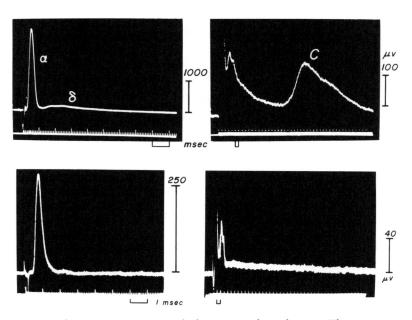

FIGURE 15.1.   *Compound nerve action potentials from excised sural nerve. The upper two panels show recordings from normal nerve displaying the A α and A δ potentials on the left and, at higher gain, the C fiber potential on the right. The lower two panels are from a patient with dominantly inherited type I amyloid neuropathy. On the left the recording shows preservation of the A α potential but loss of the A δ peak; that on the right shows loss of the C fiber potential. (From Lambert EH, Dyck PJ. Compound action potentials of sural nerve in vitro in peripheral neuropathy. In: Dyck PJ, Thomas PK, Lambert EH, eds. Peripheral neuropathy. Philadelphia: WB Saunders, 1975:427–441. With permission.)*

with an asymptomatic corneal lattice dystrophy. There was electromyographic evidence of denervation in the facial muscles and the tongue and in increased latency of the evoked response in facial muscles on stimulation of the facial nerve (Figure 15.2). The patients showed no abnormal motor signs in the limbs, but variable reflex depression and sensory impairment were present. Electromyographic studies showed mild signs of chronic denervation. Motor nerve conduction velocity in limb nerves was normal except for two instances of a mild carpal tunnel syndrome. Sensory nerve conduction velocity was normal, but the amplitude of compound sensory nerve action potentials was reduced, suggesting axonal degeneration. This was confirmed by sural nerve biopsy.

Porphyria

Peripheral neuropathy may develop in acute intermittent and variegate porphyria and at times in the rarer hereditary coproporphyria and delta-aminolevulinic acid (ALA) dehydratase. The clinical fea-

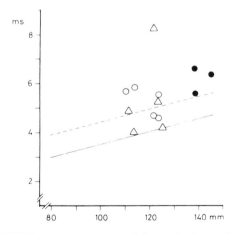

FIGURE 15.2. *Latency of the evoked muscle response (abscissa) in orbicularis oris (open circles), triangularis (open triangles) and frontalis (solid circles) on stimulation of the facial nerve in five siblings with type IV hereditary amyloid neuropathy (cranial neuropathy with corneal lattice dystrophy). The ordinate indicates the distance between the sites of stimulation and recording. The continuous line represents the regression line and the interrupted line represents the 95% confidence range for normal subjects. (From Boysen G, Galassi G, Kamieniecka Z, et al. Familial amyloid neuropathy and corneal lattice dystrophy. J Neurol Neurosurg Psychiatry 1979; 42:1020–1030. With permission.)*

tures of the neuropathy are similar in all four disorders.[98] Characteristically attacks of muscle weakness occur with a subacute onset over days or weeks. These attacks are often precipitated by drugs, in particular by barbiturates. The attacks may be preceded or accompanied by psychiatric disturbances and abdominal symptoms. The distribution of the muscle weakness and wasting is variable: it may be a generalized quadriparesis or proximal or distal in pattern. At times it may predominantly affect the upper limbs, and it may be asymmetrical. The tendon reflexes are depressed or lost, sometimes with paradoxical retention of the ankle jerks. Sensory symptoms are less frequent than motor involvement: These may be distal in distribution but can at times rather selectively affect the lower trunk and proximal lower limbs. The cranial nerves are frequently affected, most often with facial paralysis and bulbar palsy. Autonomic features are also common, including abdominal pain, vomiting, tachycardia, hypertension, and urinary retention. Cutaneous photosensitivity is an additional manifestation in variegate porphyria.

All three forms of hereditary hepatic porphyria except for δ-ALA dehydratase deficiency are considered to be of autosomal dominant inheritance. δ-ALA dehydratase deficiency is autosomal recessive. Apart from South Africa (and possible Finland), the acute intermittent variety is the most common. Variegate porphyria has a prevalence of 3 per 1000 individuals in the white population of South Africa.[99] The prevalence of acute intermittent porphyria, however, is low. The incidence in Sweden and England has been estimated as 1:13,000 and 1:18,000.[100,101] The porphyrias are disorders of heme metabolism. In the acute intermittent form, uroporphyrinogen 1 synthetase is deficient, causing a block in heme synthesis and an accumulation of δ-aminolevulinic acid and porphobilinogen, which appear in the urine in the acute attacks. Variegate porphyria is due to a deficiency in protoporphyrinogen oxidase. In hereditary coproporphyria, there is a deficiency of coproporphyrin oxidase. Coproporphyrin and protoporphyrin are excreted in large quantities in the feces. The mechanism of the damage to nervous tissues is not understood.

Early studies on small numbers of patients revealed electromyographic evidence of denervation and normal motor nerve conduction, both in acute intermittent porphyria[102] and in variegate porphyria.[103] Flügel and Druschky[104] studied 10 patients with acute intermittent porphyria, but only one was examined in the acute stage. They concluded that the changes were consistent with an axonal neuropathy. Albers et al.[105] reported a more extensive study on eight patients with an acute quadriparesis. EMG with needle electrodes revealed prominent spontaneous fibrillation potentials, especially in proximal muscles. Recruitment of MUs was reduced. In the earlier stages, the MU potentials were of normal appearance; later they tended to be polyphasic and of increased amplitude and duration. Evoked compound muscle action potentials were of reduced amplitude. Motor nerve conduction velocity was found to be normal, both for proximal and for distal muscles. This was also true for F wave latencies. Sensory conduction was normal in four of six patients in whom this was examined. In the other two individuals, sensory potentials were either absent or of reduced amplitude but with normal latencies. These findings confirm an axonal neuropathy with relative preservation of sensory fibers. This was also the conclusion reached by Wochnik-Dyjas et al.[106] and is consistent with the current neuropathologic evidence. Although earlier studies had raised the possibility of a demyelinating disorder,[107] the subsequent detailed investigation by Cavanagh and Mellick[108] established it as a distal axonopathy of the *dying-back* type. A similar conclusion has been reached for hereditary coproporphyria, where electromyographic evidence of denervation has been found, in conjunction with near-normal conduction velocity and reduced amplitude of compound sensory nerve action potentials.[109] Sural nerve biopsy showed predominant axonal damage.[110]

In vitro studies by Feldman et al.[111] raised the possibility of an interference with neuromuscular transmission produced by porphobilinogen and porphobilin, which was found to inhibit potassium-induced augmentation in the frequency of miniature end plate potentials, and reduced transmitter release with depolarization. Wochnik-Dyjas et al.[106] reported some potentiation on tetanic stimulation in patients with acute intermittent porphyria but no decrement. Albers et al.,[105] on the other hand, found no abnormalities of neuromuscular transmission.

Mustajoki and Seppäläinen[112] studied a series of patients with *latent* hereditary hepatic porphyria. These comprised patients both with acute intermittent and with variegate porphyria who either had no symptoms at the time of examination or who had never had symptoms. Maximal motor conduction velocity was found to be normal, but velocity in more slowly conducting fibers, studied by a blocking technique, was reduced in some nerves in some patients, as was upper limb sensory conduction velocity, even in individuals who had never had symptoms. It was

concluded that slight neuropathy occurs in such latent cases.

Disorders Associated with Defective DNA Repair

Ataxia telangiectasia

In ataxia telangiectasia, which is of autosomal recessive inheritance, a neurologic syndrome develops in early childhood consisting of cerebellar ataxia, oculomotor dyspraxia, and tendon areflexia. Distal weakness and sensory impairment, mainly for proprioception, develop later. These features are associated with oculocutaneous telangiectasia, immunologic incompetence, and defective DNA repair following gamma irradiation.

EMG shows signs of denervation in distal muscles. Motor conduction velocity is mildly slowed in older patients, and compound sensory nerve action potentials are diminished in amplitude or absent. This is related to loss of larger sensory myelinated fibers in the peripheral nerves.[113,114]

Xeroderma pigmentosum

Xeroderma pigmentosum constitutes a group of autosomal recessive disorders that primarily show dermatologic changes related to cutaneous photosensitivity. Skin malignancy is frequent. Excision repair following DNA damage produced by ultraviolet light is defective. Neurologic involvement may be confined to depression of the tendon reflexes. More severe involvement includes microcephaly, mental retardation, seizures, cerebellar ataxia, spasticity, choreoathetosis, and a sensorimotor neuropathy.[115]

Changes of denervation may be demonstrable on EMG.[116] Motor nerve conduction velocity is normal or slightly reduced, and compound sensory nerve action potentials are depressed or absent.[116,117] There is a loss of larger myelinated fibers in the peripheral nerves related to loss of dorsal root ganglion cells,[117,118] but with more demyelination than is usual in neuropathies that primarily give rise to axonal degeneration.

Cockayne's syndrome

This is a rare disorder in which growth retardation, progeria, cutaneous photosensitivity, mental retardation, pigmentary retinopathy, deafness, and hyporeflexia occur. DNA replication is inhibited by ultraviolet light. The changes in the central nervous system are those of a leukodystrophy.

Peripheral nerve involvement has been documented.[119–121] Motor nerve conduction velocity has been found to be markedly reduced, being 26 m per second, and 24 m per second in the median and peroneal nerves in a 4-year-old girl reported by Grunnet et al.[120] F wave latencies were correspondingly lengthened. Compound sensory nerve action potentials were found to be delayed and of reduced amplitude. The amplitudes of evoked compound muscle action potentials were normal. Nerve biopsy confirmed a demyelinating neuropathy.

Mucopolysaccharidoses and Oligosaccharidoses

Peripheral nerve involvement in the mucopolysaccharidoses is restricted clinically to entrapment neuropathies. In this group of disorders, glycosaminoglycans are stored in lysosomes in various tissues. The manifestations are mainly skeletal, with mental retardation in some forms. Entrapment neuropathies, particularly the carpal and cubital tunnel syndromes, may be encountered in the Hurler and Sheie syndromes, probably related to ligamentous thickening.[122,123] The carpal tunnel syndrome also occurs in I-cell disease (inclusion cell disease), an oligosaccharidosis.

Peripheral nerve involvement has been described in the cherry-red spot–myoclonus syndrome, an oligosaccharidosis related to a deficiency of lysosomal neuraminidase.[124] This disorder usually begins in the second or third decades of life and is dominated by action myoclonus. A nonpigmentary retinal degeneration occurs with cherry-red spots at the maculae. Affected individuals may complain of burning in the extremities.[125] A patient reported by Steinman et al.[126] who experienced intermittent tingling paresthesias in her feet and who had depressed ankle jerks showed moderate reductions of motor nerve conduction velocity but no electromyographic evidence of denervation. Sural compound sensory nerve action potentials were absent. A nerve biopsy demonstrated the presence of demyelination and inclusion material in Schwann cells thought probably to be mucopolysaccharide and lipoprotein.

Hexosaminidase Deficiency

The GM_2 gangliosidoses result from a deficiency either of hexosaminidase or of the activator protein for this enzyme. Hexosaminidase is found in human tissues as two major isozymes, hexosaminidase A and B (hex A and hex B). Hex A is composed of α-subunits and β-subunits coded for on chromosomes 15 and 5, whereas hex B is composed of only β-subunits. Thus a mutation at the alpha locus gives rise to a deficiency of hex A and a mutation at the β locus to a deficiency of hex A and hex B. Hex A deficiency is seen typically in Tay-Sachs disease and hex A and B deficiency in Sandhoff disease, both being characterized by a progressive disorder of early life with mental and motor regression. There have been descriptions of cases of juvenile or adult onset in which the salient feature has been a spinal muscular atrophy resembling Kugelberg-Welander disease associated with hex A deficiency.[127,128] Such cases have shown electromyographic evidence of denervation. Motor nerve conduction velocity has been preserved. Some individuals have had accompanying pyramidal features, ataxia, and dementia in varying combinations.[128] In one report,[129] there was a combination of an internuclear ophthalmoplegia with a mild sensory neuropathy. Nerve conduction studies and a nerve biopsy demonstrated an axonopathy. In another report[130] of a patient with hex A and B deficiency (Sandhoff disease), the clinical features resembled X-linked bulbospinal neuronopathy. There was electromyographic evidence of denervation with normal motor nerve conduction velocity and absent compound sensory nerve action potentials, although there was no clinically detectable sensory loss.

DISORDERS OF UNKNOWN CAUSATION

Neuropathies for which there is currently no known metabolic basis can conveniently be subdivided into neuronal degenerations that predominantly affect the lower motor neurons (HMNs or spinal muscular atrophies), those that affect both the lower motor and primary sensory neurons (HMSNs), and those that predominantly affect sensory and autonomic neurons (HSANs). There are also a number of miscellaneous conditions in which peripheral neuropathy exists as part of a multisystem neuronal degeneration or in association with involvement of other systems or in which distinctive neuropathologic features exist without the underlying metabolic disorder so far being apparent.

Hereditary Motor Neuronopathies (Spinal Muscular Atrophies)

The classification of HMN is still controversial but has been illuminated by advances in the molecular genetics of these disorders. The subdivisions have generally been made in terms of the age of onset, the distribution of muscle weakness, and the pattern of inheritance. The classification adopted here (Table

15.3) is that of Harding,[131] which incorporates those previously proposed by Emery[132] and Pearn.[133] Only a brief outline of the clinical features is given; more detailed aspects can be obtained by reference to these publications.

Hereditary proximal motor neuronopathies

Acute infantile SMA or Werdnig-Hoffmann disease (type I proximal SMA) is of autosomal recessive inheritance. The definition advocated by Pearn et al.[134] is currently the most acceptable, although wider delineations have been used in the past. Delayed motor development becomes apparent before 6 months of age and occasionally is evident prenatally with reduced fetal movements. Steady progression takes place and death occurs before the age of 4 years. There are other cases of autosomal recessive inheritance with an onset in infancy or childhood but with a more prolonged survival. Such cases were formerly termed *arrested Werdnig-Hoffmann*

TABLE 15.3. Hereditary motor neuronopathies (spinal muscular atrophies)

Hereditary proximal motor neuronopathies
   Type I (AR) (acute infantile, Werdnig-Hoffmann disease)
   Type II (AR) (chronic childhood)
   Type III (AR) (juvenile onset, Kugelberg-Welander disease)
   Type IV (AD) (juvenile onset)
   Type V (AD) (adult onset)
Hereditary distal motor neuronopathies (distal SMA, spinal form of CMT disease)
   Type I (AD) (juvenile onset)
   Type II (AD) (adult onset)
   Type III (AR) (mild juvenile)
   Type IV (AR) (severe juvenile)
   Type V (AD) (upper limb predominance)
Hereditary motor neuronopathies with complex distributions
   Scapuloperoneal
      Type I (AD)
      Type II (AD)
   Other forms
      Facioscapulohumeral (AD)
      Oculopharyngeal (AD)
      Bulbar (AR)

AR, Autosomal recessive; AD, autosomal dominant; SMA, spinal muscular atrophy; CMT, Charcot-Marie-Tooth.

disease and are best categorized as the chronic childhood form[135] (type II proximal SMA). The chronic form of hereditary proximal SMA (type III proximal SMA) defined by Kugelberg and Welander[136] has an onset between early childhood and adolescence. A wide range in age of onset has been described in different sibships, and the rate of advance also varies considerably.[131] The weakness tends to become generalized and, especially in cases of early onset, may lead to profound skeletal deformities, including scoliosis.

Acute infantile SMA has now been mapped to chromosome 5q12-q14.[137] More recently it has been shown that chronic childhood SMA also localizes to this region,[138,139] as does the gene in families with type III SMA (Kugelberg-Welander disease).[139,140] These disorders are therefore presumably allelic.

Autosomal dominant proximal HMN is uncommon but probably accounts for 30% of adult cases (type V SMA) but only 2% of childhood cases (type IV SMA).[141] The age of onset in the former is in the third or fourth decades.

Buchthal and Olsen[142] reported the electromyographic findings in a series of cases of spinal muscular atrophy with an onset before 2 years of age. In some patients, survival was prolonged, even up to 23 years of age; these patients are therefore likely to have been genetically heterogeneous. The most characteristic feature, both in the early and in the long survival cases, was the occurrence of spontaneous activity of a type originally described by Karlström and Wohlfart[143] and Buchthal and Clemmesen.[144] This was seen in three-quarters of the subjects studied by Buchthal and Olsen and consisted of regular discharging MU activity at a rate of 5 to 15 per second in relaxed muscles and during sleep. It differed from fasciculation in its regularity and in the fact that the units could be activated and graded voluntarily. Otherwise, needle EMG showed increased amplitude of MU potentials and, particularly in patients with longer survival, increased MU duration and territory. *Pseudomyotonia* and fasciculation were observed only in the subjects with longer survival. In comparison, juvenile-onset patients differed in displaying absence of the regular spontaneous activity; fasciculation was also observed more frequently in these subjects.

Further information has been provided by Hausmanowa-Petrusewicz and Karwanska,[145] who advocated a subdivision of the chronic SMAs with an onset in childhood or adolescence into four categories. Form Ia, the acute form, has an onset recorded at birth: affected children are never able to walk and do not survive beyond 4 years of age. In Form Ib, the onset is again recorded at birth or from the early months of life, and the children never learn to walk. Survival, however, is prolonged, being up to 30 years. In Form II, the age of onset is between the first and fifth years of life: the children become immobilized between the tenth and fourteenth years, and survival is prolonged. Finally, onset in Form III is between the first year of life and adolescence: complete immobilization does not occur, and survival is prolonged.[146] Interesting electrophysiologic differences were described between the four categories by Hausmanowa-Petrusewicz and Karwanska,[145] which may have both diagnostic and prognostic implications. The four categories were classified into three groups. Group A comprised the Form Ia cases and is equivalent to the acute infantile disease (type I as described above); group B comprised Forms Ib and II and represented *intermediate* cases; group C was the Form III cases, equivalent to chronic Kugelberg-Welander disease (type 2 proximal SMA as described above). Only groups A and B showed spontaneous rhythmically firing MUs, whereas in group C, pseudomyotonic discharges were present. MU parameters also differed. Group A showed bimodal distributions for amplitude and duration with both high-amplitude potentials of long duration and brief low-amplitude potentials. In the longer duration cases of groups B and C, the values of these parameters were shifted toward higher amplitudes and longer durations, although in the benign group C cases, there were brief low-amplitude potentials and also *linked* potentials. It is now known that these several groups probably represent allelic conditions. How many different alleles are involved has yet to be established.

Motor nerve conduction velocity is either normal or slightly reduced in patients with hereditary proximal SMA.[142,147] Moosa and Dubowitz[148] found that velocity tended to be slower in more severely affected patients, suggesting a selective loss of faster-conducting fibers. Sensory conduction was normal.

Electromyographic studies are of considerable assistance in the diagnosis of neuromuscular diseases in infancy and adolescence: in those less common cases with adult onset, such studies help in the differentiation of SMA from myopathic disorders such as limb girdle dystrophy. In case of doubt, muscle biopsy is merited, but frequently the electromyographic changes are sufficiently definite for a decision to be made without recourse to biopsy. Electromyographic studies are also helpful in the diagnosis of neonatal hypotonia, although in severe instances muscle biopsy is usually merited, particularly if a decision is required as to immediate management and genetic counseling.

Hereditary distal motor neuronopathies

The classification of HMN with a distal distribution (distal SMA) is complicated by the fact that this clinical presentation represents one form of Charcot-Marie-Tooth disease. The disorder is genetically heterogeneous, and classification is at present difficult. As for proximal SMA, the scheme advocated by Harding[131] is followed.

Type I distal SMA is an autosomal dominant disorder with an onset in childhood, usually before the age of 10 years. The lower limbs are involved to a greater extent than the upper, and foot deformity is common. The tendon reflexes, apart from ankle jerks, which are lost in one-third of the subjects, tend to be preserved. The prognosis is benign.[149,150] Late-onset cases with autosomal dominant inheritance, beginning in the third or fourth decades, are probably distinct genetically and constitute *type II distal SMA*. Such cases have been reported by Nelson and Amick[151] and McLeod and Prineas.[152] Patients with autosomal recessive inheritance may have a benign[150] or more rapidly progressive course[153] and constitute *types III and IV distal SMA*. Finally, cases occur in which the weakness begins in the upper limbs and may later involve the lower limbs. Inheritance has been autosomal dominant or sporadic.[150,154] They constitute *type V distal SMA*, although this category may not be genetically homogeneous. A further variant of distal SMA has been reported in which the onset is in infancy and in which there is early respiratory difficulty related to diaphragmatic paralysis.[155] The prognosis is poor.

EMG in all forms of distal SMA shows the customary findings of a chronic denervating process. Motor nerve conduction velocity has been found to be normal except occasionally when recordings have been made from severely denervated muscles. Compound sensory nerve action potentials have consistently been found to be of normal amplitude and latency.[150–153] Difficulty may be encountered in the differentiation between cases of SMA of adult onset and isolated nongenetic cases of chronic SMA in which the disorder remains confined to the lower motor neurons. In general, electrodiagnostic studies are not helpful in their differentiation. Prominent asymmetry of involvement is suggestive of a nongenetic cause,[156] although minor degrees of asymmetry may be present in familial cases.

Hereditary motor neuronopathies with complex distributions

Dominantly inherited scapuloperoneal muscular atrophy—*type I scapuloperoneal SMA* in the classification of Harding[131]—is a rare condition. The reported cases have been reviewed by Serratrice et al.[157] The essential clinical features have an onset in childhood, adolescence, or early adult life, usually in the legs, and the disease affects the anterolateral lower leg muscles. Proximal upper limb weakness, involving the scapular and upper arm muscles, is usually a later event. Progression is slow. Mild bulbar and facial muscle weakness may occur, and the tendon reflexes may become depressed.

EMG, including studies of the tongue muscles, has shown a neurogenic pattern with MU potentials of increased amplitude and duration and a reduced recruitment pattern. Spontaneous fibrillation potentials and fasciculation may be detected. Difficulties are sometimes encountered in deciding whether the changes are neurogenic or myopathic, as was evident in the family reported by Kaeser.[158] Motor nerve conduction velocity has been found to be normal, as have compound sensory nerve action potentials, although the latter may become depressed later in the course of the disease.[159] The neurogenic scapuloperoneal syndrome must be distinguished from myopathic disorders with this distribution, including an X-linked form with an onset in childhood[160,161] that is probably a variant of the Emery-Dreifuss syndrome,[162] dominantly inherited adult-onset cases,[163] and sporadic cases. In view of the difficulty in obtaining decisive electromyographic findings in some patients, muscle biopsy is often required for a definitive diagnosis. A neuropathic scapuloperoneal syndrome associated with distal sensory loss has also been described (Davidenkow's syndrome) (see page 410), but this may just be a phenotypic variant of HMSN type I.[164]

Scapuloperoneal SMA with autosomal recessive inheritance—*type II scapuloperonal SMA* in the classification of Harding[131]—also occurs, and such cases are probably more frequent than the dominant form. The course is more aggressive, at least at first. There again may be difficulty in deciding whether the electromyographic changes are myopathic or neurogenic.[165] Motor conduction velocity has been found to be normal or slightly reduced and sensory nerve conduction normal.

An X-linked scapuloperoneal SMA has also been described.[166] The clinical features so closely resemble the myopathic form reported by Rotthauwe et al.[160]

and Thomas et al.[161] and constituting a variant of Emery-Dreifuss muscular dystrophy that its status must remain in doubt.

X-linked bulbospinal neuronopathy was initially recognized by Kennedy et al.,[167] and subsequent descriptions were reviewed by Harding et al.[168] The onset of muscle weakness is usually during the third or fourth decades and at first generally affects proximal lower limb muscles and later proximal upper limb and bulbar muscles, with tongue wasting, dysphagia, and dysarthria. Contraction fasciculation of the facial muscles may be conspicuous. The tendon reflexes tend to be depressed, and there is frequently an antecedent history of muscle cramps and a postural tremor in the upper limbs. Mild distal sensory loss in the lower limbs may occur.[169] Gynecomastia is present in over 50% of patients, and fertility may be reduced.

The gene for this disorder was localized to the proximal long arm of the X chromosome by Fischbeck et al.,[170] and it is of considerable interest in view of the clinical manifestations that it has been shown to involve a mutation within the androgen receptor gene.[171]

EMG demonstrates denervation, and motor nerve conduction velocity is either normal or slightly reduced.[168,169] Although the disorder was initially considered to be a bulbospinal muscular atrophy, compound sensory nerve action potentials are of reduced amplitude or absent, and sensory nerve conduction velocity may be mildly reduced.[168,169] It was for this reason that Harding et al.[168] proposed the name *X-linked bulbospinal neuronopathy* for the disorder. Autopsy studies have shown loss of lower brain stem and spinal motor neurons[167,169] and loss of dorsal root ganglion cells.[169] Sural nerve biopsy reveals loss of sensory axons.[172]

Other rare inherited motor neuronopathies with complex distributions include a dominantly inherited disorder with a facioscapulohumeral distribution[173] and another of oculopharyngeal distribution.[174] The Vialetto–van Laere syndrome comprises a recessive disorder with onset in the first two decades of a progressive bulbar palsy associated with deafness, later spreading to limb and trunk muscles.[175] Fazio-Londe disease is also a progressive bulbar palsy of childhood, unassociated with deafness.[176]

Hereditary Motor and Sensory Neuropathies

Charcot-Marie-Tooth disease (peroneal muscular atrophy) is a genetically heterogeneous group of disorders, the classification of which has become easier since the introduction of nerve conduction studies and the more widespread use of nerve biopsy as a diagnostic procedure. They are also being clarified by molecular genetic studies. Current classifications are based on the subdivisions originally defined by Dyck and Lambert,[177,178] although modifications are still being introduced. The historical development of concepts concerning this group of disorders has been reviewed by Harding and Thomas.[179] As has already been stated (see page 405), one variety of Charcot-Marie-Tooth disease is represented by hereditary distal SMA. The other varieties show accompany sensory involvement, either clinically evident or detectable only by studies of sensory conduction or sensory nerve biopsy. These are designated *hereditary motor and sensory neuropathy* (HMSN) and are again divisible into several groups.

HMSN type I is distinguished by the presence of prominent peripheral nerve demyelination and often hypertrophic changes, whereas HMSN type II is characterized by predominant axonal degeneration with little demyelination. This is reflected by a bimodal distribution of motor conduction velocities for cases of HMSN as a whole[179–181] (Figure 15.3). If motor conduction velocity in index cases is plotted against that in affected relatives (Figure 15.4), two clusters are evident, one with severely reduced velocities corresponding to HMSN I and the other with normal or mildly reduced velocities corresponding

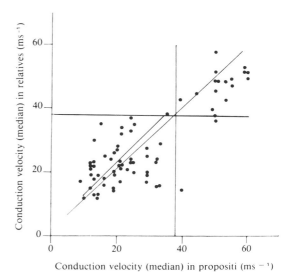

FIGURE 15-4. *Relationship between motor conduction velocity in median nerve for index cases and affected relatives in patients with hereditary motor and sensory neuropathy (HMSN). The data cluster into two groups with an approximate separation at 38 m/s (vertical and horizontal lines). There is a positive correlation (longer regression line) for the total data (r = 0.79, p < 0.001) and also for the cluster with severely reduced conduction velocity (HMSN type I; shorter regression line, r = 0.71, p < 0.001).*

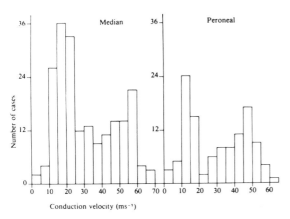

FIGURE 15.3. *Frequency distribution of motor conduction velocity in median and peroneal nerves in patients with hereditary motor and sensory neuropathy. (From Harding AE, Thomas PK. The clinical features of hereditary motor and sensory neuropathy, types I and II. Brain 1980; 103:259–280. With permission.)*

to HMSN II. The existence of genetic heterogeneity is indicated by a significant correlation coefficient between the values for the index cases and affected relatives. It must be realized that this is a statistical subdivision because some degree of overlap for motor nerve conduction velocity is evident between families, and Jones et al.[182] found discordance between motor and sensory conduction velocity values in occasional subjects. Buchthal and Behse,[183] however, found no overlap between the two groups for sural nerve conduction velocity, and complete concordance for conduction velocity was found between index patients and affected relatives in the family study on dominantly inherited HMSN I reported by Combarros et al.[184] There may be differences between the two sides of the body in some patients,[182] although overall the changes are usually generalized with a good concordance between different nerves.[183]

Hereditary motor and sensory neuropathy type I

The clinical features of HMSN I and II are similar, and it may be difficult to allocate individual cases to one or the other category. Nevertheless, broad differences exist.[179] In type I, the onset is usually in the first decade, ocasionally from birth, less frequently in the second decade, and rather rarely thereafter. Slowly progressive distal weakness and wasting occur, maximal in the lower limbs, accompanied by tendon areflexia. Postural tremor of the upper limbs may be present. Distal sensory loss occurs: this affects all modalities and is of variable severity. Foot deformity, usually pes cavus, clawing of the toes, and an equinovarus position, is common; clawing of the fingers may occur in later stages. Scoliosis may develop in severe early-onset patients. The peripheral nerves are thickened in about 50% of patients. Clinical expression is highly variable, and mild or asymptomatic patients, particularly female, are frequent. Most families show autosomal dominant inheritance, but autosomal recessive inheritance is also observed.[185] Patients with the latter form tend to be more severely affected. Isolated cases without evident family history are relatively frequent. Careful examination of relatives, however, including nerve conduction studies, may bring to light affected but asymptomatic individuals or others in whom some other diagnosis has been made, such as arthritis. The

possibility of identifying isolated patients with HMSN Ia (see later) by DNA analysis now exists.

EMG demonstrates changes of chronic partial denervation, maximal in distal muscles and greater in the lower than in the upper limbs. Buchthal and Behse[183] found that in a large series of patients with HMSN I, in muscles innervated by the common peroneal nerve, most patients showed a discrete MU potential pattern. Fibrillation potentials and positive sharp wave potentials were present in about one-half of these subjects, but fasciculation potentials were seen in less than 10%. Pseudomyotonic bursts were not recorded. In more than 50% of subjects, there was evidence of reinnervation. The duration and amplitude of MU potentials were increased, as was MU territory. Pseudomyotonic bursts were noted by Bouché et al.[181] but less frequently than in cases of HMSN II.

Motor nerve conduction velocity is usually severely reduced, usually being in the range of 15 to 35 m per second in the median and ulnar nerves (Figure 15.5). It is not possible to define a precise cutoff point from type II patients. In a large series, Harding and Thomas[179] found that a value of 38 m per second discriminated between most affected individuals. More restricted ranges have been obtained in smaller series.[182,186] Compound sensory nerve action potentials are usually absent or dispersed and of low amplitude with percutaneous recordings, but

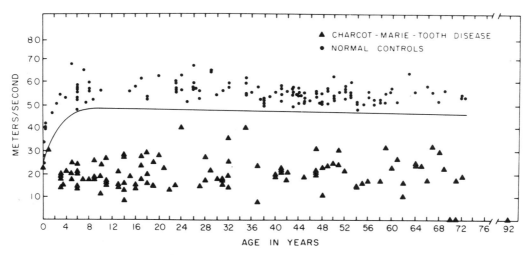

FIGURE 15.5. *Median nerve motor conduction velocities in 107 patients with hereditary motor and sensory neuropathy type I (triangles) plotted against age and compared with values for normal controls (circles). (Reprinted with permission from Gutmann L, Fakadej A, Riggs JE. Evolution of nerve conduction abnormalities in children with dominant hypertrophic neuropathy of the Charcot-Marie-Tooth type. Muscle Nerve 1983; 6:515–519.*

conduction velocity is found to be severely reduced if action potentials are collected through needle electrodes employing computer averaging of large numbers of responses[183] or estimated from cervical somatosensory potentials. Distal motor latencies may be selectively prolonged.[187] Buchthal and Behse[183] found maximum conduction velocity in the sural nerve to be 13 to 32 m per second, corresponding to 23% to 57% of normal. Amplitudes were severely reduced, being 0.3 to 0.7 μV, corresponding to 0.3% to 8% of normal. The severity of slowing of conduction in sensory fibers is, in general, less than that in motor fibers.[183]

Cases of HMSN type I with autosomal recessive inheritance tend to show a greater incidence of weakness, ataxia, tendon areflexia, and scoliosis than the dominant form, and nerve conduction velocity is significantly slower. Harding and Thomas[179] found a mean value for median motor conduction velocity was 16.5 m per second in recessive subjects, as compared with a mean of 21.1 m per second in patients with autosomal dominant inheritance.

The age of onset at which abnormalities of nerve conduction can first be detected in individuals with dominantly inherited HMSN I is uncertain, but it is probably in infancy. Combarros et al.[184] found marked slowing of nerve conduction to be present at the age of 2 to 5 years at a stage when clinical signs and symptoms were trivial, and Gutmann et al.[188] showed that it may be detectable as early as 17 months. The latter authors showed that maximal slowing of motor nerve conduction velocity evolves over the first 3 to 5 years of life (see Figure 15.5). Prolongation of the distal motor latency may be the earliest detectable change, and this abnormality evolves over 10 or more years.

The major explanation for the reduction in nerve conduction velocity is widespread demyelination and remyelination, but loss of larger and faster conducting fibers and possibly axonal atrophy may contribute.[183] The slowing of conduction in HMSN I is uniform, and significant conduction block is not a feature.[189] This may be helpful in distinguishing patients with HMSN from chronic inflammatory demyelinating polyneuropathy, in which velocity tends not to be concordant between different nerves or between different segments of the same nerve (Figure 15.6) and in which conduction block is often demonstrable.

The electrophysiologic evidence for genetic heterogeneity in HMSN[139] (see Figure 15.4) has been confirmed by genetic linkage studies. It is now clear that in the majority of families with autosomal dom-

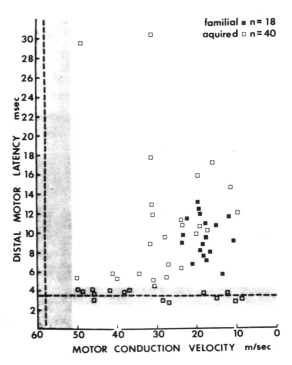

FIGURE 15.6. *Scattergram of median nerve distal motor latency and forearm conduction velocity of patients with hereditary motor and sensory neuropathy (HMSN) type I (filled squares) and chronic inflammatory demyelinating polyneuropathy (open squares). The scatter for the HMSN patients is considerably less. The shaded areas represent normal mean values ±2 SD. (Reprinted with permission from Lewis RA, Sumner AJ. The electrodiagnostic distinction between chronic familial and acquired demyelinative neuropathies. Arch Neurol 1982; 82:592–596.)*

inant HMSN I, the mutation is on chromosome 17.[190–193] This form has been designated as HMSN Ia. Studies have established that in most families with HMSN Ia so far examined, there is a segmental duplication at the site of the gene, probably amounting to greater than 500 kb.[194–195] The presence of this duplication means that it is possible to identify individual cases without a positive family history. Rarely, there is a point mutation. In other families, but much less frequently, an abnormal gene is located on the proximal arm of chromosome 1, linked to the Duffy blood group locus.[196–198] This form has been designated HMSN Ib. Finally, in other families, linkage to markers on both chromosomes 1 and 17 appears to have been excluded, suggesting the possibility of a further autosomal locus.[192,193]

Patients with prominent associated tremor are sometimes designated as having the *Roussy-Lévy syndrome*.[199] They are not genetically distinct and constitute a phenotypic variant of HMSN I, occurring in families other members of which have typical manifestations,[179] as may patients with a scapuloperoneal distribution of muscle weakness (Davidenkow's syndrome).[164]

Hereditary motor and sensory neuropathy type II

The clinical features of dominantly inherited HMSN II[178,179] differ from those of HMSN I in that the age of onset is maximal in the second rather than the first decade of life. Many patients, however, initially develop symptoms within the first decade, but, additionally, the onset is often delayed until adult life, sometimes as late as the seventh decade. In comparison with HMSN I, there is less upper limb involvement, although the calf muscles are often more severely affected, simultaneously with the anterolateral compartment lower limb muscles. Tremor and ataxia and widespread tendon areflexia are generally less evident, as is the severity of sensory loss. Foot deformity is likewise less, this presumably being related to the later age of onset. The location of the gene responsible for HMSN II has not been established.

As for HMSN I, EMG shows a reduced MU recruitment pattern with evidence of reinnervation. Fibrillation potentials and positive sharp wave potentials may be recorded, but fasciculation potentials and pseudomyotonic bursts are more frequent, both being detected in 20% to 25% of subjects in the series reported by Buchthal and Behse.[183]

Motor nerve conduction velocity is less severely reduced than in HMSN I. It may be within normal limits or moderately diminished, and, as already stated, motor nerve conduction velocity overlaps the values for HMSN I to a greater extent than does sensory conduction velocity. Maximum sensory conduction velocity in the sural nerve in the series of Buchthal and Behse[183] was 39 to 56 m per second. Compound sensory nerve action potential amplitudes are reduced, particularly in the lower limbs, where potentials were often unobtainable with percutaneous recordings. Buchthal and Behse[183] found amplitudes of 0.5 to 5 μV, corresponding to 0.7% to 59% of normal. In the median nerve, amplitudes are less severely reduced, but the proportionate degree of slowing of conduction velocity is similar.

Nerve biopsy shows loss of larger myelinated fibers, with normal numbers of small fibers, this probably being related to regeneration because regenerative clusters are frequent. It is clear that fiber loss is not confined to those of larger diameter. Segmental demyelination and remyelination and hypertrophic changes are rare or absent.[183] Autopsy studies have shown that the distal portions of both motor and sensory axons are predominantly affected and that there is loss of anterior horn and dorsal root ganglion cells.[200,201]

An interesting feature that is occasionally encountered in HMSN II is the occurrence of the continuous MU activity syndrome (neuromyotonia).[202,203] The same phenomenon may occasionally be shown by patients with HMN.[204] Affected patients complain of muscle stiffness and cramps and show persistent fascicular contractions or myokymia in distal limb muscles, together with delayed relaxation after contraction. The excessive muscular contraction is insufficient to cause postural deformity. Although distal muscle wasting is present, proximal lower limb muscles may be abnormally bulky. Signs of chronic partial denervation may be present, with spontaneous fibrillation potentials, reduced MU recruitment, and enlarged polyphasic MU potentials. The characteristic feature of neuromyotonia is the occurrence of spontaneous bursts of potentials, usually 0.5 to 1.5 mV in amplitude, with an abrupt onset and a duration of several seconds. The firing frequency of the potentials is high (200 to 250 per s), but tends to decline during the burst.[203] Discharges may be provoked by needle movement and muscle percussion. Following voluntary contraction, MU activity at high rates may persist for 10 to 20 seconds, the frequency of the discharges waxing and waning during this period. With repeated voluntary contraction, these discharges become less intense.[202] Regional neuromuscular blockade with curare has established an origin in motor nerve fibers.[202] In neuromyotonia, ectopic impulses can probably originate throughout the whole length of the axon, including its terminal arborization. Consequently the electromyographic recordings contain a range of potentials, some of which resemble MU activity, others of which are similar to fibrillation potentials. There may be accompanying evidence from intraneural recordings suggestive of ectopic impulse generation in sensory fibers, but sensory symptoms are not prominent.[202]

Autosomal recessive families with HMSN II have been described.[181,185,205,206] The onset is earlier, usually before the age of 5 years, and weakness tends to be more severe than in the dominant cases. The clinical features suggest that further genetic heterogeneity probably exists. Some cases are milder with a later onset.[185] Those described by Ouvrier et al.,[206] on the other hand, had severe paralysis by the age of 20 years, and a number of these subjects became unable to walk during adolescence. Motor nerve conduction velocities ranged from 35 m per second to the upper part of the normal range, and compound sensory nerve action potentials were small or unobtainable. Similar cases have been described by Gabreëls-Festen et al.[207] and were considered probably to represent autosomal recessive HMSN II.

X-linked hereditary motor and sensory neuropathy

Although many previous large series of patients with HMSN failed to identify X-linked pedigrees, it is clear that, although not common, the occurrence of X-linked dominant inheritance is now well established. A large pedigree, originally reported by Allan[208] in 1939, was investigated by Rozear et al.,[209] and a large Canadian kindred was reported by Hahn et al.[210] A number of other families have also been documented. The gene has been mapped to the proximal long arm of the X chromosome near Xq 13.[211]

The onset of the disorder is in early childhood, with typical features of the peroneal muscular atrophy syndrome, involving both the lower and the upper limbs. Males are severely affected, whereas females have mild or subclinical disease. Electrophysiologic studies show evidence of denervation in distal muscles with a mild reduction of motor nerve conduction velocity. Sural compound sensory nerve action potentials are of severely reduced amplitude or absent.[210] Nerve biopsies show loss of myelinated and unmyelinated axons, regenerative sprouting, and secondary demyelination.[210] It was concluded that the disorder represents a primary axonopathy.

Hereditary motor and sensory neuropathy type III

HMSN type III constitutes a rare autosomal recessive disorder that is likely to be genetically heterogeneous. It includes childhood-onset cases of mixed motor and sensory neuropathy that are sometimes referred to as Dejerine-Sottas disease.[212] It also includes congenital cases.[213] The histologic feature that these patients share is the presence of severe hypomyelination in addition to recurrent demyelination and remyelination.[212,213] Myelin sheaths of normal thickness are never achieved. They therefore differ from autosomal recessive cases of HMSN type II.[185] Hypotonic weakness may be present from birth. In other subjects, motor milestones are delayed, and

normal development is not attained. Motor nerve conduction velocity is very severely reduced, usually to less than 10 m per second and sometimes to less than 5 m per second, commensurate with the extensive lack of myelin found histologically. Conduction velocities as low as this are not usually encountered in acquired or other inherited neuropathies in children, but nerve biopsy is usually merited to achieve a definitive diagnosis. The disorder has to be distinguished from chronic inflammatory demyelinating polyneuropathy in childhood, in which nerve conduction velocity may be severely reduced and in which pes cavus or other foot deformity may occur. The occurrence of pes cavus is often erroneously taken to imply genetic neuropathy in such cases.

Complex forms of hereditary motor and sensory neuropathy

A number of publications have drawn attention to the occurrence of cases of peroneal muscular atrophy with a variety of associated features indicating involvement of the central nervous system.[183,186,214,215] In some subjects, nerve conduction velocity may be markedly reduced, comparable to HMSN I, and in others less severely so, with values similar to those of HMSN II. How many of these cases represent separate genetic entities is uncertain because extensive family studies have rarely been reported. This is required to establish the range of manifestations of individual genes. Moreover, some distal amyotrophy may be a feature of a number of recognized genetic disorders, including Friedreich's ataxia and hereditary spastic paraplegia.

Perhaps the most clearly established variant is peroneal muscular atrophy with pyramidal features[178,216] or HMSN V in the classification of Dyck.[285] Some patients with HMSN I have extensor plantar responses, which is occasionally related to spinal cord compression from enlarged spinal roots. The plantar responses are less commonly extensor in HMSN II. There are families, however, in which associated pyramidal features constitute a regular feature, in association with other manifestations of the type that occur in peroneal muscular atrophy, most closely resembling HMSN II. Harding and Thomas[216] found that the onset was usually in the first two decades with difficulty in walking. The course was benign. Distal weakness and wasting affected the lower limbs to a greater extent than the upper. The tendon reflexes tended to be increased in the arms as were the knee jerks, but the ankle jerks were often absent. Sensory loss was variable.

The degree of reduction in motor nerve conduction velocity was inconsistent, even within families, and compound sensory action potentials were reduced or absent in two-thirds of their series of 25 patients. The condition may not be genetically homogeneous. Most families showed autosomal dominant inheritance.

In a group of patients with HMSN who had accompanying pyramidal signs, Claus et al.[217] found prolonged central motor conduction time on recording from a distal upper limb muscle. The prolongation was greater for patients with HMSN I than HMSN II. Central motor conduction time was consistently normal in *uncomplicated* cases of HMSN I and II. More recently, Schnider et al.[218] studied a family with peroneal muscular atrophy with pyramidal signs (HMSN V) and assessed central motor conduction time on recording from tibialis anterior. Affected members consistently showed a prolonged central conduction time. Other types of *complicated* HMSN include association with optic atrophy, optic atrophy and deafness, and pigmentary retinal degeneration.[285] These conditions are so far poorly characterized.

Hereditary Sensory and Autonomic Neuropathies

As is true for the HMSNs, the classification of those that primarily affect sensory and autonomic function has become clearer, particularly in relation to such syndromes as *congenital indifference to pain*. There is overlap between the phenotypic manifestations of those conditions that primarily affect sensory and those that predominantly affect autonomic function. It is therefore convenient to combine them into a single category.[219]

Dominantly inherited sensory neuropathy

Sensory neuropathy with autosomal dominant inheritance was first defined by Denny-Brown[220] under the title of *hereditary sensory radicular neuropathy*. It constitutes HSAN type I in the classification of Dyck.[221] Onset is usually in the second decade with distal sensory loss in the limbs that initially affects pain and temperature sensibility and later other modalities. Spontaneous pain may be troublesome, and a mutilating acropathy is a frequent development. Apart from some distal loss of sweating and occasional vesical involvement, autonomic symptoms are not a feature. Mild distal muscle weakness and wasting are relatively frequent, and occasionally more severe distal involvement occurs.

Motor conduction velocity is usually normal or low normal. Compound sensory nerve action potentials are reduced in amplitude or absent. Signs of denervation may be present in distal lower limb muscles. Observations on the compound action potential in excised sural nerve[213] have shown a considerable decrease in the amplitude of the A α, A δ, and C fiber potentials, the diminution being least for the A α peak and greatest for the C fiber potential, with an intermediate decrease in the A δ peak. This correlates with a severe loss of unmyelinated axons and a reduction in the number of myelinated axons that is greater for those of small size.

Recessively inherited sensory neuropathy

Sensory neuropathy of autosomal recessive inheritance (HSAN type II), in contradistinction to the dominant form, affects all sensory modalities and is usually present from birth or infancy. Affected children frequently develop mutilating changes in the extremities.[222] Some autonomic deficits may occur, including vesical dysfunction and impotence, and the disorder is probably slowly progressive,[223] although some reports have claimed that neurologic progression, as distinct from the development of a mutilating acropathy, does not occur. Mild distal muscle weakness may be present.

EMG of distal muscles may reveal fibrillation potentials and a reduced MU recruitment pattern, and the amplitude of evoked compound muscle action potentials may be reduced. Motor nerve conduction velocity is at the lower limit of the normal range or is slightly reduced. Compound sensory nerve action potentials are absent.[222,223] In a study with in vitro recordings from sensory nerves, A α and A δ potentials were absent; a C fiber potential was detected in the sural nerve but not in the superficial peroneal nerve.[222]

Familial dysautonomia

Familial dysautonomia (HSAN type III) or the *Riley-Day syndrome* is a rare autosomal recessive disorder encountered most often in Jewish children. Manifestations are evident from birth and include difficulty in feeding, recurrent vomiting, and pulmonary infections, together with autonomic disturbances such as diminished lacrimation, impaired temperature regulation, postural hypotension and episodes of hypertension, and cutaneous blotching and excessive sweating provoked by emotional stimuli. Tendon areflexia and a failure to respond to painful stimuli are evident from birth. Kyphoscoliosis may develop in later childhood. Nerve biopsy demonstrates a severe loss of unmyelinated axons and a less severe depletion of small myelinated axons, probably related to neuronal aplasia.[224]

Motor nerve conduction velocity in the lower limbs has been found to be mildly reduced, and the amplitude or compound sensory nerve action potentials is greatly diminished.[225]

Other inherited sensory and autonomic neuropathies

Congenital sensory neuropathy with anhidrosis (HSAN type IV) is a further rare congenital sensory neuropathy originally delineated by Swanson et al.[226] There is a selective loss of small myelinated fibers and a virtual absence of unmyelinated axons in the peripheral nerves. Detailed results of EMG and nerve conduction studies do not appear to have been reported.

The earlier literature records patients diagnosed as *having congenital insensitivity to pain, asymbolia for pain,* and the like, in which no underlying structural changes were evident in the nervous system. One possible explanation for such patients is the disorder described by Dyck,[219] Low,[227] Donaghy[228] and their associates, which appears to represent a further type of congenital nonprogressive sensory neuropathy with a selective loss of pain sensibility. Sweating may be impaired.[219,228] Nerve biopsy shows a selective depletion of small myelinated fibers with preservation of large myelinated fibers and a relative preservation of unmyelinated axons. Such an abnormality is likely to have escaped notice before the use of contemporary morphometric methods for the study of peripheral nerve histology. An unexplained feature is the loss of pain appreciation in the face of relatively normal densities of unmyelinated axons. It is conceivable that there is a selective depletion of nociceptive C fibers or a neurotransmitter defect. Needle EMG, motor nerve conduction velocity, and compound sensory nerve action potentials are normal.[219,228] In vitro recordings of the sural compound nerve action potential have revealed a good Aα potential and a slightly reduced C fiber potential. The Aδ potential, by contrast, has been found to be small, particularly the lower velocity component.[219]

Neuropathy in Spinocerebellar Degeneration, Hereditary Spastic Paraplegia, and Inherited Extrapyramidal Disorders

Friedreich's ataxia

The observations provided by the Quebec cooperative study[229] and the extensive family study of Harding[230] have done much to clarify the definition of Friedreich's ataxia. It is now evident that it is an autosomal recessive disorder with an onset almost always before the age of 20. The diagnostic criteria have been defined in these studies. It is clear that involvement of the peripheral nervous system is an early and consistent feature of the disorder, predominantly related to loss of larger dorsal root ganglion cells, with consequent impairment of large fiber sensory modalities, that is, discriminative tactile sensibility, joint position sense, and vibration sense. In the later stages of the disease, distal amyotrophy in the limbs, because of loss of anterior horn cells, may become apparent. There has been a tendency in the past to label early-onset spinocerebellar degenerations somewhat indiscriminately as Friedreich's ataxia. If strict diagnostic criteria are applied, it is clear that it is a genetically homogeneous disorder. The gene has been mapped to the long arm of chromosome 9.[231]

Nerve conduction in Friedreich's ataxia was initially investigated by Dyck and Lambert[178] and subsequently by others.[230,232–239] Motor nerve conduction velocity is mildly but significantly reduced. Thus in the study by McLeod,[232] the mean values for the median, ulnar, and peroneal nerves were 48, 46, and 37 m per second. Evidence of denervation may be detectable in distal muscles. Compound sensory nerve action potentials are reduced in amplitude or undetectable with conventional recordings. Ouvrier et al.[240] demonstrated that abnormalities develop early in the course of the disease and are progressive. Later there is little correlation between the electrophysiologic (or histologic) changes in the peripheral nerves and the clinical state. In vitro recordings of the sural compound nerve action potentials made by Lambert and Dyck[241] demonstrated a selective loss of large myelinated fibers.

Nerve conduction studies constitute a most important aspect in the diagnosis of Friedreich's ataxia. The Roussy-Lévy variant of HMSN of I is frequently misdiagnosed as Friedreich's ataxia. The prognosis and the genetic implications of the two disorders are quite different. The distinction between them can readily be made on the basis of the substantially reduced motor nerve conduction velocity in the Roussy-Lévy syndrome. Friedreich's ataxia must also be distinguished from early-onset hereditary ataxia with retained tendon reflexes.[242] This is also an autosomal recessive disorder with clinical features that resemble Friedreich's ataxia but with a more benign prognosis. In addition to retention of the tendon reflexes, cardiomyopathy does not occur, and there is no association with diabetes. Compound sensory nerve action potentials are usually normal, as is motor conduction velocity.[242] Abetalipoproteinemia and ataxia telangiectasia may also be confused with Friedreich's ataxia but cannot be differentiated from the latter on the basis of electrodiagnostic findings.

X-linked recessive spinocerebellar degeneration

The syndrome has an onset in the first or second decades and consists of a slowly progressive disorder combining cerebellar ataxia, distal amyotrophy in the lower limbs, exaggerated tendon reflexes, and extensor plantar responses. Mild loss of vibration and joint position sense occurs in older subjects.[243] The course is benign.

Motor nerve conduction velocity is mildly reduced. Compound sensory nerve action potentials are preserved but diminish in amplitude in older subjects.[243]

Behr's syndrome

This disorder consists of the development in early childhood of a spinocerebellar degeneration in association with mental retardation and optic atrophy. It is probably genetically heterogeneous. Some subjects exhibit peripheral nerve involvement.[244] Motor nerve conduction velocity in such patients is normal. Compound sensory nerve action potentials are reduced or absent. Nerve biopsy shows loss of myelinated nerve fibers with little evidence of demyelination.

Late-onset cerebellar ataxia

The classification of hereditary ataxia in which the onset of symptoms occurs in the third decade or later is still a matter of uncertainty. The majority of these cases probably belong to a dominantly inherited disorder in which cerebellar ataxia is variably associated with dementia, extrapyramidal features, optic atrophy, disorders of eye movement, distal amyotrophy in the limbs, and depression of tendon reflexes.[245] Such patients are often referred to as having olivopontocerebellar atrophy or cerebello-olivary degeneration. McLeod and Evans[246] reported the results of nerve conduction studies in a series of patients considered on clinical grounds to have these diagnoses. Motor conduction velocity in the peroneal nerve was slowed for the group of 19 patients as a whole, no significant reduction being evident for the median or ulnar nerve. More severe changes in sensory conduction were observed with depression or loss of both upper and lower limb compound sensory action potentials. Wadia et al.[247] found normal motor conduction velocity and depression or loss of compound sensory nerve action potentials in patients

from India, along with a clinical diagnosis of olivopontocerebellar atrophy and slow eye movements.

Pollock and Kies[248] have described a late-onset cerebellar ataxia in which extensive, near global, thermoanalgesia was present. Inheritance was probably autosomal dominant. Needle EMG showed evidence of chronic partial denervation in distal muscles. Motor nerve conduction velocity was in the lower normal range, and compound sensory nerve action potentials were of reduced amplitude or absent.

Hereditary spastic paraplegias

In cases of *pure* spastic paraplegia (Strümpell's disease), both motor and sensory conduction have been found to be normal.[249] Mild distal limb wasting may occur, with electromyographic findings indicating chronic partial denervation. In *complex* forms of hereditary spastic paraplegia, more prominent distal amyotrophy related to loss of anterior horn cells may develop, as in the form described by Silver[250] with distal upper limb wasting or in the Troyer syndrome.[251] In Charlevoix-Saguenay autosomal recessive spastic ataxia,[237] signs of denervation are evident in the limbs. Motor conduction velocity is moderately reduced (24 to 16 m/s in the ulnar nerve and 22 to 36 m/s in the peroneal nerve). Compound sensory nerve action potentials are depressed or absent.

A further autosomal recessive disorder, in which spastic paraparesis is associated with disordered skin and hair pigmentation,[252] is accompanied by a mild sensory neuropathy. Lower limb compound sensory nerve action potentials are absent. Motor nerve conduction is normal. In another disorder of autosomal dominant inheritance,[253] spastic paraplegia is accompanied by a distal lower limb motor neuropathy. Motor conduction velocity in the peroneal nerve is moderately reduced. Finally, a disorder has been described marked by a combination of spastic paraplegia and severe sensory neuropathy. The onset is in childhood.[254] Motor conduction velocity was found to be normal, but sensory conduction was not recorded.

Extrapyramidal system degenerations

Neuroacanthocytosis[255] consists of a progressive disorder with an onset in adult life of a syndrome that is dominated by a movement disorder that has most often been described as choreiform, but dystonia and stereotyped tics may occur, and a rigid parkinsonism may gradually supersede an earlier hyperkinetic state. Choreiform orofacial dyskinesia is frequent, interfering with mastication and speech, and is often sufficient to cause tongue or lip biting. Involuntary vocalization may occur. Dementia develops in approximately one-third, and milder cognitive impairment has probably been underestimated in the past. Psychiatric symptoms are frequent. Distal amyotrophy and weakness, predominantly in the lower limbs, are common, and depression or loss of tendon reflexes occurs. The disorder is associated with abnormal spiny erythrocytes (acanthocytes) in the peripheral blood, although repeated sampling may be required to detect them.

The inheritance of neuroacanthocytosis is unclear. Both autosomal dominant and autosomal recessive inheritance have been described, and an association with the McLeod phenotype in some cases raises the possibility of a locus for neuroacanthocytosis on the short arm of the X chromosome.

EMG shows evidence of chronic partial denervation. Motor nerve conduction velocity is normal but compound sensory nerve action potentials are of reduced amplitude or are absent.[255] Nerve biopsies show axonal degeneration and regeneration, the appearances favoring an axonopathy, particularly affecting larger myelinated fibers.[255–257]

A dominantly inherited disorder exists combining late-onset parkinsonism, ataxia, and a sensorimotor neuropathy.[258,259] Motor conduction velocity has been found to be moderately[258] or mildly[259] reduced, and compound sensory nerve action potentials are of reduced amplitude or absent. Nerve biopsy has shown either a demyelinating neuropathy[258] or a predominant axonal loss.[259]

Miscellaneous Conditions

Inherited recurrent brachial plexus neuropathy

Recurrent episodes of neuropathy predominantly affecting the brachial plexus may occur in families with an autosomal dominant pattern of inheritance. The clinical features of this condition have been reviewed by Windebank[260] and Arts et al.[261] EMG reveals signs of denervation in affected muscles; sometimes these are also seen on the contralateral side even if it is clinically unaffected. The latency of the evoked muscle response on stimulation at Erb's point may be delayed for severely affected muscles. No evidence of denervation is detectable in paraspinal muscles, providing good evidence that the lesion is in the brachial plexus rather than in the spinal roots[262–266] Electromyographic evidence of continuing denervation may be detectable for some months after the acute attack, at the same time as reinnervation is

taking place.[261] Although minor abnormalities of nerve conduction have been reported in the lower limbs,[265] the overall conclusion reached from the reported studies is that there is no evidence of significant generalized neuropathy,[260] either from nerve conduction studies or on clinical examination, but focal neuropathies may develop elsewhere. Sural nerve biopsies from two familial cases have shown tomaculous changes, namely the presence of focal enlargements of the myelin sheath related to redundant myelin loops,[265] but not in two patients reported by Arts et al.[261] Such abnormalities are also present in some patients with IgM paraproteinemic neuropathy[267] and, more particularly, hereditary liability to pressure palsies. This is an unusual but nonspecific pathologic change.

Hereditary liability to pressure palsies

The occurrence of repeated pressure palsies in individuals with a family history of the same condition constitutes the disorder generally known as *hereditary neuropathy with liability to pressure palsies*. It is inherited as an autosomal dominant trait, and has been reviewed by Meier and Moll.[268] The first systematic electrophysiologic study was that of Earl et al.,[269] with subsequent important contributions by Mayer and Garcia-Mullin,[270] Behse et al.,[271] Bosch et al.,[272] and others. The findings have been consistent and have shown changes of denervation both in clinically affected and unaffected nerves. The findings also show evidence of focal nerve lesions superimposed on a generalized neuropathy affecting motor and sensory fibers. In vitro recording of sural compound nerve action potentials by Bosch et al.[272] demonstrated reduced amplitudes and conduction velocities for the A α and A δ peaks but preserved C fiber potentials. Behse et al.[271] first demonstrated the occurrence of focal myelin swellings related to redundant folds of myelin, which were termed tomaculi (sausages) by Madrid and Bradley.[273] Behse et al.[271] also found paranodal and segmental demyelination and related the reduced conduction velocity both to this change and to axonal narrowing in the region of the tomaculi.

Abnormalities of nerve conduction may be demonstrable in clinically unaffected relatives, possibly indicating individuals at risk of developing the overt disorder.

Giant axonal neuropathy

This disorder was originally recognized by Berg et al.[274] and Asbury et al.[275] It is probably of autosomal recessive inheritance. A sensorimotor neuropathy develops in childhood and may be accompanied by central nervous system involvement with features resembling a spinocerebellar degeneration. Most affected children have abnormally curly hair. The characteristic histologic change is the occurrence of segmental axonal enlargements containing accumulations of neurofilaments.[275] Focal demyelination occurs in relation to the axonal swellings. There is probably a generalized disorder of intermediate filaments.[276]

EMG shows changes of denervation, but motor nerve conduction velocity is normal. Compound sensory nerve action potentials are of reduced amplitude or absent.[274–277]

Chediak-Higashi syndrome

The Chediak-Higashi syndrome is a rare autosomal recessive disorder characterized by partial oculocutaneous albinism with giant melanosomes. Giant peroxidase-positive lysosomes are present in leukocytes. Symptoms begin in childhood, and affected children develop defective hair pigmentation, anemia, leukopenia, thrombocytopenia, and a tendency to lymphoreticular malignancy. Mental retardation may occur, as may peripheral neuropathy.[278] Motor nerve conduction velocity has been found to be normal, but compound sensory nerve action potentials

are reduced or absent.[279] Central motor conduction time is delayed.[279] Nerve biopsy indicates an axonopathy with loss of both myelinated and unmyelinated axons, the loss being relatively greater for larger myelinated axons.[279] Some reports have described the presence of giant lysosomes in Schwann cells[278] and inflammatory cellular infiltrates.[280]

Familial multiple symmetrical lipomatosis

This syndrome, otherwise known as Madelung's disease, is characterized by the development of large symmetrically located lipomata on the neck, shoulders, and proximal upper limbs. The disorder is probably of autosomal recessive inheritance.[281] A peripheral neuropathy develops in a proportion of these patients that affects motor, sensory, and autonomic function.[282] EMG shows evidence of denervation, and lower limb motor conduction velocity is moderately reduced. Compound sensory nerve action potentials are of reduced amplitude or are absent. Nerve biopsy indicates an axonopathy with loss of both myelinated and unmyelinated axons but particularly myelinated axons of larger size.[281,283] At one time it was suggested that the neuropathy was the result of concurrent alcoholism, but this view is no longer held. The explanation of the neuropathy is unknown.

REFERENCES

1. Hagberg B. Clinical symptoms, signs and tests in metachromatic leukodystrophy. In: Folch-pi J, Bauer HJ, eds. Brain lipids and lipoproteins. Amsterdam: Elsevier, 1963.
2. Fullerton PM. Peripheral nerve conduction in metachromatic leucodystrophy (sulphatide lipidosis). J Neurol Neurosurg Psychiatry 1964; 27:100–105.
3. Yudell A, Gomez MR, Lambert EH, et al. The neuropathy of sulfatide lipidosis (metachromatic leukodystrophy). Neurology (Minneap) 1967; 17:103–111.
4. Webster H de F. Schwann cell alterations in metachromatic leucodystrophy: Preliminary phase and electron microscope observations. J Neuropathol Exp Neurol 1962; 21:534–554.
5. Dayan AD. Peripheral neuropathy of metachromatic leucodystrophy: Observations on segmental demyelination and remyelination and the intracellular distribution of sulphatide. J Neurol Neurosurg Psychiatry 1967; 30:311–358.
6. Thomas PK, King RHM, Kocen RS, et al. Comparative ultrastructural observations on peripheral

nerve abnormalities in the late infantile, juvenile and late onset forms of metachromatic leukodystrophy. Acta Neuropathol (Berl) 1977; 39:237–245.
7. Clark JR, Miller RG, Vidgoff JM. Juvenile-onset metachromatic leukodystrophy. Biochemical and electrophysiological studies. Neurology (Minneap) 1979; 29:346–353.
8. Kolodny EH. Metachromatic leukodystrophy and multiple sulfatase deficiency. In: Scriver CR, Beaudet AL, Sly WS, et al, eds. The metabolic basis of inherited disease, ed 6. New York: McGraw-Hill, 1989:1721–1750.
9. Pilz H, Hopf HC. A preclinical case of late adult metachromatic leucodystrophy? J Neurol Neurosurg Psychiatry 1972; 35:360.
10. Martin JJ, Ceuterick C, Mercelis R, et al. Pathology of peripheral nerves in metachromatic leucodystrophy, a comparative study of 10 cases. J Neurol Sci 1982; 53:95–112.
11. Rampini S, Isler W, Baerlocher K, et al. Die Kombination von metachromatischer Leukodystrophie und Mukopolysaccharidose als selbstandiges Krankheitsbild (Mukosulfatidose) Helv Paediatr Acta 1970; 25:436–461.

12. Bischoff A. Neuropathy in leukodystrophies. In: Dyck PJ, Thomas PK, Lambert EH, eds. Peripheral neuropathy. Philadelphia: WB Saunders, 1975:891–913.

13. Shapiro LJ, Aleck K, Kaback MM, et al. Metachromatic leukodystrophy without arylsulfatase A deficiency. Pediatr Res 1979; 13:1179–1181.

14. Hahn AF, Gordon BA, Feleki V, et al. A variant form of metachromatic leukodystrophy without arylsulfatase deficiency. Ann Neurol 1982; 12:33–36.

15. Stevens RL, Fluharty AL, Kihara H, et al. Cerebroside sulfatase activator deficiency induced metachromatic leukodystrophy. Am J Hum Genet 1981; 33:900–906.

16. Dunn HG, Lake BD, Dolman CL, et al. The neuropathy of Krabbe's infantile cerebral sclerosis (globoid cell leucodystrophy). Brain 1969; 92:329.

17. Lake BD. Segmental demyelination of peripheral nerves in Krabbe's disease. Nature (Lond) 1968; 217:171–172.

18. Bischoff A, Ulrich J. Peripheral neuropathy in globoid cell leucodystrophy (Krabbe's disease): Ultrastructural and histochemical findings. Brain 1969; 92:861–870.

19. Hogan GR, Gutmann L, Chou SM. The peripheral neuropathy of Krabbe's (globoid) leukodystrophy. Neurology (Minneap) 1969; 19:1094–1100.

20. Lieberman JS, Oshtory M, Taylor RG, et al. Perinatal neuropathy as an early manifestation of Krabbe's disease. Arch Neurol 1980; 37:446–447.

21. Crome L, Hanefeld F, Patrick D, et al. Late onset globoid cell leucodystrophy. Brain 1973; 96:841–848.

22. Thomas PK, Halpern JP, King RHM, et al. Galactosylceramide lipidosis: Novel presentation as a slowly progressive spinocerebellar degeneration. Ann Neurol 1984; 618–620.

23. Skjeldal OH, Stokke O, Refsum S, et al. Phytanic acid storage disease. In: Dyck PJ, Thomas PK, Griffin JW, et al., eds. Peripheral neuropathy, ed 3. Philadelphia: WB Saunders, 1992:1149–1160.

24. Fardeau M, Engel WK. Ultrastructural study of a nerve biopsy in Refsum's disease. J Neuropathol Exp Neurol 1969; 28:278–294.

25. Eldjarn L, Try K, Stokke O, et al. Dietary effects on serum-phytanic-acid levels and on clinical manifestations in heredopathia atactica polyneuritiformis. Lancet 1966; 1:691–693.

26. Ulrich J, Esslen E, Regli F, et al. Die Beziehungen der Nervenleitgeschwindigkeit zum histologischen Befund am peripheren Nerven. Dtsch Z Nervenheilkd 1965; 187:770–786.

27. Sahgal V, Olsen WO. Heredopathia atactica polyneuritiformis (phytanic acid storage disease). A new case with special reference to dietary treatment. Arch Intern Med 1975; 135:585–587.

28. Flament-Durand J, Noel P, Rutseart J, et al. A case of Refsum's disease. Clinical, pathological, ultra-structural and biochemical study. Pathol Eur 1971; 6:172–191.

29. Barolin GS, Hodkewitsch E, Horfinger E, et al. Klinisch-biochemisch Verlaufuntersuchungen bei Heredopathia atactica polyneuritiformis (Morbus Refsum). Fortschr Neurol Psychiatr 1979; 47:53–66.

30. Salisachs P. Ataxia and other data reviewed in Charcot-Marie-Tooth and Refsum's disease. J Neurol Neurosurg Psychiatry 1982; 45:1085–1091.

31. Refsum S. Heredopathia, atactica polyneuritiformis. Phytanic acid storage disease (Refsum's disease). In: Sobue I, ed. Spinocerebellar degenerations. Tokyo: University of Tokyo Press, 1978:313–383.

32. Kark RAP, Engel WK, Blass JP, et al. Heredopathia atactica polyneuritiformis (Refsum disease): A second trial of dietary therapy in two patients. In: Bergsma D, McKusick V, eds. The nervous system. National Foundation for Birth Defects. Original Article Series, Nervous System, 1971; 7:53.

33. Laudat P. Intolerance au phytol: Maladie de Refsum. Biochimie 1972; 54:735.

34. Lundberg A, Lilja LG, Lundberg PO, et al. Heredopathia atactica polyneuritiformis (Refsum disease). Experience of dietary treatment and plasmapheresis. Eur Neurol 1972; 8:301–309.

35. Gibberd FB, Billimoria JD, Page NGR, et al. Heredopathia atctica polyneuritiformis (Refsum's disease) treated by diet and plasma-exchange. Lancet 1979; 1:575–578.

36. Pollock M, Nukuda H, Firth RW, et al. Peripheral neuropathy in Tangier disease. Brain 1983; 106:911–928.

37. Kocen RS, Lloyd JK, Lascelles PT, et al. Familial α-lipoprotein deficiency (Tangier disease) with neurological abnormalities. Lancet 1967; 1:1341–1345.

38. Haas LF, Austad WI, Bergin JD. Tangier disease. Brain 1974; 97:351–354.

39. Dyck PJ, Ellefson RD, Yao JK, et al. Adult-onset of Tangier disease. 1. Morphometric and pathologic studies suggesting delayed degradation of neutral lipids after fiber degeneration. J Neuropathol Exp Neurol 1978; 37:119–137.

40. Marbini A, Gemignani F, Ferrarini G, et al. Tangier disease. A case with sensorimotor distal polyneuropathy and lipid accumulation in striated muscle and vasa nervorum. Acta Neuropathol (Berl) 1985; 67:121–127.

41. Kocen RS, King RHM, Thomas PK, et al. Nerve biopsy findings in two cases of Tangier disease. Acta Neuropathol (Berl) 1973; 26:317–327.

42. Muller DPR, Lloyd JK, Bird AC. Long-term management of abetalipoproteinaemia. Possible role for vitamin E. Arch Dis Child 1977; 52:209–214.

43. Breslow JL. Familial disorders of high density lipoprotein metabolism. In: Scriver CR, Beaudet AL, Sly WS, et al, eds. The metabolic basis of inherited disease, ed 6. New York: McGraw-Hill, 1989:1251–1266.

44. Miller RG, Davis CJF, Ilingworth DR, et al. The neuropathy of abetalipoproteinaemia. Neurology (Minneap) 1980; 30:1286–1291.

45. Sobrevilla LA, Goodman ML, Kane CA. Demyelinating central nervous system disease, macular atrophy and acanthocytosis (Bassen-Kornzweig syndrome). Am J Med 1964; 37:821–828.

46. Schwartz JF, Rowland LP, Eder H, et al. Bassen-Kornzweig syndrome: Deficiency of serum betaprotein. Arch Neurol (Paris) 1963; 8:438–454.

47. Kott E, Delpre G, Kadish U, et al. Abetalipoproteinaemia (Bassen-Kornzweig syndrome). Acta Neuropathol (Berl) 1977; 37:255–258.

48. MacDermot KD, Morgan SH, Cheshire JK, et al. Use of closely linked RFLPs to detect the Anderson-Fabry gene. J Med Genet 1987; 24:635.

49. Cable WJL, Kolodny EH, Adams RD. Fabry's disease: Impaired autonomic function. Neurology (NY) 1982; 30:498–502.

50. Kocen RS, Thomas PK. Peripheral nerve involvement in Fabry's disease. Arch Neurol 1970; 22:81–88.

51. Ohnishi A, Dyck PJ. Loss of small peripheral sensory neurons in Fabry disease. Histologic and morphometric evaluation of cutaneous nerves, spinal ganglia and posterior columns. Arch Neurol 1974; 31:120–127.

52. Sheth KJ, Swick HM. Peripheral nerve conduction in Fabry's disease. Ann Neurol 1980; 7:319–323.

53. Oftebro H, Björkhem I, Skrede S, et al. Cerebrotendinous xanthomatosis. A defect in mitochondrial 26-hydroxylation required for normal biosynthesis of cholic acid. J Clin Invest 1980; 66:1418–1430.

54. Kuritsky A, Berginer VM, Korczyn AD. Peripheral neuropathy in cerebrotendinous xanthomatosis. Neurology (Minneap) 1979; 29:880–881.

55. Ohnishi A, Yamashita Y, Goto I, et al. De- and remyelination and onion bulb in cerebrotendinous xanthomatosis. Acta Neuropathol (Berl) 1979; 45:43–45.

56. Argov Z, Soffer D, Eisenberg S, et al. Chronic demyelinating peripheral neuropathy in cerebrotendinous xanthomatosis. Ann Neurol 1986; 20:89–91.

57. Donaghy M, King RHM, McKeran RO, et al. Cerebrotendinous xanthomatosis: Clinical, electrophysiological and nerve biopsy findings, and response to treatment with chenodeoxycholic acid. J Neurol 1990; 237:216–219.

58. Gumbinas M, Larsen M, Mei Liu M. Peripheral neuropathy in classic Niemann-Pick disease: Ultrastructure of nerves and skeletal muscles. Neurology (Minneap) 1975; 25:107–113.

59. Landrieu P, Said G. Peripheral neuropathy in Type A Niemann-Pick disease. A morphological study. Acta Neuropathol (Berl) 1984; 63:66–71.

60. Moser HW, Moser AB, Chen WW, et al. Ceramidase deficiency: Farber lipogranulomatosis. In: Scriver CR, Beaudet AL, Sly WS, et al, eds. The metabolic basis of inherited disease, ed 6. New York: McGraw-Hill, 1989:1645–1654.

61. Vital C, Battin J, Rivel J, et al. Aspectus ultrastructuraux des lésions du nerf périphérique dans un cas de maladie de Farber. Rev Neurol (Paris) 1976; 132:419–423.

62. Dyck PJ, Yao JK, Knickerbocker DE, et al. Multisystem neuronal degeneration, hepatosplenomegaly, and adrenocortical deficiency associated with reduced tissue arachidonic acid. Neurology (NY) 1981; 31:925–934.

63. Boué J, Oberle I, Heilig R, et al. First trimester prenatal diagnosis of adrenoleukodystrophy by determination of very long chain fatty acid levels and by linkage analysis to a DNA probe. Hum Genet 1985; 69:272.

64. Moser HW, Naidu S, Kumar AJ, et al. The adrenoleukodystrophies. CRC Crit Rev Neurobiol 1987; 3:29–88.

65. Moser HW, Moser AB, Kawamura N, et al. Adrenoleukodystrophy: Elevated C26 fatty acid in cultured skin fibroblasts. Ann Neurol 1980; 7:542–549.

66. Vercruysseen A, Martin JJ, Mercelis R. Neurophysiological studies in adrenomyeloneuropathy. A report on five cases. J Neurol Sci 1982; 56:327–336.

67. Scotto JM, Hadchouel M, Odievre M, et al. Infantile phytanic acid storage disease, a possible variant of Refsum's disease: Three cases including ultrastructural studies of the liver. J Inher Metab Dis 1982; 5:83–90.

68. Bolthauser E, Spycher MA, Steinman B, et al. Infantile phytanic acid storage disease: A variant of Refsum's disease? Eur J Pediat 1982; 139:317.

69. Poulos A, Pollard AC, Mitchell JD, et al. Patterns of Refsum's disease. Phytanic oxidase deficiency. Arch Dis Child 1984; 59:222–229.

70. Ogier H, Roels F, Cornelis A, et al. Absence of hepatic peroxisomes in a case of infantile Refsum's disease. Scand J Clin Lab Invest 1985; 45:767–768.

71. Budden SS, Kennaway NG, Buist NRM, et al. Dysmorphic syndrome with phytanic acid oxidase deficiency, abnormal very long chain fatty acids, and pipecolic acidemia: Studies in four children. J Pediat 1986; 108:33–39.

72. Danpure CJ, Jennings PR. Peroxisomal alanine: Glyoxylate aminotransferase deficiency in primary hyperoxaluria type I. Fed Eur Biochem Soc Lett 1986; 201:20–24.

73. Moorhead PJ, Cooper DJ, Timperley WR. Progressive peripheral neuropathy in a patient with primary hyperoxaluria. Br Med J 1975; 1:312–313.

74. Hall BM, Walsh JC, Horvath JS, et al. Peripheral neuropathy complicating primary hyperoxaluria. J Neurol Sci 1976; 29:343–349.

75. MacCollin M, De Vivo DC, Moser AB, et al. Ataxia and peripheral neuropathy: A benign variant of peroxisome dysgenesis. Ann Neurol 1990; 28:833–836.

76. Andrade C. A peculiar form of peripheral neuropathy: Familial atypical generalized amyloidosis with special involvement of the peripheral nerves. Brain 1952; 75:408–427.

77. Saraiva MJM, Birkin S, Costa PP, et al. Amyloid fibril protein in familial amyloidotic polyneuropathy, Portuguese type. J Clin Invest 1984; 74:104–109.

78. Sparkes RS, Sasaki H, Mohandas T, et al. Assignment of the prealbumin (PALB) gene (familial amyloidotic polyneuropathy) to human chromosome region 18q11.2-q.12.1. Hum Genet 1987; 75:151–154.

79. Benson MD. Inherited amyloidosis. J Med Genet 1991; 28:73–78.

80. Rukavina JG, Block WD, Jackson CE, et al. Primary systemic amyloidosis: A review and an experimental, genetic and clinical study of 29 cases with particular emphasis on the familial form. Medicine (Balt) 1956; 35:239–334.

81. Mahloudji M, Teasdall Rd, Adamkiewicz JJ, et al. The genetic amyloidoses with particular reference to hereditary neuropathic amyloidosis, type II (Indiana or Rukavina type). Medicine (Balt) 1969; 48:1–37.

82. Dwulet FE, Benson MD. Characterization of a transthyretin (prealbumin) variant associated with familial amyloidotic polyneuropathy type II (Indiana/Swiss). J Clin Invest 1986; 78:880–887.

83. Nichols WC, Liepnieks JJ, McKusick VA, et al. Direct sequencing of the gene for Maryland/German familial amyloidotic polyneuropathy type II and genotyping by allele-specific enzymatic amplification. Genomics 1989; 5:535–540.

84. Gafni J, Fischel B, Reif R, et al. Amyloidotic polyneuropathy in a Jewish family. Q J Med 1985; 55:33–41.

85. Wallace MR, Dwulet FE, Conneally PM, et al. Biochemical and molecular genetic characterization of a new variant prealbumin associated with hereditary amyloidosis. J Clin Invest 1986; 78:6–13.

86. Wallace MR, Dwulet FE, Williams EC, et al. Identification of a new hereditary amyloidosis prealbumin variant, Tyr-77, and detection of the gene by DNA analysis. J Clin Invest 1988; 81:189–193.

87. Van Allen MW, Frohlich JA, Davis JR. Inherited predisposition to generalized amyloidosis: Clinical and pathological study of a family with neuropathy, nephropathy, and peptic ulcer. Neurology (Minneap) 1969; 19:10–25.

88. Nichols WC, Dwulet FE, Liepnieks J, et al. Variant apolipoprotein A1 as a major constituent of a hereditary human amyloid. Biochem Biophys Res Commun 1988; 156:762–768.

89. Meretoja J, Teppo L. Histopathological findings of familial amyloidosis with cranial neuropathy as principal manifestation. Report on three cases. Acta Pathol Microbiol Scand A 1971; 79:432–440.

90. Boysen G, Galassi F, Kamieniecka Z, et al. Familial amyloid neuropathy and corneal lattice dystrophy. J Neurol Neurosurg Psychiatry 1979; 42:1020–1030.

91. Maury CPJ, Alli K, Baumann M. Finnish hereditary amyloidosis amino acid sequence homology between the amyloid fibril protein and human plasma gelsolin. FEBS Letts 1990; 260:85–87.

92. Sobue G, Nakao N, Murakami K, et al. Type I familial amyloid polyneuropathy. A pathological study of the peripheral nervous system. Brain 1990; 113:903–921.

93. Dyck PJ, Lambert EH. Dissociated sensation in amyloidosis. Arch Neurol 1969; 20:490–507.

94. Thomas PK, King RHM. Peripheral nerve changes in amyloid neuropathy. Brain 1974; 97:395–406.

95. Anderson R. Blom S. Neurophysiological studies in hereditary amyloidosis with polyneuropathy. Acta Med Scand 1972; 191:233–239.

96. Sales Luis ML. Electrophysiological studies in familial amyloid polyneuropathy—Portuguese type. J Neurol Neurosurg Psychiatry 1978; 41:847–850.

97. Lambert EH, Dyck PJ. Compound action potentials of sural nerve in vitro in peripheral neuropathy. In: Dyck PJ, Thomas PK, Lambert EH, eds. Peripheral neuropathy. Philadelphia: WB Saunders, 1975:427–441.

98. Becker DM, Kramer S. The neurological manifestations of porphyria: A review. Medicine (Balt) 1977; 56:411–423.

99. Dean G. The porphyrias: A story of inheritance and environment. London: Pitman Medical, 1971.

100. Wetterberg L. A neuropsychiatric and genetical investigation of acute intermittent porphyria. Stockholm: Svenska Bokförlaget, 1967.

101. Hierons R. Changes in the nervous system in acute porphyria. Brain 1957; 80:176–192.

102. Nagler W. Peripheral neuropathy in acute intermittent porphyrias. Arch Phys Med Rehab 1971; 52:426–431.

103. Maytham DV, Eales L. Electrodiagnostic findings in porphyria. South Afr Med J 1971; 45(special issue): 99–100.

104. Flügel KA, Druschky KF. Electromyogram and nerve conduction in patients with acute intermittent porphyria. J Neurol 1977; 214:267–279.

105. Albers JW, Robertson WC, Daube JR. Electrodiagnostic findings in acute porphyric neuropathy. Muscle Nerve 1978; 1:292–296.

106. Wochnik-Dyjas D, Niewiadomska M, Kostrewska E. Porphyric polyneuropathy and its pathogenesis in the light of electrophysiological investigations. J Neurol Sci 1978; 35:243–256.

107. Denny-Brown D, Sciarra D. Changes in the nervous system in acute porphyria. Brain 1945; 68:1–16.

108. Cavanagh JB, Mellick RS. On the nature of the peripheral nerve lesions associated with acute intermittent porphyria. J Neurol Neurosurg Psychiatry 1965; 28:320–327.

109. Casali C, Lo Monaco M, D'Alessandro L, et al.

Hereditary coproporphyria: Unusual nervous system involvement in two cases. J Neurol 1984; 231:99–101.

110. Di Trapani D, Casali C, Tonali P, et al. Peripheral nerve changes in hereditary coproporphyria: Light and ultrastructural studies in two sural nerve biopsies. Acta Neuropathol (Berl) 1984; 63:96–107.

111. Feldman DS, Levere RD, Lieberman JS, et al. Presynaptic neuromuscular inhibition by porphobilinogen and porphobilin. Proc Natl Acad Sci 1971; 68:383–386.

112. Mustajoki P, Seppäläinen AM. Neuropathy in latent hepatic porphyria. Br Med J 1975; 2:310–312.

113. Goodman WW, Cooper WC, Kessler GB, et al. Ataxia telangiectasia, a report of two cases in siblings presenting a picture of progressive spinal muscular atrophy. Bull Los Angeles Neurol Assoc 1969; 34:1–22.

114. Dunn HG. Nerve conduction studies in children with Friedreich's ataxia and ataxia telangiectasia. Dev Med Child Neurol 1973; 15:324–337.

115. Kanda T, Oda M, Yonezawa M, et al. Peripheral neuropathy in xeroderma pigmentosum. Brain 1990; 113:1025–1055.

116. Robbins KH, Kraemer KH, Lutzner MA, et al. Xeroderma pigmentosum. An inherited disease with sun sensitivity, multiple cutaneous neoplasms and abnormal DNA repair. Ann Intern Med 1974; 80:221–248.

117. Thrush DC, Holti G, Bradley WG, et al. Neurological manifestations of xeroderma pigmentosum in two siblings. J Neurol Sci 1974; 22:91–104.

118. Lewis PD, McLaughlin J, Thomas PK. Neurological manifestations of xeroderma pigmentosum: Case report with pathological findings. Schweiz Arch Neurol Psychiatry 1978; 113:96.

119. Mossa A, Dubowitz V. Peripheral neuropathy in Cockayne's syndrome. Arch Dis Child 1971; 45:674–677.

120. Grunnet ML, Zimmerman AW, Lewis RA. Ultrastructure and electrodiagnosis of peripheral neuropathy in Cockayne's syndrome. Neurology (Cleve) 1983; 33:1606–1609.

121. Vos A, Gabreëls-Festen A, Joosten E, et al. The neuropathy of Cockayne syndrome. Acta Neuropathol (Berl) 1983; 61:153–162.

122. Karpati G, Carpenter S, Eisen AA, et al. Multiple peripheral nerve entrapments. An unusual phenotypic variant of the Hunter syndrome (mucopolysaccharidosis II) in a family. Arch Neurol 1974; 31:418–422.

123. Neufeld EF, Muenzer J. The mucopolysaccharidoses. In: Scriver CR, Beaudet AL, Sly WS, et al, eds. The metabolic basis of inherited disease, ed 6. New York: McGraw-Hill, 1989:1565–1588.

124. Rapin I, Goldfischer S, Katzman R, et al. The cherry-red spot myoclonus syndrome. Ann Neurol 1978; 3:234–242.

125. Lowden JA, O'Brien JS. Sialidosis: A review of human neuraminidase deficiency. Am J Hum Genet 1979; 31:1–18.

126. Steinman L, Tharp BR, Dorfman LJ, et al. Peripheral neuropathy in the cherry-red spot myoclonus syndrome (sialidosis type 1). Ann Neurol 1980; 7:450–456.

127. Jellinger K, Anzil AP, Seeman D, et al. Adult GM$_2$ gangliosidosis masquerading as slowly progressive muscular atrophy. Motor neuron disease phenotype. Clin Neuropathol 1982; 1:31–44.

128. Mitsumoto H, Sliman RJ, Schafer IA, et al. Motor neuron disease and adult hexosaminidase A deficiency in two families: Evidence for multisystem degeneration. Ann Neurol 1985; 17:373–385.

129. Barnes D, Misra VP, Young EP, et al. An adult onset hexosaminidase A deficiency syndrome with sensory neuropathy and internuclear ophthalmoplegia. J Neurol Neurosurg Psychiatry 1991; 54:1112–1113.

130. Thomas PK, Young E, King RHM. Sandhoff disease mimicking adult-onset bulbospinal neuronopathy. J Neurol Neurosurg Psychiatry 1989; 52:1103–1106.

131. Harding AE. Inherited neuronal atrophy and degeneration predominantly of lower motor neurons. In: Dyck PJ, Thomas PK, Griffin JW, et al. eds. Peripheral neuropathy, ed 3. Philadelphia: WB Saunders. 1992:1051–1064.

132. Emery AEH. Review: The nosology of the spinal muscular atrophies. J Med Genet 1971; 8:481–495.

133. Pearn J. Classification of the spinal muscular atrophies. Lancet 1980; 1:919–922.

134. Pearn JH, Wilson J. Acute Werdnig-Hoffmann disease (acute infantile spinal muscular atrophy). Arch Dis Child 1973; 48:425–430.

135. Pearn JH, Gardner-Medwin D, Wilson J. A clinical study of chronic childhood spinal muscular atrophy. A review of 141 cases. J Neurol Sci 1978; 38:23–37.

136. Kugelberg E, Welander L. Heredofamilial juvenile muscular atrophy simulating muscular dystrophy. Arch Neurol Psychiatry (Chicago) 1956; 75:500–509.

137. Melki J, Sheth P, Abdelhak S, et al. Mapping of acute (type 1) spinal muscular atrophy to chromosome 5q12-q14. Lancet 1990; 336:217–223.

138. Gillam TC, Brzustowicz LM, Castilla LH, et al. Genetic homogeneity between acute and chronic forms of spinal muscular atrophy. Nature 1990; 345:823–825.

139. Melki J, Abdelhak S, Sheth P, et al. Gene for chronic proximal spinal muscular atrophies maps to chromosome 5q. Nature 1990; 344:767–789.

140. Brzustowicz LM, Lehner T, Castilla LH, et al. Genetic mapping of chronic childhood onset spinal muscular atrophy to chromosome 5q11.1-13.3. Nature 1990; 344:540–541.

141. Pearn JH. Autosomal dominant spinal muscular

atrophy. A clinical and genetic study. J Neurol Sci 1978; 38:263–275.

142. Buchthal F, Olsen PZ. Electromyography and muscle biopsy in infantile spinal muscular atrophy. Brain 1970; 93:15–30.

143. Karlström F, Wohlfart G. Klinischen and histopathologische Studien über infantile spinale Muskelatrophie (Oppenheimsche und Werdnig-Hoffmannsche Krankheit). Acta Psychiatr Neurol 1939; 14:453–488.

144. Buchthal F, Clemmesen S. On the differentiation of muscle atrophy by electromyography. Acta Psychaitr Neurol 1941; 16:143–181.

145. Hausmanowa-Petrusewicz I, Karwanska A. Electromyographic findings in different forms of infantile and juvenile spinal muscular atrophy. Muscle Nerve 1986; 9:37–46.

146. Hausmanowa-Petrusewicz I, Zaremba J, Borkowska J, et al. Chronic proximal spinal muscular atrophy of childhood and adolescence—sex influence. J Med Genet, 1984; 21:447–450.

147. Munsat TL, Woods R, Fowler W, et al. Neurogenic muscular atrophy of infancy with prolonged survival. Brain 1969; 92:9–24.

148. Moosa A, Dubowitz V. Motor nerve conduction velocity in spinal muscular atrophy of childhood. Arch Dis Child 1976; 51:974–977.

149. Davis CJF, Bradley WG, Madrid R. The peroneal muscular atrophy syndrome. Clinical, genetic, electrophysiological and nerve biopsy studies. J Genet Hum 1978; 26:311–349.

150. Harding AE, Thomas PK. Hereditary distal spinal muscular atrophy: A report on 34 cases and a review of the literature. J Neurol Sci 1980; 45:337–348.

151. Nelson JW, Amick LD. Heredofamilial progressive spinal muscular atrophy: Clinical and electromyographical study of a kinship. Neurology (Minneap) 1966; 16:306.

152. McLeod JG, Prineas JW. Distal type of chronic spinal muscular atrophy: Clinical, electrophysiological and pathological studies. Brain 1971; 94:703–714.

153. Pearn J. Hudgson P. Distal spinal muscular atrophy: A clinical and genetic study of 8 kindreds. J Neurol Sci 1979; 43:183–191.

154. O'Sullivan DG, McLeod JG. Distal chronic spinal muscular atrophy involving the hands. J Neurol Neurosurg Psychiatry 1978; 41:653–658.

155. Bertini E, Gadisseux JL, Palmieri G, et al. Distal infantile spinal muscular atrophy associated with paralysis of the diaphragm: a variant of infantile spinal muscular atrophy. Am J Med Genet 1989; 33:328–347.

156. Harding AE, Bradbury PG, Murray NMF. Chronic asymmetrical spinal muscular atrophy. J Neurol Sci 1983; 59:69–83.

157. Serratrice G, Pellisier JF, Cremieux G, et al. Scapuloperoneal myopathies, myelopathies and neutropathies. In: Serratrice G, Roux H, eds. Peroneal atro-

phies and related disorders. New York: Masson, 1976:233–252.

158. Kaeser HE. Scapuloperoneal muscular atrophy. Brain 1965; 88:407–418.

159. Thomas PK. Discussion. In: Serratrice G, Pellisier F, Cremieux G, et al. Scapuloperoneal myopathies, myelopathies and neuropathies. In: Serratrice G, Roux H, eds. Peroneal atrophies and related disorders. New York: Masson, 1976:233–252.

160. Rotthauwe H-W, Mortier W, Beyer H. Neuer Typ einer recessiv X-chromosomal vererbten Muskeldystrophie: Scapulo-humero-distale Muskeldystrophie mit Fruhzeitigen Kontrakturen und Herzrhythmusstörungen. Humangenetik 1972; 16:181–200.

161. Thomas PK, Calne DB, Elliott CF. X-linked scapuloperoneal syndrome. J Neurol Neurosurg Psychiatry 1972; 35:208–215.

162. Petty RKH, Thomas PK, Landon DN. Emery-Dreifuss syndrome. J Neurol 1986; 233:108–114.

163. Thomas PK, Schott GD, Morgan-Hughes JA. Adult onset scapuloperoneal myopathy. J Neurol Neurosurg Psychiatry 1975; 38:1008–1015.

164. Harding AE, Thomas PK. Distal and scapuloperoneal distributions of muscle involvement occurring within a family with type I hereditary motor and sensory neuropathy. J Neurol 1980; 224:17–23.

165. Mercelis R, Demeester J, Martin JJ. Neurogenic scapuloperoneal syndrome in childhood. J Neurol Neurosurg Psychiatry 1980; 43:888–896.

166. Mawatari S, Katayama K. Scapuloperoneal muscular atrophy with cardiomyopathy. An X-linked recessive trait. Arch Neurol 1973; 28:55–59.

167. Kennedy WR, Alter M, Sung JH. Progressive proximal spinal and bulbar muscular atrophy: A sex-linked trait. Neurology (Minneap) 1978; 18:671–680.

168. Harding AE, Thomas PK, Baraister M, et al. X-linked recessive bulbospinal neuronopathy: a report of ten cases. J Neurol Neurosurg Psychiatry 1982; 45:1012–1019.

169. Sobue G, Hashizume Y, Mukai E, et al. X-linked recessive bulbospinal neuronopathy. A clinicopathological study. Brain 1989; 112:209–232.

170. Fischbeck ICH, Ionasescu V, Ritter AW, et al. Localization of the gene for X-linked spinal muscular atrophy. Neurology 1986; 36:1595–1598.

171. La Spada AR, Wilson EM, Lubahn DB, et al. Androgen receptor gene mutations in X-linked spinal and bulbar muscular atrophy. Nature 1991; 353:77–78.

172. Wilde J, Moss T, Thrush D. X-linked bulbospinal neuronopathy: a family study of three patients. J Neurol Neurosurg Psychiatry 1987; 50:279–284.

173. Fenichel GM, Emery ES, Hunt P. Neurogenic atrophy stimulating facioscapulohumeral dystrophy. Arch Neurol 1967; 17:257–260.

174. Matsunaga M, Inokuchi T, Ohnishi A, et al. Oculopharyngeal involvement in familial neurogenic

muscular atrophy. J Neurol Neurosurg Psychiatry 1973; 36:104–111.

175. Van Laere J. Paralyse bulbo-pontine chronique progressive familiale avec surdite. Rev Neurol (Paris) 1966; 115:289–295.

176. Alexander M, Emery E, Koerner F. Progressive bulbar paresis in childhood. Arch Neurol 1976; 33:66–68.

177. Dyck PJ, Lambert EH. Lower motor and primary sensory neuron diseases with peroneal muscular atrophy. I. Neurologic, genetic and electrophysiologic findings in hereditary polyneuropathies. Arch Neurol 1968; 18:603–618.

178. Dyck PJ, Lambert EH. Lower motor and primary sensory neuron diseases with peroneal muscular atrophy. II. Neurologic, genetic and electrophysiologic findings in various neuronal degenerations. Arch Neurol 1968; 18:619–625.

179. Harding AE, Thomas PK. The clinical features of hereditary motor and sensory neuropathy, types I and II. Brain 1980; 103:259–280.

180. Thomas PK, Calne DB. Motor nerve conduction velocity in peroneal muscular atrophy: Evidence for genetic heterogeneity. J Neurol Neurosurg Psychiatry 1974; 37:68–75.

181. Bouché P, Gherardi R, Cathala HP, et al. Peroneal muscular atrophy. Part 1. Clinical and electrophysiological study. J Neurol Sci 1983; 61:389–399.

182. Jones SJ, Carroll WM, Halliday AM. Peripheral and central sensory nerve conduction in Charcot-Marie-Tooth disease and comparison with Friedreich's ataxia. J Neurol Sci 1983; 61:135–148.

183. Buchthal F, Behse F. Peroneal muscular atrophy and related disorders. I. Clinical manifestations as related to biopsy findings, nerve conduction and electromyography. Brain 1977; 100:41–66.

184. Combarros O, Calleja J. Figols J, et al. Dominantly inherited hereditary motor and sensory neuropathy type I. Genetic, clinical, electrophysiological and pathological features in four families. J Neurol Sci 1983; 61:181–191.

185. Harding AE, Thomas PK. Autosomal recessive forms of hereditary motor and sensory neuropathy. J Neurol Neurosurg Psychiatry 1980; 43:669–678.

186. Brust JCM, Lovelace RE, Devi S. Clinical and electrodiagnostic features of Charcot-Marie-Tooth syndrome. Uncomplicated and complicated cases. Acta Neurol Scand 1978; suppl 68:1–150.

187. Christie BGB. Electrodiagnostic features of Charcot-Marie-Tooth disease. Proc R Soc Med 1961; 54:321–324.

188. Gutmann L, Fakadej A, Riggs JE. Evolution of nerve conduction abnormalities in children with dominant hypertrophic neuropathy of the Charcot-Marie-Tooth type. Muscle Nerve 1983; 6:515–519.

189. Lewis RA, Sumner AJ. The electrodiagnostic distinctions between chronic familial and acquired demyelinative neuropathies. Neurology (NY) 1982; 32:592–596.

190. Vance JM, Nicholson GA, Yamaoaka LH, et al. Linkage of Charcot-Marie-Tooth neuropathy type Ia to chromosome 17. Exp Neurol 1989; 104:186–189.

191. Middleton-Price HR, Harding AE, Monteiro C, et al. Linkage of hereditary motor and sensory neuropathy type I to the pericentromeric region of chromosome 17. Am J Hum Genet 1990; 46:92–94.

192. Chance PF, Bird TD, O'Connell P, et al. Genetic linkage and heterogeneity in type I Charcot-Marie-Tooth disease (hereditary motor and sensory neuropathy type I). Am J Hum Genet 1990; 47:915–925.

193. Timmerman V, Raeymaekers R, De Jonghe P, et al. Assignment of the Charcot-Marie-Tooth neuropathy type I (CMT Ia) gene to 17p11.2-p12. Am J Hum Genet 1990; 47:680–685.

194. Lupski JR, De Oca-Luna RM, Slaugenhaupt S, et al. DNA duplication associated with Charcot-Marie-Tooth disease type Ia. Cell 1991; 66:219–232.

195. Raeymakers P, Timmerman V, Nelis E, et al. Duplication in chromosome 17p11.2 in Charcot-Marie-Tooth neuropathy type Ia (CMT Ia). Neuromusc Disord 1991; 1:93–98.

196. Bird TD, Ott J, Giblett ER. Evidence for linkage of Charcot-Marie-Tooth neuropathy to the Duffy locus on chromosome I. Am J Hum Genet 1982; 34:388–394.

197. Guiloff RJ, Thomas PK, Contreras M, et al. Evidence for linkage of type I hereditary motor and sensory neuropathy with the Duffy locus on chromosome I. Ann Hum Genet 1982; 46:25–27.

198. Lebo RV, Dyck PJ, Chance P, et al. Mapping of the Duffy-linked Charcot-Marie-Tooth disease locus. Cytogenet Cell Genet 1989; 51:1030.

199. Roussy G. Lévy G. Sept cas d'une maladie familiale particulière. Rev Neurol (Paris) 1926; 33:427–450.

200. Dupuis M, Brucher JM, Gonsette R. Étude anatomoclinique d'une forme neuronale de la maladie de Charcot-Marie-Tooth. Rev Neurol (Paris) 1983; 139:643–649.

201. Berciano J, Combarros O, Figols J, et al. Hereditary motor and sensory neuropathy, type II. Clinicopathological study of a family. Brain 1986; 109:817–914.

202. Lance JW, Burke D, Pollard J. Hyperexcitability of motor and sensory neurons in neuromyotonia. Ann Neurol 1979; 5:523–532.

203. Vasilescu C, Alexianu M, Dan A. Neuronal type of Charcot-Marie-Tooth disease with a syndrome of continuous motor unit activity. J Neurol Sci 1984; 63:11–25.

204. Hahn AF, Parkes AW, Bolton CF, et al. Neuromyotonia in hereditary neuropathy. J Neurol Neurosurg Psychiatry 1991; 54:230–235.

205. Hagberg B, Lyon G. Pooled European series of hereditary peripheral neuropathies in infancy and childhood. A "correspondence workshop" report of the European Federation of Child Neurology Societies (EFCNS). Neuropediatrics 1981; 12:9–17.

206. Ouvrier RA, McLeod JG, Morgan GJ, et al. Hereditary motor and sensory neuropathy of neuronal type with onset in early childhood. J Neurol Sci 1981; 51:181–197.

207. Gabreëls-Festen AAWM, Joosten EMG, Gabreëls FJM, et al. Infantile motor and sensory neuropathy of neuronal type. Brain 1991; 114:1853–1870.

208. Allan W. Relation of hereditary pattern to clinical severity as illustrated by peroneal atrophy. Arch Intern Med 1939; 63:1123–1131.

209. Rozear MP, Pericak-Vance MA, Fischbeck K, et al. Hereditary motor and sensory neuropathy, X-linked: A half-century follow-up. Neurology (Cleve) 1987; 37:1460–1465.

210. Hahn AF, Brown WF, Koopman WJ, et al. X-linked dominant hereditary motor and sensory neuropathy. Brain 1990; 113:1511–1526.

211. Beckett J, Holden JJA, Simpson NE, et al. Localization of X-linked dominant Charcot-Marie-Tooth disease (CMT 2) to Xq 13. J Neurogenet 1986; 3:225–231.

212. Dyck PJ, Lambert EH, Sanders K, et al. Severe hypomyelination and marked abnormality of conduction in Dejerine-Sottas hypertrophic neuropathy: Myelin thickness and compound action potential of sural nerve in vitro. Mayo Clin Proc 1971; 46:433–436.

213. Guzetta F, Ferrière G, Lyon G. Congenital hypomyelination neuropathy: Pathological findings compared with polyneuropathies starting later in life. Brain 1982; 105:395–416.

214. Behse F, Buchthal F. Peroneal muscular atrophy (PMA) and related disorders. II. Brain 1977; 100:67–86.

215. Ben Hamida M, Letaief F, Ben Hamida C, et al. Les atrophies en Tunésie. Étude de 70 observations pure ou associées a autres affections héredodégeneratives. J Neurol Sci 1981; 50:335–356.

216. Harding AE, Thomas PK. Peroneal muscular atrophy with pyramidal features. J Neurol Neurosurg Psychiatry 1984; 47;168–172.

217. Claus D, Waddy HM, Harding AE, et al. Hereditary motor and sensory neuropathies and hereditary spastic paraplegias: a magnetic stimulation study. Ann Neurol 1990; 28:43–49.

218. Schnider A, Hess CW, Koppi S. Central motor conduction in a family with hereditary motor and sensory neuropathy with pyramidal signs (HMSN V). J Neurol Neurosurg Psychiatry 1991; 54:511–515.

219. Dyck PJ, Mellinger JF, Reagan TJ, et al. Not "indifference to pain" but varieties of sensory and autonomic neuropathy. Brain 1983; 106:373–390.

220. Denny-Brown D. Hereditary sensory radicular neuropathy. J Neurol Neurosurg Psychiatry 1951; 14:237–252.

221. Dyck PJ. Neuronal atrophy and degeneration predominantly affecting peripheral sensory and autonomic neurons. In: Dyck PJ, Thomas PK, Griffin JW, et al, eds. Peripheral neuropathy ed 3. Philadelphia: WB Saunders, 1992: 1065–1093.

222. Ohta M, Ellefson RD, Lambert EH, et al. Hereditary sensory neuropathy, type II: Clinical, electrophysiologic, histological and biochemical studies of a Quebec kinship. Arch Neurol 1973; 29:23–37.

223. Nukuda H, Pollock M, Haas LF. The clinical spectrum and morphology of type II hereditary sensory neuropathy. Brain 1982; 105:647–665.

224. Aguayo AJ, Nair CPV, Bray GM. Peripheral nerve abnormalities in the Riley-Day syndrome: Findings in a sural nerve biopsy. Arch Neurol 1971; 24:106–116.

225. Brown JC, Johns RJ. Nerve conduction in familial dysautonomia: Riley Day syndrome. JAMA 1967; 201:200.

226. Swanson AG, Buchan GC, Alvord EC Jr. Anatomic changes in congenital insensitivity to pain. Arch Neurol 1965; 12:12–18.

227. Low PA, Burke WJ, McLeod JG. Congenital sensory neuropathy with selective loss of small myelinated nerve fibres. Ann Neurol 1978; 3:179–182.

228. Donaghy M, Hakin RN, Bamford JM, et al. Hereditary sensory neuropathy with neurotrophic keratitis. Description of an autosomal recessive disorder with a selective reduction of small myelinated fibres and a discussion of the classification of the hereditary sensory neuropathies. Brain 1987; 110:563–583.

229. Geoffroy G, Barbeau A, Breton A, et al. Clinical description and roentgenologic evaluation of patients with Friedreich's ataxia. Can J Neurol Sci 1976; 3:279–286.

230. Harding AE. Friedreich's ataxia: A clinical and genetic study of 90 families with an analysis of early diagnostic criteria and intrafamilial clustering of clinical features. Brain 1981; 104:589–620.

231. Chamberlain S, Shaw V, Rowland A, et al. The mutation causing Friedreich's ataxia maps to human chromosome 9p22.cen. Nature 1988; 334:248–250.

232. McLeod JG. An electrophysiological and pathological study of peripheral nerves in Friedreich's ataxia. J Neurol Sci 1971; 12:333–349.

233. Dunn HG. Nerve conduction studies in children with Friedreich's ataxia and ataxia-telangiectasia. Dev Med Child Neurol 1973; 15:324–337.

234. Oh SJ, Halsey JH. Abnormality in nerve potentials in Friedreich's ataxia. Neurology (Minneap) 1973; 23:52–54.

235. Salisachs P, Codina M, Pradas J. Motor conduction velocity in patients with Friedreich's ataxia. Report of 12 cases. J Neurol Sci 1975; 24:331–337.

236. Peyronnard JM, Bouchard JP, Lapointe L, et al. Nerve conduction studies and electromyography in Friedreich's ataxia. Can J Neurol Sci 1976; 3:313–317.

237. Bouchard JP, Barbeau A, Bouchard R, et al. Electromyography and nerve conduction studies in Friedreich's ataxia and autosomal recessive spastic ataxia

of Charlevoix-Saguenay (ARSACS). Can J Neurol Sci 1979; 6:185–189.

238. D'Angelo A, Di Donato S, Negri G, et al. Friedreich's ataxia in Northern Italy. I. Clinical, neurophysiological and in vivo biochemical studies. Can J Neurol Sci 1980; 7:359–365.

239. Caruso G, Santoro L, Perretti A, et al. Friedreich's ataxia: Electrophysiological and histological findings. Acta Neurol Scand 1983; 67:26–40.

240. Ouvrier RA, McLeod JG, Conchin TE. Friedreich's ataxia. Early detection and progression of peripheral nerve abnormalities. J Neurol Sci 1982; 55:137–145.

241. Lambert EH, Dyck PJ. Compound action potentials of sural nerve in vitro in peripheral neuropathy. In: Dyck PJ, Thomas PK, Griffin JW, et al, eds. Peripheral neuropathy, ed 3. Philadelphia: WB Saunders, 1992:672–684.

242. Harding AE. Early onset cerebellar ataxia with retained tendon reflexes: A clinical and genetic study of a disorder distinct from Friedreich's ataxia. J Neurol Neurosurg Psychiatry 1981; 44:503–508.

243. Spira PJ, McLeod JG, Evans WA. A spinocerebellar degeneration with X-linked inheritance. Brain 1979; 102:27–41.

244. Thomas PK, Workman JA, Thage O. Behr's syndrome: A family exhibiting pseudodominant inheritance. J Neurol Sci 1984; 64:137–148.

245. Harding AE. The hereditary ataxias and related disorders. Edinburgh: Churchill Livingstone, 1984.

246. McLeod JG, Evans WA. Peripheral neuropathy in spinocerebellar degenerations. Muscle Nerve 1981; 4:51–61.

247. Wadia N, Irani P, Mehta L, et al. Evidence of peripheral neuropathy in a variety of heredo-familial olivo-ponto-cerebellar degeneration frequently seen in India. In: Sobue I, ed. Spinocerebellar degenerations. Tokyo: Tokyo University Press, 1978:239–250.

248. Pollock M, Kies B. Benign hereditary cerebellar ataxia with extensive thermoanalgesia. Brain 1990; 113:857–866.

249. McLeod JG, Morgan JA, Reye C. Electrophysiological studies in familial spastic paraplegia. J Neurol Neurosurg Psychiatry 1977; 40:611–615.

250. Silver JR. Familial spastic paraplegia with amyotrophy of the hands. Ann Hum Genet 1966; 30:69–75.

251. Cross HE, McKusick VA. The Troyer syndrome. A recessive form of spastic paraplegia with distal muscle wasting. Arch Neurol 1967; 16:473–485.

252. Abdallat A, Davis SM, Farrage J, et al. Disordered pigmentation, spastic paraparesis and peripheral neuropathy in three siblings: A new neurocutaneous syndrome. J Neurol Neurosurg Psychiatry 1980; 43:962–966.

253. Stewart RM, Tunnell G, Ehle A. Familial spastic paraplegia, peroneal neuropathy and crural hypopigmentation: A new neurocutaneous syndrome. Neurology (Minneap) 1981; 31:754–757.

254. Cavanagh NPC, Eames RA, Galvin RJ, et al. Hereditary sensory neuropathy with paraplegia. Brain 1979; 102:79–84.

255. Hardie RJ, Pullon HWH, Harding AE, et al. Neuroacanthocytosis. A clinical, haematological and pathological study of 19 cases. Brain 1991; 114:13–49.

256. Ohnishi A, Sato Y, Nagara H, et al. Neurogenic muscular atrophy and low density of large myelinated fibres of sural nerve in chorea-acanthocytosis. J Neurol Neurosurg Psychiatry 1981; 44:645–648.

257. Sobue G, Mukai E, Fujii K, et al. Peripheral nerve involvement in familial chorea-acanthocytosis. J Neurol Sci 1986; 76:347–356.

258. Ziegler DK, Schimke RN, Kepes JJ, et al. Late onset ataxia, rigidity and peripheral neuropathy. Arch Neurol 1972; 27:52–60.

259. Byrne E, Thomas PK, Zilkha KJ. Familial extrapyramidal disease with peripheral neuropathy. J Neurol Neurosurg Psychiatry 1982; 45:372–374.

260. Windebank AJ. Inherited recurrent focal neuropathies. In: Dyck PJ, Thomas PK, Griffin JW, et al., eds. Peripheral neuropathy, ed 3. Philadelphia: WB Saunders, 1992:1137–1148.

261. Arts WFM, Busch HFM, Van Den Brand HJ, et al. Hereditary neuralgic amyotrophy. Clinical, genetic, electrophysiological and histopathological studies. J Neurol Sci 1983; 62:261–279.

262. Taylor RA. Heredofamilial mononeuritis multiplex with brachial predilection. Brain 1960; 83:113–137.

263. Jacob JC, Andermann F, Robb JP. Heredofamilial neuritis with brachial predilection. Neurology (Minneap) 1961; 11:1025–1033.

264. Geiger LR, Mancall EL, Penn AS, et al. Familial neuralgic amyotrophy: Report of three families with review of the literature. Brain 1974; 97:87–102.

265. Bradley WG, Madrid R, Thrush DC, et al. Recurrent brachial plexus neuropathy. Brain 1975; 98:381–398.

266. Dunn HG, Daube JR, Gomez MR. Heredofamilial brachial plexus neuropathy (hereditary neuralgic amyotrophy with brachial predilection) in childhood. Dev Med Child Neurol 1978; 20:28–46.

267. Rebai T, Mhiri C, Heine P, et al. Focal myelin thickening in a peripheral neuropathy associated with IgM monoclonal gammopathy. Acta Neuropathol (Berl) 1989; 79:226–232.

268. Meier C, Moll C. Hereditary neuropathy with liability to pressure palsies. Report of two families and review of the literature. J Neurol 1982; 228:73–95.

269. Earl CJ, Fullerton PM, Wakefield GS, et al. Hereditary neuropathy with liability to pressure palsies (a clinical and electrophysiological study of four families). J Med 1964; 33:4381–498.

270. Mayer RF, Garcia-Mullin R. Hereditary neuropathy manifested by pressure palsies—a Schwann cell disorder? Trans Am Neurol Assoc 1968; 93:238–240.

271. Behse F, Buchthal F, Carlsen F, et al. Hereditary neuropathy with liability to pressure palsies: Elec-

trophysiological and histopathological aspects. Brain 1972; 95:777–797.

272. Bosch EP, Chui HC, Martin MA, et al. Brachial plexus involvement in familial pressure-sensitive neuropathy: Electrophysiological and morphological findings. Ann Neurol 1980; 8:620–624.

273. Madrid R, Bradley WG. The pathology of neuropathies with focal thickening of the myelin sheath (tomaculous neuropathy). J Neurol Sci 1975; 25:415–448.

274. Berg BO, Rosenberg SH, Asbury AK. Giant axonal neuropathy. Pediatrics 1972; 49:894.

275. Asbury AK, Gale MK, Cox SC, et al. Giant axonal neuropathy: A unique case with segmental neurofilamentous masses. Acta Neuropathol (Berl) 1972; 20:237–247.

276. Prineas JW, Ouvrier RA, Wright RG, et al. Giant axonal neuropathy—a generalized disorder of cytoplasmic microfilament formation. J Neuropath Exp Neurol 1976; 35:458–470.

277. Carpenter S, Karpati G, Andermann F, et al. Giant axonal neuropathy. A clinically and morphologically distinct neurological disease. Arch Neurol 1974; 31:312–316.

278. Lockman LA, Kennedy WR, White JG. The Chediak-Higashi syndrome. J Pediatr 1967; 70:942–951.

279. Misra VP, King RHM, Harding AE, et al. Peripheral neuropathy in Chediak-Higashi syndrome. Acta Neuropathol (Berl) 1991; 81:354–358.

280. Sung JH, Meyers JP, Stadlan EM, et al. Neuropathological changes in Chediak-Higashi disease. J Neuropathol Exp Neurol 1969; 28:86–118.

281. Chalk CH, Mills KR, Jacobs JM, et al. Familial multiple symmetric lipomatosis with peripheral neuropathy. Neurology 1990; 40:1246–1250.

282. Enzi G, Angelini C, Negrin P, et al. Sensory, motor, and autonomic neuropathy in patients with multiple symmetric lipomatosis. Medicine (Balt) 1985; 64:388–393.

283. Pollock M, Nicholson GI, Nukada H, et al. Neuropathy in multiple symmetric lipomatosis: Madelung's disease. Brain 1988; 111:1157–1171.

284. Hagberg B. The clinical diagnosis of Krabbe's infantile leucodystrophy. Acta Paediatr Scand 1959; 52:213.

285. Dyck PJ, Chance P, Lebo R, et al. Hereditary motor and sensory neuropathies. In: Dyck PJ, Thomas PK, Griffin JW, et al. Periphral neuropathy, ed 3. Philadelphia: WB Saunders, 1992; 1094–1136.

16

Motor Neuron Disorders

Andrew Eisen
Alan J. McComas

CONTENTS

LIST OF ACRONYMS

ALS   amyotrophic lateral sclerosis
EDB   extensor digitorum brevis
EMG   electromyography
HMN   hereditary motor neuropathy
MEP   motor evoked potential
SFEMG   single-fiber electromyography
SMA   spinal muscular atrophy

The term *motor neuron disorders* is usually applied to those conditions thought to involve the perikaryon of the motor neuron with secondary degeneration of the axis cylinder and dendrites. The list of such conditions is long and remarkable for its clinical and etiologic diversity[1] (Table 16.1); nevertheless, this concept of motor neuron disorders is unsatisfactory for two reasons. First, with the exception of poliomyelitis, there is no irrefutable evidence that the perikaryon is the primary target of any of the etiologic factors. Second, the concept excludes that group of *peripheral* nerve disorders, the axonal neuropathies, characterized by normal impulse conduction velocities and dying-back changes in the axon, even though the perikaryon may eventually be shown to be the primary site of involvement. With these limitations in mind, the electromyographer need recognize only four categories of motor neuron disorder: amyotrophic lateral sclerosis (ALS), the spinal muscular atrophies (SMAs), and an assortment of other types (poliomyelitis, polio-like monoplegia, syringomyelia, Shy-Drager syndrome, Crutzfeld-Jakob disease, arthrogryposis multiplex congenita).

The fourth category, benign fasciculations, represents a motor neuron disorder of a different nature, the problem being one of spontaneous impulse generation rather than cell degeneration. Other syndromes of motor neuron overactivity, such as myokymia (Isaac's syndrome), tetanus, tetany, hemifacial spasm, and black widow spider bite, are not considered. The possibility that some of the muscular dystrophies contain a special form of motor neuron disorder is beyond the scope of this discussion[2]; it receives passing comment in the section on SMAs, later. Also, it should be recognized that the normal aging process is associated with a loss of motor neurons beyond the age of 60 years.[3,4]

The electromyographic features of muscle denervation are common to all disorders in which motor neurons degenerate, although with some modification in the case of infantile SMA. In most patients, conventional examination of muscles by concentric or monopolar needle electromyography (EMG), supplemented by sensory and motor nerve conduction studies, is sufficient to establish whether or not a motor neuron disorder is present. There is special interest, nevertheless, in such special examinations as single-fiber EMG, motor unit (MU) counting, motor cortex stimulation, and automatic frequency analysis. Although the last procedure increases the diagnostic power of the electromyogram, the first two combine to provide quantitative information about the sizes, numbers, and architecture of the MUs in this group of conditions.

Relevant clinical information has been added in the belief that it is incumbent on the electromyographer not only to submit a factual account of the electrophysiologic findings, but also, whenever possible, to propose, confirm, or refute a clinical diagnosis. This is especially important when patients have been sent for electrodiagnosis by primary care physicians, but even in those patients referred by specialists, the lapse of time or the changed environment may unmask a crucial physical sign.

AMYOTROPHIC LATERAL SCLEROSIS

ALS is a fatal disorder, characterized by progressive degeneration of α-motor neurons in the spinal cord and brain stem and of corticospinal neurons and their axons. It is a unique condition in that it is the only degenerative disorder to involve both upper and lower motor neurons. So far, no fully satisfactory animal model is available for study. In a typical advanced case of ALS, there is generalized muscle weakness and wasting; difficulty in swallowing, coughing, and talking; and hyperreflexia with variable spasticity. Muscle fasciculations are widespread and prominent. The annual incidence of ALS is 2 per 100,000, with the peak age of onset occurring in the sixth decade; males outnumber females 3 to 2. From the time of diagnosis, the mean life expectancy is about 3 years, although there are a minority of patients who survive for much longer; death usually results from respiratory failure and bronchopneumonia.

Clinical Considerations

Cause and pathophysiology

In 5% to 10% of cases, ALS is clearly familial, usually inherited through an autosomal dominant gene. In the remainder, the cause is unknown, although a large number of putative factors, including trauma, have been incriminated. A popular contemporary view is that ALS, in common with other neurodegenerative diseases of the aging nervous system (Parkinson's and Alzheimer's diseases), may reflect complex interactions of earlier environmental toxins, causing subclinical loss or dysfunction of relevant neuronal populations (motor neurons in the case of ALS), and natural cellular aging.[5,6] If this

TABLE 16.1.　Classification of motor neuron disorders

Conditions characterized by overactivity of motor units	Acquired disorders
Benign fasciculation—cramps	Viral
Myokymia (neuromyotonia, Isaac's syndrome)	Acute poliomyelitis
Hemifacial spasm	Acute enteroviral infection
Tetanus	Russian spring-summer encephalitis
Strychnine intoxication	Herpes zoster
Stiff man syndrome	Jakob-Creutzfeldt disease
Satoyashi syndrome	Encephalitis lethargica
Myelopathy with rigidity or spasm	Amyotrophy in asthma (?)
Black widow spider bite	AIDS
Tetany	Tropical spastic paraparesis
Spinal myoclonus	Intoxications and physical agents
Conditions characterized by weakness	Trauma
Heritable disorders	Lead
Infantile forms	X-irradiation
Infantile spinal muscular atrophy	High-voltage electric injury
(Werdnig-Hoffmann disease)	Dapsone intoxication (?)
Infantile bulbar palsy (Fazio-Londe atrophy)	Phenytoin intoxication (?)
Neurogenic arthrogryposis multiplex congenita	Immunologic
Neuraxonal dystrophy	Plasma cell dyscrasias
Juvenile and adult forms	GM_1 ganglioside antibodies
Juvenile spinal muscular atrophies(?)	Metabolic
Hereditary differences: autosomal-dominant or	Hypoglycemia
autosomal-recessive; X-linked	Hyperparathyroidism; other disorders of calcium
Topographic differences: proximal (Kugelberg-	metabolism
Welander disease) or distal limbs; scapuloper-	Hyperthyroidism
al; cranial (ocular, oropharyngeal, vocal cords)	Ischemia (?)
Enzymatic differences: hexosaminidase defi-	Syphilis (?)
ciency; hyperlipidemia	Unknown cause
Combined upper and lower motor neuron diseases	Amyotrophic lateral sclerosis and forms of motor
Familial amyotrophic lateral sclerosis or motor	neuron disease
neuron disease	Spinal muscular atrophy
Hereditary spastic paraplegia with or without dis-	Progressive bulbar palsy
tal amyotrophy	Amyotrophic lateral sclerosis
Guamanian motor neuron disease	Primary lateral sclerosis
Amyotrophy in multisystem diseases	Monomelic motor neuron disease
Spinocerebellar degenerations	Juvenile amyotrophic lateral sclerosis
Huntington's disease	Amyotrophy in Shy-Drager syndrome
Dementia	Amyotrophy with dementia
Joseph's disease	Amyotrophy in paraneoplastic syndromes
Pick's disease	Amyotrophy in myasthenia gravis
Parkinsonism	
Mental retardation	

Modified with permission from Rowland LP. Diverse forms of motoneurone diseases. Adv Neurol 1982; 36:1–11.

hypothesis is correct, it can be argued that ALS has a latency of several years or even decades predating the onset of clinical manifestations. Therefore investigative and therapeutic strategies should be directed toward early and possibly preclinical detection, when treatment is likely to be most effective. Good evidence for environmental toxicity comes from studies on the island of Guam (also the Kii peninsula of

Japan and Western New Guinea), where until recently the incidence of ALS was 100-fold that of the rest of the world. The incidence of ALS in Guam peaked in the mid-1960s, about 20 years after the Japanese invaded the island. During that time, the southern villagers, forced to retreat to the hills, resorted to *fadan* as their main staple. Fadan is made from the cycad nut, an active ingredient of which is b-N-methylamino-L-alanine (BMAA), an excitotoxic amino acid. Although the cycad story is much less convincing than when initially described, the dramatic decrease in the incidence of ALS on Guam over the last 15 years is strong supporting evidence for some kind of environmental toxicity.[6] The decrease of ALS on Guam can be contrasted with the age-specific increasing incidence of ALS (and Parkinson's disease) in the Western world.[7–9] Such epidemiologic studies further support environmental toxicity as a prime causative factor in ALS.

The role of immunologic dysfunction in ALS is difficult to evaluate.[10] Certainly there is no convincing evidence that ALS is a disease caused by disordered immunity in the conventional sense; nor has it responded to any forms of presently available immunosuppressive therapy. The possibility, however, of an *unconventional* autoimmune disease remains.[11] This concept has been strengthened by the development of an autoimmune model of anterior horn cell disease in animals.[12] Like other animal models of ALS, however, the upper motor neurons are not involved, and the resemblance is closer to progressive muscular atrophy.

The cellular mechanisms leading to cell damage and death in ALS are unknown. Accumulation of oxidants or excitants in the microenvironment, however, have been implicated in deranged axonal transport, with secondary accumulation of a variety of neurofilamentous materials within upper and lower motor neurons.[13] It is arguable as to whether any changes in axoplasmic transport are of primary importance in the pathogenesis of ALS or whether they merely serve as nonspecific markers of metabolic failure.

Differential diagnosis

In a well-established case, the diagnosis of ALS is not usually difficult. Thus the constellation of painless, progressive, upper and lower motor neuron weakness associated with fasciculation, cramps, and hyperreflexia in a previously healthy subject is almost pathognomonic. In those patients in whom the tendon reflexes are normal or depressed, consideration must also be given to the possibility of SMA, limbgirdle and facioscapulohumeral dystrophy, polymyositis, and myasthenia gravis. Peripheral neuropathy must be excluded in those ALS patients in whom there are multiple impulse conduction blocks in association with antibodies to GM_1 ganglioside. When weakness and wasting of the intrinsic muscles of the hand are the solitary features, the differential diagnosis includes ulnar neuropathy, thoracic outlet syndrome, C-8–T-1 radiculopathies, and syringomyelia. In patients in whom weakness and wasting of arm muscles are combined with upper motor neuron signs in the legs, ALS must be distinguished from the many causes of spinal cord compression. In patients presenting with footdrop, distinction must be made from peroneal neuropathies and L-5 root lesions. Cramps and fasciculations may be benign, or the former may be manifestations of a metabolic myopathy. An interesting diagnostic challenge is posed by the patient in whom there is a spastic gait in the absence of lower motor neuron findings, resulting from early involvement of the corticospinal pathways. Weakness of bulbar muscles can also be caused by lesions of the lower cranial nerves or their nuclei as well as by myasthenia gravis. Occasionally patients with ALS may present in respiratory failure. It should also be noted that ALS can sometimes be difficult to diagnose in the elderly because loss of α-motor neurons, with consequent weakness and wasting of muscles, is a normal feature of aging.[3] Indeed ALS in the older patient may possibly represent an acceleration of the normal aging process.[14]

Electromyographic Examination

The most essential initial investigative procedure required to support the clinical diagnosis of ALS is the electromyogram.[15] The electromyographic criteria for establishing the diagnosis of ALS (or other disease of the motor neuron) are as follows:

1. Widespread fibrillation potentials or positive sharp waves.
2. Fasciculations.
3. Chronic neuropathic MU potential changes in a multisegmental distribution involving at least three limbs and the paraspinal muscles.
4. Normal compound sensory nerve action potentials.
5. Normal or slightly reduced impulse conduction velocities.

Although electromyographers have their own protocols for investigating patients with, for example, weakness of an arm or a leg, the electromyographic diagnosis of ALS requires the systematic application of a battery of standard tests. In addition, there is much to be gained and learned from such special procedures as single fiber EMG, motor cortex stimulation, and MU counting. The results of each type of examination in ALS may now be considered.

Nerve conduction studies

Measurements of impulse propagation in the fastest conducting motor nerve fibers of patients with ALS have been reported by several workers. In the largest of these studies, Lambert[16] found the mean value for the forearm segment of the ulnar nerve to be 55 m per second and that for the peroneal nerve between the knee and ankle to be 44 m per second. These values were only 8% and 16% below the respective control means for that laboratory; similar observations have been made by Isch et al.[17] In those patients with few MUs remaining, however, the maximal impulse conduction velocities are undoubtedly reduced, and this is especially true for distal segments of the motor nerve fibers. Thus the distal motor latencies may be expected to increase in the median, ulnar, peroneal, and tibial nerves of severely affected patients. In most of such patients, the retention of normal conduction values for sensory fibers in the median nerve serves to exclude the presence of a carpal tunnel syndrome as a contributory factor for that nerve. Two possibilities exist for the slowed conduction velocities in distal regions of the motor nerve fibers. One is that the faster conducting axons degenerate, leaving those with lower velocities. The other explanation is that slowing accompanies *dying-back* in the more distal regions of the axons. In relation to the first possibility, it is obviously important to know the impulse velocities of the slowest conducting fibers in normal nerves; this may be done using two types of collision technique[18,19] or by highly selective recordings from single MUs.[20] Unfortunately, the data from such studies are not consistent and cannot therefore provide an answer to the cause of the lower velocities in ALS.

A more satisfactory approach has come from the study of distal motor latencies by Hansen and Ballantyne,[21] who used a computerized technique to study extensor digitorum brevis (EDB) MU populations in 32 patients with ALS. These authors found that the mean latency was significantly longer in patients than in control subjects, but they attributed this to random loss of fast conducting axons in the former. This explanation would be valid only if the graded stimulation technique was preferentially sampling the fastest conducting axons; however, the results of collision experiments[22] suggest that peroneal nerve fiber thresholds are mainly determined by their relative positions within the nerve trunk rather than by their sizes. The most plausible explanation for Hansen and Ballantyne's results is that pathologic slowing of impulse conduction may take place in surviving motor nerve fibers for a certain period

before the fibers finally become inexcitable. Such a phenomenon was observed in the sole remaining axon of an elderly but otherwise normal subject studied by Campbell et al.[3]

In the ALS-like syndrome associated with antibodies to GM_1 ganglioside, impulse conduction may be slowed not only in distal segments of motor axons, but also in a patchy manner elsewhere, and may sometimes progress to local conduction block[23] (Figure 16.1).

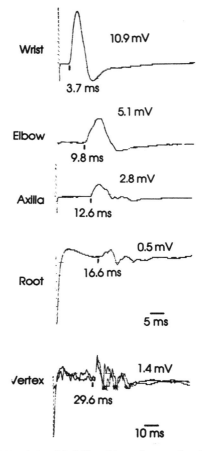

FIGURE 16.1. *Multifocal impulse conduction block in a patient with an amyotrophic lateral sclerosis syndrome associated with antibodies to GM_1 ganglioside. Recordings made from thenar muscle group with surface electrodes, following nerve stimulation at sites between wrist and motor cortex. Latencies and peak to peak amplitudes of responses shown with each trace. Note the marked drop in response amplitude as the point of stimulation is moved more proximal.*

Sensory nerve studies in ALS usually reveal normal response amplitudes and maximal impulse conduction velocities in the arm and leg.[16,24,25] In some patients with otherwise typical features of ALS, however, sensory responses are diminished, particularly in digital nerves of the hand. Although coincidental cervical radiculopathies or distal entrapment neuropathies may account for such changes in some of these patients, there are others in whom the sensory degeneration appears to be a primary event. This conclusion is borne out by the results of quantitative psychophysical testing of cutaneous sensation[26] and an appreciable incidence of abnormalities in sural nerve biopsies.[27,28]

It is probable that abnormal somatosensory cortical evoked potentials in some patients[29] may reflect degeneration in the dorsal column–lemniscal pathway as well as in peripheral nerves.

Needle studies

In a patient suspected of having ALS, the examination of muscles with a coaxial or monopolar needle electrode is the most important part of the entire diagnostic procedure. With each insertion of the needle, there are three issues to be addressed: the presence or absence of spontaneous activity; the maximal degree of MU recruitment; and the amplitudes, durations, and morphologies of the MU potentials.

There is a well-founded adage that for a firm diagnosis of ALS to be made, abnormalities on needle examination shoud be demonstrable in at least three limbs; in a patient with difficulty in swallowing, chewing, or speaking, there should also be signs of denervation in bulbar and masticatory muscles. *Fibrillation potentials and positive sharp waves* (Figure 16.2A) may be anticipated in almost all muscles with less than half the normal strength but in only one-quarter of clinically unaffected muscles.[16] The reason for this difference depends partly on the respective capacities of surviving motor neurons for reinnervation in the two situations and partly on the delay between denervation and the onset of fibrillation potentials. On the basis of observations following traumatic nerve section, it is known that 2 to 3 weeks must elapse before fibrillation potentials appear in acutely denervated human muscle fibers. If findings in small mammals,[30] however, are applicable to humans, collateral sprouting may be expected as

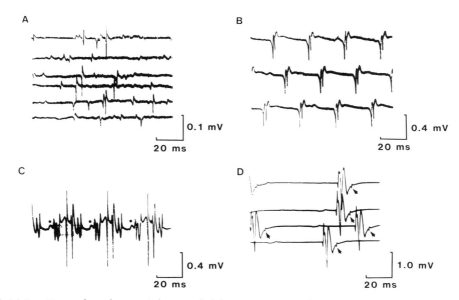

FIGURE 16.2. *Examples of potentials recorded from patients with motor neuron disorders, using a coaxial needle electrode. (A) Fibrillation potentials and positive sharp waves. (B) Complex repetitive discharges, in the form of doublets, arising spontaneously. (C) Three cycles of another complex repetitive discharge; onsets indicated by dots. Note the consistency of the components, despite the extreme complexity of each discharge. (D) Satellite potentials (arrows) forming part of the discharge of a voluntarily recruited motor unit. Potentials in (A) were recorded from a patient with amyotrophic lateral sclerosis; potentials in (B) through (D) were taken from patients with spinal muscular atrophy.*

early as 4 days. Therefore denervated muscle fibers may acquire a new innervation before fibrillation potentials can develop, provided that there are neighboring intramuscular nerve branches, belonging to *healthy* motor neurons, that can undertake sprouting. The same arguments apply to positive sharp waves, which are considered to be fibrillation potentials that are blocked at the recording site by trauma inflicted on the membranes of the denervated muscle fibers by the intramuscular electrode.

In general, the more spontaneous activity present in a muscle, the more rapidly the progress of the disease. Sometimes, especially in an older patient, there may be uncertainty as to whether cervical and lumbosacral radiculopathies, rather than ALS, are responsible for the denervation observed in limb muscles. In such cases, the thoracic paraspinal muscles shoud be examined because the thoracic spine is not usually affected by disc protrusions. If fibrillation potentials and positive sharp waves are abundant in the thoracic paraspinal muscles, it is likely that the patient will soon slip into respiratory failure.[31] In patients with bulbar involvement, the muscles examined should include the tongue, masseter, facial, and neck muscles.

Complex repetitive discharges may also occur in ALS and are even more frequent in patients with SMA[32] from whom the examples shown in Figure 16.2(B) and (C) are taken. Unlike fibrillation potentials, the majority of which arise at the site of the former neuromuscular junctions,[33,34] it is not known where the pacemakers for complex repetitive discharges are situated. It is unlikely that these potentials arise in innervated fibers because voluntary activity is incapable of provoking the same complexes once the spontaneous discharge has terminated. From single-fiber electromyographic studies (see under Single-Fiber Electromyography, Macroelectromyography, and Scanning Electromyography, later) has come evidence that these potentials may be caused by ephaptic spread of impulse activity from a spontaneously active muscle fiber to its neighbors.[35] If so, it is difficult to understand why similar discharges do not arise in normal muscles, in view of the close apposition of the fibers. A more likely explanation is that the activity originates in denervated fibers that have previously undergone splitting and that the later components represent the arrival of impulses in relatively small branches of the parent fibers.

Fasciculation potentials are the spontaneous discharges of single MUs. The site of generation of these potentials is variable because they may arise either at the level of the soma or in the intramuscular arborization of the motor axon, possibly in *irritable* collateral sprouts.[36–38] In patients with ALS, fasciculation potentials may be recorded profusely or sparsely. Their significance in ALS is not clear, and their presence and extent have little, if any, prognostic value. Indeed as the disease progresses, they may diminish in frequency as muscle fibers lose their innervation.[15]

The clinical or electrical presence of fasciculation is not synonymous with anterior horn cell disease. If restricted to a single myotome, radiculopathy is a more likely cause. Fasciculation is relevant only when associated with neurologic deficit or with other abnormalities recorded on needle EMG, such as fibrillation potentials and abnormal MU morphology or recruitment. Fasciculation is common in otherwise healthy individuals and may be associated with fatigue, excessive caffeine intake, and following sustained exercise (see under Benign Fasciculation Syndrome, later).[39] The authors, however, have encountered several patients with ALS who had been aware of fasciculation for several months before the onset of muscle wasting or weakness.

There is no definitive means of distinguishing between *benign* fasciculation and that associated with disease.[40] Features, however, suggestive of benign fasciculations include a rather higher discharge frequency,[41] the involvement of the same part of the muscle, awareness of the twitching, and the simple morphology of the potentials.

In ALS and other diseases of the anterior horn cell, fasciculation potentials are often large and multiphasic, reflecting the increased sizes of the MUs from which they arise. When the potentials are studied with a single-fiber electrode, abnormal jitter, intermittent blocking, and increased fiber density are frequently present.[42] These changes reflect the degree of collateral sprouting and also the immaturity of the new axonal twigs as well as that of the motor end plates and regenerating muscle fibers.

Motor unit potentials and recruitment

An early and progressively more striking electromyographic abnormality in ALS is the pattern of MU recruitment. Onset firing frequencies of the units are increased (normal, less than 10 c/s), and the ratio of the firing rate of a MU to the number of units already discharging is elevated; this ratio is normally less than 5:1. For example, if a MU is firing at 20 c/s and only one other unit is active, the ratio would be $20:2 = 10:1$. The increased ratio indicates that, to generate a given force, there are fewer MUs available and that these are driven at unusually high frequencies.

In ALS, the volitional MU potentials recorded during effort tend to be larger, longer, and more complex than those in normal muscles. All of these features are a result of the enlargement of the MUs that takes place following collateral reinnervation of denervated muscle fibers. During the strongest effort the patient can exert, the density of the interference pattern is reduced. Sometimes only a single MU can be recruited, and occasionally a muscle appears to be totally denervated. In a study of partially denervated brachial biceps and medial vastus muscles, including those of patients with ALS, Sica et al.[43] found that the durations of the MU potentials gave a better indication of denervation than the numbers of phases or the density and composite amplitude of the maximal interference pattern (Figure 16.3). In a later study, using the same type of automatic analyzer (Anops 101), Kopec and Hausmanowa-Petrusewicz[44] found that the mean amplitude of MU potentials during weak effort was a still more sensitive criterion for the detection of denervation.

The very large amplitudes of some volitional discharges, as recorded with an intramuscular needle electrode, find their counterparts in the increased sizes of the incremental potentials evoked by graded motor nerve stimulation (see later). The fact that

these potentials behave in an all or nothing manner during stimulation[45] proves that they are the responses of single MUs. The point is an important one because it had been repeatedly argued by Buchthal and colleagues[46,47] that the giant potentials in ALS arose from synchronous firing in two or more MUs during voluntary contractions. Figure 16.4 shows a logarithmic plot of the mean MU potential amplitudes in ALS and SMA as functions of the numbers of surviving MUs, as determined in adult patients by the MU counting technique. In both conditions, it can be seen that, as the numbers of surviving MUs decreased, their mean sizes increased. The absence of a plateau in this relationship suggested that, in many of the patients, the sizes of the surviving MUs remained proportional to the numbers of denervated fibers available for adoption by collateral sprouting. In the most extreme case, a 36-year-old woman with a 4-year history of progressive leg weakness, the sole surviving MU in EDB generated a potential of 2 mV, approximately 60 times the mean potential size in control subjects. In a study of

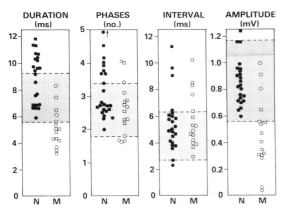

FIGURE 16.3. *Results of automatic analysis of motor unit potentials in the brachial biceps muscle of patients with chronic neuropathic or myopathic disorders (solid squares, amyotrophic lateral sclerosis; solid circles, other denervating disorders; open symbols, myopathies). Confidence limits (95%) for control subjects shown by stippling. (Reprinted with permission from Sica REP, McComas AJ, Ferreira JCD. Evaluation of an automated method for analysing the electromyogram. Can J Neurol Sci 1978; 5:275–282.)*

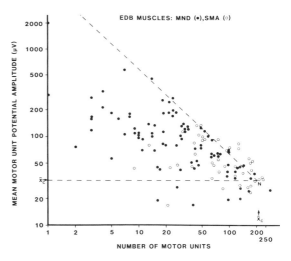

FIGURE 16.4. *Mean motor unit potential amplitudes in extensor digitorum brevis muscles of patients with amyotrophic lateral sclerosis and spinal muscular atrophy (solid and open circles). Extent of denervation shown on abscissa. Mean values for control subjects shown by arrows marked by point N. If there had been no enlargement of motor units following partial denervation, values would be scattered around the interrupted horizontal line; completely successful collateral reinnervation would be seen as values around the interrupted diagonal line. Note logarithmic axes.*

partially denervated rat anterior tibial muscles, using the glycogen depletion technique, Kugelberg et al.[48] found that the extent of collateral regeneration respected the boundaries imposed by fibrous septa within the muscle bellies. It would appear that these partitions either prevented the spread of the stimulus for sprouting, presumably a chemical one, or interfered with the successful outgrowth of axon twigs. Alternatively, the sprouting axons may conceivably respect *domains* established within the muscle bellies during embryologic development in a manner akin to that demonstrated for cutaneous mechanoreceptor fibers.[49] Other evidence for the restricted territorial spread of sprouting axons has come from the scanning EMG studies of Stalberg.[50] In considering the sizes of the MU potentials, it may be observed that the values shown in Figure 16.4 are rather larger than those found by Stalberg[50] using the macro-EMG technique (see following section).

In relation to the complexity, or polyphasicity, of the volitional MU potentials, it should be noted that careful examination, preferably assisted by the use of a window unit and delay line, will often show unusually late spike components. An example of the latter is shown in Figure 16.2(D) in a recording from a patient with SMA; these late components are also found in chronic denervation from other causes as well as in muscular dystrophy.[51] The late components are considered to be generated by muscle fibers with end plates more distant than those of other fibers in the same MU, so extra time is required for propagation of the muscle fiber action potentials toward the recording electrode. Additional delays may be introduced if some of the muscle fibers are thinner than normal, owing to atrophy, or regeneration.

In some patients with ALS, particularly those in whom the disease either is progressing rapidly or has already reached an advanced stage, the MU potentials may become small and brief. These *secondary myopathic* features reflect the inability of the residual motor neurons to undertake collateral reinnervation. The patients with ALS, however, can be distinguished from those with primary myopathies by their reduced interference patterns.

Single-fiber electromyography, macroelectromyography and scanning electromyography

Single-fiber electromyography (SFEMG) was first described in detail by Ekstedt,[52] whereas his collaborator, Stalberg,[53,54] was responsible for developing the two related techniques of macro-EMG and scanning EMG. In SFEMG, recordings are made with one or more very small lead-off areas occupying sideports in a cannula. The electrode is positioned so as to record from two fibers belonging to the same unit. One of these fibers will discharge before the other, and its action potential is used to trigger either the time-base of an oscilloscope or a digital timing device. The time elapsing before discharge of the second fiber is repeatedly measured, and the fluctuation in this interval is termed the *jitter*. Jitter is considered abnormal in a muscle if, in more than one of 20 MUs sampled, it exceeds the upper limit of normality established for the muscle. Stalberg[50] observed abnormal values in the majority of patients with ALS and noted that as many as 20% of clinically unaffected muscles yielded altered values. *Blocking* (failure of excitation) was also seen in some fibers. The increased jitter and blocking were attributed to impaired neuromuscular transmission; the latter was thought to occur both during the onset of the dying-back process in affected motor neurons and, perhaps more frequently, in newly, reinnervated fibers in which neuromuscular junctions were still functionally immature. The SFEMG technique was also used to assess fiber density within MUs; this was defined operationally as the concentration of muscle fibers belonging to one MU within a radius of approximately 300 μm. This parameter was increased in 57 of 63 muscles investigated in patients with ALS and provided a quantitative assessment of the degree of collateral reinnervation.[50] Although increased in ALS, higher values of fiber density were found in SMA, peroneal muscular atrophy, syringomyelia, and old poliomyelitis.[50]

As a practical point, it is worth trying to record single-fiber activity in an ALS patient with the same coaxial or monopolar electrode used for examination of MU potentials and their recruitment. Provided that frequencies below 500 or 1000 c/s are filtered out, it is often possible to demonstrate abnormal jitter in different components of the polyphasic potentials, as in Figure 16.5.

Scanning EMG[54] involves recording from the same MU at successive points in a track made through the muscle by a needle electrode driven by a micromanipulator; triggering of the oscilloscope is provided by a SFEMG electrode locked-in to one of the fibers in the MU. This technique yields information concerning the spatial distribution of the fibers within a MU. Because the results are mostly normal in ALS,[50,55] it would appear that collateral reinnervation usually takes place within the territory originally occupied by the sprouting motor neuron (Figure 16.6).

Macro-EMG was developed by Stalberg[53] in an

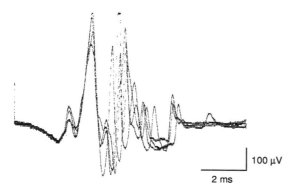

100 μV

2 ms

FIGURE 16.5. *Increased neuromuscular jitter within a polyphasic motor unit potential recorded in a patient with amyotrophic lateral sclerosis, using a monopolar needle electrode; four sweeps have been superimposed.*

attempt to obtain a relative measure of the numbers of fibers constituting single MUs. Averaged recordings are made from a large uninsulated area at the end of the needle electrode, whereas the averaging device is triggered by a single-fiber electrode mounted in a side-port. The recordings are in some respects analogous to those made by surface elec-

trodes as part of the MU counting technique (see later). The macro MU potential amplitudes were found by Stalberg[50] to be increased in more than half of the muscles studied in ALS, particularly in those patients with slowly progressive disease; even higher values were noted in SMA and old poliomyelitis. Stalberg[50] has interpreted some of his observations in ALS in the following way: When axonal sprouting takes place, the fiber density and macro MU potential amplitude increase, owing to the recently acquired fibers; however, until the newly formed neuromuscular junctions have become functionally mature, the jitter is increased.

Repetitive indirect stimulation of muscles

Even before the studies of Stalberg demonstrating increased jitter,[50] there was good evidence for defective neuromuscular transmission in ALS. Thus the amplitude and form of voluntarily recruited MU potentials were noted to fluctuate, and repetitive stimulation of muscles could evoke decremental responses indistinguishable from those of myasthenia gravis.[45,56] The resemblance to myasthenia was strengthened by the observation that the decrement in ALS was enhanced by small doses of tubocurarine and ameliorated by anticholinesterase medication.

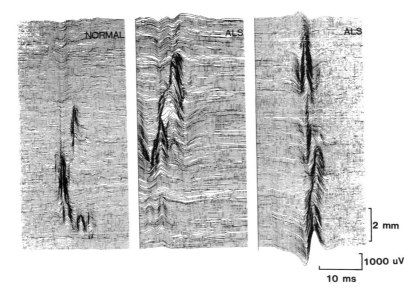

2 mm

1000 uV

10 ms

FIGURE 16.6. *Scanning EMG recordings made from tibialis anterior motor units in a normal subject (left) and in patients with amyotrophic lateral sclerosis (ALS) (middle and right). Note the territorial enlargement in the motor unit shown on the right. (Reprinted with permission from Stalberg E, Sanders DB. The motor unit in ALS studied with different neurophysiological techniques. In: Rose FC, ed. Research progress in motor neurone disease. London: Pitman, 1984:105–122.)*

The similarity between the two conditions is a superficial one, however, because although impaired neuromuscular transmission in ALS is considered to be due to immature or degenerating motor nerve terminals (see preceding section), in myasthenia there is a reduction in the numbers of acetylcholine receptors in the postsynaptic membrane.[57] Nevertheless, it is important for the electromyographer to recognize that the presence of a decremental muscle response to repetitive stimulation should not lead to a diagnosis of myasthenia gravis unless it can be shown, by other parts of the electromyographic examination, that there is no evidence of denervation (or myopathy).[58]

H wave studies

In those ALS patients with prominent upper motor neuron signs, the amplitude of the H wave in the calf muscles is increased relative to the size of the M wave. In addition, paired stimulation reveals that the recovery of excitability in the H wave loop occurs more rapidly in patients than in control subjects[59,60]; these findings reflect the partial removal of descending inhibition from the reflex circuit. The same H wave changes occur following other types of upper motor neuron lesion. It should be noted, however, that in normal subjects occasionally the entire triceps surae motor neuron population can participate in the H wave.[61] The H wave is a useful extension of the electromyographic examination in those patients with ALS who present with weakness and spasticity owing to corticospinal tract involvement. Thus a normal or enhanced reflex is clear evidence that the motor deficit is predominantly of the upper motor neuron type. Studies of F waves are of limited value in ALS but may occasionally be useful in demonstrating slowed impulse conduction in the proximal segments of motor axons in those patients having antibodies to GM_1 ganglioside.

Motor unit estimation

Motor unit estimation (counting) involves the application of weak stimuli to a motor nerve or motor point; as the stimulus intensity is gradually increased, the evoked muscle response grows in discrete increments. On the assumption that each increment is due to the excitation of an additional MU, the mean MU potential amplitude or area is measured and compared with the corresponding value for the entire muscle. Although there are limitations as well as advantages, MU estimation remains the only method capable of estimating the size of the functional motor

neuron pool[2,22]; it has also been shown to be more sensitive than coaxial needle EMG in detecting denervation in the intrinsic muscles of the hand and foot.[62] Further, the technique has been fully automated, so many of the problems previously associated with it can now be avoided.[63] Variations on the basic method include the application of Poisson analysis to examine the fluctuating responses induced by repetitive stimulation[64] and the use of spike-triggered averaging, rather than graded stimulation, to collect individual MU potentials.[65,66]

Typical recordings, made with the original manual method of McComas et al. in a patient with chronic muscle denervation, are shown in Figure 16.7 together with those from a control subject. Some of the increments evoked in the thenar muscles by graded stimulation of the median nerve are seen to be much larger in the patient than in the control subject. This enlargement is due to the increased sizes of the surviving MUs following collateral reinnervation of muscle fibers. This compensatory mechanism may be sufficient to prevent detectable weak-

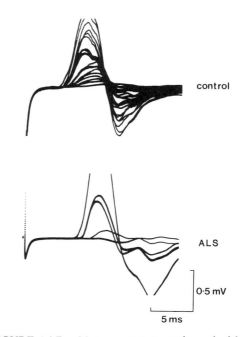

FIGURE 16.7. *Motor unit potentials evoked by graded stimulation in the median-innervated thenar muscles in a normal subject (top) and in a patient with amyotrophic lateral sclerosis (bottom). Note the larger sizes of the incremental potentials in the patient, owing to enlargement of motor units through collateral reinnervation.*

ness and wasting of muscles until late in the course of the disease, when only one-quarter of the MU population remains.[67] On the basis of averaged twitch tensions developed by single MUs, however, there is some doubt as to whether the enlarged MUs are as effective in tension generation as their sizes would suggest.[68] One reason for this discrepancy may be that, during voluntary contraction, blocking of excitation may occur at individual neuromuscular junctions or in nerve branches[50] (see later). In experimental animals, increased fatigability has been clearly demonstrated in reinnervated muscles[69] and has been shown to be due to impaired neuromuscular transmission.[70]

Figure 16.8 shows the number of functioning MUs in the EDB, thenar, and hypothenar muscles of 130 patients with ALS at the time of their first electromyographic examinations; because of the loss of units that occurs in normal subjects as part of the aging process, the results in patients beyond the age of 60 have been shown separately. It can be seen that the majority of muscles yielded abnormally low values, only 8% of the EDB muscles, 6% of the thenar muscles, and 22% of the hypothenar muscles having numbers of MUs within the respective control ranges.

Although the degree of involvement varied between muscles and between patients, there was a tendency for neighboring muscles to be similarly affected in the same individual. Thus the thenar and hypothenar muscles would be involved to similar degrees, as would the EDB and plantar muscles; there was less agreement between the intrinsic muscles of the hand as opposed to those of the foot. For example, some patients had almost total denervation of the foot with no involvement of the hand and vice versa. The heterogeneity in MU involvement was also observed when serial studies were performed on the same patient to assess the rate of MU loss. Figure 16.9 shows examples from some ALS patients; the results have been normalized for each of the muscles studied. In some muscles, there was seen to be a

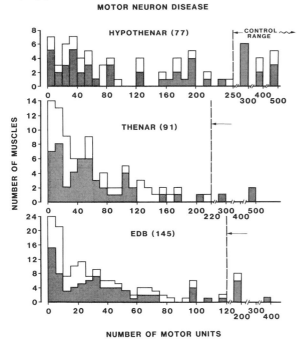

FIGURE 16.8. *Numbers of functioning motor units in extensor digitorum brevis, thenar, and hypothenar muscles of patients with amyotrophic lateral sclerosis. A total of 130 patients were investigated; the results are those obtained at the time of initial EMG. The results for patients aged 60 years and over are shown by open columns; values for younger patients indicated by solid columns.*

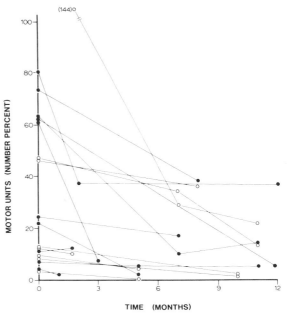

FIGURE 16.9. *Numbers of functioning motor units in patients with amyotrophic lateral sclerosis studied on two or more occasions; the values have been normalized for the muscle concerned (thenar, hypothenar, or extensor digitorum brevis). See the section on coaxial and unipolar needle studies in the text.*

steep initial drop in the number of functioning MUs, in others, the deterioration was steady, and in others, the MU population remained unchanged for up to 1 year. One remarkable patient with familial ALS, reported elsewhere (patient E.Q.[2]), has now been further studied. Over the period of observation, her MU counts have fluctuated in a striking manner, both increasing and decreasing. At the last examination of this patient, the aggregate value was not significantly different from that obtained at the time of initial EMG 6 years previously. Interestingly the fluctuations in MU counts tended to remain in step among the different muscles investigated. Our interpretation of these results is that, within the spinal cord of this patient, there was a population of motor neurons that could recover sufficient function for neuromuscular transmission to become temporarily reestablished. Additional cases of ALS, which were atypical because of their protracted course or unexpected improvement, have been reported by Engel et al.[71] In other patients of the present series, it has not been unusual to find one muscle rapidly shedding MUs, while other MU populations remained stable.

Stimulation of the motor cortex

The advent of transcranial magnetic stimulation has made it possible to study the integrity of the upper motor neuron and of the central motor pathways. It is beyond the scope of this chapter to discuss the many aspects of cortical magnetic stimulation; these have been detailed elsewhere.[72] The technique is helpful and of interest in the 10% of ALS patients in whom upper motor neuron features predominate.[73,74]

In such patients, the latency of the motor evoked potential (MEP) is only modestly prolonged. The principal abnormalities are the marked reduction in amplitude and the increased dispersions of the responses (Figure 16.10); in addition, the thresholds for magnetic stimulation appear to be raised. In patients presenting with pseudobulbar features and pyramidal tract signs, MEPs may not be detected, even when the muscle mass is preserved. In contrast, a MEP can nearly always be obtained, albeit small and dispersed, when lower motor neuron features predominate and the target muscle is weak and wasted. Finally, there are rare patients, with early ALS, in whom the MEPs are increased in amplitude.

Single motor unit contractile responses

There have been several attempts to measure the forces developed by single MUs in patients with ALS. In the first such study, McComas et al.[67] found the twitch tensions evoked by juxtathreshold stimulation of EDB axons to be increased, although the patient pool included some with muscle denervation from other causes. Using spike-triggered averaging in first dorsal interosseous muscles, Milner-Brown et al.[68] were unable to confirm these results because the averaged MU responses were diminished. The problem has now been carefully reexamined by Dengler et al.[75] using the same technique as Milner-Brown. Dengler et al. found that MU twitch tensions were increased in ALS patients with mild weakness but were decreased in those with more advanced disease. Dengler et al. considered that the *weak* responses belonged to units undergoing dying-back in their terminal axonal branches. It was more difficult to explain, in other units, the discrepancy between a small twitch and a large compound action potential; it was possible, however, that impaired neuromuscular transmission or a trophic deficiency were contributory factors.

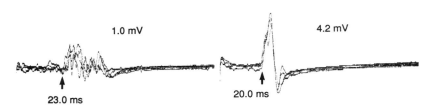

1.0 mV

4.2 mV

23.0 ms

20.0 ms

FIGURE 16.10.   *Contrasting responses evoked in thenar muscles of healthy subject (right) and patient with amyotrophic lateral sclerosis (left) by magnetic stimulation of contralateral motor cortex. Note the reduced amplitude, increased dispersion, and greater latency in the patient; the stimulus threshold was also higher, by 42%.*

SPINAL MUSCULAR ATROPHIES (HEREDITARY MOTOR NEUROPATHIES)

Clinical Considerations

The SMAs are a group of heredofamilial disorders characterized by degeneration or maldevelopment of motor neurons in the brain stem and spinal cord. The condition may present clinically at any age between infancy and late middle age, and both sexes are susceptible; a particularly large series of patients has been studied by Hausmanowa-Petrusewicz.[76] As noted by Thomas (see Chapter 15), there have been several attempts to classify these disorders on the basis of age of onset, severity, distribution of weakness, and mode of inheritance. Descriptive or eponymous terms have been replaced by numerical schemes such as that of Harding[77]; this author recognizes five types of proximal hereditary motorneuropathy (HMN), five distal types of HMN, and several forms with complex distributions of muscle involvement. In the most severe form of SMA (SMA type I; type I proximal HMN; acute Werding-Hoffman disease), an autosomal recessive gene is involved[78] and has now been localized to chromosome 5.[79] The possibility exists, however, that some cases may have resulted from an unrecognized agent, such as a viral infection, during pregnancy. Often the mother, if multiparous, will have noticed reduced fetal movements. In this type of SMA, there is widespread muscle weakness, although the extraocular muscles are spared, and some movement of the toes and fingers may be present. The limbs are hypotonic, and the poor development of the muscles is evident on palpation. The tendon reflexes are absent, and fasciculations may be seen in the tongue. The condition is associated with severe respiratory and feeding problems; the first few weeks of life are usually spent on the respirator, and there is constant danger of aspiration and cardiopulmonary collapse. The child is never able to raise the head or to sit up, but an impression of mental alertness is given by the responsive eye movements. Death, usually from pneumonia, occurs before the end of the first year. At first, the condition must be distinguished from cerebral palsy as well as from other neuromuscular disorders; the latter include infantile myotonic dystrophy, centronuclear myopathy, nemaline myopathy, myasthenia gravis, congenital muscular dystrophy, and arthrogryposis multiplex congenita.

SMA type II (type II proximal HMN; chronic infantile Werding-Hoffman disease) also presents in infancy, sometimes at birth, more commonly within the next few months, but always before 2 years of age; an autuosomal recessive gene has been traced to chromosome 5, at the same locus as that for SMA type I[80] (see earlier). The weakness and wasting are generalized in many patients, but in those who live longest there is sparing of the facial and bulbar muscles and relatively modest involvement of the intrinsic muscles of the hands and feet. The trunk and proximal muscles of the limbs are always affected, however, and this leads to the development of joint contractures. Fasciculations may be observed in the tongue but not elsewhere; upper motor neuron signs are absent. Less than one-quarter of patients are ever able to sit unsupported, and few manage to crawl or walk.[81] Some children die in their second year, but others survive into the third and fourth decades, exhibiting remarkable muscle atrophy. In such chronic cases, there are invariably severe deformities of the chest associated with scoliosis. Poor respiratory function, owing to a combination of muscular weakness and skeletal restrictions, usually leads to death from pneumonia.

SMA type III (type III proximal HMN; chronic proximal form; Kugelberg-Welander syndrome) is the most benign type of SMA. The first clear recognition of its pathologic nature was made by Kugelberg and Welander.[82] The condition typically presents as weakness in the hip, quadriceps, and trunk muscles of young adults, causing problems in walking, climbing stairs, and rising from a chair. Later, the shoulder muscles become involved, winging of the scapula appears, and there is difficulty in raising the arms above shoulder height. Distal muscles of the limbs are less commonly involved, and facial and bulbar muscles are spared. Fasciculations may be observed in the limb muscles in approximately half of the patients but not in the tongue. Tendon reflexes are usually depressed but are occasionally associated with extensor plantar responses.[83] In approximately one-third of patients, there is obvious enlargement of some muscles, particularly in the calves,[2,84] leading to a striking resemblance to limb-girdle muscular dystrophy. The close relationship between the two conditions is emphasized by the fact that adult patients, carrying the diagnosis of SMA, may show *secondary* myopathic EMG and biopsy changes in some of their muscles.[58,85] Conversely, patients with limb-girdle dystrophy may have electromyographic evidence of denervation in distal muscles.[86] Finally, in the Hamilton region of Ontario, Canada there is a sibship in which one brother and one sister woud be diagnosed as having limb-girdle dystrophy on the basis of the EMG, whereas another brother, less severely affected and exhibiting remarkable muscle hypertrophy, exhibits the electromyographic features of SMA.[2] Because limb-girdle dystrophy and SMA type III are usually inherited through autosomal recessive genes and because the two conditions progress in a similar manner, there is no practical benefit in forcing difficult cases into one diagnostic category or the other.

Distal forms of SMA are much less common than the proximal varieties described here; based on age of onset and mode of inheritance, Harding[77] has identified five types of distal HMN. It may also be remarked that some patients with a facioscapulohumeral distribution of weakness prove to have SMA on EMG. In three Hamilton families, inheritance was autosomal dominant, as in the family studied by Fenichel et al.[87] A family with a scapuloperoneal distribution of weakness and muscle wasting has been investigated in detail by Kaeser,[88] who was able to demonstrate denervation changes in distal muscles and *myopathic* features in proximal ones; losses of spinal and bulbar motor neurons were noted at autopsy in one of the patients. Among our series of patients is a man with an unusually limited form of SMA in which all the muscles of the thighs are extremely wasted and in whom other muscles are unaffected; in another patient, the gastrocnemii have atrophied completely in both legs, whereas the solei have remained strong and have retained their bulk.

Electromyographic Examination

Nerve conduction studies

The results of standard nerve conduction studies in SMA types II and III are similar to those in ALS, with normal values being found in the majority of patients.[76] Denervation of distal muscles is less severe in SMA than in ALS and prolongation of the distal motor latency less common in SMA as well. In SMA type I, conduction velocities of the slowest conducting heater fibers, when measured by special techniques are reduced relative to control children of similar ages. Further, maturation of motor nerve fibers appears to be delayed in SMA type I because adult values of maximum conduction velocities are reached at a later age than in healthy children.[76,89,90]

Sensory nerve studies in SMA type III resemble those in ALS in exhibiting normal impulse conduction velocities and response amplitudes. Among the adult patients with SMA studied by ourselves, there are two, however, in whom the radial, median, ulnar, and sural nerve responses are small; these patients

have otherwise typical features of SMA type III, including prominent fasciculations and muscle enlargement. The other exception to normality of sensory findings in SMA concerns infants with SMA type I in whom sensory responses, although present, are rather smaller than in similarly aged children with cerebral palsy (McComas AJ. Unpublished observations). Indeed, other authors have been unable to detect sural nerve responses in some of the infants with SMA type I.[91] Abnormalities in sensory nerve function would be consistent with the presence of ultrastructural changes in sensory fibers and ganglion cells.[76,92]

Needle studies

All the signs of denervation noted in ALS with needle electrodes (see earlier) are to be found in older children and adults with SMA (i.e., types II and III). There are important quantitative differences, however, in that fibrillation potentials and positive sharp waves are usually less prominent in SMA, although complex repetitive discharges are more commonly observed (see Figure 16.2). In Hausmanowa-Petrusewicz's large series[76] of patients with SMA type III, complex repetitive discharges were noted in 18% of muscles examined.

In contrast to the situation for patients with SMA type III and older children with SMA type II, the needle EMG examination is much more difficult to perform and to interpret satisfactorily in infants with SMA type I. Thus in some muscles, the volitional and reflexly elicited MU potentials may be indistinguishable from those of a normal infant. In contrast, in badly affected muscles with poorly developed bellies, there may be no detectable electromyographic activity at all. Hausmanowa-Petrusewicz[76] has drawn attention to the bimodal distribution of MU potential parameters in SMA type I. As the disease advanced, the abnormally small brief potentials persisted unchanged but were associated with an increasing incidence of large prolonged potentials. In studying infants suspected of SMA, we always include the brachial biceps, deltoid, intermediate vastus, and anterior tibial muscles in the needle examination; in the last muscle especially, it is normally possible to induce strong reflex activity by stimulation of the skin distally. Mention must be made of one electromyographic sign that appears to be specific for SMA type I; this is the occurrence of rhythmic MU discharges at a frequency of 5 to 15 c/s.[93] These potentials persist during sleep and muscle relaxation; despite their complex spontaneous activity, the discharging units are evidently functional because they can participate in voluntary movements of the infant.

Finally, in the adult form of SMA, it should be noted that there may be many muscles, particularly distal ones, that will not show any electromyographic abnormalities. This finding is in keeping with the often-normal MU counts in SMA (Figure 16.11) and with the lack of clinical involvement of the distal muscles; it stands in contrast to the results in ALS, which invariably show reduced MU counts (see Figure 16.8).

Repetitive stimulation

As in ALS, repetitive stimulation of partially denervated muscles in patients with SMA may evoke decremental responses. This abnormality is best seen with a stimulus frequency of 10 c/s and is most probably due to impaired transmission in neuromuscular junctions that have been recently established on previously denervated muscle fibers.[50,94]

Motor unit estimates

MU counting is often informative in SMA and may be carried out with equal ease in floppy neonates (SMA type I) as in adult patients (SMA type III). The results obtained at the initial examination in 45 consecutive patients with SMA are displayed in Figure 16.11. Twelve of these patients were children whose

ages ranged from 6 days to 6 years; patients with mixed myopathic and neuropathic features were excluded from the study. It can be seen that reduced MU counts were frequently observed in the muscles studied (EDB, thenar, hypothenar). The results differed from those in ALS, however, in that normal values were obtained in approximately one-third of muscles, and consequently the mean values for each muscle were significantly higher in SMA than in ALS. Figure 16.11 also shows that there was a tendency for children with SMA to have smaller MU populations than adults, a finding that would be in keeping with the more severe and generalized nature of the disorder in SMA type I and SMA type II, as opposed to SMA type III (see earlier).

Perhaps the most striking dissimilarity between SMA and ALS comes from the results of serial testing. In ALS, MU populations remain stable for a period of months, decline steadily, or rapidly diminish (see Figure 16.9). In SMA, however, the MU counts are as often found to increase as to decrease. This surprising behavior is evident in Figure 16.12, which contains first and last observations in 22 muscles of nine patients studied for 4 to 10 years (mean observation period, 6.8 ± 2.4 years). The sizes of the increases in MU counts in some muscles are too large to be accounted for on the basis of experimental error, and in one patient (see Figure 16.12, arrows), they coincided with the transition of a severely disabled 6-year-old girl into a 16-year-old adolescent

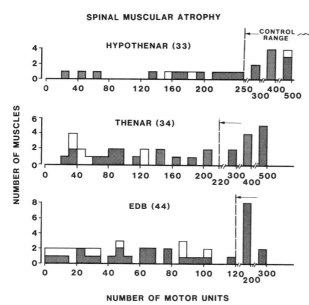

FIGURE 16.11. *Numbers of functioning motor units in the extensor digitorum brevis, thenar, and hypothenar muscles of patients with spinal muscular atrophy. A total of 45 patients were studied, and the results shown are those determined at the first electromyogram. The values for children (up to 6 years) are depicted by open bars; remaining data are indicated by stippled bars.*

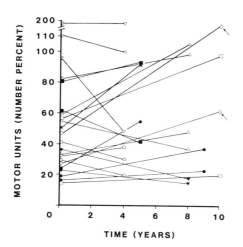

FIGURE 16.12.   *Numbers of functioning motor units in patients with spinal muscular atrophy studied on two occasions; the values have been normalized for the muscle concerned (thenar, hypothenar, or extensor digitorum brevis).*

with only mild weakness, who enjoyed a wide range of physical activities, including cycling and swimming.

The lability of the MU counts in some muscles of patients with SMA indicates that, in such instances, the motor neurons are fluctuating between *healthy* and *dysfunctional* states, so continuous remodeling of the MU territories takes place.[2] The MU counting technique has also provided data concerning the relative sizes of the surviving MUs in partially denervated muscles of patients with SMA. The results included in Figure 16.4 are those for adult patients only (SMA type III); as in ALS, there is evidence of marked enlargement of MUs, reflected in the mean amplitudes of the MU potentials. Up to a certain point, corresponding to 80% denervation, the enlargement of surviving MUs, through collateral reinnervation, appears to compensate fully for the loss of other MUs. Unlike the findings of Stalberg,[50] there is no indication that sprouting is any less vigorous in ALS than in SMA, when muscles with similar degrees of denervation are compared.

BENIGN FASCICULATION SYNDROME

Fasciculation is a term that describes twitching of part of a muscle owing to spontaneous discharges in one or more MUs. Very often the muscle contrac-

tions are visible through the skin; when the contracting units lie deeply within the muscle belly, however, their presence will be detected only by needle EMG. As already noted, fasciculations are found in the majority of patients with ALS and in half of those with the adult form of SMA (SMA type III). They may also be observed in a variety of conditions affecting either the motor neurons or, less commonly, the motor axons; these conditions include cervical spondylosis, lumbosacral radiculopathies, peroneal muscular atrophy, syringomyelia, poliomyelitis, thyrotoxicosis, tetany, anticholinesterase medication, and, infrequently, peripheral neuropathies. In the majority of subjects with fasciculation, however, no underlying neuromuscular disorder can be discovered, and the condition is then termed the *benign fasciculation syndrome*. A survey of medical personnel by Reed and Kurland[95] revealed that 70% had noticed some form of muscle twitching in themselves. It is stated that there is nothing in the oscillographic appearance of fasciculation potentials to distinguish those in ALS (malignant fasciculations) from the benign form.[41,96] Nevertheless, most electromyographers would probably accept the following statements:

1. Benign fasciculations occur at a higher frequency than malignant ones, the respective mean intervals being 0.8 and 3.5 seconds.
2. Benign fasciculations tend to involve the same part of a muscle, whereas malignant fasciculations appear unpredictably over the muscle surface.
3. Subjects are more aware of benign fasciculations than of malignant ones.
4. Benign fasciculations can usually be suppressed for a few seconds by rubbing the skin overlying the contracting part of the muscle.
5. Fasciculation potentials that appear large, prolonged, and polyphasic are more likely to be malignant.
6. Benign fasciculations are especially likely to occur in the calves and soles of the feet as well as in the lower part of the orbicularis oculi (facial myokymia). Malignant fasciculations may involve any muscle more than others.
7. Voluntary recruitment of fasciculating MUs is possible in the benign syndrome but not in ALS.

In practice, fasciculations would only be dismissed as benign if there was no clinical or electromyographic evidence of muscle denervation. In this context, it is of interest that MU estimation, perhaps the most sensitive indication of denervation, is normal in the benign fasciculation syndrome.

The uncertainty regarding the significance of fasciculations applies equally well to the site of their generation. Layzer[97] concluded that most of the experiments employing nerve block in ALS indicated a distal origin in the MU.[98] In the benign syndrome, the temporary suppression by tactile stimulation suggests that reflex inhibition of spontaneously active motor neurons is taking place. An ingenious approach to the location of the pacemaker site for fasciculations is that of Roth.[99] This author pointed out that if a fasciculation had been generated by a distal pacemaker (e.g., in the intramuscular branches of an axon), an impulse initiated in the parent axon by proximal electrical stimulation should be blocked by collision with the antidromically propagating one. In 80% of fasciculations in patients with various lower motor neuron lesions, the discharges appeared to arise distally. Wettstein,[38] however, used the same technique and concluded that the majority of fasciculations arose centrally. Part of the discrepancy may have been due to the different subject populations studied; Roth[37] also considers that excessive delay in the triggering of the interpolated stimulus may have been responsible for some of Wettstein's findings. In mice with hereditary amyelination of dorsal and ventral root fibers, Rasminsky[100] has shown that fasciculations follow ephaptic impulse transmission between neighboring motor axons; it is possible that a similar mechanism operates in those patients with fasciculations complicating focal or diffuse demyelination of axons.

OTHER MOTOR NEURON DISORDERS

Monomelic Amyotrophy or Focal Motor Neuron Disease

This is a rare motor neuron disorder, predominantly afflicting young men. The muscle wasting and weakness are insidious in onset and are usually restricted for many years to one limb (an arm more frequently than a leg). EMG of the involved limb is characterized by abnormal recruitment of MUs that are large, of long duration, and complex. Even though the other limbs are clinically normal, however, they may nevertheless exhibit similar but less marked changes. Fibrillation potentials and positive sharp waves are sparse in comparison with classic ALS, and the prognosis for monomelic atrophy is much better than for ALS. In view of the young ages of patients with

monomelic amyotrophy, the possibility of an intraspinal lesion, especially syringomyelia, should be considered in the differential diagnosis.

Motor Neuronopathy Associated with Antibodies to GM₁ Ganglioside

A motor neuronopathy closely mimicking ALS has been described.[101–104] The condition may begin asymmetrically and be associated with fasciculations. Tendon reflexes may be maintained, whereas abnormal sensory findings are either absent or minimal. The electrophysiologic hallmark is that of severe, multifocal conduction block, with or without slowing of impulse conduction (see Figure 16.1). Over a period of several years, muscle wasting can become pronounced and reflexes lost. Bulbar muscle weakness has not been described. The natural history of the condition is one of slow progression. This form of motor neuronopathy is of special interest because it is associated with the presence of antibodies to GM_1 ganglioside. There is no convincing evidence, however, that the course of the disease can be halted or reversed by cyclophosphamide, steroids, or plasmapheresis.

Although it is now apparent that anti-GM_1 ganglioside antibodies can occur in a variety of neurologic diseases (including ALS) as well as in otherwise healthy subjects,[23] the levels of antibodies are lower than in motor neuronopathy. Evidence of multifocal conduction block should be looked for in all new patients suspected of having ALS by stimulating two or more motor nerves at several sites.

Fazio-Londe Disease

This rare condition is inherited by an autosomal recessive gene and is characterized by progressive weakness of external ocular, facial, and bulbar muscles in early childhood.[105] EMG shows the presence of fibrillation potentials and positive sharp waves in bulbar and facial muscles, together with reductions in the respective interference patterns.

Arthrogryposis Multiplex Congenita

Infants born with joint contractures can usually be shown to have neuropathic features in muscles examined by coaxial needle EMG or MU counting. At autopsy, losses of anterior horn cells can be demonstrated in most if not all of the spinal cords.[95,106] These findings raise the possibility that arthrogryposis multiplex congenita is a manifestation of infantile SMA. Further, Drachman and Coulombre[107] have suggested, on the basis of experiments on the chick embryo, that the ankylosis of joints is a consequence of the lack of movements of the fetal limbs.

Poliomyelitis and Viral Infections of Motor Neurons

Owing to widespread vaccination, new cases of poliomyelitis are unlikely to be encountered by the electromyographer, although progressive paralysis has been seen following administration of the vaccine to immunodeficient children.[108] The earliest electromyographic abnormality observed in cases of poliomyelitis was a reduction in the interference pattern, followed by the appearance of fibrillation potentials and positive sharp waves. It is now considered that further muscle denervation owing to loss of terminal motor nerve branches may occur many years after an episode of paralytic poliomyelitis[109]; preceding viral infection has been incriminated as one causative agent in ALS,[110,111] although this is now doubtful. Thus no evidence of persisting viral infection can be found in such cases,[112] and it appears that the later denervation may simply reflect accelerated aging of the surviving motor neurons. These patients fare much better than those with ALS, and their electromyograms show correspondingly less spontaneous muscle fiber activity. MU counting is of great value in determining prognosis if several muscles are examined on more than one occasion, so the rate of denervation can be estimated.

A syndrome of rapidly developing muscle denervation, resembling acute poliomyelitis, may occasionally complicate infections with enteroviruses of the Coxsackie and ECHO types. Rarely an adult or child may develop a polio-like paralysis of one or more limbs without identifiable virus, and in some boys there is an association with asthma.[113] Other

viruses that may infect and destroy motor neurons are herpes zoster virus and the transmissible agent responsible for Creutzfeldt-Jakob disease. In the latter condition, postmortem studies indicate losses of motor neurons from the spinal cords of approximately half the patients.[114] Because Creutzfeldt-Jakob disease may present with weakness and wasting of muscles, fasciculations, and upper motor neuron signs (the amyotrophic form[115]), it may sometimes resemble ALS closely. If Creutzfeldt-Jakob disease is a diagnostic possibility, the intramuscular electrode must not be used again for fear of transmitting the infectious agent to another patient.

Syringomyelia

A syrinx in the central cord may mimic ALS by presenting with weakness and wasting of the intrinsic muscles of the hand and upper motor neuron signs in the legs. The similarity is heightened by the association of electromyographic features of muscle denervation and of normal sensory nerve potentials in the hands. In contrast to ALS, however, clinical examination usually reveals sensory loss of one or more modalities, and unless the syrinx has extended into the lumbosacral cord, there is no electromyographic evidence of denervation in the leg muscles.

Shy-Drager Syndrome

The full form of this condition includes wasting of distal muscles and fasciculations together with evidence of denervation in EMG and muscle biopsy.[116] Although the tendon reflexes are usually normal, the plantar responses may be extensor, increasing the similarity to ALS. The autonomic features of the Shy-Drager syndrome are sufficiently striking, however, for the correct diagnosis to be made in most instances.

REFERENCES

1. Rowland LP. Diverse forms of motor neurone diseases. Adv Neurol 1982; 1(36):1–11.
2. McComas AJ. Neuromuscular function and disorders. London: Butterworth, 1977.
3. Campbell MJ, McComas AJ, Petito F. Physiological changes in aging muscles. J Neurol Neurosurg Psychiatry 1973; 36:174–182.
4. Tomlinson BE, Irving D. The numbers of limb motor neurones in the human lumbosacral cord through life. J Neurol Sci 1977; 34:213–219.
5. Calne DB, Eisen A, McGeer et al. Alzeimer's disease, Parkinson's disease, and Motorneurone disease:

Abiotrophic interaction between aging and environment? Lancet 1986; 2:1067–1070.
6. Eisen A, Hudson AJ. Amyotrophic lateral sclerosis: Concepts in pathogenesis and etiology. Can J Neurol Sci 1987; 14:649–652.
7. Durrleman S, Alprerovitch A. Increasing trend of ALS in France and elsewhere: Are the changes real? Neurology 1989; 39:768–773.
8. Gunnarsson L, Lindberg G, Soderfelt B, et al. The mortality of motor neuron disease in Sweden. Arch Neurol 1990; 47:42–46.
9. Lilienfeld DE, Chan E, Ehland J, et al. Increasing mortality from motor neuron disease in the United States during the past two decades. Lancet 1989; 1:710–713.

10. Rowland LP. Motor neuron diseases and amyotrophic lateral sclerosis: Research progress. TINS 1987; 10:393–398.

11. Drachman DB, Kuncl RW. Amyotrophic lateral sclerosis: An unconventional autoimmune disease? Ann Neurol 1989; 26:269–274.

12. Englehardt JI, Appel SH, Killian JM. Experimental autoimmune motoneuron disease. Ann Neurol 1989; 26:368–376.

13. Murayama S, Mori H, Ihara Y, et al. Immunocytochemical and ultrastructural studies of lower motor neurons in amyotrophic lateral sclerosis. Ann Neurol 1990; 27:137–148.

14. McComas AJ, Upton AR, Sica RP. Motoneurone disease and aging. Lancet 1973; 2:1477–1480.

15. Daube JR. Electrophysiologic studies in the diagnosis and prognosis of motor neuron diseases. Neurol Clin 1985; 3:473–493.

16. Lambert EH. Electromyography in amyotrophic lateral sclerosis. In: Norris FH, Kurland LT, eds. Motor neurone diseases: Research on amyotrophic lateral sclerosis and related disorders. New York: Grune & Stratton, 1969:135–153.

17. Isch F, Isch-Treussard C, Jesel M. La mesure de la vitesse de conduction des fibres nerveuses motrices dans les atrophies neurogenes, chroniques et progressives. Rev Neurol (Paris) 1966; 115:122–129.

18. Thomas PK, Sears TA, Gilliatt RW. The range of conduction velocity in normal motor nerve fibres in the small muscles of the hand and foot. J Neurol Neurosurg Psychiatry 1959; 22:175–181.

19. Hopf HC. Untersuchungen uber die unterschiede in der leitgeschwindigkeit motorischer nervenfasern beim menschen. Deutsch Z Nervenheilk 1962; 183:579–588.

20. Freund HJ, Budingen HJ, Dietz V. Activity of single motor units from human forearm muscles during voluntary isometric contractions. J Neurophysiol 1975; 38:933–946.

21. Hansen S, Ballantyne JP. A quantitative electrophysiological study of motor neurone disease. J Neurol Neurosurg Psychiatry 1978; 41:773–783.

22. McComas AJ, Fawcett PR, Campbell MJ, et al. Electrophysiological estimation of the number of motor units within a human muscle. J Neurol Neurosurg Psychiatry 1971; 34:121–131.

23. Sadiq SA, Thomas FP, Kilidireas K, et al. The spectrum of neurological disease associated with anti-GM$_1$ antibodies. Neurology 1990; 40:1067–1072.

24. Fincham RW, Van Allen MW. Sensory nerve conduction in amyotrophic lateral sclerosis. Neurology (NY) 1964; 14:31–33.

25. Ertekin C. Sensory and motor conduction in motor neurone disease. Acta Neurol Scand 1967; 43:499–512.

26. Mulder DW, Bushek W, Spring E, et al. Motor neuron disease (ALS): Evaluation of detection thresholds of cutaneous sensation. Neurology 1983; 33:1625–1627.

27. Bradley WG, Good P, Rasool OG, et al. Morphometric and biochemical studies of peripheral nerves in amyotrophic lateral sclerosis. Ann Neurol 1983; 14:267–277.

28. Dyck RJ, Stevens JC, Mulder DW, et al. Frequency of nerve fiber degeneration of peripheral motor and sensory neurons in amyotrophic lateral sclerosis: Morphometry of deep and superficial peroneal nerves. Neurology 1975; 25:781–785.

29. Matheson JLK, Harrington HJ, Hallett M. Abnormalities of multimodality evoked potentials in amyotrophic lateral sclerosis. Arch Neurol 1986; 43:338–340.

30. Brown MC, Ironton R. Sprouting and regression of neuromuscular synapses in partially denervated mammalian muscles. J Physiol (Lond) 1978; 278:325–348.

31. Kuncl RW, Cornblath DR, Griffin JW. Assessment of thoracic paraspinal muscles in the diagnosis of ALS. Muscle Nerve 1988; 11:484–492.

32. Emeryk B, Hausmanowa-Petrusewicz I, Nowak T. Spontaneous volleys of bizzare high frequency potentials (b.h.f.p.) in neuro-muscular diseases. Part a. Occurrence of spontaneous volleys of b.h.f.p. in neuromuscular diseases. Electromyogr Clin Neurophysiol 1974; 14:303–338.

33. Belmar J, Eyzaguirre C. Pacemaker site of fibrillation potentials in denervated mammalian muscle. J Neurophysiol 1966; 29:425–441.

34. Thesleff S, Ward MR. Studies on the mechanism of fibrillation potentials in denervated muscle. J Physiol (Lond) 1975; 244:313–323.

35. Stalberg E, Trontelj JV. Abnormal discharges generated within the motor unit as observed with single-fiber electromyography. In: Culp WJ, Ochoa J, eds. Abnormal nerves and muscles as impulse generators. New York: Oxford University Press, 1982:443–474.

36. Conradi S, Grimby L, Lundemo G. Pathophysiology of fasciculations in ALS as studies by electromyography of single motor units. Muscle Nerve 1982; 5:202–208.

37. Roth G. The origin of fasciculations. Ann Neurol 1982; 12:542–547.

38. Wettstein A. The origin of fasciculations in motorneuron diseases. Ann Neurol 1979; 5:295–300.

39. Layzer RB. Diagnostic implications of clinical fasciculation and cramps. Adv Neurol 1982; 36:23–27.

40. McComas AJ. Motor neuron disorders. In: Brown WF, Bolton CF, eds. Clinical Electromyography, ed 1. Boston: Butterworths, 1987:431–451.

41. Trojaborg W, Buchthal F. Malignant and benign fasciculations. Acta Neurol Scand 1965; 41 (suppl 13):251–254.

42. Janko M, Trontelj JV, Gersak K. Fasciculations in motor neuron disease: Discharge rate reflects extent and recency of collateral sprouting. J Neurosurg Psychiatry 1989; 52:1375–1381.

43. Sica REP, McComas AJ, Ferreira JCD. Evaluation of automated method for analysing the electromyogram. Can J Neurol Sci 1978; 5:275–281.
44. Kopec J, Hausmanowa-Petrusewicz. I. 1. Computeranalyse des EMG and klinische Ergerbnisse. 2. Elektroenzeph Elektromyogr 1983; 14:28–35.
45. Kugelberg E, Taverner D. A comparison between the voluntary and electrical activation of motor units in anterior horn cell diseases. Electroencephalogr Clin Neurophysiol 1950; 2:125–132.
46. Buchthal F, Clemmesen S. On differentiation of muscle atrophy by electromyography. Acta Psychiatr Scand 1941; 16:143–181.
47. Buchthal F. The electromyogram. World Neurol 1962; 3:16–34.
48. Kugelberg E, Edstrom L, Abbruzzese M. Mapping of motor units in experimentally reinnervated rat muscle. Interpretation of histochemical and atrophic fibre patterns in neurogenic lesions. J Neurol Neurosurg Psychiatry 1970; 33:319–329.
49. Diamond J, Cooper E, Turher C, et al. Trophic regulation of nerve sprouting. Science 1976; 193:371–377.
50. Stalberg E. Electrophysiological studies of reinnervation in ALS. Adv Neurol 1982; 36:47–59.
51. Borenstein S, Desmedt JE. Electromyographical signs of collateral reinnervation. In: Desmedt JE, ed. New developments in electromyography and clinical neurophysiology. Basel: Karger, 1973:130–140.
52. Ekstedt J. Human single muscle fibre action potentials. Acta Physiol Scand 1964; 61(suppl 226):1–91.
53. Stalberg E. Macro EMG. A new recording technique. J Neurol Neurosurg Psychiatry 1980; 43:475–482.
54. Stalberg E, Antoni L. Electrophysiological cross section of the motor unit. J Neurol Neurosurg Psychiatry 1980; 43:469–474.
55. Stalberg E, Sanders DB. The motor unit in ALS studied with different neurophysiological techniques. In: Rose FC, ed. Research progress in motor neurone disease. London: Pitman, 1984:105–122.
56. Simpson JA. Disorders of neuromuscular transmission. Proc R Soc Med 1966; 59:993–998.
57. Fambrough DM, Drachman DB, Satyamurti S. Neuromuscular function in myasthenia gravis: Decreased acetylcholine receptors. Science (NY) 1973; 182:293–295.
58. McComas AJ, Campbell MJ, Sica RE. Electrophysiological study of dystrophia myotonica. J Neurol Neurosurg Psychiatry 1971; 34:132–139.
59. Teasdall RD, Park AM, Languth HW, et al. Electrophysiological studies of reflex activity in patients with lesions of the nervous system. II. Bull Johns Hopkins Hosp 1952; 91:245–256.
60. Homma I. Studies on the evoked electromyogram by stimulating peripheral nerve of man. Iryo 1956; 10:15.
61. McComas AJ, Payan JA. Motoneurone excitability

in the Holmes-Adie syndrome. In: Andrew BL, ed. Control and innervation of skeletal muscle. Edinburgh: Churchill Livingstone, 1966:182–193.
62. McComas AJ, Sica REP. Automatic quantitative analysis of the electromyogram in partially denervated distal muscles; comparison with motor unit counting. Can J Neurol Sci 1978; 5:377–383.
63. Cavasin R, de Bruin H, McComas AJ. An automated motor unit counting system. Muscle Nerve 1988; 11:957.
64. Daube JR. Statistical estimates of number of motor units in the thenar and foot muscles in patients with amyotrophic lateral sclerosis or the residual of poliomyelitis. Muscle Nerve 1988; 11:957.
65. Brown WF, Strong MJ, Snow R. Methods for estimating numbers of motor units in biceps-brachialis muscles and losses of motor units with aging. Muscle Nerve 1988; 11:423–432.
66. Brown WF, Hudson AJ, Snow R. Motor unit estimates in the biceps-brachialis in amyotrophic lateral sclerosis. Muscle Nerve 1988; 11:415–422.
67. McComas AJ, Sica RE, Campbell MJ, et al. Functional compensation in partially denervated muscles. J Neurol Neurosurg Psychiatry 1971; 34:453–460.
68. Milner-Brown HS, Stein RB, Lee RG. Contractile and electrical properties of human motor units in neuropathies and motor neurone disease. J Neurol Neurosurg Psychiatry 1974; 37:670–676.
69. Thomson JD, Morgan JA, Hines HM. Physiological characteristics of regenerating mammalian nerve and muscle. Am J Physiol 1950; 161:142–150.
70. Tonge DA. Physiological characteristics of reinnervation of skeletal muscle in the mouse. J Physiol (Lond) 1974; 241:141–153.
71. Engel WK, Hogenhuis LA, Collis WJ, et al. Metabolic studies and therapeutic trials in amyotrophic lateral sclerosis. In: Norris FH, Kurland LT, eds. Motor neurone diseases: Research on amyotrophic lateral sclerosis and related disorders. New York: Grune & Stratton, 1969:199–208.
72. Eisen A, Shtybel W. Clinical experience with transcranial magnetic stimulation. Muscle Nerve 1990; 13:995–1011.
73. Gastaut JL, Michel B, Figarella-Branger D, et al. Chronic progressive spinobulbar spasticity: A rare form of primary lateral sclerosis. Arch Neurol 1988; 45:509–513.
74. Younger DS, Chou S, Hays AP, et al. Primary lateral sclerosis: A clinical diagnosis reemerges. Arch Neurol 1988; 45:1304–1307.
75. Dengler R, Konstanzer A, Kuther G, et al. Amyotrophic lateral sclerosis: Macro-EMG and twitch forces of single motor units. Muscle Nerve 1990; 13:545–550.
76. Hausmanowa-Petrusewicz I. Spinal muscular atrophy. Infantile and juvenile type. Warsaw: National Centre for Scientific, Technical and Economic Information, 1978.

77. Harding AE. Inherited neuronal atrophy and degeneration predominantly of lower motor neurons. In: Dyck PH, Thomas PK, Lambert EH, et al, eds. Peripheral neuropathy. Philadelphia: WB Saunders, 1984:1537–1556.

78. Pearn JH. The gene frequency of acute Werdnig-Hoffman disease (SMA type 1). A total population survey in North-East England. J Med Genet 1973; 10:260–265.

79. Brzustowicz LM, Lehner T, Castilla LH, et al. Genetic mapping of chronic childhood-onset spinal muscular atrophy to chromosome 5q11.2-13.3. Nature 1990; 344:540–541.

80. Gilliam TC, Brzustowicz LM, Castilla LH, et al. Genetic homogeneity between acute and chronic forms of spinal muscular atrophy. Nature 1990; 345:823–825.

81. Pearn JH, Wilson J. Chronic generalized spinal muscular atrophy of infancy and childhood. Arch Dis Child 1973; 98:455–472.

82. Kugelberg E, Welander M. Heredofamilial muscular atrophy simulating muscular dystrophy. Arch Neurol Psychiatry 1956; 75:500–509.

83. Gardner-Medwin D, Hudgson P, Walton JN. Benign spinal muscular atrophy arising in childhood and adolescence. J Neurol Sci 1967; 5:121–158.

84. Kugelberg E. Kugelberg-Welander syndrome. In: Vinken RJ, Bruyn GW, eds. Handbook of clinical neurology. Amsterdam: North Amsterdam, 1975:67–80.

85. Gath I, Sjaastad O, Loken AC. Myopathic EMG changes correlated with histopathology in Wohlfart-Kugelberg-Welander disease. Neurology (NY) 1969; 19:344–352.

86. Sica REP, McComas AJ. An electrophysiological investigation of limb-girdle and facioscapulohumeral dystrophy. J Neurol Neurosurg Psychiatry 1971; 34:469–474.

87. Fenichel GM, Emery ES, Hunt P. Neurogenic atrophy simulating facioscapulohumeral dystrophy. Arch Neurol 1976; 17:257–260.

88. Kaeser HE. Scapulo-peroneal syndrome. In: Vinken PJ, Bruyn GW, eds. Handbook of clinical neurology. Amsterdam: North Holland, 1975:57–65.

89. Moosa A, Dubowitz V. Motor nerve conduction velocity in spinal muscular atrophy of childhood. Arch Dis Child 1976; 51:974–977.

90. Ryniewicz B. Motor and sensory conduction velocity in spinal muscular atrophy. Electromyogr Clin Neurophysiol 1977; 17:385–391.

91. Schwartz MS, Moosa A. Sensory nerve conduction in spinal muscular atrophy. Dev Med Child Neurol 1977; 19:50–53.

92. Carpenter S, Karpati G, Rothman S, et al. Pathologic involvement of sensory neurones in Werdnig-Hoffmann disease. Neurology (NY) 1975; 25:364–365.

93. Buchthal F, Olsen PZ. Electromyography and muscle biopsy in infantile spinal muscular atrophy. Brain 1970; 93:15–30.

94. Amick LD, Smith HL, Johnson WW. An unusual spectrum of progressive spinal muscular atrophy. Acta Neurol Scand 1966; 42:275–295.

95. Reed DM, Kurland LT. Muscle fasciculation in a healthy population. Arch Neurol 1963; 9:363–367.

96. Richardson AT. Muscle fasciculation. Arch Phys Med Rehab 1954; 35:281–286.

97. Layzer RB. Diagnostic implications of clinical fasciculation and cramps. Adv Neurol 1982; 36:23–27.

98. Forster FM, Alpers BJ. Site of fasciculations in voluntary muscle. Arch Neurol Psychiatry 1944; 51:264–267.

99. Roth G. Fasciculations d'origine peripherique. Electromyography 1971; 11:413–428.

100. Rasminsky M. Ectopic generation of impulses and cross-talk in spinal nerve roots of "dystrophic" mice. Ann Neurol 1978; 3:351–357.

101. Nardelli E, Steck AJ, Schleup M, et al. Motor neuropathy simulating motor neuron disease and monoclonal IgM with antibody activity against gangliosides GM1 and GD1b. J Neuroimmunol 1987; 16:131–132.

102. Parry GJ, Clarke S. Multifocal acquired demyelinating neuropathy masquerading as motor neuron disease. Muscle Neve 1988; 11:103–107.

103. Pestronk A, Adams RN, Clawson L, et al. Serum antibodies to GM1 ganglioside in amyotrophic lateral sclerosis. Neurology 1988; 38:1457–1461.

104. Pestronk A, Cornblath DR, Ilyas AA, et al. A treatable multifocal motor neuropathy with antibodies to GM1 ganglioside. Ann Neurol 1988; 24:73–78.

105. Gomez M, Clermont V, Bernstein J. Progressive bulbar paralysis in childhood (Fazio-Londe's disease). Arch Neurol 1962; 6:317–323.

106. Drachman DB. Congenital deformities produced by neuromuscular disorders of the developing embryo. In: Norris FH Jr, Kurland LT, eds. Motor neurone diseases. New York: Grune & Stratton, 1969:112–121.

107. Drachman DB, Coulombre AJ. Experimental clubfoot and arthrogryposis multiplex congenita. Lancet 1962; 2:523–526.

108. Davis LE, Bodian D, Price D, et al. Chronic progressive poliomyelitis secondary to vaccination of an immunodeficient child. N Engl J Med 1977; 297:241–245.

109. Dalakas MC, Elder G, Hallett M, et al. A long-term follow-up study of patients with post-poliomyelitis symptoms. N Engl J Med 1986; 314:959–963.

110. Salmon LA, Riley HA. Relation between chronic anterior poliomyelitis or progressive muscular atrophy and antecedent attack of acute anterior poliomyelitis. Bull Neurol Inst NY 1935; 4:35–63.

111. Zilkha KJ. Discussion. Proc R Soc Med 1962; 55:1028–1029.

112. Roos RP, Viola MV, Wollmann R, et al. Amytrophic lateral sclerosis with antecedent poliomyelitis. Arch Neurol 1980; 37:312–331.
113. Beede HE, Newcomb RW. Lower motor neuron paralysis in association with asthma. Johns Hopkins Med J 1980; 147:186–187.
114. Siedler H, Malamud N. Creutzfeldt-Jackob's disease. J Neuropathol Exp Neurol 1963; 22:381–402.
115. Van Rossum A. Spastic pseudosclerosis (Creutzfeldt-Jakob disease) In: Vinken PJ, Brunyn GW, eds. Handbook of clinical neurology. Amsterdam: North Holland, 1968:726–760.
116. Shy GM, Drager GA. A neurological syndrome associated with orthostatic hypotension. A clinical-pathologic study. Arch Neurol 1963; 2:511–527.

17

Atypical Motor Neuron Disease

David C. Preston
John J. Kelly, Jr.

CONTENTS

LIST OF ACRONYMS

ALS	amyotrophic lateral sclerosis
CIDP	chronic inflammatory demyelinating polyradiculoneuropathy
CK	creatine kinase
CMT	Charcot-Marie-Tooth polyneuropathy
CT	computed tomography
EMG	electromyography
HMSN	hereditary motor and sensory neuropathy
MND	motor neuron disease
MRI	magnetic resonance imaging
MU	motor unit
PLS	primary lateral sclerosis
PMA	progressive muscular atrophy
SMA	spinal muscular atrophies

The term amyotrophic lateral sclerosis (ALS) was first used by Charcot in 1875. The illness is characterized by selective destruction of motor neurons. Although lower motor neuron dysfunction predominates, there is usually clear evidence of upper motor neuron involvement as well. Typical cases, with widespread muscular atrophy, weakness, fasciculations, and spasticity, in the appropriate age group and clinical setting, are relatively easy to identify. In these cases, the diagnosis is usually obvious after the history and physical examination, and further laboratory testing adds little to the evaluation. Not all patients, however, are straightforward. They may present early in the course of the illness, or their symptoms may be anatomically restricted or have atypical features. Thus the electromyographer plays a central role in the evaluation of such patients and must have knowledge of the clinical and electrophysiologic features of the common variants of motor neuron disease (MND) and their early presentations. In addition, recognition of other potentially treatable disorders that can mimic MND is important (Table 17.1). Although these cases commonly present with atypical clinical features, they may resemble ALS and confuse even experienced physicians in neuromuscular diseases. It often falls to the electromyographer to evaluate these patients. The electromyogram is usually the crucial test to help decide if the patient has ALS or some other atypical, perhaps treatable MND. This chapter is presented to help the clinician-electromyographer recognize these atypical cases.

AMYOTROPHIC LATERAL SCLEROSIS VARIENTS

ALS typically presents with asymmetrical wasting and weakness in a distal arm or leg associated with fasciculations and hyperreflexia. Within weeks to months, the disease rapidly spreads to other limb or bulbar muscles. A study[1] from a large ALS clinic (Mt. Sinai, New York City) showed that although most patients had a focal limb onset, more than 80% had widespread findings of ALS at presentation (Table 17.2). Despite a restricted onset, electromyography (EMG) in early stages usually reveals widespread denervation and compensatory reinnervation. The diagnosis is straightforward in these patients, and few additional studies are needed. There are several variants, however, within the spectrum of classic ALS that can present diagnostic problems.

Progressive Bulbar Palsy

Most neurologists taking care of ALS patients recognize this variant immediately. Patients are usually elderly with severe dysarthria, dysphagia, and weight loss. In one hand, they carry a tissue to collect unswallowed saliva and, in the other hand, a notepad and pen for questions and responses. In the Mt. Sinai study, bulbar weakness was the first symptom in 25% of ALS patients. Only 9%, however, still had restricted bulbar symptoms at the time of diagnostic evaluation (Table 17.2). Most bulbar palsy patients present with a history of several months of slow and steadily progressive dysarthria with gagging, chok-

TABLE 17.1.   Atypical motor neuron disease

Amyotrophic lateral sclerosis variants
  Progressive bulbar palsy
  Primary lateral sclerosis
  Progressive muscular atrophy
Spinal muscular atrophy
  X-linked bulbospinal muscular atrophy (Kennedy's disease)
  Distal spinal muscular atrophy (spinal form of Charcot-Marie-Tooth disease)
Monomelic amyotrophy (benign focal amyotrophy)
Cervical lesions
Toxins
Hexosaminidase deficiency
Retroviral-associated syndromes
Postirradiation
Lymphoma and other malignances
Immune-mediated and demyelinating neuropathies
  Atypical chronic inflammatory demyelinating polyradiculoneuropathy
  Antiganglioside antibodies with or without conduction block

TABLE 17.2.   Amyotrophic lateral sclerosis syndromes

Locus of weakness at onset	
Leg	36%
Arm	32%
Bulbar	25%
Other	7%
Diagnosis at initial evaluation	
Amyotrophic lateral sclerosis	82%
Progressive bulbar palsy	9%
Progressive muscular atrophy	7%
Primary lateral sclerosis	2%

Reprinted with permission from Caroscio JT, Mulvihill MN, Sterling R, et al. Amyotrophic lateral sclerosis: Its natural history. Neurol Clin 1987; 5:1–8.

ing, and weight loss. Some undergo extensive neurovascular, ear, nose, and throat, or gastrointestinal evaluation before neuromuscular referral. The dysarthria is most commonly spastic with variable flaccid features, depending on the degree of lower motor neuron dysfunction. The tongue may be atrophied with fasciculations, accompanied by brisk jaw, gag, and facial reflexes. Even in those patients without clinical limb involvement, EMG usually discloses evidence of widespread denervation, as does muscle biopsy of a limb muscle. Occasional patients with bulbar onset, however, have no evidence of lower motor neuron involvement of the tongue and limb muscles on detailed electromyographic testing. In addition, follow-up for months and sometimes years reveals progression of bulbar symptoms without clear-cut evidence of glossal or limb denervation. The vast majority of these patients progress eventually to ALS. Careful quantitative study of limb muscles by EMG or biopsy eventually shows evidence of progressive, low-grade denervation with compensatory reinnervation. Rarely, despite prolonged follow-up and even autopsy, signs of lower motor neuron involvement do not appear, and the diagnosis of the bulbar form of primary lateral sclerosis (PLS) seems appropriate (see next).

Primary Lateral Sclerosis

Since its original clinical description by Erb in 1875, controversy has continued over the existence and classification of PLS.[2] Formerly a diagnosis of exclusion made only at autopsy, PLS, most now agree, represents a respectable and permissible diagnosis that can be made during life.[3] It is unknown if this illness, in its pure form, is a variant of ALS.

PLS is a progressive upper motor neuron disorder characterized by spasticity, weakness, pathologically increased reflexes, Babinski's sign, and pseudobulbar speech and affect. Atrophy (except owing to disuse), fasciculations, or other lower motor neuron signs are absent. The disease most commonly presents as a progressive paraplegia or quadriplegia. Occasionally patients present with bulbar weakness or hemiplegia.[2] Most present in the sixth and seventh decades, although one pathologically confirmed case presented at 1 year of age.[4] In general, the course tends to be prolonged with a better prognosis than ALS, and some patients live decades after the onset of illness.[2,5] Pathologically there is loss of myelin and gliosis in the corticospinal and corticobulbar tracts with preservation of anterior horn cells and cranial nerve nuclei. Betz's cells can be reduced in number

or absent, and in exceptional cases, the precentral gyrus can be grossly atrophied.[6]

EMG is an essential test in PLS. Nerve conduction studies are normal. Likewise, on needle EMG examination, motor unit (MU) potentials are normal without any evidence of denervation or reinnervation, although activation of MU potentials is decreased signifying the upper motor neuron defect. Recruitment remains appropriate for the level of activation. Many patients who present with the clinical syndrome of PLS have evidence of denervation on careful electromyographic studies or muscle biopsy and are best considered to be a predominantly upper motor neuron variant of ALS. In our experience, many of these patients have little in the way of active denervation but have large, long duration, stable MU potentials in most muscles, likely reflecting chronic low-grade anterior horn cell loss.

Imaging is required in all patients and is most useful in eliminating other diagnoses that may clinically resemble PLS (Table 17.3). Multiple sclerosis, cervical spondylosis, syringomyelia, multiple infarcts, Chiari's malformation, spinal cord tumors, and compressive foramen magnum lesions have all been confused with PLS. Nonspecific magnetic res-

TABLE 17.3.   Differential diagnosis of primary lateral sclerosis

Compressive lesions
Foramen magnum tumor
Chiari's malformation
Cervical spondylotic myelopathy
Herniated thoracic disc
Hereditary disease
Familial spastic paraplegia (Strumpell's disease)
Spinocerebellar degeneration
Joseph's disease
Adrenoleukodystrophy
Infection
Tropical spastic paraparesis (HTLV-1)
Vacuolar myelopathy (HIV)
Neurosyphilis
Vascular disease
Lacunar state
Syringomyelia
Spinal cord tumor
Multiple sclerosis

HTLV-1, Human T-cell lymphocyte virus, type 1; HIV, human immunodeficiency virus.

Adapted with permission from Younger DS, Chou S, Hayes AP, et al. Primary lateral sclerosis. Arch Neurol 1988; 45:1304–1307.

onance imaging (MRI) abnormalities can be seen in PLS. In one reported patient, increased signal intensity on T_2-weighted imaging was found along the corticospinal tract in the corona radiata, internal capsule, and basis pontis.[7]

Although imaging accurately identifies structural lesions, some diagnoses remain difficult to exclude. Plasma assay of very long-chain fatty acids may be necessary to exclude the spastic paraparetic presentation of adrenoleukodystrophy.[3] Multiple sclerosis is particularly difficult to exclude as a diagnosis, although it has been shown that with negative results from all modern screening tests (MRI, cerebrospinal fluid, and evoked potentials), there is a less than 10% chance of multiple sclerosis on prolonged follow-up.[8] In patients with a progressive paraparesis, one must consider familial spastic paraparesis (Strumpell's disease), which may be difficult to exclude without an accurate family history or examination of family members.

PLS is a rare disorder. In a large study of 672 patients with spastic paraplegia or paraparesis without other findings, more than 93% were found to have a clear diagnosis other than PLS after a thorough evaluation.[9] Of the 44 patients with no clear cause (possible PLS), only 22 had an electromyographic examination. In a more recent study from a large medical center retrospectively reviewing 4000 complete autopsies and more than 7000 neurologic in-patient admissions, only three autopsied and six living patients were found who fulfilled strict criteria for PLS.[3] Thus PLS requires thorough evaluation to exclude other alternative diagnoses, including some that are potentially treatable.

Progressive Muscular Atrophy

About 15% of ALS patients present with a pure lower motor neuron syndrome that has been referred to as progressive muscular atrophy (PMA). These patients have distal wasting of limbs, fasciculations, and cramps. There are no sensory symptoms or signs. Reflexes can be present but are generally reduced or absent in weak limbs. The clinical course is long with slow progression to proximal limb muscles. Bulbar involvement is uncommon or occurs very late. Unequivocal upper motor neuron dysfunction is lacking, although some patients have retained or slightly brisk reflexes that appear inappropriate for the level of limb weakness and atrophy. Nerve conduction studies are normal with the exception of reduced distal compound muscle action potential amplitudes. EMG discloses findings of diffuse distal denervation

and reinnervation. At autopsy, most of these patients have evidence of corticospinal tract involvement, in addition to the clinically recognized loss of lower motor neurons, and thus qualify for a pathologic diagnosis of classic ALS. The challenge is to separate these patients from whose who mimic ALS. Of all the ALS variants, patients with PMA most warrant thorough evaluation to exclude other disorders, some of which are potentially treatable.

DISTAL SPINAL MUSCULAR ATROPHY

The hereditary spinal muscular atrophies (SMAs) typically present in infancy through adolescence as proximal weakness and wasting. Classification has previously been based on age of onset, inheritance pattern, and distribution of the muscle groups involved. Although proximal muscles are most commonly involved, other anatomic variants have been described, including scapuloperoneal, facioscapulohumeral, and generalized forms.[10] In addition, there is a rare distal SMA that presents with a clinical picture similar to Charcot-Marie-Tooth (CMT) polyneuropathy.[10–17] Until the specific genetic defects in these inherited disorders are discovered, confusion and disagreement regarding their classification will likely continue.

Distal SMA has been popularly known as the *spinal or motor neuronopathy form of CMT*. Although most commonly confused phenotypically with the more frequent types of hereditary motor and sensory neuropathy (HMSN), occasionally it may be difficult to differentiate from an atypical form of MND. These patients present in their first to third decade with slowly progressive distal muscle weakness and atrophy. Incidence is slightly higher in males than in females. Inheritance can be autosomal dominant, recessive, or sporadic. The first symptom is usually gait disturbance. Cramps and fasciculations may be present. Pain and sensory loss are absent. Pes cavus is common and occurs in three-quarters of all patients.[10] Scoliosis is relatively rare. Tendon jerks are usually preserved in the upper extremities but may be depressed or lost in the lower extremities. Many patients develop profound distal tapering and atrophy of the forearm, hands, legs, and feet. In these well-developed cases that clinically resemble CMT, the diagnosis is not difficult. Similar to CMT, progression is very slow over years with a relatively benign prognosis, although an occasional patient is severely impaired. The average age requiring a walking aid is 28, with a quarter of patients being able to walk unaided as adults.[11]

Nerve conduction studies demonstrate low motor amplitudes when recording from distal atrophic muscles in the upper and lower extremities. Motor responses, when recording from intrinsic foot muscles, are commonly absent. Motor conduction velocities are normal or slightly reduced if the compound muscle action potential is very low. All sensory studies, including sural nerve biopsy, are normal, which is the key in separating this condition from the HMSNs. Although 30% of HMSN I (hypertrophic, demyelinating form of CMT) and 60% of HMSN II (neuronal or distal axonal form of CMT) have little or no sensory symptoms or findings, all have clear abnormalities on sensory nerve conduction studies, in contrast to completely normal studies in distal SMA.[10] Needle EMG in distal SMA shows a chronic neurogenic pattern in distal muscles with large-amplitude, long duration MU potentials with reduced recruitment. Abnormal spontaneous activity is uncommon.

In mild cases, especially when there is no family history, this disease can also be confused with the PMA form of ALS, especially when fasciculations and cramps are more widespread affecting the proximal arms and legs. Clues to the correct diagnosis include the subtle skeletal changes in the feet (pes cavus, hammer toes), abrupt distal symmetrical tapering, and giant MU potentials on EMG suggesting extreme chronicity along with the relative lack of weakness or acute denervation in the proximal muscles.

X-LINKED BULBOSPINAL MUSCULAR ATROPHY (KENNEDY'S DISEASE)

Adult-onset SMA is typically a slowly progressive disorder characterized by symmetrical proximal weakness, familial incidence, and lack of bulbar and long tract signs. It can be confused with ALS but is more commonly mistaken clinically for a myopathy. In 1966, Kennedy et al.[18] first described two families with an X-linked bulbospinal muscular atrophy. Over 30 additional patients have since been reported.[19–23] Because a family history is frequently not obvious in X-linked disorders, many cases may initially appear to be sporadic. Because of the prominent bulbar involvement, this disorder can be difficult to differentiate from an ALS variant.

The onset of the illness is usually between the third and fifth decades followed by a slow progres-

sion. Muscle cramps with exercise may precede the weakness by many years.[20] Proximal muscles are affected first followed by bulbar involvement, which may become marked. Dysarthria and dysphagia are associated with atrophy and weakness of facial, jaw, and glossal muscles. Rest or contraction fasciculations of the face have been reported in 90% of patients and are believed to be characteristic.[20] Distal muscles are affected later in the course. Reflexes are hypoactive or absent. There are no long tract or sensory signs. Although not universal, most patients have gynecomastia. Other endocrine abnormalities including diabetes and infertility are less commonly present. Laboratory testing is normal with the exception of a modestly elevated creatine kinase (CK) level. Some patients have had a CK level five times normal, which is higher than the mild elevation typically seen in SMAs or other MNDs.[19,20]

Motor nerve conduction studies are usually normal. Late in the course, when distal muscles are involved, motor amplitudes may be decreased with mild conduction velocity slowing. Despite lack of clinical sensory symptoms or signs, sensory studies in the majority of reported patients have shown decreased or absent responses, especially in the sural nerve.[20,22] Needle EMG shows active denervation and reinnervation, most prominent in the proximal and bulbar muscles. Olney et al.[23] studied the electrical correlate of contraction fasciculations commonly seen in the facial muscles of these patients when they purse their lips. Two different patterns of MU discharges, which were not fasciculations, were observed at the time of clinical twitching (Figure 17.1). The first were grouped repetitive MU discharges, which resembled myokymia, but differed in that they were under voluntary control. In the other pattern, a single MU fired repetitively between 20 and 40 c/s for 0.1 to several seconds and increased in discharge frequency at the time of clinically observed twitching.

Autopsy has demonstrated loss of spinal cord anterior horn cells and cranial nerve motor nuclei sparing the third, fourth, and sixth nerves.[21] Corresponding to sensory nerve studies, primary sensory neurons also are reduced in number, and sural nerve biopsies may show axonal loss.

Despite prominent bulbar weakness and the corresponding risk of aspiration, the longevity of these patients is not severely affected. Therefore the diagnosis of this disorder remains important from a prognostic point of view, in addition to its value in genetic counseling. Any daughter of a patient will be an obligate carrier with a 50% chance of passing the

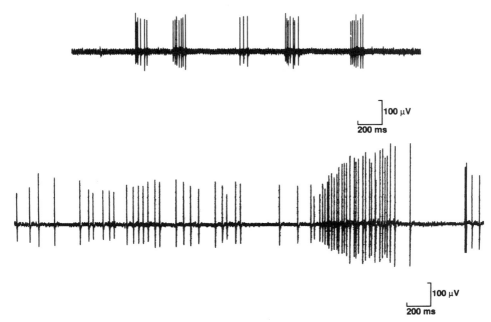

FIGURE 17.1. *Facial twitching in X-linked bulbospinal muscular atrophy. (Top trace) Grouped discharges of motor unit action potentials that resemble myokymic discharges, but occur only with mild voluntary activation. (Bottom trace) Repetitive discharges of voluntary motor unit action potentials. The period of increased firing frequency correlated with clinical twitching. (Reprinted with permission from Olney RK, Aminoff MJ, So YT. Clinical and electrodiagnostic features of X-linked recessive bulbospinal neuronopathy. Neurology 1991; 41:823–828.)*

gene to each son. The diagnosis should be suspected in any MND patient with proximal and bulbar weakness, family history, facial fasciculations, gynecomastia, or sensory abnormalities on nerve conduction studies.

MONOMELIC AMYOTROPHY

This is a rare disorder that can be confused with ALS, especially early in its course. It has been reported under a variety of names, including monomelic amyotrophy, benign focal amyotrophy, and juvenile muscular atrophy of the unilateral upper extremity.[24] More than 150 patients have been reported since it was first described by Hirayama in 1959.[24–28] Most of the patients have been from Japan or India. There have been sporadic case reports from North America, and it is not known if it is not as common or simply not reported here.

These patients are generally 15 to 30 years old and typically male. The ratio of males to females was

5:1 in one series.[25] Other family members are unaffected. Most commonly there is the insidious onset of weakness, wasting, and fasciculations of one hand. This progresses to involve the forearm flexors and extensors and in some cases the elbow extensors. The disease, as a rule, progresses in a myotomal pattern with all muscles in a given root distribution more or less equally affected. Although this is true of MNDs in general, monomelic amyotrophy may be extremely selective. The C-8–T-1 myotomes (occasional C-7 as well) typically are the most affected. Clinically there can be a striking sparing of the brachioradialis muscle (C-5–C-6) in a forearm in which all other muscles (C-7–T-1) are weak and wasted.[24–26] The illness progresses over 1 to 2 years and usually stabilizes with little subsequent change. As a rule, it does not spread to other limbs or to the bulbar muscles and is rarely severely disabling. A minority of the patients continue to progress slowly over many years or decades but not nearly as rapidly as the first couple of years. There is no pain, and the sensory system is unaffected. Although only one extremity is usually clinically affected, the illness can be bilateral in a third of the cases.[25] The dominant hand is much more frequently affected. Weakness is commonly reported to be worse in the cold but without myotonia. A coarse nonrhythmic postural tremor is common. Reflexes in the affected extremity are generally depressed or absent, although in 15% of cases they can be increased without other evidence of upper motor neuron dysfunction.[25] There are no other long tract signs. Cerebrospinal fluid studies are normal. Likewise sural nerve biopsies have been normal. Muscle biopsy of an affected muscle shows neurogenic atrophy. In some cases, computed tomography (CT) myelogram or MRI studies have shown focal cord atrophy or absence of the normal cervical enlargement.[29,30]

Although the distal upper extremity presentation is the most common, other variations have been reported. In some cases, the proximal upper extremity muscles (biceps, deltoid, spinati) are affected.[28] In others, the lower extremity is affected, with selective weakness and wasting of lower leg muscles (especially the calf) or the quadriceps.[25,27] Other than location, the disease behaves the same as with the upper extremity presentation, with progression over 1 to 2 years followed by stabilization.

Nerve conduction studies show normal sensory studies. Motor conduction velocities are normal, although motor amplitudes may be low when recording from atrophic hand muscles. Proximal conduction studies (Erb's point and root) have not been reported. Needle EMG in affected muscles usually shows a chronic neurogenic pattern with large-amplitude, long duration, polyphasic MU potentials with reduced recruitment. Abnormal spontaneous activity can be present but is typically mild when present. Of note, the homologous muscles of the clinically unaffected contralateral limb typically demonstrate qualitatively similar changes (90% in some series).[25] Likewise, contiguous more proximal muscles in the affected limb may show neurogenic changes, indicating that the disease is more widespread than can be clinically appreciated.

Because of its benign course, monomelic amyotrophy is an important condition to differentiate from other MNDs or conditions that can mimic MND. It can usually be separated from chronic distal SMA by its asymmetry, upper extremity predominance, and lack of family history. Likewise the absence of family history, lower extremity involvement, and CK elevation, in conjunction with needle EMG examination, can exclude an unusual distal myopathy (Wellander type).[24] Occasionally idiopathic bra-

chial neuritis can sometimes be mistaken for monomelic atrophy several weeks or months into an attack, especially when the proximal upper extremity is affected. The history of marked proximal pain before the onset of weakness and wasting and the nonprogressive or improving course are the important discriminating points.[31] Unfortunately, monomelic amyotrophy can be difficult to differentiate from early ALS, especially in the minority of patients with preserved or increased reflexes. Only the young age of onset, the selective myotomal involvement, and subsequent clinical follow-up can separate the two.

CERVICAL LESIONS

Cervical lesions should always be considered in the differential diagnosis of a MND syndrome. Cervical spondylosis is a relatively frequent cause of gait disturbance in the elderly and is commonly misdiagnosed by nonneurologic physicians.[32] A compressive cervical lesion can lead to a polyradiculopathy involving the cervical roots as well as a myelopathy from direct cord compression. This can create a clinical picture of lower motor neuron dysfunction in the upper extremities and upper motor neuron dysfunction in the lower extremities. The clinical picture can be further complicated by coexistent lumbar stenosis creating additional lower motor neuron signs in the lumbosacral myotomes.[33] Together the clinical picture can resemble ALS.

The history and clinical examination can usually differentiate spondylosis from MND. Cervical spondylotic myelopathy is generally asymmetrical and often has a stepwise, progressive course, sometimes with periods of improvement. It is commonly, but not always, associated with neck or radicular pain, limitation of neck motion, and sensory disturbance. Sphincter disturbance may occur late in a compressive myelopathy but is unusual in MND. The paracervical muscles are tight on palpation. A Spurling's sign may be present. There is often a gait disturbance owing to spasticity. Paresthesias and vibratory loss in the lower extremities result from posterior column compression. Romberg's sign may be present. Coexistent lumbar stenosis may limit the patient's ability to walk as pain or sensory disturbance develops after a distance, which is relieved only by the sitting position. Straight leg raising may be abnormal. Fasciculations may be present from cervical or lumbar root impingement. Rarely fasciculations in the lower extremities have been attributed to cervical compressive lesions.[34] Fasciculations over the thorax or abdomen are an important finding because they are common in MND but atypical in spondylosis. Although there are usually signs and symptoms suggesting the diagnosis of spondylosis, occasionally a patient presents with a pure motor syndrome with focal amyotrophy and spasticity, making the clinical distinction from ALS difficult.[35]

EMG in these cases can be very helpful. Although nerve conduction studies generally cannot differentiate between the two, the late responses are useful. F wave abnormalities (prolongation, impersistence, dispersion, or absence) are more likely in a polyradiculopathy. Likewise, the H wave may be absent or delayed in lumbar stenosis affecting the S-1 nerve roots. Lower extremity denervation and reinnervation on needle EMG does not occur in pure cervical compressive myelopathy unless there is coexistent lumbar stenosis. In this case, evaluation of the thoracic paraspinal muscles is important. Kuncl et al.[36] found in a prospective study of patients referred with the suspected diagnosis of ALS that 78% of all patients who were eventually proved to have that diagnosis by conventional means also had evidence of denervation in the thoracic paraspinal muscles when three or four segments were assessed. In a control group of patients with spondylosis, denervation in the thoracic region was extremely uncommon and occurred only in one of 21 patients (5%). This single patient had severe stenosis of the lumbar and adjacent thoracic spine. The thoracic paraspinal muscles were a safe and accessible site for needle EMG, and were most helpful in differentiating patients with spondylosis and MND.

Of course, clear-cut evidence of denervation and reinnervation in bulbar muscles, especially the tongue, removes the possibility of cervical spondylosis as the sole cause of the motor dysfunction. The bulbar muscles, however, are difficult to evaluate because their MU potential size and firing pattern are different from limb muscles. Difficulty with relaxation of the tongue muscle makes assessment of spontaneous activity demanding. Bulbar MU potentials are short in duration and may be misinterpreted as fibrillation potentials. It is important that the electromyographer gain familiarity with normal bulbar MU potentials before evaluating them in patients with MND.

In most cases, the combination of the history, physical examination, and EMG can differentiate between spondylosis and MND. The two conditions may coexist in elderly patients. Sometimes a repeat evaluation and EMG several months later clarify the case. In MND, the disease progresses relentlessly, and evidence of denervation and reinnervation outside the lower cervical and lumbosacral myotomes becomes evident eventually. In some cases, cervical decompression is worth a try when the diagnosis remains in doubt, but the results are seldom dramatic. The patient needs to be informed of the risks and uncertain benefits from surgery in these instances.

Complicating this issue further is the possible relationship between physical trauma and ALS.[37,38] Several epidemiologic studies have shown a statistical relationship between physical trauma and ALS. We have seen four patients over the past few years with a striking temporal relationship between cervical trauma with mild cervical cord damage and onset of an ALS-like syndrome including bulbar involvement, with electromyographic confirmation of widespread denervation.[39] Three of the four had preceding mild cervical spondylosis but without significant cord compression on myelography. Three died of progressive MND within 5½ to 9 years of the original trauma. One recovered spontaneously. Although these cases may be coincidental, they raise the important question of a causative relationship between cord trauma and ALS.

TOXINS

Since the original description of ALS, the possibility of a toxic environmental cause has been debated.[40,41] The heavy metals (lead, manganese, aluminum, mercury, selenium) have been the most investigated, with lead in particular being implicated on many occasions. The role of lead in MND remains unclear today, although no compelling evidence exists that it is an important causative factor in typical ALS. Many early investigators drew attention to the clinical similarities between ALS and chronic lead intoxication. With subsequent modern industrial control measures, the number of intoxications has fallen dramatically, and there have been few well-documented clinical reports of patients with lead intoxication and MND.[41] Even fewer detailed modern electrophysiologic studies exist. One excellent description comes from Boothby et al.,[41] who in 1974 described a lead-induced MND syndrome in a 50-year-old battery worker with the clinical picture of progressive weakness, mild fasciculations, and atrophy, affecting predominantly the intrinsic hand, finger, and wrist extensor muscles. There was no sensory loss, and reflexes were diffusely brisk. The patient, however, also had personality change, hypertension, azotemia, and hypochromic microcytic anemia with basophilic stippling, consistent with chronic lead intoxication. Blood lead level was in the *acceptable* range, whereas the urinary lead level was clearly increased, underscoring the relative insensitivity of blood levels. Nerve conductions showed normal motor studies. Sensory amplitudes were normal with slight conduction velocity slowing. Needle EMG showed no abnormal spontaneous activity. Evidence of reinnervation was seen in the hand muscles with only mild borderline changes in the quadriceps. Treatment with penicillamine resulted in a marked lead diuresis and gradual clinical and laboratory improvement.

It is clear from the study of other patients that lead can affect all parts of the nervous system.[42,43] Symptoms may vary between patients, possibly reflecting the length and dose of exposure and patient age. Chronic lead intoxication may cause an encephalopathy, myelopathy, peripheral neuropathy, motor neuronopathy, or a combination of these. A mild encephalopathy manifested by headache, dizziness, irritability, and mood change is particularly common in low-dose, subacute exposures. Gastrointestinal complaints (abdominal cramps, constipation, anorexia) are also frequent in adults.

Many investigators have looked at lead levels of different tissues in typical ALS and control patients. Most studies have shown no significant difference in blood, plasma, erythrocytes, cerebrospinal fluid, or muscle[44,46] One study of lead levels in spinal cord tissue showed a statistical difference between seven ALS patients and 11 controls.[46] Only two ALS patients, however, had spinal cord lead levels that exceeded control limits. Patients with the greatest environmental exposure during life had the highest tissue levels at autopsy. The authors noted that such results need to be interpreted cautiously because it remains possible that degenerating tissue might concentrate lead as a secondary phenomena with no role in pathogenesis.

Blood lead levels reflect only current exposure and are relatively insensitive to past exposure and total body lead burden.[42] Urinary levels are more useful and may be of greatest diagnostic value when measured after a trial of chelation therapy in high-risk patients with normal or borderline baseline blood and urinary levels.

Epidemiologic studies looking at antecedent risk factors for ALS have yielded conflicting results, although most of the larger studies have shown no relationship to lead or other heavy metal exposure.[47,48] Most now believe that heavy metals have little role in typical ALS. Nevertheless, it remains

TABLE 17.4. Clinical and laboratory clues suggesting lead intoxication

Occupational exposure
Personality or mood disturbance
Headache
Hypertension
Azotemia
Anemia, especially with basophilic stippling
Gastrointestinal disturbance
Unusual distribution of upper extremity weakness

important to obtain an accurate occupational history in all MND patients because those patients with extensive occupational exposure probably deserve greater scrutiny. In these patients, a mild encephalopathy, gastrointestinal disturbance, unusual distribution of weakness affecting the hands and forearm extensors, or abnormalities on routine laboratory tests may suggest lead intoxication (Table 17.4). These patients warrant blood and urinary lead levels and possibly a trial of chelation therapy because lead intoxication remains a treatable and potentially reversible cause of an atypical MND syndrome.

HEXOSAMINIDASE DEFICIENCY

Hexosaminidase is a lysosomal enzyme that degrades ganglioside GM_2. There are two important isoenzymes of hexosaminidase, HEX-A and HEX-B. HEX-A is composed of α-subunits and β-subunits, whereas HEX-B consists of only β-subunits. The alpha locus is on chromosome 15, and the beta locus is on chromosome 5. The most common form of GM_2 gangliosidosis is Tay-Sachs disease, which is an autosomal recessive disorder presenting in infancy. The mutation is at the alpha locus, leaving the patient devoid of HEX-A activity. It is most common in Ashkenazi Jews (carrier rate of 1:38) but also rarely occurs in non-Jews (carrier rate of 1:384).[49] Less frequent is Sandhoff's disease, which is secondary to a mutation at the beta locus, with absent or very low levels of HEX-A and HEX-B.

Juveniles or adults can also present with hexosaminidase deficiency.[49–57] These patients have low, but not absent, levels of hexosaminidase (5% to 15%), presumably owing to different allelic mutations at the alpha or beta loci. Onset is in childhood to the fifth decade with a variety of neurologic syndromes, including psychosis, dementia, atypical spinocerebellar degeneration, cerebellar ataxia, motor neuron disease, or some combination of these[49,51]

TABLE 17.5.   Clinical and laboratory clues suggesting hexosaminidase deficiency

Young age
Long temporal course
Patient or family history of psychosis
Dementia
Ataxia or tremor
Cerebellar atrophy on CT or MRI
Sensory abnormalities on nerve conduction studies
Complex repetitive discharges on EMG

CT, Computed tomography; MRI, magnetic resonance imaging.

(Table 17.5). Phenotypic expression can be diverse even within the same family.[50,53] The MND presentation takes the form of PMA or an ALS-like picture with weakness, wasting, and fasciculations. Reflexes may be decreased or increased with mild spasticity and occasional Babinski's signs. In most cases, there are mild atypical features. Psychosis or family history of psychosis is common (40% to 50% in some series).[53,56] In a patient with adult-onset SMA, the presence of ataxia, tremor, dysarthria, or slight distal sensory loss may be clues to hexosaminidase deficiency.

Nerve conduction studies are generally normal, although occasionally sural and superficial peroneal sensory amplitudes may be low or absent.[49,51,54] In rare reports of a beta locus defect (HEX-A and HEX-B deficiency), all sensory potentials have been absent.[57] Needle electrode examination usually reveals a chronic neurogenic pattern (long duration, large-amplitude MU potentials with reduced recruitment). Some patients have abnormal spontaneous activity with fibrillation potentials, positive sharp waves, fasciculation potentials, myokymic discharges, or complex repetitive discharges. Mitsumoto et al.[49] stressed the frequent occurrence of complex repetitive discharges, which were much more prominent than in patients with ALS or other diseases. Electrical evidence of chronic denervation is common in all phenotypes of hexosaminidase deficiency, including those without clinical evidence of MND.[51]

Routine laboratory testing is generally normal except for mild elevations of CK. Sural nerve biopsy may be normal or show mild axonal degeneration with increased numbers of small fiber clusters.[49] CT or MRI scanning may be helpful and commonly shows cerebellar atrophy even in the absence of clinical cerebellar signs.[50] Hexosaminidase levels in leukocytes, serum, or fibroblasts are generally low but not absent. The level of enzyme deficiency varies among patients owing to different mutations at the same locus and the different assays used to measure enzyme activity.[49]

Hexosaminidase deficiency MND is an uncommon disorder. In a study from a large ALS clinic, 350 patients with ALS were reviewed, and those with atypical features (young, positive family history, long course) were selected for HEX-A analysis.[52] No case of hexosaminidase deficiency was found among the 52 patients so identified. Thus hexosaminidase deficiency is rare but should be considered in younger patients, especially Ashkenazi Jews, if there is a family history of neurologic illness (especially psychosis), atypical features, complex repetitive discharges on EMG, or evidence of cerebellar atrophy on brain imaging.

RETROVIRAL-ASSOCIATED SYNDROMES

Human immunodeficiency virus (HIV) infection is associated with a wide variety of disorders affecting the peripheral nervous system and spinal cord.[58] These include vacuolar myelopathy, acute inflammatory demyelinating polyradiculoneuropathy (AIDP), chronic inflammatory demyelinating polyradiculoneuropathy (CIDP), sensory ataxic neuropathy, mononeuritis multiplex, distal painful predominantly sensory axonal polyneuropathy, cytomegalovirus (CMV)-related lumbosacral polyradiculopathy, and inflammatory myopathy. None of these conditions are likely to be confused with ALS.

There have been two case reports, however, of young HIV-positive patients with ALS-like syndromes. A 26-year-old man presented with cramps, fasciculations, increased reflexes, and weakness of the left arm that progressed to involve all four extremities and the bulbar muscles.[59] EMG showed evidence of widespread denervation. Nerve conduction studies were not reported. One year after the onset of the neurologic symptoms, he was found to be HIV positive. The other reported patient was a 32-year-old man with 4 months of cramps, fasciculations, and predominantly lower extremity weakness.[60] There were no sensory or sphincter symptoms. Reflexes were preserved in the presence of generalized weakness and mild atrophy. CK level was slightly elevated. Immunoprotein electrophoresis was normal. Cerebrospinal fluid protein was elevated (82 mg/dl) without cells. Nerve conductions showed normal sensory studies. Motor amplitudes were reduced, with mild slowing and no evidence of conduction block. Needle study showed widespread denervation with patchy evidence of reinnervation and MU loss. Muscle biopsy was consistent with neurogenic atrophy with some interstitial inflammation. The clinical course stabilized for several months and then slightly improved, before HIV infection was discovered. Death occurred 2 years later from opportunistic infection. Autopsy revealed marked loss of myelinated fibers in intramuscular nerve twigs and patchy loss of myelinated fibers in large nerve trunks. Muscle biopsy was consistent with an inflammatory myopathy. The anterior horn cells, pyramidal tracts, and Betz's cells were normal. The spinal cord showed increased capillary proliferation and minute hemorrhage around anterior horn cells.

Although the PLS variant of MND is rare, HIV-positive patients have also been reported in a study of PLS in two homosexual men who were otherwise well with the syndrome of PLS without other obvious cause.[4] The presentation was relatively rapid over a few months, with spastic paraparesis, hyperreflexia, and clonus. Cerebrospinal fluid showed a white blood cell (WBC) pleocytosis and elevated gamma globulins in both, with one patient having elevated cerebrospinal fluid protein (112 mg/dl). Leg somatosensory evoked potential (SSEP) studies were abnormal, suggesting subclinical sensory involvement. EMG and nerve conduction studies were normal.

Another retrovirus, human T-cell lymphotropic virus type I (HTLV-I), has been associated with spastic paraparesis and inflammatory myopathy in endemic areas. The spastic paraparesis is usually accompanied by bladder and sensory dysfunction and should not easily be mistaken for MND. When this syndrome is accompanied by an inflammatory myopathy, however, it can be confused with MND because the clinical findings may suggest both lower and upper motor neuron dysfunction.[61] In addition, nerve conduction studies are normal, and needle EMG of a chronic inflammatory myopathy can sometimes be misinterpreted as MND. Fibrillation potentials and positive sharp waves are common in both, and although MUs in myopathy are usually associated with small-amplitude, short duration, and polyphasic potentials, in chronic myopathy, large-amplitude, long duration, polyphasic MU potentials are also common. The recruitment pattern usually decides the issue because it remains normal or early in myopathy, in contrast to MND, in which it is reduced.

The relationship of retroviral disease and atypical MND remains unclear. In several studies of patients with chronic neurologic disease, the incidence of HIV and HTLV-I antibodies was not increased in patients with ALS.[62,63] Until the full spectrum of retrovirus-associated neurologic illness is defined, antibody status should probably be determined in cases of unexplained or atypical MND. Young patients (especially in high-risk groups for HIV), an abrupt and rapid onset of MND, and cerebrospinal fluid abnormalities should prompt serologic testing. Inflammation on muscle biopsy should also suggest retroviral infection.

POSTIRRADIATION MOTOR NEURON DISEASE SYNDROMES

The central nervous system is known to be more sensitive to the effects of ionizing radiation than the peripheral nervous system. Although white matter is typically more involved than gray matter, there have been several patients reported with a progressive, selective, self-limited motor neuron syndrome following irradiation of neoplasms.[64–68] Most commonly, this syndrome occurs in the treatment of testicular tumors, although it has also been seen in a variety of other tumors, including lymphoma and medulloblastoma. Typically treatment involves 4000 to 5000 cGy delivered to the pelvis or low thoracic and lumbar spine, although similar cases have been seen with total neuraxis irradiation. This is followed in 3 to 23 months by a progressive, painless weakness of the distal lower extremities. Fasciculations, atrophy, and decreased muscle tone are also present. There are no sensory symptoms, sphincter disturbance, or long tract findings, and the upper extremities are spared. The ankle reflexes are usually absent, and the knee jerks may be hypoactive or absent. Cerebrospinal fluid examination typically shows a mildly elevated protein (range 60 to 200 mg/dl) without a cellular response and a normal glucose level. Myelography and sural nerve biopsy are normal. Muscle biopsy of the gastrocnemius has shown neurogenic change (fiber type grouping, group atrophy, angulated fibers). Eventually these patients stabilize clinically (typically 3 to 12 months) and retain a variable disability.

Electrophysiology shows a restricted abnormality affecting lower lumbosacral motor fibers. Sensory nerve conduction studies are normal. Motor conduction velocities are normal, although motor amplitudes may be low when recording from distal atrophic lower limb muscles. Needle EMG shows fasciculations, fibrillation potentials, and positive sharp waves in the lower lumbosacral myotomes.

MU potentials are large and polyphasic with reduced recruitment consistent with chronic neurogenic change. The lower lumbar paraspinal muscles are abnormal as well and may demonstrate complex repetitive discharges. The upper extremities are normal.

Most authors have concluded that the site of the damage in these cases is the anterior horn cell. The self-limited course, lack of upper motor neuron dysfunction, and restricted anatomic distribution differentiate this syndrome from typical ALS. The electrophysiology is consistent with neurogenic change at or proximal to the dorsal primary ramus of the spinal nerve. The main differential exclusion is a polyradiculopathy or plexopathy, either from radiation effect or from direct recurrent neoplastic infiltration. The absence of pain, sensory symptoms, and bladder or bowel dysfunction would make a lesion in the cauda equina or lumbosacral plexus unlikely.

The mechanism underlying injury to the anterior horn cell from irradiation is not completely understood. There may be a direct toxic effect on the anterior horn cell. Ischemia remains another possibility.[67] Radiation is well known to affect vascular endothelium and can cause progressive stenosis and distal ischemia, especially in small-caliber vessels. In other well-documented cases, ischemia to the spinal cord from other mechanisms (aortic dissections, aortic clamping, cardiac arrest) has caused selective anterior horn cell loss.[67,69] The anterior horn cells may be positioned in a *watershed* area between the penetrating branches of the anterior and posterior spinal arteries and thus most susceptible to ischemia. Lower motor neuron syndromes from irradiation may have a similar pathophysiology.

LYMPHOMA AND OTHER MALIGNANCIES

The association of classic MND (ALS) with neoplasia has been suggested for a number of years. Brain et al.[70] first reviewed 11 patients with MND seen over 4 years in a population of 1465 cancer patients. They believed that a coincidence between these two illnesses was unlikely. This and other early reports led to several large case-controlled epidemiologic studies of MND, which failed to substantiate any association between neoplasia and MND.[71–73] Most now regard this occurrence as due to chance.[74,75]

Nevertheless, there continue to be small series or individual case reports of atypical MND syndromes in patients with cancer. Although many malignancies have been implicated, including lung, renal, and thy-

mus, reports are most common in patients with Hodgkin's or non-Hodgkin's lymphoma.[76–80]

In one of the early and largest series, Schold et al.[76] detailed 10 lymphoma patients. Eight had been treated with mantle and paraaortic irradiation. All developed hypotonic weakness of one or all limbs over several weeks to months. Reflexes were either depressed or absent. The weakness was commonly patchy, asymmetrical, and painless. The legs were always more involved than the arms. Two patients had moderate and unequivocal sensory abnormalities in the affected extremities, whereas the other 8 had only mild or absent sensory symptoms and signs. Only one patient had bulbar involvement. The course appeared to be independent of the underlying disease. In most patients, there was little or no clinical, laboratory, or radiologic evidence of recurrent tumor at the time of onset of neuromuscular symptoms. The weakness peaked after several months and stabilized in most. Three patients spontaneously improved to a complete recovery. The disease was seldom incapacitating in any patient. Cerebrospinal fluid was either normal or showed increased protein content, with the exception of one patient with a lymphocytic pleocytosis who subsequently received intrathecal chemotherapy for the possibility of a meningeal relapse. Sural nerve biopsies were normal and muscle biopsies showed neurogenic atrophy without signs of inflammation. Nerve conduction studies showed slight slowing of motor conduction velocity and minimal prolongation of distal sensory latency. Unfortunately, compound sensory nerve action potential amplitudes were not reported. Needle EMG followed the clinical examination with patchy evidence of acute and chronic denervation and reinnervation in the affected limbs. Pathologic examination of two patients disclosed loss of anterior horn cells and thinning with patchy demyelination of the anterior roots, brachial plexus, and lumbar plexus. Perivascular inflammation was also present in some areas.

Younger et al.[80] reported on nine patients with lymphoma and MND seen over 12 years. In contrast to earlier series, these patients had different clinical presentations and outcomes. Eight patients had unequivocal lower motor neuron signs (weakness, wasting, fasciculations) along with probable or definite upper motor neuron signs, qualifying for the diagnosis of ALS. The lymphoma preceded the MND in six patients. In the other three patients, the MND appeared first, with one having the lymphoma discovered only at autopsy. There was no correlation between tumor histology and clinical syndrome. Five patients had received radiation therapy, with two patients eventually developing lower motor neuron signs outside of the radiation ports. In seven patients, the neurologic disorder was progressive, with four patients dying of the disorder. In the other two patients, one stabilized neurologically and subsequently died of complications of chemotherapy, and the other improved with therapy for the lymphoma. This exceptional patient had a pure lower motor neuron syndrome with absent reflexes and weakness predominantly affecting the upper extremities. Nerve conduction studies in this patient and one other patient with an ALS syndrome showed multifocal conduction block. Multifocal conduction block was defined as a greater than 50% decrement in amplitude on proximal stimulation in 2 or more nerves along segments not typically affected by compression palsies. The multifocal conduction blocks resolved in the treated patient, who subsequently improved. Otherwise all other patients had normal nerve conduction studies and electromyographic studies consistent with MND. Laboratory studies showed monoclonal proteins in three patients and elevated cerebrospinal fluid protein (>50 mg/dl) in six patients. Antibodies to GM_1 and myelin associated glycoprotein (MAG) were tested only in three and six patients and were all negative. Autopsy in two patients showed loss of motor neurons. In addition, mild demyelinating features in roots and peripheral nerves were noted in one patient and scattered axonal degeneration with inflammatory infiltrates in the other.

The place of this disorder in the nosology of MND remains unclear. The clinical and electrophysiologic spectrum of these patients is heterogeneous. It remains difficult to know if the lymphoma and MND have the same underlying cause; if the lymphoma caused the MND by a known secondary effect, such as a paraprotein; or if there is some other remote or *paraneoplastic* effect on the motor neuron or axon.[80] Of course, patients with cancer are susceptible to a wide variety of neuromuscular complications by direct effect of tumor, by its therapy, or by secondary systemic effects. Tumor can infiltrate the roots or nerve or cause extrinsic compression from a mass lesion. In addition, secondary metabolic, infectious, and vascular complications can affect peripheral nerves. Chemotherapy has well-known side effects on nerve and muscle. Radiation therapy can also cause an atypical MND syndrome (see earlier). Indeed, most of the lymphoma patients reported underwent radiation therapy that included the spinal column. Some of these patients had a MND syndrome indistinguishable from that associated with radiation alone.

In many of the patients who recovered spontaneously in the earlier reports, the clinical history could also suggest an immune-mediated or demyelinating polyneuropathy. Detailed protein studies were usually not reported, and it is possible that some of these patients had one of the MND syndromes associated with antinerve antibody (see later). Although the course in most was longer than typical AIDP, an atypical acquired monophasic CIDP also remains difficult to exclude, especially considering that patients with Hodgkin's or other lymphoma are probably more susceptible to autoimmune neuropathies. Unfortunately, most of the reported cases do not contain enough detailed electrophysiology (compound sensory nerve action potential amplitudes, late responses, amplitudes on proximal stimulation) to allow the reader to exclude a peripheral neuropathy. In addition, very proximal conduction studies (Erb's point or root) or serial electrical studies over time, which might be required to demonstrate electrophysiologic evidence of demyelination, were seldom performed. More detailed electrophysiologic and morphologic studies are required before atypical MND syndromes associated with lymphoma or other malignances can be clearly differentiated from other neuromuscular syndromes.

IMMUNE-MEDIATED AND DEMYELINATING NEUROPATHIES

In the modern era, many polyneuropathies, once diagnosed as idiopathic, have been found to be inflammatory in etiology. Electrophysiology and pathologic examinations of nerve biopsy specimens have greatly contributed to the understanding of these conditions, each emphasizing the important role of demyelination. Although as a group these neuropathies are heterogeneous, there are individual syndromes, which can be well defined by their clinical course, electrophysiology, laboratory testing, and pathology. Much experimental and clinical evidence suggests that many of these neuropathies are immune-mediated. Because most polyneuropathies present with sensory symptoms or signs, there is usually little confusion with MND. An immune-mediated process, however, directed against an antigen found exclusively, or in greater abundance, in motor nerve could result in a pure motor neuropathy, a condition difficult to differentiate from a motor neuronopathy. In cases in which there is subsequent demyelination from an immune-mediated attack, electrophysiologic testing then becomes capable of separating the two conditions. Because immune-mediated, demyelinating neuropathies generally have a better prognosis and are potentially treatable, the distinction remains critical.

Chronic Inflammatory Demyelinating Polyradiculoneuropathy

This disorder typically causes a symmetrical sensorimotor polyneuropathy.[81] All ages can be affected, with most patients presenting in their fifth to sixth decades. Proximal and distal muscles are both affected. Reflexes can be hypoactive but are usually absent. Large fiber sensory symptoms and signs are frequent, although occasional patients may have prominent pain. The temporal profile is variable, with slowly progressive, stepwise progressive, monophasic, and recurrent relapsing and remitting forms described.

Nerve conduction studies demonstrate electrophysiologic evidence of demyelination with markedly prolonged distal motor latencies, absent or prolonged late repsonses, slowed conduction velocities, and temporal dispersion or conduction block on proximal motor stimulation. Sensory studies are usually abnormal, with low or absent responses and prolonged latencies. Needle EMG shows secondary axonal change with evidence of denervation and reinnervation.

Cerebrospinal fluid studies commonly show elevated protein, which may become marked, in the absence of a cellular response. Pathologic examination may demonstrate perivascular or diffuse mononuclear infiltration of nerve, without vasculitis, and segmental demyelination, although many biopsies are nonspecific.

Multiple Mononeuropathy Variant of Chronic Inflammatory Demyelinating Polyradiculoneuropathy

Typical CIDP with symmetrical weakness, areflexia, and sensory dysfunction presents no diagnostic confusion with MND. Although variants have been described that affect predominantly motor, sensory, or autonomic nerves, most are mixed, especially when studied electrically. Lewis et al.[82] described five patients with multiple mononeuropathies who were found to have multifocal conduction block on nerve conduction studies. All patients had a subacute onset of pain, numbness, and weakness in arms, usually affecting the median and ulnar nerves before spread-

ing to the legs. Although all cases were asymmetrical at onset, deficits tended to blend together over time. Reflexes were lost in the upper extremities and preserved in the lower extremities of some. Cerebrospinal fluid was normal or showed only mild elevations of protein. Sural nerve biopsies demonstrated demyelination and remyelination. Despite the presentation of multiple mononeuropathies, no patient was found to have serologic or pathologic evidence of vasculitis. Nerve conduction studies were the key and showed multifocal conduction block (defined as a loss of >40% compound muscle action potential area on proximal stimulation) in multiple nerves. Often distal motor latencies and amplitudes were normal. In addition, all patients had abnormalities on sensory nerve conductions.

These and other cases suggested that CIDP could present asymmetrically with multiple mononeuropathies, plexopathies, or radiculopathies and could be mistaken clinically for a vasculitic neuropathy.[82,83] Sensory abnormalities were prominent, however, thereby eliminating a diagnosis of MND.

Multiple Motor Mononeuropathy Variant of Chronic Inflammatory Demyelinating Polyradiculoneuropathy

Several reports subsequently have detailed patients similar to those of Lewis et al. with multifocal conduction block and multiple mononeuropathies, yet affecting only motor fibers. Most of these patients have presented with asymmetrical weakness, wasting, and fasciculations and were initially thought to have MND.

Chad et al.[84] described a 25-year-old man with multifocal cramps, asymmetrical weakness of the arms and legs, hypoactive reflexes, and fasciculations who progressed over 1 year, followed by spontaneous recovery over 3 years. Sensory symptoms and signs were absent. There was no evidence of paraproteinemia, lymphoma, or cerebrospinal fluid abnormality. Nerve conduction studies suggested a proximal demyelinating neuropathy. Corresponding to the clinically weak limbs, a conduction block was found in the right musculocutaneous nerve between the axilla and Erb's point, and F waves were greatly prolonged in the left peroneal nerve. Needle EMG showed mild denervation and reinnervation in the right C-5 and left L-5 myotomes.

Parry and Clarke[85] described five additional patients with a syndrome of slowly progressive wasting, fasciculations, cramps, and multifocal weakness, affecting the arms more than the legs. Sensory symptoms were minimal or absent. Most patients were younger (age range 25 to 58). Unlike earlier reports, reflexes in weak extremities were normal or mildly increased. No patients had areflexia or any bulbar dysfunction. Cerebrospinal fluid studies were normal. Motor nerve conduction studies showed normal distal latencies and amplitudes. Multifocal conduction block was present in multiple nerves. Sensory and mixed nerve studies were normal, even through segments that demonstrated motor conduction block. All patients had initially been diagnosed as MND.

Van den Bergh et al.[86] described a 15-year-old girl with a slowly progressive monophasic illness characterized by symmetrical proximal and distal weakness, areflexia, and absence of any bulbar or sensory

dysfunction. Cerebrospinal fluid studies were normal. Nerve conductions demonstrated normal sensory studies. Motor studies showed conduction block (defined as >20% drop in the proximal compound muscle action potential amplitude with duration not exceeding 115% of the distal response) in multiple nerves (Figure 17.2). The conduction blocks were not at usual sites of compression and were most prominent very proximally (Erb's–axilla, C-8–Erb's). F waves were dispersed, although minimal F wave latencies were normal. Clinical and electrophysiologic improvement occurred with plasma exchange and prednisone.

Each of these case reports demonstrated that a progressive, exclusively motor, demyelinating neuropathy could easily be mistaken clinically, although

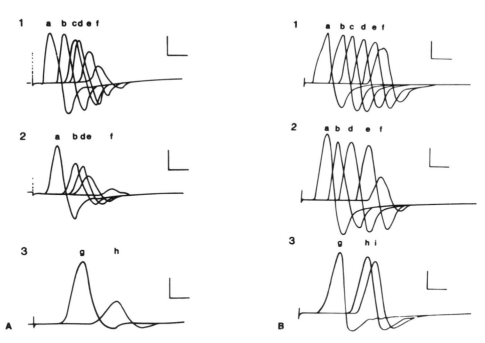

FIGURE 17.2.   *Proximal conduction blocks and temporal dispersion in a treatable pure motor neuropathy. (A) Surface recording from the abductor digiti minimi (1), abductor pollicus brevis (2), and extensor digitorum brevis (3) muscles with stimulation of the ulnar, median, and peroneal nerves at time of admission. Sites of stimulation include a = wrist; b = below ulnar groove (1) or elbow (2); c = above ulnar groove; d = axilla; e = Erb's point; f = C-8–T-1 cervical roots; g = ankle; h = below fibular head; i = above fibular head. Ordinate = 5 mV (1), 10 mV (2), 2 mV (3); abscissa = 5 ms. (B) 4½ months after treatment, conduction blocks in (1) and (3) have completely resolved. An improving conduction block is present between e and f in (2). Ordinate = 5 mV (1,2), 2 mV (3). (Reprinted with permission from Van Den Bergh P, Logigian EL, Kelly JJ Jr. Motor neuropathy with multifocal conduction blocks. Muscle Nerve 1989; 11:26–31.)*

not electrophysiologically, for the PMA variant of MND. The electrophysiology was similar in all, showing prominent conduction block on proximal motor stimulation with the absence of any sensory abnormalities. Although the electrophysiology was similar to that of CIDP, it remains unclear if these cases simply represented a pure motor variant of that disorder. At least one or many of the hallmarks of typical CIDP (areflexia, symmetry, cerebrospinal fluid protein elevation) was lacking in each of these cases. In addition, these cases were reported before the recognition of multifocal motor neuropathy associated with conduction block and antiganglioside antibody and may have represented early examples of that syndrome (see later).

Motor Neuron Disease and Antiganglioside Antibody with or without Conduction Block

A number of investigators have suggested an association between MND and monoclonal gammopathies. Early anecdotal case reports drew attention to the unusual coincidence of monoclonal gammopathies, usually gamma immunoglobulin M (IgM), and progressive lower motor neuron syndromes, resembling the PMA variant of ALS.[81–89] Rowland et al.[87] described a 48-year-old man with an IgM kappa monoclonal protein who presented with progressive distal and proximal weakness, fasciculations, cramps, and areflexia. Bulbar function and sensation were unaffected. Although clinically diagnosed as MND, several laboratory studies were atypical. Cerebrospinal fluid protein was markedly elevated (265 mg/dl), and nerve conduction studies showed low motor amplitudes with moderately slowed velocities (25 m/s in the arms). Deterioration continued despite treatment with chlorambucil and plasma exchange. Autopsy later demonstrated a predominantly motor, demyelinating radiculoneuropathy. Anterior horn cells were normal in number but had prominent chromatolysis, implying retrograde change. Motor roots were severely demyelinated, with similar but less marked changes in the posterior roots.

Parry et al.[88] described a similar patient with a progressive quadriparesis, areflexia, elevated cerebrospinal fluid protein, and polyclonal increase in IgM. Nerve conduction studies were normal, with needle EMG showing evidence of diffuse denervation and reinnervation. Unequivocal improvement followed immunosuppression on two occasions. At autopsy, anterior horn cells were only equivocally reduced in number but again showed prominent

chromatolysis. Perivascular inflammation and loss of axons were present in the ventral roots and cauda equina.

These case reports subsequently led to larger studies examining the incidence of monoclonal proteins in patients with MND. Shy et al.[90] found, in a retrospective survey, that 4.8% of patients with MND had a monoclonal protein compared with 1% of age-matched controls with other neurologic diseases. Patients with lower motor neuron syndromes more commonly had IgM gammopathies and elevated cerebrospinal fluid protein levels, whereas patients with a combination of upper and lower motor neuron signs, more typical of ALS, commonly had IgG gammopathies. The authors suggested a possible association between monoclonal gammopathies and motor neuron disease, in addition to the known relationship with polyneuropathy.

This association was further strengthened when Freddo et al.,[91] Shy et al.,[92] and Nardelli et al.[93] described individual patients with progressive lower motor neuron syndromes and IgM proteins directed against GM_1, GD_{1B}, and asialo-GM_1 gangliosides, which share the common carbohydrate epitope Gal(β1-3)GalNac. These patients presented with chronic, progressive lower motor syndromes with absent or reduced deep tendon reflexes. Bulbar muscles and sensation were spared. Two of the three cases had IgM M proteins detectable in serum. The other patient, without a M protein, had marked improvement following immunosuppression with cyclophosphamide.[92]

Schluep and Steck,[94] using indirect immunofluorescence techniques, then showed that the IgM monoclonal protein from a patient with a lower motor neuron syndrome and anti-GM_1 antibodies immunostained presynaptic nerve terminals in guinea pig neuromuscular junctions. Because GM_1 is known to be concentrated on the external surface of synaptic terminals and GD_{1B} is known to bind tetanus toxoid, both are accessible to circulating immunoglobulins.[91] It was postulated that these antibodies damaged motor nerves either by uptake and retrograde transport to the nucleus, where they may disrupt cellular function, or by peripheral action with damage to nerve terminals.[95] Santoro et al.,[96] using direct immunofluorescence, demonstrated IgM antibody deposition at the nodes of Ranvier in a sural nerve biopsy of an unusual patient with upper and lower motor neuron disease, multifocal conduction block, and anti-GM_1 antibodies. Similar findings were present in rat sciatic nerve injected with the patient's serum. Preincubation with GM_1 resulted in no binding activity. These studies suggested that the anti-GM_1 antibodies may have caused the motor dysfunction either by paranodal demyelination or interference with the sodium channels at the nodes of Ranvier.

Increasing attention to anti-GM_1 antibodies grew when Pestronk et al.[97] reported two patients with a treatable multifocal motor neuropathy, polyclonal anti-GM_1 antibodies, and multifocal conduction block on nerve conduction studies. These patients presented with asymmetrical upper extremity weakness in the distribution, more or less, of named nerves. Reflexes were reduced in one patient but in the other were inappropriately brisk for the level of weakness and wasting. No other definite upper motor neuron signs were present. Sensory symptoms were minimal or absent. Nerve conduction studies showed prolonged distal motor latencies, decreased conduction velocities, conduction block on proximal stimulation, and prolonged F waves. Sensory studies were normal. No clinical or serologic response followed either prednisone or plasma exchange. Treatment with cyclophosphamide, however, lowered anti-GM_1 titers to 10% to 30% of pretreatment levels and accompanied clinical improvement. Although these patients were initially thought to have MND clinically, the electrophysiology clearly demonstrated a disorder of motor nerve, rather than motor neuron, with changes consistent with an acquired demyelinating neuropathy, as had been most commonly seen in CIDP. The asymmetry, upper extremity predominance, normal cerebrospinal fluid, absence of sensory findings, and lack of response to prednisone, however, all suggested a disorder unique from CIDP.

Subsequent reports have continued to emphasize the triad of antiganglioside antibodies, lower motor neuron dysfunction, and multifocal motor conduction block on nerve conduction studies as a treatable syndrome that can mimic MND. It is possible that many of the early anecdotal cases of atypical MND or reversible MND were examples of this condition that were reported before the recognition of antiganglioside antibodies and the use of detailed electrophysiologic testing. Clinically these cases present with progressive, asymmetrical weakness and wasting. Distal and upper extremity muscles are often affected first. Many of the patients are younger (<50 years old) than typical MND patients. At times, it may be possible to detect weakness in the distribution of named motor nerves with sparing of others in the same myotome (clinical multifocal motor neuropathy). Definite upper motor neuron signs are absent, although some have retained or relatively brisk

reflexes in a weak and wasted limb. Bulbar function and sensation are usually spared, although some mild or transient sensory symptoms may be present.

Thorough electromyographic evaluation demonstrates electrophysiologic evidence of focal demyelination in multiple motor nerves. Compound muscle action potential amplitudes are decreased on proximal stimulation, with or without temporal dispersion. Distal motor and F wave latencies are usually prolonged. Motor conduction velocities have been slowed in some patients, down to the 20 to 30 m per second range. Sensory studies are either normal or mildly abnormal. Detailed electrophysiologic studies by Krarup et al.[98] in three patients with multifocal motor neuropathy and conduction block (two with increased anti-GM_1 antibody titers) demonstrated that the blocks selectively affected motor fibers in sharply circumscribed regions and not at the usual sites of compression. Sensory studies through segments that were blocked to motor conduction were normal (Figure 17.3).

High titers of polyclonal anti-GM_1 antibodies have been present in many reported cases. Pestronk et al.[99] reported that 84% of his patients with clinical multifocal motor neuropathy and electromyographic evidence of conduction block had high titers of anti-GM_1 antibodies. This is the important group of patients to differentiate from other MND patients because treatment with immunosuppression is most commonly associated with improvement. Antiganglioside titers have been shown to be unaffected by prednisone but response to treatment with intravenous or oral cyclophosphamide, although many months of treatment are usually needed to lower titers.[100] Reduction of antiganglioside titers by 75% or more is frequently required. Because the cumulative dose of cyclophosphamide is related to the risk of delayed malignancy, treatment is best reserved for patients with the typical clinical, electrical, and serologic syndrome who are severely disabled or have clearly progressive weakness.[99] Treatment of other patients with lower motor neuron syndromes and anti-GM_1 or other ganglioside antibodies, but without conduction block, is problematic. Most of these patients fail to respond to cyclophosphamide or other immunosuppressives. In these difficult cases, the risks of side effects and low response rate must be weighed against no treatment for a progressive and incurable disease. Serial nerve conductions over months or years may be useful in demonstrating conduction blocks in some patients.[97]

A number of workers have tried to define the frequency of antiganglioside reactivity further by

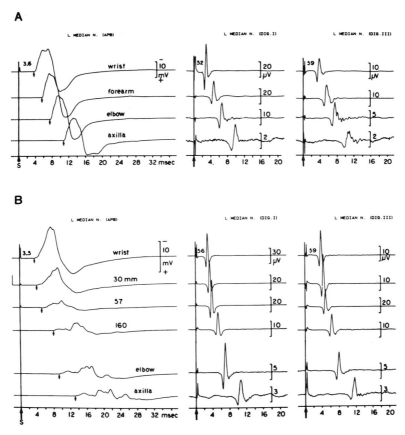

FIGURE 17.3. *Motor and sensory conduction studies of the left median nerve from a control subject (A) and a patient with multifocal motor neuropathy (B). The compound muscle action potential was recorded from the abductor pollicis brevis. The site of stimulation is indicated above the traces. In the patient, the median motor nerve was stimulated at the wrist, 30 mm, 57 mm, and 160 mm proximal to the wrist. The compound sensory nerve action potential at digit I (middle column) and digit III (right column) were recorded at the same electrode sites. (Reprinted with permission from Krarup C, Steward JD, Sumner JD, Sumner AJ, et al. A syndrome of asymmetric limb weakness with motor conduction block. Neurology 1990; 40(1):118–127.)*

studying large groups of patients with MND and other diseases. Pestronk et al.[101] initially reported that 57% of patients with ALS had polyclonal anti-GM_1 antibodies in their sera. Less than 10%, however, had high titers. Other workers have subsequently agreed that high titers of antiganglioside antibodies are rare in classical ALS.[102–105] Some of the variance in these initial studies was secondary to methodologic differences between research laboratories, patient selection, and the definition of the upper limit of normal for antiganglioside titers. Patients with pure or predominantly lower motor neu-

ron syndromes, however, do appear to have an increased frequency of high titers of antiganglioside antibodies. In most of these patients, M proteins were not present and anti-GM_1 antibodies were polyclonal, usually IgM but occasionally IgG. Although controls and patients with other neurologic diseases had low titers, patients with nonneurologic autoimmune diseases were found to have an increased frequency of high titers as well. Sadiq et al.[103] examined anti-GM_1 antibodies in various neurologic illnesses. Subpopulations of patients with lower motor neuron disease, sensorimotor neuropathy, and motor neu-

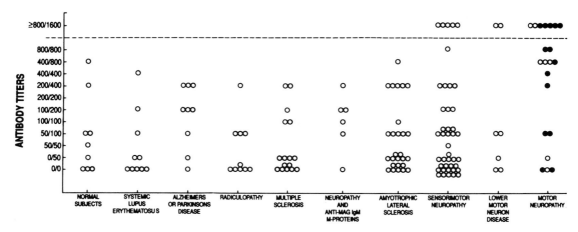

FIGURE 17.4. *Anti-GM₁ IgM antibody titers in patients with various neurologic disease and controls. Of the 21 patients with motor neuropathy (●), 11 had multifocal conduction block and 3 had coexisting upper and lower motor neuron signs. (Reprinted with permission from Sadiq SA, Thomas FP, Kilidireas K, et al. The spectrum of neurological diseases associated with anti-GM1 antibodies. Neurology 1990; 40(7):1067–1072.)*

ropathy, with or without conduction block, had high titers (Figure 17.4).

The significance of low or borderline antiganglioside titers is unclear. Normal controls, patients with nonneurologic autoimmune diseases, and those with other neurologic diseases have low titers of these antibodies in a high percentage, although not as frequent as in MND. It is likely that these antibodies, in low or borderline titers, are not of pathogenic significance but rather may be a part of the normal human immune repertoire. It is possible that, in affected individuals, specific clones that produce antibodies against peripheral nerve epitopes may escape control by unknown mechanisms and proliferate with production of high titers of antibodies producing neurologic disease. A similar mechanism had been proposed for the production of anti-MAG antibodies, which are thought to cause a form of autoimmune polyneuropathy.

It remains unclear at present how to interpret these various reports of antiganglioside antibodies and MND. These studies, however, do suggest that a lower motor neuron syndrome, with or without sensory loss, should prompt a search for anti-GM₁ antibodies. The presence of anti-GM₁ antibodies in high titers, clearly over control levels and over those of patients with other neurologic diseases and nonneurologic antoimmune diseases, raises a possible autoimmune cause for the syndrome. In addition,

the presence of conduction block or other evidence of demyelination on EMG in a lower motor neuron syndrome suggests that the patient does not have typical MND and should prompt a search for antiganglioside antibodies. The full meaning of the precise pattern of antiganglioside activity, including the definition of epitopes targeted by these antibodies, awaits further investigation. How these studies relate to ALS is less clear. There is currently no convincing evidence that classic, idiopathic ALS is an autoimmune disease. Until a clear association or benefit is demonstrated, we have not treated ALS patients with immunosuppressive drugs or plasma exchange.

CONCLUSION

The pathogenesis and treatment of typical ALS remain unknown. Immunologic, neurochemical, and electrophysiologic studies, however, have shed new light on patients with atypical MND. It is apparent that many of these patients, once formerly grouped with ALS, have separate, distinct, and definable syndromes (Tables 17.6, 17.7). Some are potentially treatable, and many others have a natural history far more benign than typical ALS. Unfortunately, the nomenclature of these syndromes, especially the autoimmune and demyelinating disorders, is complicated and is likely to change in the future. Even the

TABLE 17.6. Clinical and cerebrospinal fluid findings in motor neuron disease syndromes

Syndrome	Legs	Arms	Bulbar	Reflexes	Sensory	Sphincter	CSF Protein	CSF Cells
Amyotrophic lateral sclerosis	+++	+++	+++	I	N	N	N	N
Distal spinal muscular atrophy	+++	+	N	D	N	N	N	N
X-linked bulbospinal muscular atrophy	++	++	+++	D	N	N	N	N
Monomelic amyotrophy	+ or	++	N	D	N	N	N	N
Cervical lesions	++	++	N	I (legs)	+	+ (late)	N	N
Lead	+	++	N	I or D	N	N	N	N
Hexosaminidase deficiency	++	++	N/+	I or D	+/−	N	N	N
Retrovirus	+++	+	N	I	+	++	I	N or I
Irradiation	+++	N	N	D	N	N	N or I	N
Lymphoma	++	+	N/+	N, I, or D	N/+	N	N or I	N or I
Chronic inflammatory demyelinating polyradiculoneuropathy variants	++	++	N	D	+/−	N	N or I	N
Antiganglioside antibodies	+	++	N	D or N	+/−	N	N or I	N

Key: + = mild; + + = moderate; + + + = severe; +/− = equivocal or transient; N = normal; I = increased; D = decreased.
CSF, Cerebrospinal fluid.

471

TABLE 17.7. Electrodiagnostic findings in motor neuron disease syndromes

Syndrome	Compound SNAP Amplitude	Motor Conduction Velocity	Conduction Block/ Temporal Dispersion	Active Denervation	Chronic Reinnervation	Comment
Amyotrophic lateral sclerosis	N	N, SR	A	+++	+++	LE > UE; distal > proximal
Distal spinal muscular atrophy	N	N, SR	A	+ or A	+++	Bulbar + proximal > distal
X-linked bulbospinal muscular atrophy	D	N, SR	A	++	++	Grouped or repetitive voluntary MUAPs in facial muscles
Monomelic amyotrophy	N	N, SR	A	+ or A	++	Contralateral homonymous muscles commonly affected
Cervical lesions	N	N, SR	A	+	+	UE > LE, unless coexistent lumbar stenosis and polyradiculopathy Thoracic paraspinal spared UE > LE
Lead	N	N	A	A	++	Slight sensory conduction velocity slowing may be present
Hexosaminidase deficiency	D	N, SR	A	++	++	CRDs may be prominent
Retrovirus	N	N, SR	A	A to ++	A to ++	Coexistent inflammatory myopathy may be present
Irradiation	N	N, SR	A	++	++	LE only; CRDs may be present in lumbar paraspinals
Lymphoma	?	N, SR	A or P	+, ++	++	
Chronic inflammatory demyelinating polyradiculoneuropathy variants	N or D	N, MR	P	+, ++	++	Proximal stimulation (Erb's point or root) may be necessary to demonstrate conduction block/temporal dispersion
Antiganglioside antibodies	N or D	N, MR	A or P	+, ++	++	

Key: N = normal; I = increased; D = decreased; SR = slightly reduced (>75% lower limit of normal); MR = markedly reduced (<75% lower limit of normal); A = absent, P = present; + = mild; ++ = moderate; +++ = severe.

SNAP, Sensory nerve action potential; LE, lower extremity; UE, upper extremity; CRD, complex repetitive discharge; MUAP, motor unit action potential.

472

site of the pathology (motor neuron versus motor nerve; axon versus myelin) is not resolved. More work remains to define these syndromes fully clinically and pathologically.

Atypical clinical, laboratory, and electrophysiologic findings are commonly present. Clues suggesting the presence of an atypical and possibly treatable form of MND include the following:

Absence of definite upper motor neuron signs.
Unusual temporal course.

Absence of bulbar involvement after 1 year.
Sensory symptoms or signs.
Increased cerebrospinal fluid protein.
Unusual distribution of weakness and atrophy.
Monoclonal protein, especially IgM.
High titers of antiganglioside antibodies.
Unusual EMG with (1) abnormal sensory studies, (2) conduction block or temporal dispersion, (3) marked conduction velocity slowing, (4) delayed or absent late responses, or (5) complex repetitive discharges.

REFERENCES

1. Caroscio JT, Mulvihill MN, Sterling R, et al. Amyotrophic lateral sclerosis: Its natural history. Neurol Clin 1987; 5:1–8.
2. Gastaut JL, Michel B, Figarella-Branger D, et al. Chronic progressive spinobulbar spasticity. Arch Neurol 1988; 45:509–513.
3. Younger DS, Chou S, Haps AP, et al. Primary lateral sclerosis. Arch Neurol 1988; 45:1304–1307.
4. Grunnet ML, Leicher C, Zimmerman A, et al. Primary lateral sclerosis in a child. Neurology 1989; 39:1530–1532.
5. Russo LS. Clinical and electrophysiological studies in primary lateral sclerosis. Arch Neurol 1982; 39:662–664.
6. Beal MF, Richardson EP Jr. Primary lateral sclerosis. Arch Neurol 1981; 38:630–633.
7. Marti-Fabregas J, Pujol J. Selective involvement of the pyramidal tract on magnetic resonance imaging in primary lateral sclerosis. Neurology 1990; 40:1799–1800.
8. Geisser B, Kurtzberg D, Vaughn H, et al. Trimodal evoked potentials compared to magnetic resonance imaging in the diagnosis of multiple sclerosis. Arch Neurol 1987; 44:281–289.
9. Ungar-Sargon JY, Lovelace RE, Brust CM. Spastic paraplegia-paraparesis: A reappraisal. J Neurol Sci 1960; 46:1–12.
10. Harding AE, Thomas PK. Hereditary distal spinal muscular atrophy. J Neurol Sci 1980; 45:337–348.
11. Pearn J, Hudgson P. Distal spinal muscular atrophy. J Neurol Sci 1979; 43:183–191.
12. Bouche P, Gheradi R, Cathala HP, et al. Peroneal muscular atrophy. J Neurol Sci 1983; 61:389–399.
13. O'Sullivan DJ, McLeod JG. Distal chronic muscular atrophy involving the hands. J Neurol Neurosurg Psychiatr 1978; 41:653–658.
14. Young ID, Harper PS. Hereditary distal spinal muscular atrophy with vocal cord paralysis. JNNP 1980; 43:413–418.
15. McLeod JG, Prineas JW. Distal type of chronic spinal muscular atrophy. Brain 1971; 94:704–714.
16. Dubrovsky A, Taratuto AL, Martino R. Distal spinal muscular atrophy and opthalmoparesis. Arch Neurol 1981; 38:594–596.
17. Dyck P, Lambert EH. Lower motor and primary sensory neuron diseases with peroneal muscular atrophy. Arch Neurol 1968; 18:619–625.
18. Kennedy WR, Alter M, Sung JH. Progressive proximal spinal and bulbar muscular atrophy of late onset. Neurology 1968; 18:671–680.
19. Barkhaus PE, Kennedy WR, Stern LZ, et al. Hereditary proximal spinal and bulbar motor neuron disease of late onset. Arch Neurol 1982; 39:112–116.
20. Harding AE, Thomas PK, Baraitser M, et al. X-linked recessive bulbospinal neuronopathy: A report of ten cases. JNNP 1982; 45:1012–1019.
21. Sobue G, Hashizume Y, Makai E, et al. X-linked recessive bulbospinal neuronopathy. Brain 1989; 112:209–232.
22. Serratrice G, Pellisier JF, Pougot J. X-linked bulbospinal neuronopathy. Rev Neurol 1988; 144:756–758.
23. Olney RK, Aminoff MJ, So YT. Clinical and electrodiagnostic features of X-linked recessive bulbospinal neuronopathy. Neurology 1991; 41:823–828.
24. Oryema J, Ashby P, Spiegel S. Monomelic amyotrophy. Can J Neurol Sci 1990; 17(2):124–130.
25. Sobue I, Saito N, Iida NM, et al. Juvenile type of distal and segmental muscular atrophy of the upper extremities. Ann Neurol 1978; 3:429–432.
26. Gourie-Devi M, Suresh TG, Shankar SK. Monomelic amyotrophy. Arch Neurol 1984; 41(4):388–394.
27. Riggs JE, Schochet SS Jr, Gutman L. Benign focal amyotrophy. Variant of chronic spinal muscular atrophy. Arch Neurol 1984; 41(6):678–679.
28. Amir D, Magora A, Vatine JJ. Proximal monomelic amyotrophy of the upper limb. Arch Phys Med Rehabil 1987; 68(7):450–451.
29. Biondi A, Dormont D, Weitzner I Jr, et al. MR imaging of the cervical cord in juvenile amyotrophy of distal upper extremity. AJNR 1989; 10(2):263–268.
30. Metcalf JC, Wood JB, Bertorini TE. Benign focal

amyotrophy: Metrizamide CT evidence of cord atrophy. Muscle Nerve 1987; 10:338–345.

31. England JD, Sumner AJ. Neuralgic amyotrophy: An increasing diverse entity. Muscle Nerve 1987; 10(1):60–69.
32. Peterson DI, Dayes LA. Myelopathy associated with cervical spondylosis: A frequently unrecognized disease. J Fam Pract 1977; 4:233–236.
33. Dagi TF, Tarkington MA, Leech JJ. Tandem lumbar and cervical spinal stenosis. Natural history, prognostic indices, and results after surgical decompression. J Neurosurg 1987; 66:842–849.
34. Kasdon DL. Cervical spondylotic myelopathy with reversible fasciculations in the lower extremities. Arch Neurol 1977; 34:774–776.
35. Dorsen M, Ehni G. Cervical spondylotic radiculopathy producing motor manifestations mimicking primary muscular atrophy. Neurosurgery 1979; 5:427–431.
36. Kuncl RW, Cornblath DR, Griffin JW. Assessment of thoracic paraspinal muscles in the diagnosis of ALS. Muscle Nerve 1988; 11:484–492.
37. Gallagner JP, Sanders M. Trauma and amyotrophic lateral sclerosis: A report of 70 patients. Acta Neurol Scand 1987; 75:145–150.
38. Kondo K, Tsubaki T. Case-control studies of motor neuron disease: Association with mechanical injuries. Arch Neurol 1981; 38:220–226.
39. Sloan M, Baquis G, Munsat TL, et al. Progressive motor neuron disease after cervical spinal cord trauma. In preparation.
40. Tandan R, Bradley WG. Amyotrophic lateral sclerosis. Ann Neurol 1985; 18:271–280.
41. Boothby JA, deJesus P, Rowland LP. Reversible forms of motor neuron disease: "Lead neuritis." Arch Neurol 1974; 31:18–23.
42. Feldman RG, Hayes MK, Younes R, et al. Lead neuropathy in adults and children. Arch Neurol 1977; 34:481–488.
43. Livesley B, Sissons CE. Chronic lead intoxication mimicking motor neuron neuronal disease. Br Med J 1968; 4:387–388.
44. Stober T, Stelte W, Kunze K. Lead concentrations in blood, erythrocytes, and cerebrospinal fluid in amyotrophic lateral sclerosis. J Neurol Sci 1983; 61(1):21–26.
45. Pierce-Ruhland R, Patten BM. Muscle metals in motor neuron disease. Ann Neurol 1980; 8(2):193–195.
46. Kurlander HM, Bernard BM. Metals in spinal cord tissue of patients dying of motor neuron disease. Ann Neurol 1979; 6:21–24.
47. Gresham LS, Molgaard CA, Golbeck AL, et al. Amyotrophic lateral sclerosis and occupational metal exposure: A case-controlled study. Neuroepidemiology 1986; 5(1):29–38.
48. Deapen DM, Henderson BE. A case-control study of amyotrophic lateral sclerosis. Am J Epidemiol 1986; 123:790–799.

49. Mitsumoto H, Sliman RJ, Schafer IA, et al. Motor neuron disease and adult hexosaminidase A deficiency in two families: Evidence for multisystem degeneration. Ann Neurol 1985; 17:378–385.
50. Karni A, Navon R, Sadeh M. Hexosaminidase A deficiency manifesting as spinal muscular atrophy of late onset. Ann Neurol 1988; 24:451–452.
51. Argov Z, Navon R. Clinical and genetic variations in the syndrome of adult GM2 gangliosidosis resulting from hexosaminidase deficiency. Ann Neurol 1984; 16:14–20.
52. Gudesblatt M, Ludman MD, Cohen JA, et al. Hexosaminidase A activity and ALS. Muscle Nerve 1988; 11:227–230.
53. Argov Z, Navon R. Clinical and genetic variations in the syndrome of adult GM2 gangliosidosis resulting from hexosaminidase A deficiency. Ann Neurol 1984; 16:14–20.
54. Cashman NR, Antel JP, Hancock LW, et al. N-acetyl-B-hexosaminidase B locus defect and juvenile motor neuron disease: a case study. Ann Neurol 1986; 19:568–572.
55. Parnes S, Karpati G, Stirling C, et al. Hexosaminidase-A deficiency presenting as atypical juvenile-onset spinal muscular atrophy. Arch Neurol 1985; 42:1176–1180.
56. Specola N, Vanier MT, Goutieres F, et al. The juvenile and chronic forms of GM2 gangliosidosis: clinical and enzymatic heterogeneity. Neurology 1990; 40(1):145–150.
57. Thomas PK, Young E, King RHM. Sandhoff disease mimicking adult-onset bulbospinal neuronopathy. J Neurol Neurosurg Psychiatr 1989; 52(9):1103–1106.
58. Dalakas MC, Pezeshkpour GH. Neuromuscular diseases associated with human immunodeficiency virus infection. Ann Neurol 1988; 2(suppl):S38–S48.
59. Hoffman PM, Festoff BW, Giron LT Jr, et al. Isolation of LAV/HTLV-III from a patient with amyotrophic lateral sclerosis. N Engl J Med 1988; 313(5):324–325.
60. Verma RK, Ziegler DK, Kepes JJ. HIV-related neuromuscular syndrome simulating motor neuron disease. Neurology 1990; 40:544–546.
61. Evans BK, Gore I, Harrell LE, et al. HTLV-I-associated myelopathy and polymyositis in a US native. Neurology 1989; 39:1572–1575.
62. Provinciali L, Montroni M, Bagnarelli P, et al. Immunity assessment in early stages of amyotrophic lateral sclerosis: A study of virus antibodies and lymphocyte subsets. Acta Neurol Scand 1988; 78(6):449–454.
63. Kawanishi T, Akiguchi I, Fujita M, et al. Low-titer antibodies reactive with HTLV-I gag p19 in patients with chronic myeloneuropathy. Ann Neurol 1989; 26:515–522.
64. Gallego J, Delgrado G, Tunon T, Villaneuva JA: Delayed postirradiation lower motor neuron syndrome. Ann Neurol 1986; 19:308–309.

65. Horowitz SL, Steward JD. Lower motor neuron syndrome following radiotherapy. Can J Neurol Sci 1983; 10:56–58.

66. Kristensen O, Melgard B, Schiodt AV. Radiation myelopathy of the lumbo-sacral cord. Acta Neurol Scand 1977; 56:217–222.

67. Sadowsky CH, Sachs E Jr, Ochoa J. Postradiation motor neuron syndrome. Arch Neurol 1976; 33:786–787.

68. Lagueny A, Aupy M, Aupy M, et al. Syndrome de la corne anterieure postradiotherapique. Rev Neurol 1985; 141:222–227.

69. Herrick MK, Mills PE Jr. Infarction of spinal cord. Arch Neurol 1971; 24:228–241.

70. Brain R, Croft PB, Wilkinson M. Motor neuron disease as a manifestation of a neoplasm. Brain 1965; 88:479–500.

71. Kurtzke JF, Beebe GW. Epidemiology of amyotrophic lateral sclerosis: 1. A case-control comparison of ALS deaths. Neurology 1980; 30:453–462.

72. Jokelainen M. The epidemiology of amyotrophic lateral sclerosis in Finland. A study based on the death certificates of 421 patients. J Neurol Sci 1976; 29(1):55–63.

73. Felmus MT, Patten BM, Swanke L. Antecedent events in amyotrophic lateral sclerosis. Neurology 1976; 26:167–172.

74. Munsat TL. Adult motor neuron disorders. In: Rowland LP, ed. Merritt's textbook of neurology. Philadelphia: Lea & Febiger, 1989:682–687.

75. Barron KD, Rodichok LD. Cancer and disorders of motor neurons. In: Rowland LP, ed. Human motor neuron disease: Advances in neurology. New York: Raven Press, 1982:267–272.

76. Schold SC, Cho E, Somasundaran M, Posner JB. Subacute motor neuronopathy: A remote effect of lymphoma. Ann Neurol 1979; 5:271–287.

77. Recine U, Longi C, Pelosio A, Massini R. An unusually severe subacute motor neuronopathy in Hodgkin's disease. Acta Haematol 1984; 71:135–138.

78. Stoll DB, Lublin F, Brodovsky H, et al. Association of subacute motor neuronopathy with thymoma. Cancer 1984; 54:770–772.

79. Evan BK, Fagan C, Arnold T, et al. Paraneoplastic motor neuron disease and renal cell carcinoma: Improvement after nephrectomy. Neurology 1989; 40(6):960–962.

80. Younger DS, Rowland LP, Latov N, et al. Lymphoma, motor neuron diseases, and amyotrophic lateral sclerosis. Ann Neurol 1991; 29:78–86.

81. Dyck PJ, Lais AC, Ohta M, et al. Chronic inflammatory polyradiculoneuropathy. Mayo Clin Proc 1975; 50:621–637.

82. Lewis RA, Sumner AJ, Brown MJ, et al. Multifocal demyelinating neuropathy with persistent conduction block. Neurology 1982; 32:958–964.

83. Verma A, Tandan R, Adesina AM, et al. Focal neuropathy preceding inflammatory demyelinating polyradiculoneuropathy by several years. Acta Neurol Scand 1990; 81:516–521.

84. Chad DA, Hammer K, Sargent J. Slow resolution of multifocal weakness and fasciculations: A reversible motor neuron syndrome. Neurology 1986; 36:1260–1263.

85. Parry GJ, Clarke S. Multifocal acquired demyelinating neuropathy masquerading as motor neuron disease. Muscle Nerve 1988; 11:103–107.

86. Van Den Bergh P, Logigian EL, Kelly JJ Jr. Motor neuropathy with multifocal conduction blocks. Muscle Nerve 1989; 11:26–31.

87. Rowland LP, Defendini R, Sherman W, et al. Macroglobulinemia with peripheral neuropathy simulating motor neuron disease. Ann Neurol 1982; 11:532–536.

88. Parry GJ, Holtz SJ, Ben-Zeev D, et al. Gammopathy with proximal motor axonopathy simulating motor neuron disease. Neurology 1986; 36:273–276.

89. Rudnicki S, Chad DA, Drachman DA, et al. Motor neuron disease and paraproteinemia. Neurology 1987; 37:335–337.

90. Shy ME, Rowland LP, Smith TS, et al. Motor neuron disease and plasma cell dyscrasia. Neurology 1986; 36:1429–1436.

91. Freddo L, Yu RK, Latov N, et al. Gangliosides GM1 and GD1 are antigens for IgM M-protein in patients with motor neuron disease. Neurology 1986; 36:454–458.

92. Shy ME, Heiman-Patterson T, Parry GJ. Lower motor neuron disease in a patient with autoantibodies against Gal(beta 1-3)GalNAc in gangliosides GM1 and GD1b: Improvement following therapy. Neurology 1990; 40(5):842–844.

93. Nardelli E, Steck AJ, Barkas T, et al. Motor neuron syndrome and monoclonal IgM with antibody activity against gangliosides GM1 and GD1B. Ann Neurol 1988; 23:524–528.

94. Schluep M, Steck AJ. Immunostaining of motor nerve terminals with antibody activity against gangliosides GM1 and GD1b from a patient with motor neuron disease. Neurology 1988; 38:1890–1892.

95. Latov N, Hays AP, Donofrio PD. Monoclonal IgM with unique specificity to gangliosides GM1 and GD1B and to lacto-N-tetraose associated with human motor neuron disease. Neurology 1988; 38:763–768.

96. Santoro M, Thomas FP, Fink ME, et al. IgM deposits at nodes of Ranvier in a patient with amyotrophic lateral sclerosis, anti-GM1 antibodies, and multifocal motor conduction block. Ann Neurol 1990; 28(3):373–377.

97. Pestronk A, Cornblath DR, Ilyas AA, et al. A treatable multifocal motor neuropathy with antibodies to GM1 gangliosides. Ann Neurol 1988; 24:73–78.

98. Krarup C, Steward JD, Sumner AJ, et al. A syndrome of asymmetric limb weakness with motor conduction block. Neurology 1990; 40(1):118–127.

99. Pestronk A, Chaudhry V, Feldman EL, et al. Lower

motor neuron syndromes defined by patterns of weakness, nerve conduction abnormalities and high titers of antiglycolipid antibodies. Ann Neurol 1990; 27:316–326.

100. Pestronk A, Adams RN, Kuncl RW, et al. Differential effects of prednisone and cyclophosphamide on autoantibodies in human neuromuscular disorders. Neurology 1989; 39(5):628–633.

101. Pestronk A, Adams RN, Clausen L, et al. Serum antibodies to GM1 ganglioside in amyotrophic lateral sclerosis. Neurology 1988; 38:1457–1461.

102. Nobile-Orazio E, Carpo M, Legname G. Anti-GM1 IgM antibodies in motor neuron disease and neuropathy. Neurology 1990; 40(11):1747–1750.

103. Sadiq SA, Thomas FP, Kilidireas K, et al. The spectrum of neurological diseases associated with anti-GM1 antibodies. Neurology 1990; 40(7):1067–1072.

104. Salazar-Grueso EF, Routbort MJ, Martin J, et al. Polyclonal IgM anti-GM1 ganglioside antibody in patients with motor neuron disease and variants. Ann Neurol 1990; 27(5):558–563.

105. Shy ME, Evans VA, Lublin FD, et al. Antibodies to GM1 and GD1b in patients with motor neuron disease without plasma cell dyscrasia. Ann Neurol 1989; 25(5):511–513.

18

Diabetic Neuropathies
Asa J. Wilbourn

CONTENTS

LIST OF ACRONYMS

ADQP	abductor digiti quinti pedis
AH	abductor hallucis
CTS	carpal tunnel syndrome
CV	conduction velocity
DDSPN	diabetic distal symmetrical polyneuropathy
DM	diabetes mellitus
DPR	diabetic polyradiculopathy
DRG	dorsal root ganglion
DTR	diabetic thoracic radiculopathy
EDB	extensor digitorum brevis
ID-DM	insulin-dependent diabetes mellitus
MUP	motor unit potential
NCS	nerve conduction studies
NID-DM	non-insulin dependent diabetes mellitus
NEE	needle electrode examination
PNS	peripheral nervous system

Diabetes mellitus (DM) is the most common serious metabolic disorder having substantial peripheral nervous system (PNS) complications.[1,2] DM is an ancient disease, its symptoms having been reported in both Egyptian and Oriental medical writings as early as 1500 B.C.[3] Because of differing clinical characteristics, primary DM generally is considered under two major subgroups: (1) *insulin-dependent DM* (IDDM), also known as *juvenile-onset* or *type 1 DM,* and (2) *non–insulin dependent DM* (NIDDM), also called *adult-onset* or *type 2 DM*[2,4,5] (Table 18.1).

DM is a major public health problem, being a leading cause of death, disability, and expense. In the United States alone, it has been estimated that, during a recent year, for IDDM and NIDDM the incidence numbers were 19,000 and 586,000, whereas the prevalence cases were 435,000 and 5,069,000[6]; the total diabetic prevalence was 6.6%,[7] having increased about 10-fold over the past half century[8]; the costs (direct and indirect) of NIDDM alone were $19.8 billion.[9]

Although DM is worldwide in distribution, it is not equally distributed among persons of different ethnic groups and ages. The Eskimos, the Japanese, and some other Far East populations have the lowest prevalence rates (1% to 2%), whereas the Pima Indians of North America and the Nauru population of Micronesia have the highest (34% to 35%).[8] In the United States, blacks, hispanics, and native indians are 33%, 300%, and 1000% more likely to develop DM than are Caucasians.[9] Regarding age, the incidence of IDDM peaks near puberty, and about half the patients are diagnosed before age 21. In contrast, NIDDM is rare before age 20, but its incidence increases progressively with age, especially after age 45. Thus the rates of DM range from 2% in the 20- to 44-year age groups to 17.7% in the 65- to 74-year age groups.[7,10] This latter point is significant for electromyographers because, in many electromyography (EMG) laboratories, the ratio of older to younger aged patients studied has been increasing steadily over the past decade.

Involvement of the autonomic nervous system and the PNS represents one of the four major complications of DM, along with retinopathy, nephropathy, and vascular disease.[6] Somewhat surprisingly, PNS abnormalities were not linked to DM until 1798, although diabetic symptoms had been reported more than 3300 years earlier. Moreover, until 1864, the cause and effect relationship was miscon-

TABLE 18.1. Classification of primary diabetes mellitus

Characteristics	Insulin-Dependent Diabetes Mellitus	Non–Insulin Dependent Diabetes Mellitus
Synonyms	"Brittle" DM; juvenile-onset DM; type 1 DM	Stable DM; adult/mature-onset DM; type 2 DM
Genetic defect	High	High
HLA and autoimmune associations	Yes	No
Concordance rate for identical twins	±50%	±100%
Possible cause	Immune-mediated beta cell destruction	*Dysfunctional* beta cell, with end-organ insulin resistance
Percentage of diabetics	5–10%	90–95%
Female/male ratio	1:1	1.4:1.8/1
Age of onset (years)	usually <40–45	usually >30–40
Body habitus	Lean or normal	Obese (>80%)
Mode of onset	Often abrupt	Usually insidious
Plasma insulin levels	Low/unmeasurable	Normal to high
Major cause of death	Diabetic coma; diabetic nephropathy	Cardiovascular disease
Types of diabetic neuropathy commonly associated	All except polyradiculopathy; in young, only distal symmetric polyneuropathy and autonomic neuropathy	All; often several coexisting

Data from references 2, 4–6.

strued, and DM was attributed to the PNS disorder rather than the reverse.[11,12]

Any DM-related disorder of the PNS, as well as those of the autonomic nervous system and some cranial nerves, is grouped under the all-inclusive term *diabetic neuropathy*; although the plural form, *diabetic neuropathies,* would be more appropriate,[1,13] it seldom is used. Globally diabetic neuropathy is the second most common type of PNS affliction, following only traumatic neuropathy.[14] Nonetheless, it is a complex subject, with many of its major aspects—including definition, incidence, prevalence, and pathogenesis—enveloped in controversy and confusion. Much of the conflict stems from the fact that, in contrast to the other major complications of DM, diabetic neuropathy has no generally accepted standard definition nor set of diagnostic criteria.[12,13,15,16] Because of this, its prevalence among diabetics has been reported by various investigators to range from 0% to 93%.[15,17]

The first attempts to classify diabetic neuropathy were reported independently by Price and Layden in 1893.[12] Since then, a multitude of classifications have been proposed, with Sullivan's[18] 1958 effort probably serving as a prototype for most of the modern ones. Nonetheless, because the basic pathogenesis of diabetic neuropathy is unknown, some investigators contend that all classifications are arbitrary because they must be based primarily on nonspecific clinical criteria. Moreover, the boundaries of each syndrome often appear indistinct, and overlap is frequent.[12,19–22] Despite these admitted shortcomings, classifying diabetic neuropathy into subgroups is beneficial for several reasons: for determining natural history; for selecting the appropriate treatment regimens; and, if for nothing else, for identification purposes—any entity, or apparent entity, that lacks a name is difficult to discuss coherently.[20] Dyck et al.[20,23] have suggested a standardized approach for the detection and characterization of diabetic neuropathy. In this chapter, a classification appropriate to electromyographers is employed (Table 18.2).

ELECTRODIAGNOSTIC EXAMINATION WITH DIABETIC NEUROPATHY

Electrodiagnostic studies have been used to assess patients with possible diabetic neuropathy for approximately 40 years. The needle electrode examination (NEE) was the first of the modern techniques to be employed in this manner.[24–26] Diabetic neuropathy, however, became of prime interest to electro-

TABLE 18.2.   Classification of diabetic neuropathy

Rapidly reversible phenomena
　Hyperglycemic polyneuropathy
　Increased resistance to ischemia
DDSPN
Diabetic autonomic neuropathy
Hyperinsulinic neuropathy
DPR
　DPR involving L-2, L-3, L-4 roots: *diabetic amyotrophy*
　DPR involving T-4–T-12 roots: *diabetic thoracic radiculopathy*
　DPR involving L-5, S-1 (S-2) roots
　DPR involving C-5, C-6 (C-7–T-1) roots
Diffuse DPR plus DDSPN: *diabetic neuropathic cachexia*
Diabetic cranial mononeuropathies
Diabetic limb mononeuropathies
　Upper extremity mononeuropathies
　Lower extremity mononeuropathies
Diabetic mononeuropathy multiplex
Peripheral nervous system abnormalities indirectly caused by diabetes mellitus
Other neuromuscular abnormalities associated with diabetes mellitus

DDSPN, Diabetic distal symmetric polyneuropathy; DPR, diabetic polyradiculopathy.

myographers only after nerve conduction studies (NCS) were introduced into clinical use in the 1950s.[27] Over the next few decades, the value of electrodiagnostic studies in the evaluation of diabetic neuropathy was universally realized (Table 18.3). Although their worth in this regard is unchallenged, their use in monitoring therapeutic drug trials in patients with diabetic polyneuropathy, as advocated more recently, is of less certain benefit.[28,29]

A voluminous literature regarding electrodiagnostic studies performed on diabetic patients has now accumulated. Unfortunately, much of it is misleading, particularly those review articles in which material published decades earlier is often uncritically quoted; the information in many of them, especially that concerned with the diagnostic sensitivity of a particular procedure or component thereof, often is of more historical than practical value. Moreover, the literature is permeated with two conceptual errors:

1. Preoccupation with conduction velocities (CVs), especially motor. An inordinate amount of attention has been focused on the NCS element which (along with latencies) measures the rate of nerve impulse conduction: the conduction velocity

TABLE 18.3. Some milestones in the application of electrodiagnostic studies to the diagnosis of diabetic neuropathy

Year	Procedure	Investigator(s)
1950–1955	Needle electrode examination	Marinacci (and others)[25,26]; Garland and Taverner[24]
1960	Motor nerve conduction velocities	Ferrari-Forcade et al.[88]; Johnson and Olsen[90]
1961	Motor nerve conduction amplitudes	Mulder et al.[60]
1961	Mixed nerve conduction studies	Gilliatt et al.[219]
1961	Sensory nerve conduction studies	Downie and Newell[48]
1963	H wave	Mayer[38]
1971	Blink reflex	Kimura[183]
1975	F waves	Conrad et al.[114]
1980	Somatosensory evoked potentials	Cracco et al.[210]

(CV). (The common practice of referring to NCS as *nerve conduction velocities* demonstrates that this bias is not limited to diabetic neuropathy.) In many reports, only motor CVs alone, or motor and sensory CVs, are mentioned.[30–36] Even when the motor NCS responses are obtained with surface recording electrodes and the amplitudes of the responses are measured, they have been considered too *variable* to report.[37,38] The ultimate fixation on rate measurements occurs when unelicitable NCS (i.e., *zero* amplitudes) are considered indicative of a *rate* abnormality.[39,40] Such preoccupation in regard to diabetic neuropathy incorrectly implies that if a structural lesion is present, the predominant, if not the sole, pathophysiology is one of demyelination because generally only it is responsible for significant conduction slowing. In contrast, slowing is seldom seen with axon degeneration. When the process is complete, no NCS responses can be elicited, and therefore no rate measurements can be determined. When it is incomplete, the speed of transmission is being determined along noninvolved fibers that are conducting at their normal rate.[41] Axon degeneration, however, probably occurs more often than does demyelination with diabetic neuropathy,[12,42,43] and with axon degeneration the CV is usually normal or, at most, mildly slowed owing to loss of the fastest conducting fibers. Hence CV is extremely insensitive to axon degeneration, even when the latter has been so severe as to produce clinical weakness and fixed sensory deficits. Conversely, the NCS amplitudes are semiquantitative measures of the number of nerve fibers capable of conducting impulses from the stimulation to the recording sites. Consequently, they are helpful for demonstrating the two pathophysiologic processes that correlate highly with clinical weakness: axon loss and conduction block.[41] For this reason, Daube[28] noted that regarding electrodiagnostic studies with diabetic neuropathy, "while conduction velocity is the best known, amplitude has the most clinical significance." Moreover, the slowing in CV seen with DM can also be due to metabolic, as opposed to structural, alterations in nerves. This type of slowing may respond rapidly to treatment.[28,44–46]

2. Failure to consider confounding factors. Many articles provide no information regarding patient age, although this is often a crucial point. The results of electrodiagnostic studies (particularly those performed on the lower extremities) frequently differ significantly between patients over and under the age of 60 years. Consequently, many of the *abnormal* findings reported in elderly diabetics could actually be due to their age rather than to DM.

Also, the fact that more than one type of diabetic neuropathy may be present simultaneously often is not considered. Consequently, abnormalities actually caused by one type are attributed to another, thus generating significant confusion. For example, with diabetic amyotrophy, slowing of the peroneal F waves, recording extensor digitorum brevis (EDB) muscle, has been considered indicative of the pathophysiology affecting the peripheral L-2–L-4 fibers,[47] although it far more likely reflects that of a coexisting diabetic symmetric polyneuropathy (DDSPN).

DIABETIC MELLITUS AND THE ELECTROMYOGRAPHER

Primary DM is the source of much ambivalence for the electromyographer. On the one hand, it is by far the systemic disease most responsible for EMG laboratory referrals. On the other hand, diabetic patients require more time expenditure for adequate electrodiagnostic assessment than do any other group of patients, with the possible exception of those with mononeuropathy multiplex. Moreover, no other category of patients so often leaves the EMG laboratory with one or more inconclusive findings, primarily because DM introduces a considerable *uncertainty factor* in the electrodiagnostic data interpretation than would otherwise exist. Having electrodiagnostic studies consistently be both far more time-consuming and yet far less definitive than usual can engender considerable frustration.

There are many reasons why electrodiagnostic studies performed on diabetic patients so frequently become *worst case scenarios*. Some relate to characteristics of the patients with DM, whereas others are directly attributable to the diabetic state; many are interrelated.

Adverse Patient Characteristics

Advanced age

As previously noted, DM essentially is a disease of aging,[7,10] and its neurologic complications often are not manifest until it has been present for some years. Consequently, most diabetic patients studied in the typical EMG laboratory are elderly (e.g., at the Cleveland Clinic, the majority are over the age of 60 years). The detrimental effect of advanced age alone on the interpretation of the electrodiagnostic results is often unappreciated. Nonetheless, it can be considerable because the values for *normal* and *abnormal* overlap so much—particularly in regard to the lower extremity assessment—that many findings must be disregarded because they are of uncertain significance. Advanced age adversely affects all components of the examination. The various portions of the NCS begin to deteriorate (i.e., amplitudes decreasing, distal/peak latencies increasing, CVs decreasing) at about the age of 40.[33,38,48–54] This factor often becomes significant by the age of 60 years and beyond: Lower extremity sensory NCS (sural, superficial peroneal sensory) and H waves may be unelicitable; plantar responses often are unobtainable; lower extremity motor NCS responses typically are borderline to low in amplitude, and frequently the EDB muscles are so atrophic that peroneal motor responses cannot be recorded from them; and lower extremity motor CVs hover around the lowest limits of normal or are mildly slow. Compounding the problem, few EMG laboratories have normal NCS

values for patients over the age of 60 years because accumulating elderly control patients in sufficient numbers is difficult. Consequently, the NCS on these patients usually are judged by the normal values of the 50- to 60-year age group, supplemented by some unstandardized conversion factor. In practical terms, most changes in the plantar, sural, and superficial peroneal sensory NCS, and H waves in the elderly, excluding substantial asymmetry on bilateral studies, can be interpreted as *normal for age,* including unelicitable responses, thereby significantly diminishing their diagnostic value. The NEE is similarly affected. The motor unit potentials (MUPs) increase in duration and sometimes in amplitude with advanced age (the MUP duration almost doubles between the ages of 1 and 80 years).[55] Consequently, MUP changes considered definite evidence of a chronic neurogenic process in younger patients become equivocal findings in elderly patients, particularly when they are found in the intrinsic foot muscles. These electrophysical changes merely reflect the histologic changes occurring in the PNS, particularly in the lower extremity, with aging.[56,57] Nonetheless, they can be potent sources of confusion, forcing many electromyographic studies performed on elderly patients into the *inconclusive* category.

Obesity

Most diabetic patients studied in the typical EMG laboratory have NIDDM, and more than 80% of such patients are obese.[4] Patient obesity introduces technical problems that complicate the performance and interpretation of the electrodiagnostic examination, problems that increase almost linearly with the degree of obesity present. Because of interposed adipose tissue, the maximal output of the percutaneous stimulator may be reached before supramaximal nerve stimulation is achieved; moreover, some or all of the action potential generated in nerve and muscle may not reach the surface recording electrodes.[58] In either case, low amplitude/unelicitable responses often occur that are unrelated to intrinsic nerve pathology. For this reason, in obese patients (1) supramaximal femoral motor NCS responses often cannot be obtained; (2) posterior tibial motor responses, recording abductor hallucis, may be low or absent; (3) saphenous NCS responses generally are unelicitable; and (4) sural and superficial peroneal sensory NCS responses and H waves may be low in amplitude and sometimes unelicitable. At the least, marked patient obesity necessitates a more time-consuming study in that whenever NCS abnormalities are found in a limb, the contralateral one frequently must be assessed for comparison purposes because the normal laboratory values may or may not be applicable; this is particularly the case when only one limb is symptomatic. When bilaterally symmetric abnormalities are found, the electromyographer usually must arbitrarily choose to attribute them either to obesity-related technical factors or to pathology. Problems are encountered during the NEE portion of the study also. Extra-long needle electrodes are required. Moreover, accurately locating some of the muscles to be assessed, particularly many of the limb girdle and paraspinal muscles, can be virtually impossible because all visual and palpable anatomic landmarks are completely obscured by a sheer wall of adipose tissue.

Diabetic Factors

Normal diabetic patients

Borderline, if not definitely abnormal, electrodiagnostic changes frequently are found in diabetic patients who have no clinical evidence of diabetic neuropathy. The sensory and motor NCS amplitudes may be somewhat reduced,[48,59–61] and the motor nerve CVs usually are slower (mean of 3.7 m/s)[60] than in nondiabetic patients of the same age. In young to middle-aged patients, these changes generally are not severe enough to reach the abnormal range, but beyond age 50, the effects of age and DM frequently combine to produce equivocal to modestly abnormal NCS, based on normal laboratory values. Formerly, such changes in asymptomatic diabetes were difficult to interpret (i.e., were they sufficient for the diagnosis of subclinical DDSPN?) Because this slowing appears to be an integral component of the diabetic state, should normal diabetics have their NCS results judged against laboratory normal values established for them, just as is done for infants, rather than being expected to achieve the normal values used for the nondiabetic population? Or, conversely, should this conduction slowing be considered objective evidence of DDSPN, whether it is subclinical or not? The latter opinion now prevails substantiated by both single-fiber and pathologic evidence.[63,64]

NEE abnormalities also are seen in normal diabetics. Most often these consist of spontaneous fibrillation potentials or substantial numbers of insertional positive sharp waves in the lumbar paraspinal muscles bilaterally. Although their incidence is disputed,[65–67] the fact that they do occur means that such NEE changes are of little diagnostic value in any individual diabetic patient suspected of having a lumbar compressive radiculopathy. Occasionally, fibrillation potentials are found throughout the paraspinal muscles in otherwise normal diabetics.[68]

Focal nerve lesions and unsuspected/unappreciated diabetic distal symmetric polyneuropathy

Many patients with clinically evident DDSPN are inappropriately scheduled for electrodiagnostic examinations because either the referring physicians are unaware of the generalized PNS disorder, or they do not appreciate the likely electrophysiologic consequences of it. The typical end result is that far more extensive studies must be performed than had been anticipated. Two situations are encountered often: (1) Patients with *numb feet* are referred for a unilateral lumbosacral radiculopathy assessment. Usually, both lower extremities and at least one upper extremity ultimately must be studied so the presence of DDSPN can be confirmed, and any changes not attributable to it in the involved limb can be discovered. (2) Patients are referred for carpal tunnel syndrome (CTS) evaluation, apparently without the clinician being aware of how common upper extremity entrapment/compressive radiculopathies are with DDSPN. Typically, both upper extremities and one lower extremity must be assessed for definite diagnosis.

Coexisting lesions in presence of diabetic distal symmetric polyneuropathy

In many patients with DDSPN, the value of the electrodiagnostic examination for diagnosis or localization of coexisting neuromuscular lesions can be seriously impaired, depending on the nature and severity of the polyneuropathy. Four situations commonly are encountered:

1. Suspected superimposed median or ulnar entrapment/compressive neuropathies. When DDSPN is severe enough to alter the upper extremity NCS, via either axon loss or demyelinating slowing, a clinical suspected superimposed entrapment neuropathy, particularly CTS, sometimes cannot be confirmed by NCS; the nerve fibers are so affected by the generalized process that additional focal changes cannot be recognized.

2. Suspected superimposed radiculopathy. In the presence of a significant axon loss DDSPN, diagnosing a superimposed L-5 or S-1 radiculopathy can be difficult, if not impossible. H waves are usually un-

elicitable bilaterally because of the DDSPN and consequently are of no value. Any fibrillation potentials found in the lumbar paraspinal muscles and the more distal lower extremity muscles (all of which are innervated by the L-5–S-1 roots) must be discounted unless similar abnormalities are not seen in the corresponding, contralateral muscles. If symmetric NEE abnormalities are present in the muscles distal to the knees, a superimposed unilateral L-5 or S-1 root lesion can be diagnosed only when changes are found in the appropriate hamstrings and glutei muscles solely on the affected side. Consequently, extensive electrodiagnostic assessments of both lower extremities are almost invariably required, with particular emphasis on the more proximal L-5–S-2 innervated muscles.

Similarly, whenever DDSPN is severe enough to produce axon degeneration in the intrinsic hand muscles or whenever multiple upper extremity entrapment/compression neuropathies have been superimposed on DDSPN, diagnosing a superimposed C-8/T-1 radiculopathy can be an arduous task. Fibrillation potentials found in the abductor pollicis brevis (APB) muscle and in any of the ulnar-innervated hand muscles are of no value because they could equally be due to the generalized process or to the superimposed focal mononeuropathies. Only if fibrillation potentials are found in the flexor pollicis longus and the C-8/radial-innervated muscles (e.g., extensor indicis propius; extensor pollicis brevis) can it even be suggested that a C-8/T-1 cervical radiculopathy may also be present. Almost always extensive NEE assessments of both upper extremities must be performed for comparison purposes.

3. Differentiating root from plexus lesions. Whenever DDSPN has produced enough axon loss to alter the sensory NCS amplitudes severely, the electromyographer has lost the chief means of localizing proximal focal neurogenic lesions to either proximal to, or at/distal to, the dorsal root ganglia (DRG) (i.e., to distinguish lesions within the intraspinal canal from those located in the plexus or proximal peripheral nerve). Thus C-8/T-1 radiculopathies often cannot be differentiated from lower trunk/medial cord brachial plexopathies nor L-5 or S-1 radiculopathies from sacral plexopathies or high sciatic neuropathies.[54,67]

4. Presence of coexisting subtypes of diabetic neuropathy. Many patients are afflicted with more than one type of diabetic neuropathy simultaneously. DDSPN, for example, is so ubiquitous that it frequently coexists with diabetic polyradiculopathy or underlies diabetic-related entrapment/compression

neuropathies. Moreover, diabetic polyradiculopathy tends to become more extensive with time, yielding various subgroups. The end result is that extensive, multilimb assessments are commonplace when dealing with diabetic neuropathy. For example, in our EMG laboratory, we are almost assured of consuming three to four standard examination time slots whenever an elderly diabetic with numb feet and proximal, anterior lower extremity weakness (unilateral or bilateral) is evaluated. Almost invariably, at least three limbs must be assessed (both lower extremities and at least one upper extremity), uncommon conduction studies must be performed bilaterally (e.g., femoral motor NCS; peroneal motor NCS, recording tibialis anterior; saphenous NCS), and many muscles studied that are not sampled during the usual NEE assessment (e.g., thigh adductors, rectus femoris, iliacus, hamstrings).

For all these reasons, patients with DM, with or without diabetic neuropathy, typically require much more time-consuming electrodiagnostic examinations than do almost any other type of patient, and even then the results, far too often, are less than conclusive. To paraphrase the observations of Neel et al.[69] regarding DM and genetics: "Diabetes mellitus is in many respects an electromyographer's nightmare. As a disease, it (often) presents almost every impediment to a proper electrodiagnostic study which can be recognized."

Two other facts about the electrodiagnostic studies with DM require emphasis, one of negative and the other of positive import. First, none of the myriad of electrophysiologic changes found with diabetic neuropathy is pathognomonic. Consequently, the electromyographer cannot *confirm* that the generalized symmetric polyneuropathy found in a diabetic patient is due to DM rather than to some other cause, nor can the electromyographer distinguish diabetic amyotrophy from an L-2–L-4 compressive radiculopathy, although patients often are referred specifically for such differentiation. Second, the electromyographer sometimes proves to be of immense help in clinical management by demonstrating that a diabetic patient's symptoms are being erroneously attributed to one or more of the diabetic neuropathies. Many clinicians consider DM responsible for any neuromuscular abnormalities that develop in diabetic patients, although it is known that the diabetic population experiences the same incidence of nondiabetic neurologic disease as the general population.[17,70] These misdiagnoses most often occur when elderly diabetic patients develop bilateral distal lower extremity paresthesias. Almost reflexively, they are considered to have DDSPN, particularly by nonneu-rologists, and the electromyographer is the first to appreciate that their symptoms actually are due to bilateral S1—S-2 radiculopathies (most often a com-plication of lumbar canal stenosis). The clinical pic-ture becomes even more prone to error whenever patients present with distal paresthesias in all four limbs, with their foot symptoms caused by S-1 ra-diculopathies and their hand symptoms by CTS or by a combination of CTS and ulnar neuropathy.[67] Even neurologists, however, are not immune to such diagnostic inaccuracies; for example, a diabetic pa-tient has progressive polyneuropathy symptoms at-tributed to DDSPN and is observed for over 2 years before a belatedly obtained electrodiagnostic exam-ination reveals the actual cause: chronic inflamma-tory demyelinating polyneuropathy. Because they can prevent some of the misdiagnoses that plague diabetics who have PNS complaints, electrodiagnos-tic studies should be performed on all such patients. If diagnosis rests solely on the clinical evaluation, mistakes are inevitable, regardless of the skills of the clinician.

ELECTRODIAGNOSTIC EXAMINATION WITH DIABETIC NEUROPATHY

A vast number of PNS abnormalities are found in diabetic patients. The extent to which DM can be implicated in their cause is variable. For some, the cause and effect relationship appears secure (e.g., DDSPN, diabetic polyradiculopathy), although the exact pathogenetic mechanisms are unknown or de-bated. For others, the association is more statistical than apparent (e.g., increased incidence of Bell's palsy). In the remainder of this chapter, the electro-diagnostic features found with the various types of diabetic neuropathy are discussed, beginning with generalized disorders.

RAPIDLY REVERSIBLE PHENOMENA

Hyperglycemic *Polyneuropathy*

Some diabetic patients develop rather short-lived sensory symptoms (pain, paresthesias) in the distal extremities, either following an episode of ketotic coma or immediately before their DM is diagnosed. They promptly become asymptomatic as soon as the hyperglycemia responds to treatment.

Apparently no detailed electrophysiologic studies have been reported. The fact that the symptoms sub-side so quickly following onset of treatment indicates that the cause is primarily, if not solely, some meta-bolic disturbance of nerve, rather than a structural lesion.[71,72]

Increased Resistance to Ischemia

The peripheral nerves of patients with DM (either IDDM or NIDDM), with or without DDSPN, man-ifest a *peculiar resistance to ischemia,* compared with the nerves of nondiabetic patients.[73] This phenome-non was first described by Steiness in 1959 in regard to vibratory perception,[74] but it also affects the sen-sory NCS amplitudes and the motor CVs.[73,75,76] The cause is uncertain, although several theories have been proposed.[71,75] This abnormal ischemic toler-ance correlates highly with the HbA_{1c} level and can be partly reduced by aldose reductase inhibitors.[75] Also, it is found not only in patients with DM, but also in those with uremia, chronic liver disease, and motor neuron disease.[12,71]

This phenomenon apparently has no clinical sig-nificance, at least not at this time. Consequently, any NCS performed to assess it are done primarily for research purposes.

DIABETIC DISTAL SYMMETRIC POLYNEUROPATHY

This is the most common subgroup of diabetic neu-ropathy, constituting almost three-fourths of it.[12,77,78] For this reason, many physicians incorrectly assume that the term *diabetic neuropathy* is synonymous with DDSPN. Historically DDSPN was the first type of diabetic neuropathy to be recognized.[16]

Pathogenesis

Despite enormous amounts of research, the cause of DDSPN remains unknown. Several theories regard-ing the mechanism of peripheral nerve damage in DDSPN have focused on the metabolic abnormalities known to occur in diabetic nerves. The most obvious etiologic factor is hyperglycemia. Nonetheless, al-though improved glycemic control benefits periph-eral nerve function, there is little convincing evidence that it prevents, halts, or reverses the clinical features of DDSPN.[44] Hyperglycemia produces at least three chemical defects, however, that may have adverse consequences on peripheral nerves. These include increased sorbitol pathway activity, decreased myo-inositol content, and increased nonenzymatic protein glycosylation; the first two are causally interrelated. Unfortunately, attempts to treat some of these metabolic abnormalities in patients with DDSPN, for example, by administering aldose reductase inhibitors or myoinositol, have yielded disappointing results.[79]

One of the initial theories regarding the pathogenesis of DDSPN, which is receiving renewed interest in modified form, is the vascular/ischemic mechanism.[11] Some postmortem studies performed on patients with DDSPN have suggested that the nerve fibers in the proximal nerve trunks are lost in a multifocal fashion, with the cumulative effect responsible for the distal limb symptoms and signs.[63,80]

An allied theory proposes that endoneurial hypoxia results from capillary pathology caused by the hyperglycemia, and the endoneurial hypoxia, in turn, causes abnormalities of axonal transport and enzymatic compromise, which produce nerve dysfunction.[81]

Pathology and Pathophysiology

The nerve fiber lesions in DDSPN consist of both axon degeneration and demyelination. Whether the demyelination, however, is a dependent or independent change (i.e., represents primary or secondary demyelination) and which process is predominant, are controversial[12,42,63,77,82]; the latter may be determined by the duration of the DM.[83] From the electromyographer's viewpoint, DDSPN is classified under both *axon loss* and *demyelination* whenever symmetric polyneuropathies are categorized according to the electrodiagnostic changes found with them.[84,85]

Electrodiagnostic Findings with Diabetic Distal Symmetric Polyneuropathy

DDSPN apparently was the first diabetic neuropathy to be assessed in the EMG laboratory.[26,86] Those initial studies were performed in the 1950s, before NCS came into clinical use. Consequently they were limited to the NEE, and the first reported results were the presence of fibrillation potentials in the distal lower extremity muscles.[25,26] Since the advent of NCS, however, a large body of literature has accumulated regarding the electrophysiologic changes seen with DDSPN. Most of these studies have focused on the NCS—often NEEs were not performed or not reported—and until fairly recently, they concentrated almost solely on CVs.[31–34,37,38,60,87–92] This is true even for papers published in the 1980s, a decade in which the

marked limitations of CV alone to assess polyneuropathy became widely known.[93–95]

Two major misconceptions regarding motor (and, to a lesser extent, sensory) CV slowing in patients with DDSPN has dominated much of the literature on the topic for more than 30 years. (1) Slowing of CV is an inevitable finding with DDSPN. In fact, even the most ardent supporters of this view report that slowing is present in only 80% of patients with DDSPN,[96] and the percentage is significantly lower in our experience. (2) Whenever slowing is present, it is invariably due to demyelination. In fact, such slowing is typically only modest in degree electrically, usually falling into the *gray zone,* where it can equally be due to mild demyelination or to loss of the fastest conducting fibers owing to axon degeneration.[85,97–99] In most of the patients we assess with DDSPN, any slowing of motor CV usually is less than 40% of the normal mean for age and is often accompanied by fibrillation potentials in the intrinsic foot muscles. Hence axon loss appears to be the main underlying pathophysiology, a conclusion shared by others.[42,77] Nonetheless, modest slowing of the motor CVs, especially in the lower extremities, occasionally is the sole abnormality found, suggesting that demyelination alone may be responsible at times.

Motor nerve conduction studies

The use of motor NCS to assess patients with DDSPN was first reported in 1960.[88,90] The rate of conduction along motor nerves, expressed as motor CVs, has been the prime, if not the sole, topic of interest in the majority of reports on DDSPN since then. Numerous investigators have noted that motor CVs are significantly slower (by approximately 5 to 13 meters per second) in patients with DDSPN than in age-matched normal controls.[33,37,38,48,60,61,100,101] The slowing is more severe in degree than that seen in normal diabetics (those with subclinical DDSPN), often by a factor of two or more. In one study, the average motor CV slowing was 3.7 meters per second in normal diabetics and 8.6 meters per second in those with DDSPN.[60] This conduction abnormality appears to begin early in the course of DM, commonly within the first year of recognition of the disorder, and frequently is present in a generalized distribution.[33,38] Thus, the upper extremity (median, ulnar) motor CVs may be slowed in patients with DDSPN whose symptoms are limited to the distal lower extremities. Many investigators have found a correlation between the degree of motor conduction slowing and poor control of DM, the clinical severity of DDSPN, or both. Much disagreement can be found in the literature, however, regarding CV slowing and its relationship to the duration of DM or to advancing age (or both), whether it is diffuse along the nerve or affects the proximal or distal segments most severely, and exactly which nerves it involves most consistently and severely. Although some reports describe upper and lower extremity nerves affected equally, in our experience and probably that of most investigators, the motor CVs of the peroneal and posterior tibial nerves are more often outside the range of normal than are those of median and ulnar nerves.

The majority of studies have been concerned with adults with DDSPN, reflecting (1) the relative prevalence of DM among the various age groups, (2) the fact that the incidence of overt DDSPN is less in juvenile than in adult diabetics, and (3) the fact that motor CV slowing is seldom apparent in diabetic children less than 5 years of age. Nonetheless, just as with adults, the mean motor CV in children with DDSPN is significantly slowed (especially of the peroneal nerve, according to some reports),[45] and the slowing seen is more severe in degree than that found in asymptomatic diabetic children of the same age. The degree of motor CV slowing in diabetic children and adolescents is more often linked to the severity and poor control of DM than to its duration.[30,32,37,40,87,93,103]

Although motor NCS amplitude changes are described in relatively few reports,[60,91,101] they characteristically are present when significant axon loss occurs, particularly with the peroneal and posterior tibial NCS. Ironically the significance of low amplitudes or unelicitable (i.e., zero) amplitudes sometimes is unappreciated, and they are mentioned only to explain why motor CVs cannot be determined along the affected nerves.[34] The motor distal latencies also may be abnormal with DDSPN, but often they are within the normal range even when CVs assessed along the same fibers more proximally are abnormal.[28]

Sensory nerve conduction studies

The results of sensory NCS performed on patients with DDSPN were first reported in 1961.[48] It is now appreciated that sensory NCS responses overall tend to be the most sensitive NCS parameter with this disorder. As with polyneuropathies in general, they often are absent, low in amplitude, dispersed, or slowed at a time when the motor NCS results are

still within the normal range. The sensory NCS abnormalities are found more often in the lower than in the upper extremity nerves.[28,30–32,45,104,105]

NCS of the plantar nerves reportedly are most often abnormal with DDSPN, probably because those nerves (which are actually mixed, rather than sensory, nerves) are the most distally situated.[106] Depending on the particular NCS techniques used, either the sural or the superficial peroneal sensory response is the next most sensitive. Unelicitable responses are the most common finding seen with all axon loss DDSPN except very mild ones. With the latter, the sensory NCS amplitudes may be low in amplitude, the sensory rate measurements (peak latencies/CVs) may be slowed, or both.[107] An important point is that low amplitude or unelicitable lower extremity sensory NCS responses in patients under the age of 60 usually are due to polyneuropathy; these NCS characteristically are unaltered with lumbosacral radiculopathies, regardless of the severity of sensory fiber loss, because the L-5 and S-1 root involvement is occurring proximal to the DRG, causing axon degeneration to progress centrally rather than peripherally.[67]

The main limitation of lower extremity sensory NCS is that they may be absent bilaterally in normal persons age 60 years and over. The upper extremity sensory NCS responses, however, are never unelicitable in normal persons of any age if antidromic techniques are used. Consequently, although they are less often abnormal with DDSPN than are the lower extremity sensory NCS responses, when they are abnormal, and not attributable to a focal process, they provide definite evidence of DDSPN. This is one of the many reasons why upper extremity sensory NCS are indicated in patients with suspected DDSPN and also why performing radial as well as median and ulnar sensory NCS often is helpful. (In comparison with the median and ulnar sensory NCS responses, the radial sensory NCS responses seldom are affected by entrapment/compression neuropathies.)

Late responses (H waves, F waves)

The H wave studies were first demonstrated to be of value in assessing patients with DDSPN in 1963.[38] In fact, they are one of the most sensitive electrodiagnostic procedures for polyneuropathies in general, usually being unelicitable bilaterally or, much less often, being of low amplitude or prolonged in latency.[38,108–113] Unfortunately, they frequently are absent bilaterally in normal persons over the age of 60, similar to the lower extremity sensory NCS responses. Unlike the latter, however, they are also sensitive indicators of S-1 radiculopathies. This proves to be a major limiting factor in using H wave testing to diagnose DDSPN because in elderly diabetic patients, lumbar canal stenosis occurs with about the same frequency as DDSPN, causing bilateral S-1 radiculopathies with resultant bilaterally absent H waves.[67]

An often unappreciated component of the H wave study is the M response—the direct motor response recorded from the gastrocnemius/soleus muscles. Its amplitude can be compared with the peroneal motor NCS amplitude, recorded over the tibialis anterior muscle, to provide a semiquantitative measure of the amount of axon loss affecting the major muscle groups located between the knee and ankle. Generally, with DDSPN, as with other polyneuropathies, the responses recorded from the tibialis anterior and the gastrocnemius/soleus muscles are affected to approximately the same degree, i.e., if one is low in amplitude, the other is usually equally low in amplitude. In contrast, in patients with cauda equina lesions, these responses often are dissimilar, with the tibialis anterior recording being of reduced amplitude or unelicitable with severe L-5 root compromise and the gastrocnemius/soleus recording being similarly affected with severe S-1 radiculopathies.

F waves have been used in the diagnosis of DDSPN since 1975.[114] The most common reported finding has been diffuse F wave slowing, although disproportionate F wave slowing along the proximal and distal segments of the nerves has been described by various investigators.[115–118] F waves elicited by stimulating the lower extremity nerves reportedly are abnormal more often with DDSPN than are those elicited by stimulating upper extremity nerves.[109] In general, posterior tibial nerve F waves are thought to yield more reliable findings than peroneal nerve F waves; the EDB muscle so frequently is at least partially denervated, especially in older patients, that peroneal F wave recordings made from it may be unreliable.[119] Some investigators have reported that F waves are more sensitive indicators of nerve dysfunction than are conventional NCS. Such statements must be viewed with caution, particularly in regard to DDSPN, for two reasons. First, F waves tend to be affected in the same manner as the routine motor nerve CVs, and consequently they usually just provide unneeded supporting evidence of slowing; conversely, only rarely in our experience are F waves slowed with DDSPN in the presence of normal motor CVs. Second, in many patients, DDSPN is an axon loss, rather than a demyelinating, disorder. Conse-

quently, in the lower extremities, the sensory NCS responses and the H waves may be low in amplitude or unelicitable bilaterally, the motor NCS responses low in amplitude, and fibrillation potentials and MUP loss found in the intrinsic foot muscles, and yet the F waves may still be within normal limits.[120]

Needle electrode examination

The NEE was the first electrodiagnostic procedure used to assess patients with DDSPN,[25,26] and it remains a helpful one. Nonetheless, the results of the NEE in patients with DDSPN are mentioned rather infrequently, and the changes reported have varied from one study to another.[60,61,87,92,100,121]

Whether fibrillation potentials or MUP abnormalities (or both) are detectable in patients with DDSPN depends on a number of factors, including: (1) the severity of axon loss, (2) its rate of progression, (3) the duration of the process, and (4) the particular muscles assessed. In occasional patients, the absence of NEE findings coupled with modest slowing of CV on NCS suggests that demyelination is the only process operative. Far more often, however, at least some evidence of axon loss is detectable during the electrodiagnostic examination, particularly during the NEE. With rapidly evolving DDSPN, fibrillation potentials typically are seen, their density reflecting the rapidity of fiber loss. With slowly progressive lesions, particularly those of long duration, chronic neurogenic MUP changes and MUP loss tend to overshadow any fibrillation potentials present. Curiously in some IDDM patients with long-standing DDSPN, the only abnormalities seen may be those of MUP dropout. As with other symmetric polyneuropathies, the most distal muscles, i.e., the intrinsic foot muscles, such as the EDB, abductor hallucis, and abductor digiti quinti pedis, are the muscles most consistently abnormal with DDSPN. If the NEE is restricted to lower extremity muscles no further distal than the midleg, for example, the tibialis anterior and medial gastrocnemius, many mild axon loss DDSPNs will be overlooked. The contention that intrinsic foot muscles should not be assessed by NEE in diabetic patients for fear of causing infection, although well meaning, appears unwarranted. To my knowledge, such a complication has never been reported.

With severe DDSPN, the intrinsic foot muscles may be completely atrophic and, therefore, the most active NEE changes found in the immediately more proximally situated limb muscles. The incidence of fibrillation potentials in the intrinsic hand muscles is considerably lower than for the intrinsic foot muscles. Generally until fibrillation potentials are detected as far proximal as the hamstrings and vasti, they usually are not found in the upper extremity.

Special electrodiagnostic studies

Several specialized electrophysiologic procedures have been performed on patients with known or suspected DDSPN for a variety of reasons, probably most often to detect subclinical disease. These tests include evoked responses, motor unit counting, single-fiber electromyographic studies, macro-electromyographic studies, assessing the refractory period, and determining the resistance of nerve conduction to ischemia (discussed earlier).[28]

Electrodiagnostic changes seen with diabetic distal symmetric polyneuropathy

Because DDSPN varies from patient to patient in predominant nerve fiber involvement (e.g., motor, sensory), in main pathophysiology present, and in severity, its electrophysiologic presentation is quite diverse. Certain of its features, however, are predictable: (1) Nerves in the lower extremity are affected before those of the same type in the upper extremity. Thus unlike the situation seen with some of the acquired demyelinating polyradiculoneuropathies, if the upper extremity sensory NCS responses are abnormal owing to DDSPN, the lower extremity ones will always be affected as well, typically more so. (2) The motor CVs are not markedly slow, unless one or more entrapment/compressive mononeuropathies are superimposed. The major exception to this is the occasional patient with rather severe, very chronic DDSPN in whom the lower extremity motor NCS responses recording intrinsic foot muscles are both very low in amplitude and very slow in CV. The fact that the upper extremity motor amplitudes and CVs are normal/near normal, however, speaks against this being a generalized change; more likely it reflects very severe prior axon loss along the lower extremity motor nerves, with subsequent reinnervation. (3) The NEE abnormalities are most prominent in the distal lower extremities until the intrinsic foot muscles lack viable muscle fibers owing to chronic denervation. Also, in the upper extremity, fibrillation potentials appear first in the intrinsic hand muscles and only after they are found proximal to the knee in the lower extremity. An exceptional patient is seen, however, in whom active denervation is surprisingly severe and yet is essentially restricted to the hands and

feet, that is, the typical distoproximal gradient of change is lacking in the lower extremities.

With mild DDSPN, the abnormalities seen, either alone or in various combinations, consist of: (1) bilaterally unelicitable H waves; (2) low amplitude/unelicitable medial plantar, sural, and superficial peroneal sensory responses (if low amplitude, with or without prolonged peak latencies); (3) fibrillation potentials in the intrinsic foot muscles (EDB, abductor hallucis, abductor digiti quinti pedis); and (4) mild slowing of the peroneal or posterior tibial motor CVs. A study just completed in our laboratory of over 100 patients under the age of 60 with DDSPN suggests that bilaterally absent H waves is the single most common finding, being seen in nine out of 10 patients.

Upper extremity assessment in DDSPN yields evidence of a generalized disorder in approximately two-thirds of patients; in the other one-third, the DDSPN is so mild that electrophysiologic changes are detectable only in the lower extremities. Low amplitude sensory (median, ulnar, radial) NCS responses are the most common abnormality. Less often, fibrillation potentials are found in the intrinsic hand muscles, and the forearm median and ulnar motor CVs are mildly slowed.

A common problem compounding upper extremity NCS in DDSPN is the presence of superimposed entrapment/compression neuropathies. In our experience, median neuropathy distal to the wrist (CTS) is detectable bilaterally in approximately one-third of patients with DDSPN under the age of 60 and in about two-thirds of those over that age. Moreover, bilateral ulnar neuropathies, probably located at the elbow but often solely axon loss in type and therefore poorly localizable by electrodiagnostic studies, are found in an appreciable number of patients as well (approximately 15% of patients under the age of 60 years with DDSPN), usually coexisting with bilateral CTS.

Although DDSPN has numerous electrodiagnostic presentations, certain patterns rarely, if ever, are found with it, including those seen with *pure* sensory polyneuropathy and acquired demyelinating polyradiculoneuropathy.

Many patients with DDSPN present with sensory symptoms alone; hence it is often referred to as *diabetic sensory polyneuritis*.[12,17] Nonetheless, on electrodiagnostic examination, some evidence of associated asymptomatic motor nerve dysfunction is found in the vast majority of patients. Thus although the occasional diabetic patient presents with NCS and late response findings suggestive of a pure sensory polyneuropathy (i.e., low-amplitude/unelicitable upper and lower extremity sensory responses, unelicitable H waves, normal upper and lower extremity motor NCS responses, and normal F waves[122]), usually some NEE abnormalities, particularly fibrillation potentials, can be found in the intrinsic foot muscles. Over the past few years, however, we have encountered a few patients with a pure sensory polyneuropathy on electrodiagnostic studies, in whom the only underlying cause appeared to be DM. Thus in contrast to Daube's view,[28] we believe that DM can cause a pure sensory polyneuropathy, although rarely.

Occasionally a diabetic patient develops a Guillain-Barré–type syndrome. This combination probably represents no more than chance association.[12,77] Of note is that certain changes sometimes seen with acquired demyelinating polyradiculoneuropathies never occur with DDSPN, including (1) sensory NCS responses that are normal in the lower extremity but low amplitude or unelicitable in the upper extremity; (2) severe slowing of lower extremity motor CVs in the absence of abundant axon loss; and (3) generalized marked slowing of motor CVs with normal motor distal latencies, or the reverse.

Diagnostic Approach to Diabetic Distal Symmetric Polyneuropathy

As with all generalized neuromuscular disorders, electrodiagnostic studies are performed not only to demonstrate abnormalities, but also to prove, if possible, their widespread distribution. To accomplish this satisfactorily, one side of the body—one upper and one lower extremity—should be assessed by both NCS and NEE. It is pointless to routinely evaluate corresponding nerves in the lower extremities or those in one lower extremity and the contralateral upper extremity, as described in some reports.[30,31,61] With many patients, however, particularly those over the age of 60, the other lower extremity must be studied as well, and under certain conditions, at least a limited assessment of the contralateral upper extremity must be done. Depending on the results as the examination proceeds, additional studies often are required. The standard *polyneuropathy evaluation* used in our laboratory is listed in Table 18.4.

Value of Electrodiagnostic Studies in Diabetic Distal Symmetric Polyneuropathy

The value of performing electrodiagnostic examinations on patients with known or suspected DDSPN must be stressed. If the disorder is present and if sufficient studies are performed on at least one upper and lower extremity, the electrodiagnostic evaluation is highly likely to be abnormal. It is sensitive enough to uncover subclinical cases, and in both asymptomatic and symptomatic patients with DDSPN, it can be used to determine the type and severity of pathophysiology present; the latter can then serve as a baseline for longitudinal studies. We have never seen a completely normal electrodiagnostic examination in a patient with clinically unequivocal DDSPN, even when the *predominantly small fiber* type was suspected.[42,106] Because there is little to no clinical evidence of larger myelinated fiber involvement in these patients and because those are the only fibers assessed in the EMG laboratory, a logical assumption is that the electrodiagnostic study would be normal. Yet some large fibers are compromised, because electrodiagnostic changes to some degree are consistently detectable.

By demonstrating findings suggestive of a generalized polyneuropathy, the electrodiagnostic examination often proves valuable for distinguishing DDSPN from other PNS conditions with which it may be clinically confused: tarsal tunnel syndrome, chronic inflammatory polyradiculoneuropathy, and, very often in the elderly patients, bilateral S-1 radiculopathies or more extensive cauda equina lesions. Conversely, in patients with distal sensory symptoms suspected of having DDSPN, a completely normal electrodiagnostic study may shift the clinician's attention from the PNS to other diagnoses, such as multiple sclerosis or hysteria.

The value of electrodiagnostic studies to monitor various therapies proposed for DDSPN, that is, to determine the efficacy of various drugs and treatment regimens, is somewhat controversial. Although various components of the electrodiagnostic examination, particularly motor nerve CVs, have been described as being helpful in this regard, questions can be raised about the validity of many of the reports. Problems include the design of some of the clinical trials, the choice of electrodiagnostic tests employed and the parameter(s) assessed, and the lack of rigorous standardization of the studies. Even when abnormalities are reported, they often are so minute that they become apparent only after extensive statistical manipulation of the raw data. Moreover, they are more likely to be due to temporary fluctuations in nerve osmolality than to an actual arrest or reversal of the basic process injuring the nerve fibers.[16,29,96,123,124] Further details on this point are available.[28]

TABLE 18.4. Electrodiagnostic evaluation for suspected diabetic distal symmetric polyneuropathy*

Component	Upper Extremity	Lower Extremity
Nerve conduction studies		
Sensory	Median (with CV)	Sural (with CV)
	Ulnar	Medial plantar
	Radial	(Superficial peroneal)
Motor	Median (APB)	Peroneal (EDB)
	Ulnar (ADM)	Posterior tibial (AH)
Late responses	Median F waves	H wave
	Ulnar F waves	Posterior-tibial F waves
Needle electrode examination (muscles assessed)	First dorsal interosseous; abductor pollicis brevis (more proximal ones [e.g., flexor carpi ulnaris, flexor pollicis longus] if necessary)	Abductor hallucis; extensor digitorum brevis; tibialis anterior, flexor digitorum longus/tibialis posterior; gastrocnemius medialis; vastus lateralis; gluteus medius/maximus; high sacral paraspinals (hamstrings, if necessary)

* Performed on one upper extremity and ipsilateral lower extremity.

CV, Conduction velocity; APB, abductor pollicis brevis; ADM, abductor digiti minimi; EDB, extensor digitorum brevis; AH, abductor hallucis.

DIABETIC AUTONOMIC NEUROPATHY

Autonomic neuropathy has been classified as one type of diabetic neuropathy since 1945.[12] It can appear in clinical isolation, usually in young patients with IDDM who have electrodiagnostically proved subclinical DDSPN.[28,42] Much more often, however, it occurs in patients with overt DDSPN. In fact, as autonomic tests have become more refined and widespread, the high association between autonomic neuropathy and DDSPN has been appreciated.[125] Because any tissues that receive autonomic fibers can be involved, the systems and mechanisms that may be adversely affected by autonomic neuropathy are widespread: cardiovascular, alimentary, genitourinary, sweating, and pupillary.[16] Nonetheless, this type of diabetic neuropathy is of less interest to electromyographers than most others because few of its manifestations can be assessed in the EMG laboratory. Sympathetic skin conduction can be recorded, but the test has not been standardized.[28] One clinical disorder that has been studied to some extent is impotence. This complication of DM is reported to occur in 30% to 60% of diabetic men, and its incidence increases with age.[12] It usually begins gradually, is accompanied by other evidence of autonomic dysfunction, and once established is typically permanent. Some electrodiagnostic studies used to assess patients with impotence include cortical and spinal pudendal evoked responses, bulbocavernosus reflex responses, and CV determinations along the dorsal nerve of the penis.[126–129] Unfortunately, none of these studies evaluates autonomic nerve fibers directly. Instead pelvic somatic nerves are assessed, and any abnormalities detected are assumed to be affecting autonomic fibers as well. Moreover, although conduction slowing has been the most frequent abnormality sought, it is likely that slowing along surviving fibers is an epiphenomenon, and the clinically important feature is the failure of many fibers to conduct at all because of axonal degeneration. Because DDSPN, either overt or subclinical, so frequently is associated with autonomic neuropathy, electrodiagnostic studies should be performed on every patient with suspected diabetic autonomic neuropathy, including diabetics with impotence.

HYPERINSULINIC NEUROPATHY

A rare disorder, variously entitled *hyperinsulin neuronopathy, hyperglycermic peripheral neuropathy,* and *polyneuritis hyperglycemia,* can occur following episodes of insulin excess. Although this entity is mentioned in reviews of diabetic neuropathy,[28] its relationship to DM is speculative. Theoretically it could develop in diabetics following severe insulin-provoked hypoglycemia, just as it could in psychiatric patients subjected to insulin coma,[28,50,77] but apparently this has never occurred or at least has never been reported. Instead all the published cases have developed in patients with pancreatic neoplasms, particularly islet cell adenomas.[130,131] The PNS lesions with this disorder have been variably localized to the peripheral nerves (i.e., a symmetric polyneuropathy), the anterior horn cells (i.e., a myelopathy), and both areas simultaneously.[102] Electrodiagnostic studies have not pinpointed the location of the lesion, mainly because the reported studies have not been extensive, or they were performed before sensory NCS came into clinical use.[102,130–132]

DIABETIC POLYRADICULOPATHY

That diabetic neuropathy can affect the proximal limb and trunk fibers of the PNS, often in an asymmetric fashion, has long been recognized by clinicians. Nonetheless, no serious attempt was made to consider any of these presentations as distinct entities until 1953, when Garland and Taverner[24] described diabetic amyotrophy (which they first called diabetic myelopathy). In 1958, Sullivan[18] grouped many of the non-DDSPN diabetic disorders of the PNS under the term *asymmetric (motor) proximal neuropathy*, and variations of this title appear in most of the current classifications of diabetic neuropathy.

Until rather recently, this subgroup defied all attempts to view it coherently because of both its apparent lack of a common cause and its markedly polymorphic presentation. Thus in different patients, it (1) affects primarily motor nerves or sensory nerves or both equally; (2) affects solely nerves to trunk muscles, proximal limb muscles, more distal limb muscles, or various combinations of these; (3) is unilateral, bilateral but asymmetric, or bilaterally symmetric in presentation; and (4) if bilateral, is either of simultaneous or sequential onset. For these reasons, some investigators questioned grouping these non-DDSPN manifestations of diabetic neuropathy under a single title, whereas others questioned their very existence, suggesting that the symptoms attributed to them actually were due to a number of diverse entities.[22,133]

Several authors, however, including Garland,[134] saw common threads linking the components of this subgroup,[135–137] and in 1981 a unifying concept for them, based in large part on their electrodiagnostic findings, was formulated by Bastron and Thomas.[65]

They proposed that all these non-DDSPN types of diabetic neuropathy affecting the PNS are subgroups of *diabetic polyradiculopathy*; that is, they are merely different presentations of the same basic process: diabetic involvement, often sequential, of various lumbar, thoracic, and, occasionally, cervical roots.[65,138] This subdivision of diabetic neuropathy therefore includes entities that previously have been labeled *diabetic amyotrophy* and *diabetic thoracic radiculopathy*; it also includes the neuropathic processes responsible for some of the distal or diffuse lower extremity weaknesses associated with DM (e.g., some diabetic footdrop); some of the upper extremity abnormalities, particularly those involving the shoulder girdle muscles; and most components of diabetic neuropathic cachexia. With Bastron and Thomas' hypothesis serving as a frame of reference, considerable order can be perceived in what initially appears to be a bewildering number of independent neurogenic abnormalities connected only by underlying DM. Moreover, certain tentative conclusions can be drawn based on this concept:

1. DM often attacks the PNS at the root level, typically one root very severely or two or more contiguous roots rather severely.
2. The lesion is predominantly, if not completely, axon degeneration in type.
3. Although the root involvement may remain isolated, frequently additional roots are involved, cephalad, caudally, or, particularly, contralaterally. Such *territorial extension* (a term coined by Bastron and Thomas) occurs in approximately two-thirds of patients.
4. Some roots are affected frequently, sometimes in isolation, whereas others are affected infrequently and typically only when preceded by involvement of more frequently involved roots. Diabetic radiculopathy most often affects the L-2, L-3, and L-4 roots, producing the clinical syndrome of diabetic amyotrophy. This may be strictly unilateral, but similar root abnormalities often develop contralaterally, sometimes almost simultaneously but usually after a variable interval, and the resulting bilateral diabetic amyotrophy may be asymmetric or symmetric. The mid and lower thoracic roots also may be affected in isolation, particularly the T-8 to T-12 segments, producing the clinical syndrome of diabetic thoracic radiculopathy, which has a similar tendency to spread contralaterally. The same diabetic patient may have both diabetic amyotrophy and diabetic thoracic radiculopathy, and

such concurrent involvement of the L-2–L-4 roots and the T-8–T-12 roots usually results from *territorial extension* from the former, with the lesions thus developing sequentially rather than simultaneously. The L-5–S-2 roots are sometimes affected, but they are seldom compromised initially or in isolation; much more often their involvement is due to territorial extension from ipsilateral L-2–L-4 root compromise. Consequently, many patients with diabetic amyotrophy who initially have weakness only of the anterior (and medial) thigh muscles eventually develop footdrop or even *global involvement of the leg muscles*, a fact noted by Garland[134] as early as 1957. Occasionally the process spreads to the upper extremities, usually in a bilaterally symmetric fashion, and involves the C-5, C-6 roots, producing bilateral shoulder girdle weakness. The C-7–T-1 roots appear to be the ones least likely to be affected by diabetic polyradiculopathy.

5. The majority of patients with diabetic polyradiculopathy have coexisting DDSPN, a separate process but one that, by affecting SNAP amplitudes and producing NEE abnormalities in the more distal limb muscles, often prevents electromyographic localization of the diabetic polyradiculopathy to the root level.

6. Rarely diabetic polyradiculopathy is almost diffuse in distribution, affecting the L-2–S-2 roots bilaterally, most of the thoracic roots bilaterally, and in the upper extremities at least the C-5–C-6 roots bilaterally. Typically this process is associated with a severe, axon loss DDSPN, an autonomic neuropathy, depression, and considerable weight loss, culminating in the syndrome of diabetic neuropathic cachexia. Supporting this concept is the fact that all entities included under diabetic polyradiculopathy have many similarities in regard to their clinical and electrodiagnostic presentations. (Table 18.5)

Nonetheless, this concept is not universally accepted. Most investigators who reject it do so because they localize the lesion(s) causing diabetic amyotrophy to some point other than the root level, either because of pathologic or electrophysiologic findings. The status of the L-2–L-4 roots, however, is not specifically mentioned in the single published report of an autopsy performed on a patient with diabetic amyotrophy,[139] and most of the electrodiagnostic results considered inconsistent with diabetic polyradiculopathy are seriously flawed: Either they focus on conduction slowing, which has no real relevance to either the clinical or the major electrophysiologic changes seen with diabetic polyradiculopathy, or their conclusions are based on extrapolation from the electrophysiologic changes caused by the patient's coexisting DDSPN, a separate process. Many of these reports localize the responsible lesion to the lumbar plexus or peripheral nerve rather than to the roots. To explain the presence of fibrillation potentials in the limb muscles, however, as well as the appropriate paraspinal muscles requires lesions to develop simultaneously along two or more peripheral nerves. It seems far more reasonable to attribute denervation appearing simultaneously in the posterior and anterior rami distributions to a single lesion at the root level.

TABLE 18.5. Features common to various subgroups of diabetic polyradiculopathy

Elderly men with NIDDM most often affected
Pain typically the outstanding complaint (often with nocturnal persistence)
Weakness/atrophy usually prominent in distribution of 1 or more (contiguous) roots
Pronounced tendency for process to become more widespread with time (*territorial extension*)
Axon loss conspicuous on electrodiagnostic studies
DDSPN frequently coexisting
Weight loss often associated
Clinical course characteristically prolonged ($\pm$ 8–12 mo)
Spontaneous regression the norm; ultimate recovery usually striking

NIDDM, Non–insulin dependent diabetes mellitus; DDSPN, diabetic distal symmetric polyneuropathy.

Diabetic Polyradiculopathy Involving the L-2, L-3 (L-4) Roots: Diabetic Amyotrophy

Diabetic amyotrophy was not recognized as a distinct entity until Garland's publications appeared, beginning in 1953.[24,134,140–142]

Among the diabetic neuropathies involving the PNS, diabetic amyotrophy is second only to DDSPN in prevalence and is by far the most controversial. Opinions differ regarding its clinical presentation, pathogenesis, and site of motor unit involvement.[22,59,115,143–153] Following the old aphorism "the more confusion, the more names," this entity has acquired many synonyms[12,24,42,47,65,144,145,152,154,155] (Table 18.6).

Diabetic amyotrophy has been variously attributed to lesions of the anterior horn cells, lumbar roots, lumbar plexus, femoral nerve, distal (intra-

TABLE 18.6.   Synonyms for diabetic
polyradiculopathy involving the L-2–L-4 roots

Diabetic amyotrophy
Diabetic anterior neuropathy
Diabetic anterior neuronopathy
Diabetic asymmetric proximal motor neuropathy
Diabetic femoral neuropathy
Diabetic femoral-sciatic neuropathy
Diabetic ischemic mononeuropathy multiplex (of
    proximal lower extremity)
Diabetic lumbar plexopathy
Diabetic lumbosacral plexus neuropathy
Diabetic myelopathy
Diabetic myopathy
Diabetic plexus neuropathy
Diabetic polyradiculoplexopathy
Diabetic proximal amyotrophy
Diabetic proximal motor neuropathy
Diabetic radiculoplexus neuropathy
Diabetic symmetric proximal motor neuropathy
Diabetic (thoraco)lumbar polyradiculopathy
Garland's syndrome
Proximal diabetic neuropathy
Subacute proximal diabetic neuropathy

Data from Alderman JE. Anterior neuropathy in
diabetes. Arch Neurol Psych 1938; 39:194; and references
12, 24, 42, 47, 65, 77, 145, 152, 155, 156.

muscular) femoral nerve fibers, and the quadriceps muscles. Adding to the confusion, each of these localizations has been *substantiated* by results of electrodiagnostic examinations.

Whether diabetic amyotrophy even exists as a discrete entity has been questioned. Some investigators have viewed the entire syndrome with considerable skepticism, attributing its findings to DDSPN, the *femoral neuropathy of diabetes*, and polymyositis.[133] Others believe the term *diabetic amyotrophy* should be discarded because it encompasses two separate entities, each with a different pathogenesis and clinical presentation: (1) a rapid-onset, asymmetric proximal lower extremity neuropathy caused by ischemia and (2) a chronic, slow-onset symmetric proximal lower extremity neuropathy caused by metabolic derangement.[143,144,145,156] Neither of these criticisms is convincing. Denying that a proximal lower extremity syndrome occurs in diabetics that is separate from DDSPN and that definitely is not femoral neuropathy or polymyositis runs counter to a wealth of clinical and electrodiagnostic evidence to the contrary. Conversely, dividing diabetic amyotrophy into two separate subgroups emphasizes the difference between two of its presentations while ignoring their many similarities. In fact, the clinical features in the individual limbs are identical except for their tempo of development. Thus pain, particularly in the anterior thighs, is ultimately present in both, as is anterior and medial thigh weakness. Moreover, the motor nerve fibers that bear the brunt of insult in both subgroups are affected identically, a fact readily confirmed by electrodiagnostic studies. With both types, axon loss is found in essentially identical patterns in the symptomatic limbs. Hence the two entities cannot be separated from one another by their ultimate clinical and electrodiagnostic findings. Finally, in many patients, as emphasized by Bastron and Thomas,[65] a third presentation is seen in which the symptoms begin in one lower extremity, either abruptly or gradually, and subsequently spread to the contralateral limb. Thus what begins as a unilateral lesion eventually presents as a bilateral, sometimes symmetric disorder. Consequently, to accept the concept that diabetic amyotrophy is actually two separate entities, one has to believe that the nerve fibers supplying the vasti, thigh adductors, and iliacus muscles are compromised by two completely separate mechanisms, one ischemic and the other metabolic, and yet this occurs in such a fashion that the clinical and electrophysiologic findings resulting from either cause ultimately are identical. It seems far more probable that the same process, whatever it may be, is operative in both cases but is merely unilateral or bilateral at onset and progressing at different rates. Such variations in distribution and tempo are not unique to the radicular involvement that occurs with diabetic amyotrophy. Cauda equina lesions owing to lumbar canal stenosis, for example, can present either suddenly or gradually and be either unilateral or bilateral, with the latter being present from onset or developing subsequently. Yet these different clinical and electrodiagnostic presentations are not attributed to different pathogenetic mechanisms.

A number of concepts concerning diabetic amyotrophy have been proposed by electromyographers, based on studies of nerve fibers derived from other than the L-2, L-3, and L-4 roots, that is, by performing NCS or F waves on distal lower extremity nerves and NEE on muscles distal to the knee.[22,47,156] These studies have no relevance to diabetic amyotrophy per se because any abnormalities found are likely to be due to an associated DDSPN, a separate disorder. Nonetheless, the results of both electrodiagnostic examinations and nerve and muscle biopsies have been extrapolated in this manner, with confusing results.[47]

How often DDSPN is associated with diabetic amyotrophy is somewhat controversial. Most investigators have found this relationship to be a common, although not an inevitable, one.[65,108,148,150,151,153] The majority of the patients we have studied with diabetic amyotrophy have also had DDSPN, particularly those with gradual onset and bilateral findings.[153]

Electrodiagnostic findings with diabetic amyotrophy

The electrodiagnostic features of diabetic amyotrophy vary considerably from limb to limb and person to person, but almost invariably they indicate that the pathophysiology is axon loss rather than demyelination.[153] This is not an unexpected finding, considering that patients present with significant weakness and wasting of the quadriceps muscles, a clinical picture inconsistent with any type of demyelinating lesion except possibly very prolonged, profound conduction block. Certainly, mere demyelinating conduction slowing cannot produce such clinical findings.

Femoral motor conduction studies often are abnormal. Because the underlying process is axon loss, surface recording electrodes must be used if pertinent information is to be obtained, because the only consistently abnormal component is the amplitude of the response. In most patients, one or both quadriceps muscles have been denervated enough that femoral motor responses recording from them are unelicitable or low in amplitude (below 4 mV, or less than 50% of the amplitude obtained when the same procedure is performed on the contralateral limb). With recent-onset lesions, the femoral motor amplitude accurately reflects the degree of quadriceps denervation. Thus it is unelicitable or quite low when marked wasting is present and NEE reveals severe denervation in all heads of the quadriceps. Occasionally, however, it is still within normal limits; this occurs whenever the quadriceps muscle's denervation is only moderate in severity overall, either because all heads are involved to a moderate degree or, as frequently happens, because the process is patchy and causing severe denervation in one or two heads while relatively sparing the others. With chronic lesions, the femoral motor amplitude often is deceptively higher than the severe atrophy, and the prominent MUP loss seen on NEE suggests it should be. This is because marked collateral sprouting has occurred, which is obvious on NEE of the quadriceps:

The MUPs, although severely reduced in number, are substantially increased in duration and often in amplitude as well (up to two or three times normal). These surviving axons, although relatively few in number, can generate a normal or near-normal amplitude following a single supramaximal stimulus to the femoral nerve, as occurs during NCS, but often are incapable of conducting trains of stimuli repeatedly, as clinical use demands.

The NEE invariably is abnormal with diabetic amyotrophy. The presentation from limb to limb is quite diverse, however, being significantly influenced by both the severity and the duration of the lesion. Fibrillation potentials are found in variable numbers in the involved muscles. They are abundant with severe lesions of recent onset but tend to be less prominent with less severe lesions and with those of long duration, in which the process is resolving. The latter explains why Garland and Taverner[24] reported a "striking absence of fibrillation potentials" in the first five patients they studied, most of whom had been symptomatic for at least 2.5 years.

The MUP changes seen also are quite variable. With severe lesions reduced recruitment, or a *neurogenic MUP firing pattern*, is always present, regardless of duration: The MUPs fire in decreased numbers, often severely so, at a moderate to rapid rate. In contrast, the MUP configuration can vary substantially, being influenced by the duration and severity of the lesion. With recent-onset lesions, the MUPs often are of relatively normal configuration. Later in the course, they frequently reflect various stages of reinnervation, being of variable duration but complexly polyphasic in configuration and unstable on repetitive firing. In the past, such MUP changes were erroneously interpreted as being indicative of a myopathy.[92,149] With chronic lesions, the MUPs frequently are of increased duration and sometimes increased amplitude as well. Such chronic neurogenic MUP changes have been considered evidence of an anterior horn cell disorder, i.e., a myelopathy, particularly when accompanied by some sporadic fasciculations, as happens occasionally.[22,24,156]

The NEE abnormalities typically are found in the vasti, rectus femoris, iliacus, and thigh adductor muscles, although the severity of the process (as judged by the density of fibrillation potentials and amount of MUP loss) varies greatly from one patient to another and from one muscle to another in any given patient; for example, the vastus lateralis and adductor magnus may be severely denervated, whereas only minimal denervation can be found in the vastus intermedius and iliacus and then only after a diligent search.

Fibrillation potentials usually are detectable in the ipsilateral, and often contralateral, lumbar paraspinal muscles as well, the exact incidence depending partly on the extensiveness of the study. Nonetheless, as with compressive radiculopathies, occasionally none is seen, even after an extensive search. Their absence, however, never excludes a root lesion. Because of the "cascade" effect of paraspinal muscle innervation, fibrillation potentials with L-2 and L-3 radiculopathies are often found in the lower lumbar levels along with, or instead of, changes at the mid-lumbar paraspinal muscle level.

In any particular patient, diabetic amyotrophy may have one of many electrodiagnostic presentations, including the following.

1. The electrophysiologic abnormalities are strictly unilateral and restricted to the L-2–L-4 root distributions. Probably only a minority of patients present in this manner.

2. The abnormalities are found in L-2–L-4 distributions in both lower extremities; that is, the patient has bilateral diabetic amyotrophy. (Sometimes this fact is not apparent clinically because of markedly different degrees of severity in the two limbs). When the processes in the two limbs develop at about the same time, the electrodiagnostic findings, as the clinical, often are similar. Nonetheless, the NEE abnormalities in the two limbs are seldom identical (e.g., the vastus lateralis may be the muscle most severely involved on one side and the rectus femoris on the other.) Whenever the two limbs are affected sequentially, rather than simultaneously, the electrodiagnostic findings in the two limbs usually are dissimilar, particularly if the processes are of *very* different duration, and the studies are performed fairly soon after onset of symptoms in the second limb. In the most recently involved extremity, active denervation is prominent: The femoral motor NCS amplitude is usually lower than that on the contralateral side, fibrillation potentials are present in abundant numbers, a neurogenic MUP firing pattern is common, and the MUPs are normal in configuration or consist of a mixture of normal and highly polyphasic *reinnervational* MUPs. In contrast, residuals of active denervation are more prominent in the more remotely involved limb: The femoral motor NCS amplitude may be only modestly low or even within the normal range; fibrillation potentials usually are sparse; and chronic neuro-

genic MUP changes are prominent, with or without a neurogenic MUP firing pattern.

3. In some patients, with either unilateral or bilateral diabetic amyotrophy, the process extends caudally to involve the L-5 and sometimes even the S-1/S-2 roots. Occasionally this is prominent and apparent on both clinical and electrodiagnostic examinations. The peroneal motor NCS amplitude, recording tibialis anterior, may be low (with L-5 involvement), and the M component of the H wave may be low (if the S-1, S-2 roots are involved); NEE shows fibrillation potentials, chronic neurogenic or nonspecific MUP changes, and sometimes a neurogenic MUP firing pattern in most or all of the muscles of the affected myotome(s), including the hamstrings and glutei. In contrast, in many patients, territorial extension to the L-5 and S-1 roots is only modest in degree, and in some it is so mild as to be clinically inapparent. Nonetheless, on NEE, fibrillation potentials are found in modest numbers in some of the L-5, S-1 myotomal muscles, often so few muscles that a definite diagnosis cannot be made. This is probably the reason why fibrillation potentials are occasionally seen in the hamstrings and other muscles outside the L-2–L-4 myotomes in patients with diabetic amyotrophy.

4. In some patients, the process extends cephalad, and abnormalities are found not only in the L-2–L-4 root distributions, but also in the lower thoracic (T-8–T-12) distributions. Thus the patient has both diabetic amyotrophy and diabetic thoracic radiculopathy. This can occur with unilateral diabetic amyotrophy but is more common when the disorder is bilateral.

5. In about two-thirds of patients, DDSPN is also present, particularly when the diabetic amyotrophy is of gradual onset and bilateral. The DDSPN is usually axon loss in type and frequently is severe electrically. When diabetic amyotrophy and an axon loss DDSPN coexist, a bimodal peak of abnormality typically is seen on NEE as the involved limb is assessed in a distal to proximal manner or vice versa: Fibrillation potentials are prominent in the intrinsic foot muscles because of the DDSPN, less plentiful in the tibialis anterior, while once again prominent in the vasti, thigh adductors, and iliacus because of the diabetic amyotrophy. Territorial extension to the L-5 and S-1, S-2 roots also can occur in these patients, causing fibrillation potentials to be found not only throughout the lumbar paraspinal muscles bilaterally,

but also in the hamstrings and glutei. Involvement of the latter muscles proves confusing and difficult to localize to a root level because muscles distal to the knees within the same myotomes already contain fibrillation potentials caused by the coexisting DDSPN.

6. Rarely, bilateral diabetic amyotrophy is associated with bilateral involvement of the shoulder gridle muscles (i.e., bilateral C-5, C-6 root involvement). This is discussed later.

The differential diagnosis of diabetic amyotrophy includes intraspinal canal lesions involving the L-2, L-3 and L-4 segments/roots (either compressive lesions such as lumbar canal stenosis or diffuse lesions such as motor neuron disease); lumbar plexopathies (often caused by neoplasms); myopathies, particularly polymyositis; and femoral neuropathies.

L-2–L-4 root lesions caused by ischemia (e.g., diabetic amyotrophy) cannot be distinguished from those caused by compression (e.g., lumbar canal stenosis). Although the electrodiagnostic examination is sensitive for detecting axon loss, its ability for determining the cause of such axon loss is extremely limited. Nonetheless, the electromyographer can make some useful inferences based on statistics alone. In our EMG laboratory, at least, elderly male diabetics with bilateral L-2–L-4 radiculopathies are far more likely to have their symptoms caused by diabetic amyotrophy than multiple root compression.

Distinguishing L-2, L-3 (L-4) radiculopathies from lumbar plexopathies by electrodiagnostic studies is often difficult and can be virtually impossible in patients with diabetic amyotrophy because the two main electrodiagnostic features used in such differentiation are negated: the presence of lumbar paraspinal fibrillation potentials and involvement or noninvolvement of the appropriate sensory NCS.[67]

Because the paraspinal muscles are innervated by the posterior primary rami, they often contain fibrillation potentials, along with the limb muscles, with root lesions. Conversely, they never contain fibrillation potentials when axon loss affects solely plexus fibers because the latter do not innervate paraspinal muscles. Unfortunately, fibrillation potentials can be seen in the lumbar paraspinal muscles in all diabetic patients, and consequently their presence in a patient with diabetic amyotrophy may merely reflect the diabetic state, rather than being indicative of diabetic polyradiculopathy. Moreover, the absence of paraspinal fibrillation potentials *never* excludes a radiculopathy. Hence lumbar plexus lesions cannot be diagnosed by default whenever fibrillation potentials are found in the quadriceps, thigh abductors, and iliacus but not in the mid or low lumbar paraspinal muscles.

With axon loss of the magnitude often seen in diabetic amyotrophy, differentiation between root and plexus involvement usually is readily made by the sensory NCS. The sensory NCS amplitudes are affected only by those proximal axon loss lesions located at or distal to their DRG, which are situated within the intervertebral foramen. Thus they are unaltered by intraspinal canal lesions, such as radiculopathies, but are low in amplitude or unelicitable with plexus and peripheral nerve lesions. Unfortunately, this extremely helpful localization technique is useless with diabetic amyotrophy because no reliable sensory NCS is available for evaluating the fibers that originate from the L-2–L-4 DRG and traverse the lumbar plexus. Both saphenous and lateral cutaneous nerve of thigh NCS have been proposed for this purpose, but responses can be consistently obtained in only a minority of persons, usually those who are young and lean. Patients with diabetic amyotrophy, however, are almost always middle-aged or older and obese. Moreover, the majority of patients with diabetic amyotrophy also have an associated DDSPN, and that alone can render saphenous NCS responses unelicitable because, similar to the sural and superficial peroneal sensory NCS responses, they are being elicited in the distal portion of the limb.

For the aforementioned reasons, the electrodiagnostic examination in diabetic amyotrophy is much less helpful in differentiating between radiculopathy and plexopathy than it usually is in other conditions. Nonetheless, none of the electrophysiologic findings in diabetic amyotrophy is inconsistent with diabetic polyradiculopathy affecting the L-2–L-4 roots.

Patients with diabetic amyotrophy often are erroneously reported to have *diabetic femoral neuropathy*, presumably because the motor fibers that supply the iliopsoas and quadriceps muscles are often the most severely affected clinically.[135,157–159] Unfortunately, many clinicians and electromyographers do not assess the thigh adductor muscles when examining patients with diabetic amyotrophy. Consequently, they do not appreciate that abnormalities are rarely restricted to the femoral nerve distribution; the obturator-innervated thigh adductor muscles almost always are involved as well. Isolated femoral neuropathies caused by DM must be extremely rare; we have never encountered one.

Sometimes the iliopsoas and quadriceps muscle weakness caused by diabetic amyotrophy is erroneously attributed to a myopathic process. Moreover, if only one or two quadriceps muscles are sampled on NEE, and reinnervation is occurring, the combination of fibrillation potentials and complexly polyphasic MUPs seen can be misinterpreted as evidence of a necrotizing myopathy, such as polymyositis.[92,149] The correct diagnosis is usually readily made in the EMG laboratory if the examination is extensive enough.

Electrodiagnostic approach to diabetic amyotrophy

The standard polyneuropathic assessment should be performed on all patients because the majority have an associated DDSPN that can complicate the lower extremity evaluation. Femoral motor NCS should be performed bilaterally. If they are low or unelicitable, peroneal motor NCS, recording tibialis anterior, are indicated. The standard NEE for polyneuropathies should be done, supplemented by examination of several L-2–L-4 innervated muscles. The latter muscles are assessed bilaterally, both for comparison purposes and because diabetic amyotrophy so often affects both lower extremities, sometimes with one side

TABLE 18.7.   Electrodiagnostic evaluation for suspected diabetic amyotrophy

Standard polyneuropathy evaluation (performed on side of symptomatic or more symptomatic limb)
Additional procedures:
  Nerve conduction studies (bilaterally):

Motor	Sensory
Femoral (quadriceps)	Saphenous*
(if femoral motor nerve conduction study response low or unelicitable: peroneal (tibialis anterior))	

  Needle electrode examination (bilaterally):
  Vastus lateralis, rectus femoris (or other muscles innervated by femoral nerve)
  Adductor magnus (or other muscles innervated by obturator nerve)
  Iliacus
    (if fibrillation potentials are found in above, some hamstring muscles—biceps femoris, long or short head, and semitendinosus/semimembranosis—should be studied)

Note. The L-2–L-4 roots are assessed bilaterally because diabetic amyotrophy is so often bilateral, and several quadriceps and thigh adductor muscles are assessed because the findings in a symptomatic limb are often variable among the L-2–L-4 innervated muscles.

* Rarely elicitable in typical patient with diabetic amyotrophy.

clinically inapparent. Depending on the findings, NEE of other lower extremity muscles (e.g., the hamstrings) may be indicated (Table 18.7).

Diabetic Radiculopathy Involving the T-4–T-12 Roots: Diabetic Thoracic Polyradiculopathy

The association between DM and thoracic or abdominal pain (and sometimes weakness) has been recognized by clinicians and electromyographers for years.[140,160,161] This type of diabetic neuropathy, however, was not considered a distinct entity until 1966.[162] Unfortunately, it is referred to by a different name in almost every report (Table 18.8). The term *diabetic thoracic radiculopathy* (DTR) is used throughout this discussion because it appears to be the most anatomically exact.

Nominally DTR is readily confused with *diabetic truncal polyneuropathy*, a term coined by Waxman and Sabin[163] in 1981 to describe the symmetric sensory loss found over the anterior trunk in patients with severe DDSPN. That this finding merits a specific name seems questionable, and its designation as *diabetic truncal polyneuropathy* is doubly unfortunate. First, it is not limited to diabetic patients, as its authors concede; instead, because it is due to progressive centripetal degeneration of axons that occurs with any length-related symmetric polyneuropathy, it can be seen with any severe axon loss symmetric polyneuropathy. Second, the name is so similar to some of the synonyms for DTR, particularly *diabetic truncal mononeuropathy* and *diabetic truncal neuropathy*, that inevitably much confusion

TABLE 18.8.   Synonyms for diabetic polyradiculopathy involving the T-4–T-12 roots

Acute thoracic sensory mononeuropathy
Acute thoracic sensory radiculopathy
Diabetic intercostal neuralgia
Diabetic pseudovisceral syndrome
Diabetic thoracic mononeuropathy
Diabetic thoracic radiculitis
Diabetic thoracic radiculopathy
Diabetic thoracoabdominal neuropathy
Diabetic truncal mononeuropathy
Diabetic truncal neuropathy
Thoracic truncal mononeuropathy

Not a synonym: Diabetic truncal polyneuropathy (see text)

Data from references 77, 164–171.

is generated. This was vividly illustrated when two experts on DTR reported that its clinical picture could be *variable*, while referring to an article on diabetic truncal polyneuropathy.[164]

DTR affects the mid and lower thoracic roots ($\pm$ T-4 through T-12), with a predilection for the lower four. It may be unilateral or bilateral. With clinically unilateral lesions, NEE abnormalities often are found on the asymptomatic side. When bilateral, the two sides are usually involved sequentially rather than simultaneously, and often the findings are asymmetric. Both abrupt and gradual onset have been described, in various reports, as typical.[165–171] Although DTR can occur in isolation, it often coexists with other types of diabetic neuropathy, particularly DDSPN and other subgroups of diabetic polyradiculopathy, especially diabetic amyotrophy. When DTR is unilateral and is associated with unilateral diabetic amyotrophy, both disorders usually are on the same side, and the diabetic amyotrophy is the first to be symptomatic.

Unlike the situation with diabetic amyotrophy, the location of the lesion causing DTR is not particularly controversial. Primarily because the symptoms are so overwhelmingly sensory in character, no one has seriously attributed it to a myopathy, and because the involved fibers do not traverse an intervening plexus, the question of it being a plexopathy is moot. Consequently, either the lesion is at the root (or mixed spinal nerve) level or two separate lesions coexist, one involving the thoracic posterior primary rami and the other simultaneously affecting the intercostal or abdominal nerves or both. The former possibility seems by far the most likely and is consistent with Bastron and Thomas'[65] concept that DTR merely represents one type of diabetic polyradiculopathy.

Just as with diabetic amyotrophy, the pathogenesis of DTR is unclear. Those of rapid onset and limited to one or two roots are most easily explained on a vascular basis, whereas those of gradual onset and involving multiple roots, particularly when bilateral, are more readily attributed to a metabolic process.[166] Once the process is established, however, neither clinical nor electrodiagnostic examination can distinguish the rapid-onset from the gradual-onset variety, making it probable that one pathologic process underlies both.

Electrodiagnostic findings with diabetic thoracic radiculopathy

As early as 1962, Marinacci and Courville[161] reported that the electromyographic examination was "vital" for detecting a diabetic radicular syndrome that could simulate a surgical intra-abdominal condition. Nonetheless, difficulties are encountered in diagnosing thoracic radiculopathies of any cause in the EMG laboratory, for several reasons.

First, for practical purposes, the involved fibers cannot be evaluated by NCS. Sensory NCS cannot be performed on intercostal nerves, nor have any motor NCS using surface recording electrodes been described. The intercostal motor nerve fibers can be assessed by NCS, using a needle recording electrode.[172] The procedure, however, is not only potentially hazardous (requiring general anesthesia and producing pneumothorax in 9% of patients in one series),[173] but also it is unlikely to yield useful information because DTR causes axon degeneration, which affects the amplitude (as recorded with surface electrodes), rather than the latency, of the response.

Because of these NCS limitations, thoracic radiculopathies are detected in the EMG laboratory almost solely during the NEE. The typical NEE findings with DTR are fibrillation potentials, often abundant; when found in the thoracic paraspinal muscles with DTR, their distribution often corresponds to the area of maximal pain.[166] Although chronic neurogenic MUP changes may be present as well, they are of relatively little help in diagnosis.

Second, compared with most of the cervical and lumbosacral myotomes, the mid and lower thoracic myotomes are composed of few muscles—for practical purposes, only intercostal, abdominal, and paraspinal—each of which can be difficult to examine satisfactorily, for various reasons.

During NEE of the intercostal or abdominal muscles, a needle inserted too deeply may enter the pleural or peritoneal cavity. This is particularly likely to occur in obese patients, whose overlying adipose tissue requires extra long needles to be used and prevents identification of anatomic landmarks, even by palpation. The intercostal muscles are considered "off limits" by many electromyographers for this reason. In contrast, and despite the potential hazards, NEE of the abdominal muscles is often performed and proves informative. In some patients with DTR, fibrillation potentials can be found in the abdominal muscles, although undetectable in the thoracic paraspinal muscles. For this reason, Streib et al.[66a] recommend studying the abdominal muscles whenever there is a question of DTR and have devised a standardized procedure for doing so.

During NEE of the thoracic paraspinal muscles, achieving adequate relaxation often proves impossible, regardless of effort and time expended; when this occurs, the presence or absence of spontaneous activity cannot be determined.[66a] Moreover, even with sufficient relaxation of the thoracic paraspinal muscles, problems remain. First, low-amplitude potentials with brief negative or positive components, volume conducted from respiratory muscles, are frequently encountered. These not only can obscure fibrillation potentials, but also are easily mistaken in turn for showers of fibrillation potentials. To avoid this pitfall, any *spontaneous activity* seen in the thoracic paraspinal muscles should be considered significant only after its relationship, if any, to the patient's inspiration or expiration has been determined. In addition, fibrillation potentials are not restricted to the lower lumbar paraspinal muscles in a certain percentage of patients with diabetes but, instead, extend as far cephalad as the midthoracic region and sometimes are found diffusely throughout the paraspinal muscles.[68] For this reason, whenever fibrillation potentials are found in the thoracic paraspinal muscles, the boundaries of the affected segment must be defined by studying paraspinal muscles ipsilaterally proximal and distal to it as well as contralaterally at the same level.

The NEE of the thoracic paraspinal muscles can be falsely negative when the study is too limited or when inappropriate areas are examined. Moreover, even with extensive NEEs, fibrillation potentials are not detectable in a certain proportion of patients with DTR, either because the root fibers supplying the posterior primary rami were not affected owing to subtotal root involvement or because the study is being performed so long after the onset of symptoms that the paraspinal muscles, although once denervated, have become reinnervated in the interim because of their proximal location.

DTR can mimic a number of intraabdominal and intrathoracic conditions as well as other intraspinal canal lesions, so the differential diagnosis is formidable. Electrodiagnostic studies, at least, can separate those affecting PNS fibers from those affecting other structures. Diagnosing a thoracic radiculopathy, however, based on clinical and electromyographic abnormalities, is not synonymous with diagnosing DTR. When fibrillation potentials are found in the thoracic paraspinal or abdominal muscles, they have no special characteristics that identify their cause. Compressive radiculopathies, focal intraspinal tumors, and other lesions involving the thoracic cord segments or roots may all have NEE features identical to DTR.[161,166] Because DM is such a common disorder, particularly in the elderly, a thoracic radiculopathy found in a diabetic patient may

be due to an independent lesion rather than to DTR. For this reason, neuroimaging procedures are often performed on patients with suspected DTR even when both the clinical and the electrodiagnostic features appear typical.

Electrodiagnostic approach to diabetic thoracic radiculopathy

Although NCS and NEE routinely are performed on all patients referred to the EMG laboratory, the value of the former with suspected DTR is debatable because the affected nerve fibers cannot be assessed. Consequently, we perform NCS on one limb ipsilateral to the symptomatic, or more symptomatic, side. Lower limb assessment often reveals evidence of a coexisting DDSPN, which may or may not cause the study to be expanded to include a polyneuropathy evaluation. An extensive, bilateral NEE of the paraspinal muscles is indicated, extending from the midthoracic to the midlumbar regions and even further if fibrillation potentials are found at the margins. Multiple needle insertions should be performed along the longitudinal axis of the entire region that is most painful or that the patient's trunk symptoms suggest should be involved. Each of the four quadrants of the abdomen also should be studied. Obviously, if a more widespread polyradiculopathy is suspected, e.g., an associated diabetic amyotrophy, more extensive NCS and NEE are indicated.

Diabetic Polyradiculopathy Involving the L-5, S-1, (S-2) Roots

The L-5–S-1 (S-2) roots are affected by diabetic polyradiculopathy much less often than the L-2, L-3, (L-4) roots. For this reason, their involvement is not recognized as a discrete entity, nor has it merited a specific name. Nonetheless, weakness and wasting of muscles supplied by the L-5 and S-1 (S-2) roots, such as the tibialis anterior, peronei, gastrocnemii, hamstrings, and glutei, alone or in various combinations, have been reported in diabetic patients.[47,59,146,147,149,][151,174,175] Diabetic footdrop figured prominently in some early reports.[11] These were variously attributed to very asymmetric DDSPN, an expanded type of diabetic amyotrophy and to DM-caused lower extremity mononeuropathies.[176] The actual location of the lesions causing the symptoms was more often assumed than proved, however, and none was confirmed by detailed electrodiagnostic studies. In fact, in many instances, it seems likely that the site of nerve fiber injury was at the root level, particularly in those patients whose weakness developed with, or subsequent to, ipsilateral diabetic amyotrophy, an evolution consistent with territorial extension of polyradiculopathy to involve the L-5 and S-1 roots.

Little can be found in the literature regarding the electrodiagnostic findings with these lesions. Bastron and Thomas[65] provide few details in their report. Child and Yates[177] described a diabetic with pain in both lower extremities, which they attributed to bilateral diabetic L-5 radiculopathies. They had found fibrillation potentials in L-5 root distributions bilaterally, including the paraspinal muscles, and a myelogram was normal.[177] Such isolated involvement of the L-5 (or S-1) root, however, is probably far less common than their involvement by territorial extension from preexisting L-2, L-3 (L-4) lesions. Nonetheless, we have studied several diabetic patients with isolated L-5 radiculopathies and a few with S-1 radiculopathies in whom root compression could never be implicated as the cause, even after extensive neuroimaging studies and sometimes even surgical exploration. Consequently, diabetic polyradiculopathy should be considered whenever neuroimaging studies are normal in a diabetic patient with a L-5 or S-1 radiculopathy, particularly when the pain is unusually severe and persistent (e.g., especially if it is not improved by bed rest and persists during the night).

Diabetic Polyradiculopathy Involving the C-5, C-6 (C-7, C-8, T-1) Roots

Extension of diabetic polyradiculopathy to the upper extremities is rare. Nonetheless, changes suggestive of this process have been briefly noted in a number of reports dealing with diabetic amyotrophy.[59,146,149,151,156] Characteristically proximal (shoulder girdle) muscles innervated by the C-5, C-6 roots, such as the deltoid, supraspinatus, and infraspinatus, are affected. The only muscle that receives substantial innervation with any frequency from other than those roots mentioned is the triceps. Typically the abnormalities are bilateral, although sometimes asymmetric. The electrodiagnostic features of diabetic C-5, C-6 radiculopathies were almost unreported[156] until Riley and Shields[178] described the findings in four patients. All had C-5, C-6 radiculopathies causing axon loss and producing fibrillation potentials in the appropriate shoulder girdle muscles, and all had bilateral diabetic amyotrophy.[178]

The lower cervical roots appear to be the ones least affected by diabetic polyradiculopathy; their involvement is rarely mentioned in the literature. Child and Yates[177] described a patient with unilateral arm pain, fibrillation potentials in the C-7 root distribution, and a negative myelogram. Also, several authors have made brief reference to DM causing hand wasting, presumably on other than a severe DDSPN basis; these seem unlikely to be due to C-8/T-1 radiculopathies based on the information provided.[62,140,179]

DIFFUSE DIABETIC POLYRADICULOPATHY PLUS DIABETIC DISTAL SYMMETRIC POLYNEUROPATHY: DIABETIC NEUROPATHIC CACHEXIA

Quite infrequently, diabetic polyradiculopathy becomes diffuse, or nearly so, in distribution. The L-2 through S-2 myotomes are involved bilaterally as well as the C-5 through C-6 roots bilaterally and usually most or all of the thoracic roots bilaterally. Almost invariably, a severe DDSPN coexists. Profound weight loss, depression, and impotence usually complete the clinical presentation. This particular combination of diabetic neuropathies and associated symptoms merits the term *diffuse diabetic polyradiculoneuropathy*.

Although probable examples of this entity were reported earlier,[150,180] it was first well described by Ellenberg. Initially he designated it as *diabetic myeloradiculoneuropathy*,[181] but later he gave it the more nondescriptive name *diabetic neuropathic cachexia*.[62]

From the electromyographer's viewpoint, studies performed on these patients, who are mostly elderly men, are an exercise in frustration. With few exceptions, the *EMG overload syndrome* is invariably encountered: So many severe electrophysiologic abnormalities are present, each with many possible causes, that few definite conclusions can be drawn, regardless of the time expended. Typically despite extensive evaluations of multiple limbs and the paraspinal muscles, not a single NCS result nor a single muscle on NEE appears normal. On NCS, no sensory NCS responses can be elicited, whereas the motor NCS responses, recording distally, are low in amplitude or unelicitable. Even the motor NCS responses recording from proximal muscles are often low in amplitude. Motor CVs, when they can be calculated, usually are significantly slow, at least in the lower extremities. Although many of the NCS findings can be attributed to unusually severe DDSPN, other superimposed neurogenic lesions, such as radiculopathies, plexopathies, and mononeuropathies, cannot be excluded. Similarly, on NEE, not only are fibrillation potentials and MUP loss prominent in the more distal muscles, presumably because of the severe DDSPN, but even most or all of the proximal limb muscles contain fibrillation potentials and nonspecific or chronic neurogenic MUP changes. Characteristically fibrillation potentials also are abundant throughout the paraspinal muscles bilaterally. Consequently, most of the NEE findings in the limb muscles can be attributed to lesions situated at almost any point along the peripheral neuraxis, from the spinal cord to the terminal nerve fiber, and are therefore unhelpful for localization. Sometimes such diffuse NEE changes are interpreted as being indicative of a diffuse *neuromyopathy* or a *severe polyneuropathy plus polymyositis*. In keeping with the concepts described in this section, these changes are most likely attributable to a diffuse diabetic polyradiculopathy and a coexisting DDSPN.

DIABETIC CRANIAL MONONEUROPATHIES

An association between DM and various cranial mononeuropathies has been recognized for more than 100 years. Cranial nerves supplying the extraocular muscles (oculomotor, trochlear, abducens) are the ones most often affected in diabetic patients.[16,17,135,158,160] These cranial nerves cannot be evaluated in most EMG laboratories, however, and therefore are of little interest to the electromyographer. In contrast, facial nerve involvement with DM has attracted the attention of electromyographers for more than 25 years, both in regard to diabetic patients with DDSPN and those with Bell's palsy.

In patients with DDSPN, slowing of conduction along the facial nerve fibers often can be demonstrated on both the facial motor NCS and blink response testing; that is, the latencies for both the direct M response and the R-1 component of the blink response are increased.[182,183] Such studies are of little practical value, however, because the NCS performed on the limb nerves invariably will be abnormal and sufficient for diagnosis.

Patients with Bell's palsy have DM more often than would be expected by chance alone.[184,185] Some investigators believe the facial mononeuropathy associated with DM is not *idiopathic* at all but rather a specific diabetic cranial mononeuropathy caused by ischemic insult to the facial nerve.[186,187] It is known that the Bell's palsy occurring in diabetics often differs in certain respects from that affecting

nondiabetics. Diabetic patients with Bell's palsy, compared with nondiabetics, (1) are far more likely to lack a taste disturbance (suggesting the sites of nerve injury differ between the two groups), (2) are more likely to have bilateral or recurrent Bell's palsy, and (3) are more prone to cluster in the 10% to 15% of patients who have axon loss rather than demyelinating conduction block as the underlying pathophysiology.[185,186] Consequently, the following electrodiagnostic features, indicative of severe Bell's palsy (i.e., a severe axon loss facial mononeuropathy), are more likely to be found in diabetic than in nondiabetic patients: (1) very low or unelicitable facial motor NCS amplitudes on studies performed 1 week or more after onset, (2) absent R1 and R2 responses on blink reflex testing, and (3) substantial numbers of fibrillation potentials and severe or total MUP loss on NEE of the affected facial muscles 3 or more weeks after onset. Patients with these features are far more likely to have no recovery or unsatisfactory recovery (e.g., incomplete reinnervation, misdirection of fibers) than the average patient with Bell's palsy.[188] From the clinical viewpoint, every patient referred to the EMG laboratory with Bell's palsy who is found to have an axon loss facial mononeuropathy probably should be screened for DM.

DIABETIC LIMB MONONEUROPATHIES

Various types of mononeuropathies are commonly seen in patients with DM. Of 103 nonselected diabetic patients, Mulder et al.[60] found that 16 had one or more mononeuropathies. In contrast, over 30 had DDSPN.[60] Brown and Greene[77] reported that 40% of 38 diabetic patients had clinical or electrophysiologic evidence of an entrapment mononeuropathy.

The electrodiagnostic findings typically seen with focal mononeuropathies of any type, including those associated with DM, have been the source of much confusion. An extremely prevalent misconception is that all mononeuropathies affect the rate of conduction along involved nerves.[96,189] This erroneous idea probably arose from extrapolation of the typical NCS changes found with CTS. Conduction slowing, owing to focal demyelination and manifested as prolonged peak (sensory) or distal (motor) latencies, is a characteristic finding with that disorder unless or until the process becomes severe, and the median nerve fibers degenerate. Such changes, however, are not at all representative of mononeuropathies as a group. Instead the type of electrophysiologic changes seen depend primarily on the particular nerve affected and the severity of the lesion.

With acute-onset mononeuropathies, regardless of the nerve involved or its location, almost always electrodiagnostic examinations demonstrate axon loss or conduction block. One or both of these processes invariably is present whenever the recorded muscles are clinically weak. In either case, amplitudes are the NCS parameter affected. Such lesions rarely produce conduction slowing, and when it is seen, it usually is due to loss or block of the fastest conducting fibers and has no clinical and little electrodiagnostic significance.[41]

With chronic mononeuropathies, the electrodiagnostic presentation is much more variable. As noted, CTS characteristically presents with conduction slowing along the sensory fibers, followed, in more severe cases, by slowing along the motor fibers as well. Focal slowing, however, is detectable in only about half the patients with ulnar mononeuropathy at the elbow. In the remainder, the prominent or sole findings are amplitude alterations caused by axon loss or, less often, demyelinating conduction block.[190] With peroneal mononeuropathies at the fibular head and radial mononeuropathies at the spiral groove, both of which typically present with clinical weakness, the electrodiagnostic examination reveals significant axon loss, demyelinating conduction block, or a combination of the two. Slowing across the fibular head or about the spiral groove occasionally is found, owing to loss or block of the fastest conducting fibers, but it is an epiphenomenon, having no relationship to the clinical findings and rarely being necessary for either detecting or localizing the lesions.[191]

Although focal mononeuropathies can result from a multitude of causes, with DM the cause almost always is one of two basic mechanisms: (1) nerve entrapment/compression or (2) nerve infarction. The clinical and electrophysiologic features vary significantly, depending on which of these is operative. Of the two, nerve infarction has by far the most stereotyped clinical and electrodiagnostic presentation.

With nerve infarction, regardless of the particular nerve affected, the onset typically is abrupt, and axon loss is the sole process operative. Pain usually is prominent, and depending on the percentage of infarcted motor fibers, variable amounts of weakness and subsequent atrophy occur. As with all lesions caused by focal axon loss, recovery tends to be slow and is influenced by the severity of the lesion, its location, and the patient's age. Recovery is often suboptimal with diabetic infarction mononeuropa-

thies because (1) most or all of the nerve fibers are affected, (2) the lesions typically occur in the proximal or mid portions of main nerve trunks, and (3) the patients usually are elderly.

In contrast, mononeuropathies in diabetic patients caused by entrapment/compression occur at predictable sites and have variable clinical and electrical presentations, depending primarily on the nerve affected. In diabetics with CTS, just as in nondiabetics, slowing of conduction owing to localized demyelination is a characteristic electrophysiologic feature. Thus the median sensory peak latencies and, less frequently, the median motor distal latencies are prolonged. With more severe lesions, the sensory NCS responses may be unelicitable, owing either to demyelinating conduction block or differential slowing or to axon loss. Nonetheless, seldom does axon loss supervene to the extent that the motor NCS responses become unelicitable and abundant fibrillation potentials and severe/total MUP dropout are found in the median-innervated thenar muscles. Conversely, in diabetic patients with ulnar mononeuropathy at the elbow, the pathophysiology is quite variable: Axon loss, demyelinating focal slowing, demyelinating differential slowing, and demyelinating conduction can all be seen, either alone or in various combinations. Finally, compressive lesions of the peroneal nerve at the fibular head have a different presentation. Axon loss, demyelinating conduction block, or a combination of both is invariably found when footdrop is present. In contrast, focal slowing or differential slowing is almost never seen, reports in the literature to the contrary notwithstanding. The ultimate recovery with entrapment/compression radiculopathy is also variable. If demyelination is the sole or predominant process, recovery is often excellent, although surgery may be required for some lesions (e.g., CTS).

Upper Extremity Mononeuropathies

Many patients with upper extremity mononeuropathies have underlying DM. In the vast majority, the median or ulnar nerves, especially the former, are involved. Most are entrapment/compression mononeuropathies; they are of gradual onset, affect the median nerve at the wrist or ulnar nerve at the elbow, and frequently are bilateral.[60,192]

The relationship between CTS and DM is somewhat confusing. Up to 12% of patients with CTS are diabetic.[193–196] Nonetheless, most authorities deny that a cause and effect relationship exists, and DM is not listed as one of the many causes of CTS in several sources concerned solely with entrapment neuropathies.[197–200] Instead, this association is thought by many to be due to chance alone because both DM and CTS are relatively common, and both predominantly occur in the same *over 40* age group. Moreover, CTS has been found in only a small percentage (1.3%) of a large series of diabetic patients followed over a prolonged period.[78] (This percentage has been misquoted in some subsequent sources as being *12%*.[201]) According to one investigator, the CTS found in diabetic patients may reflect obesity more than DM[200] because in a large series of patients with CTS, 12% were diabetic, whereas 37% were obese.[193] The major source of confusion on this point probably is the failure to distinguish clearly those patients with DM and overt DDSPN from those with DM alone. The incidence of CTS in the latter may not be increased. Those diabetic patients, however, with overt DDSPN have a markedly increased incidence of CTS, usually bilateral. In our EMG laboratory, about one-third of patients under the age of 60 with DDSPN have associated CTS, whereas almost two-thirds of those over the age of 60 do. Although DM may not be responsible for CTS per se, it is the most common underlying condition detected by far in patients studied in our EMG laboratory who have bilateral CTS coexisting with bilateral ulnar neuropathy at the elbow, with or without associated DDSPN.

The electrodiagnostic features seen with upper extremity entrapment neuropathies in diabetic patients do not differ from those seen in nondiabetics, but the studies are complicated, often substantially so, by the presence or possible presence of a coexisting DDSPN. This is a problem in two different situations.

First, when bilateral CTS is found in diabetic patients, particularly elderly diabetics in whom coexisting DDSPN is not clinically suspected, sometimes bilateral ulnar neuropathy at the elbow is also present. Frequently all the upper extremity NCS amplitudes and motor NCS CVs are borderline abnormal, but often these changes could be due to the patient's age. Even though only the upper extremities are symptomatic, at least one lower extremity must be assessed to determine whether the upper extremity abnormalities are due to a combination of mononeuropathies and advanced age or to mononeuropathies superimposed on a clinically unappreciated DDSPN. In practical terms, this means that a patient referred for a "simple" CTS evaluation ultimately requires a far more extensive evaluation, a scenario that plays havoc with patient scheduling in the EMG laboratory.

Second, when diabetic patients with known DDSPN are referred with a question of possible superimposed CTS or ulnar neuropathy at the elbow, determining this can be difficult when the generalized process is producing slowing along most or all of the upper extremity nerves. Typically one lower extremity must be assessed so the upper extremity abnormalities can be placed in perspective. In these situations, a superimposed CTS can be diagnosed with reasonable confidence only when: (1) the median NCS changes (e.g., increased latencies) are more prominent in one limb than the other; (2) one or both median latencies but no other upper extremity NCS latencies are prolonged; (3) the latencies of all the upper extremity nerves are prolonged, but one or both of the median nerve latencies are disproportionately prolonged. It can also be suspected, but not confirmed, whenever only the median (one or both), of the various upper extremity NCS responses, are unelicitable. On the other hand, if the DDSPN is causing such severe axon loss that substantial denervation is present in the distal upper extremities, diagnosing a superimposed CTS usually is impossible; when all, or nearly all, the median nerve fibers have degenerated, no evidence of focal slowing can be detected on the NCS. Because of the anatomy of the median nerve, CTS cannot be diagnosed by NEE alone. Whenever fibrillation potentials and MUP loss are found in the median-innervated hand muscles but in no other muscles of the limb (including the median-innervated forearm muscles), the responsible lesion may be located at any point along the main trunk of the median nerve, from the palm to the proximal forearm, where the anterior interosseus branch originates. Hence when only axon loss is present, regardless of severity, localization of median neuropathies by electrodiagnostic examination becomes much less precise.

Infrequently upper extremity mononeuropathies develop in diabetic patients because of nerve infarcts, usually as a component of diabetic mononeuropathy multiplex (described in a later section). The median, ulnar, and radial nerves essentially are the only ones so involved. Sometimes more than one mononeuropathy occurs in the same upper extremity, although they usually are of sequential rather than simultaneous onset.[12,17,60,189] Typically the underlying cause of these lesions is clinically obvious. Occasionally, however, their actual cause is not appreciated, particularly when (1) their rapid evolution is not determined, (2) they are confined to a single upper extremity, or (3) they are bilateral, but affecting only corresponding nerves in the two limbs. Under such circumstances, these mononeuropathies often are mistakenly attributed to entrapment/compression, and patients may undergo needless surgical procedures (e.g., CTS release, ulnar nerve transposition) in vain attempts to treat them.

Differentiating between nerve entrapment/compression and infarction is usually relatively simple in regard to median nerve involvement because axon loss is a primary event with infarction but a very late event with entrapment (i.e., CTS). Moreover, with median nerve infarction, the lesion is often situated at or proximal to the elbow, so NEE changes (fibrillation potentials, MUP loss) are found in the median-innervated forearm muscles, and CTS is therefore excluded. With ulnar nerve involvement, however, such distinctions can be much more difficult because axon degeneration is the sole abnormality seen not only with infarctions, but also with many compressive lesions. Consequently, only when focal demyelination is detected, manifested as focal slowing, differential slowing, or conduction block along the elbow segment, can ulnar lesions confidently be attributed to compression. If only axon degeneration is seen, as in virtually all ulnar lesions caused by infarction and in approximately half of those caused by entrapment/compression, the responsible process cannot be determined.[190] Nonetheless, an infarction etiology should be considered whenever severe axon loss ulnar neuropathies are found, particularly when the onset was abrupt and fibrillation potentials are abundant in the forearm ulnar-innervated muscles. The latter seldom is seen with compressive ulnar neuropathies at the elbow but is almost a constant finding with those that are due to infarction because the responsible lesion generally is located quite proximally, along the upper arm/axilla segment.

For completeness, the *diabetic hand* or *diabetic hand syndrome* must be mentioned. A few investigators have reported that the appearance of the hands in some diabetics is so characteristic that it virtually leads to a diagnosis of DM. The clinical manifestations described, however, are quite variable, whereas the electrodiagnostic findings reported are too fragmentary to be of any benefit.[1,181,202] Consequently, it is not at all clear what is meant by these titles nor, if the process is neurogenic, the responsible cause and the nerve or nerves (median? ulnar? both?) involved.

Although it is highly unlikely that DM produces unique hand abnormalities, there are several known causes for hand changes in patients with DM: (1) upper extremity involvement by severe axon loss DDSPN; (2) ulnar mononeuropathies of the axon loss type, owing to either compression or infarction; (3) severe CTS, which has progressed to the terminal axon loss stage; (4) C-8–T-1 root involvement as a component of diabetic polyradiculopathy (this is by far the rarest cause); (5) combinations of these mechanisms, the most frequent being bilateral CTS and bilateral ulnar neuropathy.

Lower Extremity Mononeuropathies

Depending on the series, 33% to 50% of diabetic mononeuropathies involve lower extremity nerves.[60,192] Although femoral neuropathies are most often mentioned in the literature, peroneal neuropathies are the most common.

The widely held belief that there is an association between femoral neuropathy and DM[12,16,77,117,135,157,189,197,199,203] is likely fallacious. This concept is based mainly on two articles, both published more than 30 years ago; neither substantiates the reputed relationship. Goodman,[204] in 1954, described 17 patients with what he labeled femoral neuropathy, 16 of whom also had DM. From the brief case histories he provided, however, the diagnosis of *femoral neuropathy* appears unjustified in almost all of them: Only a small fraction of the patients had convincing evidence of femoral nerve fiber involvement, and that subgroup may well have had diabetic amyotrophy, which had just been described by Garland and Taverner[24] the preceding year. In 1960, Calverley and Mulder[154] mislabeled cases of diabetic amyotrophy as femoral neuropathy. Both noted in later publications that the lesions were usually located more proximally, at the root or plexus level.[60,145] In fact, although lesions of the L-2–L-4 roots, from which the femoral nerve fibers are derived, are not uncommon in diabetics (i.e., diabetic amyotrophy), lesions of the femoral nerve proper owing to DM are extremely rare. The femoral nerve shares this attribute with most other nerves (e.g., musculocutaneous, axillary) supplying primarily proximal muscles.

A link between DM and peroneal mononeuropathies is well established.[60,192,205] These typically arise at or near the fibular head and may be unilateral or bilateral. The cause is either compression or nerve infarction. The main difference is that compressive lesions may cause demyelinating conduction block, axon loss, or a combination of the two, whereas infarction produces solely axon loss.[191] Consequently, recovery with some compressive lesions may be rapid, whereas it is always prolonged following infarction.

Sciatic mononeuropathies have been attributed to DM,[176] but as already discussed, many reported cases of *diabetic sciatic neuropathy* actually could be examples of diabetic L-5/S-1 radiculopathy. None of the nontraumatic sciatic mononeuropathies studied in our EMG laboratory over a 20-year period has been associated with DM. Occasionally, lateral femoral cutaneous neuropathy is symptomatic in a diabetic patient.[189] The same question arises with these patients as with those diabetics who have CTS: Is the cause DM, or is it obesity?

Diabetic footdrop

Unilateral or bilateral weakness of foot dorsiflexion is encountered with some frequency in patients with DM.[11,187] The cause of *diabetic footdrop* is often unclear, with possibilities including: (1) proximal extension of severe axon loss DDSPN to involve the peroneal fibers near the knees (always bilateral and usually symmetric); (2) peroneal mononeuropathy at the fibular head, caused by either compression or infarction (unilateral or bilateral); (3) diabetic polyradiculopathy, either with isolated involvement of the L-5 root or, much more often, by extension to the L-5 root of L-2–L-4 lesions, that is, diabetic amyotrophy (unilateral or bilateral); and (4) a coexisting, independent disorder, such as a L-4 or L-5 compressive radiculopathy or a severe necrotizing myopathy extending distally enough in the limbs to involve the tibialis anterior muscles bilaterally.

Electrodiagnostic studies can be extremely helpful in evaluating patients with footdrop. The single most useful NCS, as would be expected from the clinical presentation, is the peroneal motor response, recording for the tibialis anterior muscle; with stimulations proximal and distal to the fibular head, lesions at the fibular head caused by axon loss can readily be differentiated from those caused by demyelinating conduction block. The next most helpful NCS is the superficial peroneal sensory, which is normal with uncomplicated L-5 radiculopathies and demyelinating conduction block along the peroneal nerve at the fibular head but low in amplitude or unelicitable with axon loss lesions involving the sacral plexus, sciatic nerve, or peroneal nerve. The NEE of the limb must be rather extensive, including not only the peroneal-innervated muscles, particularly the tibialis anterior, peroneus longus, and biceps femoris (short head), but also the more distal muscles innervated by the L-5 root via the tibial nerve, for example, the tibialis posterior and flexor digitorum longus muscles as well as the intrinsic foot muscles.[206] Unfortunately, the electrodiagnostic results often are less definite in diabetic patients because so many of them are elderly or have DDSPN; thus, the superficial

peroneal sensory NCS responses (as well as the other lower extremity sensory NCS responses) may be unelicitable bilaterally because of either. Generally when DDSPN is present, fibrillation potentials frequently are found in the intrinsic foot muscles bilaterally and can extend as far proximal as the knees or beyond if axon loss is severe. Consequently, in these situations, relative findings become significant: If fibrillation potentials and MUP loss are found in all the muscles distal to the knee but are much more prominent in the muscles of the anterior and lateral compartments, an axon loss peroneal mononeuropathy at or proximal to the fibular head probably is superimposed on an axon loss DDSPN. Also helpful in this regard is comparing the peroneal motor NCS amplitudes recorded from the tibialis anterior muscles bilaterally with each other, and with the posterior tibial motor amplitudes recorded off the gastrocnemius/soleus muscles, as the M components of the H-responses. With typical DDSPN, all of these should be affected to about the same degree. Conversely, if an axon loss peroneal mononeuropathy is superimposed, unilateral, or bilateral, the peroneal motor NCS amplitude on the affected limb(s) will be disproportionately involved, compared with the others.[42,139,144]

DIABETIC MONONEUROPATHY MULTIPLEX

Collagen vascular disease and DM are the two systemic disorders most often responsible for nerve infarctions occurring along two or more nerve trunks owing to occlusion of the vasa nervorum. Diabetic mononeuropathy multiplex presents as peripheral nerve deficits that appear abruptly, usually sequentially, and at irregular intervals, affecting two or more peripheral nerves (often nerves of different limbs). Some investigators, as previously noted, consider unilateral diabetic amyotrophy of abrupt onset a type of diabetic mononeuropathy multiplex.[42,139,144] Mononeuropathy multiplex is discussed in another chapter, so this discussion focuses on a few points concerning the electrodiagnostic examination with diabetic mononeuropathy multiplex.

1. Lesions caused by nerve infarcts are almost solely of the axon degeneration type; demyelinating features are not seen on NCS, as with multifocal demyelinating neuropathy.[207] Consequently, the only NCS components affected to any appreciable extent are the amplitudes of the sensory and motor responses; CVs and distal/

peak latencies are usually within or near the normal range as long as some responses can be elicited to permit their determination. On NEE performed 3 or more weeks after onset, abundant fibrillation potentials are found in the distribution of the affected motor fibers, along with variable but often severe (sometimes total) MUP loss.

2. NCS performed for suspected diabetic mononeuropathy multiplex can be misleading if done within the first 10 days of onset, before all the degenerating fibers composing the distal stump have ceased to conduct impulses.[206] This is true for all acute axon loss lesions, but it is particularly relevant with mononeuropathy multiplex because the clinical presentation often results in the patient being referred to the EMG laboratory exceptionally soon after onset.

3. In many instances, only some nerve fascicles are affected, with other fibers at the lesion site escaping injury. For this reason, both clinical and electrodiagnostic evidence of partial axon loss lesions are seen. Different muscles innervated by the same involved nerve may show different degrees of denervation; for example, with ulnar nerve infarction at or near the elbow, the motor NCS amplitude recorded from the forearm ulnar-innervated muscles may be 50% of normal, whereas that recorded over the ulnar-innervated hand muscles may be only 5% to 10% of normal.

4. Because of the multifocal nature of diabetic mononeuropathy multiplex, adequate electrodiagnostic studies invariably are extensive and therefore time-consuming.

PERIPHERAL NERVOUS SYSTEM ABNORMALITIES INDIRECTLY CAUSED BY DIABETES MELLITUS

In addition to the various types of diabetic neuropathy discussed, DM can compromise the PNS indirectly in a variety of ways. Two disorders of this nature with serious import are uremic distal symmetric polyneuropathy and ischemic monomelic neuropathy. Both of these are discussed in other chapters and therefore merit only brief comments in this section.

Diabetic nephropathy is one of the major complications of DM and a leading cause of death among diabetic patients with IDDM.[2,4] It often causes chronic renal failure, and 25% of patients with the latter develop uremic polyneuropathy.[96] Whenever a symmetric polyneuropathy develops in a diabetic patient who is uremic, both DM and uremia are possible causes. Clinicians often refer such patients to the EMG laboratory, with the mistaken belief that the electrophysiologic findings with DDSPN and uremic polyneuropathy are sufficiently different that they can be distinguished from one another. Unfortunately, this is not possible. Although some differences between their electrodiagnostic features have been reported for both conventional NCS and F waves,[96,116,117] these are mainly statistical in nature; in the individual patient, generally they cannot be separated by either conventional or single-fiber electrodiagnostic studies.[208] Patients with uremia, caused by DM as well as other conditions, also have abnormal susceptibility to entrapment/compression neuropathies.[201]

The arteriovenous shunts placed in the upper extremities of uremic patients for dialysis purposes can also be responsible for PNS disorders.

Ischemic monomelic neuropathy (IMN) is a type of ischemic neuropathy in which acute, noncompressive occlusion of a proximal limb artery, or shunt placement in it, produces multiple distal axon loss mononeuropathies in the limb. It seldom occurs in the upper extremities and then almost solely in patients whose uremia resulted from diabetic nephropathy. IMN occurs much more frequently in the lower extremities, often in diabetics, either because of spontaneous thrombosis in, or surgical manipulation of, the femoral artery.[209] The clinical and electrodiagnostic features of IMN are discussed in another section.

Also, in patients who require dialysis because of uremia, DM-induced or otherwise, CTS often develops in the upper extremity that contains the arteriovenous shunt.[201]

OTHER NEUROMUSCULAR CONDITIONS ASSOCIATED WITH DIABETES MELLITUS

Most reports concerned with neuromuscular abnormalities related to DM have focused on PNS disorders. Occasionally, however, abnormalities of some other component of the neuromuscular unit have been mentioned, including the spinal cord, neuromuscular junctions, and muscle fibers. These are briefly discussed.

Some investigators have found slowing along the central pathways in diabetic patients, using evoked potentials.[74a,210,211] Also, neuromuscular transmission defects in asymptomatic diabetic patients, detectable on repetitive stimulation, have been mentioned in a single report.[212] Finally, both focal and generalized myopathies associated with DM have been reported, although only evidence for the former is conclusive.[213–217]

Focal myopathies occur in diabetic patients in two separate contexts. First, muscle atrophy can be seen at the site of previous protamine zinc insulin injections.[213] This same mechanism probably explains the unexpected presence of fibrillation potentials, limited to a discrete area, in muscles underlying sites of previous insulin injections. Second, diabetic patients can experience abrupt thigh pain, swelling, and tenderness because of thigh muscle infarction; these rare lesions may occur bilaterally. No electrodiagnostic studies have been reported.[214,215]

At least two reports have suggested that DM can cause a generalized myopathy, but the evidence for this, particularly the electrodiagnostic changes reported, is both meager and unconvincing.[216,217] This possibility probably is raised most often when bilateral diabetic amyotrophy goes unrecognized. Every year a few elderly diabetic men with bilateral iliopsoas and quadriceps muscle weakness and pain are referred to our EMG laboratory with the diagnosis of inflammatory myopathy. Inexplicably, diabetic amyotrophy is not even included in the differential diagnosis. The problem is not limited to clinicians. As noted, some early electromyographers labeled diabetic amyotrophy a myopathic disorder partly because they mistook the highly polyphasic MUPs seen in the quadriceps muscle during reinnervation for *myopathic* MUPs.[92,149] The situation becomes even more complex when diabetic polyradiculopathy is more diffuse and has affected not only the hip, but also the shoulder girdle muscles. The fibrillation potentials and nonspecific MUP changes found in the involved muscles are readily mistaken for evidence of a necrotizing myopathy. Also noteworthy is that nonspecific MUP changes, consisting of MUPs of borderline to increased duration that are moderately polyphasic, are frequently found in the proximal muscles of both the upper extremities and the lower extremities in patients with severe, axon loss DDSPN. The cause of these MUP abnormalities is unclear, but it seems far more likely that they are due to a neurogenic, rather than a myopathic, process.

CONCLUSIONS

A great variety of PNS disorders are associated with DM. This fact, combined with the age and habitus of the average patient studied, often means that assessing diabetic patients challenges both the skills and the patience of the electromyographer. No other group of patients in our EMG laboratory requires greater time expenditure than do diabetics. Often the very extensive studies are mandated not by a lack of sufficient changes being found consistent with a particular diagnosis, as is often the case when patients are being evaluated for evidence of other disorders (e.g., motor neuron disease), but rather because of an overabundance of electrical abnormalities that defy all efforts at localization and classification. For this reason, when studying diabetic patients, the electromyographer often must resist the premature invocation of *Swift's rule* (Swift T. Personal communication): "There comes a time in every EMG examination when you might as well stop, because no matter how much more you do, you'll never get the answer."

Both the incidence and the prevalence of DM—and therefore of diabetic neuropathy—are likely to increase in the future for the following reasons: (1) More diabetics with IDDM are living long enough to have children and thus transmit the diabetic gene(s); (2) the life expectancy of treated diabetics, both with IDDM and NIDDM, is increasing; (3) the population is aging, and therefore more persons consequently are at risk to develop NIDDM; (4) obesity, which often precipitates NIDDM, is becoming more common in the general population; and (5) progressive modernization of lifestyle is occurring, among both some endemic and some immigrant populations; this transition leads not only to a greater incidence of obesity via both lack of physical activity and increased caloric intake, but also to increased carbohydrate consumption, reduction in dietary fiber, and increased psychosocial stress (which alters the central nervous system's release of various neurotransmitters)—NIDDM increases as a result.[8,218] Because diabetic neuropathy will be more common, the number of diabetic patients studied yearly in the EMG laboratory is likely to increase. Consequently, every electromyographer must be familiar with the PNS disorders that affect diabetics, the optimal electrodiagnostic methods for evaluating them, and the myriad of problems that can be encountered while undertaking evaluation of the diabetic patient.

REFERENCES

1. Ellenberg M. The clinical aspects of diabetic peripheral neuropathy. In: Canal N, Pozza G, eds. Peripheral neuropathies. Amsterdam: Elsevier/North Holland Biomedical Press, 1978: 225–237.
2. Foster DW. Diabetes mellitus. In: Petersdorf RG, Adams RD, Braunwald E, et al, eds. Harrison's Principles of Internal Medicine, ed 10. New York: McGraw-Hill, 1983: 661–679.
3. Marble A. Current concepts of diabetes. In: Marble A, White P, Bradley R, et al, eds. Joslin's diabetes mellitus, ed 11. Philadelphia: Lea & Febiger, 1971: 1–9.
4. Halter JB, Porte D. The clinical syndrome of diabetes mellitus. In: Dyck PJ, Thomas PK, Asbury AK, et al, eds. Diabetic neuropathy. Philadelphia: WB Saunders, 1987: 3–26.
5. National Diabetes Data Group. Classification and diagnosis of diabetes mellitus and other categories of glucose intolerance. Diabetes 1979; 28:1039–1057.
6. Herman WH, Teutsch SM, Geiss LS. Closing the gap: The problem of diabetes mellitus in the United States. Diab Care 1985; 8:391–406.
7. Harris MI, Hadden WC, Knowler WC, et al. Prevalence of diabetes and impaired glucose tolerance and plasma glucose levels in U.S. population aged 20–74 years. Diabetes 1987; 36:523–534.
8. Zimmet P. Type 2 (non-insulin-dependent) diabetes—an epidemiological overview. Diabetologia 1988; 22:399–411.
9. Anderson RM. Editorial. Diab Care 1991; 14:416–421.
10. Marks HH, Krall LP, White P. Epidemiology and detection of diabetes. In: Marble A, White P, Bradley R, et al, eds. Joslin's diabetes mellitus, ed 11. Philadelphia: Lea & Febiger, 1971: 10–34.
11. Martin MM. Diabetic neuropathy; a clinical study of 150 cases. Brain 1953; 76:594–624.
12. Thomas PK, Eliasson SG. Diabetic neuropathy. In: Dyck PJ, Thomas PK, Lambert EH, et al, eds. Peripheral neuropathy, ed 2. Philadelphia: WB Saunders, 1984: 1773–1810.
13. Harati Y. Diabetic peripheral neuropathies. Ann Intern Med 1987; 107: 546–559.
14. Thomas PK (in discussion). Differential diagnosis of peripheral neuropathies. In: Refsum S, Bolis CL, Portera Sanchez A, eds. International Conference on Peripheral Neuropathies. (International Congress Series 592.) Amsterdam: Excerpta Medica, 1982: 76–84.
15. Melton LJ, Dyck PJ. Epidemiology. In: Dyck PJ, Thomas PK, Asbury AK, et al, eds. Diabetic neuropathy. Philadelphia: WB Saunders, 1987: 27–36.
16. Thomas PK, Ward JD, Watkins PJ. Diabetic neuropathy. In: Keen H, Jarrett J, eds. Complications of diabetes, ed 2. London: Edward Arnold, 1982: 109–136.
17. Bruyn GW, Garland H. Neuropathies of endocrine origin. In: Vinkin PJ, Bruyn GW, eds. Handbook of clinical neurology. Vol 8 (Diseases of nerves, Part 2). Amsterdam: Elsevier/North Holland, 1970: 29–56.
18. Sullivan JF. The neuropathies of diabetes. Neurology 1958; 8:243–249.
19. Asbury AK, Brown MJ. Clinical and pathological studies of diabetic neuropathies. In: Goto Y, Horiuchi A, Kogure K, eds. Diabetic neuropathy. Amsterdam: Excerpta Medica, 1982: 50–57.
20. Dyck PJ, Karnes J, O'Brien PC. Diagnosis, staging and classification of diabetic neuropathy and associations with other complications. In: Dyck PJ, Thomas PK, Asbury AK, et al, eds. Diabetic Neuropathy. Philadelphia: WB Saunders, 1987: 36–45.
21. Green DA, Pfeifer MA. Diabetic neuropathy. In: Olefsky JM, Sherwin RS, eds. Diabetes mellitus: Management and complications. New York: Churchill Livingstone, 1985: 223–225.
22. Gregersen G. Diabetic amyotrophy—a well-defined syndrome? Acta Med Scand 1969; 185:303–310.
23. Dyck PJ, Karnes J, Daube J, et al. Clinical and neuropathologic criteria for the diagnosis and staging of diabetic polyneuropathy. Brain 1985; 108:861–880.
24. Garland H, Taverner D. Diabetic myelopathy. Br Med J 1953; 1:1405–1408.
25. Marinacci AA. Clinical electromyography. Los Angeles: San Lucas Press, 1955.
26. Marinacci AA. The value of electromyography in neurology. Calif Med 1954; 80:314–315.
27. Lambert E. Electromyography and electrical stimulation of peripheral nerves and muscles. In: Mayo Clinic staff (eds). Clinical evaluation in neurology. Philadelphia: WB Saunders, 1955:287–317.
28. Daube JR. Electrophysiological testing in neuropathy. In: Dyck PJ, Thomas PK, Asbury AK, et al, eds. Diabetic neuropathy. Philadelphia: WB Saunders, 1987: 162–176.
29. Greene DA, Brown MJ, Braunstein SN, et al. Comparison of clinical course and sequential electrophysiological tests in diabetics with symptomatic polyneuropathy and its implications for clinical trials. Diabetes 1981; 30:139–147.
30. Eng GD, Hung W, August GP, et al. Nerve conduction velocity determinations in juvenile diabetics: Continuing study of 190 patients. Arch Phys Med Rehab 1976; 57:1–5.
31. Gallai V, Massi-Beneditti F, Firenze C, et al. Diabetic neuropathy in children. In: Canal N, Pozza G, eds. Peripheral neuropathies. Amsterdam: Elsevier/North Holland Biomedical Press, 1978: 291–294.
32. Gamstorp I, Shelburne SA, Engleson G, et al. Peripheral neuropathy in juvenile diabetics. Diabetes 1966; 15:411–418.

33. Gregersen G. Diabetic neuropathy: Influence of age, sex, metabolic control, and duration of diabetes on motor conduction velocity. Neurology 1967; 17:972–980.

34. Kraft GH, Guyton JD, Huffman JD. Follow-up study of motor nerve conduction velocities in patients with diabetes mellitus. Arch Phys Med Rehab 1970; 51:207–209.

35. Lawrence DG, Locke S. Neuropathy in children with diabetes mellitus. Br Med J 1963; 1:784–785.

36. Negrin P, Fardin P, Fedele D, et al. Clinical and electromyographic observation on 83 cases of diabetic neuropathy. In: Canal N, Pozza G, eds. Peripheral neuropathies. Amsterdam: Elsevier/North Holland Biomedical Press, 1978:281–285.

37. Lawrence DG, Locke S. Motor nerve conduction velocity in diabetes. Arch Neurol 1961; 5:483–489.

38. Mayer RF. Nerve conduction studies in man. Neurology 1963; 13:1021–1030.

39. Braddom RL, Hollis JB, Castell DO. Diabetic peripheral neuropathy: A correlation of nerve conduction studies and clinical findings. Arch Phys Med Rehab 1977; 58:308–313.

40. Takeuchi H, Nonaka K, Takahashi M. et al. Diabetic neuropathy in children and adults: Clinical and electroneuromyographic studies. In: Goto Y, Horiuchi A, Kogure K, eds. Diabetic neuropathy. Amsterdam: Excerpta Medica, 1982: 139–145.

41. Wilbourn AJ. Nerve conduction studies in axonopathies and demyelinating neuropathies. In: 1989 AAEE Course A: Fundamentals of Electrodiagnosis. American Association of Electromyography and Electrodiagnosis, Rochester, Minn, 1989: 7–20.

42. Brown MJ, Asbury AK. Diabetic neuropathy. Ann Neurol 1984; 15:2–12.

43. Greene DA, Sima AAF, Albers JW, et al. Diabetic neuropathy. In: Rifkin H, Porte D, eds. Diabetes mellitus: Theory and practice, ed 4. New York: Elsevier, 1990.

44. Greene DA. Metabolic control. In: Dyck PJ, Thomas PK, Asbury AK, et al, eds. Diabetic neuuropathy. Philadelphia: WB Saunders, 1987: 177–187.

45. Kraft GH. Peripheral neuropathies. In: Johnson EW, ed. Practical electromyography, ed 2. Baltimore: Williams & Wilkins, 1988: 246–318.

46. Ward JD, Fisher DV, Barnes CG, et al. Improvement in nerve conduction velocity following treatment in newly diagnosed diabetics. Lancet 1971; 1:428–430.

47. Chokroverty S. Proximal nerve dysfunction in diabetic proximal amyotrophy. Arch Neurol 1982; 39:403–407.

48. Downie MB, Newell MA. Sensory nerve conduction in patients with diabetes and controls. Neurology 1961; 11:876–882.

49. Drechsler F. Sensory action potentials of the median and ulnar nerves in aged persons. In: Kuze K, Desmedt JE, eds. Studies on neuromuscular disease. Basel: S Karger, 1975: 232–235.

50. Goodgold J, Eberstein A. Electrodiagnosis of neuromuscular diseases, ed 3. Baltimore: Williams & Wilkins, 1983.

51. Kaeser HE. Nerve conduction velocity measurements. In: Vinken PJ, Bruyn GW, eds. Handbook of clinical neurology. Vol 7(Diseases of nerve, Part I). Amsterdam: North Holland, 1970: 116–196.

52. Ma DM, Wilbourn AJ, Kraft GH. Unusual sensory conduction studies. An American Association of Electromyography and Electrodiagnosis workshop. American Association of Electromyography and Electrodiagnosis, Rochester, Minn, 1984: 1–10.

53. Norris AH, Shock NW, Wagman IH. Age changes in the maximal conduction velocity of the motor fibers of human ulnar nerves. J Appl Physiol 1953; 5:589.

54. Wilbourn AJ. Uncommon cutaneous nerve studies. Special Course No. 16: Clinical electromyography. American Academy of Neurology, Minneapolis, 1979: 67–82.

55. Buchthal F. An introduction to electromyography (Minimonograph No. 15). Rochester, MN: American Association of Electromyography and Electrodiagnosis, 1981: 1–21.

56. Jacobs JM, Love S. Qualitative and quantitative morphology of human sural nerve at different ages. Brain 1985; 108:879–924.

57. Swallow M. Fiber size and content of the anterior tibial nerve of the foot. J Neurol Neurosurg Psychiatry 1966; 29:205–213.

58. Brown WF. The physiological and technical basis of electromyography. Boston: Butterworth, 1984.

59. Locke S, Lawrence DG, Legg MA. Diabetic amyotrophy. Am J Med 1963; 34:775–785.

60. Mulder DW, Lambert EH, Bastron JA, et al. The neuropathies associated with diabetes mellitus. Neurology 1961; 11:275–284.

61. Skillman TG, Johnson EW, Hamwi GW, et al. Motor nerve conduction velocity in diabetes mellitus. Diabetes 1961; 10:46–51.

62. Ellenberg M. Diabetic neuropathic cachexia. Diabetes 1974; 23:418–423.

63. Dyck PJ. Pathology. In: Dyck PJ, Thomas PK, Asbury AK, et al, eds. Diabetic neuropathy. Philadelphia: WB Saunders, 1987:223–236.

64. Shields RW. Single-fiber electromyography in diabetic polyneuropathy. Neurology 1984; 34(suppl 1):172.

65. Bastron JA, Thomas JE. Diabetic polyradiculopathy. Mayo Clin Proc 1981; 56:725–732.

66. Streib E, Daube JR. Electromyography of paraspinal muscles. Neurology 1975; 25:386.

66a. Streib EW, Sun SF, Panstrain FF, et al. Diabetic thoracic radiculopathy: Diagnostic study. Muscle Nerve 1986; 9:548–553.

67. Wilbourn AJ, Aminoff MJ. AAEE Minimonograph #32: The electrophysiological examination in pa-

tients with radiculopathy. Muscle Nerve 1988; 11:1099–1114.

68. Bicknell JM, Johnson SF. Widespread electromyographic abnormalities in spinal muscles in cancer, disc disease and diabetes. U Mich Med Center J 1976; 42:124–127.

69. Neel JV, Fejans SS, Conn JW, et al. Diabetes mellitus. In: Neel JV, Shaw MW, Schull WV, eds. Genetics and the epidemiology of chronic diseases. Washington, D.C.: Department of U.S. Public Health Services Publication No. 1163, 1965:105–132.

70. Locke S. The peripheral nervous system in diabetes mellitus. Diabetes 1964; 13:307–311.

71. Thomas PK, Brown MJ. Diabetic polyneuropathy. In: Dyck PJ, Thomas PK, Asbury AK, et al, eds. Diabetic neuropathy. Philadelphia: WB Saunders, 1987: 56–65.

72. Thomas PK. Human and experimental diabetic neuropathy. In: Canal N, Pozza G, eds. Peripheral neuropathies. Amsterdam: Elsevier/North Holland Biomedical Press, 1978:239–246.

73. Gregersen G. A study of the peripheral nerves in diabetic subjects during ischemia. J Neurol Neurosurg Psychiatry 1968; 31:175–181.

74. Steiness IB. Vibratory perception in diabetes during arrested blood flow to the limb. Acta Med Scand 1959; 163:195–205.

74a. Gupta P, Dorfman L. Spinal somatosensory conduction in diabetics. Neurology 1981; 31:844–845.

75. Price DE, Alani SM, Wales JK. Effect of aldose reductase inhibition on resistance to ischemic conduction block in diabetic patients. Diab Care 1991; 14:411–413.

76. Seneviratne KN, Peiris OA. Effect of ischaemia on the excitability of sensory nerves in diabetes mellitus. J Neurol Neurosurg Psychiatry 1968; 31:348–353.

77. Brown MJ, Greene DA. Diabetic neuropathy: Pathophysiology and management. In: Asbury AK, Gilliatt RW, (eds.): Peripheral nerve disorders. London: Butterworths, 1984: 126–153.

78. Palumbo PJ, Elveback LR, Whisnant JP. Neurological complications of diabetes mellitus: Transient ischemic attack, stroke, and peripheral polyneuropathy. In: Schoenberg BS, ed, Neurological epidemiology: Principles and clinical applications. (Advances in neurology. Vol 19.) New York: Raven Press, 1978: 593–601.

79. Pfeifer MA, Greene DA. Diabetic neuropathy. Current concepts. Kalamazoo, MI: Upjohn Co, 1985.

80. Sugimura K, Dyck PJ. Multifocal fiber loss in proximal sciatic nerve in symmetric distal diabetic neuropathy. J Neurol Sci 1982; 53:501–508.

81. Low PA, Tuck RR, Takeuchi M. Nerve microenvironment in diabetic neuropathy. In: Dyck PJ, Thomas PK, Asbury AK, et al, eds. Diabetic neuropathy. Philadelphia: WB Saunders, 1987: 266–278.

82. Thomas PK, Lascelles RG. The pathology of diabetic neuropathy. Quart J Med NS 1966; 35:489–509.

83. Dyck PJ, Sherman WR, Hallcher LM, et al. Human diabetic endoneurial sorbitol, fructose and myoinositol related to sural nerve morphometry. Ann Neurol 1980; 8:590–596.

84. Daube JR. Nerve conduction studies. In: Aminoff MJ, ed. Electrodiagnosis in clinical neurology, ed 2. London: Churchill-Livingstone, 265–306, 1986.

85. Gilliatt RW. Nerve conduction in human and experimental neuropathies. Proc Royal Soc Med 1966; 59:989–993.

86. Huddleston O, Golseth JG, Marinacci AA, et al. The use of electromyography in the diagnosis of neuromuscular disorders. Arch Phys Med Rehabil 1950; 31:378–387.

87. Eeg-Olofsson O, Petersen I. Childhood diabetic neuropathy; a clinical and neurophysiological study. Acta Paediatr Scand 1966; 55:163–176.

88. Ferrari-Forcade A, Temesio P, Gomensoro JB. Estudio de la velocidad de conduccion nerviosa en la diabetes. Acta Neurol Lat Am 1960; 6:43–48.

89. Hudson CH, Dow RS. Motor nerve conduction velocity determination. Neurology 1963; 13:982–988.

90. Johnson EW, Olsen KJ. Clinical value of motor nerve conduction velocity determination. JAMA 1960; 172:2030–2035.

91. Kuribayashi T, Kurihawa T, Tanaka M, et al. Diabetic neuropathy and electrophysiological studies: Evoked muscle action potentials, nerve conduction and short latency SEP. In: Goto Y, Horiuchi A, Kogure K, eds. Diabetic neuropathy. Amsterdam: Excerpta Medica, 1982:120–124.

92. Lamontagne A, Buchthal F. Electrophysiological studies in diabetic neuropathy. J Neurol Neurosurg Psychiatry 1970; 33:442–452.

93. Gallai V, Firenze C, Mazzotta G, et al. Neuropathy in children and adolescents with diabetes mellitus. Acta Neurol Scand 1988; 78:136–140.

94. Kaar ML, Saukkonen AL, Pitkanen M. Peripheral neuropathy in diabetic children and adolescents. Acta Paediatr Scand 1983; 72:373–378.

95. Rendell MS, Katims JJ, Richter R. A comparison of nerve conduction velocities and current perception thresholds as correlates of clinical severity of diabetic sensory neuropathy. J Neurol Neurosurg Psychiatry. 1989; 52:502–511.

96. Oh SJ. Clincal electromyography. Baltimore: University Park Press, 1984.

97. Behse F, Buchthal F, Carlsen F. Nerve biopsy and conduction studies in diabetic neuropathy. J Neurol Neurosurg Psychiatry 1977; 40:1072–1082.

98. Buchthal F, Behse F. Sensory action potentials and biopsy of the sural nerve in neuropathy. In: Canal N, Pozza G, eds. Peripheral neuropathies. Amsterdam: Elsevier/North Holland Biomedical Press, 1978:1–22.

99. McLeod JC, Prineas JW, Walsh JC. The relationship of conduction velocity to pathology in peripheral nerves. A study of the sural nerve in 90 patients. In:

Desmedt J, ed. New developments in electromyography and clinical neurophysiology. Vol 1. Basel: S Karger, 1973: 248–259.

100. Fagerberg SE, Petersen I, Steg G, et al. Motor disturbances in diabetes mellitus: A clinical study using electromyography and conduction velocity determination. Acta Med Scand 1963; 174:711–716.

101. Gregersen G. Motor-nerve function and duration of diabetes. Lancet 1964; 1:733.

102. Mulder DW, Bastron JA, Lambert EH. Hyperinsulin neuronopathy. Neurology 1956; 6:627–635.

103. Duck SC, Wei F, Parke J, et al. Role of height and glycosylated hemoglobin in abnormal nerve conduction in pediatric patients with Type 1 diabetes mellitus after 4–9 years of disease. Diab Care 1991; 14:386–392.

104. Buchthal F, Rosenfalck A. Sensory potentials in polyneuropathy. Brain 1971; 94:241–262.

105. Teckemann W, Kaeser HE, Berger W, et al. Sensory and motor parameters in leg nerves of diabetics: Intercorrelations and relationship to clinical symptoms. Eur Neurol 1981; 20:344–350.

106. Levy DM, Abraham RR, Abraham RM. Small and large fiber involvement in early diabetic neuropathy: A study with the median plantar response and sensory thresholds. Diab Care 1987; 10:441–447.

107. Izzo KL, Sobel E, Demopoulos JT. Diabetic neuropathy: Electrophysiological abnormalities of distal lower extremity sensory nerves. Arch Phys Med Rehabil 1986; 67:7–11.

108. Harada N, Imanishi H, Iwasaki M, et al. Nerve conduction study in diabetic neuropathy by Buchthal's method and by the H-reflex method. In: Goto Y, Horiuchi A, Kogure K, eds. Diabetic neuropathy. Amsterdam: Excerpta Medica, 1982: 135–138.

109. Kaplan JG, Shahani BT, Young RR. Electrophysiological studies in diabetic neuropathy. Muscle Nerve 1981; 4:443–444.

110. Lachman T, Shahani BT, Young RR. Late responses as aids in the diagnosis in peripheral neuropathy. J Neurol Neurosurg Psychiatry 1980; 43:156–162.

111. Noel P. Diabetic neuropathy. In: Desmedt JE, ed. New developments in electromyography and clinical neurophysiology. Vol 2. Basel: S Karger, 1973: 318–332.

112. Shahani BT, Sumner AJ. Electrophysiological studies in peripheral neuropathy. Early detection and monitoring. In: Stalberg E, Young R, eds. Clinical neurophysiology. London: Butterworths, 1981: 117–144.

113. Shahani BT, Young RR. Studies of reflex activity from a clinical viewpoint. In: Aminoff MJ (ed). Electrodiagnosis in clinical neurology. London: Churchill Livingstone, 1980: 290–304.

114. Conrad J, Aschoff J, Fisher M. Der Diagnostishe Wert der F-Welen—Latemz. J Neurol 1975; 210:391–418.

115. Chokroverty S. Diabetic proximal amyotrophy. In:

Canal N, Pozza G, eds. Peripheral neuropathies. Amsterdam: Elsevier/North Holland Biomedical Press, 1978: 257–268.

116. Fierro B, Modica A, D'Arpa A, et al. Analysis of F-wave in metabolic neuropathies: A comparative study in uremic and diabetic patients. Acta Neurol Scand 1987; 75:179–185.

117. Kimura J. Electrodiagnosis in diseases of nerve and muscle: Principles and practice, ed 2. Philadelphia: FA Davis, 1989.

118. Narita S, et al. F-wave studies in patients with diabetes mellitus. In: Goto Y, Horiuchi A, Kogure K, eds. Diabetic neuropathy. Amsterdam: Excerpta Medica, 1982: 125–130.

119. Troni W, Bergamini L, Lacquaniti F. F and H responses in the evaluation of conduction velocity in the proximal tracts of peripheral nerves in diabetic and alcoholic patients. In: Canal N, Pozza G, (eds), Peripheral Neuropathies. Amsterdam: North Holland Biomedical Press, 1978: 295–301.

120. Mysiw WJ, Colachis SC, Vetter J. F-response characteristics in Type I diabetes mellitus. Am J Phys Med 1990; 69:112–116.

121. Thage O, Trojaborg W, Buchthal F. Electromyographic findings in polyneuropathy. Neurology 1963; 13:273–278.

122. Massarweh W, Wilbourn AJ, Campbell J. The EMG examination with "pure" sensory polyneuropathies: A study of 36 cases. Muscle Nerve 1983; 6:529.

123. Dyck PJ, O'Brien PC. Meaningful degrees of prevention or improvement of nerve conduction in controlled clinical trials of diabetic neuropathy. Diabetes Care 1989; 12:649–652.

124. Troni W, Carta Q, Cantello R, et al. Peripheral nerve function and metabolic control in diabetes mellitus. Ann Neurol 1984; 16:178–183.

125. Canal N, Comi G, Saibene V, et al. The relationship between peripheral and autonomic neuropathy in insulin-independent diabetes: A clinical and instrumental evaluation. In: Canal N, Pozza G, eds. Peripheral neuropathy. Amsterdam: Elsevier North Holland Biomedical Press, 1978, 247–255.

126. Bradley WE, Lin JT. Assessment of diabetic sexual dysfunction and cystopathy. In: Dyck PJ, Thomas PK, Asbury AK, et al, eds. Diabetic neuropathy. Philadelphia: WB Saunders, 1987: 146–154.

127. Ertekin C, Reel F. Bulbocavernosus reflex in normal men and in patients with neurogenic bladder and/or impotence. J Neurol Sci 1976; 28:1–15.

128. Haldeman S, Bradley WE, Bhatia NN, et al. Neurogenic evaluation of bladder, bowel and sexual disturbance in diabetic men. In: Goto Y, Horiuchi A, Kogure E, eds. Diabetic neuropathy. Amsterdam: Excerpta Medica, 1982: 298–301.

129. Haldeman S, Bradley WE, Bhatia NN. Pudendal evoked responses. Arch Neurol 1982; 39:280–283.

130. Danta G. Hypoglycemic peripheral neuropathy. Arch Neurol 1969; 21:121–132.

131. Jaspan JB, Wollman RL, Berstein L, et al. Hypoglycemic peripheral neuropathy in association with insulinoma: Implication of glucopenia rather than hyperinsulinism. Medicine 1982; 61:33–44.

132. Harrison MJG. Muscle wasting after prolonged hypoglycemic coma: Case report with electrophysiological data. J Neurol Neurosurg Psychiatry 1976; 39:465–470.

133. Rowland LP, Layzer RB. Muscular dystrophies, atrophies, and related diseases. In: Baker AB, Baker LH, eds. Clinical neurology. Vol 3. New York: Harper & Row, 1974: 14.

134. Garland H. Diabetic amyotrophy. In: Williams D, ed. Modern trends in neurology, ser. 2. New York: Paul B Hoeber, 1957: 229–239.

135. DeJong RN. The neurologic manifestations of diabetes mellitus. In: Vinkin PJ, Bruyn GW, eds. Handbook of clinical neurology. Vol 27. Amsterdam: North Holland Publishing Co, 1976: 99–142.

136. Simpson JA. The neuropathies, series 3. In: Williams D, ed. Modern trends in neurology. London: Butterworths, 1972: 245–291.

137. Treanor WJ. Diabetic polyradiculopathy: A syndrome in need of definition. Arch Phys Med Rehab 1974; 55:592–593.

138. Thomas JE, Bastron JA. Clinical recognition of diabetic polyradiculopathy. Pract Cardiol 1984; 10:135–142.

139. Raff MC, Sangalang V, Asbury AK. Ischemic mononeuropathy multiplex associated with diabetes mellitus. Arch Neurol 1968; 18:487–499.

140. Garland H. Diabetic amyotrophy. Br Med J 1955; 2:1287–1290.

141. Garland H. Neurological complications of diabetes mellitus: Clinical aspects. Proc Royal Soc Med 1960; 53:137–146.

142. Garland H. Diabetic amyotrophy. Br J Clin Pract 1961; 15:9–13.

143. Asbury AK. Focal and multifocal neuropathies of diabetes. In: Dyck PJ, Thomas PK, Asbury AK, eds. Diabetic neuropathy. Philadelphia: WB Saunders, 1987:45–55.

144. Asbury AK. Proximal diabetic neuropathy. Ann Neurol 1977; 2:179–180.

145. Calverley JR. Lumbosacral plexus lesions. In: Dyck PJ, Thomas PK, Lambert EH, eds. Peripheral neuropathy. Philadelphia: WB Saunders, 1975: 682–687.

146. Casey EB, Harrison MJG. Diabetic amyotrophy: A follow-up study. Br Med J 1972; 1:656–659.

147. Chokroverty S, Reyes MG, Rubino FA, et al. The syndrome of diabetic amyotrophy. Ann Neurol 1977; 2:131–194.

148. Donovan WH, Sumi SM. Diabetic amyotrophy—a more diffuse process than clinically suspected. Arch Phys Med Rehab 1976; 57:397–403.

149. Hamilton CR, Dobson HL, Marshall J. Diabetic amyotrophy: Clinical and electron-microscopic studies in 6 patients. Am J Med Sci 1968; 256:81–90.

150. Issacs H, Gilchrist G. Diabetic amyotrophy. S Afr Med J 1960; 134:501–505.

151. Leedman PJ, Davis S, Harrison LC. Diabetic amyotrophy: Reassessment of the clinical spectrum. Aust NZ J Med 1988; 18:768–773.

152. Skanse B, Gydell K. A rare type of femoral-sciatic neuropathy in diabetes mellitus. Acta Med Scand 1956; 155:463–468.

153. Subramony SH, Wilbourn AJ. Diabetic proximal neuropathy. Clinical and electromyographic studies. J Neurol Sci 1982; 53:293–304.

154. Calverley JR, Mulder DW. Femoral neuropathy. Neurology 1960; 10:963–967.

155. Stevens JC. Lumbar plexus lesions. In: Dyck PJ, Thomas PK, Lambert EH, et al, eds. Peripheral neuropathy, ed 2. Vol 2. Philadelphia: WB Saunders, 1984:1425–1434.

156. Williams IR, Mayer RF. Subacute proximal diabetic neuropathy. Neurology 1976; 26:108–116.

157. Biedmond A. Femoral neuropathy. In: Vinkin PJ, Bruyn GW, eds. Handbook of clinical neurology. Vol 8, Part 2. Amsterdam: North Holland, 1970:303–310.

158. Brown MR, Dyck PJ, McClearn GE, et al. Central and peripheral nervous system complications. Diabetes 1982; 32 (suppl 1):65–70.

159. Kimura J, Yamada T, Stevland NP. Distal slowing of motor nerve conduction velocity in diabetic polyneuropathy. J Neurol Sci 1979; 42:291–302.

160. Locke S. The nervous system and diabetes. In: Marble A, White P, Bradley R, et al. eds. Joslin's diabetes mellitus, ed 11. Philadelphia: Lea & Febiger, 1971:562–580.

161. Marinacci AA, Courville CB. Radicular syndromes simulating intraabdominal conditions. Am Surg 1962; 28:59–63.

162. Schulz A. Diabetische Radiculopathie der unteren Thorakalsegmente mit Bauchdeckenparesen. Verh Dtsch Ges Inn Med 1966; 72:1171–1175.

163. Waxman SG, Sabin TD. Diabetic truncal polyneuropathy. Arch Neurol 1981; 38:46–47.

164. Sun SF, Streib EW. Reply to letter: Diabetic thoracoabdominal neuropathy. Ann Neurol 1981; 10:496.

165. Ellenberg M. Diabetic truncal mononeuropathy—a new clinical syndrome. Diab Care 1978; 1:10–13.

166. Kikta DG, Breuer AC, Wilbourn AJ. Thoracic root pain in diabetes: The spectrum of clinical and electromyographic findings. Ann Neurol 1982; 11:80–85.

167. Kikta DG. Diabetic truncal neuropathy: A distinct and frequently overlooked syndrome. Pract Cardiol 1984; 10:103–108.

168. Longstreth GF, Newcomer AD. Abdominal pain caused by diabetic neuropathy. Ann Intern Med 1977; 86:166–168.

169. Massey EW. Diabetic truncal mononeuropathy: Electromyographic evaluation. Acta Diabet Lat 1980; 17:269–272.

170. Massey EW. Diabetic thoracoabdominal neuropathy (letter). Ann Neurol 1981; 10:496.

171. Sun SF, Streib EW. Diabetic thoracoabdominal neuropathy: Clinical and electrodiagnostic features. Ann Neurol 1981; 9:75–79.

172. Caldwell JW, Crane CR, Boland GL. Determinations of intercostal motor conduction time in the diagnosis of nerve root compression. Arch Phys Med Rehab 1968; 49:515–518.

173. Johnson ER, Powell J, Caldwell J, et al. Intercostal nerve conduction and posterior rhizotomy in the diagnosis and treatment of thoracic radiculopathy. J Neurol Neurosurg Psychiatry 1974; 37:330–332.

174. Bloodworth JMB, Epstein M. Diabetic amyotrophy: Light and electron microscopic investigation. Diabetes 1967; 16:181–190.

175. Redwood DR. Diabetic amyotrophy. Br Med J 1962; 2:521–522.

176. Jacobs EM. Diabetic sciatic mononeuropathy: Report of a case. Diabetes 1958; 7:493–494.

177. Child DL, Yates DAH. Radicular pain in diabetes. Rheumatol Rehab 1978; 17:195–196.

178. Riley DE, Shields RW. Diabetic amyotrophy with upper extremity involvement. Neurology 1984; 34(suppl 1):216.

179. Spritz N. Nerve disease in diabetes mellitus. In: Prodolsky S, ed. Diabetes mellitus. Med Clin North Am 1978; 62:787–798.

180. Gilliatt RW, Willison RG. Peripheral nerve conduction in diabetic neuropathy. J Neurol Neurosurg Psychiatry 1962; 25:11–18.

181. Ellenberg M. Diabetic neuropathy of the upper extremities. J Mt Sinai Hosp 1968; 35:134–148.

182. Johnson EW, Waylonis GW. Facial nerve conduction delay in patients with diabetes mellitus. Arch Phys Med Rehab 1964; 45:131–139.

183. Kimura J. An evaluation of the facial and trigeminal nerves in polyneuropathy: Electrodiagnostic study in Charcot-Marie-Tooth disease, Guillain-Barré syndrome, and diabetic neuropathy. Neurology 1971; 21:745–752.

184. Karnes WE. Diseases of the seventh cranial nerve. In: Dyck PJ, Thomas PK, Lambert EH, Bunge R, eds. Peripheral neuropathy, ed 2. Vol 2. Philadelphia: WB Saunders, 1984; 1266–1299.

185. Pecket P, Schatter A. Concurrent Bell's palsy and diabetes mellitus: A diabetic mononeuropathy? J Neurol Neurosurg Psychiatry 1982; 45:652–655.

186. Adour KK, Wingerd JW, Doty HE. Prevalence of concurrent diabetes mellitus and idiopathic facial paralysis (Bell's palsy). Diabetes 1975; 24:449–451.

187. Korczyn AD. Bell's palsy and diabetes mellitus. Lancet 1971; 1:108–110.

188. Moldaver J. The problem of Bell's palsy: Etiology and analysis of therapeutic approach. In: Moldaver

J, Conley J, eds. The facial palsies. Springfield, IL: Charles C Thomas, 1980:65–73.

189. Winkelman AC. Peripheral neuropathy. In: Kryston LJ, Shaw RA, eds. Endocrinology and diabetes. New York: Grune & Stratton, 1975:419–426.

190. Jabre JF, Wilbourn AJ. The EMG findings in 100 consecutive ulnar neuropathies. Acta Neurol Scand 1979; (suppl 73):91.

191. Katirji MB, Wilbourn AJ. Common peroneal neuropathy: A clinical and electrophysiological study of 116 cases. Neurology 1988; 38:1723–1728.

192. Fraser DM, Campbell IW, Ewing DJ, et al. Mononeuropathy in diabetes mellitus. Diabetes 1979; 28:96–101.

193. Czeuz KA, Thomas JE, Lambert EH, et al. Long-term results of operation for carpal tunnel syndrome. Mayo Clin Proc 1966; 41:232–241.

194. Frymoyer JW, Bland J. Carpal-tunnel syndrome in patients with myxedematous arthropathy. J Bone Joint Surg 1973; 55A:78–82.

195. Leach RE, Odom JA: Systemic causes of carpal tunnel syndrome. Postgrad Med J 1968; 44:127–131.

196. Loong SC. The carpal tunnel syndrome: A clinical and electrophysiological study in 250 patients. In: Tyler JH, Eadie MJ, eds. Clinical and experimental neurology. Baltimore: University Park Press, 1977:51–65.

197. Dawson DM, Hallett M, Millender LH. Entrapment neuropathies, ed 2. Boston: Little, Brown, 1990.

198. Kopell HP, Thompson WAL. Peripheral entrapment neuropathies. Baltimore: Williams & Wilkins, 1963.

199. Nakano KK. The entrapment neuropathies. Muscle Nerve 1978; 1:264–279.

200. Staal A: The entrapment neuropathies. In: Vinkin PJ, Bruyn GW, eds. Handbook of clinical neurology. Vol 7. Amsterdam: Elsevier/North Holland, 1970: 285–325.

201. Layzer RB. Neuromuscular manifestations of systemic disease. Philadelphia: FA Davis, 1985:117–126.

202. Jung Y, Holmann TC, Gerneth JA, et al. Diabetic hand syndrome. Metabolism 1971; 20:1008–1015.

203. Schaumburg HH, Spencer PS, Thomas PK. Disorders of peripheral nerves. Philadelphia: FA Davis, 1983:41–55.

204. Goodman JI. Femoral neuropathy in relation to diabetes mellitus. Diabetes 1954; 3:266–273.

205. Shahani B, Spalding JMK. Diabetes mellitus presenting with bilateral foot-drop. Lancet 1969; 2:930.

206. Wilbourn AJ. AAEE Case report No. 12: Common peroneal mononeuropathy at the fibular head. Muscle Nerve 1986; 9:825–836.

207. Lewis RA, Sumner AJ, Brown MJ, et al. Multifocal demyelinating neuropathy with persistent conduction block. Neurology 1982; 32:958–964.

208. Thiele B, Stalberg E. Single fibre EMG findings in

polyneuropathies of different aetiology. J Neurol Neurosurg Psychiatry 1975; 38:881–887.

209. Wilbourn AJ, Furlan AJ, Hulley W, et al. Ischemic monomelic neuropathy. Neurology 1983; 33:447–451.

210. Cracco J, Costells S, Mark E. Conduction veolocity in peripheral nerve and spinal afferent pathways in juvenile diabetics. Neurology 1980; 30:370–371.

211. Donald M, Bird C, Laevon J. Delayed auditory brainstem responses in diabetes mellitus. J Neurol Neurosurg Psychiatry 1981; 44:641–644.

212. Miglietta O. Neuromuscular transmission defect in diabetes. Diabetes 1973; 22:719–723.

213. Gilmore CM. Muscle atrophy from sensitivity to Protamine zinc insulin. S Med Surg 1947; 109:394.

214. Angervall L, Steiner B. Tumoriform focal muscular degeneration in two diabetic patients. Diabetologia 1965; 1:39–42.

215. Banker BQ, Chester S. Infarction of thigh muscle in the diabetic patient. Neurology 1978; 23:667–676.

216. Kito S, Tokinobu H, Itoga E, et al. A clinical study of skeletal muscle disorders in diabetes. In: Goto Y, Horiuchi A, Kogure K, eds. Diabetic neuropathy. Amsterdam: Excerpta Medica, 1982; 179–184.

217. Swash M, Van den Noort S, Craig JW. Late-onset proximal myopathy with diabetes mellitus in four sisters. Neurology 1970; 20:694–699.

218. Steinke J, Soeldner JS. Diabetes mellitus. In: Thorn GW, Adams RD, Braunwald E, et al, eds. Harrison's principles of internal medicine, ed 8. New York: McGraw-Hill, 1977:563–583.

219. Gilliatt RW, Goodman HV, Willison RG. The recording of lateral popliteal nerve action potentials in man. J Neurol Neurosurg Psychiat 1961; 24:305–318.

220. Bolton CF, Driedger AA, Lindsay RM. Ischemic neuropathy in uremic patients caused by bovine arteriovenous shunt. J Neurol Neurosurg Psychiatry 1979; 42:810–814.

221. Williams AJ. Diabetic neuralgic amyotrophy. Postgrad Med J 1981; 57:450–452.

19

Peripheral Neuropathies Associated with Plasma Cell Dyscrasias

John J. Kelly, Jr.

CONTENTS

LIST OF ACRONYMS

ALS	amyotrophic lateral sclerosis
CIDP	chronic inflammatory demyelinating polyneuropathy
CMAP	compound muscle action potential
GHCD	gamma heavy chain disease
IEP	immunoelectrophoresis
IF	immunofixation
MG	monoclonal gammopathy
MGUS	monoclonal gammopathy of undetermined significance
PCD	plasma cell dyscrasia
SNAP	sensory nerve action potential
SPEP	serum cellulose acetate protein electrophoresis
WM	Waldenström's macroglobulinemia

The finding of a serum monoclonal protein (M-protein) in a patient with an idiopathic polyneuropathy is an important diagnostic clue. If patients with idiopathic polyneuropathy are screened with cellulose acetate electrophoresis of serum, about 10% are found to have an M-protein.[1] Further studies in these patients lead to a diagnosis of a specific plasma cell dyscrasia, such as monoclonal gammopathy of undetermined significance, multiple myeloma, osteosclerotic myeloma, Waldenström's macroglobulinemia, gamma-heavy chain disease, amyloidosis (light-chain type), or other rare disorders (Table 19.1). These neuropathies often present in a distinctive fashion, so a combination of clinical and electrophysiologic signs may allow recognition of a specific syndrome and help direct the subsequent evaluation.[2] These signs may even allow the clinician to predict the nature of the underlying hematologic disease. For this reason, a detailed presentation and thorough understanding of the clinical and electrodiagnostic findings in patients with polyneuropathy associated with monoclonal gammopathy are useful. Because patients with individual plasma cell dyscrasias are more likely to present with distinctive polyneuropathies than are patients with other malignancies,[2] these neuropathic syndromes are discussed in the context of the underlying plasma cell dyscrasia, which can usually be diagnosed by appropriate hematologic screening of all idiopathic polyneuropathy patients.

EPIDEMIOLOGY

Although early case reports suggested an association between plasma call dyscrasias and polyneuropathies, the first solid statistical evidence linking the two came in a study of idiopathic polyneuropathy patients screened prospectively for monoclonal gammopathy (MG).[1] In this large series, about 10% of idiopathic polyneuropathy patients had a MG, as compared with 2.5% of patients with polyneuropathy secondary to other diseases. The latter percentage is slightly higher than that in the normal population because the frequency of MG in a population survey ranged from 0.1% in the third decade to 3% in the eighth decade.[3] This and other studies strongly suggested an etiologic association between MG and polyneuropathy.

Other studies also appeared that supported such an association. These consisted of studies of the natural history and etiopathogenesis of subcategories of polyneuropathy associated with MG. Amyloid in sporadic or primary systemic amyloidosis, for example, was found to consist of the variable portion of a monoclonal light chain.[4] A distinctive polyneuropathy was found to accompany osteosclerotic myeloma,[5,6] possibly owing to the monoclonal light chain, although the mechanism remains uncertain. Anti–myelin associated glycoprotein (MAG) antibody activity (and other antinerve antibodies) were found in a substantial proportion of patients with MG of undetermined significance, especially of immunoglobulin M (IgM) type.[7,8] These studies augmented epidemiologic studies and supported the concept that plasma cell dyscrasias are overrepresented in patients with idiopathic polyneuropathy and, at least in some cases, are clearly etiologically linked.

It can be estimated that there is such an association in approximately 5% of all polyneuropathy patients and 10% of idiopathic polyneuropathy patients.[1] Latov et al.[9] have estimated that the prevalence of anti-MAG polyneuropathy is roughly one to five per 10,000 adults. Other studies have shown that approximately 16% of patients with MG have a polyneuropathy.[10] If the frequency of MG in a community study was 1.25% in subjects greater than 50 years of age,[3] the prevalence of polyneuropathy associated with MG can be estimated as approximately two per 1000 in patients over 50. Roughly one-half of these will be monoclonal gammopathy of undetermined significance (MGUS)–associated polyneuropathies, 25% amyloid-associated, and the rest smaller percentages of other syndromes.[1] These, of course, are rough estimates but show that polyneuropathies associated with MG are frequent and underdiagnosed.

HEMATOLOGIC EVALUATION

A plasma cell dyscrasia (PCD) or MG (Table 19.2) is defined as a proliferation of a single clone of plasma cells, either neoplastic or nonneoplastic, usually associated with the production of a serum M-

TABLE 19.1. Final hematologic diagnosis in 28 patients with polyneuropathy and M proteins

Monoclonal gammopathy of undetermined significance	16
Amyloidosis, light-chain type	7
Multiple myeloma	3
Waldenström's macroglobulinemia	1
Gamma heavy-chain disease	1

TABLE 19.2.　Classification of plasma cell dyscrasias

Malignant plasma cell dyscrasias
　Multiple myeloma (IgG, IgA, IgD, IgE, and free light chains)
　　Overt multiple myeloma
　　Smoldering multiple myeloma
　　Plasma cell leukemia
　　Nonsecretory myeloma
　　Osteosclerotic myeloma
　Plasmacytoma
　　Solitary plasmacytoma of bone
　　Extramedullary plasmacytoma
　Malignant lymphoproliferative diseases
　　Waldenström's macroglobulinemia or primary macroglobulinemia (IgM)
　　Malignant lymphoma
　　Chronic lymphocytic leukemia
　　Other malignant lymphoproliferative processes
　Heavy chain diseases (HCD)
　　γ HCD
　　α HCD
　　μ HCD
　　δ HCD
　Amyloidosis
　　Primary Amyloidosis, light chain type (AL)
　　With myeloma (AL)
　　(Secondary, localized, and familial amyloidosis have no monoclonal protein)
Plasma cell dyscrasias of undetermined significance
　Benign (IgG, IgA, IgD, IgM, and, rarely, free light chains)
　Associated with neoplasms of cell types not known to produce monoclonal proteins
　Biclonal gammopathies

Reprinted with permission from Kelly JJ Jr, Kyle RA, Latov N. Polyneuropathies associated with plasma cell dyscrasias. Boston: Martinus-Nijhoff, 1987.

protein which can be measured in the serum, urine, or both.[10–12] M-proteins, or more properly monoclonal immunoglobulins, consist of a single heavy chain (IgM, IgG, IgD, or IgA) and a single light chain (kappa or lambda) as opposed to polyclonal gammopathies, which consist of both light chains and generally more than one heavy chain.[11] Occasionally only the light chain or heavy chain may be secreted by the clone of plasma cells. It was formerly thought that the M-protein was abnormal and had no biologic activity. It is now known that these proteins derive from the expansion of clones of immunoglobulin-secreting cells with activity directed at specific antigens, and M-proteins often have idiotypically specific biologic activity, probably accounting for many of the remote effects of these monoclonal gammopathies.[12]

The M-protein in most commonly detected by screening patients with serum cellulose acetate protein electrophoresis (SPEP). The spike can occur in the gamma, beta, or even the alpha-2 area. A mini-

monoclonal spike may be obscured by the normal components of the electrophoretic pattern in some disorders[6,50] and occasionally may be broad and resemble a polyclonal increase in immunoglobulins. Other clues to a possible PCD on the SPEP include a low total gamma globulin level, an elevated alpha-2 globulin level, and a low albumin level, usually in the presence of the nephrotic syndrome. In cases in which a spike is seen on SPEP and in all cases in which a monoclonal gammopathy is suspected but not seen on SPEP, such as idiopathic polyneuropathy or atypical motor neuron disease, immunoelectrophoresis (IEP) or immunofixation (IF) should be performed. These tests are more sensitive for the presence of a small M-protein and allow characterization of the single heavy and light chain, thus verifying the monoclonal nature of the protein. Of the two, IF is more sensitive and detects M-proteins occasionally where IEP is negative but is more expensive and technically more demanding.[11,12] Urine should also be examined for the presence of monoclonal light

TABLE 19.3.   Laboratory tests for multiple myeloma

Hemoglobin/hematocrit
Leukocytes with differential
Platelets
Serum calcium, creatinine, phosphorus, alkaline phosphatase, and uric acid
Serum protein electrophoresis
Quantitation of immunoglobulins
Immunoelectrophoresis and/or immunofixation of serum
Tests for cryoglobulin and viscosity
Bone marrow aspirate and biopsy
Routine urinalysis
Electrophoresis, immunoelectrophoresis, and/or immunofixation of aliquot from a 2 h urine specimen
Roentgenographic skeletal survey including humeri and femurs

Reprinted with permission from Kelly JJ, Kyle RA. Polyneuropathies associated to plasma cell dyscrasias. Martinus-Nijhoff, Boston, 1987.

chains (Bence-Jones proteinuria) because their presence suggests either a malignant plasma cell dyscrasia or light chain amyloidosis. The total protein concentration should be determined in a 24-hour collection. Urine PEP and IEP or IF should then be performed even if the 24-hour collection shows no appreciable proteinuria. The concentrations of serum and urine M-protein should be followed longitudinally because they correlate directly with the body plasma cell burden, and an increase can herald relapse of a ma-

lignancy or the malignant conversion of MGUS syndrome.[10]

After identification and characterization of a M-protein in serum, urine, or both, further studies should be done to classify the PCD (Table 19.3). Following these studies, PCD can be classified into one of the major diagnostic categories based on hematologic criteria[1,12] (Table 19.4). Close cooperation with a hematologist who is familiar with these neurologic syndromes is important. Although general

TABLE 19.4.   Hematologic diagnostic criteria of M-protein syndromes

Syndrome	Anemia	M-protein, Serum	M-protein Urine	Bone Marrow	Skeletal Survey	Tissue Diagnosis
Monoclonal gammopathy of undetermined significance	No	+ *	±	±	Normal	—
Amyloidosis, light-chain type	+/+ +	+ +	+	+	Normal	+ + (amyloid)
Multiple myeloma	+ + +	+ + +†	+ +	+ + +	Abnormal (lytic)	+ + + (myeloma)
Osteosclerotic myeloma	No	+‡	No	±	Abnormal (sclerotic)	+ + + (sclerotic myeloma)
Waldenström's macroglobulinemia	+ + +	+ + +†	±	+ +/+ + +	±	—
Gamma heavy-chain disease	+ + +	+	+	+ +	Normal	—

± = Equivocal or occasional; + = rare or mildly abnormal; + + = common or moderately abnormal; + + + = almost always or severely abnormal.
* Less than 3 g/dl.
† More than 3 g/dl.
‡ Almost always lambda light chain.

TABLE 19.5. Features of polyneuropathy in M-protein syndromes

Type of Polyneuropathy	Topography	Weakness	Sensory Loss	Autonomic Loss	Course	Cerebrospinal Fluid Protein	Pathology	EMG
Monoclonal gammopathy of undetermined significance (IgG, IgA)	Distal, rarely proximal	++	++	+	Chronic	++	SD AD	Mildly slow CV
Amyloidosis, light-chain type	Distal symmetric	+/++	+++	+	Chronic	+	AD	Mildly slow CV
Multiple myeloma	Variable							
Osteosclerotic myeloma	Distal, symmetric	+++	++	0	Chronic	++/+++	SD (AD)	Slow CV
Monoclonal gammopathy of undetermined significance	Distal symmetric	++	++	0	Chronic	++	SD	Slow CV
Waldenström's macroglobulinemia	Distal, symmetric	++	++	0	Chronic	++	SD	Slow CV

AD, Axonal degeneration; CV, conduction velocity; SD, segmental demyelination.

± = Equivocal or occasional; + = rare or mildly abnormal; + + = common or moderately abnormal; + + + = almost always or severely abnormal.

knowledge of these disorders is increasing, often hematologists are conservative in their evaluation of these patients, especially those with low levels of M-protein and no other feature to suggest serious hematologic disease. Hematologists must be encouraged to evaluate these patients aggressively. More detailed information on the hematologic characteristics of these syndromes can be found in other sources.[11,12]

TYPES OF POLYNEUROPATHY

Monoclonal Gammopathy of Undetermined Significance

Most polyneuropathy patients with a M-protein have no evidence of a serious underlying PCD after hematologic evaluation, and their disorder is called *MGUS.*[1] Although formerly known as benign monoclonal gammopathy, prolonged follow-up of these patients reveals that 19% eventually convert to a malignant PCD; hence the new designation.[10,11]

The polyneuropathy of MGUS (Table 19.5), although heterogeneous, resembles that of chronic inflammatory demyelinating polyradiculoneuropathy (CIDP)[13] in many patients, with distal or proximal muscle weakness, large-fiber sensory loss, high cerebrospinal fluid protein levels, and moderate slowing of conduction velocities[14] (Tables 19.6 and 19.7). These patients have variable degrees of axonal loss

on electromyography (EMG), as evidenced by low-amplitude or absent compound muscle action potentials and compound sensory nerve action potentials and acute and chronic denervation predominantly in distal muscles.[17] Histopathologic studies of biopsied peripheral nerves reveal a mixture of demyelination and axonal degeneration, with the former usually predominating.[14,16] Other patients have a neuropathy that electrophysiologically and morphologically appears to be primarily due to axonal degeneration, with distal, symmetric involvement; low amplitude compound muscle action potentials and compound sensory nerve action potentials on nerve stimulation; minimal slowing of conduction velocities; and prominent evidence of distal denervation on needle EMG.[14,17]

It has been discovered that a large number of patients with MGUS-associated polyneuropathy, almost all IgM-MG, display antinerve activity in their M-protein fraction.[7,8] The most frequent of this group is the antibody activity against MAG, a glycoprotein with neural adhesion properties located on the myelin sheaths of peripheral nervous system and central nervous system myelin.[7–9,18] In several studies, about 50% or more of the polyneuropathies associated with IgM M-proteins have had anti-MAG activity.[9,19,20,22] Other antinerve antibodies are much less common.[8,22,23]

The anti-MAG antibody syndrome, originally described by Latov et al.,[7] is now well characterized. These patients present with the slow and insidious

TABLE 19.6. Nerve conduction studies in monoclonal gammopathy polyneuropathy

Type Polyneuropathy	Conducting Velocity <60%†	DL‡	Block	CTS§	F wave >F Est	Axonal	Demyelinated	Indeterminate
MGUS-PN (n = 9)*	3/9	6/9	2/9	2/9	2/7‖	1	3	5
SM-PN (n = 15)	13/15	11/15	10/15	3/15	8/9‖	0	14	1
PSA-PN (n = 27)	3/27	6/27	0/27	8/27	0/0‖	21	2	4

* n = Number of patients in group.

† 2 or more motor nerves with CV < 60% mean normal CV for nerve.

‡ DL of 2 or more motor nerves prolonged.

§ Median motor DL > 1.8 ms longer than ulnar motor DL.

‖ = Number in denominator had measurable F wave elicited.

MGUS-PN, Monoclonal gammopathy of undetermined significance; Reprinted with permission from Kelly JJ Jr. The electrodiagnostic findings in peripheral neuropathy associated with monoclonal gammopathy. Muscle Nerve 1983; 6:504–509.

onset, after months to years, of progressive ascending numbness and gait ataxia, usually without pain.[9,19] Intention tremor may be prominent in some. Weakness is usually much less pronounced, and indeed, early on, the clinical picture may resemble the sensory neuronopathy syndrome, with predominant discriminatory sensory loss with preserved power. Areflexia is the rule. Clues to the diagnosis in this setting are palpably thickened and enlarged nerves,[19] best felt over the neurovascular bundle in the upper arm, and slowing of motor conduction velocity (with prolonged distal latencies) in the *demyelinating* range,[15,24] despite the fact that strength is relatively preserved in these patients. Indeed, a detailed study of electromyographic findings in patients with IgM-MG associated polyneuropathy showed that although anti-MAG polyneuropathy patients presented with a demyelinating picture, MAG-nonreactive patients had more diverse findings with an axonal pattern most commonly[15] (Table 19.8; Figure 19.1). Others, however, have had difficulty separating these two groups electrophysiologically or clinically.[57,58] Cerebrospinal fluid examination may disclose increased protein (>100 mg/dl) in advanced cases of anti-MAG polyneuropathy. The keys of diagnosis in laboratory studies include nerve biopsy and serologic studies. Nerve biopsy shows combined axonal degeneration and demyelinating features, and

TABLE 19.7. Major electrodiagnostic features of monoclonal gammopathy polyneuropathy

	Demyelinating	Axonal	CTS*	Pure Sensory	Other†
MGUS-PN	+ +	+			+ +
SM-PN	+ + +	±			±
PSA-PN	+	+ + +	+ +		±
MM-PN	+	+ +	+ +	+	+ +

MGUS-PN = Monoclonal gammopathy of undetermined significance with polyneuropathy

SM-PN = Osteosclerotic myeloma with polyneuropathy

PSA-PN = primary systemic amyloidosis

MM-PN = Multiple myeloma

* Carpal tunnel syndrome superimposed on polyneuropathy.

† Other findings and nonclassifiable electromyographic studies.

± = possible but unlikely; + = can occur; + + = occurs moderately frequently; + + + = the rule in this disorder.

Reprinted with permission from Kelly JJ Jr. The electrodiagnostic findings in peripheral neuropathy associated with monoclonal gammopathy. Muscle Nerve 1983; 6:504–509.

TABLE 19.8.   Median motor nerve conduction values in demyelinative range*

	Conduction velocity slow	Increased DL	Increased F	Disp/block	Demyel. study†
MAG-reactive	3/7	6/7	2/7 0/7	2/7	7/7
MAG-nonreactive	1/7	1/7	1 = NR	1/7	1/7

CV = conduction velocity
DL = Distal latency
F = F-wave
Disp = Dispersion
Demyel = demyelinating
Reprinted with permission from Kelly JJ Jr. The electrodiagnostic finidings in polyneuropathies associated with IgM monoclonal gammopathies. Muscle Nerve 1990; 13:113–117.

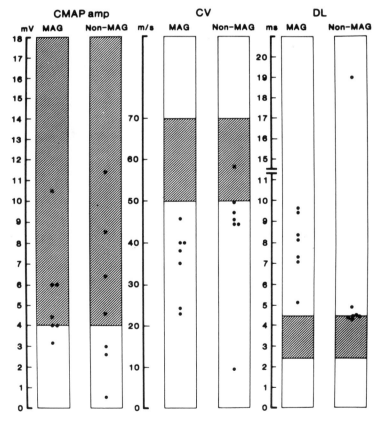

FIGURE 19.1.   *Median motor nerve conduction study results are presented and contrasted in the myelin associated glycoprotein (MAG)–reactive (MAG) group and the MAG-nonreactive (non-MAG) group. The normal range for each function is shown by the shaded area. Note that although the compound muscle action potential amplitudes are relatively similar, at least in mean value, the conduction velocities and distal latencies are much more abnormal in the MAG group. (Reprinted with permission from Kelly JJ Jr. The electrodiagnostic findings in polyneuropathies associated with IgM monoclonal gammopathies. Muscle Nerve 1990; 13:113–117.)*

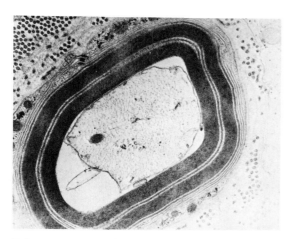

FIGURE 19.2. *Splitting of the outer lamellae of the myelin sheath of a myelinated nerve fiber in a case of anti-MAG polyneuropathy. (Courtesy of Lester S. Adelman, M.D.)*

most patients display positive immunostaining of the nerve for the M-protein, which is deposited on the surface of the myelin sheaths.[20,21,25] Ultrastructural studies show splitting and widening of the outer lamellae of myelin (Figure 19.2), presumably owing

to complement-dependent[26] myelin disadhesion activity of the anti-MAG antibodies.[9,20] Immunoblot and enzyme-linked immunosorbent assay (ELISA) studies demonstrate the anti-MAG antibodies in high titers in serum.[18] Recognition of these patients is important because aggressive treatment aimed at lowering anti-MAG levels with plasmapheresis or cytotoxic drugs promotes recovery in most[7,9,19] (Figure 19.3).

As already mentioned, most of the IgMMAG-nonreactive patients have axonal polyneuropathy by EMG,[15] but some have a demyelinating pattern and are difficult to distinguish from anti-MAG polyneuropathy.[57,58] In a minority, the M-protein may react with other nerve antigens.[22,23] In most, no antinerve antibody activity can be demonstrated, immunofluorescent studies are negative, and myelin splitting is not observed. These patients may, however, respond to treatment with steroids, plasmapheresis, or immunosuppressants/cytotoxics[19] and may represent variants of CIDP.

The nature of IgG and IgA M-proteins associated with polyneuropathy is much less clear. Many of these patients have axonal polyneuropathies that are chronic and mild.[1,27] Antinerve antibody activity is rarely demonstrated,[8,27,28] and these patients do not respond to therapy. It is important to exclude amy-

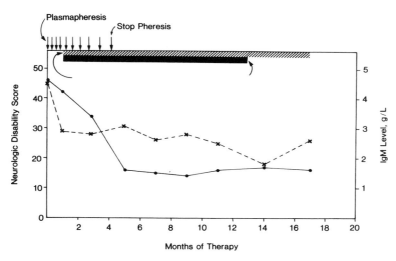

FIGURE 19.3. *Results of treatment in a 62-year-old man with anti-MAG polyneuropathy. At the beginning of treatment, he was moderately disabled with a Neurologic Disability Score (•) of 46. Plasmapheresis was performed at each vertical arrow and medication began as indicated. He rapidly improved concomitant with lowering of the IgM level (x), which remained low on medication after plasmapheresis was stopped. The shaded bar indicates prednisone (100 mg every other day) and the solid bar cyclophosphamide (125 mg/day). (Reprinted with permission from Kelly JJ Jr, Adelman LS, Berkman E, et al. Polyneuropathies associated with IgM monoclonal gammopathies. Arch Neurol 1988; 45:1355–1359.*

loidosis (see later), however, in these patients, especially those with recent onset, rapid progression, pain, autonomic symptoms, or systemic features. Less commonly, these patients have a CIDP-like picture with evidence of demyelination on EMG. In these, osteosclerotic myeloma and the Crow-Fukase syndrome (see later) should be excluded by appropriate tests.

Amyloidosis (Light-Chain Type)

Amyloidosis is a devastating disease and extremely variable in its clinical presentation.[29,30] It typically affects elderly men past the sixth decade of life and can present with pure neurologic involvement, with involvement of multiple organ systems, or both.[29–32] Involvement of multiple organ systems (Table 19.9), which typically affects renal, gastrointestinal, cardiac, and hematologic systems, often suggests an underlying malignancy or collagen vascular disease. The discovery of the serum M-protein, which is present in most patients, or the recognition of the distinctive neuropathy, which occurs in about 15% of these patients, often aids diagnosis.

The neuropathy[30,31] is sensory dominant with prominent early loss of small fiber function (nociceptive, thermesthetic, and autonomic) followed by progressive weakness and large fiber (discriminative sensation) loss. Autonomic symptoms are often severe and disabling, as is the pain associated with degeneration of the small unmyelinated nociceptive fibers. Diagnosis is confirmed by discovery of amyloid on tissue biopsy.[29] Pathology reveals amyloid deposition in peripheral nerve, although the exact mechanism of nerve fiber degeneration is unclear.[2,12,30,31] The prognosis for these patients is poor, with progressive decline leading to death in 1 to 3 years (Figure 19.4),[29–32] unaffected by therapy with steroids, plasmapheresis, or cytotoxic drugs.[30,33]

EMG is useful in the evaluation of these patients.[27,30] The pattern of findings is often distinctive, and in the appropriate setting, it can help to suggest

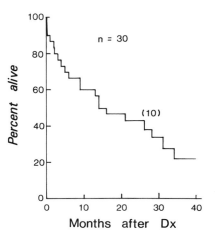

FIGURE 19.4.   *Mortality in patients with amyloid polyneuropathy. (Reprinted from Kelly JJ Jr, Kyle RA, O'Brien PC, et al. The natural history of peripheral neuropathy in primary systemic amyloidosis. Ann Neurol 1979; 5:271–287.)*

the diagnosis. Typical findings on EMG show evidence of symmetric axonal degeneration (Figure 19.5) with minimal slowing of conduction velocities and low-amplitude compound muscle action potentials with absent or severely reduced compound sensory nerve action potentials.[27,30] Needle EMG examination findings are those of distal chronic and acute denervation with variable reinnervation. Occasionally amyloid can also infiltrate proximal muscles and cause a myopathy with characteristic motor unit action potential changes.[34] The picture of distal axonal neuropathy and proximal myopathy can mimic the syndromes occurring with malignancies, but sural nerve and proximal muscle biopsies with appropriate histochemical preparation and staining for amyloid are diagnostic. In vivo intraneural recordings of small fiber and autonomic axon action potentials can be valuable in these patients, but such recordings are usually not of practical diagnostic assistance because the findings are not yet well established, and the technique is available only in a few centers. Another helpful clue to diagnosis, which occurs in 25% of the amyloid patients, is the carpal tunnel syndrome caused by amyloid infiltration of the flexor retinaculum of the wrist.[29–31]

Multiple Myeloma

The neuropathy of multiple myeloma is heterogeneous and rare, occurring in less than 5% of cases.[5] Most patients have a mild, distal axonal polyneu-

TABLE 19.9.   Medical syndromes in amyloid polyneuropathy

Orthostatic hypotension	42%
Nephrotic syndrome	23%
Cardiac failure	23%
Malabsorption	16%

Reproduced with permission from Kelly JJ Jr, Kyle RA, Latov N. Polyneuropathies associated with plasma cell dyscrasias. Boston: Martinus-Nijhoff, 1987.

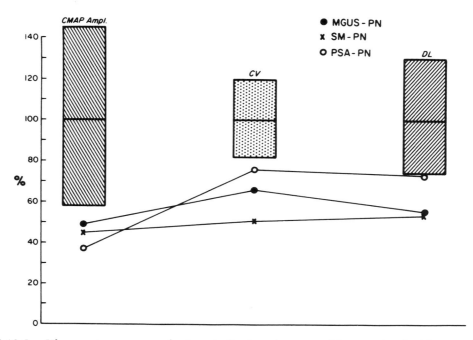

FIGURE 19.5. *Ulnar motor nerve conduction studies in polyneuropathies associated with monoclonal gammopathies: Group mean values and range of normal values are expressed as a percentage of the normal mean value except for DL, where reciprocals were used. SM, Osteosclerotic myeloma; PSA, primary systemic amyloidosis. (Reprinted with permission from Kelly JJ Jr. The electrodiagnostic findings in peripheral neuropathy associated with monoclonal gammopathy. Muscle Nerve 1983; 6:504–509.)*

ropathy. Rare patients have an acute or chronic demyelinating polyradiculoneuropathy or a sensory neuronopathy. These neuropathies and their electromyographic findings seem similar to those occurring with other cancers. In one series of patients with multiple myeloma and polyneuropathy,[5] about two-thirds of the patients had amyloid neuropathy, and in these cases, the clinical and electromyographic findings for the most part resembled those in amyloidosis without myeloma.[30,31] In all cases of multiple myeloma and polyneuropathy, superimposed root or polyradicular syndromes can overshadow or confuse the clinical picture and have to be carefully delineated by EMG and other studies. The frequency of asymmetric root lesions in these patients probably accounts for the often mentioned occurrence of mononeuropathy multiplex in myeloma, which we have rarely seen in our patients except for the median neuropathy associated with amyloidosis.

Osteosclerotic Myeloma

These patients have a neuropathy and clinical course radically different from typical multiple myeloma

patients.[6,35–37] The underlying hematologic disease is often indolent and is discovered fortuitously by an alert radiologist or neurologist. The osteosclerotic lesions (solitary and multiple) affect only the truncal skeleton and proximal limbs, sparing the skull, and are often mistaken for benign lesions (Figure 19.6). The diagnosis can also be suggested by discovery of a serum M-protein, discovery of IgG or IgA and nearly always lambda light chain, and recognition of the distinctive polyneuropathy. Some of these patients develop a dramatic syndrome of organomegaly and polyendocrinopathy, which can also suggest the diagnosis (Table 19.10). This is often referred to as the POEMS syndrome (polyneuropathy, organomegaly, endocrinopathy, M-protein, skin involvement)[36] or, perhaps more properly, the Crow-Fukase syndrome.[39] Confirmation requires biopsy of suspicious bony lesions. Recognition of this syndrome is important because treatment of the majority of solitary lesions with radiation therapy[6,37] and of some of the multiple-lesion patients with chemotherapy can result in dramatic improvement. Most investigators believe that the monoclonal immunoglobulin causes the syndrome.[6,42]

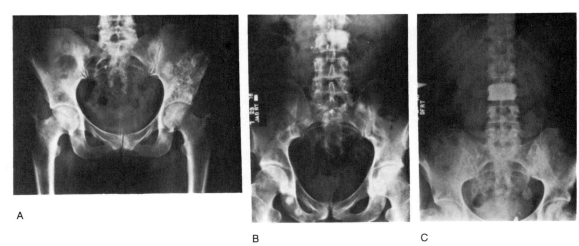

FIGURE 19.6.   *Bone lesions from three patients with osteosclerotic myeloma. (A) Patient has a mixed sclerotic and lytic solitary lesion of the iliac wing. (B) Patient has multiple sclerotic lesions affecting the L-1 and L-2 vertebra and the right pubic ramus. (C) Patient has a solitary sclerotic lesion affecting the L-3 vertebra (ivory vertebra). (Reprinted with permission from Kelly JJ Jr, Kyle RA, Miles JM, et al. Osteosclerotic myeloma and peripheral neuropathy. Neurology (NY) 1983; 33:202–210.)*

The neuropathy of osteosclerotic myeloma is chronic and symmetric, with a distal to proximal spread.[6] It is slowly and relentlessly progressive and affects large fiber populations, causing severe weakness and large fiber discriminative sensory loss. Cerebrospinal fluid protein levels are usually high (>100 mg/dl), and nerve biopsies reveal a combination of demyelination and axonal degeneration. Electromyographic studies[6,27] reveal marked slowing of motor and sensory conduction velocities with prolonged distal latencies and reduced compound muscle action potential and compound sensory nerve action potential amplitudes (Figure 19.5). Needle electrode examination reveals distal and symmetric acute and chronic neurogenic changes. This disorder is probably a polyradiculoneuropathy because cerebrospinal fluid protein levels are high and somatosensory evoked potential studies[38] have shown slowing proximally across root segments. Histopathologic data, unverified as yet, however, suggest that axonal degeneration may be primary with secondary demyelination.[40] For practical purposes, however, this is a demyelinating polyneuropathy.

Miscellaneous Syndromes

Waldenström's macroglobulinemia

It is sometimes difficult to separate Waldenström's macroglobulinemia from IgM-MGUS, and the latter may evolve into Waldenström's macroglobulinemia over time.[10] Thus similar polyneuropathy syndromes occur.[9,20,41] The most frequent polyneuropathy encountered is that associated with anti-MAG antibodies.[9,20] This syndrome has the same features and clinical course as in nonmalignant IgM-MGUS. Other patients have a CIDP-like picture, a distal axonal neuropathy, typical amyloid polyneuropathy, or even the sensory neuronopathy syndrome usually seen with small cell cancer of the lung.

Cryoglobulinemia

Cryoglobulins are immunoglobulins that precipitate in cool blood often in association with immune complexes, usually in blood vessels of distal limbs.[43] This disorder is divided into three types.[43] In type 1, the M-protein itself is a cryoglobulin in the setting of a PCD. In type 2, the cryoglobulin is a mixture of a M-protein, usually IgM, and polyclonal immunoglobulins, usually occurring in the setting of a lymphoproliferative disorder. Type 3 occurs in the setting of a collagen vascular or other chronic inflammatory disease, and the cryoglobulin consists wholly of polyclonal immunoglobulins. The polyneuropathy in all these syndromes is painful, symmetric or asymmetric, sensorimotor and axonal in nature. Purpura occurs in distal limbs in a high percentage of patients, and the neuropathy is generally considered to be due to a vasculopathy or vasculitis

TABLE 19.10. Nonneurologic abnormalities in patients with osteosclerotic myeloma

	Patient															
	1	2	3	4	5	6	7	8	9	10	11	12	13	14	15	16
Sex	M	M	M	F	M	F	M	M	F	F	M	F	M	M	M	F
Abnormality																
Gynecomastia	+												+			
Hepatomegaly		+	+	+		+	+						+			
Splenomegaly			+			+										
Hyperpigmentation		+						+	+				+			+
Edema		+	+					+								
Lymphadenopathy		+		+												
Papilledema			+	+			+							+		
Digital clubbing		+									+		+			
White nails													+			
Hypertrichosis		+						+					+			+
Atrophic testes								+					+	+		
Impotence		+						+					+	+		
Polycythemia	+					+			+			+				+
Leukocytosis	+										+			+		
Thrombocytosis	+		+			+	+		+	+	+	+	+	+	+	+
Low plasma testosterone		+		+				+					+	+		
High serum estrogen		+						+					+			
Low serum thyroxine		+												+		
Hyperglycemia			+													

Reprinted with permission from Kelly JJ Jr, Kyle RA, Miles JM, et al. Osteosclerotic myeloma and peripheral neuropathy. Neurology (NY) 1983; 33:202–210.

of skin and vasa nervorum. These is one case report, however, of a patient with polyneuropathy and IgM M-protein with anti-MAG activity and cryoglobulinemia with vasculitis.[9]

Gamma-heavy chain disease

This condition, often referred to as Franklin's disease, is a rare malignant PCD that has been associated with the Guillain-Barré syndrome.[44]

Lymphoma, leukemia, cancer

These disorders can be associated with MG and polyneuropathy. In lymphoma with IgM M-protein, the IgM may have anti-MAG activity with the usual clinical and pathologic features. Other syndomes without clear antinerve activity in the M-protein fraction may respond to ablation of the malignancy.[19] Still others have an unclear relation to lowering of the M-protein concentration in serum.

Angiofollicular lymph node hyperplasia (Castleman's disease)

This is a peculiar, nonmalignant syndrome with lymphatic hyperplasia that can be localized to one site

(usually thoracic) or generalized.[45] The generalized type may be associated with polyclonal or monoclonal gammopathy and systemic features. There are occasional reports of a polyneuropathy in some cases with systemic features characteristic of the POEMS or Crow-Fukase syndrome.[46,47,50] The neuropathy resembles closely that seen in osteosclerotic myeloma, with prominent slowing of conduction velocities suggesting a prominent demyelinating component. Treatment by resection of localized hyperplastic tissue or treatment with chemotherapy can yield remission.

Motor neuropathy with antiganglioside antibodies

Antiganglioside antibodies in increased titers have been found in a high percentage of patients with syndromes variously termed *motor neuropathy, motor neuronopathy,* or *motor neuron disease.*[48–51] Some of these patients have M-proteins,[50] but the majority have polyclonal antibody activity directed at ganglioside epitopes.[48,49] This syndrome, as opposed to classic ALS, has generally no bulbar or upper motor neuron findings.[51] Patients are normoreflexic or areflexic and have a peculiar, asymmetric, at times mononeuropathic distribution to their weakness, mainly affecting the arms, with little or no sensory findings.[51] Elevated antiganglioside antibodies, however, have also been described in some patients with a clinical picture said to be consistent with amyotrophic lateral sclerosis.[99] EMG is of great importance in the detection of these patients. Typically there is normal or near-normal conduction in most motor and sensory nerves.[51,53–56] With proximal stimulation, especially in the arms, there is a marked drop in compound muscle action potential amplitude with or without dispersion of the potential, suggesting either a focal conduction block or demyelination without block.[51,54–56] The cases we have seen would not be mistaken for classic amyotrophic lateral sclerosis,[51] although others report that some are indistinguishable. Not all patients with this clinical and electromyographic picture have antiganglioside antibodies, however. This syndrome is important to recognize because some of these patients respond to immunosuppression.

CONCLUSION

The area of PCD and neuromuscular disease has been a field of active research over the last decade or so. These patients are of great importance to recognize because treatment may lead to remission. Also, careful study of these patients may lead to a better understanding of the pathogenesis of polyneuropathies and possibly motor neuron disease, which may bring about effective treatment for conditions for which there are now no effective treatments. The neuromuscular electrophysiologist clearly has a prominent role in the recognition and management of these patients.

REFERENCES

1. Kelly JJ Jr, Kyle RA, O'Brien PC, Dyck PJ. Prevalence of monoclonal protein in peripheral neuropathy. Neurology 1981; 31:1480–1483.
2. Kelly JJ Jr. Peripheral neuropathies associated with monoclonal proteins: A clinical review. Muscle Nerve 1985; 8:138–150.
3. Kyle RA, Finkelstein S, Elveback LR, Kurland LT. Incidence of monoclonal proteins in a Minnesota community with a cluster or multiple myeloma. Blood 1972; 40:719–724.
4. Glenner GG, Terry W, Harada M, et al. Amyloid fibril proteins: Proof of homology with immunoglobulin light chains by sequence analysis. Science 1971; 172:1150–1151.
5. Kelly JJ Jr, Kyle RA, Miles JM, et al. The spectrum of peripheral neuropathy in myeloma. Neurology (NY) 1981;31:24.
6. Kelly JJ Jr, Kyle RA, Miles JM, et al. Osteosclerotic myeloma and peripheral neuropathy. Neurology (NY) 1983; 33:202–210.
7. Latov N, Sherman WH, Nemni R, et al. Plasma cell dyscrasia and peripheral neuropathy with a monoclonal antibody to peripheral nerve myelin. N Engl J Med 1980; 303:618–621.
8. Steck AJ, Murray N, Dellagi K, et al. Peripheral neuropathy associated with monoclonal IgM autoantibody. Ann Neurol 1987; 22:764–767.
9. Latov N, Hays AP, Sherman WH. Peripheral neuropathy and anti-MAG antibodies. CRC Crit Rev Neurobiol 1988; 3:301–332.
10. Kyle RA. Monoclonal gammopathy of undetermined significance: Natural history in 241 cases. Am J Med 1978; 64:814–826.
11. Kyle RA. Plasma cell dyscrasias. *In* Spitell JA Jr, ed. Clinical medicine. Philadelphia: Harper & Row; 1981:1–35.
12. Kelly JJ Jr, Kyle RA, Latov N. Polyneuropathies associated with plasma cell dyscrasias. Boston: Martinus-Nijhoff, 1987.
13. Dyck PJ, Lais AC, Ohta M, et al. Chronic inflammatory polyradiculoneuropathy. Mayo Clin Proc 1975; 50:621–637.
14. Dalakas MC, Engel WK. Polyneuropathy with monoclonal gammopathy. Ann Neurol 1981; 10:45–52.
15. Kelly JJ Jr. The electrodiagnostic findings in polyneuropathies associated with IgM monoclonal gammopathies. Muscle Nerve 1990; 13:113–117.
16. Donofrio PD, Kelly JJ Jr. AAEE Case Report #17: Peripheral neuropathy in monoclonal gammopathy of undetermined significance. Muscle Nerve 1989; 12:1–8.
17. Kelly JJ Jr. The electrodiagnostic findings in peripheral neuropathy associated with monoclonal gammopathy. Muscle Nerve 1983; 6:504–509.
18. Nobile-Orazio E, Francomano E, Daverio R, et al. Antimyelin-associated glycoprotein IgM antibody titers in neuropathy associated with macroglobulinemia. Ann Neurol 1989; 26:543–550.
19. Kelly JJ Jr, Adelman LS, Berkman E, et al. Polyneuropathies associated with IgM monoclonal gammopathies. Arch Neurol 1988; 45:1355–1359.
20. Vital A, Vital C, Julien J, et al. Polyneuropathy associated with IgM monoclonal gammopathy: Immu-

nological and pathological study in 31 patients. Acta Neuropathol 1989; 79:160–167.

21. Nemmi R, Galassi G, Latov N, et al. Polyneuropathy in nonmalignant IgM plasma cell dyscrasia: A morphological study. Ann Neurol 1983; 14:43–54.

22. Pestronk A, Li F, Griffin J, et al. Antibodies to myelin-associated glycoprotein and sulfatide in predominantly sensory polyneuropathy (abstr.). Ann Neurol 1990; 28:239.

23. Sherman WH, Latov NH, Hays AP, et al. Monoclonal IgMk antibody precipitating with chondroitin sulfate C from patients with axonal polyneuropathy and epidermolysis. Neurology (NY) 1983; 33:192–201.

24. Nobile-Orazio E, Marmiroli P, Baldini L, et al. Peripheral neuropathy in macroglobulinemia: Incidence and antigen specificity of M-proteins. Neurology 1987; 37:1506–1514.

25. Takatsu H, Hays AP, Latov N, et al. Immunofluorescence study of patients with neuropathy and IgM M-proteins. Ann Neurol 1985; 18:173–181.

26. Monaco S, Benette B, Ferrari S, et al. Complement-mediated demyelination in patients with IgM monoclonal gammopathy and polyneuropathy. N Engl J Med 1990; 52:322.

27. Nemni R, Foltri ML, Fazio R, et al. Axonal neuropathy with monoclonal IgG kappa that binds to a neurofilament protein. Ann Neurol 1990; 28:361–364.

28. Sadiq SA, Thomas FP, Kilidreas K, et al. The spectrum of neurologic disease associated with anti-GM1 antibodies. Neurology 1990; 40:1067–1072.

29. Kyle RA, Bayrd ED. Amyloidosis: Review of 236 cases. Medicine (Balt) 1975; 54:271–299.

30. Kelly JJ Jr, Kyle RA, O'Brien PC, et al. The natural history of peripheral neuropathy in primary systemic amyloidosis. Ann Neurol 1979; 5:271–287.

31. Trotter JL, Engel WK, Ignaszak TF. Amyloidosis with plasma cell dyscrasia: An overlooked cause of adult onset sensorimotor neuropathy. Arch Neurol 1977; 34:209–214.

32. Duston MA, Skinner M, Anderson J, et al. Peripheral neuropathy as an early marker of amyloidosis. Arch Intern Med 1989; 149:358–360.

33. Dalakas MC, Gertz MA, Olson LJ, et al. Cardiac amyloidosis. N Engl J Med 1988; 318:641–642.

34. Whitaker JN, Hashimoto K, Quinones M. Skeletal muscle hypertrophy in primary amyloidosis. Neurology 1977; 27:47–54.

35. Iwashita H, Ohnishi A, Asada M, et al. Polyneuropathy, skin hyperpigmentation, edema and hypertrichosis in localized osteosclerotic myeloma. Neurology 1977; 27:675–681.

36. Bardwick PA, Zvaifler NJ, Gill GN, et al. Plasma cell dyscrasia with polyneuropathy, organomegaly, endocrinopathy, M-protein and skin changes: The POEMS syndrome. Medicine (Balt) 1980; 59:311–322.

37. Davis LE, Drachman DB. Myeloma neuropathy: Successful treatment of two patients and review of cases. Arch Neurol 1972; 27:507–511.

38. Shibasaki H, Ohnishi A, Kuroiwa Y. Use of SEP's to localize degeneration in a rare polyneuropathy: Studies on polyneuropathy associated with pigmentation, hypertrichosis, edema and plasma cell dyscrasia. Ann Neurol 1982; 12:355–360.

39. Nakanishi T, Sobue I, Toyokura Y, et al. The Crow-Fukase syndrome: A study of 102 cases in Japan. Neurology 1984; 34:712–720.

40. Ohi T, Nukada H, Kyle RA, et al. Detection of an axonal abnormality in myeloma neuropathy (abstr.). Ann Neurol 1983; 14:120.

41. Dayan AD, Lewis PD. Demyelinating neuropathy in Waldenström's macroglobulinemia. Neurology (Minn) 1966; 16:1141–1144.

42. Reulecke M, Dumas M, Meier C. Specific antibody activity against neuroendocrine tissue in a case of POEMS syndrome with IgG gammopathy. Neurology 1988; 38:614–616.

43. Chad O, Pariser K, Bradley WG, et al. The pathogenesis of cryoglobulinemic neuropathy. Neurology (NY) 1982; 32:725–729.

44. Kyle RA, Greipp PR, Banks PM. The diverse picture of gamma heavy-chain disease. Mayo Clin Proc 1981; 56:439–451.

45. Yood RA, Fienberg R. Case studies of the Massachusetts General Hospital: Case #42-1989. N Engl J Med 1989; 321:1103–1118.

46. Hineman VL, Phyliky RL, Banks PM: Angiofollicular lymph node hyperplasia and peripheral neuropathy: Association with monoclonal gammopathy. Mayo Clin Proc 1982; 57:379–382.

47. Donaghy M, Hall P, Jawler J, et al. Peripheral neuropathy associated with Castleman's disease. J Neurol Sci 1989; 89:253–267.

48. Pestronk A, Adams RN, Cornblath D, et al. Serum antibodies to GM$_1$ ganglioside in ALS. Neurology 1988; 38:1457–1461.

49. Pestronk A, Cornblath DR, Ilyas AA, et al. A treatable multifocal motor neuropathy with antibodies to GM1 ganglioside. Ann Neurol 1988; 24:73–78.

50. Freddo L, Yu RK, Latov N, et al. Gangliosides GM1 and GD1b are antigens for IgM M-protein in a patient with motor neuron disease. Neurology 1986; 36:4554–4558.

51. Hollander D, Kelly JJ. EMG findings in anti-GM$_1$ motor neuropathy (Abstr). Muscle Nerve 1990; 13:854.

52. Feigert JM, Sweet DL, Coleman M, et al. Multicentric angiofollicular lymph node hyperplasia with peripheral neuropathy, pseudotumor cerebri, IgA dysproteinemia and thrombocytosis in women: a distinct syndrome. Ann Intern Med 1990; 113:362–367.

53. Parry GJ, Holtz SJ, Ben-Zeev D, et al. Gammopathy with proximal motor axonopathy simulating motor neuron disease. Neurology 1986; 36:273–276.

54. Lange DJ, Blake DM, Hirano M, et al. Multifocal conduction block motor neuropathy: Diagnostic value of stimulating cervical roots (abstr.). Neurology 1990; 40(suppl 1):182.

55. Trojaborg W, Lange DJ, Sumner AJ, et al. Conduction

block and other abnormalities of nerve conduction in motor neuron disease: A review of 110 patients (abstr.). Neurology 1990; 40:(suppl):182.

56. Krarup C, Stewart JD, Sumner AJ, et al. A syndrome of asymmetric limb weakness with motor conduction block. Neurology 1990; 40:118–127.

57. Gosslin S, Kyle RA, Dyck PJ. Neuropathy associated with monoclonal gammopathy of undetermined significance. Ann Neurol 1991; 30:54–61.

58. Surarez G, Kelly JJ Jr. Polyneuropathy associated with monoclonal gammopathy of undetermined significance. Neurology (in press).

20

Acute and Chronic Inflammatory Demyelinating Neuropathies

William F. Brown

CONTENTS

LIST OF ACRONYMS

GBS	Guillain Barré syndrome
M	surface recorded maximum compound action potential
MDL	motor distal latency
MMCV	maximum motor conduction velocity
MSCV	maximum sensory conduction velocity
DL	distal latency
SNAP	sensory nerve action potential

Demyelinating neuropathies are neuropathies in which the primary attack is on the myelin sheath. Causes include hereditary defects in laying down or maintaining the myelin sheath, biochemical defects, and immunologic and toxic mechanisms (Table 20.1) Many are associated with some degree of axonal degeneration. The pathophysiology of these neuropathies is best understood by reviewing the normal biophysical role of the myelin sheath.[1]

Conduction is saltatory in normal myelinated nerve fibers, generation of action potentials being confined to successive nodes of Ranvier. The high transverse resistance and low capacitance characteristics of the internode, conferred by the myelin sheath, greatly reduce transverse leakage of the internal longitudinal current. The latter precedes the action potential, and if conduction is to proceed, sufficient internal longitudinal current must remain to depolarize the next node or two of Ranvier beyond threshold for generating an action potential. The cable properties of the internode impose a delay of 20 µs between the times at which action potentials are generated at successive nodes of Ranvier in large myelinated nerve fibers.

Paranodal and internodal demyelination increase the transverse capacitance and reduce the resistance of the internode, resulting in some instances in greatly increased transverse leakage of the internal longitudinal current preceding the action potential.[1,2] Such increased transverse current leakage may delay generation of the impulse at the next node of Ranvier by as much as 10 times. Beyond the latter point, insufficient internal longitudinal current may remain to depolarize the next node of Ranvier beyond threshold, resulting in impulse block at the preceding node. Paranodal demyelination may be especially important because potassium channels underlie the paranodal myelin sheath.[3,4] Exposure of these channels further reduces the safety factor transmission, an effect that may be reversed by 4-aminopyridine.

TABLE 20.1.   Causes of demyelinating neuropathies

Guillain-Barré syndrome or acute idiopathic inflammatory
   polyneuropathy
Diphtheritic polyneuritis
Chronic inflammatory demyelinating polyneuropathy
Inherited demyelinating neuropathies (see Chapter 15)
Demyelinating neuropathies in association with
   Malignancies (see Chapter 17)
   Plasma cell disorders (see Chapter 19)
   Lupus erythematosis

It should not be surprising therefore to find that most demyelinating neuropathies are characterized by reduced conduction velocities and sometimes conduction block. The latter is uncommon in hereditary demyelinating neuropathies, and the former may be absent early in acute demyelinating neuropathies. Ectopic impulse generation in demyelinated nerve fibers may be responsible for the prickling, tingling, and pain sensations; increased sympathetic activity; occasional fasciculation; and myokymia in human demyelinating neuropathies (see Chapter 5). The inability to transmit high-frequency trains of impulses, another characteristic of demyelinating neuropathies, probably produces no clinical deficit in human demyelinating neuropathies.

Of all the pathophysiologic abnormalities that characterize human demyelinating neuropathies, the most important, from a clinical point of view, are conduction block and axonal degeneration. These two readily account for the paralysis, slowed conduction, and sometimes loss of sensation in these neuropathies. Losses of tendon reflexes and vibratory sense, phenomena probably highly dependent on relatively high degrees of synchronization in their respective afferent volleys, are probably explained by slowed conduction and increased temporal dispersion of the requisite afferent impulses.

GUILLAIN-BARRÉ SYNDROME

Clinical Features

Guillain-Barré syndrome (GBS) is a monophasic, primarily motor polyradiculoneuropathy accompanied by an increase in cerebrospinal fluid protein but usually not cells. For the purposes of clinical trials and multicenter studies, clinical and laboratory criteria have been proposed.[5,6,7,8,9] The paralytic phase is often preceded by an antecedent illness. In some cases, viruses, including Epstein-Barr, cytomegalovirus, hepatitis, and human immunodeficiency virus (HIV), or other infectious agents, such as toxoplasmosis, *Mycoplasma* pneumonia, Lyme disease, and *Campylobacter jejuni* enteritis, have been identified. In still other cases, immunosuppression, Hodgkin's disease,[10] vaccination including rabies vaccine,[11] and even recent surgery[12] have preceded the onset of GBS. By the onset of the paralysis, fever is usually absent.

The course of GBS varies from fulminant, reaching complete paralysis within 1 to 2 days, to more gradual, with over 90% of cases reaching peak paralysis within 4 weeks, before beginning to improve after plateauing for 1 to 14 days. Ten percent to 30% of patients become temporarily respirator dependent. Extraocular muscles may be involved in 10%, facial muscles in over 50%, and bulbar muscles in 10% to 30%. Autonomic involvement is common and featured primarily by fluctuating, sometimes abrupt, hypertension or hypotension; arrhythmias; and disordered sweating. Although sensory symptoms and signs tend to be relatively minor features, pain may be severe in as many as one-third of patients.

The outcome for full clinical recovery is good in most cases, but some residual weakness is common. At 6 months, most patients are able to walk, although 10% are still confined to bed or a wheelchair at this point. In the *axonal* form of the disease, persistent, widespread severe paralysis and wasting usually follow in the wake of the acute paralysis.[13–19] Poor prognostic signs include prolonged delays to recovery, initially rapid evolution, and ventilator dependence,[17] although it must be stressed that these and even severely reduced distal maximum compound muscle action potentials (M potentials) do not preclude satisfactory recovery in some cases.

Five percent of patients relapse. Some of these relapses follow an initial course of plasma exchange, whereas in others the initial event turns out to be the first of several relapses of chronic inflammatory demyelinating polyneuropathy (CIDP). GBS variants are listed in Table 20.2 and described as follows.
1. Mild cases. These are cases in which paralysis is mild, recovering often within a few days, autonomic involvement is absent, and bulborespiratory muscles are spared. Sensory involvement may be limited to minor paresthesia. A high index of suspicion is necessary, but cerebrospinal fluid analysis after 7 to 10 days usually reveals the characteristic albumino-cytologic association. Electrophysiologic studies normally reveal no reduction in conduction velocity in the early brief paretic stage. Conduction slowing, evident at 2 to 4 weeks, is often missed because the

patient recovers and is lost to follow-up.
2. Acute axonal GBS. This uncommon variant is usually ushered in by fulminant development of complete or nearly complete paralysis of all skeletal muscles, including oculobulbar and respiratory muscles, within 1 to 7 days; very reduced or absent distal M potentials, and poor subsequent clinical recovery.[13–19]
3. Painful GBS. Severe pain, often in the back but sometimes more widespread, is a prominent feature in about one-third of cases. The severity of the pain may be so dominant as to confuse and delay the diagnosis for several hours or even days and, if persistent, present a major therapeutic challenge in patients all too often unable to report their pain adequately.
4. Asymmetric or focal onset of paralysis. Strikingly asymmetric or focal onset of paralysis is occasionally seen in GBS. Again, although the paralysis usually evolves in a more symmetric and widespread pattern, the initial asymmetry or focal paralysis broadens the differential diagnosis at the outset and may delay recognition of these cases.
5. Limitation of paralysis to craniobulbar muscles. Patients in whom the paralysis initially involves eyelid, extraocular, facial, and bulbar muscles are sometimes seen with little or no obvious extension to limb or trunk muscles.[7,8,20] Such patients present major clinical and electrodiagnostic challenges because conventional electrodiagnostic tests applied to the limbs may be entirely normal and the tendon reflexes preserved.
6. Miller-Fisher Variant. This syndrome, comprised of external ophthalmoplegia, areflexia, and ataxia, is uncommon in the author's experience.[8]
7. Acute Sensory Polyneuropathy. This form of polyneuropathy is probably an axonal rather than a demyelinating neuropathy.[21]

Cerebrospinal fluid

The protein is raised generally within a week of the onset of the paralysis, but the cell count of the cerebrospinal fluid should not exceed 10 mononuclear cells per mm³. Higher cell counts should prompt a search for HIV infection.

Differential diagnosis

The differential diagnosis includes other causes of acute polyneuropathy, including porphyria,[22] hexa-

TABLE 20.2.   Guillain-Barré variants

Mild GBS
Acute axonal GBS
Painful GBS
Strikingly asymmetric or focal onset GBS
Restricted oculofacial bulbar GBS
Acute sensory neuropathy
Miller-Fisher variant

TABLE 20.3.   Pathology of Guillain-Barré Syndrome

Demyelination—paranodal—segmental and later remyelination[24,25,27]
Axonal shrinkage in demyelinated regions[24]
Distribution[23,24,25]
  Multifocal
  Widespread—uniform or nonuniform
    Involving roots, dorsal root ganglia, plexuses, peripheral nerve trunks, and intramuscular nerve
      preterminals and terminal branches
Axonal degeneration—chromatolysis and/or loss of motor neurons[18,22,24]
Involvement of the sympathetic chains and ganglia
Inflammatory cell infiltrates[24,27]
  Lymphocytic infiltration of epineural and endoneural venules and invasion of endoneurium
  Macrophage mediated myelin breakdown
Edema with no accompanying cellular reaction[25]
  Absent or minimal cellular infiltrates despite myelin breakdown
Axonal variant[18,23]
  Severe—widespread wallerian degeneration with little or no accompanying primary demyelination
    or inflammatory cell infiltrates
  Severe—inflammatory infiltrates and presumed secondary axonal breakdown

---

carbon abuse, dapsone, nitrofurantoin, arsenic poisoning, poliomyelitis, myasthenia gravis, botulism, acute lead poisoning, leukemic infiltration of peripheral nerves, and paraneoplastic syndrome.[7,8,9]

Pathology

The pathology of GBS is summarized in Table 20.3. Early descriptions of the pathology of GBS emphasized edema of nerve roots evident as early as 4 days with little or no cellular reaction.[23] Some swelling and irregularity of the myelin sheaths was present as early as 3 to 5 days, and evidence of chromatolysis of motor neurons was observed as well in some cases.

Asbury et al.[24] extensively examined the peripheral nervous system and found the lesions, in most cases, to be widespread involving motor and sensory roots, dorsal root ganglion, plexuses, peripheral nerve trunks, and even intramuscular branches. Involvement of sympathetic chains in ganglia was also shown. These authors emphasized the widespread multifocal character of the lesions as well as the inflammatory infiltration by macrophages. The latter were shown to invaginate the interperiod line with subsequent breakdown of myelin and demyelination. Axonal shrinkage in demyelinated regions was shown as well as axonal degeneration and in some cases swelling and chromatolysis of motor neurons.

One recently reported study, of a single fulminant patient who died within 6 days of the onset, showed lesions maximally present in the roots, vagus nerve, and median nerve at the elbow and to a much lesser extent in the sciatic nerve and sural nerves.[25] Inflammatory cell reactions were absent or at the most mild, despite clear evidence of breakdown of the myelin sheath. Nerve biopsies from three cases of the acute axonal form of GBS have shown evidence of severe axonal degeneration without any indications of primary demyelination.[15] A fourth case, however, revealed extensive severe demyelination and axonal degeneration, the latter perhaps secondary to the former.

The relative importance of humeral versus cellular factors in the pathogenesis of GBS is unknown. Regions where the blood-nerve or perineural barriers are broken as at sites of focal compression or are naturally deficient may, at the outset of the disease at least, determine the topography of the lesions. The fact that maximum motor and sensory conduction velocities (MMCVs, MSCVs) are often normal early in the course of the disease suggests that segmental demyelination is not widespread but focal or multifocal and, although severe enough at one or more points to block transmission, is not so widespread as to slow conduction noticeably.

Electrophysiologic Features

The clinical and electrophysiologic features of the inflammatory demyelinating neuropathies been thoroughly reviewed.[17,25] Electrodiagnostic studies in GBS are most important early in the course of the disease, when most of the important diagnostic and therapeutic decisions are made that may influence the outcome of the neuropathy. Table 20.4 summarizes the main electrophysiologic abnormalities in

TABLE 20.4. Electrophysiologic findings in Guillain-Barré syndrome

Motor
Conduction block
  Decreased M size >> temporal dispersion
    pattern*
      Maximal—plexus/roots
      Entrapment/compression sites
      Distal
      Uniform—distal—proximal
  Decreased motor unit recruitment*
  Decreased numbers/loss F waves*
Axonal degeneration
  Decreased M size distal
    ? Distinguish ⟨ Demyelinating block
                 Axonal block
  Decreased motor unit recruitment
  Decreased numbers/loss F waves
  Fibrillation potentials
Conduction slowing
  Increased MDL
  Increased F latencies*
  Decreased MMCVs
    Pattern
      Proximal—plexus root
      Entrapment/compression sites
      Uniform—distal—proximal
Hyperexcitability
  Myokymia
  Fasciculation
Sensory
Decreased SNAP size   median, ulnar > sural*
Conduction slowing
  Increased DL
  Decreased MSCV
    Pattern
      Proximal—plexus/roots
      Intermediate
      Distal
      Uniform—distal—proximal

* Common abnormalities within the first 1 to 2 weeks.
M, Maximum compound muscle action potential—surface recorded; MDL, motor distal latency.
SNAP, sensory nerve action potential.

GBS. Points with asterisks (*) indicate abnormalities found most often early in GBS. Unfortunately, electrodiagnostic studies emphasizing conduction velocities and latencies and concentrating on the peripheral one-third and one-half of the peripheral nervous system may be normal at this stage, although F waves and sensory evoked potentials[28–30] may be abnormal. Representative current diagnostic criteria for GBS are outlined in Table 20.5. These criteria for an *acute demyelinating* neuropathy, although relatively simple and within the technical capabilities of most laboratories, with the exception of F waves, assess only the peripheral one-third to one-half of the peripheral nervous system and place too much emphasis on conduction times and velocities rather than conduction block and axon losses. Further, only 10% to 30% of GBS patients may meet these criteria for *significant demyelination* within the first 2 weeks.[17] The criteria of Asbury and Cornblath[6] are even more stringent and, although intended for use in clinical

TABLE 20.5.   Electrophysiologic criteria for acute Guillain-Barré polyneuropathy*

	Albert and Kelly, 1989[14]	Asbury and Cornblath, 1990[6]
	Must have three of	*Must have three of*
MMCV	2 or more nerves <90%LLN, M >50% LLN <80%LLN, M <50% LLN	2 or more nerves <80% LLN, M >80% LLN <70% LLN, M <80% LLN

MDL	2 or more nerves
	    >115% ULN, M >LLN
	    >125% ULN, M <LLN
		2 or more nerves
		    >125% ULN, M >80% LLN
		    >150% ULN, M <80% LLN

Temporal dispersion/
    conduction block
	? number of nerves
	    $\dfrac{M_{Prox}}{M_{Distal}}<0.7$
		1 or more nerves
		    partial conduction block
		    >20% reduction in negative·
		    peak area or peak to peak ampli-
		    tude of M between distal and
		    proximal sites accompanied by
		    <15% increase in negative peak
		    duration
		Temporal dispersion
		    >15% increase in negative peak
		    duration and >20% reduction in
		    negative peak area or peak to
		    peak amplitude of M

F waves	1 or more nerves
	    latency >125% ULN
		2 or more nerves
		    absent or latency
		    >120% ULN, M >80% LLN
		    >150% ULN, M <80% LLN

MDL, motor distal latency; LLN, lower limit of normal; ULN, upper limit of normal.

* Motor nerves include peroneal nerve between ankle and fibular head, median nerve between wrist and elbow, or ulnar nerve between wrist and below elbow.

trials, often fail to detect the essential electrophysiologic abnormalities, especially conduction block, within the first 1 to 2 weeks.

The single most important hallmark of GBS is paralysis. Paralysis must indicate conduction block or axonal degeneration or some combination of the two. These must, *a priori*, be evident somewhere between the ventral roots and motor point in motor fibers supplying clinically weak muscles.[30,31] Of course, early in the course of GBS, conduction block in primarily demyelinated but otherwise intact motor nerve fibers cannot be distinguished reliably from conduction block in nerve fibers undergoing active degeneration in which portions of the axons remain excitable and capable of impulse transmission for a few days. Other consequences of demyelination, such as the inability to transmit high-frequency trains of impulses or slowed conduction, probably make little, if any, contribution in the case of the former and no

contribution in the case of the latter to weakness. Because motor conduction velocities are often normal early in GBS, every attempt should be made to identify and assess conduction block and possible axonal degeneration, especially because extensive axonal degeneration portends such a poor prognosis for recovery.

Conduction block

For electrodiagnosticians, the most convenient way to assess conduction block is to assess the changes in M size as recorded with surface electrodes from convenient clinically weak muscles in response to successively more proximally displaced stimulus sites, including in some cases the spinal nerves (Figures 20.1 and 20.2). In all instances, stimuli must be supramaximal to ensure that the resultant M potentials represent the true compound sum of all motor units whose axons are capable of transmitting im-

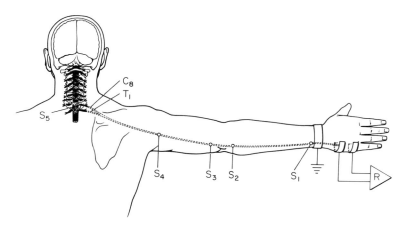

FIGURE 20.1.   *Motor conduction technique. Sites of motor nerve stimulation (S_1 through S_5) correspond-ing to stimulation of the ulnar nerve at the wrist, at least 2 cm distal to the cubital tunnel, 2 to 3 cm proximal to the elbow, and as high in the axilla as possible. The latter stimuli were delivered by a bipolar percutaneous electrode. A DEVICES D-180 high-voltage stimulator was employed to stimulate the spinal roots. The anode was positioned 1 to 2 cm lateral to the tip of the C-6 spine and the cathode directly inferiorly. Manually triggered single pulses were used to minimize the number of stimuli required to estab-lish a supramaximal response (five or fewer usually) and were well tolerated by most subjects.*

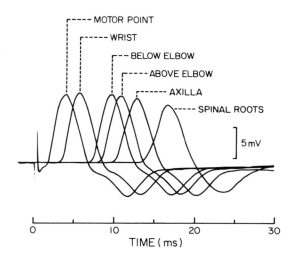

FIGURE 20.2.   *Maximum hypothenar M poten-tials recorded with surface electrodes in response to supramaximal percutaneous stimulation at the wrist, below the elbow, above the elbow, axilla, and spinal roots in a control. Additionally, a mon-opolar needle electrode was inserted as close to the hypothenar motor point as possible and a supra-maximal stimulus delivered through the needle (an-ode was a surface plate over the back of the hand). No significant differences between maximum M potentials elicited by stimulation at the motor point and wrist were seen in this or other controls.*

pulses, without failure, between the site of stimula-tion and the motor point.

Suitable muscles include distal muscles such as the thenar, hypothenar, extensor digitorum brevis, plantar foot, and anterior and lateral compartment muscles. It is also important to position the stigmatic (G_1) electrode over the innervation zone or motor point. Some muscles make better choices than others for assessing changes in M potentials. For example, hypothenar recording sites see little activity from median-supplied intrinsic hand muscles. This makes hypothenar recordings ideal for stimulation at the level of the spinal roots, brachial plexus, or in some cases the axilla because spread of the stimulus to median motor fibers supplying intrinsic hand muscles at such sites is unavoidable if the stimulus is to be supramaximal for all hypothenar motor fibers.

Thenar muscles offer the advantage that nine of 10 surface-recorded motor unit action potentials (S-MUAPs) recorded from the innervation zone are simple biphasic negative positive potentials. For hy-pothenar, plantar foot, and anterior and lateral com-partment muscles, however, where it is simply im-possible to cover with a single recording electrode the innervation zone for all or in some cases even most of the motor units, higher proportions of bi-phasic, positive-negative, triphasic, and even more complex S-MUAPs are encountered. The latter in-crease the chances of cancellations between opposite phases of S-MUAPs that together sum to make the

TABLE 20.6.   Problems interpreting changes in M size in controls and patients with Guillain-Barré syndrome

---

Anatomic—physiologic
   Relative numbers of motor units of differing conduction velocities and S-MUAPs sizes
   Conditional nature of conduction proximal to any sites of conduction block
Distance between the motor point and site of stimulation
Technical factors
   Ensuring the stimulus is supramaximal
   Band width of the recording system
   Temperature of the muscle
   Way in which the negative peak area is calculated
   Shapes of the S-MUAPs and interpotential phase cancellations
      Most S-MUAPs are biphasic negative-positive
      Some are biphasic positive-negative, triphasic positive-negative positive, or even more complex
Pathophysiologic
   Any change in conduction velocities of motor units and especially in the relation between motor
      unit size (S-MUAP size) and conduction velocity
   Changes in the sizes of motor units (and S-MUAP size) as a result of reinnervation

---

S-MUAP, Surface-recorded motor unit action potential.

M potential. This and other theoretical and technical problems complicating the interpretation of the M potential are summarized in Table 20.6. The highest proportion of simple negative-positive S-MUAPs are recorded from extensor digitorum brevis and thenar muscles with strip electrodes positioned over the respective innervation zones.

The M potential in normal subjects is dominated by a relatively small number of rapidly conducting motor axons, the motor units of which generate the largest twitches and S-MUAPs.[32,33] This probably explains the relatively modest reduction (<25%) in the negative peak ($-p$) area of the M potential over the several hundred millimeters that separate the usual most distal sites of stimulation of motor nerves in humans and the most proximal sites of stimulation such as the ventral roots or spinal nerves (Figure 20.2). Such modest reductions in $-p$ area of the M potential are accompanied by relatively modest increases in $-p$ duration (<50%).

The extent to which the size of the maximum M potential can be reduced by temporal dispersion and summation of opposite phases of component S-MUAPs depends on several factors, including:

1.   The relative sizes, durations, shapes, and latencies of the component S-MUAPs.
2.   The distance between the site of stimulation and the motor point.

If, for the purposes of modeling, two S-MUAPs of identical shape, size, and negative peak duration (5 ms) are chosen and one assigned a conduction velocity of 60 m/s, representative of the fastest, and the other a conduction velocity of 40 m/s, representative of the slowest conducting motor axons, the impact of phase cancellation on the size and shape of the summation M potential may be assessed at various stimulus sites proximal to the motor point (Figure 20.3 and 20.4). Maximum phase cancellation occurs when the latency of the slower of the two S-MUAPs exceeds that of the faster S-MUAP by a value equal to the negative peak duration. This point would lie near the spinal roots in this example (Figure 20.3) but phase cancellation would begin much closer to the motor point (Figures 20.3 and 20.4) and taper off to zero, theoretically at some point well proximal to the spinal roots where the two S-MUAPs no longer overlap. The greater the duration of the negative peaks of the two S-MUAPs, the more proximally situated will be the site where maximum phase cancellation occurs. If the duration of the negative peaks is increased enough, phase cancellation between the motor point and roots should be minimized and perhaps even nonexistent.

At 30° to 32°C, the negative peak durations of thenar S-MUAPs lie between 1.0 to 11.8 ms (mean 5.5 ± 1.7 1 S.D.), whereas that of the maximum M potential lies between 4.5 and 8.1 ms (mean 6.3 ± 1.0 1 S.D.). These negative peak durations may be increased by opening the high pass filter and cooling the muscle (Figure 20.5), the combination effectively doubling and even tripling the negative peak durations of S-MUAPs and displacing the site where maximum phase cancellation might be expected to some theoretical point well proximal to the roots.

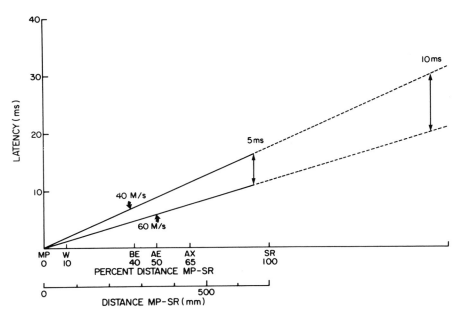

FIGURE 20.3.   *Plot of the cumulative latencies of two surface-recorded motor unit action potentials (S-MUAPs) of identical negative peak duration (5 ms), one conducting at 60 m/s and the other at 40 m/s. The latencies for these stimulated S-MUAPs are plotted over a distance corresponding to 100% of the distance between the motor point (MP) and spinal roots (SR) for hypothenar motor fibers. Stimulus sites at the wrist (W), below elbow (BE), above elbow (AE), and axilla (AX) would, in most cases, correspond to 10%, 40%, 50%, and 65% of this distance. The overall distance between the MP and SR sites is approximately 600 to 800 mm, depending on the size of the subject. A latency difference of 5 ms corresponding to the negative peak duration of these S-MUAPs would represent the stimulus point at which maximum phase cancellation would occur. In this example, maximum phase cancellation would be expected close to the spinal roots. Doubling or even tripling the negative peak duration would set the point at which maximum phase cancellation occurs well proximal to the spinal roots in this example.*

Of course, real S-MUAPs differ in size and shape and systematically in size with conduction velocity, faster conducting motor axons generating larger amplitude and often longer duration S-MUAPs.[33,34,35] Despite the relatively greater numbers of the small S-MUAPs, their impact on the size and shape of the maximum M potential is much less than the impact of the relatively fewer but larger sized S-MUAPs (see Chapter 4). On the other hand, slowed conduction in some of the normally more rapidly conducting motor axons generating relatively large S-MUAPs could produce much greater phase cancellation, especially if there was any appreciable overlap between the negative phases and positive phases of the larger S-MUAPs. Some authors have suggested that reductions in M potential size by as much as 50% could be produced through desynchronization and phase cancellation alone.[35,36,37] It should be pointed out as

well that commercial electromyography (EMG) systems take no account of baseline displacements produced by stimulus artifact or the positive phase of preceding M potential (as when collision is used to block activity from one nerve) in calculating the negative peak areas of M potentials.

The shape of successively more proximally evoked M potentials is also dramatically influenced by the *conditional* nature of conduction in the presence of conduction block.[38,39] To understand this concept, it is useful to examine a model of conduction block in which conduction block affects nerve fibers randomly, the chance of conduction failure being the same throughout the course of constituent nerve fibers between the motor point and spinal roots and between motor fibers. To examine the impact on the size of the M potential in response to successively more proximally displaced sites of stimulation,

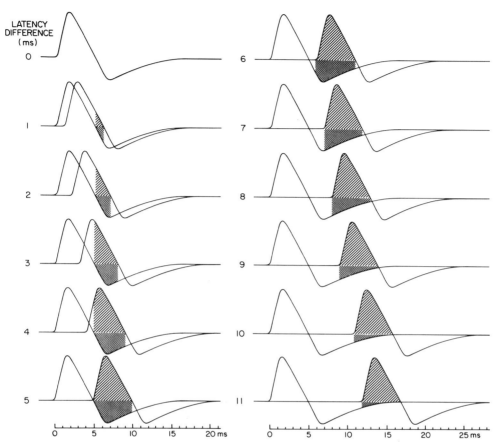

FIGURE 20.4. *Two modeled surface-recorded motor unit action potentials (S-MUAPs) of identical size and negative peak duration (−p dur); here 5 ms are shown. One of the two S-MUAPs is shown displaced in ever-increasing latency with respect to the first S-MUAP. The crosshatching highlights the overlapping portions of the positive phase of the earlier S-MUAP and the negative phase of the successively delayed second S-MUAP. Note that in this example, maximum cancellation of opposite phases and therefore reduction in the sum of the negative phases of the two S-MUAPs occurs when one S-MUAP is delayed with respect to the other S-MUAP by a time difference equal to the negative peak duration.*

the model may usefully be simplified by assuming that all motor nerve fibers generate monophasic S-MUAPs of equal size. The former precludes any phase cancellations between S-MUAPs (Figure 20.6).

In such a model in which conditions exist sufficient to block conduction of the impulse at two or more sites throughout the distal-proximal course of the nerve fibers, the pattern of changes in M size produced by successively more proximal stimuli will reflect the following:

• The frequency of conduction block per unit length of nerve.

• The distance between the motor point and site of stimulation.

• The conditional nature of such a study.

In the case of the last-mentioned it is the most distal sites of conduction failure in the constituent nerve fibers that determine the pattern of changes in M size, not any additional more proximally situated sites of conduction failure. Of course, the latter contribute to the overall frequency of conduction failures in the segment in which they reside, but their contributions to the M potential are masked by the most distal sites of conduction failure in the same

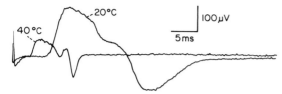

FIGURE 20.5.   *Single thenar surface-recorded single motor unit action potential at 40° and 20°C. In this example, the negative peak duration almost tripled at 20°C and was almost triple that at 40°C.*

fibers. It is the latter, most distal sites of conduction failure in each nerve fiber that *condition* the actual pattern of M potential changes observed as the sites of stimulation are displaced proximally.

In the preceding model, reductions in M size per unit length of nerve, expressed as a percent of the M size at the motor point, progressively diminish over successively more proximal but equidistant segments. It follows that the maximum reduction in M size will be in the most distal or terminal segment between the motor point and the first site of stimulation proximal to the motor point.

Such a model may also be used to predict changes in M size corresponding to actual sites of stimulation in humans. For example, for hypothenar motor fibers, stimulus sites at the wrist, below elbow, above elbow, axilla, and spinal roots correspond approxi-

mately to 10%, 40%, 50%, 65%, and 100% of the distance between the motor point and spinal roots (Figure 20.6). In this model for probabilities of conduction block exceeding 50% per 10% length of nerve, reductions in M size as a percent of the motor point value progressively diminish across the terminal, forearm, elbow, proximal arm, and axilla to spinal root segments. For probabilities of conduction block of less than 50% per 10% length of nerve, however, the reduction in M size across the forearm exceeds reductions across other segments. Such a pattern is sometimes seen in GBS.

Of course, such a model takes no account of differences in conduction velocities and sizes of S-MUAPs or the impact of phase cancellations. The impact of the latter factors would be to reduce further the $-p$ amplitude and $-p$ area while increasing the $-p$ duration of successively more proximally evoked M potentials.

The precise relative contributions of temporal dispersion and phase cancellations relative to conduction block in GBS cannot be determined with any accuracy, but the impact of the former is unlikely to be important early in the course of GBS before conduction velocities change much or there is any increase in $-p$ duration.[34,35] Reductions in M size exceeding normal values in early GBS are therefore likely to provide reasonable guides to the quantitative contribution of conduction block and possibly axonal losses in GBS. Special confidence in reductions in M size as accurately reflecting conduction

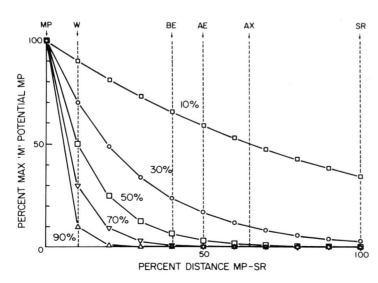

FIGURE 20.6.   *Progressive reductions in M size as a percent of the motor point M as the stimulus site is moved further from the motor point toward the spinal roots (SR). Changes in M size were calculated for percent reductions in M size per 10% length of nerve of 10%, 30%, 50%, 70%, and 90%. Shown also are the approximate locations for stimulation at the wrist (W), below elbow (BE), above elbow (AE), axilla (AX), and spinal roots (SR) levels.*

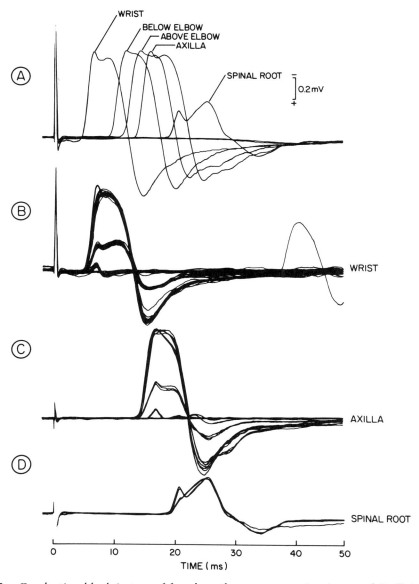

FIGURE 20.7. *Conduction block in two of four hypothenar motor units. A case of Guillain-Barré syndrome studied at 10 days when only four hypothenar surfaced-recorded motor unit action potentials (S-MUAPs) could be identified by their successive all or nothing incremental responses to increases in the stimulus intensity at the wrist, below and above elbow, and axillary stimulus sites (A, B, C). Only two of these S-MUAPs, however, could be identified by stimulation at the level of the spinal roots (D). Surprisingly maximum motor conduction velocities (MMCVs) were normal between the wrist and axilla, and the motor distal latency was also normal. The MMCV between the axilla and spinal roots, however, was <45 m/s and below the lower limit of normal.*

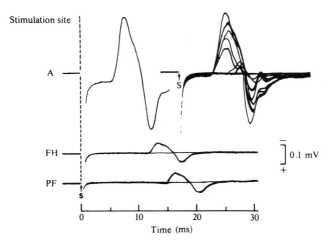

FIGURE 20.8.   *Guillain-Barré polyneuropathy 10 days after the onset of paralysis. The changes in the maximum M potentials in extensor digitorum brevis (EDB) elicited by stimulation at the ankle (A), fibular head (FH), and popliteal fossa (PF) are illustrated. The amplitude of the maximum M potential evoked by stimulation at the ankle was less than 10% of the control mean value for this muscle. Incremental stimulation at the ankle above threshold evoked only seven successive motor unit potentials, only one of which could be elicited by stimulation at the more proximal levels, indicating conduction block in six out of seven motor axons between the FH and A stimulus sites. The conduction velocity between the popliteal fossa and fibular head was therefore based on conduction in a single motor axon and was 27 m/s, whereas the velocity between the fibular head and ankle was higher at 41 m/s. The lower proximal velocity suggested a possible local injury to the common peroneal nerve between the fibular head and popliteal fossa. It was not clear whether the apparent block in the impulses of six of the motor axons proximal to the ankle was the result of demyelination or ongoing axonal degeneration in these fibers, whose excitability and conductivity had not yet been lost distal to the ankle.*

block is justified where conduction block in single units can clearly be identified, as illustrated by Figures 20.7 and 20.8.

Later in the course of the disease, however, when conduction velocities are characteristically reduced, the usual relations between S-MUAPs size and conduction velocity might well be disturbed and prejudice reductions in M size as reasonable guides to the extent of conduction block. Even so, whether reduced by conduction block or increased temporal dispersion and phase cancellations, reductions in M size and increases in M −p duration are still of considerable diagnostic value because they help to confirm the presence of a demyelinating neuropathy.

That substantial reductions in M size may occur with little or no reductions in conduction velocity should not be surprising. Even probabilities of conduction block as low as 10% per 10% length of nerve are capable of reducing M size by more than

60% between the motor point and spinal roots. Because the minimum requirement for conduction block is an increase in internodal conduction time by approximately 10 times or more, over two or possibly three successive internodes, the increase in latency between the wrist and thenar or hypothenar motor points (a distance of 60 to 80 mm) for nerve fibers close to block might be only 0.5 ms. Such an increase is well within control limits. The apparent discrepancy then between paralysis and substantial reductions in M size on the one hand and normal or nearly normal conduction velocities on the other hand may simply lie in the presence of relatively scattered, infrequent lesions in the peripheral nervous system, severe enough at a few sites to block conduction but not slow conduction velocities overall.

How then might conduction across successively more proximal segments be studied in GBS? To assess the quantitive extent of conduction block or axonal degeneration properly, a reference value for the motor point M size may be adopted.[35] Because we have found no significant differences between M potentials evoked by stimulation at the wrist for intrinsic hand and ankle for extensor digitorum brevis muscles and stimulation as close to the motor point as possible (within 10 to 15 mm) in normal subjects, we adopted the conservative expedient of applying the control means -2 S.D. value for the M potential in response to stimulation at the wrist or ankle, as the *stand-in* value for the motor point M in GBS patients. Overall reductions in M size between the motor point and most proximal site of stimulation may then be calculated by:

$$\frac{M_{MP} - M_{Prox}}{M_{MP}} \times 100$$

where M_{MP} = control mean $-$ 2 S.D. value for M at the usual most distal site of stimulation (e.g., the wrist or ankle) and M_{Prox} = M size at the most proximal site of stimulation employed (e.g., axilla, brachial plexus, or in some cases spinal or ventral roots).

Quantitative assessment of reductions in M size in the terminal segment may be calculated by:

$$\frac{M_{MP} - M_{(Wrist/Ankle)}}{M_{MP}} \times 100$$

and for any segment in between as:

$$\frac{M_{Distal} - M_{Proximal}}{M_{MP}} \times 100$$

The application of the preceding method to the hypothenar muscles in GBS revealed the following:
1. Overall reductions in M size between the motor point and spinal roots of more than 90% in one-third and more than 50% in 85% of patients.[39]
2. Reductions in M size in the terminal segment exceeding 50% in one-third and 20% in almost two-thirds of patients.
3. Disproportionately greater reductions in M size, often accompanied by disproportionately slowed MMCVs across the elbow and between the axilla and spinal roots relative to adjacent segments and in the case of the terminal segment by an increase in MDL relative to controls in one-half of our patients (Figure 20.9 and 20.10). Disproportionately greater reductions in M size between the axilla and spinal roots were also usually accompanied by slowed sensory conduction between the axilla and spinal cord as well (Figure 20.11). One practical method for assessing sensory conduction between the digits and spinal cord is shown in Figure 20.12. The reasons for such preferential involvement at these sites is not clear but may in some way be related to natural deficiencies in the blood-nerve and perineural barriers at the terminal ends of nerve fibers or at the root level or perhaps acquired deficiencies at common sites of chronic compression, as in the case of the ulnar nerve at the elbow.
4. Patterns of reductions in M size in one-third of cases more in keeping with a uniformly distributed conduction block, as proposed by Van der Meche and others.

The relative contributions of axonal degeneration and conduction block to reductions in M size in the terminal segment early in the disease cannot be assessed with current techniques. Reductions in MMCV and MSCV are usually apparent by the sec-

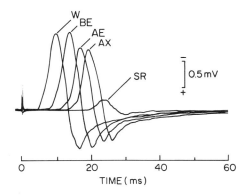

FIGURE 20.9. *Hypothenar maximum M potential recording from a patient with Guillain-Barré syndrome studied at 5 days. At this stage, the overall reduction in M $-p$ area between the motor point (control -2 SD value at wrist) and spinal roots (SR) was 96.9%, whereas that between the motor point and wrist (W) was 68%. In this case, the condition abnormalities were greatest across the terminal, elbow, and axillary to spinal root segments. The maximum motor conduction velocity (MMCV) between the axilla and spinal roots was 37.2 m/s, a value clearly slowed relative to the proximal arm 58.8 m/s and the relatively normal MMCVs for the elbow and forearm of 44.3 and 49.8 m/s. Note also the conduction block across the elbow.*

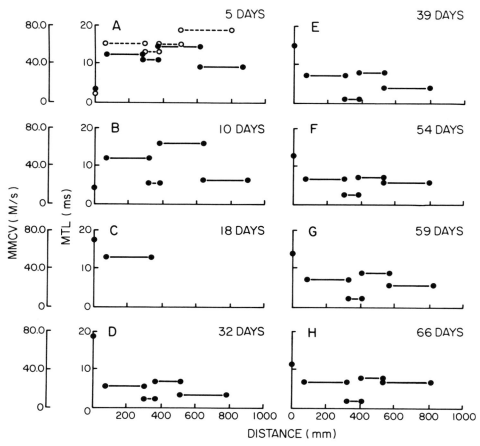

FIGURE 20.10.   *Plots of successive changes in maximum motor conduction velocity (MMCV) and motor distal latency (MDL) in the same patient as illustrated in Figure 20.9. Peak clinical paralysis was reached at 10 days. The ulnar nerve was stimulated at the wrist, below the elbow, above the elbow, axillary, and spinal root sites. Studies were carried out at 5, 10, 18, 32, 39, 54, 59, and 66 days following the onset of paralysis. By 54 days, the first flicker of recovery in abductor digiti minimi was observed. The relative lengths of the various segments as a percent of the total distance between the hypothenar motor point and spinal roots are shown on the X axis and closely correspond to real values in human subjects. The MMCVs in meters per second for the corresponding examinations are indicated by the solid lines connecting closed circles for each of the forearm, elbow, proximal arm, and axillary to spinal root segments. MDLs in milliseconds are plotted on the Y axis. The control mean values for the MMCVs for each segment are indicated by the dotted lines connecting open circles. The control mean value for the MDL is shown by the open circles on the Y axis and patient values by the closed circles. At 5 days, the forearm and proximal arm MMCVs were normal, as was the MDL, but the MMCV between the axilla and spinal roots was clearly reduced. At 10 days, the MMCVs across the elbow and axillary to spinal root segments were both disproportionately reduced with respect to the adjacent forearm and proximal arm segments. By 18 days, there was no response to stimulation proximal to the elbow. At 39 days, the M potential at the wrist was well within the normal range, but almost no response could be evoked by stimulation at the spinal roots. By 66 days, conduction block was clearly recovering, but the MMCVs showed little sign of recovery.*

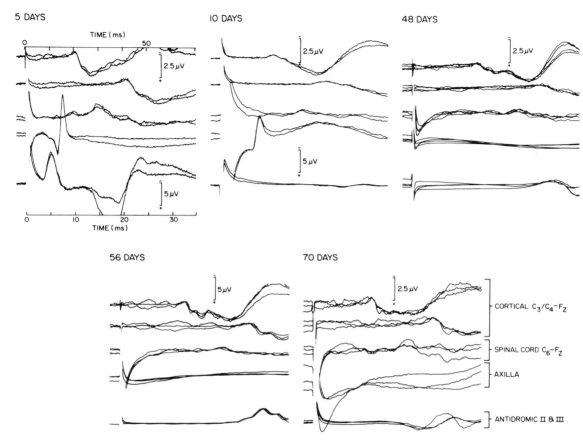

FIGURE 20.11.   *Serial changes in sensory conduction in the patient shown in Figures 20.9 and 20.10. The cortical potential is shown at 2 sweeps speeds. Only at 5 days was an antidromic potential detected. At this time, the distal latency and maximum sensory conduction velocity (MSCV) between the wrist and axilla were normal (69.2 m/s), but the MSCV between the axilla and spinal cord was clearly reduced (42.4 m/s). In all subsequent antidromic recordings, there was only a very delayed volume conducted thenar-lumbrical electromyographic potential, which itself was barely detectable at 10 days. Note also the temporally dispersed cortical potential was 5 days. At 48 and 56 days, the gains were identical for all channels, but at 5 and 10 days, the gain was higher for the cortical channel. Control values for the MSCVs between the wrist and axilla and axilla and spinal cord are 63.9 m/s +5.3 1 S.D. and 60.9 m/s ±7.6 1 S.D.*

ond week and most reduced by the third to fifth weeks at a stage when most patients have plateaued and others begun to recover (Figures 20.10 and 20.11; Table 20.7). Signs of denervation in the form of fibrillation potential activity and positive sharp waves are also late, appearing at the earliest between 2 and 3 weeks and reaching a peak by 4 to 5 weeks.

Sensory conduction is relatively spared in GBS, especially in the sural nerve.[17,42,43] Elsewhere reductions in amplitude and distal latency parallel changes

in distal M size and MDL usually, although abnormalities are usually more striking in the latter. Somatosensory evoked potential studies often reveal proximal slowing between the axilla and spinal cord[30,39] (Figures 20.11 and 20.13).

Axonal degeneration

Some axonal degeneration in GBS is common and evident in both pathologic studies of GBS and needle

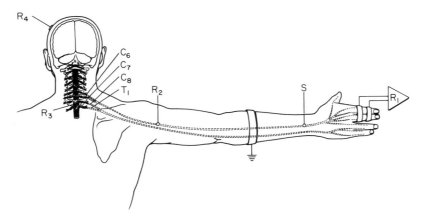

FIGURE 20.12.   *Somatosensory evoked potential technique. Percutaneous stimuli at the wrist were adjusted to evoke maximal antidromic compound nerve action potentials from the second and third digits combined, or when absent, a maximal M potential. From the foregoing technique, amplitudes for all potentials and maximum sensory conduction velocities between the wrist and digits, wrist to axilla, and axilla to spinal cord as well as the latency to the N_{20} potentials were measured. Orthodromic nerve trunk potentials were recorded as high in the axilla as possible with the reference electrode positioned over the lateral deltoid. The cervical potential was recorded over the C-6 spine with FZ as reference. Additionally, the cortical potential was recorded over the primary sensory area for the hand, again with FZ as reference. Surface electrodes were used throughout to record these potentials except for a bare needle electrode for the hand area recording. The latter provided a convenient low-resistance (less than 2k ohms), relatively painless electrode with which to record from the hairy scalp. The ground site is indicated by the band about the proximal forearm.*

EMG examinations. The latter reveal some fibrillation potential activity occasionally as early as the second week but more often after the third week in both proximal and distal muscles, persisting longer in the latter.[17] Sometimes moderate to abundant fibrillation potential activity develops in muscles supplied by a compressed nerve. This is most common in the motor innervation territory of the common peroneal nerve but is common as well in the motor innervation territories of the median nerve in the hand and ulnar nerve in the hand and forearm and usually correlates with other electrophysiologic and clinical evidence of focal nerve injury to the median nerve in the carpal tunnel or elbow in the case of the ulnar nerve.

Electrophysiologic Changes in Guillain-Barré Syndrome Variants

Acute axonal Guillain-Barré syndrome

Large multicenter trials have clearly shown that the parameter that best correlates with outcome is the size of the distal M potential, especially when the distal M potential is severely reduced in two or more motor nerves.[13–19,38,44] M potentials may be severely reduced (less than 5% of the lower limit of normal) and even absent (Figure 20.14). In some of the latter cases, advancing the site of stimulation closer to the motor point reveals a small M potential, but over successive days often even this small potential is lost (Figure 20.15). Sensory conduction may be relatively spared in such cases but not always.

Miller-Fisher variant

The Miller-Fisher variant is characterized by normal or nearly normal MMCVs and MDL's, reductions in M size, and normal blink reflex latencies but reduced or absent compound sensory nerve action potentials.[45,46]

Acute pure sensory neuropathy

This neuropathy is characterized in at least one report by modest reductions in MMCVs and MSCVs and segmental demyelination in the biopsy.

TABLE 20.7. Conduction velocity and motor terminal latency changes in patients with GBS at various times following the onset of the paralysis

Days	Subject	Motor Distal latency	Forearm	Elbow	Axilla	Axilla to Ventral Root
1–7	1	−	−	−	−	−
	2	+	+	−	−	+ +
	3	−	−	−	−	+
	4	+ +	−	+ + + +	−	?
8–14	5	+	+ +	−	+	Complete block
	2	+ + + +	+ + +	+ + + +	+ + +	+ + + +
	6	+ +	+	−	+	+ +
	3	−	−	−	−	−
	4	−	−	−	−	+
15–21	7	+ + +	+	+	−	+ + +
	2	+ + + +	+	?	?	?
	3	−	−	−	−	−
	8	−	−	−	−	−
22–28	9	+ + +	+ + +	+ + +	+ +	?
	10	+ +	−	+ + +	+	+ + +
	11	+ +	+ +	+ + +	+	+
	4	+ + +	+ +	+ + + +	+	+ + + +
>28						
29	1	+ +	+ + +	+ + + +	+ +	+ + + +
31	7	+ +	+ + +	+ + + +	−	?
32	2	+ + + +	+ + +	+ + + +	+ + +	+ + + +
34	9	+ +	+ + + +	+ + +	+ + + +	+ + + +
39	2	+ + +	+ + +	+ + + +	+ +	+ + + +
42	9	+ +	?	?	?	?
44	10	+ +	+	+ + + +	+	+ +
47	3	+ +	−	−	−	+ +
49	9	+ +	+ + +	+ + + +	+	+ + +
50	2	+ + +	+ + +	+ + + +	+ + +	+ + +
56	9	+ +	+ + + +	+ + + +	?	?
59	2	+ + +	+ + +	+ + + +	+ +	+ + +
67	2	+ + +	+ + +	+ + + +	+	+ + +
73	11	+ +	+ + +	+ + +	+ +	+ + +
78	10	+ +	−	+ + +	+	+
17	2	+	+	+ + + +	−	+ +
125	4	+	−	−	+ +	+ + +
196	3	+	−	+	−	+

Motor distal latency (ms)		Maximum motor conduction velocity (m/s)	
Normal	−	Normal	−
3.5–5	+	< − 2 SD	+
5.1–10	+ +	30–40	+ +
10.1–15	+ + +	20–20	+ + +
>15	+ + + +	<20	+ + + +

Question marks indicate instances where the precise onset of potentials could not be reliably identified enough to calculate a conduction velocity.

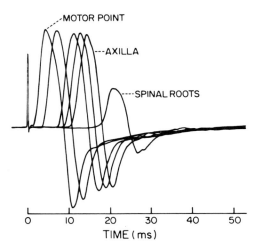

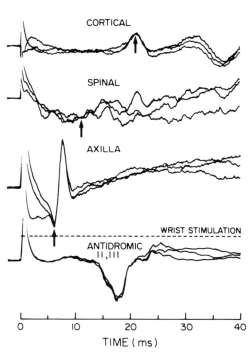

FIGURE 20.13.   *Electrophysiologic studies at 9 days after the onset of paralysis in a 32-year-old patient with Guillain-Barré syndrome. At the top are shown hypothenar maximum M potentials in response to stimulation at the motor point, wrist, below elbow, above elbow, axilla, and spinal root levels. At this time, there was a 34% reduction in M negative peak area between the wrist and the* stand-in *value for the motor point (see text), no significant reduction in M negative peak area between the wrist and axilla, but a further 36% reduction in M size between the axilla and spinal root stimulus sites. The motor point value, here obtained by needle electrode stimulation of the ulnar nerve at least 15 mm proximal to the motor point, was well below the expected control stand-in value, and this suggests that the 34% reduction in M size was in the terminal 15 mm of the nerve. At this stage, the maximum motor conduction velocities were entirely normal between the wrist and axilla (61.3, 59.4, and 56.9 m/s over the forearm, elbow, and proximal arm segments) but clearly slowed (43.7 m/s) between the axilla and spinal roots. At the bottom are shown (from bottom to top) the antidromic II and III digit, axillary, cervical spinal, and contralateral cortical recordings in response to supramaximal stimulation of the median nerve at the wrist. In the bottom trace only, a volume-recorded small and delayed response from the lumbrical and thenar muscles was recorded. The axillary potential, however, was normal in size and the maximum conduction velocity between the wrist and axilla also normal (65.8 m/s), whereas the maximum conduction velocity was slowed between the axilla and cervical cord (45.8 m/s and less than the control 3 S.D. lower limit.) This study has therefore shown that conduction in this case at this time was most abnormal in the distal and proximal segments of the peripheral nervous system.*

Recommendations for Electrodiagnostic Studies

1. To be most useful for formulating the diagnosis and prognosis, electrodiagnostic studies should be carried out as early as possible and repeated serially as necessary to clarify the involving clinical and electrophysiologic picture.

2. Electrodiagnostic studies should concentrate on weak muscles and preferably those most readily studied, such as distal limb muscles.
3. Abnormalities should be demonstrable in at least one motor nerve each in the upper and lower extremities.
4. Changes in M potential size should, where pos-

STIMULUS

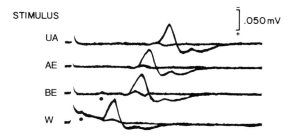

FIGURE 20.14. *Guillain-Barré patient examined 4 days after the onset of paralysis. This patient had only two remaining excitable hypothenar motor unit potentials at 1 week and throughout subsequent examinations at 2, 4, and 28 weeks. The figure illustrates these two hypothenar motor unit potentials as elicited by stimulation at the wrist (W), below the elbow (BE), above the elbow (AE), and upper arm (UA) levels. In this muscle group and in the thenar and extensor digitorum brevis muscles, where there were zero and two excitable motor unit potentials, abundant fibrillation potentials developed. Despite this, conduction velocities in the two remaining hypothenar motor axons were within the 2 S.D. lower limit of control maximum motor conduction velocity for this nerve except on the earliest occasion (1 week), when maximum velocity across the forearm was 36 m/s. On all four subsequent tests over the next 50 days, the distal motor latencies were prolonged (beyond 3 S.D. of the upper limits of controls). A prepotential (see dot marker), originating in an underlying cutaneous branch of the ulnar nerve, is seen in the BE and W records.*

sible, be assessed at successively more proximal sites of stimulation, including, at least for the median nerve, the wrist, elbow, and axilla, and for the ulnar nerve, the wrist, below elbow, above elbow, and axillary stimulus sites. If the preceding studies are normal, optional stimulus sites should include the spinal roots. For the last, high-voltage electrical surface stimulation (DEVICES D-180) or needle electrical stimulation[47] may profitably be employed. For the lower limb, the common peroneal nerve can be studied while recording from extensor digitorum brevis and anterior and lateral compartment muscles and stimulating at the fibular head, popliteal fossa, and optionally at the L-1–2 level, the last-mentioned employing high-voltage percutaneous

electrical stimulation. For L-1–2 stimulation, collision may be employed by stimulating the medial popliteal nerve in the popliteal fossa at the same time. Alternatively, motor conduction in the posterior tibial nerve may be studied while recording from plantar foot and calf muscles and stimulating the posterior tibial nerve at the ankle, popliteal fossa, and possibly at L-1–2, the last-mentioned employing stimulation of the common peroneal nerve at the fibular head for collision at the same time.

5. F waves should be assessed using the criterion as laid out by Asbury and Cornblath.[6]
6. There is no need to do extensive (if any) needle EMG within the first 1 to 2 weeks unless there is reason to suspect another disorder in which needle EMG would be indicated.
7. In some cases, for example, those in which the dominant abnormalities are in the craniobulbar territory, trigeminal facial reflexes and motor stimulation studies of the VII cranial nerve should be carried out.

Miller-Fisher variant

MMCVs are often normal or only slightly reduced, and EMG is either normal or shows some evidence of denervation. More strikingly, compound sensory nerve action potentials are often reduced in size. Reductions in the M potential size may also be present.[46,47,49]

Acute pure sensory neuropathy

A case of acute pure sensory neuropathy accompanied by segmental demyelination in 10% of nerve fibers and some reductions in MMCVs and MSCVs has been described.[21,49,50]

Diphtheritic polyneuritis

Studies of diphtheritic polyneuritis[51–53] have shown, in some cases, normal or at the most, modest reductions in MMCVs within the first 2 weeks. Clinical recovery is often paradoxically accompanied by further reductions in MMCVs for a few weeks.

CHRONIC INFLAMMATORY DEMYELINATING NEUROPATHY

Clinical Features

CIDP is a sensorimotor neuropathy characterized by a slowly progressive, stepwise progressive, or relaps-

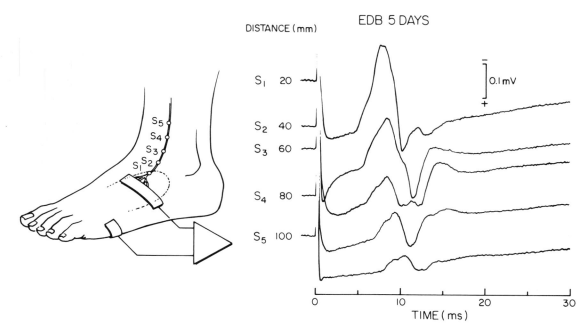

FIGURE 20.15.   *Patient with acute axonal form of Guillain-Barré syndrome. Maximum M potentials recorded from extensor digitorum brevis (EDB) in response to supramaximal stimulation of the anterior tibial nerve at 20, 40, . . . 100 mm proximal to the motor point. The maximum motor conduction velocity was 22.9 m/s.*

ing and remitting course.[54,55,56] The onset is usually slower than GBS, although the first attack may be similar. Sensory symptoms and signs are usually minor and involve large fiber more than small fiber functions.[17] The neuropathy is usually symmetric, rarely multifocal, and almost invariably associated with loss of tendon reflexes, especially during relapses. Autonomic disturbances are minimal,[57] but cranial nerves may become involved, and some patients may become respirator dependent during a relapse.

Some patients exhibit a striking action tremor during relapses that stops or is very much reduced with remission. Spontaneous or treatment-induced relapses are usually not associated with any particular preceding event, although relapses in pregnancy are well described. Of 53 patients studied by Albers and Kelly,[17] nine died and six became wheelchair bound or bedridden, with only two completely recovering.

Cerebrospinal fluid

The cerebrospinal fluid protein is almost invariably raised, but no more than 10 mononuclear cells per mm³ are present in the cerebrospinal fluid. Higher cell counts should prompt suspicion of HIV infection, although seronegative HIV cases may have lower cell counts.

Pathology

Pathologic studies of affected nerves characteristically reveal both segmental demyelination and remyelination as well as segmental axonal narrowing of as much as 30% to 40% in CIDP.[54,55] Axonal degeneration is common, but mononuclear cell inflammatory infiltrates are present in only about one-half of nerve biopsy specimens.[58] Other features sometimes include onion bulb formation and subperineural or endoneural edema.

Two cases of a chronic relapsing idiopathic polyneuropathy with primary axonal lesions have been reported by Julien et al.[59] In one case, the MMCV was as low as 25 m/s in the median nerve. In the other case, however, MMCVs were at or just below the lower limit of normal.

Cases indistinguishable from CIDP may be associated with HIV infection, Lyme disease, paraproteinemias, malignancies including lymphoma, lupus, and Castleman's disease. The neuropathies associated with malignancies, plasma cell disorders, and amyotrophic lateral sclerosis variants are discussed in chapters 17 and 19. Leukemia infiltration of peripheral nerves may rarely simulate the clinical presentation of CIDP.

All patients presenting with clinical courses and features suggestive of CIDP should have serum protein electrophoresis as well as electrodiagnostic studies. Any abnormalities in the former, especially where electrodiagnostic studies suggest the presence of a demyelinating neuropathy, should have immunoelectrophoresis of serum and urine and, if a M (monoclonal) protein is found, a radiologic skeletal survey and biopsy of any suspicious lesion carried out to look for evidence of osteosclerotic myeloma. The latter cases constitute 3% of all multiple myeloma cases but cause two-thirds of the neuropathies associated with this disease. The M protein may be immunoglobulin IgM, IgG or even IgA and associated with lambda light chains or less often kappa light chains. If the investigations for osteosclerotic myeloma are normal, the diagnosis should be considered as monoclonal gammopathy of undetermined significance, over one-half of which are associated with an IgM M protein. Where no M protein is found but electrodiagnostic studies suggest a demyelinating neuropathy, consideration should still be given to a search for a possible carcinoma or lymphoma or, if the cell count in the cerebrospinal fluid is elevated, HIV infection.

Electrophysiologic Diagnosis

Albers and Kelly in 1989[17] and Cornblath in 1990[60] have proposed electrodiagnostic criteria for CIDP. The latter criteria are the same as for GBS. In general, patients with CIDP exhibit much greater and sometimes severe reductions in MMCVs with corresponding increases in F wave latencies and often substantially greater temporal dispersion as compared with GBS, although the electrophysiologic findings in the two disorders may be indistinguishable (Figures 20.16 and 20.17). The chronic progressive, steadily or stepwise progressive, and relapsing forms cannot be distinguished electrophysiologically from one another.

The pattern of the electrophysiologic changes in CIDP varies from more or less uniform distribution of the conduction abnormalities among various motor and sensory nerves to a more uneven pattern in which some nerves in a limb are more affected than neighboring nerves, whereas other cases show evidence of multifocal conduction abnormalities often accompanied by conduction block. From 40 cases of CIDP, Lewis and Sumner[61] in 1982 isolated five cases, which they termed *multifocal demyelinating neuropathy with persistent conduction block*. These cases were subacute in onset and involved the upper more than the lower extremities. In these cases, there were regions where conduction velocities were normal or nearly normal accompanied by other often focal regions of reduced conduction velocities and sometimes conduction block often at unusual sites for any entrapment neuropathy. Parry and Clarke[62] in 1988 described a form of multifocal acquired demyelinating neuropathy masquerading as amyotrophic lateral sclerosis. Five patients had fasciculations, normal cerebrospinal fluid, multifocal conduction block, and normal compound sensory nerve action potentials and somatosensory evoked potentials.

CIDP must be distinguished from hereditary sensory motor neuropathies characterized by reduced MMCVs and MSCVs to within the demyelinating range. In the latter, hereditary, so-called primary demyelinating neuropathies, the onset is insidious. Skeletal abnormalities such as pes cavus, hammer toes, and scoliosis are common; sensory and motor levels are often sharp; and the mode of transmission is usually autosomal dominant. Conduction velocities are usually uniformly reduced, affecting all nerves more or less to the same degree, values for conduction velocity varying by no more than 30% between nerves.[63] Familial cases also exhibit very little if any increased temporal dispersion and no conduction block, but conduction velocities are often severely reduced. These findings contrast with CIDP cases in which more nonuniform reductions in maximum conduction velocities may be present, often accompanied by appreciable differences in MMCVs between nerves of the same limb or between different limbs. Increased temporal dispersion and conduction block are often present as well. Conduction slowing is often more modest than present in hereditary sensorimotor neuropathy type I, al-

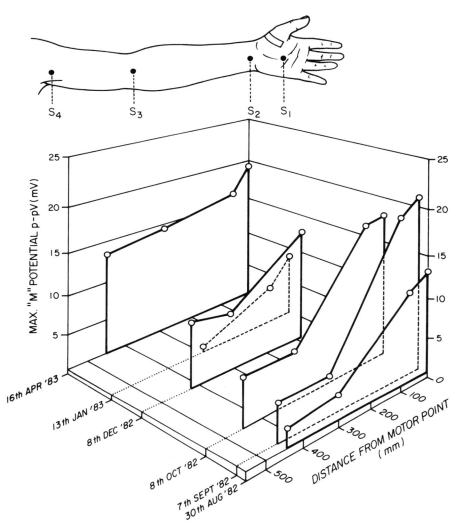

FIGURE 20.16.   *Patient with chronic, relapsing, biopsy-proved inflammatory and demyelinating polyneu-ropathy. Shown are successive plots of the peak to peak amplitude of the maximum thenar compound action potentials as recorded with surface electrodes and elicited by supramaximal stimuli delivered to the median nerve at the proximal upper arm,[52] elbow,[51] just proximal to the wrist,[50] and, in all but one instance, just distal to the flexor retinaculum. The studies were carried out at irregular intervals but clearly illustrate not only the steep decline in amplitude (paralleled by changes in the area of the respective M potential) as the distance increased between the site of stimulation and the motor point, indicating conduc-tion block (examples being 30 Aug. 1982, 7 Sept. 1982, 8 Oct. 1982, and 13 Jan. 1983), but also the changes in the degree of block apparent at successive studies. The study on 16 April 1983 was recorded when the patient was at his best and on 13 January when he was the most weak in the period of study embraced by these recordings.*

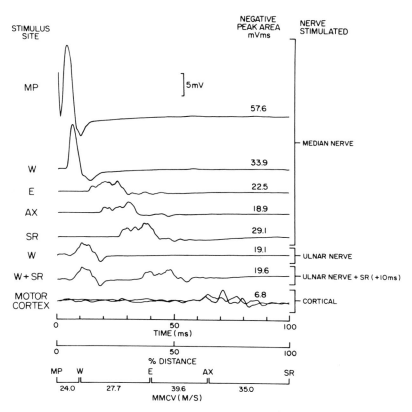

FIGURE 20.17. *Patient with chronic inflammatory demyelinating polyneuropathy (CIDP) illustrating peripheral and central conduction abnormalities. All recordings were carried out using surface electrodes from the thenar muscles in response to stimulation just proximal to the motor point (MP), wrist (W), elbow (E), axilla (AX), and spinal roots (SR). The top four recordings were in response to stimulation of the median nerve alone, whereas recording 5 was in response to surface stimulation of the spinal roots using a DE-VICES D-180 electrical stimulator. On the right are shown the respective negative peak areas of the maximum M potentials in millivolt milliseconds. Note that the M potential in response to spinal root stimulation is significantly larger than in response to stimulation of the median nerve in the axilla alone. The larger M potential with SR stimulation probably reflects inescapable stimulation of some ulnar motor fibers to the thenar muscles. To exclude the latter, collision was employed by stimulating the ulnar nerve at the wrist and spinal roots together (W and SR). This successfully removed any ulnar contribution to the thenar recording and produced a thenar M potential almost identical to that with median stimulation at the axilla.[4] Note that for the purposes of this and similar studies, we usually delay the spinal root stimulus by 10 ms or so to allow for more complete recovery from the after-following positive phase from the ulnar stimulus evoked thenar M potential. In this case, the maximum reduction in M size and increased temporal dispersion occurred between the motor point and elbow but not proximal to the elbow. This pattern is common in CIDP despite the fact that the maximum motor conduction velocities were uniformly reduced. Finally, magnetoelectrical stimulation (motor cortex) evoked an M potential that was very delayed (60.8 m/ s). The central motor conduction time was very prolonged (34.7 ms), exceeding by four times the upper limit of normal. The alternative explanation, very severe reductions in the conduction velocities in the ventral roots of the order of 1 to 2 m/s, would be required to explain such an apparently very prolonged increase in the conduction time between the cortex and spinal roots. The case had magnetic resonance imaging evidence suggestive of central demyelination.*

though severe reductions in conduction velocities may be present.

Occasionally patients with hereditary sensorimotor neuropathy type I exhibit conduction block, elevation of the cerebrospinal fluid protein, and inflammation and edema in the nerve biopsy, findings suggestive of an acquired inflammatory demyelinating neuropathy superimposed on the hereditary neuropathy. Some of these patients improve with corticosteroids.

Although single-fiber EMG adds little to the diagnosis of CIDP, studies in 19 patients have shown increased fiber densities and jitter as well as blocking, changes that no doubt reflect reinnervation.

REFERENCES

1. Brown WF. The physiological and technical basis for electromyography. Boston: Butterworths, 1984.
2. Koles ZJ, Rasminsky M. A computer simulation of conduction in demyelinated nerve fibers. J Physiol 1972; 227:351–364.
3. Bostock H, Sears TA, Sherratt RM. The effects of 4-aminopyridine and tetraethylammonium ions on normal and demyelinated mammalian nerve fibers. J Physiol 1981; 313:301–315.
4. Chiu SY, Ritchie JM. Evidence for the presence of potassium channels in the paranodal region of acutely demyelinated mammalian single nerve fibers. J Physiol 1981; 313:415–437.
5. Asbury AK. Diagnostic considerations in Guillain-Barre syndrome. Ann Neurol 1981; 9(suppl):1–5.
6. Asbury AK, Cornblath DR. Assessment of current diagnostic criteria for Guillain-Barre syndrome. Ann Neurol 1990; 27(suppl):S21–S24.
7. Ropper AH. The Guillain-Barre Syndrome. NEJM 1992 326:1130–1136.
8. Ropper AH, Wijdicks EFM, Truax BT. Guillain-Barre Syndrome. Philadelphia: F.A. Davis 1991.
9. Hughes RAC. Guillain-Barre Syndrome. London: Springer-Verlag 1990.
10. Lisak RP, Mitchell M, Zweiman B, et al. Guillain-Barre syndrome and Hodgkin's disease: Three cases with immunological studies. Ann Neurol 1977; 1:72–78.
11. Hemachudha T, Phanuphak P, Johnson RT, et al. Neurologic complications of Semple-type rabies vaccine: Clinical and immunologic studies. Neurology 1987; 37:550–556.
12. Arnason BGW, Asbury AK. Idiopathic polyneuritis after surgery. Arch Neurol 1968; 18:500–517.
13. Feasby TE, Gilbert JJ, Brown WF, et al. An acute axonal form of Guillain-Barre polyneuropathy. Brain 1986; 109:1115–1126.
14. Miller RG, Peterson C, Rosenberg NL. Electrophysiologic evidence of severe distal nerve segment pathology in the Guillain-Barre syndrome. Muscle Nerve 1987; 10:524–529.
15. Cornblath DR, Mellits ED, Griffin JW, et al. and the Guillain Barre Study Group. Motor conduction studies in Guillain-Barre syndrome: Description and prognostic value. Ann Neurol 1988; 23:354–359.
16. Miller RG, Peterson GW, Daube JR, Albers JW. Prognostic value of electrodiagnosis in Guillain-Barre syndrome. Muscle Nerve 1988; 11:769–774.
17. Albers JW, Kelly JJ. Acquired inflammatory demyelinating polyneuropathies: Clinical and electrodiagnostic features. Muscle Nerve 1989; 12:435–451.
18. Brown WF, Feasby TE, Hahn AF. Electrophysiological Changes in Acute 'Axonal' Form of Guillain Barre Syndrome. Muscle Nerve—in press.
19. Van der Meche FGA, Meulstee V, Kleyweg RP. Axonal Damage in Guillain-Barre Syndrome. Muscle Nerve 1991; 14:997–1002.
20. Ropper AH. Unusual clinical variants and signs in Guillain-Barre syndrome. Arch Neurol 1986; 43:1150–1152.
21. Dawson DM, Samuels MA, Morris J. Sensory form of acute polyneuritis. Neurology 1988; 38:1728–1731.
22. Abers JW, Robertson WC, Daube JR. Electrodiagnostic findings in acute porphyric neuropathy. Muscle Nerve 1978; 1:292–296.
23. Haymaker W, Kernohan JW. The Landry-Guillain-Barre syndrome. Medicine 1949; 28:59–141.
24. Asbury AK, Arnason BG, Adams RD. The inflammatory lesion in idiopathic polyneuritis. Medicine 1969; 48:173–215.
25. Kanda T, Hayashi H, Tanabe H, et al. A fulminant case of Guillain-Barre syndrome: Topographic and fiber size related analysis of demyelinating changes. Neurolo Neurosurg Psychiatry 1989; 52:857–864.
26. Albers JW. Inflammatory demyelinating polyradiculoneuropathy. In: Brown WF, Bolton CF, eds. Boston: Butterworths, Clinical Electromyography. 1987:211–244.
27. Prineas JW. Pathology of the Guillain-Barre syndrome. Ann Neurol 1981; 9(suppl):6–19.
28. Kimura J. Proximal versus distal slowing of motor nerve conduction velocity in the Guillain-Barre syndrome. Ann Neurol 1978; 3:344–350.
29. King D, Ashby P. Conduction velocity in the proximal segments of a motor nerve in the Guillain-Barre syndrome. J Neurol Neurosurg Psychiatry 1976; 39:538–544.
30. Brown WF, Feasby TE. Sensory evoked potentials in Guillain-Barre polyneuropathy. J Neurol Neurosurg Psychiatry 1984; 47:197–200.
31. Mills KR, Murray NMF. Proximal conduction block

in early Guillain-Barre syndrome. Lancet 1985; 2:659.

32. Brown WF. Clinical electromyography. Boston: Butterworths, 1987.

33. Dengler R, Stein RB, Thomas CK. Axonal conduction velocity and force of single human motor units. Muscle Nerve 1988; 11:136–145.

34. Milner-Brown HS, Stein RB. The relation between the surface electromyogram and muscular force. J Physiol (Lond) 1975; 246:549–569.

35. Kimura J, Sakimura Y, Machida M, et al. Effect of desynchronized inputs on compound sensory and muscle action potentials. Muscle Nerve 1988; 11:694–702.

36. Rhee EK, England JD, Sumner AJ. A computer simulation of conduction block: Effects produced by actual block versus interphase cancellation. Ann Neurol 1990; 28:146–156.

37. Cornblath DR, Sumner AJ, Daube J, et al. Conduction block in clinical practice. Muscle Nerve 1991; 14:869–871.

38. Brown WF, Feasby TE. Conduction block and denervation in Guillain-Barre polyneuropathy. Brain 1984; 107:219–239.

39. Brown WF, Snow R. Patterns and severity of conduction abnormalities in Guillain-Barre syndrome. J Neurol Neurosurg Psychiatry 1991; 54:768–774.

40. Van der Meche FGA, Meulstee J. Guillain-Barre syndrome: A model of random conduction block. J Neurol Neurosurg Psychiatry 1988; 51:1158–1163.

41. Van der Meche FGA, Meulstee J, Vermeulen M, Kievit A. Patterns of conduction failure in the Guillain-Barre syndrome. Brain 1988; 111:405–416.

42. Murray NMF, Wade DT. The sural sensory action potential in Guillain-Barre syndrome (letter). Muscle Nerve 1980; 3:444.

43. Albers JW, Donofrio PD, McGonagle TK. Sequential electrodiagnostic abnormalities in acute inflammatory demyelinating polyradiculoneuropathy. Muscle Nerve 1985; 8:528–539.

44. The Guillain-Barre Study Group. Plasmapheresis and acute Guillain-Barre syndrome. Neurology 1985; 35:1096–1104.

45. Sauron B, Bouche P, Cathala HP, et al. Miller Fisher syndrome: Clinical and electrophysiological evidence of peripheral origin in 10 cases. Neurology 1984; 34:351–364.

46. Fross RD, Daube JR. Neuropathy in the Miller Fisher syndrome: Clinical and electrophysiologic findings. Neurology 1987; 37:1493–1498.

47. Berger AR, Logigian EL, Shahani BT. Reversible proximal conduction block underlies rapid recovery in Guillain-Barre syndrome. Muscle Nerve 1988; 11:1039–1042.

48. Weiss JA, White JC. Correlation of 1A afferent conduction with the ataxia of Fisher syndrome. Muscle Nerve 1986; 9:327–332.

49. Vallet JM, Leboutet MJ, Hugon J, et al. Acute pure sensory paraneoplastic neuropathy with perivascular endoneurial inflammation: Ultrastructural study of capillary walls. Neurology 1986; 36:1395–1399.

50. Vallat KM. Sensory Guillain-Barre syndrome (letter). Neurology 1989; 39:879.

51. Solders G, Nennesmo I, Persson A. Diphtheritic neuropathy, an analysis based on muscle and nerve biopsy and repeated neurophysiological and autonomic function tests. J Neurol Neurosurg Psychiatry 1989; 52:876–880.

52. Kurdi A, Abdul-Kader M. Clinical and electrophysiological studies of diphteritic neuritis in Jordan. J Neurol Sci 1979; 42:243–250.

53. Kazemi B, Tahernia C, Zandian K. Motor nerve conduction in diphtheria and diphtheritic myocarditis. Arch Neurol 1973; 29:104–106.

54. Thomas PK, Lascelles RG, Hallpike JF, et al. Recurrent and chronic relapsing Guillain-Barre polyneuritis. Brain 1969; 92:560–589.

55. Prineas JW, McLeod JG. Chronic relapsing polyneuritis. J Neurol Sci 1976; 27:427–458.

56. Dalakas MC, Engel WK. Chronic relapsing (dysimmune) polyneuropathy: Pathogenesis and treatment. Ann Neurol 1981; 9(suppl):134–144.

57. Ingall TJ, McLeod JG, Tamura N. Autonomic function and unmyelinated fibers in chronic inflammatory demyelinating polyradiculoneuropathy. Muscle Nerve 1990; 13:70–76.

58. Dyck PJ, Lais AC, Ohta M, et al. Chronic inflammatory polyradiculoneuropathy. Mayo Clin Proc 1975; 50:621–637.

59. Julien J, Vital C, Lagueny A, et al. Chronic relapsing idiopathic polyneuropathy with primary axonal lesions. J Neurol Neurosurg Psychiatry 1989; 52:871–875.

60. Cornblath DR. Electrophysiology in Guillain-Barre syndrome. Ann Neurol 1990; 27(suppl):S17–S20.

61. Lewis RA, Sumner AJ. The electrodiagnostic distinctions between chronic familial and acquired demyelinative neuropathies. Neurology (Minneap) 1982; 32:592–596.

62. Parry GJ, Clarke S. Multifocal acquired demyelinating neuropathy masquerading as motor neuron disease. Muscle Nerve 1988; 11:103–107.

63. Buchthal F, Behse F. Peroneal muscular atrophy and related disorders: Clinical manifestations as related to biopsy findings, nerve conduction, and electromyography. Brain 1977; 100:41–66.

21

Metabolic Neuropathy

Charles F. Bolton

CONTENTS
_____

LIST OF ACRONYMS

BUN   blood urea nitrogen
CAPD   continuous ambulatory peritoneal dialysis

For the modern physician, peripheral neuropathy resulting from metabolic disturbances is a common problem. In North America, the neuropathy associated with diabetes mellitus is a particularly prevalent disorder of peripheral nerve. This is only one example of a situation in which treatment of dysfunction of a specific organ, that is, insulin to replace failing secretion by the islets of Langerhans in the pancreas, has resulted in survival, but survival often accompanied by distressing complications such as peripheral neuropathy. There are other examples. In chronic renal failure, despite improvements in methods of hemodialysis, approximately 50% of patients so treated show some evidence of uremic neuropathy. The syndrome of multiple organ failure, that is, critical illness, now occurring with increasing frequency as more patients are being rescued from death in critical care units, is associated with a significant incidence of polyneuropathy.

Clinical electromyography (EMG) should play a prominent role in the investigation and management of metabolic neuropathies. It may detect neuropathy before it has produced either symptoms or signs. It can determine, with reasonable accuracy, whether the underlying pathology is predominantly a segmental demyelination or an axonal degeneration, and it can estimate the severity of that pathology. Finally, follow-up studies provide relatively objective methods of determining the course of the polyneuropathy and the results of treatment.

Unfortunately, too often studies of metabolic neuropathies have been limited, relying only on measurements of conduction velocity of distal segments of limb nerves. More comprehensive testing provides valuable additional information. H and F waves measure the speed of conduction in proximal as well as distal segments. Somatosensory evoked potential techniques measure conduction along central and peripheral somatosenory pathways. Measurements of the amplitude of compound muscle and sensory nerve action potentials estimate not only the total number of fibers that are conducting, but also, when correlated with action potential duration, show disproportionate slowing among different-diameter myelinated fibers. The degree of conduction block of nerve impulse propagation may be determined by comparing the amplitude and duration of compound action potentials evoked by proximal stimulation to those evoked by distal stimulation. Because of their normal variation, amplitude measurements are often discounted, but when factors contributing to this variation are taken into account,[1] such measurements become valuable. Computer analysis of com-

pound action potential size and configuration may in the future provide even more valuable information.[2] Concentric needle EMG of muscle gives important information on the degree of muscle denervation and reinnervation and its distribution among the various muscles of the body. Finally, single-fiber EMG techniques allow more accurate quantitation of such denervation and reinnervation. The various neuropathies caused by metabolic disturbances are classified in Table 21.1. All are discussed in this

TABLE 21.1. Metabolic disturbances causing neuropathy

Inherited metabolic defects[a]
  Neuropathies associated with specific metabolic defect
    Disturbances of lipid metabolism
    Peroxisomal disorders
    Hereditary amyloid neuropathies
    Porphyria
    Disorders associated with defective DNA repair
    Mucopolysaccharidoses and oligosaccharidoses
    Hexosaminidase deficiency
  Disorders of unknown causation
    Hereditary motor and sensory neuropathies
    Hereditary sensory and autonomic neuropathies
    Hereditary proximal motor neuronopathies
    Hereditary distal motor neuronopathies (*spinal* form of Charcot-Marie-Tooth disease)
    Hereditary motor neuronopathies with complex distributions
Specific organ dysfunction
  Diabetes mellitus[b]
  Hypothyroidism
  Acromegaly
  Renal failure
  Hepatic failure
Nutritional disturbances
  Vitamin deficiencies
    Thiamine
    Vitamin B_{12}
    Pyridoxine (B_6)
    Niacin
    Vitamin E
  Hypophosphatemia
Nonspecific or multiple deficiencies
  Adult celiac disease
  Tropical myeloneuropathies
  Protein calorie malnutrition in children
  Postgastrectomy polyneuropathy
  Neuropathy associated with weight reduction
  Critical illness polyneuropathy
  Alcoholic polyneuropathy

---

  [a] See Chapter 15.
  [b] See Chapter 18.

chapter except for neuropathies caused by inherited metabolic defects (see Chapter 15) and diabetes mellitus (see Chapter 18).

NEUROPATHY DUE TO SPECIFIC ORGAN DYSFUNCTION

Hypothyroidism

Thyroid deficiency causes widespread effects on peripheral nerve and muscle, these effects worsening the longer the deficiency persists. The clinical features of hypothyroid neuropathy were described with considerable detail and accuracy by Gull in 1874[3] and by Ord in 1878.[4] Since then, it has been recognized that the most common neuropathy is carpal tunnel syndrome, mononeuropathies at other sites of compression being less common. Severe, diffuse polyneuropathy is, fortunately, rare.

Electrophysiology has played a prominent part in the development of our knowledge on this subject. In 1958, Murray and Simpson[5] documented the clinical and electrophysiologic features of carpal tunnel syndrome associated with myxedema, 2 years after Simpson[6] had first observed the characteristic nerve conduction defect in carpal tunnel syndrome. Nerve conduction studies have shown that polyneuropathy may occur at an early stage, while signs and symptoms are still equivocal,[7] and have documented improvement in the neuropathy after treatment with thyroid hormone.

Mononeuropathy

Carpal tunnel syndrome. Before the study by Murray and Simpson in 1958,[5] ill-defined paresthesias were recognized as a common complaint in myxedema, but the cause was unknown. In the Murray and Simpson study, 26 of 35 patients suffering from hypothyroidism complained of paresthesias of the fingers. Eleven had nerve conduction studies, seven showing abnormal prolongation of the median nerve motor distal latency (6 to 14 ms) (Figure 21.1) but not of the ulnar nerve distal latency. In follow-up studies, 30 of 35 patients became euthyroid, and in all but three of these patients, the signs and symptoms of carpal tunnel syndrome disappeared. Follow-up nerve conduction studies were performed in one patient, in whom the median distal latency decreased from 16 to 7.5 ms as the myxedema resolved.

Three years later, Purnell et al.[9] at the Mayo Clinic showed that seven of nine hypothyroid pa-

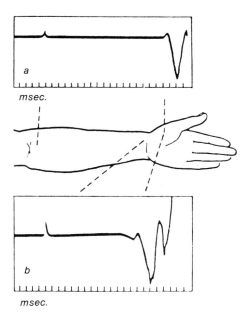

FIGURE 21.1.   *Original observation by Murray and Simpson of prolonged motor distal latency (12 ms) in a patient who had carpal tunnel syndrome associated with myxedema. The median nerve was stimulated at the elbow (A) and wrist (B) and the compound muscle action potential recorded with coaxial needle electrodes inserted into the abductor pollicis brevis muscle. (Reprinted with permission from Murray IPC, Simpson JA. Acroparaesthesia in myxoedema: A clinical and electromyographic study. Lancet 1958; 1:1360.)*

tients had clinical and electrophysiologic indications of carpal tunnel syndrome. Adequate follow-up after treatment with desiccated thyroid was possible in eight of the nine patients, in four of whom there was complete disappearance of the symptoms and signs of the carpal tunnel syndrome, whereas in the remaining four there was incomplete resolution of the symptoms. Five of these patients underwent repeat nerve conduction studies at intervals of 1 to 18 months. The latency of the response returned to normal in two patients who had an abnormal response before treatment and shortened in the remaining patients whose latency was at the upper limits of normal initially. In two patients, surgery was performed because of the severity of the carpal tunnel syndrome, and improvement occurred subjectively, but repeat nerve conduction studies were not carried out.

Biopsy in two patients revealed edematous tissue surrounding the median nerve.

These pioneering studies, which were devoted exclusively to the clinical and electrophysiologic studies of carpal tunnel syndrome and myxedema, have not, to my knowledge, been repeated using comprehensive electrophysiologic techniques, detailed clinical examinations, and systematic follow-up. The clinical features appear to be similar to carpal tunnel syndrome associated with other conditions except in myxedema, in which they are more likely to occur bilaterally.

The mechanism of carpal tunnel syndrome in myxedema is related to the accumulation of mucopolysaccharides in the extracellular connective tissue at several locations within the perineurium and endoneurium of the nerve itself but also outside the nerve, in the tendon sheaths and synovial membranes within the carpal tunnel. These mucopolysaccharides are osmotically active, and the increased edema at these sites accounts for increased pressure and a resulting compression dysfunction of the median nerve. An additional factor is a disturbance of the metabolism of the nerve itself, rendering it susceptible to compression.[5,10,11]

Other mononeuropathies.   Other nerves are subject to focal compression in hypothyroidism, particularly the ulnar nerve. None of these, however, have been studied electrophysiologically, other than compression of the tibial nerve in the tarsal tunnel.[12] Four of nine patients who had myxedema and carpal tunnel syndrome had an associated tarsal tunnel syndrome demonstrated electrophysiologically.

Polyneuropathy

Both nerve and muscle are involved commonly, and in a diffuse fashion, in hypothyroidism. In 25 myxedematous patients, Nickel et al.[13] showed that almost all had tingling, numbness, and muscular weakness. Two-thirds had objective evidence of diminished peripheral sensation, and one-third had objective muscle weakness. The majority showed prolongation of the relaxation phase of the deep tendon reflexes. Half of the patients had muscle cramps, and a third exhibited the mounding phenomenon (prolonged contraction of muscle induced by direct percussion). Muscle weakness, muscle cramps, and ataxia occurred in two-thirds, likely predominantly as a result of cerebellar dysfunction but perhaps also as a result of polyneuropathy. The

spinal fluid protein, including the gamma globulin fraction, tended to be increased.

Muscle weakness, muscle cramps, and slowness in the relaxation phase of the deep tendon reflexes are all likely due to a primary metabolic disturbance within the muscles itself. Morphologic changes indicate variations in the size of muscle fibers, enlargement of some of them, and necrotic changes in others. Greatly increased amounts of glycogen are deposited in a focal reticular fashion between the myofibrils. All of these changes disappear after thyroid replacement therapy.[10]

In hypothyroid polyneuropathy, pathologic changes[10,14] consist of reductions in the total numbers of myelinated fibers as well as reductions in the mean diameter of such fibers. Teased fiber preparations reveal segmental demyelination and remyelination. Degenerating fibers are also seen. Segmental demyelination may be secondary to a primary axonal degeneration.[14] Quantitative study of unmyelinated fibers reveals a relative increase in their number, suggesting a primary degeneration followed by regeneration. As in muscle, electron microscopy discloses an excess of glycogen granules that are in either aggregate or diffuse distributions. Such accumulations are found within the cytoplasm of Schwann cells, within their nuclei or outside the myelin sheaths, at the nodes of Ranvier. Mitochondria within Schwann cells show abnormal clustering, abnormal enlargement, and degenerative changes. All of these morphologic changes have been noted to disappear when the polyneuropathy improved after replacement therapy.[10]

Nerve conduction studies may be abnormal at a stage when symptoms of peripheral neuropathy are equivocal. Fincham and Cape[15] noted that in 13 of 16 patients with myxedema who reported paresthesia, the mean values for sensory conduction velocities were mildly but significantly reduced, as compared with control values. Yamamoto et al.[16] showed mild reduction in motor and sensory conduction velocities and prolongation of distal latencies in seven of 15 patients with primary hypothyroidism, only two of whom had symptoms of polyneuropathy. Dick et al.[19] reported such mild conduction abnormalities in a single patient whose values returned to normal following hormonal replacement therapy.

Rarely in prolonged and severe hypothyroidism, a more severe polyneuropathy occurs. The symptoms and signs are most marked distally and in the lower limbs, with variable muscle weakness; reduced or absent deep tendon reflexes; spontaneous pain; impairment of all sensory modalities, particularly of touch-pressure, vibration sense, and position sense; and ataxia of gait.[10,14,17,18] This polyneuropathy may antedate other evidence of hypothyroidism and definitive diagnosis by months or years.

In the classic study by Dyck and Lambert,[10] two such patients were described. Motor and sensory conduction velocities were moderately reduced, and distal latencies were considerably prolonged. Stimulation of the digital nerves of the index finger failed to evoked a detectable potential from the median nerve at the wrist. Compound muscle action potentials were severely reduced in amplitude and considerably dispersed (Figure 21.2). From sural nerve biopsies in each patient, in vitro nerve conduction studies revealed that the A alpha and A delta potentials were reduced in amplitude, and their conduction velocities were considerably reduced. The size of the C potential was reduced, although its conduction

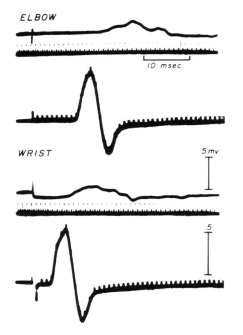

FIGURE 21.2.   *Ulnar nerve conduction studies before and after treatment in a patient who had severe hypothyroid polyneuropathy. Note the markedly prolonged latency and dispersion of the compound muscle action potential recorded with surface, belly-tendon electrodes over hypothenar muscles on both elbow and wrist stimulation. The potentials are nearly normal (lower traces of each pair) after treatment. (Reprinted with permission from Dyck PJ, Lambert EH. Polyneuropathy associated with hypothyroidism. J Neuropathol Exp Neurol 1970; 29:631–658.)*

velocity was normal (Figure 21.3). Dyck and Lambert concluded, based on their electrophysiologic and morphologic data, that segmental demyelination and remyelination were the primary underlying abnormalities in hypothyroid neuropathy. The electrophysiologic abnormalities improved in both patients after treatment (see Figure 21.2). For example, in one patient, 7 months following the treatment of the hypothyroidism, the peroneal maximum motor conduction velocity rose from 35 to 44 m per second, the extensor digitorum brevis (EDB) compound muscle action potential rose from 0.5 to 2.8 mV, and digital compound nerve action potential amplitude rose from 0 to 13 μV. In the same patient, a repeat of the nerve biopsy at 4 months revealed a resolution of the pathologic changes. Further reports largely supported these observations[14,17,18] except that Pollard et al.[14] concluded from their electrophysiologic and morphologic studies that the predominant feature was a primary axonal degeneration.

Myopathy

Muscle cramps, stiffness, and weakness, experienced by patients with hypothyroidism, are due to a primary myopathy.[22] Hofmann and Denys[21] have clearly shown there is no defect in neuromuscular transmission. There is a delay in the relaxation phase of the deep tendon reflex,[20] and a mounding phenomenon may occur when the muscle is directly percussed (myoedema). In rare circumstances, the muscles may become hypertrophied, weak, and slow in their movement (Hofmann's syndrome).[22] Serum creatine kinase levels and the myoglobin concentration in the serum may both be elevated. Needle EMG reveals no abnormal spontaneous activity and a normal recruitment pattern, although the potentials may be diminished in amplitude and duration. With an increased proportion of polyphasic units and with full interference pattern, the overall amplitude of the potentials is decreased.[23] Muscle biopsy reveals type II fiber atrophy and some predominance of type I fibers.[23] In one patient, central *cores* were seen in type I fibers with oxidative enzyme preparations.[24] Studies of the mechanical properties of the muscles have shown the speed of muscular contraction is slowed, and the isometric tension is reduced. Thyroid replacement may cause improvement in hypothyroid myopathy,[24] but such improvement may be incomplete in severe cases.[26]

Severe hypothyroidism caused respiratory muscle weakness in one patient. Phrenic nerve conduction times were mildly prolonged. Considerable improvement occurred with treatment.[27]

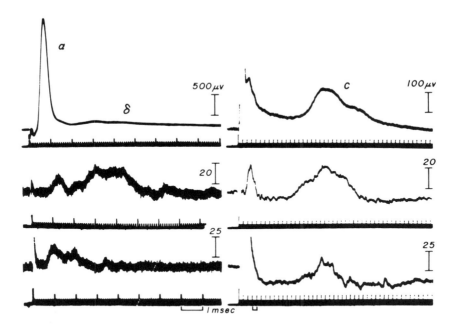

FIGURE 21.3. *In vitro nerve conduction studies in a 21-year-old healthy person (upper traces) and in two patients with severe hypothyroid polyneuropathy, a 55-year-old man (middle traces) and a 71-year-old woman (lower traces). In the patients, the A alpha and A delta potentials were reduced in amplitude and conduction velocity and the unmyelinated C fiber potential was reduced in amplitude but not in velocity. The stimulating and recording electrodes were 2 mm apart. (Reprinted with permission from Dyck PJ, Lambert EH. Polyneuropathy associated with hypothyroidism. J Neuropath Exp Neurol 1970; 29:631–658.)*

Neuromuscular Disorders Associated with Hyperthyroidism

Despite reports suggesting that polyneuropathy may be a complication of hyperthyroidism,[28–31] the issue is still in doubt. There is no doubt, however, Guillain-Barré syndrome may rarely occur as a complication of hyperthyroidism.[32,33] The incidence of myasthenia gravis is increased, occurring in approximately 5% of patients with hyperthyroidism, about the same frequency as in hypothyroidism.[34] Myasthenia gravis may appear before, during, or after the development of the thyroid dysfunction. Primary myopathy has been a well-documented complication of hypothyroidism. Neurotoxic periodic paralysis is also a well-defined entity that occurs in patients of Asian descent but not as a familial condition.[22]

Acromegaly

Among the widespread effects of excessive growth hormone are carpal tunnel syndrome and polyneuropathy. Typical and often severe bilateral carpal tunnel syndrome occurs in one-third of patients suffering from acromegaly.[35,36] It occurs as a result of proliferation of cartilage, bone, connective tissue, and synovial membranes in the area of the carpal tunnel.[37] Treatment by radiation[8] or surgery[38] results in subsidence of both the acromegaly and carpal tunnel syndrome, whereas surgical section of the carpal ligament alone may or may not bring about improvement in the carpal tunnel–related symptoms and signs.[8,36,38]

In a definitive study of 11 acromegalic patients by Low et al.,[39] a longstanding and relatively mild motor and sensory polyneuropathy was noted in five patients. The ulnar and peroneal nerves were enlarged on palpation. Mild reductions in motor conduction velocities of median, ulnar, and peroneal nerves and mild to severe reduction in the amplitude of median and ulnar compound sensory nerve action potentials and of ulnar and peroneal mixed compound sensory nerve action potentials was noted. Sural nerve biopsy in four patients showed an increase in fascicular size and subperineurial and endoneurial tissue, a reduction in the density of myelinated and unmyelinated fibers, segmental demyelination, and small onion bulb formations. Nine patients had clinical and electrophysiologic evidence of carpal tunnel syndrome. Jamal et al.[40] confirmed these observations and noted that thermal and vibratory thresholds were abnormal in two-thirds of acromegalic patients. The polyneuropathy appeared unrelated to associated diabetes mellitus, but the precise mechanism is not known. There appears to be little information on the course of the neuropathy after treatment of the pituitary tumor.

Khaleeli et al.[42] focused on muscle dysfunction in acromegaly. Six patients had no convincing evidence of polyneuropathy (sensory and motor conduction were performed), but most patients had decreased values for quadriceps force in the presence of normal muscle bulk (as measured by computed tomography [CT] scan), *myopathic* features on needle EMG, raised creatinine kinase levels, and a variation in fiber size and type 2 fiber atrophy on needle biopsy of quadriceps muscle. The mechanism of these changes is not yet understood.

Uremic Neuropathy

Clinical features

Descriptions given by both Charcot and Osler before the turn of the century were too fragmentary to be regarded as convincing descriptions of uremic polyneuropathy.[41,43] Moreover, cerebral manifestations, coma, and seizures dominated the clinical picture, and death often occurred early, so for many years the clincial signs of uremic polyneuropathy were overlooked. With the advent of chronic hemodialysis 30 years ago, many patients were rescued from early death, and it was then that uremic polyneuropathy became obvious. Hegstrom et al.[44,45] in Seattle observed progressing polyneuropathy during hemodialysis, which improved when the dialysis was intensified. At the same time, Asbury et al.[46] provided detailed clinical and pathologic descriptions of severe uremic polyneuropathy in four patients. Because none had received hemodialysis, it was concluded that this procedure was not the culprit, and the as yet ill-defined uremic toxins were the presumed cause. In a series of articles published in *Acta Medica Scandinavica* between 1971 and 1974, Nielsen provided a remarkably detailed and comprehensive account of the clinical and physiologic features of this condition.[47–55] Since than, modern methods of management have largely eliminated the more severe forms of uremic neuropathy.

Uremic polyneuropathy is a common complica-

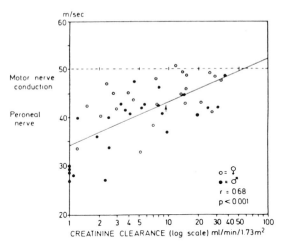

FIGURE 21.4.   *Fall in conduction velocity as kidney function declined in 56 patients before institution of hemodialysis. The arrow indicates when 50% of patients will show pathologic values. The conduction velocities tended to be lower in males than females (P<0.02). (Reprinted with permission from Nielsen VK. The peripheral nerve function in chronic renal failure. I. Sensory and motor conduction velocity. Acta Med Scand 1973; 194:446.)*

tion of chronic renal failure but for some reason seems not to occur in acute renal failure. When kidney function slowly deteriorates, however, as measured by creatinine clearance values, nerve conduction velocities progressively fall[52] (Figure 21.4). These and other nerve conduction abnormalities precede signs and symptoms. The earliest clinical manifestations include the restless legs syndrome, distal numbness and tingling, distal weakness, and, later, unsteadiness in walking. Loss of vibration sense in the toes and reduced deep tendon reflexes are early clinical signs[48,56] (Figure 21.5). The restless legs syndrome and muscle cramps may not be strictly a result of the neuropathy per se.[48] Rarely the polyneuropathy is quite severe, with marked involvement of the legs, causing the patient to be bedridden. Overt clinical signs of autonomic neuropathy are usually absent.[52] Physiologic measurements, however, are often abnormal (see section on electrophysiologic testing, later).

Mononeuropathy as well as polyneuropathy frequently occurs. Carpal tunnel syndrome is now recognized to arise commonly distal to arteriovenous fistulas implanted into the forearm for access during hemodialysis.[57] Distal ischemia and edema in the

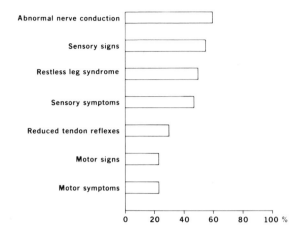

FIGURE 21.5. *Incidence of signs and symptoms of uremic polyneuropathy in 30 unselected patients on chronic hemodialysis at Victoria Hospital, London, Ontario, 1973. (Reprinted with permission from Bolton CF. Peripheral neuropathies associated with chronic renal failure. Can J Neurol Sci 1980; 7:89–96.)*

region of the carpal tunnel are the presumed mechanisms. Surgical decompression, closure of the fistula, or both may improve symptoms and signs.

Patients who have been receiving hemodialysis for more than 10 years with a machine using a cuprophan membrane almost invariably develop carpal tunnel syndrome as just one manifestation of generalized amyloidosis. It arises because β_2-microglobulin accumulates systemically, a form of amyloidosis peculiar to renal failure. Electrophysiologic tests disclose carpal tunnel syndrome, and biopsy and special stains for β_2-microglobulin should be instituted at the time of surgery.[58]

Bovine shunts, implanted in the upper arm, may rarely induce excessive arteriovenous shunting and a severe ischemic neuropathy affecting radial, median, and ulnar nerves.[59] Uremic patients who are bedridden and cachectic have a tendency to compressive palsies of both the ulnar nerve at the elbow and the common peroneal nerve at the fibular head.

Other types of neuropathies must be considered in the differential diagnosis. The most common is diabetes mellitus, particularly when renal failure develops as a complication of the diabetes. In this and other conditions, however, in which the primary disease may affect both the kidneys and the peripheral nerves, the clinical features of the neuropathy usually allow the clinician to distinguish between a primary

diabetic and uremic peripheral neuropathies. In diabetes mellitus, for example, cranial nerve palsies, compressive palsies, and autonomic neuropathies are much more frequent and prominent features than is the case in uremic polyneuropathy. A more difficult problem is presented by drug-induced polyneuropathies in which the clinical signs and symptoms may be identical to uremic polyneuropathy. Nitrofurantoin, however, is the only drug that has been conclusively shown to produce polyneuropathy in renal failure, and its use is now avoided in this situation.

Hemodialysis or chronic ambulatory peritoneal dialysis halts the progress of uremic polyneuropathy, but unfortunately in most instances, significant improvement may not occur, despite various manipulations of the dialysis schedules. Successful renal transplantation, however, invariably brings satisfactory resolution of the neuropathy, although mild residual clinical signs may remain.[55,60–62]

Pathologic studies of the spinal cord and peripheral nerves were carried out in the original report by Asbury et al.[46] Peripheral nerves showed a predominantly distal segmental demyelination and axonal degeneration, and there was chromatolysis of anterior horn cells of the spinal cord, consistent with primary damage to peripheral nerve axons. In severe polyneuropathy, however, demyelination in lumbosacral nerve roots has been noted.[63] Comprehensive studies of peripheral nerves by Dyck et al.[64] and Thomas et al.[65] have revealed a combination of paranodal demyelination, segmental demyelination, axonal degeneration, and segmental remyelination. Dyck et al.,[64] however, noted that the ratio of the circumference of the axis cylinders to the number of myelin lamellae was decreased in distal nerve fibers, suggesting axonal shrinkage. Moreover, segmental demyelination tended to occur only on certain fibers, completely sparing others, suggesting that demyelination was secondary to axonal disease. Consistent with this argument was the observation that demyelination and axonal degeneration were much more marked distally.

A number of electrophysiologic studies by Nielsen,[66] however, have suggested a more generalized effect on the nerve axon membrane, specifically an inhibition of sodium-activated and potassium-activated adenosine triphosphatase (ATPase). Conduction is slowed in both proximal and distal portions of peripheral nerves in the early stages of uremic neuropathy. Uremic nerves, when ischemic, demonstrate both an electrodecremental response and a failure of vibration sense and the evoked sensory action potential to disappear as quickly as they do in normal nerve—so-called ischemia resistance. Thus the first effect of the uremic toxins may be on the two membrane barriers that normally limit access of higher molecular weight substances to individual peripheral nerves, that is, the perineurial barrier and the capillary barrier within the endoneurium. Castaigne et al.[67] have observed that this *resistance* of compound sensory nerve action potentials to ischemia can be enhanced by a single hemodialysis procedure and abolished by macromolecular perfusion. Because the amplitude of compound sensory nerve action potentials is positively related to the density of myelinated fibers,[68] a fluctuation in endoneurial volume, secondary to *leaky* diffusion barriers, which allow osmotically active substances to leave or enter the endoneurial spaces, might account for this observation. Thus the as yet unknown uremic toxins might diffuse through the leaky barriers and cause direct nerve damage.[56]

Brismar and Tegner[69] have shown in the sciatic nerve of rats rendered acutely uremic that the sodium permeability of the nodal membrane is decreased, as determined by potential recordings and potential clamp of myelinated fibers; this explained the reduced conduction velocity.

The nature of the uremic toxin or toxins is still unknown. Either urea or creatinine are the most obvious offenders because they are effectively removed by adequate hemodialysis. In fact, studies by Teschan et al.[70] indicate that uremic neuropathy is more likely to develop under hemodialysis schedules in which each hemodialysis procedure was of short duration and the blood urea nitrogen (BUN) became markedly elevated. On the other hand, Nielsen[66] noted a poor relationship between nerve conduction abnormalities and serum concentrations of creatinine and urea.

The *middle molecule* theory, although controversial, still remains the most plausible and is still being actively investigated. These substances, of molecular weight 300 to 2000 daltons, are normally elevated in end-stage renal failure and are most effectively reduced by parallel plate (Kiil) dialyzing units rather than coil (Kolff) dialyzers.[71] The observation that successful renal transplantation invariably causes improvement in uremic neuropathy[55,62] fits well with this theory because it is known that the functioning kidney can deal effectively with substances of varying molecular weights, including middle molecules. Bergstrom et al.[72] have noted that progressive peripheral neuropathy is associated with an elevation of several fractions of middle molecules, and Faguer et al.[73] believe that the B42 peak correlated with the incidence of uremic neuropathy in 43 uremic patients. Moreover, they noted that continuous ambulatory peritoneal dialysis, which in a separate study at the Mayo clinic[74] was associated with a progressing neuropathy in several subjects, was associated with particularly large elevations of the B42 middle molecule peak. Finally, Braguer et al.[75] from culture studies of the microtubules of nerve axons, have shown that middle molecules have an inhibiting effect on the growth of these microtubules and that this effect appears to be reversed by a new drug, isaxonine phosphate.

Electrophysiologic testing of the peripheral nervous system

Electrophysiologic studies are particularly valuable in assessing the peripheral nervous system in chronic uremia. Conduction velocities in peripheral nerves become reduced before either signs or symptoms of peripheral neuropathy have developed. In individual patients, the function of large myelinated fibers of the peripheral nervous system can be tested both proximally and distally, repeatedly, and in a noninvasive way. Thus objective measurements of nerve function can be obtained to assess the wide variety of methods that are currently used to treat chronic renal failure: that is, diet, vitamin supplementation, various forms of dialysis, and renal transplantation.

As in all forms of metabolic neuropathy, electrophysiologic techniques must be carefully and consistently performed to give reliable results. It is wise to test conduction in both motor and sensory fibers of upper and lower limbs. Because axonal degeneration predominates, the most marked abnormality is a reduction in the amplitude of compound muscle and sensory action potentials. Attention to the various factors that normally affect this amplitude, sex, limb circumference, and temperature in particular, reduces the variability of this measurement.[1] It is most important to apply the recording electrodes in precisely the same position from one examination to the next and to use a standard method. Temperature measurement is important because these patients often are catabolic, and distal limb temperature is often elevated in comparison to control subjects. We have avoided the use of needle EMG as much as possible because uremic patients are already being subjected to repeated venipuncture through blood tests, chronic hemodialysis, and so on, and they are unlikely to return for repeat studies if the electrophysiologic test is too uncomfortable. Thus we use surface instead of needle electrodes for recording in nerve conduction studies and perform concentric needle EMG of muscle only in clinically apparent and more severe polyneuropathies. Finally, owing to the frequent occurrence of carpal tunnel syndrome distal to forearm arteriovenous shunts or fistulas, nerve conduction studies should be performed in both upper limbs, to detect carpal tunnel syndrome in the limb containing the fistula and as a way of further studying the general pattern and severity of the polyneuropathy.

Three years after regular hemodialysis had been instituted, Chaumont et al.[76] in France, Versaki et al.[77] in the United States, and Preswick and Jeremy[78] in Australia reported reduced conduction velocities in uremic patients, often preceding clinical signs. Since then, this and other neurophysiologic mea-

surements have been used extensively in uremia. The subject has been reviewed by Bolton and Young.[79]

Both motor and sensory conduction velocities are reduced[51] and distal latencies prolonged. Conduction velocity changes during the various stages of renal failure, largely reflecting its severity (Figure 21.6). Amplitudes of muscle and sensory compound action potentials are considerably reduced, the reduction being due partly to a dispersion of the action potential as a result of disproportionate slowing of conduction in some nerve fibers (Figure 21.7). The main reason for the reduction, however, is axonal degeneration and loss of conduction in affected fibers and denervation of muscle. Of the various nerve conduction measurements, reduction of the amplitude of both muscle and sensory nerve compound action

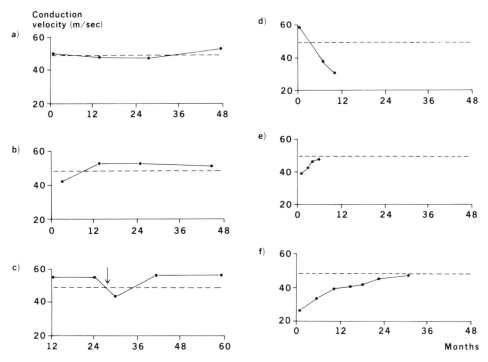

FIGURE 21.6. *Variations in the course of uremic neuropathy in individual patients as reflected in median motor conduction velocity. (dashed line = 2 S.D. below mean control value). Other nerves tested showed similar results. (A) A stable course in a 54-year-old man on three times weekly home dialysis. (B) Improvement in uremic neuropathy in a 55-year-old man on three times weekly home dialysis. (C) Transient worsening in uremic neuropathy in a 48-year-old woman during intercurrent illness (↓ = hysterectomy, septicemia, and uremic encephalopathy). (D) Rapidly progressing neuropathy in a 21-year-old man on twice weekly hemodialysis with a Kolff twin-coil unit. (E) Rapid recovery after successful renal transplantation in a 43-year-old man with a subclinical neuropathy. (F) Gradual recovery after successful renal transplantation in a 21-year-old man with severe, quadriplegic neuropathy. (Reprinted with permission from Bolton CF. Peripheral neuropathies associated with chronic renal failure. Can J Neurol Sci 1980; 7:89–96.)*

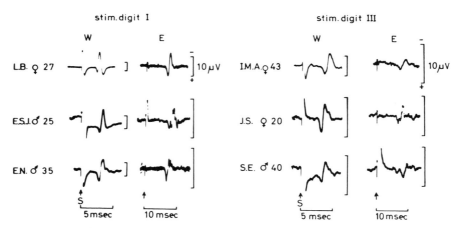

FIGURE 21.7. *Compound sensory nerve action potentials recorded at the wrist (W) and elbow (E) in uremic patients. Note the dispersion of the action potentials on proximal recording at the elbow. (Reprinted with permission from Nielsen VK. The peripheral nerve function in chronic renal failure. VI. The relationships between sensory and motor nerve conduction and kidney function, azotemia, age, sex and clinical neuropathy. Acta Med Scand 1973; 194:456.)*

potentials is the most marked.[80] Needle EMG shows abnormalities only when the neuropathy has become moderate or severe. At this time, positive sharp waves and fibrillation potentials appear mainly in distal muscles, and the number of motor unit potentials on voluntary recruitment becomes moderately decreased in number.[56,62] The sural nerve, a purely sensory nerve, is possibly the site of the earliest abnormality.[81,82] In general, the degree of slowing of nerve conduction in proximal segments is at least equal to or perhaps more marked than in distal segments.[52,83] Moreover, van der Most Van Spijck et al.[84] demonstrated that there was slowing in conduction in small as well as large myelinated fibers. The excitation threshold to peripheral nerve stimulation is increased in comparison to controls,[85] but the variability in this test is too great to make it of any clinical value.

In Nielsen's[52] comprehensive studies of 56 patients with chronic renal failure who were not yet receiving regular hemodialysis, he demonstrated that nerve conduction was significantly slowed once the 24-hour creatinine clearance fell below 10 ml per minute for a 1.73-m² membrane area. In fact, there was a linear relationship between reduced peroneal nerve conduction velocity and creatinine clearance[52] (Figure 21.4). Slowing of nerve conduction was more marked in males than females, but age was not a factor when the degree of renal failure was taken into account. There was a relatively poor correlation

between the prevalence of clinical signs and abnormalities of nerve conduction, the latter often being present when clinical signs were absent.

Standard nerve conduction as well as H waves and F waves (late responses) reveals abnormalities in 60% of children.[80,86,87] Nerve conduction values tend to stabilize during chronic hemodialysis but consistently improve after successful renal transplantation.[86]

Hansen and Ballantyne,[88] using a computer technique, found that the total number of units in the EDB muscle was one-third the normal value. Single-fiber EMG[89,90] showed the fiber density was normal, suggesting a failure of reinnervation. There was an abnormality, however, in the variation in the interval between the firing of two single fibers, so-called jitter, likely related to peripheral demyelination. Thus these investigations point to significant peripheral demyelination and failure of collateral reinnervation, both presumably secondary to axonal degeneration.

There is general agreement[91–96] that conduction is slowed along both the peripheral segment and the central segments of primary sensory neurons, but only through the spinal cord, not higher in the brain stem or cerebral hemispheres. The only exception to this was the observation by Serra et al.[91] that trans-callosal conduction time was increased. Lewis et al.[93] and Serra et al.[91] reported that the amplitude of the evoked potentials recorded over the cerebral hemispheres was abnormally increased in comparison to controls, suggesting excessive synchronization of the traveling impulse.

Several studies[81,97–99] have shown that the F wave latency is abnormally prolonged in up to 86% of patients in chronic renal failure. The latency has been shown to shorten toward normal in some patients during the course of hemodialysis and in all patients after successful renal transplantation. The H wave response is abnormal in an equally high percentage of patients and may be abnormal in approximately 20% of the patients who have normal nerve conduction studies.[81]

Tests of the autonomic nervous system

Solders et al.[100] have performed comprehensive testing on uremic patients. Almost all patients have abnormalities of the cardiac beat to beat variation (R-R interval). This abnormality is more marked in relationship to the severity of the renal failure. A single hemodialysis treatment had no effect on the R-R variation. The abnormality was more marked in those patients who had abnormal lowering of the amplitude of the sensory compound action potential of the sural nerve, suggesting that the axonal degeneration of peripheral nerve affects both the somatic and the autonomic nerves. Thus Dyck et al.[64] noted a degeneration of nonmyelinated as well as myelinated fibers in nerve biopsies in patients who had uremic polyneuropathy. Signs of autonomic dysfunction are more marked in the elderly. Using a battery of tests, Solders et al.[101] found abnormalities of the parasympathetic system to be the most frequent.

Despite the well-documented evidence for autonomic neuropathy in uremia, in an earlier study, Bolton[56] found that few patients exhibited overt symptoms or signs of severe autonomic insufficiency at any time during the course of chronic renal failure: that is, orthostatic hypotension, impotence, or bowel or bladder disturbance. In the ill uremic patient, however, orthostatic hypotension could be erroneously attributed to volume depletion or antihypertensive drugs, impotence to a variety of other causes, bladder problems to decreased urine volumes from renal failure, and bowel problems and constipation to aluminum-containing antacids. Thus the incidence and type of autonomic disturbance are difficult to assess in the uremic patient on a purely clinical basis.

Treatment and prevention

Hemodialysis. Electrophysiologic tests provide an objective and quantitative assessment of peripheral nerve function. As already noted, a remarkable number of tests, most of them electrophysiologic, have since been devised in an attempt to accomplish this objective. In particular, it had been hoped that these tests would provide one method of assessing the adequacy of the various types of dialysis. Unfortunately, the results have been controversial, the discussion centering around two main problems. Initially, it was assumed that electrophysiologic measurements, notably nerve conduction velocity, were much more precise than they actually are. When the variability was realized, opinion shifted too far in the opposite direction, and many centers have now entirely discarded this method of patient assessment. The second problem has been that even when nerve conduction studies are properly evaluated, they have borne a poor relationship, so it seemed, to the course of the neuropathies assessed by symptoms and signs or by other methods of measuring uremic toxicity. Thus it was the recommendation in one review[102] that nerve conduction studies are of little value in assessing patients during long-term hemodialysis.

Although there is little doubt that long-term hemodialysis halts the progression of uremic polyneuropathy and that modern methods are associated with an extremely low incidence of moderate or severe polyneuropathy, electrophysiologic tests still disclose an incidence of approximately 60%[103] in patients receiving long-term hemodialysis. There would seem little doubt therefore that this complication remains a significant contributing factor to the morbidity associated with this group of patients. Thus it is our view that objective methods of measuring peripheral nerve function should continue to be regularly used in patients receiving long-term hemodialysis, and such methods should be taken into account in evaluating a dialysis method that claims to be an improvement. Nerve conduction measurements have been strongly correlated with underlying pathologic changes[64,104] and are, in our opinion, still the best method of peripheral nerve assessment.

Jebsen et al.[105] emphasized that uremic neuropathy could potentially be prevented by starting hemodialysis earlier in the course of chronic renal failure and by intensifying hemodialysis should evidence of polyneuropathy develop. They also emphasized that nerve conduction values were an important method of detecting the neuropathy in its early stages and following its course.

As various refinements in the hemodialysis techniques have taken place over the years, it has been noted that the incidence of uremic polyneuropathy, certainly the clinical symptoms and signs of such a neuropathy, have fallen dramatically. Overt uremic polyneuropathy must now be considered a relatively rare entity.[101,106] As is noted later, alterations in dialysis methods are unlikely to be the only reason. Others to be considered are institution of long-term hemodialysis earlier in the course of renal failure, when there is still some residual renal function and more severe peripheral nerve damage has not yet occurred (Figure 21.8) and earlier renal transplantation when uremic *toxicity* cannot be controlled.

Rapidly progressive and ultimately severe polyneuropathy seems to develop in association with critical illness: that is, sepsis and malfunction of other organs of the body, in addition to the kidney. We have noted in the last 15 years that an acute axonal type of polyneuropathy is a specific complication of sepsis and multiple organ failure.[107,108] Thus one would anticipate that in a patient with advanced renal failure, any episodes of sepsis or injury such as surgery might be particularly harmful to peripheral nerves. This was noted by Tenckhoff et al.[109] Williams et al.[110] observed worsening in polyneuropathy during an epidemic of hepatitis in their renal unit. Thus it is possible that the improvement in polyneuropathy over the years is due not to refinements in the type of dialyzer but to the advent of the Brescia-

Cimino fistula, which has dramatically reduced the incidence of recurring sepsis.

A study in Japan[111] disclosed improvement in the beat to beat cardiac interval when patients in hemodialysis were treated with mecobolamin, an analog of vitamin B_{12}, suggesting improvement in uremic autonomic neuropathy. The results, however, need confirmation.

Dialysis schedules. After the first 10 years of experience with regular hemodialysis, there was the general feeling that uremic polyneuropathy was an indication of the adequacy of hemodialysis. It was thought that if signs of polyneuropathy developed during hemodialysis, particularly as detected by changes in nerve conduction results, improving the dialysis would result in improvement in the uremic neuropathy.[105,112-114] If one could measure the adequacy of dialysis by various techniques and then adjust the type of dialysis accordingly, theoretically an ideal dialysis method would eventually result. Uremic polyneuropathy was regarded as a major index of the adequacy of dialysis.

It has been difficult, however, to prove that optimal hemodialysis regularly improves uremic polyneuropathy.[62,115] In his study of 14 patients, Nielsen[53] observed only a stabilization in nerve con-

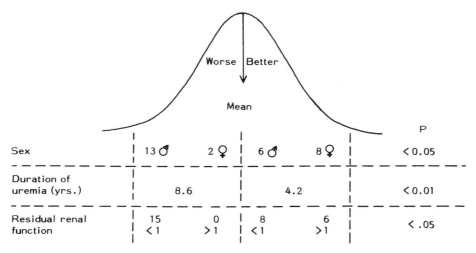

FIGURE 21.8. *Factors influencing peripheral nerve function during chronic hemodialysis. Twenty-nine patients on a three times weekly home dialysis program in London, Ontario, Canada, were tested by nerve electrophysiologic methods at yearly intervals for 3 years. Electrophysiologic values remained constant over this period. Based on the results, the patients were classified as having better or worse peripheral nerve function. Those with better function tended to be females, had had uremia a shorter period of time, and had better residual renal function based on creatinine clearance values. (Reprinted with permission from Bolton CF, Young GB. The neurological complications of renal disease. Boston: Butterworths, 1990.)*

duction studies, although symptoms improved. In a much larger study of 213 patients, Cadilhac et al.[116] again found mainly a stabilization, a few patients improving or worsening.

Deliberately manipulating the dialysis schedule also seems to have little effect. In 1975, Dyck et al.[117] at the Mayo Clinic, using a crossover method halfway through the 1-year trial period, found that patients treated with restricted intake of protein and fluid and infrequent dialysis had no worsening of peripheral nerve function compared with a conventional hemodialysis treatment schedule. Of all patients initially entered in the study, however, only five were able to complete it for various reasons. Thus despite the use of sensitive and comprehensive methods of testing, it is difficult to draw firm conclusions from this study.

In 1977, Bolton et al.[118] chose six adult patients who had been treated for 2 years on a Gambro 17 dialyzer, twice weekly for a total of 15 m² hours per week and switched them while still on hospital dialysis to three times per week, 18 m² hours per week, using the same type of dialyzer. There were no significant changes in nerve conduction measurements in individual patients or in the mean values of these measurements for the group when assessed every 4 months for a year. Six healthy controls were tested at the same time by the same methods. In this study, each patient served as his or her own control.

Bolton and colleagues[115,119] have also found no convincing differences in incidence or severity while managing patients on either home or hospital dialysis. Some preservation of residual renal function, perhaps induced by starting regular hemodialysis earlier, is associated with less severe uremic polyneuropathy[106,120] (Figure 21.8).

A concept that is still in vogue arose from Babb et al.[71] They believed that patients on peritoneal dialysis did not have the same tendency to uremic polyneuropathy as those on hemodialysis. They theorized that the peritoneal membrane was much more permeable to middle-molecule substances than the artificial membrane in dialysis machines. It might also explain the observation that patients being dialyzed by the Kiil machine, in which there would theoretically be a greater clearance of middle molecules, had a lower incidence of uremic neuropathy than those being dialyzed by the Kolff twin-coil machine. Clearance of these middle molecules, or higher molecular weight than urea and creatinine, or approximately 500 to 3000 daltons, could be calculated by multiplying the number of hours of dialysis per week by the surface area of the dialyzing membrane and dividing this by the body weight in kilograms—the so-called square-meter-hours per kilogram body weight. This middle-molecule concept was then subject to intensive investigation.[121]

Funck-Brentano et al.[106] treated four uremic patients with a dialysis machine containing a polyacrylonitrile membrane that had a high clearance for vitamin B_{12}, which is in the same molecular range as the middle molecules. Dramatic improvement in uremic polyneuropathy was claimed by this treatment. Lowrie et al.,[122] however, assessed, among other factors, peripheral nerve function, measuring the ulnar nerve conduction velocity and distal latency in a carefully randomized study. They reported improvement in nerve conduction measurements when small-molecule clearance had no effect on the neuropathy. Results in the 1983 study by Lindsay et al.[123] also failed to substantiate the middle-molecule theory. In 14 patients with end-stage renal disease who had been established on hemodialysis, treatment was compared with a conventional hemodialyzer and an experimental device that combined hemodialysis and hemoperfusion in such a way that *in vitro* vitamin B_{12} clearances and hence middle-molecule clearances were improved. A crossover design was used, switching between these two techniques every 2 months. Although there was an improvement in the velocity of platelet aggregation in response to 10 μM adenosine diphosphate and to standard collagen preparation associated with treatment with the experimental device, there was no demonstrable influence on nerve conduction studies (Figure 21.9). Thus enhanced middle-molecule clearance seemed to improve platelet, but not peripheral nerve, function. Alternatively, the crossover may have been too often (every 2 months) to allow sufficient time for measurable changes in peripheral nerve function to have occurred.

The arguments, however, for middle molecules as factors in the production of peripheral neuropathy are strong. Asaba et al.[124] by using the technique of gel chromatography followed by ion exchange gradient lucent chromatography, were able to separate various middle-molecule fractions. Among 65 regularly hemodialyzed patients, six had significantly elevated plasma concentrations of middle molecules, including 7C, 7B, and 7D fractions. These patients had a high incidence of acute infections, which seemed to be associated with elevation of the 7C fraction. Three of these patients developed a progressive peripheral neuropathy. Finally, Braguer et al.[75] have shown by *in vitro* methods that tubulin, an intracellular protein that polymerizes microtu-

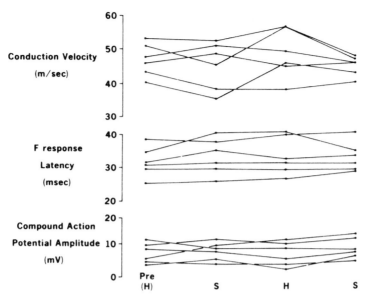

FIGURE 21.9.   *The effect of altering uremic retention products on peripheral nerve function. Fourteen patients were studied at 2-month intervals in a crossover trial. Treatment with a conventional Cuprophan membrane dialyzer, the Hemoclear (H) (Medical Incorporated, Minneapolis, MN) was compared with a Sorbiclear (S) dialyzer (Medical Incorporated), which had better clearance of middle, but not smaller, molecular weight substances. There was no significant change in peripheral nerve function, and the same result occurred when the sequence of treatments was reversed. Thus there was no evidence for improved peripheral nerve function with enhanced removal of middle molecules. (Reprinted with permission from Lindsay RM, Bolton CF, Clark WF, Linton AL. The effect of alterations of uremic retention products upon platelet and peripheral nerve function. Clin Nephrol 1983; 19:110–115.)*

bules, essential components of the axons of nerve cells, is inhibited by the middle molecules of uremia.

Effect of treatment by a single hemodialysis procedure.   Studies on this subject have provided somewhat conflicting results. Jebsen et al.[105] in 1967 reported that a single hemodialysis procedure had no effect on peripheral nerve conduction studies. Solders et al.,[100] however, reported a rise in the amplitude of the sensory compound action potential. The most detailed study has been by Lowitzsch et al.[125] These authors studied several neurophysiologic conditions in 18 patients 1 hour before and 2 hours after a single hemodialysis procedure. There was an increase in the conduction velocity and the duration of the sensory nerve compound action potential but not its amplitude. The most striking abnormality, however, was a decrease in the refractory period of the nerve immediately after this procedure. There was no change in vibratory perception or in visual evoked potentials. The pattern of changes suggested that

there is a decreased resting membrane potential in uremia that is reversible by a single hemodialysis procedure.

Peritoneal dialysis.   There is now at least 10 years' experience with peritoneal dialysis. The subject was reviewed by Gokal.[126] In the United Kingdom, this form of treatment is now used twice as often as it was 5 years ago, accounting for one-third of all dialysis patients. Patients on hemodialysis who are then started on peritoneal dialysis immediately notice an improved sense of well-being, and there is a rise in hemoglobin concentration. Hypertension is easier to control, and there is improvement in renal osteodystrophy. Patients who were previously thought unacceptable for hemodialysis can now be treated by this method. They include patients who are elderly, very small children, and those who suffer from diabetes mellitus or cardiovascular disease. The patient who has just developed end-stage renal failure is now often placed on continuous ambulatory peritoneal dialysis (CAPD) first, if he or she is a good candidate for transplantation.

The main problems are recurring attacks of peritonitis, poor catheter function, and damage to the peritoneal membrane. The infecting organisms are often skin contaminants. A peritonitis rate of at least one episode per 24 patient-months of treatment occurs. One-third of all CAPD patients, however, remain peritonitis-free over several years. Rarely sclerosing encapsulating peritonitis may develop that ultimately proves fatal.

Initial observations suggested a low incidence of polyneuropathy.[127] It was theorized that the higher permeability of the peritoneal membrane compared with the dialysis membrane would allow more efficient removal of middle molecules. This originally helped form the basis of the middle-molecule hypothesis.[71] Progressive uremic polyneuropathy, however, was subsequently observed during peritoneal dialysis.[74,128] Tegner and Lindholm[129] compared CAPD and hemodialysis in 21 and 22 patients. Motor nerve conduction and vibration sensation decreased, more in CAPD patients. Paradoxically clinical testing suggested improvement. A similar paradox was noted by Nielsen[54] in relationship to long-term hemodialysis, apparent clinical improvement occurring but only a stabilization in electrophysiologic tests. Pierratos et al.[130] found no significant change in nerve conduction velocities during peritoneal dialysis, perhaps because most of their patients were women, in whom the incidence of polyneuropathy is quite low.

Amair et al.[131] studied 20 diabetic patients with end-stage renal disease who were treated for 36 months with CAPD. Although 15 of the 20 patients (75%) had clinical evidence of polyneuropathy before treatment, follow-up for 1 year revealed no change in the clinical signs or in the nerve conduction velocities of median, ulnar, and peroneal nerves. Polyneuropathy in diabetic patients, however, may not improve even after successful renal transplantation, suggesting that the neuropathy in these patients may be due to diabetes mellitus. Thus despite the theoretical advantages of CAPD, uremic polyneuropathy seems to behave the same for this procedure as it does for long-term hemodialysis; that is, it mainly stabilizes, worsening or improving in a few patients or with various methods of assessment.

Kidney transplantation. Kidney transplantation has been the centerpiece of transplantation development. So successful has this procedure been that in the United States it is being performed at an increasingly rapid rate: from 4697 per year in 1980 to 7695 per year in 1985, approximately a 10% annual increase.[132]

The 1-year survival of cadaveric transplants has improved, partly due to the use of cyclosporine, from 53% in 1977 to 68% in 1984. The quality of life is better than with dialysis. Moreover, the procedure is much more cost-effective. Thus there is a great pressure to use this procedure for the management of end-stage renal disease, particularly in patients under 65 years of age.

Versaki et al.[77] stated that nerve conduction studies failed to improve after renal transplantation. Several systematic studies clearly showed the beneficial effects of successful renal transplantation on uremic polyneuropathy. Using both clinical observation and electromyographic techniques, Dinapoli et al.,[133] Tenckhoff et al.,[109] Dobblestein et al.,[60] in Germany, and Funck-Brentano et al.[106] in France reported consistent improvement in the polyneuropathy, even in severe forms, following successful renal transplantation.

The first symptoms to improve, within a few days or weeks, are distal numbness and tingling.[54] Even patients who have had no signs or symptoms of polyneuropathy, however, have a greater feeling of well-being soon after the transplantation, and this coincides with improvement in nerve conduction velocities.[7] Moreover, during this early stage, Nielsen[54] noted a dramatic improvement in previously elevated thresholds to vibratory perception.

Clinical recovery seems to occur in two phases:[54,60] initial rapid improvement over days or weeks and then more protracted improvement over months. The rate of improvement is related mainly to the severity of the neuropathy, being more protracted in severe cases.[62] Even in these severe cases, walking may be possible within 2 to 3 months, and reasonably satisfactory function may eventually occur. Patients will then be able to perform fine movements with their hands, such as buttoning their clothes or writing. In severe neuropathy, a disabling action tremor may develop during the recovery phase, but this eventually disappears and allows normal function of the hands (Casano. Personal Communication, 1972).

In severe polyneuropathy, however, residual clinical signs often remain. Ankle jerks may remain absent, and distal muscles may be moderately weak and wasted, particularly in the lower limbs. Despite evidence of impotence and signs of autonomic dysfunction during regular hemodialysis, potency and fertility virtually return to normal.[62,134]

Improvement in these various manifestations of polyneuropathy occurs only if the transplanted kidney continues to function successfully for a matter of months. Should acute or chronic rejection occur, not only will uremic polyneuropathy fail to improve, but also progressive worsening will likely occur.[60,62] With successful renal transplantation, however, clinical and electrophysiologic improvement prevails for a second time.[119] This observation provides strong evidence that immunosuppressive methods such as irradiation, steroids, and azathioprine, which are used following successful renal transplantation, are not, in themselves, responsible for the recovery from uremic polyneuropathy. There is little doubt that the restoration of near-normal function is responsible for this improvement.

Mononeuropathies, particularly of a compressive nature, of the ulnar nerve at the elbow and the peroneal nerve at the fibular head, occasionally occur during terminal renal failure, particularly if the patient is cachectic and bedridden for any length of time. Successful renal transplantation restores the function of these individually damaged nerves, as it does the more general polyneuropathy.[119] Mallamaci et al.[135] observed that autonomic nervous system function was equally impaired in patients on hemodialysis and peritoneal dialysis but was essentially normal in patients who had successfully received a renal transplantation.

Studies of the effects of transplantation on diabetics with end-stage renal disease have been of great interest. Gonzales-Carrillo et al.[136] and Van der Vliet et al.[137] noted no convincing improvement in the polyneuropathy of such patients after successful renal transplantation. In a careful, well-controlled study, Solders et al.[138] observed that polyneuropathy failed to improve not only in 15 diabetics who had renal transplantation, but also in a further 13 diabetics who had combined kidney and pancreatic transplantation; a third group of nondiabetic patients evinced complete recovery from *pure* uremic polyneuropathy after renal transplantation alone. Thus the polyneuropathy in diabetic patients who are in renal failure would seem to be due mainly to the diabetes mellitus, this type of neuropathy being relatively resistant to even combined kidney and pancreatic transplantation.

Kidney transplantation is a successful method of managing end-stage renal disease in children. In Canada, approximately 2% of all new patients entering the dialysis transplantation program are children, and of all transplants performed, 9% are performed on children.[87] Uremic polyneuropathy fails to improve during long-term hemodialysis but improves regularly after each successful renal transplantation, although the recovery phase may be somewhat more protracted than in adults.[86]

Electrophysiologic changes after successful renal transplantation

Chaumont et al.,[76] Funck-Brentano et al.,[106] and Dobblestein et al.[60] were the first to report that nerve conduction studies consistently improved after successful renal transplantation. Dobblestein et al.[60] emphasized the clinical improvement along with the electrophysiologic improvement and indicated that, as with the clinical signs, recovery occurred in two phases. Funck-Brentano et al.[106] indicated, however, that electrophysiologic recovery might be incomplete:

In all 10 cases, tracings definitely showed denervation of a number of motor units despite apparent complete motor recovery. This observation suggests that the healing process occurs only in fibers which are partially functional at the time of transplantation.

These observations were largely substantiated and then expanded by more detailed studies by Bolton[62,119] and Nielsen.[53,54]

Just how early electrophysiologic changes begin following the transplant is debatable. Neither Nielsen nor Bolton systematically tested nerve conduction in the days and weeks immediately before and then after the transplantation procedure. Bolton, however, did perform nerve conduction studies in nine patients at least once in the 2 months before and once within 2 months after transplantation. No significant change was demonstrated in either median or peroneal nerve conduction velocities. Ibrahim et al.[139] and Oh et al.,[140] however, measured nerve conduction velocity at frequent intervals immediately before and then after transplantation. They noted statistically significant rises in the conduction velocity within a week following the transplantation. This suggested a rapidly reversible metabolic effect on the peripheral nerve. In fact, Oh et al. demonstrated that the rise in conduction velocities coincided with a fall in the previously abnormally elevated levels of myoinositol.

A word of caution should be introduced in interpreting these last results. Ibrahim et al.[139] failed to measure limb temperature. Oh et al.[140] recorded limb temperature and applied a correction factor to their nerve conduction results. The correction factor, however, was one based on changes in normal nerve.[139] Bolton et al.[141] have demonstrated that in peripheral neuropathy, specifically uremic neuropathy, the speed of impulse conduction tends to rise more rapidly with increasing limb temperature than in normal nerve. Thus the results following transplantation may be spurious if limb temperature rose, as it often does postoperatively, and appropriate correction factors were not applied.

There is little doubt that the more definitive rise in conduction velocities that occurs in the weeks after transplantation[142] (see Figure 21.6) parallels the significant clinical recovery and likely represents segmental remyelination. The later, less rapid, more protracted rise in conduction velocities may represent axonal regeneration, a slower process.[54,142] A rise in the amplitude of muscle and sensory compound action potentials, however, also occurs. In observing the change in the shape of the action potential when comparing proximal and distal stimulation, Nielsen[54] and Bolton et al.[142] (Figure 21.10) noted

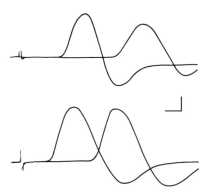

FIGURE 21.10. *Return of nerve conduction to normal after successful renal transplantation. Upper trace: Three months before transplantation when the patient had a severe uremic polyneuropathy. Lower trace: Twenty-seven months after transplantation, when almost complete recovery had occurred. The median nerve was stimulated at the wrist and elbow, and the recording was made from the thenar muscle. Conduction velocity rose from 39 to 55 m/s, and the previously dispersed compound action potential became normal, consistent with segmental remyelination. (See the case report in this chapter). Calibration: vertical, 2 mV; horizontal, 2 ms. (Reprinted with permission from Bolton CF, Young GB. The neurological complications of renal disease. Boston: Butterworths, 1990.)*

that the reversal of dispersed action potentials occurs as a result of segmental remyelination. The action potentials, however, do not recover to the same degree as conduction velocities, particularly in more severe neuropathies,[62,119] indicating that recovery may be incomplete, as originally suggested by Funck-Brentano et al.[106] Presumably axons have been irreversibly damaged. The improvement in speed of nerve conduction occurs in distal segments as well as more proximal sgements, as indicated by the shortening of distal latencies. Needle EMG shows eventual disappearance of fibrillation potentials and positive sharp waves. The number of motor unit potentials, which was previously decreased, increases toward normal values. The potentials assume a more polyphasic form, an indication of the reinnervation process.[54,142]

Should the kidney graft that was initially successful later show evidence of rejection and deteriorating renal function, the polyneuropathy again appears. This phenomenon was originally noted by Dobblestein et al.[60] Bolton[119] confirmed this observation by systematic studies in four patients, noting the deterioration of clinical and electrophysiologic studies as the first transplant failed and then noting with a second successful renal transplantation the subsequent partial recovery.

Conclusions

Uremic polyneuropathy still occurs, although mild in degree, in about one-half of patients on dialysis. Carpal tunnel syndrome frequently occurs distal to forearm arteriovenous fistulas. Hemodialysis or peritoneal dialysis halts the progress of the polyneuropathy, but improvement fails to occur. Improvement, however, is invariably accomplished by successful renal transplantation.

A variety of electrophysiologic techniques may be used to assess peripheral nerve function in uremia, each testing a different component of the peripheral nervous system but none clearly superior to the other in overall assessment. The following have proved to be abnormal: motor and sensory conduction velocities, distal latencies, F and H wave latencies, central and peripheral conduction as assessed by somatosensory evoked potential technique, amplitudes of the maximum compound sensory nerve and muscle action potentials, degree of dispersion of such action potentials, excitation thresholds of peripheral nerve, refractory periods of peripheral nerve, and concentric and single-fiber needle EMG of muscle. These results suggest a diffuse metabolic disturbance of nerve, of poorly understood pathophysiology, in which axonal degeneration and secondary segmental demyelination have been shown to occur.

Hepatic Neuropathy

There are a number of diseases in which liver failure and polyneuropathy coexist. In most cases, the mechanism is simply that the primary disease has widespread effects that involve both liver and peripheral nerve. Examples are infectious mononucleosis, acute intermittent porphyria, polyarteritis nodosa, celiac disease, a wide variety of toxic chemicals, and alcoholism, which is the best example.[143] There are three instances, however, in which liver disease occurs as a primary event, and polyneuropathy is a direct complication, the mechanism in each of these instances being quite different.

In the rare, painful sensory neuropathy that complicates biliary cirrhosis,[144] middle-aged women show evidence of hepatomegaly, jaundice, pruritus, and xanthomatosis. There are clinical signs of a mild sensory neuropathy. Nerve biopsy reveals small yellow swellings that are visible to the naked eye. Microscopy reveals that the appearance is due to the accumulations of large globular cells filled with sudanophilic lipids. These cells are present in the greatest concentrations in the perineural space but are found also in the epineurium, where they appear to involve the nerve fibers directly. There is a moderate reduction in the myelinated fiber population. In electrophysiologic studies, motor conduction studies are normal, but sensory conduction studies reveal compound sensory nerve action potentials that are either absent or, if present, are of low amplitude and of relatively normal latency, suggesting a relatively pure axonal degeneration of sensory fibers.[144,145] Charron et al.[146] reported a high incidence of circulating immune complexes in this and other cases of primary biliary cirrhosis. They postulated that these complexes played a role in the cause of the neuropathy.

Typical Guillain-Barré syndrome rarely complicates viral hepatitis and then usually late in the course of this illness.[143] This is another example of Guillain-Barré syndrome following a presumed viral infection. This mechanism may have been operative in 11 patients reported by Davison et al.[137] All were being treated by long-term hemodialysis for renal failure and developed serum hepatitis during the course of this treatment. Nerve conduction velocities worsened at that time but later improved when evidence of hepatitis had disappeared.

In the final group, the polyneuropathy is due to a direct effect of parenchymal liver failure. A major problem has been to exclude the effects of alcoholism from that of liver failure. When this was done by Thulworth et al.[148] 22% of patients with nonalcoholic liver disease had clinical signs of a polyneuropathy, predominantly sensory and involving the lower limbs. Sixty-eight percent of these patients had an autonomic neuropathy, chiefly parasympathetic. Sural nerve biopsy has shown segmental demyelination and remyelination. Electrophysiologic studies have shown mild reductions in conduction velocity and compound sensory nerve action potential amplitude, a mild temporal dispersion of the action potential, and an elevated excitation threshold. Nielsen and Kardel[149] observed the phenomenon of *resistance* to nerve excitability previously reported in 50 patients with chronic liver disease by Seneviratne and Peiris.[152] In this phenomenon, the upper limbs are rendered ischemic by a tourniquet, during which time sensory nerve conduction studies are performed repeatedly. In a normal person, after 30 minutes, the compound sensory nerve action potential disappears entirely. In nerve *resistance*, however, the compound action potential remains for a number of minutes afterward, as does vibratory perception. The mechanism for this phenomenon is unknown. Moreover, it is nonspecific, having been observed in diabetes mellitus,[150–153] uremia,[154,155] and motor neuron disease.[156] Chopra et al.[157] found that 90% of patients who had idiopathic portal fibrosis with portal systemic shunting but no evidence of hepatocellular damage had, on sural nerve biopsy, evidence of demyelination and remyelination but minimal electrophysiologic abnormalities. In animal experiments in the rat, portocaval anastomosis resulted in reduced motor nerve conduction velocities that were thought to be secondary to hepatocellular failure.[158]

NUTRITIONAL DISTURBANCES

Vitamin Deficiencies

Neuropathy due to thiamine deficiency (beri-beri)

This subject has been extensively reviewed by Victor.[159] In 1611, the Governor-General of the Dutch West Indies, Vaelz, recorded the occurrence of beri-beri and speculated that it was due to a degeneration of the peripheral nerves. Pekelharing and Winkler[160] gave the first, and remarkably comprehensive, clinical description in 1877. The neuropathy almost always began in a chronic or subacute fashion. These authors noted that before symptoms or signs, the *reaction of degeneration* occurred as a result of galvanic and faradic stimulation of limb muscles. This was apparently the first electrophysiologic test of this condition. Then, paresthesias or anesthesias developed in the distal parts of the limbs, beginning in the lower limbs. Tibial edema and palpitations were due to associated cardiac disease. Staggering, difficulty in standing on tip-toe, weakness of extensors of the fingers and hands, loss of deep tendon reflexes, and distal impairment of touch and temperature sensation followed. Pain or *unbearable formication in the hands and feet* was often a prominent manifestation. It was recognized that the *neuritis* could become extremely severe.

The cranial nerve abnormalities of deafness, numbness around the lips, weakness of the tongue, bilateral facial weakness, and central and cecocentral scotomas were also described. Ocular disorders such as lateral rectus palsy and nystagmus, often accompanied by confusional states and memory disorders, were probably on the basis of Wernicke's disease. Weakness and hoarseness of the voice, owing to laryngeal involvement, is particularly common in infantile beri-beri.

The pathology has been considered to be a combination of both axonal degeneration and segmental demyelination. As a result of more recent studies by Takahashi and Nakamura[161] of sural nerve biopsies, however, there seems little doubt that the primary change is axonal degeneration and that segmental demyelination is secondary. The distal parts of the nerves, both motor and sensory, are most severely involved. There are secondary changes in the dorsal root ganglia and anterior horn cells. Degenerative changes of the dorsal columns in the spinal cord are likely secondary to disease of the dorsal root ganglia. Unmyelinated fibers undergo degeneration, and both myelinated and unmyelinated fibers show evidence of regeneration. The earliest axonal changes, revealed by microscopy, appear as flattened sacs or tubuli in the axoplasm of large myelinated fibers.

The cause was established in a classic series of experiments that initiated the vitamin era. A landmark discovery was made by Williams in 1936[162] when he first synthesized and established the chemical structure for thiamine, which he had named. Deprivation experiments have produced polyneuropathy in dogs, rats, pigeons, and chicks.[159] Prineas[163] observed in thiamine-deficient rats an accumulation of flattened membrane-bound sacs and a depletion of neurotubules and neurofilaments in the distal axons of motor neurons and the central terminations of sensory neurons. Electrical stimulation of healthy nerve releases thiamine. Thiamine has been shown to play a role in the transfer of ions such as sodium across the axolemmal membrane, and it is through the blocking of thiamine diphosphate or triphosphate that pyrothiamine, a thiamine antagonist, may impair conduction in peripheral nerve.[164–166]

Biochemical methods of documenting thiamine deficiency in humans have been fraught with problems.[159] The amount excreted in the urine does not correlate well with signs of deficiency, and blood levels show only small differences in control subjects and patients with beri-beri. The blood pyruvate estimation, although showing high levels in florid cases of beri-beri, is relatively nonspecific because it may also be elevated in a variety of other illnesses. The erythrocyte transketolase assay, however, is quite sensitive but does not distinguish acute from chronic states of thiamine deficiency.

Modern epidemiologic studies have shown that beri-beri may be prevalent not only in underdeveloped countries, but also in developed ones in which the nutrition of the population is thought to be good.[167] Such a situation occurred in Japan among young adult men, particularly athletes who ate large amounts of carbohydrates but little green vegetables.

Seven patients with this interesting complication were studied comprehensively by Ohnishi et al.[168] Sural nerve biopsies showed a predominantly axonal degeneration, mild degrees of segmental demyelination occurring as a secondary phenomenon. Electron microscopy of the sural nerves revealed accumulations of flattened sacs or tubuli within the axoplasma similar to what had been noted by Prineus[163] in experimental animals. The subperineural spaces were large, presumably owing to endoneurial edema. The polyneuropathy was symmetric, with motor and sensory involvement and predominantly distal findings. The cerebrospinal fluid was normal. Blood levels of thiamine were low. Nerve conduction studies showed relatively normal conduction velocities and distal latencies, but the amplitude of the compound muscle and sensory nerve action potentials was severely reduced or absent. Needle EMG revealed findings consistent with denervation of muscle. Administration of thiamine resulted in clinical recovery, and nerve biopsy showed signs of active regeneration of nerves.

Cyanocobalamin deficiency (vitamin B$_{12}$)

Deficiency of this essential vitamin may cause dysfunction of the spinal cord and peripheral nerves as well as the hematologic and gastrointestinal systems. The neurologic aspects have been reviewed by

Pallis[169] and Victor[159] and the general aspects by Babior and Bunn.[170] The commonly used vitamin preparation, and that contained in animal products, contains cyanocobalamin, but this must be converted to biologically active forms in human tissue. Normally dietary cyanocobalamin binds with intrinsic factor, a thermolabile glycoprotein produced by the parietal cells of the stomach. It is then absorbed in the terminal ileum.

Thus vitamin B_{12} deficiency may arise from dietary lack, a pure vegetarian diet, or breast milk deficient in vitamin B_{12}; lack of intrinsic factor, a thermolabile glycoprotein, likely owing to an autoimmune gastritis (pernicious anemia); extensive resections of the stomach or ileum; and a variety of forms of malabsorption from the intestine (i.e., nontropical and tropical sprue). In pernicious anemia, in addition to neurologic manifestations, the patient may not have anemia if folic acid has been present in sufficient quantities in the diet. The present discussion concentrates on pernicious anemia; other causes of vitamin B_{12} deficiency are discussed later in this chapter.

The precise mechanism by which vitamin B_{12} deficiency affects the nervous system has been the subject of considerable debate over the years. Current evidence would indicate that vitamin B_{12} (methylcobalamin) is essential to the action of the enzyme methionine synthetase in converting homocystine to methionine through the process of methylation.[159] In experimental animals, the administration of nitrous oxide inactivates methionine synthetase and results in the production of a megaloblastic bone marrow and a sensory and motor polyneuropathy.[171,172]

Further controversy centers on the precise incidence of spinal cord involvement, peripheral nerve involvement, or both. For many years, it was believed that dysfunction of the spinal cord, termed *subacute combined degeneration,* could account for all of the clinical features. Unfortunately, this conclusion was based on outdated methods of examining the peripheral nervous system morphologically. From their review of the literature, Pallis and Lewis[169] concluded that polyneuropathy was a common, perhaps invariable, complication of pernicious anemia. These conclusions were largely based on electrophysiologic studies because until recently study of peripheral nerves by modern methods was lacking and because, as Victor[159] points out, the entire nervous system has not yet been studied systematically at autopsy. Victor further quotes studies of vitamin B_{12} deficiency in baboons and Rhesus monkeys that failed to produce lesions of the peripheral nerves even though central nervous system changes were observed.

Fortunately, a study reported by McCombe and McLeod[173] settled the issue. Three patients who had typical clinical and laboratory features of vitamin B_{12} deficiency owing to pernicious anemia exhibited a polyneuropathy in which nerve conduction studies suggested a predominantly axonal degeneration. This was confirmed by sural nerve biopsy studied by bright field and electron microscopy, quantitation of myelinated and unmyelinated fibers, and teased fiber preparation. In earlier days when subacute combined degeneration of the spinal cord was untreated, many cases came to autopsy and the spinal cord was usually examined. The typical pathologic changes in the spinal cord were initial separation of myelin sheaths and formation of vacuoles within myelin. The lesions coalesced, producing a sieve-like appearance to the tissue. Both myelin sheaths and axis cylinders were involved. The degree of gliosis was variable. The lesions were scattered throughout the white matter and were not necessarily limited to the posterior and lateral columns, as implied by the name.[174]

As is noted later, electrophysiologic findings in particular provide strong evidence for frequent occurrence of peripheral neuropathy in pernicious anemia. The presence of an associated myelopathy gives an important clue as to the diagnosis in an individual case; that is, spinal cord and peripheral nerve signs and symptoms coexist, a situation that considerably narrows the differential diagnosis in individual patients. In addition to the anemia and other systemic symptoms, patients complain of distal numbness and tingling in all four extremities and severe unsteadiness in walking. Sensory testing reveals a stocking-glove loss to light touch, pain, and temperature, and impairment of vibration sense and position sense distally, particularly in the lower limbs. Vibration sense may be lost out of proportion to position sense. Deep tendon reflexes are usually reduced, especially ankle jerks. Thus all of the signs and symptoms suggest peripheral neuropathy and tend to *mask* spinal cord signs. The only exception to this is a bilaterally positive Babinski sign. In rare circumstances, such peripheral nerve signs and symptoms are absent or minor, and the predominant picture is that of spinal cord dysfunction, with spasticity and hyperreflexia dominating the clinical picture.

Thus the differential diagnosis may be quite extensive, involving a variety of conditions that may develop in a subacute fashion and produce evidence of peripheral neuropathy, myelopathy, or both. As noted later, electrophysiologic studies should aid greatly in verifying the neurologic localization. Then hematologic investigations and assessment of vitamin B_{12} absorption through use of the Schilling test will, in almost all instances, provide not only confirmatory evidence of vitamin B_{12} deficiency, but also, in observing the response to ingested intrinsic factor, will serve to distinguish pernicious anemia from intestinal causes of vitamin B_{12} deficiency. When the myelopathy predominates, in extremely rare instances a magnetic resonance imaging scan may be necessary to rule out a compressive lesion of the spinal cord.

The intramuscular injection of 1000 μg of cyanocobalamin in association with the Schilling test provides the necessary therapeutic loading dose. Thereafter, 2000 μg is given intramuscularly in total during the first 6 weeks and then 100 μg at monthly intervals.[170] Many have assumed that this results in satisfactory resolution of the problem. This is rarely the case, however, and it is the experience of many neurologists that patients are left with significant residual symptoms and signs. This fact is emphasized in the report by McCombe and McLeod.[173]

Electrophysiologic abnormalities

The first study to give clear indication of the presence of the polyneuropathy was that of Gilliatt et al.[175] In this pioneering investigation of the utility of sensory nerve conduction studies, specifically of the lateral popliteal nerve in the investigation of a variety of polyneuropathies, these authors noted their findings in four patients who had evidence of subacute combined degeneration of the spinal cord. The anterior tibial nerve was stimulated at the ankle and the compound sensory nerve action potential recorded near the fibular head using needle electrodes. The electrophysiologic events were photographed from the oscilloscope after the traces from 100 stimuli had been superimposed (Figure 21.11). In one patient, no action potential could be recorded, and in a second patient, a low-voltage compound sensory nerve action potential of prolonged latency was recorded (conduction velocity 29 m/s). In a third patient, a low-voltage action potential of normal latency was recorded, and in the fourth patient, a normal action potential of normal latency was recorded. The first three patients had signs suggesting an associated polyneuropathy, but in the last patient, there were signs only of spinal cord disease.

Since then, a number of studies have been performed but with marked inconsistencies in the elec-

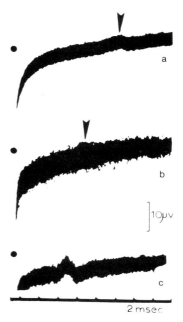

FIGURE 21.11. *Compound sensory nerve action potentials recorded with needle electrodes near the lateral popliteal nerve at the fibular head in three patients with subacute combined degeneration of the spinal cord. In each study, the traces on the oscilloscope screen induced by 100 stimuli were superimposed. The conduction velocity in the upper trace was 29 m/s. The patient with this tracing had signs of an associated polyneuropathy. The patient with the lower tracing had only spinal cord signs. (The arrow indicates low-voltage compound action potential.) (Reprinted with permission from Gilliatt RW, Goodman HV, Willison RG. The recording of lateral popliteal nerve action potentials in man. J Neurol Neurosurg Psychiatry 1961; 24:305–318.)*

trophysiologic approach.[176–178] Nonetheless, the combined results indicated conduction velocities are only mildly reduced, and there is a more marked reduction in conduction velocity, consistent with a primary axonal degeneration of peripheral nerve fibers.[179] This was confirmed in the fine study by McCombe and McLeod.[173] Motor and sensory conductions are both abnormal, and fibrillation potentials may be found on needle EMG.[180]

Somatosensory evoked potential studies have shown abnormalities of conduction, both centrally and peripherally in sensory pathways.[181–183] The involvement, however, may be predominantly central or peripheral. Lower limb stimulation studies produce the most marked abnormalities. Mid and short latency responses may both be affected. In two patients reported by Jones et al.,[183] somatosensory evoked potential studies showed improvement in central and peripheral conduction.

A remarkably similar clinical and electrophysiologic picture may be produced by nitrous oxide abuse, which interferes with cobalamin-dependent enzyme reactions.[184] The diagnosis can be made only by history and should be suspected in younger patients presenting with symptoms of vitamin B_{12} deficiency.

To illustrate a classic case of pernicious anemia involving a patient with both subacute combined degeneration of the spinal cord and polyneuropathy, who had comprehensive electrophysiologic studies initially and in follow-up, plus biopsy of a peripheral motor and sensory nerve and muscle, the following case report from our own department is included.

A 63-year-old furniture salesman experienced, over a period of 3 years, cramps in the calves, a sensation of pins and needles in the hands and feet, and numbness that began distally and spread proximally to the level of the wrists and mid-calves. He had noted difficulty in fastening buttons and had become more unsteady on his feet. He has lost approximately 30 lb despite a good appetite. On examination, it was noted that he walked with a broad-based, ataxic gait and moved from one piece of furniture to the next for support. He did not outwardly appear anemic, and general physical examination disclosed no

pertinent abnormality. Examination of the mental status and cranial nerves was normal. The only weakness was in dorsiflexion of the feet. The triceps and biceps reflexes were moderately depressed, and all other deep tendon reflexes were absent. The plantar responses were upgoing. He had sensory ataxia in all four limbs. There was a moderate loss of vibration sense at the fingertips and a total loss in the lower limbs to the level of the knees. Position sense was moderately impaired in the toes. Two-point discrimination was lost in the fingers and toes. Pinprick sensation was impaired to the level of the wrists and mid-calves.

The hemoglobin was 11.3 g and the white blood cell count 4500 mm³. A blood smear revealed 3 + macrocytes and large numbers of hypersegmented neutrophils. The serum vitamin B_{12} level was 24 (150 to 850) pg/ml. In the Schilling test, he was given radioactive cobalt and vitamin B_{12} orally, followed 1 hour later by 1000 μg of vitamin B_{12} intramuscularly. The percentage of vitamin B_{12} excreted on days 1 and 2 was 1.8% and 3.1% (normal >6%). The test was repeated giving intrinsic factors orally, and the percentage excreted rose to 23.7% the first day and fell to 2.5% 1 day later.

Nerve conduction studies were performed according to standard techniques for surface electrodes (Table 21.2). These revealed motor and sensory conduction velocities that were at the lower limbs of normal or mildly reduced. Compound muscle and sensory nerve action potential amplitudes were reduced or absent, particularly

TABLE 21.2. Nerve conduction studies in a patient with polyneuropathy and pernicious anemia[a]

Month[b]	CONDUCTION VELOCITIES[c] (m/s)				CAP DISTAL LATENCIES (ms)			CAP AMPLITUDES				F-RESPONSE LATENCIES[d] (ms)	
	Median Motor	Median Sensory	Peroneal Motor	Sural Sensory	Thenar Muscle	Digital Nerve	EDB Musle	Thenar Muscle (mV)	Digital Nerve (uV)	EDB Muscle (mV)	Sural Nerve (uV)	Median Nerve	Peroneal Nerve
0	49.0	42.0	—[e]	—	4.7	3.5	—	3.2	12.0	0	0	34.2	—
6	52.3	48.4	—	—	4.3	3.2	—	2.6	10.0	0	0	33.8	—
18	55.9	48.5	—	—	5.1	3.4	—	3.3	4.0	0	0	32.4	—

Abbreviations: CAP, compound (sensory nerve) action potential; EDB, extensor digitorum brevis; SD, standard deviation.

[a] These studies, along with neurologic signs, failed to improve despite parenteral treatment with vitamin B_{12}.

[b] After treatment started.

[c] Conduction velocity nerve segments: median—elbow to wrist; peroneal—knee to ankle; sural—mid-calf to ankle.

[d] F-wave stimulation sites: median—wrist; peroneal—ankle.

[e] Not measured.

in the lower limbs. Compound sensory nerve action potentials were particularly affected. These amplitudes were somewhat more reduced on proximal stimulation, suggesting a degree of conduction block. F wave and distal latencies were prolonged, commensurate with the degree of reduction of conduction velocity, suggesting diffuse slowing of conduction along the length of the limb nerves. Needle EMG revealed active denervation only in distal lower limb muscles, where there was also some evidence for collateral reinnervation. Needle EMG of upper limbs and lumbar paraspinal muscles was normal. Follow-up studies (Table 21.2) showed no significant changes at 6 and 18 months.

Somatosensory evoked potential studies were performed by stimulating the median nerve at the wrist 2048 times and averaging the response from recording electrodes placed over the median nerve at the elbow, brachial plexus, C-7 spine, and the opposite sensory cortex. In the lower limbs, the tibial nerve was stimulated 2048 times at the ankle, and averaged recordings were made from the knee, T-12 spine, C-7 spine, and opposite sensory cortex. These studies were performed bilaterally. The results, shown in Table 21.3, are consistent with a peripheral neuropathy, most marked in the lower limbs, but also a neuropathy of central somatosensory pathways, again involving particularly those from the lower limbs.

Biopsy specimens of a fascicle of the right deep peroneal nerve and a portion of adjacent anterior tibialis muscle were obtained. The nerve fascicle was embedded in epon and then stained in toluidine blue. Cross-sections and longitudinal sections were examined. There was a marked loss of myelinated fibers, both large and small, consistent with ongoing wallerian degeneration. The occasional fiber was thinly myelinated and showed abortive onion bulb formation. No active demyelination was seen. There was a moderate loss of myelinated fibers. Schwann cell nuclei were slightly increased in number, and endoneurial collagen was increased. Several sections showed large Raynaud bodies, which took up to one-third of the endoneurial fascicular area. In other sections, an unusual nerve trabeculation was noted.

Muscle biopsy was examined by frozen sections and paraffin sections, both in cross and longitudinal orientation. There were large groups of small atrophic fibers and of well-preserved fibers. The toluidine blue staining confirmed this observation. Some of the fibers showed cytoarchitectural disorganization.

Teased fiber preparation revealed that 25% of the fibers had undergone acute wallerian degeneration. There was mild evidence of secondary segmental demyelination and remyelination.

Electron microscopy confirmed the marked loss of fibers. Numerous fibers had undergone acute wallerian degeneration. Other axons, myelinated and unmyelinated, showed relative loss of axonal organelles such as neurofilaments. There was no active demyelination or remyelination. Raynaud's bodies appeared to be formed by whorls of disorganized collagen.

This patient received 1000 μg of vitamin B_{12} parenterally at the outset and then at monthly intervals thereafter. Unfortunately, there was only mild improvement. His unsteadiness improved to the point that he could walk without support but was somewhat unsteady. There was no other clinical improvement, and the electrophysiologic abnormalities failed to improve (see Table 21.2). Despite this, his hemoglobin rose to 148 g/L and evidence for macrocytosis disappeared on the peripheral blood smear. At 2 years, the serum vitamin B_{12} level was 519 (>150) pmol/L, and serum folate was 42 (>6) nmol/L.

Conclusions

Deficiency of vitamin B_{12} usually causes a myelopathy and a polyneuropathy, both of which may be quite severe. Electrophysiologic studies aid greatly in establishing the presence of a polyneuropathy. Motor and sensory conduction velocities are mildly reduced, and compound muscle and sensory nerve action potentials are severely reduced. Needle EMG revealed denervation of distal lower limb muscles. These results, taken in conjunction with information on peripheral nerve pathology, suggest the polyneuropathy is primarily an axonal degeneration. Somatosensory evoked responses reveal delays of latencies from peripheral nerves and central somatesthetic pathways, particularly those involving the lower limbs. A Schilling test determines in most instances if the vitamin B_{12} malabsorption is of gastric or intestinal origin. Long-term treatment with parenteral vitamin B_{12} results in equivocal clinical improvement. Nitrous oxide abuse should always be considered in the differential diagnosis, particularly in younger patients.

Neuropathy owing to pyridoxine (vitamin B_6) deficiency

This condition develops as a side effect of the drugs, isoniazed or hydralazine (Apresoline).[151] It is manifest as symmetric motor and sensory loss with pain

TABLE 21.3.   Somatosensory evoked potential studies in a patient with polyneuropathy owing to pernicious anemia

Nerve	Stimulation Site	Recording Site	Latency (ms)	Conduction Velocity (ms)
Right median	Wrist	Elbow	5	53
		Brachial plexus	11	60.6
		C-7 spine (N14)	19.5	
		Cortical		
		(P15)	21	
		(N20)	24.5	
		(P25)	31	
		(N35)	36	
		(P40)	49	
Left median	Wrist	Elbow	5	53.4
		Brachial plexus	11.5	55.8
		C-7 spine (N14)	18.5	
		Cortical		
		(P15)	Not clearly defined	
		(N20)	24	
		(P25)	26.5	
		(N35)	36	
		(P40)	49	
Right tibial	Ankle	Knee	Not clearly defined	
		T-12 spine	Not clearly defined	
		C-7 spine	Not clearly defined	
		Cortical		
		(P30)	56	
		(N30)	62	
		(P40)	74	
		(N50)	81	
		(P60)	96	
Left tibial	Ankle	Knee	Not clearly defined	
		T-12 spine	Not clearly defined	
		C-7 spine	Not clearly defined	
		Cortical		
		(P30)	56	
		(N30)	63	
		(P40)	72	
		(N50)	84	
		(P60)	96	

and burning in the limbs. Recovery usually occurs after the discontinuation of the drugs. To my knowledge, no electrophysiologic studies on these patients have been performed.

Neuropathy owing to niacin deficiency

Pellagra is the result of this deficiency, and it is still common among vegetarian, maize-eating people, particularly in the black populations of South Africa.[159] The classic triad involves dermal, gastrointestinal, and neural symptoms. The skin is erythematous, then reddish-brown and hyperkeratotic, notably over the face, neck, sternum, dorsal surfaces of the hands and feet, shins, and back of the forearms. Gastrointestinal symptoms consist of anorexia, dysphagia, abdominal discomfort, and diarrhea. The neurologic lesions occur to a variable extent in the brain, spinal cord, and peripheral nerve. In developed countries, this occurs most commonly in chronic alcoholics. In this situation, the skin lesions are often absent, and the cerebral signs are quite similar to delirium tremens. Thus pellagra is often missed during life and may be discovered only at autopsy, where the characteristic distribution of central chromatolysis is found throughout the central nervous system.[185] Unfortunately, the electrophysiologic studies have not been performed, to my knowledge, in such patients.

Neuropathy owing to folate deficiency

It is still debated whether pure folate deficiency will produce a polyneuropathy.

Neuropathy owing to vitamin E deficiency

Investigations indicate that vitamin E deficiency may arise in a variety of states of chronic fat malabsorption, notably longstanding cholestatic liver disease, exocrine pancreatic failure,[186] acquired intestinal malabsorption[187] and in association with A-betalipoproteinemia.[188–190] These patients show evidence of dysarthria, cerebellar ataxia, and peripheral nerve signs of loss of proprioception and reduced deep tendon reflexes. Motor and sensory conduction studies have been normal but may show mild delays in impulse conduction and reduced or absent compound sensory nerve action potential amplitude. Needle EMG has been normal. Two patients reported by Harding et al.[189] showed central delay in somatosensory evoked potential studies, consistent with dysfunction of the posterior columns. Electrophysiologic results improved after treatment with vitamin E.

Analysis of sural nerve biopsy specimens and adipose tissue has revealed deficiency of vitamin E.[191] This causes degeneration of neuronal membrane by disturbing lipid peroxidation because of a deficiency of the major lipid-soluble secondary antioxidant.[192]

Hypophosphatemia

This condition has been attributed to decreased intake, increased loss, or transcellular shift of phosphorus.[193] Diabetic ketoacidosis, chronic alcoholism or alcohol withdrawal, nutritional repletion and hyperalimentation, and recovery from burns are all predisposing conditions. There may be confusion, seizures, and coma. Both a nonspecific peripheral neuropathy and Gullain-Barré paralysis[193–195] have been described, but unfortunately, electrophysiologic studies have not been sufficiently detailed to draw any conclusions.

NONSPECIFIC OR MULTIPLE DEFICIENCIES

Adult Celiac Disease

Glutin in the diet may be the major initiating factor, and the result is malabsorption of a number of substances: fat causing steatorrhea, protein causing hyperproteinemia, iron and folic acid causing anemia, vitamin D and calcium causing osteomalacia and tetany, vitamin E causing cerebellar ataxia and polyneuropathy (see earlier), vitamin K causing hemorrhages, and potassium causing hypokalemia. Vitamin B_{12} levels are not as reduced as in pernicious anemia, and the relationship of these levels as well as folic acid levels to neuropathy is less well defined. Moreover, the neuropathy is much less frequent. Electrophysiologic studies[196,197] have revealed either normal results or findings consistent with a mild axonal degeneration of motor and sensory fibers, as is seen in pernicious anemia. Proximal muscle weakness in these patients may be due to an associated osteomalacia.

Tropical Myeloneuropathies

This subect has been reviewed by Roman et al.[198] These conditions are quite frequent in certain developing countries and consist mainly of either a tropical ataxic neuropathy or tropical spastic paraparesis. Single or multiple nutrient deficiencies may be responsible in individual instances. The cause is still poorly understood and may be multifactorial, relating to malnutrition, particularly thiamine,[199] malabsorption, and infection. In fact, there is growing evidence that tropical spastic paraparesis (even nontropical varieties) is an autoimmune reaction to human T-cell lymphotropic virus Type I (HTLV-I) viral infection.[200,201]

Electrophysiologic studies have shown either normal findings, suggesting the manifestations are due to myelopathy, or some reduction in conduction velocity and in the amplitude of compound muscle and sensory nerve action potentials; needle EMG findings may suggest a myopathy.[197]

Protein Calorie Malnutrition in Children

This subject has been reviewed by Dastur et al.[202] Work, both in experimental animals and in clinical studies in children, indicates that the basic abnormality may be a retardation in the myelination of peripheral nerves, particularly the larger myelinated fibers. A similar situation may occur in muscles, in which muscle biopsies have shown a relatively uniform reduction in the diameter of muscle fibers. Clinically this produces weakness and hypotonia, which is most marked proximally and is accompanied by reduced or absent deep tendon reflexes. Sensory findings may be difficult to interpret. Electrophysiologically there is simply a mild reduction in motor and sensory conduction velocities and distal latencies as well as some reduction in the amplitude of compound muscle and sensory nerve action potentials. Fibrillation potentials and positive sharp waves may be present in muscles and motor unit potentials and at times may have a *myopathic* pattern. Although this condition appears to be most prevalent in underdeveloped countries, it is now being observed in certain of the developed countries, including the United States, in children who live in poverty. With proper treatment, however, the peripheral neuropathy and myopathy associated with this type of malnutrition may be reversed relatively completely. It is of interest that this type of malnutrition also has an effect on the brain and may produce mental retardation.

Polyneuropathy of the Postgastrectomy State

Vitamin B_{12} deficiency invariably develops following total gastrectomy owing to the lack of intrinsic factor, the manifestation being megaloblastic anemia.[203,204] Subacute combined degeneration of the spinal cord, however, appears to be a rare complication.[205] Moreover, in gastric lesions other than gastrectomy, such as carcinoma or chronic gastritis, vitamin B_{12} deficiency appears not to occur.

The issue of neuropathy following partial gastrectomy remains quite controversial. If it does occur, it is usually delayed, after a period of several years in about 15% of patients.[206,207] The findings clinically are those of a combined motor and sensory neuropathy, mainly distally, with some reduction of deep tendon reflexes, again particularly distally. Motor and sensory conduction studies show moderate reduction of conduction velocities and more severe reduction of the amplitude of compound muscle and sensory nerve action potential amplitudes. Sural nerve biopsies[208] reveal a combination of segmental and paranodal demyelination, but it would seem that these changes are more likely secondary to a primary axonal degeneration. In addition to deficiency of vitamin B_{12}, other vitamins and nutrients may be deficient through malabsorption. Moreover, the measurements of these substances in the blood often do not correlate with the incidence and severity of the neuropathy. Also, it has been theorized that *toxic* absorption from a blind loop may damage the nervous system.[209,210]

Neuropathy Associated with Weight Reduction

This type of neuropathy may occur as a result of being on a reducing diet or as a result of a complication of gastric stapling for morbid obesity. With a reducing diet, the neuropathy is most likely to develop in excessively rigorous weight reduction programs and may be clinically manifest as generalized polyneuropathy but often one in which there is particular involvement of the common peroneal nerve.[211] The neuropathy usually develops 2 to 4 months after the onset of dieting. Electrophysiologic studies reveal normal or slightly reduced conduction velocities, and needle EMG reveals signs of denervation of muscle. There is no evidence of conduction block at the fibular head, nerve compression alone therefore being an unlikely factor. Thus the neuropathy would appear to be a relatively pure motor and sensory axonal degeneration. Institution of a nutritious diet results in satisfactory resolution of the neuropathy.

Nutritional problems following gastric surgery for morbid obesity are particularly prevalent. The deficiency may be relatively specific and produce typical Wernicke-Korsakoff psychosis due to acute thiamine deficiency. Early reports also indicated that there may be severe polyneuropathy, ataxia, and pseudochorea.[212,213] An excellent study by Abarbanel et al.[214] indicated subacute or chronic polyneuropathy was most common, with burning foot syndrome, myotonia, meralgia paresthetica, and myelopathy being less common. The precise mechanism of these neurologic manifestations is still incompletely understood because, although there may be variable reductions in various nutrients in the blood, including certain vitamins, these measurements usually do not correlate well with the clinical manifestations.[215] Nerve conduction and morphologic studies indicate that this is a primary, predominantly distal, axonal degeneration of motor and sensory fibers. Despite attempts at improved nutrition, recovery is often incomplete.

Critical Illness Polyneuropathy

Critical illness is the term currently used for the combination of sepsis and multiple organ failure. This condition developed in the majority of patients who had been in our critical care unit for longer than 1 week, and it carried a mortality of at least 50%. We have observed that in at least half of these patients, a polyneuropathy develops.[216] The first sign is often a difficulty in weaning from the ventilator when the sepsis and multiple organ failure seem to be coming under control. Because of the often associated septic encephalopathy and the presence of an endotracheal tube, clinical assessment is often difficult. In about half of the cases, however, there are clear-cut signs of a polyneuropathy consisting of weakness of limb muscles, particularly distally; reduced or absent deep tendon reflexes; and inconstant signs of distal sensory loss. In severe neuropathy, quadriplegia may occur, but it will be noted that movements of the cranial nerve musculature are strong.[107,217]

Electrophysiologic abnormalities,[108] as expected, are the earliest and most reliable signs of this polyneuropathy. These can, with a good portable unit, be demonstrated in the critical care unit. Because this is a relatively pure axonal degeneration of motor and sensory fibers, conduction velocities and distal latencies are relatively preserved, but the amplitudes of compound muscle and sensory nerve action potentials are reduced or absent. Needle EMG (Figure 21.12) reveals fibrillation potentials and positive sharp waves with considerable abundance in more severe cases but at times in a multifocal fashion, so comprehensive needle EMG studies should be done. Motor unit potentials may be recruited poorly, owing either to the neuropathy or septic encephalopathy. Such units, when they do appear, may have a relatively normal appearance or appear somewhat polyphasic. Phrenic nerve conduction studies may disclose an absent response from either leaf of the diaphragm in severe cases and a reduced amplitude in less severe cases. Thus neuropathy of the phrenic

nerve is the major reason for difficulty in weaning from the ventilator.[216] Needle EMG studies of chest wall muscles may show abnormal spontaneous activity, as in the limb muscles. Needle EMG studies of the diaphragm are safe and often revealing. (See Chapter 26.)

There may be relatively complete recovery from critical illness polyneuropathy, unless it is exceptionally severe, should the patient survive the sepsis and multiple organ failure syndrome. Recovery often occurs unusually rapidly for primary axonal degeneration of peripheral nerve, so we have speculated it may be the distal nerve segments that are predominantly affected.

The precise cause of critical illness polyneuropathy is not known. We had originally suspected that nutritional deficiency might be the cause because our first five patients seemed to show some improvement after the institution of total parenteral nutrition.[107] Subsequent studies, however, have shown no evidence for a specific nutritional deficiency. Moreover, these patients are routinely given enteral and total parenteral nutrition soon after admission to the critical care unit, and yet polyneuropathy continues to develop and progresses while under such treatment. We have largely excluded other possible causes, notably Guillain-Barré syndrome.[108] It is now our view that critical illness polyneuropathy is due to the same

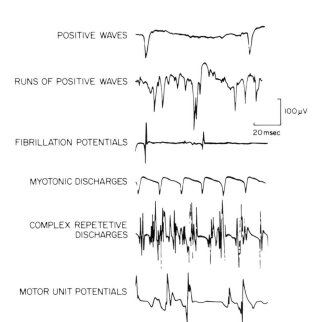

FIGURE 21.12. *Needle electrode findings in the acute polyneuropathy associated with critical illness. Positive sharp waves and fibrillation potentials were more numerous than shown here in severe neuropathy and might be recorded from intercostal as well as limb muscles. Myotonic and complex repetitive discharges, although less common in this condition, were more common than in most neuropathies. Motor unit potentials were decreased in number and seemed of rather low amplitude and more polyphasic than is normally seen, suggesting an associated primary myopathy.*

fundamental defect, still unknown, that affects all body systems in this condition.

Alcoholic Polyneuropathy

Victor's extensive personal observations[217a] have indicated that polyneuropathy complicates chronic alcoholism in 9% of cases. Dietary deficiencies are well-documented predisposing factors and consist of excessive weight loss, generalized dryness and scaliness of the skin, pigmentation of the face, thinness and glossiness of the skin, and weakness of the limbs. There may be anemia owing to folic acid deficiency and evidence of attendant liver disease and hepatic encephalopathy. Alcoholic polyneuropathy may develop acutely, in association with Wernicke-Korsakoff syndrome, and consist of reduction or absence of deep tendon reflexes. There may be considerable return of these reflexes and also muscle strength, with treatment by intravenous thiamine. Most commonly, however, the neuropathy develops in a chronic fashion, in association with chronic alcoholism, and is often an accompaniment of alcoholic cerebellar degeneration. Electrophysiologic signs, as described next, are the earliest manifestations. Clinical signs consist of thinness and tenderness of leg muscles, depression of deep tendon reflexes (which occasionally may be normal or increased), and impairment of sensation distally. Sensory disturbances are often prominent and consist of dull, constant, aching, sharp, lancinating pains and coldness or intermittent burning. In some patients, the weakness seems to be mainly proximal, and in this situation, a myopathy may be suspected. The muscles may be tender. Alcoholic myopathy may develop in association with acute alcoholic rhabdomyolysis, but there is some evidence now that myopathy of gradual onset is due to denervation atrophy or to a primary effect of alcohol on muscle metabolism or both in conjunction.[218–223] Alcoholic polyneuropathy may progress to severe paraplegia.

Electrophysiologic abnormalities are often the earliest manifestations.[224] They may show only normal or mild abnormalities of conduction velocity and distal latency in motor and sensory fibers. Compound muscle and sensory nerve action potentials, however, are considerably reduced. There may be prolongation of the latency of the H wave and the ankle jerk, consistent with involvement of large group (IA) afferent fibers and possibly the finer motor fibers that supply muscle spindles.[225] Needle EMG reveals fibrillation potentials and positive sharp waves and abnormalities of recruitment, con-

sisting of discrete activity with full effort, diminished amplitude of the recruitment pattern (<2 mV), and, at times, an increased incidence of polyphasic motor unit potentials.[208] There may be clinical or subclinical evidence of compressive neuropathies, particularly of the ulnar nerve at the elbow, the radial nerve in the upper arm, and the common peroneal nerve at the fibular head. Computer techniques by Ballantyne and Hansen[226] suggest that reinnervation in alcoholic polyneuropathy may be poor. These electrophysiologic studies therefore strongly indicate that there is a relatively pure, primary axonal degeneration of motor and sensory fibers. This has been quite clearly demonstrated in the comprehensive studies by Walsh and McLeod[227] and Behse and Buchthal,[208] which correlate electrophysiologic and morphologic studies. Although overt autonomic disturbances are uncommon, studies of the R-R cardiac interval reveal a vagal neuropathy in one-third of chronic alcoholics, and this may contribute to their mortality.[228]

With the cessation of alcohol and the institution of proper nutrition, it is possible for alcoholic polyneuropathy to resolve completely. In this regard, electrophysiologic studies are quite valuable in documenting such recovery, as demonstrated in the investigations by Hillbom and Wennberg.[229]

Conclusions

It can be seen that virtually all of the polyneuropathies associated with nutritional deficiency are characterized by a primary axonal degeneration of motor and sensory fibers, predominantly distally. Thus the neuropathy may be readily detected by standard electromyographic techniques. Motor and sensory nerve conduction velocities and latencies are usually normal or only mildly abnormal. Thus particular attention must be paid to the compound muscle and sensory nerve action potential measurements. These measurements are considerably affected by limb temperature, reduced temperature tending to increase the amplitude.[1] Thus skin temperature should be routinely monitored and taken into account in interpreting the results. In making a correction factor, it should be kept in mind, however, that this correction factor may be different for neuropathy than for healthy nerve.[141] Needle EMG studies are particularly valuable and should, at a minimum, include sampling of proximal and distal muscles in upper and lower limbs. There may be abnormalities in resting muscle and during recruitment of motor unit potentials. Because recovery from all nutritional polyneuropathies is quite possible, it is important to look for needle EMG signs of reinnervation, notably the development of long duration, highly polyphasic motor unit potentials. Studies of central conduction, in particular recording of somatosensory evoked potentials, may be worthwhile because most nutritional neuropathies cause degeneration of the dorsal columns of the spinal cord, and in some instances, this may be the predominant site of involvement. It should be emphasized again, however, that because the electrophysiologic abnormalities are remarkably similar for all nutritional polyneuropathies, the clinical features and other investigations supply the correct diagnosis.

REFERENCES

1. Bolton CF. Factors affecting the amplitude of human sensory compound action potentials. Minimonograph No. 17. Rochester, MN: American Association of Electromyography and Electrodiagnosis, 1981.
2. Dorfmann LJ. The distribution of conduction velocities (DCV) in peripheral nerve: A review. Muscle Nerve 1984; 7:2–11.
3. Gull WW. On a cretinoid state supervening in adult life in women. Trans Clin Soc Lond 1874; 7:180.
4. Ord WM. On myxoedema, a term proposed to be applied to an essential condition in the "chretinoid" affection occasionally observed in middle-aged women. Med-Chir Trans Lond 1878; 61:57.
5. Murray IPC, Simpson JA. Acroparaesthesia in mxoedema: A clinical and electromyographic study. Lancet 1958; 1:1360–1363.
6. Simpson JA. Electrical signs in the diagnosis of carpal tunnel and related syndromes. J Neurol Psychiatry 196; 19:275.
7. Rao SN, Katiyar BC, Nair KRP, et al. Neuromuscular status in hypothyroidism. Acta Neurol Scand 1980; 61:167.
8. Schiller F, Kolb FO. Carpal tunnel syndrome in acromegaly. Neurology (Minneap) 1954; 4:271.
9. Purnell DC, Daly DD, Lipscomb PR. Carpal-tunnel syndrome associated with myxedema. Arch Intern Med 1961; 108:751–756.
10. Dyck PJ, Lambert EH. Polyneuropathy associated with hypothyroidism. J Neuropath Exp Neurol 1970; 29:631–658.
11. Golding DN. Hypothyroidism presenting with musculoskeletal symptoms. Ann Rheum Dis 1970; 29:10.
12. Schwartz MS, Mackworth-Young CG, McKeran RO. The tarsal tunnel syndrome in hypothyroidism. J Neurol Neurosurg Psychiatry 1983; 46:440–442.
13. Nickel SN, Frame B, Bebin J, et al. Myxedema, neuropathy and myopathy. A clinical and pathologic study. Neurology (Minneap) 1961; 11:125–137.
14. Pollard JD, McLeod JG, Angel Honnibtal TG, et al. Hypothyroid polyneuropathy. Clinical, electrophysiological and nerve biopsy findings in two cases. J Neurol Sci 1982; 53:461–471.

15. Fincham RW, Cape CA. Neuropathy in myxedema: A study of sensory nerve conduction in the upper extremities. Arch Neurol 1968; 19:464–466.
16. Yamamoto K, Saito K, Takai T, et al. Unusual manifestations in primary hypothyroidism. In: New concepts in thyroid disease. New York: Alan R. Liss, 1983:163–187.
17. Meier C, Bischoff A. Polyneuropathy in hypothyroidism. Clinical and nerve biopsy study of four cases. J Neurol 1977; 215:103–114.
18. Martin J, Tomkin GH, Hutchinson M. Peripheral neuropathy in hypothyroidism—an association with spurious polycythaemia (Gaisbock's syndrome). J Roy Soc Med 1983; 76:87–89.
19. Dick DJ, Nogues MA, Lane RMJ, et al. Polyneuropathy in occult hypothyroidism. Posgrad Med J 1983; 59:518–519.
20. Lambert EH, Underdahl LO, Beckett S, et al. A study of the ankle jerk in myxedema. J Clin Endocrinol Metab 1951; 11:1186.
21. Hofmann WW, Denys EH. Effects of thyroid hormone at the neuromuscular junction. Am J Physiol 1972; 223:283.
22. Kendall-Taylor P, Turnbull DM. Endocrine myopathies. Br Med J 1983; 287:705–708.
23. Khaleeli AA, Griffith DG, Edwards RHT. The clinical presentation of hypothyroid myopathy and its relationship to abnormalities in structure and function of skeletal muscle. J Clin Endocrin 1983; 19:365–376.
24. Evans RM, Watanabe I, Singer PA. Central changes in hypothyroid myopathy: A case report. Muscle Nerve 1990; 13:952–956.
25. Maurer K, Hopf HC, Lowitzsch K, et al. Mechanomyographische Veranderungen bei Schilddrussenfunktionsstorungen. Z EEG-EMG 1981; 12:94–99.
26. Torres CF, Moxley RT. Hypothyroid neuropathy and myopathy: Clinical and electrodiagnostic longitudinal findings. J Neurol 1990; 237:271–274.
27. Laroche CM, Cairns T, Moxham J, Green M. Hypothyroidism presenting with respiratory muscle weakness. Am Rev Respir Dis 1988; 138(2):472–474.
28. Arnould G, Tridon P, Andre M, et al. A propos des neuropathies peripheriques survenant au cours des hyperthyroidies (letter). Presse Med 1971; 79:634.

29. Chollet PH, Rigal J-P, Pignide L. Une Complication meconnue de l'hyperthyroidie: la neuropathie peripherique (letter). Presse Med 1971; 79:145.

30. Gluckman JC, Guy-Grand B, Roger M, et al. Neuropathie centrale et peripherique associee a une hyperthyroidie chez un home. Sem Hop Paris 1968; 44:2661.

31. Ludin HP, Spiess H, Koenig MP. Neuropathie et hyperthyreose. Rev Neurol (Paris) 1969; 120:424.

32. Bronsky D, Kaganiec GI, Waldstein SS. An association between the Guillain-Barre syndrome and hyperthyroidism. Am J Med Sci 1964; 247:196.

33. Feibel JH, Campa JF. Thyrotoxic neuropathy (Basedow's paraplegia). J Neurol Neurosurg Psychiatry 1976; 39:491.

34. Osserman KE, Tsairis P, Weiner LB. Myasthenia gravis and thyroid disease: Clinical and immunologic correlation. J Mt Sinai Hosp NY 1967; 34:469.

35. O'Duffy JD, Randall RV, MacCarty CS. Median neuropathy (carpal-tunnel syndrome) in acromegaly. Ann Intern Med 1978; 78:379–383.

36. Davidoff LM. Studies in acromegaly. III. The anamnesis and symptomatology in one hundred cases. Endocrinology 1926; 10:461.

37. Sullivan CR, Jones DR, Bahn RC, et al. Clinics on endocrine and metabolic diseases. 9. Biopsy of the costochondral junction in acromegaly. Mayo Clin Proc 1963; 38:81.

38. Skanse B. Carpal-tunnel syndrome in myxedema and acromegaly. Acta Chir Scand 1961; 121:476.

39. Low PA, McLeod JE, Turtle JR, et al. Peripheral neuropathy in acromegaly. Brain 1974; 97:139–152.

40. Jamal GA, Kerr DJ, McLellan AR, et al. Generalized peripheral nerve dysfunction in acromegaly: A study by conventional and novel neurophysiological techniques. J Neurol Neurosurg Psychiatry 1987; 50:886–894.

41. Charcot JM. Lecons sur les maladies due systeme nerveux. XVI des paraplegies urinaires. Ed 3. Paris; 1880:295.

42. Khaleeli AA, Levy RD, Edwards RHT, et al. The neuromuscular features of acromegaly: A clinical and pathological study. J Neurol Neurosurg Psychiatry 1984; 47:1009–1015.

43. Osler W. The principles and practice of medicine, ed 7. London: Appleton, 1909:685.

44. Hegstrom RM, Murray JS, Pendras JP, et al. Hemodialysis in the treatment of chronic uremia. Trans Am Soc Artif Intern Organs 1961; 7:136.

45. Hegstrom RM, Murray JS, Pendras SP, et al. Two years' experience with periodic hemodialysis in the treatment of chronic uremia. Trans Am Soc Artif Intern Organs 1962; 8:266.

46. Asbury AK, Victor M, Adams RD. Uremic polyneuropathy. Arch Neurol 1963; 8:413–428.

47. Nielsen VK. The peripheral nerve function in chronic renal failure. I. Clinical symptoms and signs. Acta Med Scand 1971; 190:105–111.

48. Nielsen VK. The peripheral nerve function in chronic renal failure. II. Intercorrelation of clinical symptoms and signs and clinical grading of neuropathy. Acta Med Scand 1971; 190:113–117.

49. Nielsen VK, Winkel P. The peripheral nerve function in chronic renal failure. III. A multivariate statistical analysis of factors presumed to affect the development of clinical neuropathy. Acta Med Scand 1971; 190:119–125.

50. Nielsen VK. The peripheral nerve function in chronic renal failure. IV. An analysis of the vibratory perception threshold. Acta Med Scand 1972; 191:287–296.

51. Nielsen VK. The peripheral nerve function in chronic renal failure. V. Sensory and motor conduction velocity. Acta Med Scand 1973; 194:445–454.

52. Nielsen VK. The peripheral nerve function in chronic renal failure. VI. The relationship between sensory and motor nerve conduction and kidney function, azotemia, age, sex, and clinical neuropathy. Acta Med Scand 1973; 194:455–462.

53. Nielsen VK. The peripheral nerve function in chronic renal failure. VII. Longitudinal course during terminal renal failure and regular hemodialysis. Acta Med Scand 1974; 195:155–162.

54. Nielsen VK. The peripheral nerve function in chronic renal failure. VIII. Recovery after renal transplantation. Clinical aspects. Acta Med Scand 1974; 195:163–170.

55. Nielsen VK. The peripheral nerve function in chronic renal failure. IX. Recovery after renal transplantation, electrophysiological aspects (sensory and motor nerve conduction). Acta Med Scand 1974; 195:171–180.

56. Bolton CF. Peripheral neuropathies associated with chronic renal failure. Can J Neurol Sci 1980; 7:89–96.

57. Harding AE, Le Fanu J. Carpal tunnel syndrome related to antebrachial Cimino-Brescia fistula. J Neurol Neurosurg Psychiatry 1977; 40:511–513.

58. Bolton CF, Young GB. The neurological complications of renal disease. Boston: Butterworths, 1990:108–113.

59. Bolton CF, Driedger AA, Lindsay RM. Ischaemic neuropathy in uremic patients due to a bovine arteriovenous shunt. J Neurol Neurosurg Psychiatry 1979; 42:810–814.

60. Dobblestein H, Altmeyer B, Edel H, et al. Periphere Neuropathie bei chronische Niereninsuffizienz, bei Dauerdialyse—behandlung und nach Nierentransplantation. Med Klin 1968; 63:616.

61. Funck-Brentano JL, Cueille GF, Man NK. A defense of the middle molecule hypothesis. Kidney Int 1978; 13(suppl 8):531–535.

62. Bolton CF, Baltzan MA, Baltzan RB. Effects of

renal transplantation on uremic neuropathy. N Engl J Med 1971; 2844:1170–1175.

63. Bolton CF, Rozdilsky B. Electrophysiological and structural changes in uremic neuropathy. Read before the Sixth Canadian Congress of Neurological Sciences, St. John's, Newfoundland, 1971.

64. Dyck PJ, Johnson WJ, Lambert EH, et al. Segmental demyelination secondary to axonal degeneration in uremic neuropathy. Mayo Clin Proc 1971; 46:400.

65. Thomas PK, Hollinrake K, Lascelles RG, et al. The polyneuropathy of chronic renal failure. Brain 1971; 94:761.

66. Nielsen VK. Pathophysiological aspects of uraemic neuropathy. In: Canal N, Pozza G, eds. Peripheral neuropathies. Amsterdam: Elsevier/North Holland Biomedical Press, 1978:197–210.

67. Castaigne P, Cathala HP, Beaussart-Boulenge L, et al. Effect of ischaemic on peripheral nerve function in patients with chronic renal failure undergoing dialysis treatment. J Neurol Neurosurg Psychiatry 1972; 35:631–637.

68. Lambert EH, Dyck PJ. Compound action potentials of sural nerve in vitro in peripheral neuropathy. In: Dyck PJ, Thomas PK, Lambert EH, eds. Peripheral neuropathy. Vol 1. Philadelphia: WB Saunders, 1975:430–431.

69. Brismar T, Tegner R. Experimental uremic neuropathy. Part 2. Sodium permeability decrease and inactivation in potential clamped nerve fibers. J Neurol Sci 1984; 65:37–45.

70. Teschan PE, Bourne JR, Reed RB, et al. Electrophysiological and neurobehavioral responses to therapy: The National Cooperative Dialysis Study. Kidney Int 1983; 23(suppl 13):558–565.

71. Babb AL, Popovich RP, Christopher TG, et al. The genesis of the square meter-hour hypothesis. Trans Am Soc Artif Intern Organs 1971; 17:81.

72. Bergstrom J, Asaba H, Alvestrand A, et al. Clinical implications of uremic middle molecules in regular hemodialysis patients. Clin Nephrol 1983; 19(4):179–187.

73. Faguer P, Man N-K, Cueille G, et al. Improved separation and quantification of the "middle molecule" b4-2 in uremia. Clin Chem 1983; 29(4):703–707.

74. Kurtz SB, Wong VH, Anderson CF, et al. Continuous ambulatory peritoneal dialysis. Three years' experience at the Mayo Clinic. Mayo Clin Proc 1983; 58:633–639.

75. Braguer D, Chauvet-Monges AM, Sari JC, et al. Inhibition in vitro of the polymerization of tubulin by uremic middle molecules: Corrective effect of isaxonine. Clin Nephrol 1983; 20(3):149–154.

76. Chaumont PJ, Lefevre J, Lerique JL. Explorations electrologiques au cours des insuffisances renales graves. Rev Neurol 1963; 108:199–201.

77. Versaki AA, Olsen KJ, McMain PB. Uremic polyneuropathy: Motor nerve conduction velocities. Trans Am Soc Artif Intern Organs 1964; 10:328–330.

78. Preswick G, Jeremy D. Subclinical polyneuropathy in renal insufficiency. Lancet 1964; 2:731–732.

79. Bolton CF, Young GB. The neurological complications of renal disease. Boston, Butterworths, 1990:81–86.

80. Ackil AA, Shahani BT, Young RR. Sural nerve conduction studies and late responses in children undergoing hemodialysis. Arch Phys Med Rehabil 1981; 62:487–491.

81. Ackil AA, Shahani BT, Young RR, Rubin NE. Late response and sural conduction studies. Usefulness in patients with chronic renal failure. Arch Neurol 1981; 38:482–485.

82. D'Amour ML, Dufresne LR, Morin C, Slaughter D. Sensory nerve conduction in chronic uremic patients during the first six months of hemodialysis. Can J Neurol Sci 1984; 11:269–271.

83. Chokroverty S. Proximal vs. distal slowing in renal failure treated by long-term hemodialysis. Arch Neurol 1982; 39:53–54.

84. van der Most van Spijk D, Hoogland RA, Dijkstra S. Conduction velocities and related degrees of renal insufficiency. In: Desmedt JE, ed. New developments in electromyography and clinical neurophysiology. Vol 2. Basel: Karger, 1973:381–389.

85. Wright EA, McQuillen MP. Hypoexcitability of ulnar nerve in patients with normal conduction velocity. Neurology 1973; 23:78–83.

86. Alderson K, Seay A, Brewer E, Petajan J. Neuropathies in children with chronic renal failure treated by hemodialysis. Neurology 1985; 35(suppl 1):94.

87. Arbus GS, Geary DF, McLorie GA, et al. Pediatric renal transplants: A Canadian perspective. Kidney Int 1986; 30:S31–S34.

88. Hansen S, Ballantyne JP. A quantitative electrophysiological study of uraemic neuropathy. Diabetic and renal neuropathies compared. J Neurol Neurosurg Psychiatry 1978; 41:128–134.

89. Thiele B, Stalberg E. Single fibre EGM findings in polyneuropathies of different aetiology. J Neurol Neurosurg Psychiatry 1975; 38:881–887.

90. Konishi T, Hiroshi N, Motomura S. Single fiber electromyography in chronic renal failure. Muscle Nerve 1982; 5:458–461.

91. Serra C, D'Angelillo A, Facciolla D, et al. Somatosensory cerebral evoked potentials in uremic polyneuropathy. Acta Neurol (Napoli) 1979; 34:1–14.

92. Ganji SS, Mahajan S. Changes in short-latency somatosensory evoked potentials during hemodialysis in chronic renal failure. Clin Electroencephalogr 1983; 14:202–206.

93. Lewis EG, Dustman RE, Beck EC. Visual and somatosensory evoked potential characteristics of patients undergoing hemodialysis and kidney trans-

plantation. Electroencephalogr Clin Neurophysiol 1978; 44:223–231.

94. Obeso JA, Marti-Masso JF, Asin AL, et al. Conduction velocity through the somesthetic pathway in chronic renal failure. J Neurol Sci 1979; 43:439–445.

95. Rossini PM, Treviso M, Di Stefano E, Di Paolo B. Nervous impulse propagation along peripheral and central fibres in patients with chronic renal failure. Electroencephalogr Clin Neurophysiol 1983; 56:293–303.

96. Vaziri D, Pratt H, Saiki JD, Starr A. Evaluation of somatosensory pathway by short latency evoked potentials in patients with end-stage renal disease maintained on hemodialysis. Int J Artif Organs 1981; 4:17–21.

97. Guihneuc R, Ginet J. The use of the H-reflex in patients with chronic renal failure. In: Desmedt JE, ed. New developments in electromyography and clinical neurophysiology. Vol 2. Basel: Karger, 1973:400–403.

98. Panayiotopoulous CP, Scarpalezos S. F-wave studies in the deep peroneal nerve. J Neurol Sci 1977; 31:331–341.

99. Panayiotopoulous CP, Laxos G. Tibial nerve H-reflex and F-wave studies in patients with uremic neuropathy. Muscle Nerve 1980; 3:423–426.

100. Solders G, Persson A, Guitierrez A. Autonomic dysfunction in non-diabetic terminal uraemia. Acta Neurol Scand 1985; 71:321–327.

101. Solders G. Autonomic function tests in healthy controls and in terminal uraemia. Acta Neurol Scand 1986; 73:638–639.

102. Jennekens FGI, Kemmelems-Schinkel AJ. Neurological aspects of dialysis patients. In: Drukker W, Parsons FM, Maher JF, eds. Replacement of renal function by dialysis, ed 2. Amsterdam: Martinus Nijhoff, 1983:732–741.

103. Bolton CF. Chronic dialysis for uremia. N Engl J Med 1980; 302:1980.

104. Dyck PJ, Johnson WJ, Lambert EH, et al. Detection and evaluation of uremic peripheral neuropathy in patients on hemodialysis. Kidney Int 1975; 7:S201–S205.

105. Jebsen RH, Tenckhoff H, Honet JC. Natural history of uremic polyneuropathy and effects of dialysis. N Engl J Med 1967; 277:327–332.

106. Funck-Brentano JL, Chaumont P, Vantelon J, Zingraff J. Polyneuritis during the course of chronic uremia. Follow-up after renal transplantation (10 personal observations). Nephron 1968; 5:31–42.

107. Bolton CF, Gilbert JJ, Hahn AF, Sibbald WJ. Polyneuropathy in critically ill patients. J Neurol Neurosurg Psychiatry 1984; 47:1223–1231.

108. Bolton CF, Laverty DA, Brown JD, et al. Critically ill polyneuropathy: Electrophysiological studies and differentiation from Guillain-Barré syndrome. J Neurol Neurosurg Psychiatry 1986; 49:563–573.

109. Tenckhoff HA, Boen FST, Jebsen RH, Spiegler JH. Polyneuropathy in chronic renal insufficiency. JAMA 1965; 192:1121–1124.

110. Williams IR, Davison AM, Mawdsley C, Robson JS. Neuropathy in chronic renal failure. In: Desmedt JE, ed. New developments in electromyography and clinical neurophysiology. Vol 2. Basel: Karger, 1973:390–399.

111. Taniguchi H, Ejiri K, Baba S. Improvement of autonomic neuropathy after mecobalamin treatment in uremic patients on hemodialysis. Clin Therapeut 1987; 9:607–614.

112. Konotey-Ahulu FID, Baillod R, Comty CM, et al. Effect of periodic paralysis on the peripheral neuropathy of end-stage renal failure. Br Med J 1965; 2:1212–1215.

113. Curtis JR, Eastwood JB, Smith EK. Maintenance hemodialysis. Q J Med 1969; 38:49–59.

114. Pendras JP, Erickson RV. Hemodialysis: A successful therapy. Ann Intern Med 1966; 64:293–311.

115. Bolton CF, Lindsay RM, Linton AL. The course of uremic neuropathy during chronic hemodialysis. Can J Neurol Sci 1975; 2:322–333.

116. Cadilhac J, Mion CH, Duday H, et al. Motor nerve conduction velocities as an index of the efficiency of maintenance dialysis in patients with end-stage renal failure. In: Canal N, Pozz G, eds. Peripheral neuropathies. New York: Elsevier/North-Holland, 1978:372–380.

117. Dyck PJ, Johnson WJ, Nelson RA, et al. Uremic neuropathy. III. Controlled study of restricted protein and fluid diet and infrequent hemodialysis versus conventional hemodialysis treatment. Mayo Clin Proc 1975; 50:641–649.

118. Bolton CF, Lindsay RM, Linton AAL. Uremic neuropathy in patients on different hemodialysis schedules. Neurology 1977; 27:396.

119. Bolton CF. Electrophysiologic changes in uremic neuropathy after successful renal transplantation. Neurology 1976; 26:152–161.

120. Del Campo M, Bolton CF, Lindsay RM. The value of electrophysiological studies in assessing peripheral nerve function during optimal hemodialysis. Muscle Nerve 1983; 533–534.

121. Bergstrom J, Furst P. Uraemic toxins. In: Drukker W, Parsons FM, Maher JF, eds. Replacement of renal function of dialysis. Amsterdam: Martinus Nijhoff, 1983:368–372.

122. Lowrie EG, Steinberg SM, Galen MA, et al. Factors in the dialysis regimen which contribute to alterations in the abnormalities of uremia. Kidney Int 1976; 10:409–422.

123. Lindsay RM, Bolton CF, Clark WF, Linton AL. The effect of alterations of uremic retention products upon platelet and peripheral nerve function. Clin Nephrol 1983; 19:110–115.

124. Asaba H, Alvestrand A, Furst P, Bergstrom J. Clinical implications of uremic middle molecules in reg-

ular hemodialysis patients. Clin Nephrol 1983; 19:179–187.

125. Lowitzsch K, Gohring U, Hecking E, Kohler H. Refractory period, sensory conduction velocity and visual evoked potentials before and after hemodialysis. J Neurol Neurosurg Psychiatry 1981; 44:121–128.

126. Gokal R. Continuous ambulatory peritoneal dialysis (CAPD)—ten years on. Q J Med (New Ser 63) 1987; 242:465–472.

127. Tenckhoff HA, Curtis FF. Experience with maintenance peritoneal dialysis in the home. Trans Am Soc Artif Intern Organs 1970; 16:90–95.

128. Lindholm B, Tegner R, Tranaeus A, Bergstrom J. Progress of peripheral uremic neuropathy during continuous ambulatory peritoneal dialysis (CAPD). Trans Am Soc Artif Intern Organs 1982; 28:263–268.

129. Tegner R, Lindholm B. Uremic polyneuropathy: Different effects of hemodialysis and continuous ambulatory peritoneal dialysis. Acta Med Scand 1985; 218:409–416.

130. Pierratos A, Blair G, Khanna R, et al. Nerve electrophysiological parameters in patients undergoing continuous ambulatory peritoneal dialysis (CAPD) over two years. Ann CRMCC 1981; 14:231.

131. Amair P, Khanna R, Liebel B, et al. Continuous ambulatory peritoneal dialysis in diabetics with end-stage renal disease. N Engl J Med 1982; 306:625–630.

132. Eggers PW. Effect of transplantation on the medicare end-stage renal disease program. N Engl J Med 1988; 318:1223–1229.

133. Dinapoli RP, Johnson WJ, Lambert EH. Experience with a combined hemodialysis-renal transplantation program: Neurologic aspects. Mayo Clin Proc 1966; 41:809–820.

134. Phadke AG, Mackinnon KJ, Dossetor JB. Male fertility in uremia: Restoration by renal allografts. Can Med Assoc J 1970; 102:607–608.

135. Mallamaci F, Zoccali C, Ciccarelli M, Briggs JD. Autonomic function in uremic patients treated by hemodialysis in CAPD and in transplant patients. Clin Nephrol 1986; 25:175–180.

136. Gonzales-Carrilo M, Moloney A, Bewick M, et al. Renal transplantation in diabetic neuropathy. Brit Med J 1982; 285:1713–1716.

137. Van der Vliet J, Navarro T, Kennedy WR, et al. Diabetic polyneuropathy and renal transplantation. Transplant Proc 1986; 19:3597–3599.

138. Solders G, Wilczek H, Gunnarsson R, et al. Effects of combined pancreatic and renal transplantation on diabetic neuropathy: A two year follow-up study. Lancet 1987; 2:1232–1235.

139. Ibrahim MM, Crossland J, Honigsberger L, et al. Effect of renal transplantation on uraemic neuropathy. Lancet 1974; 2:739–742.

140. Oh SJ, Clements R, Lee YW, Diethelm AG. Rapid improvement in nerve conduction velocity following renal transplantation. Ann Neurol 1978; 4:369–373.

141. Bolton CF, Carter K, Koval JJ. Temperature effects on conduction studies of normal and abnormal nerve. Muscle Nerve 1982; 5:S145–S147.

142. Bolton CF, Sawa GM, Carter K. The effects of temperature on human compound action potentials. J Neurol Neurosurg Psychiatry 1981; 44:407–413.

143. Thomas PK, Lambert EH, eds. Diseases of the peripheral nervous system. Philadelphia: WB Saunders, 1974:1826.

144. Thomas PK, Walker JG. Xanthomatous neuropathy in primary biliary cirrhosis. Brain 1965; 88:1079–1088.

145. Ludwig J, Dyck PJ, LaRusso NF. Xanthomatous neuropathy of liver. Human Pathol 1982; 13(11):1049–1051.

146. Charron L, Peyronnard J-M, Marchand L. Sensory neuropathy associated with primary biliary cirrhosis. Arch Neurol 1980; 37:84–87.

147. Davison AM, Williams IR, Mawdsley C, et al. Neuropathy associated with hepatitis in patients maintained on haemodialysis. Br Med J 1972; 1:409.

148. Thuluvath PJ, Triger DR. Autonomic neuropathy and chronic liver disease. Quart J Med 1989; 72(268):737–747.

149. Nielsen WK, Kardel T. Delayed decrement of the nerve in pulse propagation during induced limb ischaemia in chronic hepatic failure. J Neurol Neurosurg Psychiatry 1975; 38:966–976.

150. Castaigne P, Cathala H-P, Dry JR, et al. Les reponses des nerfs et des muscles a des stimulations electriques au cours d'une epreuve de garrot ischemique chez l'homme normal et chez le diabetique. Rev Neurol (Paris) 1966; 155:61.

151. Gregersen G. A study of the peripheral nerves in diabetic subjects during ischaemia. J Neurol Neurosurg Psychiatry 1968; 31:175.

152. Seneviratne KN, Peiris OA. The effect of ischaemia on the excitability of sensory nerves in diabetes mellitus. J Neurol Neurosurg Psychiatry 1968; 31:348–353.

153. Steiness IB. Vibratory perception in diabetes during arrested blood flow to the limb. Acta Med Scand 1959; 163:195–205.

154. Nielsen VK. Pathophysiological aspects of uraemic neuropathy. In: Canal N, Pozza G, eds. Peripheral neuropathies. Amsterdam: Elsevier/North Holland Biomedical Press, 1978:197–210.

155. Christensen NJ, Orskov H. Vibratory perception during ischemia in uremic patients with mild carbohydrate intolerance. J Neurol Neurosurg Psychiatry 1969; 32:519–524.

156. Shahani B, Russell WR. Motor neuron disease. An abnormality of nerve metabolism. J Neurol Neurosurg Psychiatry 1969; 32:1–5.

157. Chopra JS, Samanta AK, Murthy JMK, et al. Role of porta-systemic shunt and hepatocellular damage in the genesis of hepatic neuropathy. Clin Neurol Neurosurg 1980; 82:37.

158. Hindfelt B, Holmin T. Experimental portacaval anastomosis and motor nerve conduction velocity in the rat. J Neurol 1980; 223:171.

159. Victor M. Polyneuropathy due to nutritional deficiency and alcoholism. In: Dyck PJ, Thomas PK, Lambert EH, et al, eds. Peripheral neuropathy. Philadelphia: WB Saunders, 1984:1899–1940.

160. Pekelharing CA, Winkler C. Mitteilung uber die Beriberi. Dtsch Med Wochenschr 1887; 13:845–848.

161. Takahashi K, Nakamura H. Axonal degeneration in beriberi neuropathy. Arch Neurol 1976; 33:836–841.

162. Williams RR. Structure of vitamin B1. J Am Chem Soc 1936; 58:1063.

163. Prineas J. Peripheral nerve changes in thiamine-deficient rats. Arch Neurol 1970; 23:541.

164. Armett CJ, Cooper JR. The role of thiamine in nervous tissue: Effect of antimetabolites of the vitamin on conduction in mammalian non-myelinated nerve fibers. J Pharmacol Exp Ther 1965; 148:137.

165. von Muralt A. The role of thiamine in neurophysiology. Ann NY Acad Sci 1962; 98:499.

166. Itokawa Y, Cooper JR. Ion movements and thiamine. II. The release of the vitamin from membrane fragments. Biochim Biophys Acta 1970; 196:274.

167. Dastur DK, Manghani DK, Osuntokun BO, et al. Neuromuscular and related changes in malnutrition. J Neurol Sci 1982; 55:207–230.

168. Ohnishi A, Tsuji S, Igisu H, et al. Beriberi neuropathy. Morphometric study of sural nerve. J Neurol Sci 1980; 45:177–190.

169. Pallis CA, Lewis PD. The neurology of gastrointestinal disease. In: Walton JN, ed. Major problems in neurology. Philadelphia: WB Saunders, 1974:30–97.

170. Babior BM, Bunn HF. Megaloblastic anemias. In: Petersdorf RG, Adams RD, Braunwell E, et al, eds. Harrison's principles of internal medicine. New York: McGraw-Hill, 1983:1853–1860.

171. Dinn JJ, Weir DG, McCann S, et al. Methyl group deficiency in nerve tissue. A hypothesis to explain the lesion of subacute combined degeneration. Irish J Med Sci 1980; 149:1.

172. Layzer RB. Myeloneuropathy after prolonged exposure to nitrous oxide. Lancet 1978; 2:1227.

173. McCombe PA, McLeod JG. The peripheral neuropathy of vitamin B12 deficiency. J Neurol Sci 1984; 66:117–126.

174. Adams RD, Victor M. Diseases of the nervous system due to nutritional deficiency. In: Adams RD, Victor M, eds. Principles of neurology. New York: McGraw-Hill, 1985:718.

175. Gilliatt RW, Goodman HV, Willison RG. The recording of lateral popliteal nerve action potentials in man. J Neurol Neurosurg Psychiat 1961; 24:305–318.

176. Mayer RF. Peripheral nerve function in vitamin B12 deficiency. Arch Neurol 1965; 13:355–362.

177. Lockner D, Reisenstein P, Wennberg A, et al. Peripheral nerve function in pernicious anemia before and after treatment. Acta Haematol 1969; 41:257–263.

178. Kayser-Gatchalian MC, Neundorfer B. Peripheral neuropathy with vitamin B12 deficiency. J Neurol 1977; 214:183–193.

179. Hahn A, Gilbert JJ, Brown WF. A study of the sural nerve in pernicious anemia. Can J Neurol Sci 1976; 3:217.

180. Fine EJ, Soria E, Paroski MW, et al. The neurophysiological profile of vitamin B12 deficiency. Muscle Nerve 1990; 13:158–164.

181. Fine EJ, Hallett M. Neurophysiological study of subacute combined degeneration. J Neurol Sci 1980; 45:331–336.

182. Krumholz A, Wiess HD, Goldstein PJ, et al. Evoked responses in vitamin B12 deficiency. Ann Neurol 1981; 9:407–409.

183. Jones SJ, Yu YL, Rudge P, Kriss A, et al. Central and peripheral SEP defects in neurologically symptomatic and asymptomatic subjects with low vitamin B12 levels. J Neurol Sci 1987; 82:55–65.

184. Vishnubhakat SM, Beresford HR. Reversible myeloneuropathy of nitrous oxide abuse: Serial electrophysiological studies. Muscle Nerve 1991; 14:22–26.

185. Ishii N, Nishihara Y. Pellagra among chronic alcoholics. Clinical and pathological study of 20 necropsy cases. J Neurol Neurosurg Psychiatry 1981; 44:209–215.

186. Davidai G, Zakaria T, Goldstein R, et al. Hypovitaminosis E induced neuropathy in exocrine pancreatic failure. Arch Dis Child 1986; 61:901–903.

187. Palmucci L, Doriguzzi C, Orsi L, et al. Neuropathy secondary to vitamin E deficiency in acquired intestinal malabsorption. Ital J Neurol Sci 1988; 9:599–602.

188. Muller DPR, Lloyd JK, Wolff OH. Vitamin E and neurological function. Lancet 1983; 1:225–227.

189. Harding AE, Muller DPR, Thomas PK, et al. Spinocerebellar degeneration secondary to chronic intestinal malabsorption: A vitamin E deficiency syndrome. Ann Neurol 1982; 12:419–424.

190. Werlin SL, Harb JM, Swick H, et al. Neuromuscular dysfunction and ultrastructural pathology in children with chronic cholestasis and vitamin E deficiency. Ann Neurol 1983; 13:291–296.

191. Traber MG, Sokol RJ, Ringel SP, et al. Lack of tocopherol in peripheral nerves of vitamin E-deficient patients with peripheral neuropathy. N Engl J Med 1987; 30:262–265.

192. Muller DP, Goss-Sampson MA. Neurochemical, neurophysiological, and neuropathological studies in vitamin E deficiency. Crit Rev Neurobiol 1990; 5:239–263.

193. Berkelhammer C, Bear RA. A clinical approach to common electrolyte problems: 3. Hypophosphatemia. Can Med Assoc J 1984; 130:17–23.

194. Silvis SE, Paragas PD. Paresthesias, weakness, seizures and hypophosphatemia in patients receiving hyperalimentation. J Gastroenterol 1972; 62:513–520.

195. Weintraub MI. Hypophosphatemia mimicking acute Guillain-Barre-Strohl syndrome. JAMA 1976; 235:1040–1041.

196. Morris JS, Ajdukiewicz AB, Read AE. Neurological disorders and adult coeliac disease. Gut 1970; 11:549.

197. Iyer G, Taori GM, Kapadia CR, et al. Neurologic manifestations in tropical sprue. Neurology 1973; 23:959–966.

198. Roman GC, Spencer PS, Schoenberg BS. Tropical myeloneuropathies: The hidden endemias. Neurology 1985; 35:1158–1170.

199. Osuntokun B, Aladetoyinbo A, Bademosi O. Vitamin B nutrition in the Nigerian tropical ataxic neuropathy. J Neurol Neurosurg Psychiatry 1985; 48:154–156.

200. Gessain A, Barin F, Vernant JC, et al. Antibodies to human T-lymphotropic virus type-I in patients with tropical spastic paraparesis. Lancet 1985; 2:407–410.

201. Grimaldi LME, Roos RP, Devare SG, et al. HTLV-1-associated myelopathy: Oligoclonal immunoglobin G bands contain anti-HTLV-1 p24 antibody. Ann Neurol 1988; 24:727–731.

202. Dastur DK, Manghani DK, Osuntokun BO, et al. Neuromuscular and related changes in malnutrition; A review. J Neurol Sci 1982; 55:207–230.

203. Paulson M, Harvey JC. Hematological alterations after total gastrectomy. JAMA 1954; 156:1556–1560.

204. MacLean LD, Sundberg RD. Incidence of megaloblastic anemia after total gastrectomy. N Engl J Med 1956; 254:885–893.

205. Pallis CA, Lewis PD. The neurological complications of coeliac disease in tropical sprue. In: Pallis CA, Lewis PD, eds. The neurology of the gastrointestinal system. Philadelphia: WB Saunders, 1974: 138–156.

206. Chanarin I. The megaloblastic anaemias. Oxford: Blackwell, 1969.

207. Hoffbrand AV. The megaloblastic anaemias. In: Goldberg A, Brain MC, eds. Recent advances in haematology. London: Longman Group Limited, 1971:1–76.

208. Behse F, Buchthal F. Alcoholic neuropathy: Clinical, electrophysiological, and biopsy findings. Ann Neurol 1977; 2:95.

209. Williams JA, Hall GS, Thompson AG, et al. Neurological disease after partial gastrectomy. Br Med J 1969; 3:210.

210. Naissh J, Capper W. Intestinal cul-de-sac phenomena in man. Lancet 1953; 2:597.

211. Sotaniemi KA. Slimmer's paralysis—peroneal neuropathy during weight reduction. J Neurol Neurosurg Psychiatry 1984; 47:564–566.

212. Feit H, Glasberg M, Ireton C, et al. Peripheral neuropathy and starvation after gastric partitioning for morbid obesity. Ann Intern Med 1982; 96:453–455.

213. Paulson M, Harvey JC. Hematological alterations after total gastrectomy. JAMA 1954; 156:1556–1560.

214. Abarbanel JM, Berginer VM, Osimani A, et al. Neurologic complications after gastric restriction surgery for morbid obesity. Neurology 1987; 37:196–200.

215. MacLean LD, Rhode BM, Shizgal HM. Nutrition following gastric operations for morbid obesity. Ann Surg 1983; 198:347–355.

216. Witt NJ, Zochodne DW, Bolton CF, et al. Peripheral nerve function in sepsis and multiple organ failure. Chest 1991; 99:176–184.

217. Zochodne DW, Bolton CF, Wells GA, et al. Polyneuropathy associated with critical illness: A complication of sepsis and multiple organ failure. Brain 1987; 110:819–842.

217a. Victor M. Polyneuropathy due to nutritional deficiency and alcoholism. In: Dyck PJ, Thomas PK, Lambert EH, et al., eds. Peripheral neuropathy. Philadelphia: WB Saunders, 1984; 2:1899–1940.

218. Ekbom K, Hed R, Kustein L, et al. Muscle affections in chronic alcoholism. Arch Neurol 1964; 10:449–458.

219. Perkhoff GT. Alcoholic myopathy. Ann Rev Med 1971; 22:125–132.

220. Martin FC, Slavin G, Levi J. Alcoholic muscle disease. Br Med Bull 1982; 38:53–56.

221. Faris AA, Reyes MG, Abrams BM. Subclinical alcoholic myopathy: Electromyographic and biopsy study. Trans Am Neurol Assoc 1967; 92:102–106.

222. Faris AA, Reyes MG. Reappraisal of alcoholic myopathy. Clinical and biopsy study on chronic alcoholics without muscle weakness or wasting. J Neurol Neurosurg Psychiatry 1971; 34:8–92.

223. Roussos JE, Keeton RG, Hewlett RH. Chronic proximal weakness in alcoholics. S Afr Med J 1976; 50:2095–2099.

224. Shields RW. Alcoholic polyneuropathy. Muscle Nerve 1985; 8:183–187.

225. Blackstock E, Rushworth G, Gath D. Electrophysiological studies in alcoholism. J Neurol Neurosurg Psychiatry 1972; 35:326–334.

226. Ballantyne JP, Hansen S. A quantitative assessment of reinnervation in the polyneuropathies. Muscle Nerve 1982; 5:S127–S134.

227. Walsh JC, McLeod JG. Alcoholic neuropathy: An electrophysiological and histological study. J Neurol Sci 1970; 10:457–469.

228. Johnson RH, Robinson BJ. Mortality in alcoholics with autonomic neuropathy. J Neurol Neursurg Psychiatry 1988; 51:476–480.

229. Hillbom M, Wennberg A. Prognosis of alcoholic peripheral neuropathy. J Neurol Neurosurg Psychiatry 1984; 47:699–703.

22

Toxic Neuropathies

Viggo Kamp Nielsen

CONTENTS

ACRONYMS

ALS	amyotrophic lateral sclerosis
ATPase	adenosine triphosphatase
CNS	central nervous system
CoA	coenzyme A
CS	carbon disulfide
DMAPN	dimethylaminoproprionitrile
EMG	electromyography
K	potassium
Na	sodium
OP	organophosphorus
PNS	peripheral nervous system
SSEP	somatosensory evoked potential
TOCP	triorthocresyl phosphate

In 1984, a revised and greatly expanded list classi-fying all known neurotoxic substances was pub-lished.[1] It reflects the unprecedented rapid expansion of our knowledge about the pathology of toxic neu-ropathy that has taken place since the early 1960s, in part on the basis of human nerve electrophysiol-ogy and biopsy studies but to a much larger extent thanks to the significant contributions from the ex-perimental neurosciences. For further consultation, several comprehension reviews have appeared over the past decade.[2–9]

In keeping with the scope of this book, toxic neuropathies are approached from the point of view of the clinical neurophysiologist, for whom the topic at first sight may seem deceptively simple, inasmuch as the majority of toxic neuropathies produce an *axonal degeneration*, one way or the other, with a rather stereotyped electrophysiologic pattern. As it subsequently appears, this is indeed an unwarranted simplification. As a matter of fact, toxic neuropathies exhibit quite a variety of individual, more or less subtle, electrophysiologic differences, which should constitute a constant challenge to the clinical neu-rophysiologist. Myopathies, with or without neurop-athy, have also been recognized as a response to toxic chemicals and as an important side effect to certain drugs. This topic is not included in this chapter, but readers are referred to a recent review.[10]

Toxic neuropathies have always existed. During the second half of this century, however, we have witnessed an alarming growth in the number of toxic substances, their complexity, and potential hazard for the public health. This has not only coincided with the often incriminated explosive evolution of the chemical and pharmaceutical industries, but also with equally significant changes in lifestyle, working habits, and communication. Toxic neuropathies tend to appear as isolated cases or in local outbreaks, related to local industrial procedures, hygienic prob-lems, or water and food pollution. Therefore it is virtually impossible to produce realistic figures for the prevalence of a toxic neuropathy. As a result, the clinical neurophysiologist may not see the dimension of the problem reflected in the daily routine of the laboratory, where the confrontation with a toxic neuropathy may be a rare event.

PATHOPHYSIOLOGY

Next to the clinical and epidemiologic picture of toxic neuropathies, the pathologic manifestations in the central and peripheral nervous system are by far the most extensively studied aspects.[11] A detailed account of neuropathologic findings is outside the scope of this chapter, but the principal findings are reviewed under the description of individual neuro-toxic substances. For the purpose of the subsequent discussion, suffice it to state that peripheral neurop-athies of toxic origin can be classified into three distinctive pathologic classes: (1) *neuronopathies*, where the target is the neuronal cell body, usually in the dorsal root ganglion; (2) *myelinopathies*, with impairment of the Schwann cell function resulting in primary paranodal and segmental demyelination, eventually with secondary axonal degeneration; and (3) *axonopathies*, usually in the form of the so-called distal axonopathy, with primary degeneration of mo-tor or sensory axons, in some cases with secondary demyelination.

The pathophysiologic basis for our current inter-pretation of clinical neurophysiologic studies has emerged from two lines of experimental research, both initiated in the early 1960s through the pioneer-ing work by Kaeser and Lambert[12] on axonal degen-eration and by McDonald[13] on segmental demyeli-nation. In the present context, it is of particular interest to note that these and most of the subsequent experimental studies have been conducted on ani-mals with induced toxic neuropathy.

Axonal Degeneration

Using thallium-induced toxic neuropathy in guinea pigs as a model, Kaeser and Lambert[12] studied changes in nerve conduction velocity and amplitude of the evoked muscle response. They observed that the amplitude gradually decreased toward zero in the course of days, whereas the conduction velocity remained practically unaltered. Apart from differ-ences in the time course, they demonstrated that the dissociation between changes in amplitude and ve-locity had principal similarities with that in wallerian axonal degeneration, the unaffected conduction ve-locity indicating that some fast conducting fibers were preserved. The amplitude/velocity dissociation is probably the most significant observation for the pathophysiology of toxic neuropathies. In 1966, Ful-lerton and Barnes[14] introduced acrylamide as a neu-rotoxin for experimental studies of pure axonal de-generation. In rats[14] and baboons,[15] it could be shown that conduction velocities in compound nerve might eventually become reduced by up to 20%, and from correlative histometric measurements, it was argued that this was due to a selective degeneration of large-diameter fibers.

In a series of experiments performed on single myelinated fibers in acrylamide-intoxicated cats, Sumner[16,17] addressed the question of selective susceptibility of fibers. He made a clear distinction between the influence of fiber length versus fiber diameter and showed that for the same fiber length, large-diameter fibers were about two to three times more vulnerable than small-diameter fibers. Further, comparing ventral root motor unit fibers with dorsal root muscle afferent fibers in the same animal (i.e., the same degree of intoxication), he also observed that sensory afferent fibers were several times more susceptible than motor efferent fibers. This is a demonstration of the *neuron size principle*, stating that the larger the total cytoplasmic volume, the more susceptible is the neuron to axonal degeneration. This principle was introduced by Schaumburg et al.[18] based on the observation in cats that the earliest structural signs of axonal degeneration were seen in plantar nerve fibers supplying pacinian corpuscles in the foot. These fibers belong to the largest neurons.

Of further interest to clinical neurophysiology, Sumner[19] demonstrated that the electrical threshold to stimulation was elevated distally in fibers undergoing axonal degeneraton and that these fibers might show a slowing of conduction in their most terminal segments. This applies to the common experience that an increased distal motor latency may be the only sign of impaired nerve conduction in toxic neuropathy. Finally, an interesting observation was that of paradoxic recruitment of fibers, in which by gradually increasing the stimulus strength, slow conducting fibers are recruited before fast conducting fibers.[19]

Not all axonotoxic substances have shown the same selective fiber affinity as described for acrylamide. Hern[20] studied triorthocresyl phosphate (TOCP) neuropathy in baboons and observed a severe drop in amplitude of compound muscle action potentials with preserved normal conduction velocity. Histometric measurements showed that TOCP affects fibers of all diameters equally, that is, sparing enough large-diameter fibers to preserve a normal conduction velocity.

Pathologic studies have shown that although axonal degeneration primarily affects distal portions of axons, it does not always begin in the terminal segment but rather as a multifocal process. Similarly, the progression toward the cell body is multifocal rather than continuous. For these reasons, it has become widely accepted that the often used term *dying-back neuropathy* should be replaced with the more precise term *distal axonopathy*.[21] Further, it is

recognized that toxic substances causing distal axonopathy affect central as well as peripheral nerve tracts according to the principles just described. The central involvement may become apparent as residual central nervous system symptoms, ataxia and spasticity, during recovery from a neuropathy because central nerve tract lesions seem to be more resistant to regeneration than peripheral axons.[22] For a detailed review of the sequential steps in progressive axonal degeneration, see Spencer and Schaumburg.[22]

Axonal Degeneration with Secondary Demyelination

In 1962, Asbury et al.[23] described a new pathologic abnormality in nerves, giant axonal neuropathy, which electron microscopically features segmental axonal swelling with densely packed masses of 10-nM neurofilaments, especially proximal to the nodes of Ranvier. In more severe cases, a secondary feature appears, with thinning of the myelin sheath and paranodal retraction of myelin producing a marked widening of the nodal gap. This has been shown to be the typical pathologic picture in hexacarbon-induced neuropathies[11,24] and in experimental carbon disulfide neuropathy.[25] Electrophysiologically these neuropathies are characterized by amplitude reduction accompanied by severe slowing of nerve conduction, the expected correlate to paranodal demyelination.

Segmental Demyelination

Diphtheria neuropathy is the classic example of a neuropathy in which segmental demyelination is the primary nerve pathology. Although still encountered in the Middle East and Asian countries,[26] it is virtually nonexistent in the Western world. Among modern toxic neuropathies, perhexiline neuropathy is the only other example in which segmental demyelination is the primary pathology. This was observed in sural nerve biopsy specimens from patients with nerve conduction velocities around 20 m per second.[27] Perhexiline neuropathy, however, has not been reproduced in experimental animals.[28] The electrophysiologic correlates to segmental demyelination, slowing of impulse propagation and eventually conduction block, were first described in animals with diphtheria toxin–induced polyneuropathy.[12,13] This has since been the preferred model for extensive electrophysiologic studies on impulse propagation,[29] as described elsewhere in this book.

Traditionally toxic neuropathies are divided into those caused by heavy metals, nonmetal drugs, and industrial agents. As in any classification, borders between classes are blurred; for instance, neuropathy induced by gold or platinum is only known from therapeutic applications. If not for other reasons, however, there is a historical perspective in this subdivision in that heavy metals belong to the oldest known neurotoxins, pharmaceutical agents appeared in the 19th century, and industrial agents encompass neurotoxins of today and tomorrow. Further, there are general features regarding the epidemiology and the clinical picture that warrant this subdivision to be maintained.

NEUROPATHIES OWING TO HEAVY METALS

As a class, heavy metals stand between *drugs* and *industrial compounds*. Except for lead, they all have had clinical therapeutic applications in the past or presently, and for centuries lead has been an inevitable part of our environment in all civilized cultures. Heavy metals are key examples of the general rule that *neurotoxic* substances rarely affect the nervous system selectively. In fact, the neurotoxic component may be the least conspicuous or significant part of the total clinical picture, and the diagnosis is usually made from the involvement of other organ systems, simultaneously or in a characteristic sequence.

Arsenic

Throughout history, arsenic has been a popular poison for homicide and suicide, and this is still the cause in most cases of arsenic neuropathy. The metal, however, also constitutes an environmental hazard[30] even though its use as an antisyphilitic remedy and an agricultural pesticide has been abandonded. In 1975, it was estimated that 1.5 million American workers were chronically exposed to arsenic, especially in copper smelting industries, in which arsenic trioxide is a by-product.[31] Thus, arsenic neuropathy is stated to be the most common of all heavy metal–induced neuropathies.[4,32–35] The traditional distinction between a chronic and a subacute form seems to rest on a difference in dose and time course of clinical development, rather than a difference in the clinical, pathologic, and electrophysiologic findings. Clinically the picture is dominated by sensory symptoms, severely burning feet being the most prominent and also the most resistant to treatment. Vibratory perception and joint position sense are more severely affected than other sensory modalities. Motor symptoms are usually mild and a clinical problem only in

chronic intoxication. In the subacute form, symptoms typically develop 1 to 3 weeks after a single exposure. At that time, acute gastrointestinal and other systemic symptoms have abated, and the proper diagnosis can be made only if the suspicion is raised and elevated tissue levels of arsenic are found in urine or keratin. In unsuspected cases, clinical and electromyographic findings may indistinguishably mimic a Guillain-Barré syndrome.[36] Recovery is slow both in the chronic and in the subacute form and complete only in mild cases.[32,34]

Arsenic interferes with neuronal energy metabolism by inhibition of pyruvate dehydrogenase, which blocks the conversion of pyruvate to acetyl CoA. This is presumed to account for the distal degeneration of axons, the predominant pathologic finding. Sural nerve biopsies show a marked decrease in the number of myelinated fibers over the whole diameter spectrum, although one study showed a predominant loss of large-diameter fibers,[34] which may account for the mild slowing of nerve conduction reported by several authors because segmental demyelination does not seem to occur. There are few neurophysiologic studies, but in all a severe reduction of the amplitude to complete disappearance of sensory potentials in upper and lower extremities was the most conspicuous finding, both in the subacute and the chronic type.[33,34,37] Compound muscle action potentials are low in amplitude, but motor conduction velocity is normal or modestly slowed. In patients with subacute neuropathy after a single dose of arsenic, longitudinal studies showed a slow increase in nerve conduction over years, compatible with axonal regeneration.[34,38,39]

Gold

Gold-induced neuropathy is known only as a side effect to chrysotherapy in rheumatoid arthritis and is extremely rare considering the extensive use of this treatment for several years. Endtz[40] analyzed 72 case reports and argued that gold neuropathy should be considered a separate entity independent of the underlying disease, among other reasons because neuropathic symptoms and signs disappeared on drug withdrawal. Gold neuropathy is a symmetric sensorimotor affliction in patients without other evidence of arteritis, which distinguishes it from the malignant mononeuritis multiplex of rheumatoid arthritis, in which widespread necrotizing arteritis involves vasa nervorum with patchy fascicular nerve degeneration.[41] Gold-induced neuropathy should be recognized in time because one clinical feature is a rapidly progressive motor involvement, which may result in severe pareses in the course of days, in one case leading to tetraplegia.[42] The motor symptoms distinguish gold neuropathy from the predominantly sensory neuropathy associated with rheumatoid arthritis.[43] In the few sural nerve biopsies studied, a mixture of axonal degeneration and segmental demyelination was described.[44,45]

Some patients with gold neuropathy also present with clinical signs of myokymia, which have been misinterpreted as fasciculations suggestive of motor neuron disease.[45–47] This is of special interest to the clinical neurophysiologist because myokymia can be diagnosed with certainty only by the presence of spontaneous repetitive discharges on electromyography (EMG). This has not been described in other toxic neuropathies. The pattern consists of regular repetitive grouped discharges, *multiplets*, of two to many motor unit potentials[48] or continuous trains of spontaneously firing motor units.[49] In two patients, myokymia in the anterior tibial muscle persisted in sleep and after local conduction block of the peroneal nerve but was stopped by succinylcholine, suggesting that the activity is generated in the peripheral segment of the nerve.[46] Other electrophysiologic findings are incompletely described and do not contribute to elucidate the pathophysiology of the neuropathy.

Lead

There is hardly any more confusing toxic neuropathy than that caused by lead. In experimental animals, lead intoxication produces a purely segmental demyelination in adult rats[50,51] but an encephalomyelopathy in suckling rats[52] and mixed axonal degeneration and segmental demyelination in guinea pigs,[53] whereas baboons do not show morphologic alterations.[54] In humans, pathologic findings in lead neuropathy are difficult to evaluate because most data are old. The conclusion from the classic study of Gombault[55] from 1880 that lead causes a segmental demyelination has been very hard-lived. Recent reviews, on the contrary, conclude that the primary lesion in humans is that of an axonal degeneration.[4,33,56] The clinical picture is equally confusing. In adults, the peripheral neuropathy is almost purely motor, with a predominance of symptoms and signs located to the upper extremities, and even more specifically wth a predilection for one single nerve, the radial, with forearm extensor paresis (*drop-hand*) as the typical sign. In children, the motor neuropathy more often affects the legs, apart from the fact that children usually develop an encephalopathy,[57] which is a rare presentation in adults (compare with the difference between suckling and adult rats).

From an environmental point of view, it is a peculiar but fortunate fact that typical lead-induced clinical neuropathy has become increasingly rare during this century despite our heavily industrialized and urbanized society. In England, the number of new cases of lead intoxication showed an impressive drop from 1000 in 1900 to 50 in 1960.[58] This is no doubt due to effective hygienic precautions in lead-contaminated industries.[59] Thus typical examples of clinical lead neuropathy are to be found among single case reports.[60,61] It is the general consensus, however, that the constant accumulation of lead through ages represents a real hazard for public health but probably more by its effects on nonnervous tissues and organ systems (e.g. hematologic changes). Opinions differ widely as to the significance of environmental lead exposure, in industry or community, for the nervous system. There have been plenty of large-scale field studies, some of which have demonstrated a statistically significant *subclinical* lead *neuropathy* in exposed groups of the population.[62–69] Many of these studies, however, have employed nerve conduction velocities as the only electrophysiologic test. With our revised view on the primary pathology, it is probably fair to state that the menace to public health and employment of a borderline low conduction velocity, not to say the risk for subsequent development of clinical neuropathy, has yet to be demonstrated. Moreover, many field studies have been contaminated by data from competitive causes of neuropathy, such as chronic alcoholism.

Because classic overt lead neuropathy belongs to a time before the development of clinical neurophysiologic techniques, the paucity of detailed studies is hardly surprising. The patient studied by Oh,[61] however, essentially illustrates the expected findings with axonal degeneration of motor nerves as the primary pathology: fibrillation potential activity in distal muscles, low amplitudes of evoked muscle responses, normal or subnormal motor conduction velocities, evidence of a predominant affliction of the radial nerve. A sural nerve biopsy showed evidence of axonal degeneration, which may be surprising in face of the predilection for upper extremity motor nerves in lead neuropathy. In a larger study of sural nerve biopsies from occupationally lead-exposed subjects with elevated blood lead levels but without clinical neuropathy, no histologic abnormalities were found except for slight signs of paranodal remyelination in teased fibers.[56]

The question about a possible causal relationship between lead intoxication and amyotrophic lateral sclerosis (ALS) continues to appear in the literature at intervals since it was first mentioned by Aran[70] in 1850 that three of his 11 patients with Aran-Duchenne atrophy has been exposed to lead, two of them with symptoms of intoxication. Campbell et al.[71] found statistical evidence for a correlation from a retrospective and prospective study of the history in 74 cases and noted that the lead-exposed patients had a milder form of ALS with a longer 5-year survival. However, this could not be confirmed by others.[60] Boothby et al.[60] tabulated the existing electromyographic evidence (six cases), all of them displaying fasciculations, which is not considered to be pathognomonic today. Boothby et al. appear to be the only ones who have provided electromyographic evidence in favor of an anterior horn cell lesion, observing a 50% increase in the mean territory and increased amplitude of motor units in an eight-lead multielectrode study of the extensor digitorum communis muscle. The patient improved clinically after treatment with penicillamine, but unfortunately there is no follow-up electromyographic examination. This is, of course, insufficient evidence to warrant a general conclusion to such an important problem.

Mercury

Elemental and organic mercury compounds have different effects on the nervous system and are treated separately. The neurotoxic effects of *organic* mercury compounds, methyl and ethyl mercury, have attracted worldwide public attention because of two large pollution catastrophes. The first occurred in the 1950s around Minamata Bay in Japan and was traced down to water pollution by industrial chemical waste products containing inorganic mercury, which was transformed into methyl mercury and taken up by fish, with a resulting large-scale intoxication of fish-eating birds, animals, and humans. A similar chain of pollution has been demonstrated in heavily industrialized countries of North America and Europe and has caused growing public attention and concern. The second catastrophe took place in Iraq in 1971-72, where wheat grain intended for sowing was prepared with an ethyl mercury—containing fungicide but inadvertently used for baking bread. The intoxication of the population had dramatic dimensions, with more than 6500 hospital admissions and about 450 deaths. Organic mercury is primarily neurotoxic to the central nervous system because distal paresthesia usually is the presenting and a prominent symptom, a peripheral toxic neuropathy was also suspected and has not yet been ruled out with certainty. It is known that methyl mercury in rats affects the dorsal root ganglion with secondary degeneration of sensory axons, whereas ventral roots are not or only minimally affected.[72] Murai et al.[73] studied the sural nerve function in rats and showed a significant decrease in compound sensory nerve action potential amplitude after 32 days. After 54 days, an action potential could no longer be evoked. Until the potential disappeared, sensory conduction velocity remained normal, consistent with axonal degeneration. In monkeys, however, motor and sensory nerve function remained normal, but somatosensory evoked potentials and visual evoked potentials showed a progressive slowing *of the major components*, and the monkeys developed ataxia. In humans, studies are somewhat conflicting. Japanese studies of patients with *Minamata disease* have shown degeneraton of both axon and myelin sheath of sensory nerves, posterior root, or dorsal root ganglion (quoted by Murai et al.[73]), whereas electrophysiologic studies of patients from Iraq[74–76] showed normal compound sensory nerve action potential amplitudes and conduction velocities (median and sural nerves), although all patients had sensory abnormalities on clinical examination, which suggested a pathologic condition in the central nervous system. Tokuomi et al.[77] recorded somatosensory evoked potentials in five patients with Minamata disease and found a normal N-11 peak latency, but the N-20 peak, representing the sensory cortex, was absent. Thus it seems that in humans organic mercury primarily produces a central nervous system disease with predilection to the sensory cortex.

Inorganic mercury is neurotoxic both as mercury salts, absorbed through the gastrointestinal tract, and as elemental mercury, which is volatile at room temperature and lipid soluble and absorbed through the lungs and the skin. It is primarily neurotoxic to the central nervous system, with tiredness, mental alteration, and tremor as typical symptoms. Eventually after prolonged exposure, distal paresthesia may develop, signaling impairment of the peripheral nerves, which, however, is mainly motor and usually mild and reversible after removal from exposure. The only available pathologic data are from sural nerve biopsies from two children with severe, predominantly motor neuropathy. Both cases showed "a slight increase in the frequency of teased fibers undergoing axonal degeneration."[4]

Several reports describe electrophysiologic findings in patients with clinical neuropathy after accidental[4,78] and occupational[79–81] exposure to mercury vapor and in asymptomatic, potentially exposed, workers in chlor-alkali plants[82] and in dental offices.[83] The most consistent findings are electromyographic evidence of denervation in distal muscles and less frequently reduced amplitudes of compound sensory nerve and motor action potentials, consistent with axonal degeneration. In a detailed study with quantitative sensory testing and electrophysiologic examination, Albers et al.[82] found evidence of a subclinical neuropathy in 13% of 138 chlor-alkali workers, the severity being related to the degree of exposure. Adams et al.[78] studied a patient who was initially suspected of having ALS because of prominent fasciculations clinically and on EMG, with positive sharp waves and normal motor and sensory conduction velocities. As it turned out, the patient had been exposed to mercury vapors 3½ months earlier, and symptoms and signs gradually disappeared, but findings indicate that anterior horn cells may be involved in mercury intoxication.

Platinum

In 1972, platinum was taken into use in the chemotherapy of solid cancers in the form of cis-diamminedichloroplatinum (*cisplatin*). It soon showed several serious side effects,[84] however, among which toxic neuropathy is probably the least important because it produces neither pain nor motor dysfunction. It was long questioned whether platinum had neurotoxic effects at all. Symptoms alleged to cisplatin, paresthesias and distal sensory loss, are similar to those of cancer neuropathy and were often present before onset of treatment,[85] and besides many patients had already received other potentially neurotoxic chemotherapeutic drugs. Case reports have appeared, however, demonstrating that development and remission of clinical and electrophysiologic signs of neuropathy was temporally related to the onset and cessation of cisplatin therapy.[86–88]

The well-documented case report by Reinstein et al.[88] may serve as an example. A 52-year-old man with a left anticubital malignant fibrous histiocytoma presented with symptoms and signs of compression of the left median nerve, but the left ulnar and right median nerves were normal. After seven courses of cisplatin therapy, he developed paresthesias in both hands and both feet, and 5 months after onset, a repeat nerve conduction study showed that the previously normal compound sensory nerve action potentials were either unobtainable or severely reduced in amplitude. Cisplatin was continued for another 6 months, when ulnar and median compound sensory nerve action potentials were unobtainable in both arms. Potentials reappeared 1 month after cessation of therapy but now showed increased latency and reduced amplitude, both of which returned toward normal in the subsequent 10-month follow-up period. This was accompanied by improvement of sensory symptoms. The distal motor latency and motor conduction velocity in arm nerves were unaffected throughout, but both peroneal nerves showed a reversible increase in the distal motor latency (muscle potential amplitudes were not reported). In another study, 18 patients were examined before and after treatment with high-dose cisplatin. All of them developed clinical and electrophysiologic signs of peripheral sensory neuropathy, and three patients also showed central conduction defects in evoked potential studies.[89] A local chemical reaction, however, might be involved in patients who developed symptoms and signs of plexopathy or mononeuropathies within a few days after intraarterial infusion of cisplatin. The suspected mechanism was chemical small vessel injury with subsequent plexus and nerve infarction.[90] Furthermore autonomic neuropathy has also been suggested as a side effect to cisplatin treatment to account for long-lasting gastroparesis in a patient induced by cisplatin but only disappearing 5 weeks after withdrawal of the drug.[91]

In recent years, tetany has been described in several patients as a result of the nephrotoxic action of cisplatin leading to impairment of the tubular reabsorption of magnesium and calcium.[92–94] Thus one study showed that electromyographic signs of tetany were present in 75% of patients who developed hypomagnesemia during cisplatin therapy.[93]

Pathologic findings are conflicting; axonal degeneration, segmental demyelination, and mixed alterations have all been described.[95,96]

Thallium

Thallium is a contender for the position as the most neurotoxic substance, but being a much *younger* metal (discovered in 1861) than arsenic, it does not share the historical reputation of arsenic in the public. The medical application of two of its toxic effects, as a depilator in the treatment of ringworms and as an autonomic neurotoxin in the treatment of hyperhidrosis in tuberculosis, has been abondoned long ago. Today thallium neuropathy is encountered only in acute intoxications resulting from accidental ingestion (rodenticides) or in a homicidal/suicidal intent, and reported cases in the medical literature are few and far between.[97–99]

The early diagnosis of a thallium intoxication mainly rests on the neurotoxic symptoms because the more conspicuous and well-known feature of alopecia does not appear until 2 or more weeks after ingestion.[98] Neurotoxic symptoms include manifestations from the central nervous system, the autonomic, and the peripheral sensorimotor nerves, all of them characterized by a rapid onset within hours. Central nervous system symptoms include confusion and psychosis, convulsions, and coma. Cranial nerves are involved, with ptosis and retrobulbar neuritis. Autonomic symptoms are tachycardia, hypertension, and dry skin. Peripheral nerve involvement appears as a polyneuropathy with painful paresthesia, numbness and hypalgesia, and distal weakness progressing central-ward, with widespread pareses to paralysis that may also effect respiratory muscles. Characteristic and distinguishing features are first of all the preserved, maybe even brisk, deep reflexes and the normal or only mildly impaired vibratory perception and position sense.[98] The progressive pathologic changes were studied at autopsy in three patients, who died 8 days, 19 days, and 1 month after exposure.[98] From a pathophysiologic point of view, considering the rapid onset of severe neurologic symptoms, it is of interest that significant pathologic changes were first seen after 19 days in the second patient, who displayed severe axonal degeneration in the sural and vagus nerves and in intramuscular nerves. After 1 month, severe axonal degeneration was present in all nerves examined. This discrepancy between acute symptoms and delayed pathology suggests that thallium interferes biochemically with the cell membrane function. It is known that thallium is interchangeable with potassium in its action on the myocardium.[100] Thallium has a 10-fold higher affinity for sodium/potassium–activated ATPase than potassium in renal tissue[101] and human erythrocytes,[102] and a thallium-induced dephosphorylation of the sodium/potasium–activated ATPase has been described in brain tissue.[103] Thus although thallium is known to produce a *pure* axonal degeneration of the distal axonopathy type, it is likely that the pathophysiologic mechanism is in fact primarily biochemical.

Few electrophysiologic findings have been re-

ported in human subjects.[97–99,104–106] In a longitudinal study of one patient, the earliest electrophysiologic abnormality was signs of profound axonopathy in the plantar nerves, which subsequently became demonstrable in more proximal nerves also.[106] Nonetheless, clinical neurophysiologists owe much of their knowledge about the typical electrophysiology of axonal degeneration to the classic experimental study by Kaeser and Lambert,[12] who employed thallium intoxication as a model for axonal degeneration.

DRUG-INDUCED NEUROPATHIES

The toxic effects of heavy metals and industrial compounds almost always affect *normal* subjects. In drug-induced neuropathies, however, one must always recognize the possible influence of the primary disease itself on the neuromuscular function. Pharmaceutical toxicity testing in animals is an important step before the drug is released. This is usually an effective precaution although not a guaranteed tight control, among other things owing to species variations in susceptibility. Other factors include uncalculated clinical dose and time applications of the drug, preconditioning or synergistic factors residing with the primary disease, impaired excretion of the drug (renal failure), and individual hypersensitivity. Moreover, in quite a few instances, a potentially neurotoxic drug is used none the less with a *calculated risk*. The risk may be small when neurotoxic symptoms are insignificant, preventable by dose regulation or supplementation (isoniazid and pyridoxin), or high but acceptable because the primary effect of the drug is considered to be of greater importance (chemotherapy in patients with cancer). In the latter situation, the clinical neurophysiologist should be able to offer valuable assistance in the clinical control of patients and in the planning of therapeutic strategies.

Chloramphenicol

Chloramphenicol may cause optic neuritis and mild distal sensory symptoms of peripheral neuropathy, especially in children, which disappear after cessation of treatment.[107,108] The main toxic side effects of the antibiotic, however, are hematologic, and the current practice of intermittent use, neuropathic complications have become rare. There are no reports on electrophysiologic abnormalities.

Dapsone

The polyneuropathy in leprosy may be seriously aggravated when tuberculoid patients are treated with dapsone (4,4'-sulfonylbisbenzenamine), but this side effect is reversible, as illustrated by a highly significant increase of distal motor latencies and motor conduction velocities only 4 months after withdrawal of the drug.[109] Dapsone has caused neuropathy in a few patients, when used in high doses over several weeks in the treatment of other dermatologic disorders.[110–113] Acute neuritis has also been described as a result of an overdose of dapsone.[114,115] The neuropathy is interesting by its predominant or isolated affection of motor fibers. Symptoms include symmetric weakness and wasting of distal muscles.

Electrophysiologic studies are consistent with a distal, purely motor axonopathy with widespread fibrillation potential activity in the presence of normal or mildly reduced motor conduction velocities. In severe cases, the muscle may be nonresponsive to supramaximal nerve stimulation. In one study, the severely reduced potential amplitude of thenar muscles returned to normal over 5 years after withdrawal of the drug.[111] The amplitude of sensory potentials was normal in all studies. It has not been possible to reproduce dapsone neuropathy experimentally in rats and guinea pigs.[111]

Diphenylhydantoin

In opposition to earlier reports,[116,117] it has been questioned whether diphenylhydantoin (phenytoin) causes a clinical neuropathy at all.[118,119] The controversy relates to the selection of patients, possible effects of other antiepileptic drugs, lack of adequate control groups, and lack of prospective studies. Taking these problems into account, Swift et al.[118] found a prevalence of peripheral neuropathy (distal hypesthesia and reduced Achilles reflexes) of 16.7% in 186 epileptic patients. A multivariate statistical analysis, however, failed to demonstrate a relationship with phenytoin treatment, phenytoin serum levels, or duration of treatment. Shorvon and Reynolds[119] followed previously untreated epileptic patients for 1 to 5 years, 32 patients on phenytoin and 19 on carbamazepine. None of the groups developed clinical evidence of neuropathy. In the phenytoin group, six patients (18%) had *abnormal* sural compound sensory nerve action potentials, thought to be caused by previous high phenytoin serum levels.

The picture seems less confounded as regards the effect of phenytoin on the peripheral nerve conduc-

tion. Conduction velocities were mildly slowed in normal volunteers given high doses of phenytoin,[120] and motor conduction velocity was also reduced in patients with phenytoin serum levels over 120 μmol/l. This became normal when serum phenytoin was reduced to therapeutic levels.[121] The same was seen in rabbits after intravenous injection of phenytoin[122] and in guinea pigs fed high doses of phenytoin, but only if serum levels exceeded 200 μmol/l.[123] Acutely intoxicated rats showed increased membrane instability and decreased nerve potential amplitude.[124] Thus there is evidence of reversible impairment of the nerve function in humans and experimental animals but only with excessively high phenytoin levels. Within therapeutic levels, phenytoin does not appear to produce signs of acute or chronic neuropathy.

Disulfiram

Disulfiram (Antabuse) neuropathy is rare but has been established beyond doubt as a clinical entity, although it may be difficult to assert its presence because the underlying disease, chronic alcoholism, is a much more common cause of similar symptoms and clinical and electrophysiologic signs. The predominant symptoms are paresthesia and sensory loss in the feet, and there is often evidence of optic neuritis.[125] Motor symptoms, dropfoot and ascending pareses, and upper extremity symptoms may develop in severe cases.[126] Cessation of treatment leads to remission of symptoms and electrophysiologic signs in weeks.[126–128] Nerve biopsies show a primary axonal degeneration of the neurofilamentous giant axonal type,[128–130] similar to findings in carbon disulfide–intoxicated animals. Disulfiram is converted enzymatically to carbon disulfide, which may be the actual toxic agent.

EMG and nerve conduction studies are consistent with a distal axonopathy with profuse fibrillation potential activity, reduced potential amplitudes to absent muscle, and nerve potentials with normal or mildly slowed nerve conduction, when obtainable. In favor of a distal axonopathy, Olney and Miller[131] found complete denervation of intrinsic foot muscles and absent or severely reduced sural nerve potentials as opposed to mild abnormalities or normal findings in the upper extremities. Their patients showed a slow and incomplete improvement after drug withdrawal, but more complete remission of clinical and electrophysiologic signs has been described by others.[126,127,129] In a well-controlled study, 42 alcoholic patients were followed before and during a 6-month course on disulfiram. Overt clinical neuropathy did not appear, but electrophysiologic variables showed a statistically significant deterioration, although only in patients treated with a daily dose of 250 mg, whereas those on 125 mg were unaffected.[132] Careful supervision and monitoring of neurologic side effects during disulfiram treatment are recommended.[133]

Isoniazid

By inhibition of pyridoxal phosphokinase, isoniazid interferes with the metabolism of the coenzyme, pyridoxine (vitamin B_6). The neurotoxic effect shows great innerspecies variation.[134] In humans, it is linked to a genetically determined impaired capacity to acetylate isoniazid,[5] and neuropathy can be prevented by pyridoxine supplementation. Neuropathic symptoms, essentially sensory, develop slowly and are rapidly reversible in the early stages, whereas recovery from more severe stages is considerably more protracted. The pathologic picture is characterized by multifocal axonal degeneration with wallerian degeneration of the axon. Isoniazid was introduced before clinical electrophysiologic methods were fully developed. This and the early recognition of the preventive effect of pyrodixine and the disappearance of tuberculosis explain the absence of electrophysiologic studies of isoniazid neuropathy in humans.

Misonidazole

Misonidazol (2-nitroimidazol) was introduced in the mid-1970s as a radiosensitizer in cancer chemotherapy, but its use has been limited by a dose-related interval-related sensory neuropathy, dominated by painful burning sensations in the feet. The neuropathy is of the distal axonopathy type and develops within weeks after onset of therapy. Clinical findings are predominantly sensory: impaired touch and pain sensation, impaired vibratory perception and position sense, and disappearance of ankle jerks with only mild muscle weakness and no atrophy.[135–137] In rats, pathologic studies show distal axonal degeneration, primarily affecting sensory terminals in intramuscular fibers.[138] Sural nerve biopsies in three patients with neuropathy[136] showed a reduction of the total number of myelinated fibers, especially large-diameter fibers. The myelin was fragmented with debris and clumps of disorganized myelin and paranodal demyelination, which contrasted with the normal conduction velocity in the same nerves. A biopsy from the anterior tibial muscle showed groups of atrophic fibers, but necrotic fibers were absent.

Mamoli et al.[135] studied electrophysiologic changes in 13 patients before and after treatment with misonidazole. Six developed neuropathy, but they were not distinguished from patients without neuropathy, and the full protocol was not applied to all, which makes interpretation of their results difficult. A marked reduction of the sural nerve potential amplitude was seen *in some cases,* which tended to improve 6 months after the end of therapy.

Melgaard et al.[136] studied eight patients, all with neuropathy. The median nerve was normal except for severely reduced compound sensory nerve action potential amplitudes in two patients. The sural nerve conduction was mildly slowed in two patients, whereas the amplitude was severely reduced in all but one. In one patient, the amplitude dropped from 17 μV to 2.2 μV after 11 weeks of treatment (near-nerve recordings). Similar findings were seen in the superficial peroneal and posterior tibial nerves. EMG was performed only in the anterior tibial muscle. The recruitment pattern was reduced in four patients, with abundant fibrillation potential activity in two. In a new prospective study,[137] 14 out of 36 patients treated with misonidazole (39%) developed clinical polyneuropathy, whereas this was seen in only two out of 34 patients in the placebo group (6%). The most consistent sign was a rise in vibratory perception threshold.

Nitrofurantoin

Nitrofurantoin is a dangerous antibiotic because it may cause an insidious and often severe polyneuropathy.[139] The presenting symptom is paresthesia in the feet, but the neuropathy is predominantly motor, sometimes with rapid development of severe pareses, which are only partially reversible. Nitrofurantoin is concentrated and excreted through the kidneys and commonly used to treat ordinary lower urinary tract infections. Therefore it proved to be particularly dangerous in patients with mild or moderate renal failure, now considered as an absolute contraindication. Neuropathy, however, may also appear in patients with a normal kidney function. This was indicated by a high incidence of electromyographic signs of denervation,[140] and administration of nitrofurantoin to normal volunteers resulted in subclinical changes of motor and sensory nerve conduction.[141] Nitrofurantoin neuropathy may be confused with uremic neuropathy, but in the latter, neurologic symptoms and signs are encountered only in patients with severe, terminal uremia.[142] Therefore when patients with mild to moderately impaired kidney function present with symptoms of neuropathy, an exogenous intoxication should be suspected.

There are no recent pathologic or electrophysiologic studies, but older data are consistent with a distal axonopathy. Thus motor nerve conduction was only mildly reduced in a patient with severe muscle weakness.[143]

Perhexiline

Perhexiline maleate is used in the treatment of angina pectoris, one of its presumed actions being a slowing of conduction at the sinoauricular node. Toxic neuropathy may develop with a prevalence of one out of 1000 treated patients.[144] This neuropathy has attracted special attention as being the only modern example of a toxic neuropathy owing to segmental demyelination, as shown in sural nerve biopsies, where primary segmental demyelination, predominantly of large-sized fibers, was accompanied by mild secondary axonal degeneration.[27] Concordantly nerve conduction is severely slowed to the order of 20 per second in symptomatic patients.[27,145–147] The neuropathy develops slowly after months to years of treatment and seems to be more generalized than usual in toxic neuropathies, involving both proximal and distal nerve segments and also cranial nerves with facial diplegia.[27] Asymptomatic patients, however, showed normal motor and sensory conduction velocities,[144] and segmental demyelination has not been reproduced in experimental animals.[28]

Pyridoxine

Toxic neuropathies may appear from the most unsuspected sources. The neuropathy caused by intake of pyridoxine (vitamin B_6) in megadoses is a good example. Although the normal daily minimal requirement of vitamin B_6 is 2 to 4 mg, pyridoxine in high doses has gained reputation for some unproved effects, ameliorating premenstrual edema and advancing physical fitness. In 1983, seven patients were described who developed serious neurotoxic symptoms, ataxia and sensory dysfunction, after intake of pyridoxine in doses of 2 to 6 g per day for months to years.[148] Clinical findings included profound distal impairment of position sense and vibratory perception and ataxia, whereas the muscle function was well preserved. Pathologic studies have shown a selective degeneration of sensory neurons of the dorsal root and gasserian ganglia and their central and peripheral extensions. Distal sensory nerve conduction

was absent in all nerves, but the motor conduction velocity was normal throughout.

Since the first description in 1983, several papers on this issue have appeared, and pyridoxine polyneuropathy was the topic of an international conference in 1987.[149] The duration of intake rather than the dose seems to be a significant factor in chronic cases. Among 172 women with a daily ingestion of 117 mg (which is certainly far from the megadoses described in the original paper) for 2.9 years, an average 60% showed symptoms and signs of neuropathy, which disappeared in all when medication was stopped.[150] Severe polyneuropathy of rapid onset has also been described following high doses of vitamin B_6 parenterally.[151,152] Symptoms were consistent with that of a sensory ganglion neuropathy, in keeping with the pathologic[153] and pathophysiologic[154] findings in experimental animals.

Thalidomide

Thalidomide was withdrawn from the market in 1961 because of its teratogenic side effects. Before its withdrawal, however, several studies had demonstrated a peripheral neurotoxic effect as well.[155] Although only of historical interest today, it deserves mentioning because there was clinical and pathologic evidence that thalidomide exerts its toxic effect on the sensory nerve cell body in the dorsal root ganglia with secondary distal axonal degeneration. Hence thalidomide belongs to the relatively few neuronotoxic agents. As a consequence, many patients have obtained only partial remission of neuropathic symptoms and signs with persisting sensory deficits and low-amplitude compound nerve action potentials present several years after intake of the drug had been stopped.[5,156,157]

Vinca Alkaloids

The vinca alkaloids, vinblastine, vincristine, and vindesine, are all neurotoxic. Vincristine is a good example of a drug in which toxic neuropathy is a calculated, and high, risk. It is the most potent of the three in the chemotherapy of hematologic oncology, one of the major advantages being the low degree of bone marrow depression. All patients, however, develop some degree of sensorimotor neuropathy, the severity of which is dose and time related. Major symptoms and signs are usually reversible on a lowering of the dosage alone without complete discontinuation of therapy. Hence the proper dosage becomes an important balance for which a clinical and electrophysiologic evaluation of the peripheral nerve function may be useful. The initial stages of the neuropathy are dominated by the usual distal sensory symptoms with loss of ankle jerks as the presenting neurologic sign. In more severe cases, a motor neuropathy with marked weakness and muscle atrophy may ensue. Patients may become unable to walk.[158–160] Motor impairment usually shows a predilection for upper extremity muscles, especially the forearm extensor muscles, and motor signs are also reversible on drug withdrawal. In sural nerve biopsies, axonal degeneration is the dominant finding, but mild segmental demyelination has also been described.[158,161] Muscle biopsy specimens are normal in light microscopy, but many fibers showed myofibrillar disruption under the electron microscope.[158,162] Two independent papers point to the higher susceptibility to vincristine neurotoxicity in patients with Charcot-Marie-Tooth disease, hereditary motor and sensory neuropathy type I, and the authors advocate that "vincristine should be used with caution in patients with a family history of polyneuropathy."[163,164]

The study by Casey et al.[159] may serve as a prototype for a clinical electrophysiologic evaluation of a drug-induced neuropathy. Their patients were studied before onset of treatment, permitting them to assess the influence of the underlying disease, a basic problem in drug-induced neuropathies. Patients were followed longitudinally with closely spaced examinations that provided information about the relationship between drug dosage and duration of treatment and neurologic findings. In patients followed after drug withdrawal, special attention was paid to the relative recovery of clinical and electrophysiologic abnormalities. The electrophysiologic protocol was specifically designed to study distal axonopathies with a balanced combination of invasive and noninvasive techniques, a necessary consideration to maintain patient compliance in a longitudinal study. Results were typical for distal axonopathies. Electromyographic signs of axonal degeneration, fibrillation potential activity and reduced recruitment pattern, were present in intrinsic hand and foot muscles of all patients as well as in more proximal muscles when clinically weak. The amplitude of compound muscle action potentials decreased rapidly after institution of therapy, whereas motor nerve conduction velocity remained normal or mildly decreased. One patient showed a decrease of 94% in amplitude of the extensor digitorum brevis muscle potential with un-

changed conduction velocity. The distal motor latency was increased in less than half the patients. The amplitude ratio between proximal and distal stimulation remained unchanged, pointing to the predominantly distal affection. With a special technique, developed by the authors,[165] compound sensory nerve action potentials were recorded at the base of the third digit following stimulation of the tip of the finger. All patients showed a reduction of the finger potential amplitude within 4 to 6 weeks after onset of treatment, and the maximal decrease was a function of dose and duration of treatment. The amplitude reduction was less pronounced for compound sensory nerve action potentials recorded at the wrist. When the dose was reduced or the drug stopped, recovery of the compound sensory nerve action potential amplitude was poor, on average 15%, despite a marked improvement of clinical sensory symptoms and signs. Similar results were reported by Guiheneuc et al.,[160] who stated that the most sensitive index of peripheral nerve impairment was a reduction of the ratio between the soleus muscle potential amplitude elicited by ankle reflex and H wave stimulation, in keeping with a predominantly distal affection.

NEUROPATHIES OWING TO INDUSTRIAL COMPOUNDS

Usually neurotoxic industrial compounds are first discovered when a sufficient number of subjects presents with sufficiently alarming symptoms. This is the time when the toxic agent has to be identified. It is often an unsuspected, maybe even unknown, intermediary substance in a technical process. Neuropathies owing to industrial compounds, as opposed to drugs, tend to cluster in local outbreaks, some of which have taken *epidemic* proportions. By occupational exposure, they usually affect normal and healthy subjects without preexisting peripheral nerve lesions, although alcoholic neuropathy should always be taken into consideration. Individual cases may appear as accidental intoxications owing to our increasingly domestic coexistence with potent chemicals in modern households, owing to addiction (glue sniffing), or owing to suicidal attempts. Industrial compounds such as acrylamide have provided some of the most important model substances for experimental neurobiologic research. This has been discussed in a previous section. The present section therefore focuses on clinical problems. All chemicals discussed in this section cause axonal degeneration, but in addition, hexacarbons produce prominent secondary demyelination, giving rise to a *mixed pattern*.

Acrylamide

Acrylamide-induced neuropathy hits workers engaged in the polymerization process of the neurotoxic monomer to the nontoxic polymers, used in several industries. Peripheral neuropathy in humans as a result of exposure to acrylamide was first described in Japan in 1960, and the first reports in the English literature appeared in 1967.[166,167] Clinical symptoms include numbness but no paresthesia; excessive sweating of hands and feet, often with exfoliative neurodermatitis; and severe ataxia but initially only mild distal weakness. Clinical findings characteristically show severe impairment of vibratory perception and loss of distal and *proximal* deep reflexes, clumsiness, and atactic gait, the pronounced ataxia being out of proportion to the sensory loss.[168] There are no reliable methods to detect acrylamide in urine or blood, so a careful occupational history is mandatory to confirm the diagnosis.[3] Only two sural nerve biopsies from patients have been reported, both showing a reduction of the large fiber density with no evidence of demyelination.[169] However, the pathology of nerves in experimental acrylamide neuropathy in rats, cats, and baboons has been extensively studied, as discussed previously in this chapter.[18]

The clinical electrophysiologic findings have been outlined in a few reports,[169–171] and their significance for the detection of subclinical neuropathy is emphasized. Absent or low-amplitude sensory responses and a marked dispersion and low amplitude of evoked muscle potentials were characteristic features, sometimes with isolated late components. The conduction velocity of surviving fibers was normal or only mildly reduced. These findings are identical to nerve conduction data from experimental animal studies.[14,15,172] In acrylamide-intoxicated monkeys, somatosensory potentials recorded over the spinal cord after stimulation of the peroneal nerve showed changes in latency and amplitude before any alterations could be detected in the peripheral nerve conduction,[173] for which reason the authors advocate that somatosensory evoked potentials should be employed as a clinical screening procedure. The merits of vibratory perception threshold measurements are emphasized as a screening method for subclinical acrylamide neuropathy.[3] This applies in particular to field studies in areas where electrophysiologic studies are not readily available.[174]

Carbon Disulfide

Carbon disulfide is a highly volatile liquid used in the production of viscose rayon fiber and cellophane. Workers are intoxicated by inhalation of vapors, and the clinical picture of the neurotoxic effects is dose dependent.[175] After acute, high-dose exposure, patients present with a picture of encephalopathy (carbon disulfide has a high lipid solubility). Chronic, low-dose exposure may produce numbness and distal weakness and sensorimotor signs of peripheral neuropathy. There are no nerve biopsy studies from human subjects, but experimental studies in animals have shown a primary axonal degeneration with marked 10-nm neurofilament accumulation and giant axonal swelling.[176] Besides the ultrastructure and sensory nerve supply to pacinian corpuscles was studied in rats after 6 months of exposure to carbon disulfide vapors. Thirty percent of corpuscles were denervated, but 60% showed signs of reinnervation with terminal sprouting of axons with the formation of new terminals in the inner core.[177]

Electrophysiologic studies have shown fibrillation potential activity in leg muscles and mild slowing of conduction velocities in motor and sensory nerves, most pronounced in the legs.[178,179] The reduction in motor conduction velocity was related to the length of exposure.[180] Vasilescu[181] studied 81 workers with symptoms of carbon disulfide neuropathy. Thirty patients also presented clinical signs: *glove and stocking* hypesthesia, weakness and wasting of distal muscles, and absent knee and ankle reflexes. Among the 51 patients without clinical signs of neuropathy, 30 had significantly reduced motor conduction velocities in the peroneal, median, and ulnar nerves, whereas these values were within normal limits in the remaining 21 patients. From the thoroughly documented study, however, it appears that the most significant change, not discussed by the author, was a marked reduction in the distal compound muscle action potential amplitudes to less than half the control values, whereas amplitudes of mixed compound nerve action potentials, recorded at the knee and elbow after stimulation at the ankle and wrist, were not significantly reduced. Compound sensory nerve potential amplitudes were not significantly changed either, although they were generally lower than in the control group. These data illustrate a predominantly distal affection of motor nerves, compatible with axonal degeneration.

Hexacarbons

The neuropathy caused by 2,5-hexanedione, the presumed toxic metabolite of the hexacarbon solvents, n-hexane and methyl n-butyl ketone, is the classic example in our time of a toxic neuropathy owing to industrial agents. The neuropathy was first described in a large-scale outbreak among workers in the sandal industry in Nagoya, Japan,[182] and detailed epidemiologic studies have been reported from similar outbreaks in Italian shoe and leather industries[183-185] and in a fabric-producing plant in Ohio.[186,187] Isolated cases were studied from various other industries.[188] The fluid n-hexane may be absorbed through the skin, but owing to its low boiling point, inhalation of vapors in poorly ventilated rooms is a more common exposure. This was discovered to have an euphoric effect, and very serious cases of neuropathy have been reported in addicted *glue-sniffers*.[24,189,190] In mild cases, numbness of toes and fingers, distal sensory loss, and absent ankle jerks may be the only clinical findings, but more heavy exposure produces a subacute sensorimotor neuropathy, gradually dominated by motor symptoms, with weakness and wasting of intrinsic foot and hand muscles progressing to wheelchair invalidity. It is a general experience that the neuropathy may continue to progress for months after the patient has been removed from exposure, but recovery, although slow, is usually complete except for the most severe cases. As described previously, the pathologic picture is the typical example of a *giant axonal neuropathy*, as demonstrted in human nerve biopsies and in extensive animal studies.[11]

Clinical electrophysiologic procedures, nerve conduction and visual evoked responses, have proved of great value in identifying subclinical and mild cases in epidemiologic studies.[187,191] EMG shows signs of chronic partial denervation, fibrillation potential activity, increased duration and polyphasia of single motor unit potentials, and loss of motor units on maximal contraction.[185] As in other distal axonopathies, compound muscle action potentials are low in amplitude, and sensory potentials are small or absent. Normal conduction velocities may be found in mild cases, but the distinguishing feature in hexacarbon neuropathies is that of a disproportionately severe reduction in conduction velocity to about 50% to 60% of the normal value in only moderately severe cases, often progressing to conduction block. This has been ascribed to the widening of the Ranvier nodes caused by secondary paranodal demyelination.[24]

Thirteen years after his first publication,[182] Iida[192] reexamined 21 of his 44 patients from the outbreak of n-hexane neuropathy in Nagoya, Japan. He used exactly the same electrophysiologic protocol in both studies. The patients had not been totally removed from exposure to n-hexane, but hygienic conditions had been improved through better ventilation. This resulted in clinical recovery in 92% of patients after 4 years. It should be noted, however, that the patients still complained of distal numbness *especially in the winter time*. After 13 years, fibrillation potential activity was no longer present, but more than 50% of patients still showed reduced interference pattern on EMG, and 15% had increased incidence of polyphasic units. The number of patients with slowed motor nerve conduction in the peroneal nerve (less than 40 m/s) had fallen from 70% in 1968 to 28% in 1981. No information, however, is given about the incidence of clinical and subclinical neuropathy among *new* workers employed *after* establishment of improved hygienic conditions. This would have been of interest to evaluate whether these figures represent permanent sequelae reflecting the true capacity of regeneration. In any event, the study exemplifies the value of maybe even suboptimal hygienic precautions and is an illustration of the value of electrophysiologic methods for quantifiable screening and control purposes.

In 1983–85, a new outbreak of n-hexane polyneuropathy took place in printing factories in Taipei, Taiwan. Patients were followed for about 5 years with serial electrophysiologic, in particular evoked potential, studies. These showed evidence of central nervous system involvement with prolonged latency of visual and somatosensory evoked potentials, an increase of the central conduction time, and of the interpeak latency between the I and V peak in auditory brain stem evoked potentials. Fortunately, the n-hexane–induced neuropathy had a good prognosis. All patients, including one with tetraplegia, regained full motor control within 1 to 4 years, and the central nervous system affection was also functionally reversible.[193-195]

Organophosphorus Compounds

Among the organophosphorus compounds (OP esters), the best known is TOCP. It has become the most important single substance causing a toxic neuropathy in the 20th century, at least in terms of the number of afflicted persons. Several large-scale outbreaks are known, and two of them will retain their position in the medical history owing to their epidemic-like dimension. The largest occurred in the United States in 1929–30, following ingestion of adulterated ginger ale ("Ginger Jake"), and caused paralysis in about 20,000 persons. Of similar proportion was the outbreak in Morocco in 1959, where TOCP-contaminated cooking oil resulted in about 10,000 cases of severe motor neuropathy. Since then, there have only been reports of sporadic cases.[196–200] The neuropathy is characterized by a delayed onset of 1 to 3 weeks after ingestion, after the acute cholinergic symptoms, caused by the OP-ester inhibition of acetylcholinesterase, have subsided. Progressive muscle weakness, usually maximal 2 weeks after onset of neurologic symptoms, dominates the picture to the degree that ALS comes to mind unless the preceding history is known. In comparison, the accompanying sensory findings are inconspicuous. The final picture includes signs of both upper and lower motor neuron affection, and during the remission persistent central nervous system symptoms, in particular spasticity, become more apparent. The pathology of TOCP neuropathy has been studied in experimental animals and consists of symmetric nonselective distal axonal degeneration of both ascending and descending fibers.[201]

As with pathologic studies, modern neurophysiologic studies in typical cases of OP ester–induced neuropathy in humans are rare. In workers occupationally exposed to OP esters, Roberts[196] found a decrease in evoked muscle potential amplitudes, whereas Lotti et al.[199] did not observe any consistent changes. The only detailed electrophysiologic study was done in the patient reported by Hierons and Johnson[197] (cited by LeQuesne[172]). Only one motor unit could be detected in the hand, which had a normal conduction velocity of the forearm segment of its axon. Paradoxically despite absence of sensory loss in the upper extremities, sensory potentials in median and ulnar nerves had abnormally low amplitudes (2 μV), and no potential could be recorded in the sural nerve. As discussed in the section on pathophysiology, these findings are compatible with severe and nonselective diffuse axonal degeneration, sparing some of the largest fibers.[172]

Rare Industrial-Compound Neuropathies

The list of neurotoxic industrial compounds has grown steadily for several years. Most of them, however, are rare and have been discussed only in isolated case reports, which of course is not a measure of their prevalence. A few examples are given, selected mainly because of their electrophysiologic data.

Dimethylaminoproprionitrile[202,203] causes urologic symptoms with sexual dysfunction and sensory loss in sacral dermatomes. This may be accompanied by mild sensory loss in the feet and mild weakness of intrinsic hand and foot muscles. Urodynamic studies revealed a flaccid neurogenic bladder. Sacral nerve latencies were prolonged, and motor conduction velocities were mildly slowed, but compound sensory nerve action potentials had severely reduced amplitudes. A sural nerve biopsy showed a diminished number of fibers with signs of wallerian-like degeneration. Experimental studies in rats showed filamentous swelling in proximal, but not distal, segments of peripheral nerves.

Ethylene oxide has caused a subacute, predominantly motor neuropathy with bilateral footdrop in some of the nine reported cases.[204–206] Sural nerve biopsy showed axonal degeneration with mild changes of the myelin sheath. EMG showed abundant fibrillation potential activity in affected muscles. Motor and sensory responses had low amplitudes, but motor conduction velocity was normal when recordable. As a curiosity, ethylene oxide has been used for years to sterilize monopolar EMG needles, apparently without any adverse side effects.

Polychlorinated biphenyls caused a local outbreak of toxic neuropathy in Japan, affecting 21 workers.[207] It seems to be a predominantly sensory neuropathy, with slowed sensory nerve conduction in about half the patients, whereas motor conduction velocity was slowed only in one. There is no information about amplitudes of evoked responses and no pathologic studies in patients.

Trichlorethylene has been reported as being a neurotoxic substance.[108–212] It affects cranial nerves with symptoms and signs of trigeminal neuropathy, the electrophysiologic findings being an increased latency of the blink reflex and the masseter reflex, and of the trigeminal somatosensory evoked response. Neurogenic changes of the facial nerve and optic neuritis have also been reported. Cavanagh and Buxton,[213] however, suggest that the neuropathy associated with heavy exposure to trichlorethylene may be due to reactivation of latent orofacial herpes simplex virus caused by the chemical, which readily gains entrance into the nervous system.

CONCLUSION

This chapter has demonstrated that the simple sequence of events—intoxication, axonal degeneration, clinical neuropathy—with the well-known electrophysiologic pattern—fibrillation potential activity, reduced amplitude of evoked responses, normal or subnormal conduction velocity—can be varied in a multitude of ways. The variations encompass the time course of development of symptoms and the relative affection of motor and sensory fibers, of upper and lower extremity, of large and small diameter fibers, and of the peripheral and central nervous system. Of diagnostic importance are concomitant symptoms and signs from other organs and tissues, not discussed here. Add to this the history of exposure, and it is warranted to conclude that there are hardly two toxic neuropathies with an identical clinical picture. From this also follows that the ultimate diagnosis of a toxic neuropathy rests with the clinician. Albeit certain discriminative features can be documented, a final evaluation of neurophysiologic findings can be made only in context with the clinical picture and history.

Several of the examples of electromyographic findings presented here, however, were chosen to demonstrate that clinical neurophysiology has often provided information for the elucidation of diagnostic, prognostic, and first of all pathophysiologic problems that could not be achieved without such information. It has contributed in translating pathologic observations into clinically functional correlates. Providing sensitive and quantifiable methods, it has proved indispensible for the detection of mild or subclinical cases in screening studies. A limited battery of relatively simple electrophysiologic tests can be tailored for field studies, for dose regulation of neurotoxic drugs, and for an objective assessment of the development of a neuropathy and its remission. Thus clinical electrophysiology provides the methods of choice in longitudinal studies.

The literature on clinical electrophysiology in toxic neuropathy is mainly composed of case reports and incidental studies prompted by local outbreaks of environmental, usually industrial, episodes. It is definitely too optimistic to hope that the rare appearance of reports in the literature on toxic neuropathies induced by certain chemicals should reflect the true prevalence, especially in a global context. A major practical problem is the fact that clinical electrophysiology often has only limited opportunities to develop and test appropriate techniques and protocols for the study of individual toxic neuropathies. The discipline relies more heavily than usual on results from experimental research, which for natural reasons tends to be delayed by years from the actual event. When confronted with a new outbreak of a suspected neurotoxic neuropathy in the community, however, it seems logical, from experiences in the past, to tailor the study protocol on the preconception of a distal axonopathy, the electrophysiologic correlates of which are well described.

REFERENCES

1. Spencer PS, Schaumburg HH. An expanded classification of neurotoxic responses based on cellular targets of chemical agents. Acta Neurol Scand 1984; 70(suppl 100):9–19.
2. Spencer PS, Schaumburg HH. Experimental and clinical neurotoxicology. Baltimore: Williams & Wilkins, 1980.
3. Schaumburg HH, Spencer PS. Human toxic neuropathy due to industrial agents. In: Dyck PJ, Thomas PK, Lambert EH, Bunge R, eds. Peripheral neuropathy, ed 2. Philadelphia: WB Saunders, 1984: 2115–2132.
4. Windebank AJ, McCall JT, Dyck PJ. Metal neuropathy. In: Dyck PJ, Thomas PK, Lambert EH, Bunge R, eds. Peripheral neuropathy, ed 2. Philadelphia: WB Saunders, 1984:2133–2161.
5. LeQuesne PM. Neuropathy due to drugs. In: Dyck PJ, Thomas PK, Lambert EH, Bunge R, eds. Peripheral neuropathy, ed 2. Philadelphia: WB Saunders, 1984:2162–2179.
6. Sahenk Z. Toxic neuropathies. Semin Neurol 1987; 7:9–17.
7. Arezzo JC, Schaumburg HH. Screening for neurotoxic disease in humans. J Am Coll Toxicol 1989; 8:147–155.
8. Asbury AK, Brown MJ. Sensory neuronopathy and pure sensory neuropathy. Curr Opin Neurol Neurosurg 1990; 3:708–711.
9. Schaumburg HH. Toxic and metabolic neuropathies. Curr Opin Neurol Neurosurg 1991; 4:438–441.
10. Le Quintrec JS, Le Quintrec JL. Drug-induced myopathies. Baillieres Clin Rheumatol 1991; 5:21–38.
11. Spencer PS, Schaumburg HH. Pathobiology of neurotoxic axonal degeneration. In: Waxman SG, ed. Physiology and pathobiology of axons. New York: Raven Press, 1978:265–282.
12. Kaeser HE, Lambert EH. Nerve function studies in experimental polyneuritis. Electroencephalogr Clin Neurophysiol 1962; 22(suppl):29–35.
13. McDonald WI. The effects of experimental demyelination on conduction in peripheral nerve. A histological and electrophysiological study. II. Electrophysiological observations. Brain 1963; 86:501–524.
14. Fullerton PM, Barnes JM. Peripheral neuropathy in rats produced by acrylamide. Br J Ind Med 1966; 23:210–221.
15. Hopkins AP, Gilliatt RW. Motor and sensory nerve

conduction in the baboon. Normal values and changes during acrylamide neuropathy. J Neurol Neurosurg Psychiatry 1971; 34:415–426.

16. Sumner AJ. Early discharge of muscle afferents in acrylamide neuropathy. J Physiol (Lond) 1975; 246:277–288.

17. Sumner AJ, Asbury AK. Physiological studies of the dying-back phenomenon. Muscle strength afferents in acrylamide neuropathy. Brain 1975; 98:91–100.

18. Schaumburg HH, Wisniewski HM, Spencer PS. Ultrastructural studies of the dying-back process. I. Peripheral nerve terminal and axon degeneration in systemic acrylamide intoxication. J Neuropathol Exp Neurol 1974; 33:260–284.

19. Sumner AJ. Axonal polyneuropathies. In: Sumner AJ, ed. The physiology of peripheral nerve diseases. Philadelphia: WB Saunders, 1980:340–357.

20. Hern JEC. Tri-orthocresyl phosphate neuropathy in the baboon. In: Desmedt JE, ed. New developments in electromyography and clinical neurophysiology. Vol 2. Basel: Karger, 1973:181–187.

21. Schaumburg HH, Spencer PS. Toxic neuropathies. Neurology 1979; 29:429–431.

22. Spencer PS, Schaumburg HH. Ultrastructural studies of the dying-back process. IV. Differential vulnerability of PNS and CNS fibers in experimental central-peripheral distal axonopathies. J Neuropathol Exp Neurol 1977; 36:300–320.

23. Asbury AK, Gale MK, Cox SC, et al. Giant axonal neuropathy—a unique case with segmental neurofilamentous masses. Acta Neuropathol 1972; 20:237–247.

24. Korobkin R, Asbury K, Sumner AJ, Nielsen SL. Glue-sniffing neuropathy. Arch Neurol 1975; 32:158–162.

25. Seppäläinen AM, Haltia M. Carbon disulfide. In: Spencer PS, Schaumburg HH, eds. Experimental and clinical neurotoxicology. Baltimore: Williams & Wilkins, 1980:356–373.

26. Kurdi A, Abdul-Kader M. Clinical and electrophysiological studies of diphtheritic neuritis in Jordan. J Neurol Sci 1979; 42:243–250.

27. Said G. Perhexiline neuropathy. A clinicopathological study. Ann Neurol 1978; 3:259–267.

28. Fardeau M, Tome FMS, Simon P. Muscle and nerve changes induced by perhexiline malleate in man and mice. Muscle Nerve 1979; 2:24–36.

29. Rasminsky M. Physiology of conduction in demyelinated axons. In: Waxman SG, ed. Physiology and pathobiology of axons. New York: Raven Press, 1978:361–376.

30. Franzblau A, Lilis R. Acute arsenic intoxication from environmental arsenic exposure. Arch Environ Health 1989; 44:385–390.

31. U.S. Department of Health, Education, and Welfare, National Institute for Occupational Safety and Health. Criteria for a recommended standard. Occupational exposure to inorganic arsenic. New

criteria, 1975, (NIOSH) 75-149. Washington, DC: United States Government Printing Office, 1975.

32. Chhuttani PN, Chawla LS, Sharma TD. Arsenical neuropathy. Neurology 1967; 17:269–274.

33. Goldstein NP, MacCall JT, Dyck PJ. Metal neuropathies. In: Dyck PJ, Thomas PK, Lambert EH, eds. Peripheral neuropathy. Philadelphia: WB Saunders, 1975:1227–1262.

34. LeQuesne PM, McLeod JG. Peripheral neuropathy following a single exposure to arsenic. J Neurol Sci 1977; 32:437–451.

35. Feldman RG, Niles CA, Kelly-Hayes M, et al. Peripheral neuropathy in arsenic smelter workers. Neurology 1979; 29:939–944.

36. Wilbourn A, Rogers L, Salanga V. Acute arsenic intoxication producing a segmental demyelinating polyradiculoneuropathy. Electroencephalogr Clin Neurophysiol 1984; 57:85P.

37. Oh SJ. Abnormality in sensory nerve conduction. A distinct electrophysiological feature in arsenic polyneuropathy. Electroencephalogr Clin Neurophysiol 1980; 49:21P.

38. O'Shaughnessy E, Kraft GH. Arsenic poisoning. Long-term follow-up of a nonfatal case. Arch Phys Med Rehab 1976; 57:403–426.

39. Murphy MJ, Lyon LW, Taylor JW. Subacute arsenic neuropathy. Clinical and electrophysiological observations. J Neurol Neurosurg Psychiatry 1981; 44:896–900.

40. Endtz LJ. Complications nerveuses du traitement aurique. Rev Neurol 1958; 99:395–410.

41. Dyck PJ, Conn DL, Okazaki H. Necrotizing angiopathic neuropathy. Three dimensional morphology of fiber degeneration related to sites of occluded vessels. Mayo Clin Proc 1972; 47:461–475.

42. Gilg G, Vraa-Jensen G. Histological examination of the central nervous system after gold treatment. Acta Psychiatr Neurol Scand 1958; 33:174–180.

43. Chamberlain MA, Bruckner FE. Rheumatoid neuropathy. Clinical and electrophysiological features. Ann Rheum Dis 1970; 29:609–616.

44. Walsh JC. Gold neuropathy. Neurology 1970; 20:455–458.

45. Katrak SM, Pollock M, O'Brian CP, et al. Clinical and morphological features of gold neuropathy. Brain 1980; 103:671–693.

46. Meyer M, Haecki M, Ziegler W, et al. Autonomic dysfunction and myokymia in gold neuropathy. In: Canal N, Pozza G, eds. Peripheral neuropathies. Amsterdam: Elsevier, 1978:475–480.

47. Mitsumoto H, Wilbourn AJ, Subramony SH. Generalized myokymia and gold therapy. Arch Neurol 1982; 39:449–450.

48. Denny-Brown D, Foley JM. Myokymia and the benign fasciculations of muscular cramps. Trans Assoc Am Phys 1948; 61:88–96.

49. Gamstorp I, Wohlfart G. A syndrome characterized by myokymia, myotonia, muscular wasting and in-

creased perspiration. Acta Psychiat Neurol Scand 1959; 34:181–194.

50. Lampert PW, Schochet SS. Demyelination and re-myelination in lead neuropathy—electron micro-scopic studies. J Neuropath Exp Neurol 1968; 27:527–544.

51. Ohnishi A, Schilling K, Brimijoin WS, et al. Lead neuropathy. 1. Morphometry, nerve conduction, and choline acetyltransferase transport. New finding of endoneurial edema associated with segmental de-myelination. J Neuropathol Exp Neurol 1977; 36:499–518.

52. Pentschew A, Garro F. Lead-encephalo-myelopathy of the suckling rat and its implications on the por-phyrinopathic nervous diseases. Acta Neuropathol 1966; 6:266–278.

53. Fullerton PM. Chronic peripheral neuropathy pro-duced by lead poisoning in guinea-pigs. J Neuropa-thol Exp Neurol 1966; 25:214–236.

54. Hopkins A. Experimental lead poisoning in the ba-boon. Br J Ind Med 1970; 27:130–140.

55. Gombault PM. Contribution a l'etude anatomique de la nevrite parenchymateuse subaique et chronique—nevrite segmentaire peri-axile. Arch Neurol 1880; 1:11–38.

56. Buchthal F, Behse F. Electrophysiology and nerve biopsy in men exposed to lead. Br J Ind Med 1979; 36:135–147.

57. Seto DS, Freeman JM. Lead neuropathy in child-hood. Am J Dis Child 1964; 107:337–342.

58. Lane RE. Health control in inorganic lead industries. Arch Environ Health 1964; 8:243–250.

59. Nielsen CJ, Nielsen VK, Kirkby H, Gyntelberg F. Absence of peripheral neuropathy in long-term lead-exposed subjects. Acta Neurol Scand 1982; 65:241–247.

60. Boothby JA, deJesus PV, Rowland LP. Reversible forms of motor neurone disease. Lead "neuritis." Arch Neurol 1974; 31:18–23.

61. Oh SJ. Lead neuropathy. Case report. Arch Phys Med Rehab 1975; 56:312–317.

62. Catton MJ, Harrison MJG, Fullerton PM, Kazantzis G. Subclinical neuropathy in lead workers. Br Med J 1970; 2:80–82.

63. Seppäläinen AM, Hernberg S. Sensitive technique for detecting subclinical lead neuropathy. Br J Ind Med 1972; 29:443–449.

64. Araki S, Honma T. Relationship between lead ab-sorption and peripheral nerve conduction velocities in lead workers. Scand J Work Environ Health 1976; 4:225–231.

65. Melgaard B, Clausen J, Rastogi SC. Electromyo-graphic changes in automechanics with increased heavy metal levels. Acta Neurol Scand 1976; 54:227–240.

66. Triebig G, Weltle D, Valentin H. Investigations on neurotoxicity of chemical substances at the work-place. V. Determination of the motor and sensory nerve conduction velocity in persons occupationally exposed to lead. Int Arch Occup Environ Health 1984; 53:189–204.

67. He FS, Zhang SL, Li G, et al. An electroneurographic assessment of subclinical lead neurotoxicity. Int Arch Occup Environ Health 1988; 61:1–6.

68. Schwartz J, Landrigan PJ, Feldman RG, et al. Threshold effect in lead-induced peripheral neurop-athy. J Pediatr 1988; 112:12–17.

69. Murata K, Araki S, Aono H. Effects of lead zinc and copper absorption on peripheral nerve conduction in metal workers. Int Arch Occup Environ Health 1987; 59:11–20.

70. Aran F. Recherches sur une maladie non encore de-crite de systeme musculaire (atrophie musculaire progressive). Arch Gen Med 1850; 24:4–35.

71. Campbell AMG, Williams ER, Barltrop D. Motor neurone disease and exposure to lead. J Neurol Neu-rosurg Psychiatry 1970; 33:877–885.

72. Somjen GG, Herman SP, Klein R. Electrophysiology of methyl mercury poisoning. J Pharmacol Exp Ther 1973; 186:579–592.

73. Murai Y, Shiraishi S, Yamashita Y, et al. Neurophys-iological effects of methyl mercury on the nervous system. In Buser PA, Cobb WA, Okuma T, eds. Kyoto Symposia (EEG Suppl. no 36). Amsterdam: Elsevier Biomedical Press, 1982:682–687.

74. Bakir F, Damluji SF, Amin-Zaki L, et al. Methyl mercury poisoning in Iraq. Science 1973; 181:230–242.

75. LeQuesne PM, Damluji SF, Rustam H. Electrophysi-ological studies of peripheral nerves in patients with organic mercury poisoning. J Neurol Neurosurg Psy-chiatry 1974; 37:333–339.

76. Von Burg R, Rustam H. Electrophysiological inves-tigations of methylmercury intoxication in humans. Electroencephalogr Clin Neurophysiol 1974; 37:381–392.

77. Tukuomi H, Uchino M, Imamura M, et al. Mina-mata disease (organic mercury poisoning). Neuro-radiologic and electrophysiologic studies. Neurology 1982; 32:1369–1375.

78. Adams CR, Ziegler DK, Lin JT. Mercury intoxica-tion simulating amyotrophic lateral sclerosis. JAMA 1983; 250:642–643.

79. Vroom FQ, Greer M. Mercury vapour intoxication. Brain 1972; 95:305–318.

80. Iyer K, Goodgold J, Eberstein A, Berg P. Mercury poisoning in a dentist. Arch Neurol 1976; 33:788–790.

81. Singer R, Valciukas JA, Rosenman KD. Peripheral neurotoxicity in workers exposed to inorganic mer-cury compounds. Arch Environ Health 1987; 42:181–184.

82. Albers JW, Cavender GD, Levine SP, Langolf GD. Asymptomatic sensorimotor polyneuropathy in workers exposed to elemental mercury. Neurology 1982; 32:1168–1174.

83. Shapiro IM, Sumner AJ, Spitz LK, et al. Neurophys-iological and neuropsychological function in

mercury-exposed dentists. Lancet 1982; 1:1147–1150.

84. Talley RW, O'Bryan RM, Gutterman JU, et al. Clinical evaluation of toxic effects of cis-diamminedichloroplatinum (NSC-119875)—phase I, clinical study. Cancer Treat Rep 1973; 57:465–471.

85. Cowan JD, Kies MS, Roth JL, Joyce RP. Nerve conduction studies in patients treated with cis-diamminechloroplatinum. II. A preliminary report. Cancer Treat Rep 1980; 64:1119–1122.

86. Kedar A, Cohen M, Freeman A. Peripheral neuropathy as a complication of cis-dichlorodiammineplatinum (II) treatment. A case report. Cancer Treat Rep 1978; 62:819–821.

87. Hadley D, Herr H. Peripheral neuropathy associated with cis-dichloro-diammine-platinum (II) treatment. Cancer 1979; 44:2026–2028.

88. Reinstein L, Ostrow S, Wiernik P. Peripheral neuropathy after cis-platinum (II) (DDP) therapy. Arch Phys Med Rehab 1980; 61:280–281.

89. Daugaard GK, Petrera J, Trojaborg W. Electrophysiological study of the peripheral and central neurotoxic effect of cis-platin. Acta Neurol Scand 1987; 76:86–93.

90. Castellanos AM, Glass JP, Yung WKA. Regional nerve injury after intra-arterial chemotherapy. Neurology 1987; 37:834–837.

91. Cohen SC, Mollman JE. Cisplatin-induced gastric paresis. Neuro-oncol 1987; 5:237–240.

92. Smart-Harris R, Ponder BA, Wrigley PF. Tetany associated with cis-platin. Lancet 1980; 2:1303.

93. Ashraf M. Cis-platin-induced hypomagnesemia and peripheral neuropathy. Gynecol Oncol 1983; 16:309–318.

94. Hayes FA, Green AA, Senzer N, Pratt CD. Tetany. A complication of cis-dichlorodiammine-platinum (II) therapy. Cancer Treat Rep 1979; 63:547–548.

95. Roelofs RI, Hrushesky W, Rogin J. Peripheral sensory neuropathy and cis-platin chemotherapy. Neurology 1984; 34:934–938.

96. Von Hoff DD, Schilsky R, Reichert CM, et al. Toxic effects of cis-dichlorodiammine-platinum (II) in man. Cancer Treat Rep 1979; 63:1527–1531.

97. Bank WJ, Pleasure DE, Suzuki K, et al. Thallium poisoning. Arch Neurol 1972; 26:456–464.

98. Cavanagh JB, Fuller NH, Johnson HRM, Rudge P. The effects of thallium salts, with particular reference to nervous system changes. Q J Med 1974; 43:293–319.

99. Davis LE, Standefer JC, Kornfeld M, et al. Acute thallium poisoning. Toxicological and morphological studies of the nervous system. Ann Neurol 1981; 10:38–44.

100. Bank WJ. Thallium. In: Spencer PC, Schaumburg HH, eds. Experimental and clinical neurotoxicology. Baltimore: Williams & Wilkins, 1980:570–577.

101. Britten JS, Blank M. Thallium activation of the (Na$^+$- and K$^+$-) activated ATPase of rabbit kidney. Biochim Biophys Acta 1968; 159:160–166.

102. Cavieres JD, Ellory JC. Thallium and the sodium pump in human red cells. J Physiol 1974; 243:243–266.

103. Inturrisi CE. Thallium activation of K$^+$-activated phosphatases from beef brain. Biochim Biophys Acta 1969; 173:567–569.

104. Labauge R, Pages M, Tourniaire D, et al. Neuropathie peripherique recidivante par intoxication au thallium. Rev Neurol (Paris) 1991; 147:317–319.

105. Yokoyama K, Araki S, Abe H. Distribution of nerve conduction velocities in acute thallium poisoning. Muscle Nerve 1990; 13:117–120.

106. Dumitru D, Kalantri A. Electrophysiologic investigation of thallium poisoning. Muscle Nerve 1990; 13:433–437.

107. Joy RJT, Scalettar R, Sodee DB. Optic and peripheral neuritis. Probable effect of prolonged chloramphenicol therapy. JAMA 1960; 173:1731–1734.

108. Ramilo O, Kinane BT, McCracken GH Jr. Chloramphenicol neurotoxicity. Pediatr Infect Dis J 1988; 7:358–359.

109. Sebille A, Cordoliani G, Raffalli M-J, et al. Dapsone-induced neuropathy compounds Hansen's disease nerve damage: An electrophysiological study in tuberculoid patients. Int J Lepr Other Mycobact Dis 1987; 55:16–22.

110. Rapoport AM, Guss SB. Dapsone-induced peripheral neuropathy. Arch Neurol 1972; 27:184–185.

111. Gutmann L, Martin JD, Welton W. Dapsone motor neuropathy—an axonal disease. Neurology 1976; 26:514–516.

112. Helander I, Partanen J. Dapsone-induced distal axonal degeneration of the motor neurones. Dermatologica 1978; 156:321–324.

113. Koller WC, Gehlmann K, Malkinson FD, Davis FA. Dapsone-induced peripheral neuropathy. Arch Neurol 1977; 34:644–648.

114. Abhayambika K, Chacko A, Mahadevan K, Najeeb OM. Peripheral neuropathy and haemolytic anaemia with cherry red spot on macula in dapsone poisoning. J Assoc Phys Ind 1990; 38:564–565.

115. Navarro JC, Rosales RL, Ordinario AT, et al. Acute dapsone-induced peripheral neuropathy. Muscle Nerve 1989; 12:604–606.

116. Lovelace RD, Horwitz SJ. Peripheral neuropathy in long-term diphenylhydantoin therapy. Arch Neurol 1968; 18:69–77.

117. Eisen AA, Woods JF, Sherwin AL. Peripheral nerve function in long-term therapy with diphenylhydantoin. A clinical and electrophysiological correlation. Neurology 1974; 24:411–417.

118. Swift TR, Gross JA, Ward LC, Crout BO. Peripheral neuropathy in epileptic patients. Neurology 1981; 31:826–831.

119. Shorvon SD, Reynolds EH. Anticonvulsant peripheral neuropathy. A clinical and electrophysiological study of patients on single drug treatment with phenytoin, carbamazepine or barbiturates. J Neurol Neurosurg Psychiatry 1982; 45:620–626.

120. Hopf HC. Über die Veränderung der Leitfunktion peripherer motorischer Nervenfasern durch Diphenylhydantoin. Dtsch Z Nervenheilkd 1968; 193:41–56.

121. Birket-Smith E, Krogh E. Motor nerve conduction velocity during diphenylhydantoin intoxication. Acta Neurol Scand 1971; 47:265–271.

122. Morrell F, Bradley W, Ptashne M. Effect on diphenylhydantoin on peripheral nerve. Neurology 1958; 8:140–144.

123. LeQuesne PM, Goldberg V, Vajda F. Acute conduction velocity changes in guinea-pigs after administration of diphenylhydantoin. J Neurol Neurosurg Psychiatry 1976; 39:995–1000.

124. Markus D, Swift TR, McDonald T. Acute effects of phenytoin on peripheral nerve function in the rat. Muscle Nerve 1981; 4:48–50.

125. Gardner-Thorpe C, Benjamin S. Peripheral neuropathy after disulfiram administration. J Neurol Neurosurg Psychiatry 1971; 34:253–259.

126. Bradley WG, Hewer RL. Peripheral neuropathy due to disulfiram. Br Med J 1966; 2:449–450.

127. Moddel G, Bilboa JM, Ohnishi A, Dyck PJ. Disulfiram neuropathy. Arch Neurol 1978; 35:658–660.

128. Bergouignan FX, Vital C, Henry P, Eschapasse P. Disulfiram neuropathy. J Neurol 1988; 235:382–383.

129. Mokri B, Ohnishi A, Dyck PJ. Disulfiram neuropathy. Neurology 1981; 31:730–735.

130. Ansbacher LE, Bosch EP, Cancilla PA. Disulfiram neuropathy. A neurofilamentous distal axonopathy. Neurology 1982; 32:424–428.

131. Olney RK, Miller RG. Peripheral neuropathy associated with disulfiram administration. Muscle Nerve 1980; 3:172–175.

132. Palliyath SK, Schwartz BD, Gant L. Peripheral nerve function in chronic alcoholic patients on disulfiram: A six month follow up. J Neurol Neurosurg Psychiatry 1990; 53:227–230.

133. Wright C, Moore RD. Disulfiram treatment of alcoholism. Am J Med 1990; 88:647–655.

134. Blakemore WF. Isoniazid. In: Spencer PS, Schaumburg HH, eds. Experimental and clinical neurotoxicology. Baltimore: Williams & Wilkins, 1980:476–489.

135. Mamoli B, Wessely P, Kogelnik HD, et al. Electroneurographic investigation of misonidazole polyneuropathy. Eur Neurol 1979; 18:405–414.

136. Melgaard B, Hansen HS, Kamieniecka Z, et al. Misonidazole neuropathy. A clinical, electrophysiological and histological study. Ann Neurol 1982; 12:10–17.

137. Melgaard B, Kohler O, Sand-Hansen H, et al. Misonidazole neuropathy. A prospective study. J Neuro-oncol 1988; 6:227–230.

138. Griffin JW, Price DL, Kuerthe DO, Goldberg AM. Neurotoxicity of misonidazole in rats. I. Neuropathology. Neurotoxicology 1979; 1:299.

139. Olivarius B de F. Polyneuropathy due to nitrofurantoin therapy. Ugeskr Læger 1956; 118:753–755.

140. Lindholm T. Electromyographic changes after nitrofurantoin (furadantin) therapy in non-uremic patients. Neurology 1967; 17:1017–1020.

141. Toole JF, Gergen JA, Hayes DM, Felts JH. Neural effects of nitrofurantoin. Arch Neurol 1968; 18:680–687.

142. Nielsen VK, Winkel P. The peripheral nerve function in chronic renal failure. III. A multivariate statistical analysis of factors presumed to affect the development of clinical neuropathy. Acta Med Scand 1971; 190:119–125.

143. Honet JC. Electrodiagnostic study of a patient with peripheral neuropathy after nitrofurantoin therapy. Arch Phys Med Rehab 1967; 48:209–212.

144. Sebille A. Prevalence of latent perhexiline neuropathy. Br Med J 1978; 1:1321–1322.

145. Bousser MG, Bouche P, Brochard C, Herreman G. Neuropathies peripheriques au maleate de perhexiline. A propos de 7 observations. Coeur Med Interne 1976; 15:181.

146. Lhermitte F, Fardeau M, Credru F, Mallecourt J. Polyneuropathy after perhexiline maleate therapy. Br Med J 1976; 1:1256.

147. Bouche P, Bousser MG, Peytour MA, Cathala HP. Perhexiline malleate and peripheral neuropathy. Neurology 1979; 29:739–743.

148. Schaumburg HH, Kaplan J, Windebank A, et al. Sensory neuropathy from pyridoxine abuse. A new megavitamin syndrome. N Engl J Med 1983; 309:445–448.

149. Leklem JE, Reynolds RD, eds. Current topics in nutrition and disease. Vol 19. Clinical and physiological applications of vitamin B-6; third international conference on vitamin B-6, Gosler-Hahnenklee, West Germany, 1987. New York: Alan Liss, Inc., 1987.

150. Dalton K, Dalton MJ. Characteristics of pyridoxine overdose neuropathy syndrome. Acta Neurol Scand 1987; 76:8–11.

151. Albin RL, Albers JW. Acute sensory neuropathy-neuronopathy from pyridoxine overdose. Neurology 1987; 37:1729–1732.

152. Albin RL, Albers JW. Long-term follow-up of pyridoxine-induced acute sensory neuropathy-neuronopathy. Neurology 1990; 40:1319.

153. Montpetit VJ, Clapin DF, Tryphonas L, Dancea S. Alteration of neuronal cytoskeletal organization in dorsal root ganglia associated with pyridoxine neurotoxicity. Acta Neuropathol (Berl) 1988; 76:71–81.

154. Bowe CM, Veale K. Sensitivity to 4-aminopyridine observed in mammalian sciatic nerves during acute pyridoxine-induced sensory neuropathy and recovery. Exp Neurol 1988; 100:448–458.

155. Fullerton PM, Kremer M. Neuropathy after intake of thalidomide (Distaval). Br Med J 1961; 2:855–858.

156. Fullerton PM, O'Sullivan DJ. Thalidomide neuropathy. A clinical, electrophysiological and histological follow-up study. J Neurol Neurosurg Psychiatry 1968; 31:543–551.

157. Powell RJ, Jenkins JS, Smith NJ, Allen BR. Peripheral neuropathy in thalidomide treated patients. Br J Rheumatol 1987; 26 (suppl 2):12.

158. Bradley WG, Lasman LP, Pearce GW, Walton JN. The neuromyopathy of vincristine in man—clinical, electrophysiological and pathological studies. J Neurol Sci 1970; 10:107–131.

159. Casey EB, Jellife AM, LeQuesne PM, Millett YL. Vincristine neuropathy—clinical and electrophysiological observations. Brain 1973; 96:69–86.

160. Guiheneuc P, Ginet J, Grouleau JY, Rojuan J. Early phase of vincristine neuropathy in man. J Neurol Sci 1980; 45:355–366.

161. McLeod JG, Penny R. Vincristine neuropathy. An electrophysiological and histological study. J Neurol Neurosurg Psychiatry 1969; 32:297–304.

162. Hildebrand J, Coërs C. Etude clinique, histologique et electrophysiologique des neuropathies associees au traitement par la vincristine. Eur J Cancer 1965; 1:51–58.

163. Geny C, Gaio JM, Mallaret M, et al. Charcot-Marie-Tooth disease revealed by vincristine treatment of familial Hodgkin's disease. Ann Med Int 1990; 141:709–710.

164. McGuire SA, Gospe SM Jr, Dahl G. Acute vincristine neurotoxicity in the presence of hereditary motor and sensory neuropathy type I. Med Pediatr Oncol 1989; 17:520–523.

165. Casey EB, LeQuesne PM. Digital nerve action potentials in healthy subjects, and in carpal tunnel and diabetic patients. J Neurol Neurosurg Psychiatry 1972; 35:612–623.

166. Auld RB, Bedwell SF. Peripheral neuropathy with sympathetic overactivity from industrial contact with acrylamide. Can Med Assoc 1967; 96:652–654.

167. Garland TO, Patterson MWH. Six cases of acrylamide poisoning. Br Med J 1967; 4:134–138.

168. LeQuesne PM. Acrylamide. In: Spencer PS, Schaumburg HH, eds. Experimental and clinical neurotoxicology. Baltimore: Williams & Wilkins, 1980:309–325.

169. Fullerton PM. Electrophysiological and histological observations on peripheral nerves in acrylamide poisoning in man. J Neurol Neurosurg Psychiatry 1969; 32:186–192.

170. Takahashi M, Ohara T, Hashimoto K. Electrophysiological study of nerve injuries in workers handling acrylamide. Int Arch Arbeitmed 1971; 28:1–11.

171. Nagymajtenyi L, Desi I, Lorencz R. Neurophysiological markers as early signs of organophosphate neurotoxicity. Neurotoxicol Teratol 1988; 10:429–434.

172. LeQuesne PM. Neurophysiological investigation of subclinical and minimal toxic neuropathies. Muscle Nerve 1978; 1:392–395.

173. Arezzo J, Schaumburg HH, Vaughan HC, et al. Short latency somatosensory evoked potentials to peroneal stimulation in the monkey. Specific changes in distal axonopathy. Ann Neurol 1982; 12:24–32.

174. Myers JE, Macun I. Acrylamide neuropathy in a South African factory: An epidemiologic investigation. Ann J Ind Med 1991; 19:487–493.

175. Aaserud O, Hommeren OJ, Tvedt B, et al. Carbon disulfide exposure and neurotoxic sequelae. Am J Ind Med 1990; 8:25–38.

176. Seppäläinen AM, Haltia M. Carbon disulfide. In: Spencer PS, Schaumburg HH, eds. Experimental and clinical neurotoxicology. Baltimore: Williams & Wilkins, 1980:356–373.

177. Jirmanova I. Pacinian corpuscles in rats with carbon disulfide neuropathy. Acta Neuropathol (Berl) 1987; 72:341–348.

178. Seppäläinen AM, Tolonen M. Neurotoxicity of long term exposure to carbon disulfide in the viscose rayon industry. A neurophysiological study. Work Environ Health 1974; 11:145–153.

179. Gilioli R, Bulgheroni C, Bertazzi PA, et al. Study of neurological and neurophysiological impairment in carbon disulfide workers. Med Lav 1978; 69:130–143.

180. Knave B, Kolmodin-Hedman B, Persson HE, Goldberg JM. Chronic exposure to carbon disulfide. Effects on occupationally exposed workers with special reference to the nervous system. Work Environ Health 1974; 11:49–58.

181. Vasilescu C. Sensory and motor conduction in chronic carbon disulfide poisoning. Eur Neurol 1976; 14:447–457.

182. Iida M, Yamamura Y, Sobue I. Electromyographic findings and conduction velocity in n-Hexane polyneuropathy. Electromyography 1969; 9:247–261.

183. Buiatti E, Cesshini S, Ronchi O, et al. Relationship between clinical and electromyographic findings and exposure to solvents, in shoe and leather workers. Br J Ind Med 1978; 35:168–173.

184. Cianchetti C, Abbritti G, Perticoni G, et al. Toxic polyneuropathy of shoe-industry workers. A study of 122 cases. J Neurol Neurosurg Psychiatry 1976; 39:1151–1161.

185. Caruso G, Santoro L, Perretti A, et al. Electrophysiological findings in the polyneuropathy of leather cementing workers. In: Persson A, ed. Symposia, Sixth International Congress of Electromyography, Stockholm, 1979:219–223.

186. Allen N, Mendell JR, Billmaier DJ, et al. Toxic polyneuropathy due to methyl n-butyl ketone. An industrial out-break. Arch Neurol 1975; 32:209–218.

187. Allen N. Identification of methyl n-butyl ketone as the causative agent. In: Spencer PS, Schaumburg HH, eds. Experimental and clinical neurotoxicity. Baltimore: Williams & Wilkins, 1980:834–845.

188. Herskowitz A, Ishii N, Schaumburg H. n-Hexane neuropathy. A syndrome occurring as a result of industrial exposure. N Engl J Med 1971; 285:82–85.

189. Shirabe T, Tsuda T, Terao A, Araki S. Toxic polyneuropathy due to glue-sniffing. Report of two cases with a light and electron microscope study of the peripheral nerves and muscles. J Neurol Sci 1974; 21:101–113.

190. Altenkirch H, Mager J, Stoltenberg G, Helmbrecht J. Toxic polyneuropathies after sniffing a glue thinner. J Neurol 1977; 214:137–152.

191. Seppäläinen AM, Raitta C, Huuskonen MS. n-Hexane-induced changes in visual evoked potentials and electroretinograms of industrial workers. Electroencephalogr Clin Neurophysiol 1979; 47:492–498.

192. Iida M. Neurophysiological studies of n-Hexane polyneuropathy in the sandal factory. In: Buser PA, Cobb WA, Okuma T, eds. Kyoto Symposia (EEG Suppl No 36). Amsterdam: Elsevier Medical Press, 1982:671–681.

193. Chang YC. Neurotoxic effects of n-hexane on the human central nervous system: Evoked potential abnormalities in n-hexane polyneuropathy. J Neurol Neurosurg Psychiatry 1987; 50:269–274.

194. Chang YC. An electrophysiological follow-up of patients with n-hexane polyneuropathy. Br J Ind Med 1991; 48:12–17.

195. Chang YC. Patients with n-hexane induced polyneuropathy: A clinical follow-up. Br J Ind Med 1990; 47:485–489.

196. Roberts DV. A longitudinal electromyographic study of six men occupationally exposed to organophosphorous compounds. Int Arch Occup Environ Health 1977; 38:221–229.

197. Hierons R, Johnson M. Clinical and toxicological investigations of a case of delayed neuropathy in man after acute poisoning by an organophosphorous pesticide. Arch Toxicol (Berl) 1978; 40:279–284.

198. Senanayaka N, Johnson MK. Acute polyneuropathy after poisoning by a new organophosphate insecticide. N Engl J Med 1982; 306:155–157.

199. Lotti M, Becker CE, Aminoff MJ, et al. Occupational exposure to the cotton defoliants DEF and merphos. A rational approach to monitoring organophosphorous-induced delayed neurotoxicity. J Occup Med 1983; 25:517–522.

200. Wadia RS, Chitra S, Amin RB, et al. Electrophysiological studies in acute organophosphate poisoning. J Neurol Neurosurg Psychiatry 1987; 50:1442–1448.

201. Davis CS, Richardson RJ. Organophosphorus compounds. In: Spencer PS, Schaumburg HH, eds. Experimental and clinical neurotoxicology. Baltimore: Williams & Wilkins, 1980:527–544.

202. Pestonk A, Keogh JP, Griffin JW. Dimethylaminopropionitrile. In: Spencer PC, Schaumburg HH, eds. Experimental and clinical neurotoxicology. Baltimore: Williams & Wilkins, 1980:422–429.

203. Kreis K, Wegman D, Niles CA, et al. Neurological dysfunction of the bladder in workers exposed to dimethylaminopropionitrile. JAMA 1980; 243:741–745.

204. Gross JA, Haas ML, Swift TR. Ethylene oxide neurotoxicity. Report of four cases and review of the literature. Neurology 1979; 29:978–983.

205. Finelli PF, Morgan TF, Yaar I, Granger CV. Ethylene oxide-induced polyneuropathy. A clinical and electrophysiological study. Arch Neurol 1983; 40:419–421.

206. Kuzuhara S, Kanazawa I, Nakanishi T, Egashira T. Ethylene oxide polyneuropathy. Neurology 1983; 33:377–380.

207. Murai Y, Kuroiwa Y. Peripheral neuropathy in chlorobiphenyl poisoning. Neurology 1971; 21:1173–1176.

208. Buxton PH, Hayward M. Polyneuritis cranialis associated with industrial trichlorethylene poisoning. J Neurol Neurosurg Psychiatry 1967; 30:511–518.

209. Feldman RG, Mayer RM, Taub A. Evidence of peripheral neurotoxic effect of trichlorethylene. Neurology 1970; 20:599–606.

210. Dogui M, Mrizak N, Yacoubi M, et al. Potentiels evoques somesthesique du trijumeau chez des travailleurs manipulant le trichlorethylene. Neurophysiol Clin 1991; 21:95–103.

211. Feldman RG, Chirico-Post J, Proctor SP. Blink reflex latency after exposure to trichlorethylene in well water. Arch Environ Health 1988; 43:143–148.

212. Ruijten MW, Verberg MM, Salle HJ. Nerve function in workers with long term exposure to trichloroethene. Br J Ind Med 1991; 48:87–92.

213. Cavanagh JB, Buxton PH. Trichloroethylene cranial neuropathy: Is it really a toxic neuropathy or does it activate latent herpes virus? J Neurol Neurosurg Psychiatry 1989; 52:297–303.

III

Disorders of Neuromuscular Transmission and Muscles

23

Electrical Testing in Disorders of Neuromuscular Transmission

Michael H. Rivner
Thomas R. Swift

CONTENTS

LIST OF ACRONYMS

ACh	acetylcholine
AChE	acetylcholinesterase
AMP	adenosine monophosphate
AP	action potential
ATP	adenosine triphosphate
cAMP	cyclic adenosine monophosphate
CMAP	compound muscle action potential
EDC	extensor digitorum communis
EOM	extraocular eye movements
EPP	end plate potential
FIM	familial infantile myasthenia
Hz	hertz
IPI	interpotential interval
IV	intravenous
LEMS	Lambert-Eaton myasthenic syndrome
MAP	muscle action potential
MCD	mean consecutive difference
μs	microseconds
ms	milliseconds
mV	millivolts
MEPP	miniature end plate potentials
MG	myasthenia gravis
MP	muscle membrane potential
NMJ	neuromuscular junction
NMT	neuromuscular transmission
SRI	stimulus to response interval

The neuromuscular junction (NMJ) is the interface between the nerve and muscle. At this location, a nerve impulse leads to the release of quanta of acetylcholine (ACh) that traverse the NMJ producing an end plate potential and resultant action potential in the muscle.[1–3] Although in most people the safety margin of neuromuscular transmission (NMT) is high and an action potential in the nerve always leads to a contraction of the muscle fiber, certain diseases, drugs, and toxins can interfere with NMT. The autoimmune disorders myasthenia gravis (MG) and Lambert-Eaton myasthenic syndrome (LEMS) are the most common causes of NMT failure, owing to autoimmune reactions either at the postjunctional receptor (MG) or at prejunctional active zones (LEMS) where ACh is released. Various drugs, most notably aminoglycoside antibiotics, calcium channel blockers, and agents containing divalent cations such as magnesium sulfate, interfere with NMT. Snake and insect venoms act at the NMJ both prejunctionally and postjunctionally. Botulinum toxin interferes with the release of ACh, and organophosphates interfere with the elimination of ACh at the NMJ. Finally, there are rare congenital defects of NMT. In this chapter, we discuss these disorders and methods used to study them in the clinical neurophysiology laboratory. To begin, it is necessary to outline the mechanisms of NMT and then the electrophysiologic techniques used clinically.

NEUROMUSCULAR TRANSMISSION

The axon terminal is the site of ACh release (Figure 23.1). ACh (the transmitter at the NMJ) is synthesized in the axon terminal and packaged in vesicles. A quantum is the amount of ACh packaged in a single vesicle, which contains approximately 10^4 molecules of ACh.[4] There are three mechanisms for the release of ACh[5]. The first is spontaneous quantal release of ACh that occurs continuously independently of the activity of the nerve. Quanta of ACh undergo exocytosis at active specialized release sites called *active zones*. A second, minor type of release is nonquantal leakage of ACh that occurs across the prejunctional axon terminal membrane at sites other than the active zones. The third type of ACh release occurs at the active zones of the terminal in response to compound nerve action potentials. In a process requiring energy, voltage-sensitive calcium channels are opened, producing an influx of calcium. During this process, adenyl cyclase catalyzes the conversion of adenosine triphosphate (ATP) to cyclic adenosine monophosphate (cAMP).[6,7] cAMP is the link between voltage changes and the opening of the calcium channels.[6–8] The amplitude and duration of the depolarization produced by the compound nerve action potential depend on both sodium (Na^+) and potassium (K^+) channels. If Na^+ channels are blocked, release of ACh is reduced.[9] K^+ channels act to repolarize the axon at the end of an action potential.[10–14] Inhibiting the K^+ channels prolongs the duration of the action potential, enhancing transmitter release.[15] Calcium binds with and activates calmodulin, an intracellular protein. Activated calmodulin binds with an intracellular receptor protein, which causes the release of transmitter.[16] These events result in the release of many quanta of transmitter. The number of quanta released depends on several factors, among them (1) the amplitude and duration of depolarization; (2) the number of vesicles available for release; and (3) a probability factor, which depends on the concentration of calcium at the release site.[1] Vesicles at the axon terminal may be classified as those immediately available for release and those that are not.[17,18] Approximately 1000 to 2000 vesicles make up this immediately releasable store. Additional vesicles in the nerve terminal are not positioned to be released immediately. As the releasable vesicles are used up, this reserve is used to replenish the supply of immediate available vesicles. It is believed that ACh receptors located on the axon terminal are responsible for this process.[19–23]

After release, ACh diffuses across the NMJ, where it either is inactivated by acetylcholinesterase (AChE) or attaches to the ACh receptor[24] (Figure 23.1). If it binds with AChE, it is broken down into acetic acid, which is metabolized, and choline, most of which is taken up by the axon terminal and used to make more ACh through the action of the enzyme choline acetyl transferase.[17,25] If two molecules of ACh bind with the ACh receptor located at the end plate, ion channels open, and the end plate is depolarized.[26,27] This depolarization is dependent on the amount of time ACh is bound to the receptor, channel kinetics, and membrane factors. If the channels remain open excessively long, repetitive discharges occur at the end plate.[28] If the end plate potential is large enough, the membrane is depolarized above threshold, and an action potential is generated in the muscle. The compound muscle action potential propagates along the muscle membrane and invades and depolarizes the T tubule system of the muscle, which results in release of calcium from adjacent sarcoplasmic reticulum stores, and muscles contraction occurs.

Much of what we know about NMT has been

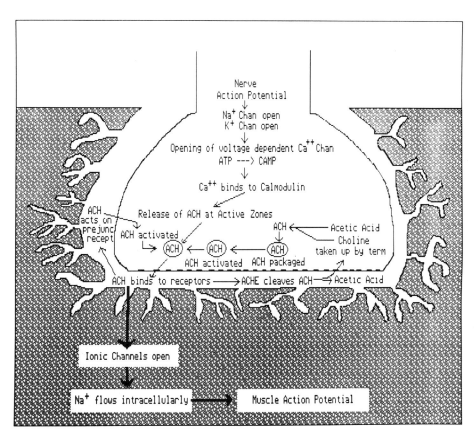

FIGURE 23.1.   *The neuromuscular junction. The steps linking the mononeuron action potential to the compound muscle action potential are outlined. The nerve action potential is produced by the opening of both the sodium (Na^+) and potassium (K^+) channels in the axon. The Na^+ channels produce membrane depolarization, whereas the K^+ channels produce hyperpolarization. The influx of K^+ limits the duration of the axon action potential. Depolarization activates the voltage-sensitive calcium (Ca^{++}) channels, causing an influx of calcium. This step involves the conversion of adenosine triphosphate (ATP) to cyclic adenosine monophosphate (cAMP) using energy. The intracellular calcium binds to calmodulin, which leads to the release of acetylcholine (ACh) at the terminal's active zones. ACh diffuses across the neuromuscular junction either binding to a receptor on the muscle or nerve terminal or binding to acetyl cholinesterase (AChE). If ACh binds to the muscle membrane receptor, postjunctional membrane channels open, allowing sodium and other ions to enter the muscle. If above threshold, a compound muscle action potential is produced, which ultimately leads to the contraction of the muscle. ACh binding to nerve terminal receptors is responsible for the conversion of reserve stores of ACh to readily releasible stores of ACh (activation). If bound to AChE, ACh is dissociated to acetic acid, which diffuses out of the neuromuscular junction, and choline. Choline is taken up by the terminal and used to make more ACh, which is packed into vesicles. As ACh is used, reserve stores of ACh are made available to enter the readily available pool (activation).*

learned by microelectrode recording of end plate potentials intracellularly from frog muscle, rat phrenic nerve–diaphragm preparations, or human intercostal muscles[18,29,30] (Table 23.1). To measure the end plate potential accurately, it is necessary to record from an undamaged muscle cell. The normal muscle membrane potential (MP) is about -90 mV (inside of the cell negative with respect to the outside). The

TABLE 23.1. Prejunctional and postjunctional disorders*

Laboratory Findings	Clinical Electromyography
Prejunctional Disorders	
Decreased quantal content	Low-amplitude CMAP at rest
Normal MEPP size	Increment after exercise
Reduced MEPP frequency	Increment with high-frequency stimulation
	Jitter improved with high-frequency stimulation
Postjunctional Disorders	
Normal quantal content	Normal CMAP
Decreased MEPP size	Decrement to low-frequency stimulation
Normal MEPP frequency	Decrement corrected after exercise
	Jitter improved with low-frequency stimulation

* Most diseases of this type follow this pattern, but there are exceptions.
MEPP, Miniature end plate potentials; CMAP, compound muscle action potential.

MP experiences small (about 1 mV) fluctuations when the muscle is at rest.[31,32] These fluctuations in potential are called *miniature end plate potentials* (MEPP). A MEPP is the voltage change resulting from the spontaneous release of a single synaptic vesicle with one quantum of ACh. The frequency of MEPPs is reduced in certain prejunctional NMT disorders. The magnitude of the MEPP amplitude is reduced in postjunctional NMT disorders but is normal in most prejunctional disorders.[33] When the nerve is stimulated, a large voltage change, the end plate potential, occurs at the NMJ. The end plate potential size is, in principle, a multiple of the MEPP size. The number of quanta that make up the end plate potential is known as the quantal content, identical to the number of quanta released by the compound nerve action potential. Quantal content is diminished in prejunctional NMT disorders such as LEMS but is normal in postjunctional disorders such as MG.

As already mentioned, when a compound nerve action potential reaches the axonal terminal, a certain number of vesicles are released into the NMJ. This number is dependent on the quantity of vesicles immediately available for release, degree and duration of terminal depolarization, and local concentration of calcium. It is believed that transmitter is released at specialized sites known as active zones containing the voltage-sensitive calcium (Ca^{++}) channels and ACh release sites.[5] If the nerve is stimulated at a rate slow enough so releasable vesicles may be replenished, the number of vesicles released with each nerve impulse remains constant. If the

nerve is stimulated at a higher rate, the number of ACh vesicles available for release progressively declines; therefore the number of vesicles released per stimulus also decreases. If a train of stimuli are given to the nerve, after a lag of about a second, the terminal starts replenishing the number of vesicles available for release and the number of vesicles released per impulse levels off. If the nerve is continually stimulated, more vesicles are made available for immediate release, and the level of intracellular calcium increases. This leads to an increased quantal content released with each stimulus. If the subject were to exercise for a period of 10 to 15 seconds, immediately after this period the quantal content released with each stimulus would increase. After a period of rest of about 60 seconds, quantal content released with each stimulus would decline. This decline lasts for several minutes. This initial increase in quantal content is known as postactivation facilitation, whereas the subsequent decrease is known as postactivation exhaustion. Activation of ACh receptors at the axonal terminal is believed to be linked to the mobilization of transmitter at the axon terminal. The cause for postexercise exhaustion is unknown.

PHYSIOLOGIC TECHNIQUES FOR EVALUATION OF NEUROMUSCULAR TRANSMISSION

There are several methods available to evaluate NMJ function. Each has its advantages and disadvantages. Not infrequently, a battery of these tests must be employed to determine whether or not an abnormality exists and, if so, the nature of the abnormality.

Pharmacologic Testing

Perhaps the easiest diagnostic test to perform for NMT disorders is the edrophonium (Tensilon) test. Edrophonium is a rapid-acting cholinesterase inhibitor.[34] Edrophonium binds to the anionic site of the enzyme AChE, making it unable to hydrolyze and thereby deactivate ACh.[2,35] Because the combination of edrophonium with AChE is relatively unstable, its effects last only about 5 minutes. Also, because edrophonium is active at both muscarinic (in the autonomic nervous system) and nicotinic synapses (NMJ and ganglion), patients develop muscarinic side effects from this test.[36] These symptoms can be disturbing and include bradycardia, bronchorrhea, salivation, nausea, sweating, diarrhea, and abdominal cramps. To prevent these symptoms, patients may be pretreated with atropine, which selectively blocks muscarinic receptors. We generally give 0.4 mg of atropine intravenously slowly 5 minutes before or intramuscular 30 minutes before administering edrophonium. To perform a valid test, the patient needs to have demonstable weakness. This weakness may be seen either clinically or electrophysiologically. The patient is given a test dose of 2 mg edrophonium intravenously. During this dose, the heart rate should be monitored for bradycardia. In addition, the patient should be observed for clinical improvement. If clear-cut improvement is seen, the test is said to be *positive* and may be terminated at this point. If no significant muscarinic effects are seen and the test is not conclusive, the remaining 8 mg edrophonium should then be injected intravenously. Clinical improvement should be seen in about 30 seconds and should last from 3 to 5 minutes. A more prolonged response, however, is sometimes seen.[37] In doubtful cases, or on suggestible patients, the test may be done in a double blind fashion in which neither the patient nor examiner knows whether edrophonium or normal saline is administered. The double blind test has limited value because most patients develop fasciculation and tearing during edrophonium administration, which are signs that the active agent has been used. Unfortunately, false-positive and false-negative test results occur, limiting the value of this test. This is particularly true when weakness is minimal.[38,39]

A second pharmacologic test that is rarely used is the regional curare test.[40] Curare is a nondepolarizing nicotinic receptor blocker. In patients with NMT disorders, a small dose of curare, which usually does not produce effects, produces profound weakness. Because curare can cause respiratory embarrassment if diaphragmatic and intercostal muscles are affected, one must be prepared to ventilate these patients. To limit the effects of the curare, a blood pressure cuff is inflated above systolic pressure in the arm to be tested. This limits the effects of curare to the injected limb. A dose of 0.2 mg of curare is given intravenously, and the arm is checked for weakness. Normally this dose is not sufficient to produce weakness, but in patients with NMT disorders weakness may develop. Often the injection of curare is used in conjunction with electophysiologic testing. We do not perform this test because other safer and just as effective tests are available.

Ice Pack Test

The ice pack test has been designed to take advantage of the finding that NMT improves with cooling and worsens with increased temperature because of inhibition of AChE and other factors.[41] In patients with ptosis, a glove filled with ice is applied to one eye for 2 minutes. In positive tests, the ptosis is temporarily improved. The advantage of this test is that it is safe and easy to perform.

Repetitive Stimulation

Repetitive nerve stimulation recording compound muscle action potentials has been widely used to test for NMT disorders for about 40 years and was based on observations by Jolly in 1855 that muscle contractions in MG become progressively reduced during a train of stimuli. Any muscle may be studied electrophysiologically, but proximal muscles are more likely to be abnormal than distal muscles in MG.[42] The most common locations studied are (1) stimulating the ulnar nerve at the wrist and recording responses at the hypothenar muscles, (2) stimulating the median nerve at the wrist and recording over the thenar muscles, (3) stimulating the accessory nerve in the posterior triangle of the neck and recording over the trapezius muscle,[43] and (4) stimulating the facial nerve at the angle of the jaw and recording over the orbicularis oculi. Other less-studied nerves are the musculocutaneous and axillary nerves. They are harder to stimulate and generally do not give more information than the ones already mentioned.

The nerve is first stimulated in the standard manner to find the stimulus necessary to produce a compound muscle action potential of maximum size. It is important to provide supramaximal stimulation because the interpretation of the test depends on the fact that the nerve is maximally stimulated so any change in the amplitude of the muscle response is due to failure of NMT and not due to failure to stimulate the nerve fully. Once a maximal response is obtained, either the voltage or current stimulus (depending on whether a constant current or voltage stimulator is being used), is increased to a value 150% of that necessary to produce a maximal response (supramaximal stimulus). This ensures that even if the stimulating electrode is moved slightly, the nerve will still be fully stimulated.

Trains of four to 10 stimuli are given at a rate of 2 to 5 c/s (Figure 23.2). Either the amplitude or the area of the first response is compared with that of the fourth. In normal subjects at these stimulation frequencies, the amplitude of the first response is the same as the fourth. In postjunctional NMT disorders such as MG (Figure 23-2), the amplitude of the fourth response is lower than that of the first. Surface recordings are produced by the summed electrical activity of all the muscle fibers contained in the muscle. When there is failure of NMT, certain muscle fibers do not produce action potentials. If this occurs in enough muscle fibers, the amplitude of the compound muscle action potential is reduced. The percent decrement can be calculated using the following formula:

$$\%Dec = \frac{Amp_{1st\ resp} - Amp_{4th\ resp}}{Amp_{1st\ resp}} \times 100$$

Where $\%Dec$ is the percent decrement, and Amp is the amplitude of either the first or fourth response.

A decrement of greater than 10% is significant. In prejunctional NMT disorders (Table 23.1), the amplitude of the first response is reduced, and a decrement is seen at low stimulation frequencies. In this case, progressive NMT failure is occurring in many muscle fibers. Normally the safety factor, which is the difference between the end plate potential amplitude and the minimum depolarization necessary for a compound muscle action potential, is about four, meaning that roughly four times more transmitter is released at the NMJ than is needed to develop an action potential.[44] In patients with disorders of NMT, this value becomes lower, often approaching one. As explained earlier, with repetitive stimulation, fewer vesicles of ACh are released with the subsequent stimuli compared with the first. In a normal subject, this reduction would not cause a failure of NMT. If the safety factor were close to one, however, this slight difference in the number of ACh vesicles may mean the difference between success and failure of NMT. To see significant decre-

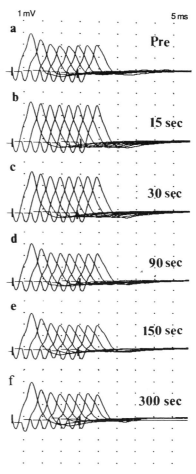

FIGURE 23.2. *Accessory nerve repetitive stimulation study in a patient with myasthenia gravis. In all traces, the time base is 5 ms/division, and voltage is 1 mV/division. The accessory nerve is stimulated in the posterior triangle in the neck by a train of 8 stimuli at a rate of 3 c/s. The response is recorded from the trapezius muscle. Before exercise (A), a 35% decrement is seen. Then the trapezius muscle is exercised for 15 seconds and the test repeated. The number of seconds following exercise is displayed for each trace. At 15 seconds (B), the decrement partially corrects to 9%. At 300 seconds (F), the decrement returns to baseline.*

ment, NMT failure must occur in a large percentage of muscle fibers, making this technique relatively insensitive in mild NMT disorders.[45]

To increase the sensitivity of the repetitive stimulation technique, a number of ancillary procedures have been added. The first is the effect of exercise. Repetitive stimulation is repeated before and after exercise. Our protocol for this technique is to give two trains of eight stimuli each at a rate of 3 c/s before exercise (see Figure 23.2). The patient exercises the muscle in question for 15 to 20 seconds and is then told to rest. To exercise the muscle, we have the patient push against resistance. If the patient is unable to exercise voluntarily, we give the patient a 40- to 60-second train at 30 c/s to exercise the muscle. We then stimulate the patient (using a train of eight stimuli at 3 c/s) at 3 seconds, 15 seconds, 30 seconds, 60 seconds, 90 seconds, 120 seconds, 150 seconds, and 180 seconds and then every 60 seconds for 5 minutes if no change in the response is seen or until any change in the response that is seen following exercise returns to the baseline preexercise state.

In postjunctional NMT disorders, the decrement seen before exercise improves at the 3-second and 15-second time interval after exercise[46] (see Figure 23.2). This phenomenon is known as *postactivation facilitation* and is due to a temporary excess of ACh quanta available for release at the axon terminal and increased concentration of calcium at the release sites, resulting in a greater number of ACh vesicles being released with nerve stimulation. This is followed by a period where the decrement may worsen.[47] This is known as postexercise exhaustion and is usually maximal at 3 to 4 minutes following exercise. The exact cause of this is not known but is believed to be due to reduced availability of ACh vesicles during this time, receptor desensitization, or other factors.

In prejunctional NMT disorders the amplitude of the compound muscle action potential dramatically increases 3 to 15 seconds after exercise[48] (Figure 23.3). Often the amplitude is 200% to 400% higher than the initial response. This indicates that there is significant failure of transmitter release at rest, which is corrected by the increased concentration of calcium occasioned by exercise.

Heating the muscle exacerbates preexistent decrements or may even produce abnormalities in repetitive responses that were initially normal. Virtually all NMT disorders worsen with increased temperature. In cases with equivocal results to repetitive stimulation, the tested limb should be heated to at least 35°C to bring out the abnormalities. Another method to increase the sensitivity of this test is to do a two-step repetitive stimulation test.[49] First, repetitive stimulation is done in the standard manner. Then a blood pressure cuff is applied to the arm and inflated to above systolic pressure. The arm is then

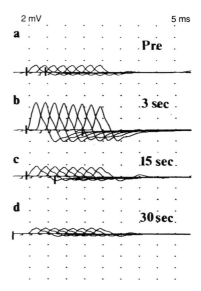

FIGURE 23.3. *Ulnar nerve repetitive stimulation study in a patient with myasthenic syndrome. In all traces, the time base is 5 ms/division and the amplitude 2 mV/division. The ulnar nerve at the wrist is stimulated by a train of 8 pulses at 3 c/s. Before exercise (A), the response is of low amplitude with only a negligible decrement of 8%. Following 15 seconds of exercise, the response amplitude increases by 400% (B). This response returns to baseline within 30 seconds (D).*

stimulated at 3 c/s for 4 minutes, and the repetitive study is repeated. We do not perform this test because it only marginally increases the test's sensitivity. Repetitive stimulation may also be combined with either the regional curare or Tensilon test.[37,40]

Higher stimulation rates are used in the investigation of patients suspected of having presynaptic abnormalities. We usually stimulate at rates ranging from 10 to 50 c/s using stimuli trains varying from eight to 500 stimuli. In prejunctional NMT disorders, the amplitude of the response increases at high stimulation rates (20 to 50 c/s) (Figure 23.4). It may take trains of 20 to 30 stimuli to observe this response. It is believed that this increase is due to the increased amount of calcium at the NMJ, which enhances transmitter release. Following a nerve impulse, calcium is increased at the NMJ for about 100 to 200 ms. Therefore 10 c/s is the minimum stimulation rate in which this response is seen. Usually 20 c/s is needed to produce an incremental response. In postjunctional NMT disorders, a slight increment

2 mV   **200 ms**

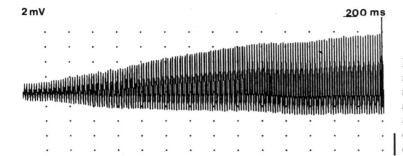

FIGURE 23.4. *High-frequency repetitive stimulation in a patient with myasthenic syndrome. The ulnar nerve is stimulated with a train of 150 pulses at a rate of 50 c/s. A marked increment is seen during this train.*

may occur, but in many patients the only response may be a leveling off of the decrement.

Single-Fiber Electromyography

Single-fiber electromyography (EMG) is used to evaluate fiber density, which is useful in situations in which denervation and sprouting are suspected, and to evaluate jitter and blocking, which is useful for the evaluation of NMT disorders. The technique of single-fiber EMG was developed by Stålberg et al.[50] using voluntary activated muscles.

Single-fiber EMG is more sensitive than repetitive stimulation for detecting defects in NMT.[50–52] NMT failure need not occur to detect abnormalities in this test. A special recording electrode is used that allows the activity of only a small area of the muscle to be examined, thus making it possible to record the activity of a single muscle fiber. This electrode is a concentric bipolar needle with a side port that contains a recording electrode of about 25 mm in diameter. The low-frequency filter is set to 500 c/s, filtering out most low-frequency signals that may interfere with the baseline.

There are two types of single-fiber EMG studies, voluntary and stimulated. In voluntary single-fiber EMG, the patient is told to activate the tested muscle slightly so only one motor unit near the needle is activated. The single-fiber needle is advanced until the activity of at least two muscle fibers innervated by the same motor neuron can be recorded. The time interval between the peaks of both responses, the interpotential interval (IPI), is measured for 50 to 100 successive firings of this muscle fiber pair (Figure 23.5). This information is used to calculate the mean consecutive difference for this fiber pair using the following formula:

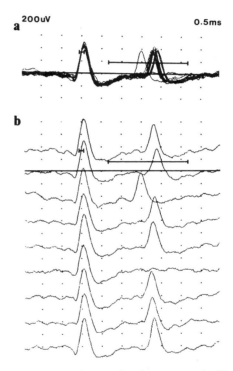

a **200uV**   **0.5ms**

b

FIGURE 23.5. *Abnormal voluntary single-fiber EMG in the extensor digitorum communis muscle. The sweep is being triggered by the first potential. (A) Fifty traces are superimposed. (B) Nine sequential traces are displayed in a raster mode. Increased jitter and blocking are seen (fourth trace from the bottom). The mean consecutive difference is calculated by measuring consecutive interpotential intervals (see equation in text). The interpotential interval is the interval between the triggered potential and the second fiber potential.*

$$MCD = \frac{\sum\limits_{1}^{n-1} k \ (|x_k - x_{k+1}|)}{n-1}$$

where x is either the IPI or stimulus to response interval (SRI) of a muscle fiber pair, n is the number intervals studied, k is the current interval, and *MCD* is the mean consecutive difference.[51]

MCD is also known as jitter. If NMT is normal, the IPI is due to differences in the axonal length to the two muscle fibers plus the slight variability it takes for the end plate to reach threshold. In the case of NMT disorders, successive IPIs may show increased variability because fibers with compromised NMT take a longer time to reach threshold. Jitter varies depending on the muscle studied. In the extensor digitorum communis muscle, the average MCD of 20 fiber pairs should be less than 34 μs, and no more than 10% of the units should have MCDs of greater than 55 μs.[51] These values are lower for more proximal muscles such as the frontalis or deltoid muscle. One muscle fiber of a fiber pair may fail to fire. This is known as *blocking* (Figure 23.5) and represents a NMT failure. Obviously it is important that the patient cooperate to perform an accurate voluntary single-fiber study. If the two fibers studied are not innervated by the same motor unit, one cannot evaluate jitter or blocking because these fibers will fire independently of each other.

Stimulated single-fiber EMG allows less cooperative patients to be studied.[53,54] In this test, an intramuscular nerve twig is stimulated by another needle electrode inserted into the muscle. Because the motor unit is stimulated directly, it is not necessary to record from a fiber pair. Rather, the study may be performed on a single muscle fiber. Instead of measuring the interval between two fiber potentials, the SRI is measured (Figures 23.6, and 23.7). Jitter values are reduced compared with those of voluntary single-fiber EMG because only the variability of a single NMJ is studied. Normal MCD in the extensor digitorum communis muscle using stimulated single-fiber EMG is 25 μs.[53]

There are three major pitfalls that need to be avoided when doing stimulated single-fiber EMG. First, direct stimulation of the muscle fibers must be avoided. If the muscle fiber itself rather than the nerve is accidentally stimulated, the MCD calculated would be very low, usually less than 9 μs. In these cases, either the recording or stimulating electrodes should be moved. Second, it is important to ensure that a large enough stimulus current is being used. If not, it would appear that NMT failure is occurring when these findings are due to incomplete nerve stimulation. A final caveat is to ensure that the current is not spreading to other segments of the nerve.

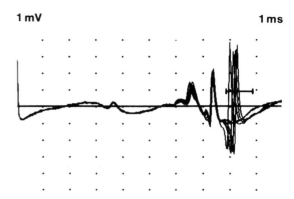

1 mV   **1 ms**

FIGURE 23.6.   *Abnormal stimulated single-fiber EMG of the extensor digitorum communis muscle. The intramuscular branch of the radial nerve innervating the extensor digitorum communis muscle is stimulated at 15 c/s. In this trace, three units are identified. The stimulus response interval is measured from the stimulus to the peak of the response. The amount of jitter varies with each unit on this trace: The first unit shows a moderate amount of jitter (78 μs). The second unit shows a normal amount of jitter (21 μs). The third unit shows a large amount of jitter (165 μs) with blocking 30% of the time.*

If this happens, it will appear that the patient is having increased jitter when in fact the potential is skipping by a fixed internodal interval (Figure 23.8). This is due to current spreading to an adjacent node of Ranvier. When this occurs, the stimulus response interval is reduced by the time the nerve impulse conducts down this segment.

We generally favor using stimulated single-fiber EMG because this technique can be performed more rapidly than a voluntary study and is less dependent on patient cooperation. In addition to the extensor digitorum communis muscle, techniques have been developed to study the biceps, deltoid, and orbicularis oculi muscles.[55] Often only abnormalities in these proximal muscles are seen in postjunctional NMT disorders. A different population of muscle fibers is studied by stimulated single-fiber EMG compared with single-fiber EMG. Single-fiber EMG preferentially studies larger motoneurons with small cell bodies, whereas stimulated single-fiber EMG studies motor units of all sizes.[53] In addition to calculating the MCD, the standard deviation of either the IPIs (in the case of single-fiber EMG) or SRIs (in the case of stimulated single-fiber EMG) may be calculated.

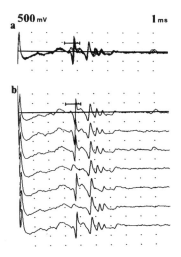

FIGURE 23.7. *Stimulated single-fiber EMG of the orbicularis oculi muscle. The intramuscular nerve innervating this muscle is stimulated at 15 c/s. (A) Twenty traces are superimposed. (B) Seven sequential traces are displayed in the raster mode. Four units are seen. The first unit shows a moderate amount of jitter (mean consecutive difference = 46 μs) and occasionally shows blocking. The second unit has normal jitter (mean consecutive difference = 20 μs) with no blocking. The third unit displays increased jitter and blocking, whereas the fourth unit shows only a moderate degree of jitter.*

We recommend using the MCD because it factors out variations owing to fluctuations secondary to needle position.

Examining the change in jitter with different motor unit firing rates may assist the evaluator in dis-

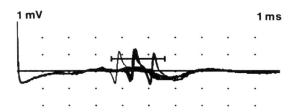

FIGURE 23.8. *This is a stimulated single-fiber EMG from the extensor digitorum communis muscle demonstrating the effect of improper stimulation. In this case, the unit fires at three different intervals. This occurs because the nerve is being stimulated at three different sites, skipping successive nodes of Ranvier.*

tinguishing between prejunctional and postjunctional NMT disorders. Because high-frequency stimulation depletes transmitter in a postjunctional defect but facilitates release in a prejunctional defect, the MCD in a prejunctional defect becomes shorter with increases in firing rate, whereas the opposite is true in a postjunctional defect[56] (Figure 23.9).

Stapedial Reflex Decay

The stapedial reflex is a multisynaptic reflex mediated by the seventh and eighth cranial nerves. Loud sounds will cause contraction of the stapedius muscle in both ears. A method has been devised to record the contraction of this muscle in response to pulsed sounds.[57–59] An earphone is placed over one ear and an acoustic impedance bridge over the other to re-

A. MYASTHENIA GRAVIS

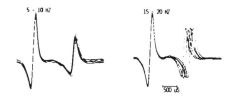

B. LAMBERT - EATON SYNDROME

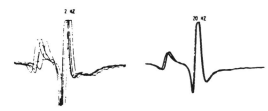

FIGURE 23.9. *The effect of firing rate on jitter in myasthenia gravis (A) and myasthenic syndrome (B). (A) Recordings made from one pair of potentials in a motor unit in the extensor digitorum communis muscle during voluntary activation of the muscle at different firing rates. (B) Recordings made from two muscle fibers in the hypothenar muscle during stimulation of the ulnar nerve at two different rates. Each figure contains five superimposed oscilloscope sweeps. (Reprinted with permission from Sanders DB. Electrophysiologic study of disorders of neuromuscular transmission. In: Aminoff MJ, ed. Electrodiagnosis in clinical neurology, ed 2. New York: Churchill Livingstone, 1986:321.)*

cord the activity of the stapedius muscle. Generally, 500 c/s sounds are pulsed at rates of either 1 or 2.5 c/s. The *off* interval is equal to the *on* interval of the pulses. Normally there is no decay in the amplitude of the stapedial response to pulsed times, but in patients with NMT disorders, the response decays, so 30 seconds after the onset of the tone, the amplitude of the stapedial response is reduced. The administration of edrophonium reduces this decay. The response to continuous tones is less useful than pulsed tones. Most centers are not doing this study at this time because the equipment necessary is not readily available in the usual EMG laboratory, and its reliability is no greater than that of other tests.

NEUROMUSCULAR TRANSMISSION DISORDERS

Myasthenia Gravis

This is the most common NMT disorder, with a prevalence rate varying from 1 in 10,000 to 1 in 50,000.[60,61] In this disorder, autoantibodies attack the postjunctional ACh receptors, ultimately destroying them.[62] There are two populations of patients afflicted: predominantly women in their teens and twenties and predominantly men in their fifties and sixties.[60,63] MG is often associated with thymic abnormalities. Thymic hyperplasia often occurs in younger patients, whereas thymomas often occur in older patients.[62,64] In addition, MG is frequently associated with other autoimmune diseases, such as rheumatoid arthritis, pernicious anemia, polymyositis, thyroiditis, scleroderma, Sjögren's syndrome, and lupus erythematosus.[65]

Ptosis and ophthalmoplegia are often the first symptoms of the disease, followed by difficulty swallowing liquids and nasal, slurred speech.[66] Palatal weakness may result in nasal regurgitation. Later neck and shoulder weakness and finally respiratory weakness occur. It is unusual to see distal limb weakness, unless proximal weakness is severe. The legs are much less often affected. Characteristic of the weakness is its tendency to vary in severity during the day or even during the examination. This is known as *fatigue*.

The initial examination determines which muscles, if any, are clinically weak. Then the patient should be checked for signs of fatigability. If ptosis is present, it is useful to have the patient gaze upward for 90 to 180 seconds to see if it worsens. An ice pack test can be performed.[41] This test is based on the fact that NMT disorders improve with cool temperature. A pack of ice is gently held to the patient's closed eye for a period of 2 minutes to see if the ptosis is ameliorated. In a positive test, the ptosis is improved.

Next an edrophonium test as described earlier should be performed (Table 23.2). Thyroid functions should be evaluated because thyroid disease may be associated with these symptoms. A careful clinical history should be taken to rule out exposure to any of the drugs and toxins mentioned later in this chapter. In particular, the patient should be questioned about home canning (a possible source of botulinum toxin exposure) and exposure to aminoglycosides or penicillamine. Serum ACh receptor antibodies and antistriatal muscle antibodies should be obtained. Binding ACh receptor antibodies are found in 85% of patients with MG.[67,68] In general, patients with a higher titer of ACh receptor antibodies have more severe disease.[69–71] Antistriatal muscle antibodies are seen in about 10% of patients but more often in patients with thymoma.[64] A computed tomography (CT) scan of the chest should be performed to eval-

TABLE 23.2.　Myasthenia gravis and Lambert-Eaton myasthenic syndrome workups

Myasthenia gravis	Lambert-Eaton myasthenic syndrome
Tensilon test	Tensilon test
Ice pack test	Repetitive nerve stimulation
Repetitive nerve stimulation	Single-fiber EMG
Single-fiber EMG	CT scan of the chest
Acetylcholine receptor antibody, antistriatal antibody	Malignancy workup
Thyroid functions	Workup for other autoimmune diseases
CT scan of the chest	
Workup for other autoimmune diseases	
Pulmonary function testing	

uate the patient for either thymic hyperplasia or thymoma.[72] A complete blood count (CBC) should be checked for the rare association of thymoma with primary red cell aplasia.

The initial electrophysiologic test that we perform on patients suspected of having MG is repetitive stimulation (see Table 23.2). Even though it is less sensitive than single-fiber EMG and stapedial reflex decay, it is easy to perform and, if positive, helpful. In patients with ocular MG, we omit repetitive stimulation because it is rarely positive. To increase the yield of this procedure, we warm the tested muscle to 35°C. Our first study is usually an accessory nerve repetitive study. The reason we do this is that it is more likely to be positive than an ulnar repetitive study and is relatively painless. We find that if performed properly this test can usually be done with a stimulus intensity of less than 20 μA. If this is negative, we do a facial repetitive study. We have found this study to be more sensitive than an accessory, but it is technically more difficult to perform and is more uncomfortable for the patient because a relatively high stimulus intensity is needed. We always exercise the patient when doing repetitive stimulation unless the patient is unable to cooperate with the study. Abnormal studies show a normal or near-normal amplitude compound muscle action potential that shows a decremental response of greater than 10% (see Figure 23.2). The decrement is reduced 3 and 15 seconds after exercise. The decrement usually increases 1 to 5 minutes after exercise. In some patients, we do an edrophonium test during the repetitive study to see if the abnormality in NMT may be corrected.

We perform single-fiber EMG on all patients having normal or borderline repetitive studies. We may also perform it on patients with abnormal repetitive studies because it can be used to monitor the magnitude of the NMT disorders. We usually do stimulated single-fiber EMG of the extensor digitorum communis muscle because we have found this to be an easy, reliable, and relatively painless test. In patients with only mild ocular symptoms having normal stimulated single-fiber EMG of the extensor digitorum communis, we do stimulated single-fiber EMG of the orbicularis oculi muscle. Stimulated single-fiber EMG is abnormal in approximately 85% to 95% of patients with MG.[51] The jitter in single-fiber EMG increases with increased firing rate in MG (see Figure 23.9). The combination of stimulated single-fiber EMG and ACh receptor antibodies is able to diagnose correctly 95% of patients with this disease.[45]

We treat patients symptomatically with pyridostigmine, a long-acting anticholinesterase.[36] We use an initial dose of 60 mg every 4 hours while awake and increase by 30 mg as needed to control symptoms. Although blood levels of this drug may be obtained, we do not routinely get them.[73,74] If the patient develops muscarinic side effects, we treat the patient with tincture of belladonna, starting at a dose of 5 to 8 drops three times a day and titrating the dose to relieve symptoms. In patients with ocular MG, this is usually the extent of our therapy. Patients with generalized MG undergo thymectomy.[64,75,76] We recommend a complete thymic exenteration through a midsternal incision. In patients with mild generalized MG, we thymectomize without any additional treatment. In patients with mild bulbar symptoms, we pretreat with either plasma exchange (three exchanges of 3 L each)[77,78] or high-dose gamma globulin (0.4 g intravenously a day for 5 days) therapy before thymectomy.[79–83] We examine all patients before thymectomy and cancel the surgery of any patient with bulbar symptoms.

In patients with more severe symptoms, we begin immunosuppressive therapy in an effort to improve their symptoms before thymectomy. Patients who cannot tolerate the surgery because of age or other medical problems are maintained on immunosuppressive therapy. We start patients either on prednisone or azathioprine.[36,66] The advantage of prednisone is that it is relatively fast acting and is an effective drug. Unfortunately, the drug has many side effects. The initial dose is 60 mg a day. After a month of therapy, we gradually taper the dose and place the patient on an alternate-day regimen. Side effects are usually seen in virtually all patients treated with prednisone. These include but are not limited to weight gain, edema, depression, infection, gastric ulcer, and bone demineralization. Avascular necrosis of the hips and other bones is a serious complication. Azathioprine takes longer (usually 3 to 6 months) to have an effect but usually has fewer side effects.[84,85] We usually start the patient on a dose of 50 mg three times a day. Side effects of azathioprine include anemia, hepatic abnormalities, and, on rare occasions, malignancy. For these reasons, a CBC and liver enzymes should be measured frequently. In patients who do not improve with these drugs, we use cyclosporine at a dose of 5 mg/kg (2.5 mg/kg two times a day).[86] Side effects of cyclosporine are predominately renal. Some patients can be controlled only with periodic immunoglobulin therapy or plasma exchange.

Patients who present with profound weakness or

respiratory insufficiency are treated with either plasma exchange[77,78,87] or immunoglobulin therapy.[79–83] We exchange the patient three times, exchanging 3 to 4 L each exchange. Improvement usually occurs after 7 days and lasts for about a month. Immunoglobulin therapy is given at a dose of 0.4 g/kg per day for 5 days. We check pulmonary functions on all patients whom we suspect of having respiratory difficulties. We have found that blood gases are not of much value in this population unless these patients have underlying pulmonary disease. We advocate intubating all patients with myasthenia gravis who are complaining of respiratory difficulty and have a forced vital capacity of less than 1L. In our experience, with immunotherapy including plasma exchange and the addition of immunosuppressive therapy, most patients can live normal or near-normal lives with this disease.

Myasthenic Syndrome

LEMS is an autoimmune disorder in which antibodies attack the active release zones in the axon terminal.[88,89] As a result, the voltage-dependent release of transmitter at the NMJ is defective.[33] In addition to physiologic evidence supporting the defect in the release of ACh at the axon terminal, there is anatomic evidence by freeze fracture techniques of degradation of the active sites at the NMJ in this syndrome.[90] Clinically the symptoms of LEMS are quite different from MG.[91,92] These patients develop proximal limb weakness that is often manifested by difficulty climbing stairs. In addition, they may develop dry mouth, impotence, and other symptoms of autonomic insufficiency owing to impaired transmitter release in autonomic nerves.[93] They almost never develop ptosis or ophthalmoplegia. This syndrome is often associated with small cell carcinoma of the lung and may be the first sign of this disease. Other autoimmune diseases such as lupus erythematosus,[94] MG,[95] polymyositis, and thymoma[96] have been associated with LEMS. One characteristic sign of the disease is the so-called vise-like grip. As the patient grips the examiner's hand, the tension increases. Often the patient may just be complaining of generalized weakness.

In contrast to MG, this disease is often not diagnosed before EMG. Because these patients have difficulty releasing a normal amount of ACh at the NMJ, there may be considerable NMT failure present at rest. Nerve conduction studies reveal low-amplitude motor evoked responses but normal sensory action potentials.[91,97] If these are found at

several sites, the clinician should have a high index of suspicion for LEMS, particularly if the patient has pulmonary problems.

Repetitive nerve stimulation results make the diagnosis (see Table 23.2). It is usually not as critical that a proximal muscle be used as it is for MG because the characteristic abnormalities are seen in distal muscles as often as in proximal ones. A muscle that has a low-amplitude compound muscle action potential should be studied because there is evidence that this muscle is abnormal. With low-frequency stimulation (2 to 3 c/s), a low-amplitude response is seen with a slight decrement. At 3 to 15 seconds after exercise, the amplitude of the compound muscle action potential is markedly increased (200% to 300%) compared with the preexercise value (see Figure 23.3). Later the response once again becomes reduced in amplitude. The cause of this low-amplitude response is NMT failure as a result of reduction of ACh release at the axon terminal. Following exercise, transmitter release is facilitated, and less NMT failure is seen. This pattern, although highly suggestive of prejunctional NMT failure, may occasionally be seen in severe MG. However, the improvement in the amplitude after exercise is less marked.

With higher rates of stimulation (20 to 30 c/s), the amplitude of the compound muscle action potential is increased owing to enhanced release of ACh at the nerve terminal active zones stimulated by an increased concentration of calcium (see Figure 23.4). Often the stimulus train must be prolonged (20 to 50 pulses) before a noticeable increment is seen. Edrophonium administration improves the amplitude of the motor response but has less effect than in MG.

In some instances, single-fiber EMG is desirable to quantify the defect of NMT, particularly in borderline states. Once again, increased jitter and blocking are seen. If the muscle's firing rate is increased, there is improvement in the single-fiber EMG with shortening of the MCD (see Figure 23.9). Patients with LEMS often have occult pulmonary neoplasms; therefore they should be carefully checked for a lung lesion with a chest CT scan.

Treatment usually has two components. The symptoms of patients discovered to have neoplasms may improve with treatment of the tumor.[98,99] Patients without detectable neoplasms usually respond to immunosuppressive therapy with plasma exchange,[100] prednisone,[101] or azathioprine (Imuran).[102,103] Patients are also given symptomatic treatment. Anticholinesterase inhibitors such as pyridostigmine (Mestinon) are often effective in ameliorating the symptoms. Other agents effective in the symptomatic therapy of this syndrome are 4-aminopyridine[103,104] and 3,4-diaminopyridine.[105] These drugs enhance the release of ACh at the axon terminal by interfering with the voltage-sensitive K^+ channels. Their effectiveness is limited by central nervous system toxicity, most notably seizures. The dose of 3,4-diaminopyridine is 30 to 60 mg divided into three daily dosages. 4-Aminopyridine is given at a dose of 40 to 200 mg a day. Guanidine[106] is another drug that enhances ACh release at the NMJ. It should not be used because of bone marrow and liver toxicity.

Childhood Neuromuscular Transmission Disorders

Three NMT disorders affect infants and children (Table 23.3). The first, juvenile MG, is essentially an autoimmune disorder of the NMJ that behaves like adult-onset MG and is treated similarly.[107–110] The second is neonatal MG. This disorder results from transplacental transport of antibodies and possibly antibody-producing cells from the mother to the fetus.[110–112] Infants with this disorder usually develop weakness, hypotonia, and feeding difficulties within the first 4 days of life. The disease usually improves on its own 2 to 4 weeks after its onset but has been reported for longer periods. Because this disease is caused by the passive transport of antibodies from the mother, she, of necessity, invariably has MG. The severity of the disease in the mother and her antibody level are not well correlated with the severity of the disease in the infant. Infants of asymptomatic mothers with MG may develop neonatal MG. Affected infants should receive symptomatic treatment by slowly increasing the initial dose of 0.05 mg/kg of pyridostigmine or 0.04 mg/kg of neostigmine until symptoms improve. Repetitive stimulation reveals a decrement at low stimulus frequencies (2 to 3 c/s). Injection of 0.1 mg of edrophonium during the repetitive study may help make this diagnosis. Elevated

TABLE 23.3. Childhood neuromuscular transmission disorders

Neonatal myasthenia gravis
Juvenile myasthenia gravis
Congenital myasthenia gravis
　Congenital absence of acetylcholinesterase
　Slow channel syndrome
　Familial infantile myasthenia
　Acetylcholine receptor decrease
　Defect in acetylcholine resynthesis and mobilization

ACh receptor antibodies are seen in both the infant and mother.

The third group of NMJ disorders in childhood are the congenital myasthenia syndromes, which are hereditary diseases of NMT.[113,114] Several prejunctional and postjunctional defects have been described. Familial infantile myasthenia is an autosomal recessive disorder of NMT.[110,115] This syndrome is characterized by hypotonia and difficulty with feeding and breathing in the infant, along with absence of myasthenia in the mother. These patients have periodic apneic spells, and this syndrome may be a cause of sudden infant death. Because inheritance is autosomal recessive, neither parent has the disorder, but siblings have a 25% chance of being affected. Symptoms generally improve as patients get older. Patients older than 2 years of age usually do not have significant problems. Symptoms in older children may vary from mild weakness with easy fatigability to moderate weakness. It is believed that this syndrome is due to a defect in the packaging of ACh at the axon terminal. The number of ACh molecules contained in a vesicle becomes progressively reduced with continued transmitter release.

Patients with familial infantile myasthenia have no ACh receptor antibodies but respond to edrophonium. In infants, the recommended dose of edrophonium is 0.1 mg. A decrement is seen with low-frequency repetitive stimulation (2 to 10 c/s). Treatment is supportive care along with AChE inhibitors. As mentioned earlier, these patients improve gradually with increasing age, and most show only mild fatigability during adolescence.

Another form of congenital MG is deficiency of AChE.[114,116] This autosomal recessive disorder is characterized by weakness at birth, combined with a poor suck, poor cry, and respiratory distress. The weakness usually then stabilizes until patients are approximately 10 years of age at which point they become increasingly weak. Patients have weakness of the face, neck, shoulder, and limbs. Electron microscopy shows a marked decrease in the size of the nerve terminals. AChE is absent from the end plates, and total muscle AChE level is markedly reduced. Because these patients have congenital absence of AChE, edrophonium does not produce symptomatic improvement and may cause an exacerbation of the symptoms. In addition to the absence of AChE, nerve terminal size is reduced, and there is degeneration of the junctional folds. In response to a single stimulus, a repetitive compound muscle action potential is seen (Figure 23.10). The second component is smaller than the first and represents a second action potential

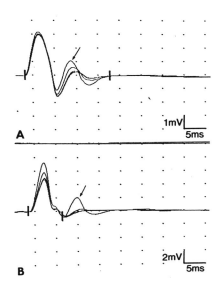

1mV|
5ms

A

2mV|
5ms

B

FIGURE 23.10.   *Neuromuscular junction acetyl-cholinesterase deficiency. Repetitive compound muscle action potential recorded from extensor digitorum brevis muscle (A) and thenar muscle (B) during 2 c/s stimulation of peroneal and median nerve. The second response (arrow) decrements more rapidly than the first response. (Reprinted with permission from Engel AG. Congenital disorders of neuromuscular transmission. Semin Neurol 1990; 10:12–26.)*

of some muscle fibers owing to the prolonged duration of the end plate potential. A decremental response is seen with 2 c/s repetitive stimulation. The second component decays faster and to a greater extent than the first component. Usually the second component disappears completely at stimulation frequencies greater than 0.2 c/s. Treatment is symptomatic because there is no effective therapy for this condition.

The slow channel syndrome is an autosomal dominant disorder with variable expressivity.[114,117] The age of onset of this condition is variable and can occur both in infancy and in adulthood. Muscle involvement is patchy with weakness and atrophy of affected muscles. It may progress in either a gradual or an episodic manner with the patient having episodic weakness. ACh receptor antibodies are not found, and edrophonium is ineffective. The disorder is caused by defective postjunctional channels that remain open longer than they should. The end plate potential is prolonged, resulting in multiple action

potentials to a single nerve impulse. Similar to the previous disorder, a single stimulus produces multiple compound muscle action potentials with the second response being of reduced size. A decrement is produced with 2 c/s nerve stimulation but only in affected muscles. Treatment is supportive. Although both this and the previous disorder have an abnormally increased duration and half decay time of the MEPP, this disorder differs from the former by having normal MEPP frequency and normal quantal content at 1 c/s. Treatment is supportive.

Another form of congenital myasthenia is due to a reduction in the number of ACh receptors.[114,118,119] These patients have variable clinical presentations, but they usually are weak at birth, with hypotonia, feeding difficulties, and respiratory distress. ACh receptor antibodies are not present, but patients do respond to edrophonium. These patients have abnormal repetitive studies in affected muscles. About half of the patients with this disorder show an abnormal decrement with low-frequency (3 c/s) stimulation, but all have abnormal single-fiber EMG. On histologic analysis, they have simplification of the junctional folds. The inheritance of this disease is autosomal recessive. Treatment is with the use of AChE inhibitors and supportive care.

In a final form of congenital myasthenia, there is a defect in ACh resynthesis, storage, and mobilization without abnormality of ACh release.[120] Motor nerve conductions have low amplitude and a decrement with low-frequency repetitive stimulation. Postexercise facilitation is seen. Cholinesterase inhibitors are ineffective, as is guanidine. This disease is probably inherited in an autosomal recessive manner. Clinical findings are hypotonia and areflexia with intact extraocular movements. There was slight improvement with age, but the patient described with this disease died at 8 months of age.

Clostridial Toxins

Botulinum toxin is a potent presynaptic toxin that is manufactured by the anaerobic bacterium, *Clostridium botulinum*.[121] This toxin acts on the axon terminal in a three-step process.[122] The first step is the binding of botulinum toxin to the axonal terminal. At this step, the toxin may be disassociated from the nerve. The next step is the calcium-dependent transport of the toxin across the terminal membrane. The final step is the destruction of the axon terminal. Failure of NMT occurs because the toxin renders the axon terminal no longer capable of releasing ACh initially by a process possibly interfering with exocytosis of vesicles.[123,124] Later the axon terminal undergoes destruction. Recovery is by regrowth of the nerve terminal. Only five of the eight subtypes of toxin have produced human disease.[125–127] Subtypes A, B, and E are the ones most often associated with human disease. Type A is the most potent and is found mainly west of the Mississippi River. Type B is found mainly east of the Mississippi River and in Europe. Type E is found in contaminated shellfish and is found in Alaska, the upper midwestern United States, and Asia. Types F and G rarely cause human disease.

Foods contaminated as a result of defective canning are the most common cause of botulism.[126] Patients present 16 to 60 hours after ingestion of the toxin with symptoms caused by interference with ACh transmission both at the NMJ and parasympathetic nervous system.[128] The first signs are usually due to autonomic involvement and include dry mouth, abdominal cramps, diarrhea, and constipation. Generalized weakness most prominent in bulbar and ocular musculature then occurs. In contrast to MG, pupillary constriction is almost always but not invariably impaired. The weakness than spreads to involve the remainder of the body. Respiratory muscles can be affected. Because more than one person usually ingests the tainted food, there is characteristically clustering of cases. The severity of the symptoms are related to both the amount of toxin ingested and host factors. Patients who develop symptoms early in the course of the disease are destined to develop more severe disease than those that develop symptoms later.

Diagnosis is easy after the index case has been identified, but diagnosis of the initial patient may be difficult unless botulism is considered. The toxin may be identified and typed from serum and stool samples. In addition, the organism may be cultured from the stool. Unfortunately, treatment cannot wait for the confirmation of the disease in this manner. Electrophysiologic tests are quite helpful. The disease is often spotty, with some muscles being quite affected, whereas others are normal. Usually clinically involved muscles are abnormal electrophysiologically.[129,130] An affected muscle has a low compound muscle action potential to nerve stimulation. Little or no decrement usually is seen to low-frequency repetitive stimulation (2 to 5 c/s). Following exercise, the amplitude of the response usually but not invariably increases. With high-frequency repetitive stimulation (20 to 50 c/s), an increment of 125% to 200% is usually seen.[131] This increment is lower than that seen in LEMS. In addition, only selected muscles

show this abnormal repetitive response; other muscles may be normal. Single-fiber EMG reveals increased jitter and blocking of fiber potentials. As in LEMS, jitter is reduced with an increased muscle firing rate. Standard needle EMG reveals brief, low-amplitude, irregular potentials.

The goals of treatment are to support the patient and neutralize the toxin. Botulinum antitoxin is administered as soon as botulism is suspected. Trivalent antitoxin (A, B, E) is usually given. It is important to give the toxin as early as possible because after the toxin is internalized by the terminal, it can no longer be neutralized by the antitoxin. Emetic agents and enemas are not recommended because the toxin is already absorbed from the digestive tract by the time the diagnosis is made. The respiratory status of the patient should be observed carefully, and artificial ventilation should be given if necessary. Agents that enhance release of ACh such as 4-aminopyridine, and 3,4-diaminopyridine may be of value in the treatment of this condition.[132,133]

In wound botulism, the organism grows in a wound and slowly releases the toxin in the body.[134,135] The wound is usually caused by trauma and may be contaminated by *C. botulinum* even though it appears well healed. Diagnosis of this condition is more difficult than food-borne botulism because patients with this syndrome are not clustered. Abdominal symptoms do not occur, and the weakness may progress more slowly because the toxin is slowly released into the body. The electrophysiologic response is similar to that described earlier for food-borne botulism. Botulinum toxin is present in the serum but not in the stool. The treatment of this condition is to support the patient, administer trivalent antitoxin, and débride the wound.

Infantile botulism is due to weakness from toxin released by *C. botulinum* colonizing the gut of an infant from 1 to 6 months of age.[136,137] These patients usually have severe constipation, hypotonia, feeding difficulties, and ophthalmoplegia. Toxin cannot usually be found in the serum, but the organism can be grown from the stool. It is believed that the immature gastrointestinal tract provides the environment that allows *C. botulinum* to grow. The toxin is then released in the gut and absorbed into the blood stream causing disease. Honey is believed to contain *C. botulinum* spores and should be avoided in infants.[138] Breast milk is believed to be protective against it.[139] Botulism was identified in some patients who developed sudden infant death and may be responsible for some of these cases.[140] Electrophysiologically EMG is characterized by brief, low-amplitude irregular potentials.[141] Abnormal insertional activity is seen about 50% of the time. The initial amplitude of the response is diminished. A small incremental response is usually seen to high-frequency repetitive stimuli, and often a decrement is seen to low-frequency repetitive stimulation. Treatment is symptomatic because there are no effective drugs for this disease. Penicillin and enemas, although effective, are not recommended because they would lead to destruction of the organism in the gut and produce an influx of toxin that would harm the infant. Antitoxin is to be avoided because it may lead to a harmful allergic reaction.

Tetanus toxin from the anaerobic bacteria *Clostridium tetani* acts similarly to botulinum toxin at the NMJ.[121,142] Tetanus toxin also reduces the release of many neurotransmitters in the central nervous system, including gamma-aminobutyric acid, glycine, norepinephrine, and ACh. Tetanus usually begins with facial muscle spasms and trismus. EMG shows spontaneous motor unit firing, which occurs in bursts. Single-fiber EMG shows increased jitter and blocking with an improvement when the muscle is fired at a faster rate.[143] Treatment is symptomatic.

OTHER NEUROMUSCULAR TOXINS AND DRUGS

As discussed at the beginning of this chapter, there are many steps involved in the generation of a compound muscle action potential in response to a nerve stimulus. For each step, toxins occur in nature that interfere with the function of the NMJ (Table 23.4). In addition to their medical interest, these toxins are important because much of what we know about NMT is derived from the study of these toxins. Most of the active toxins in the NMJ have been isolated from snake, snail, spider, or scorpion venom. As explained earlier, the mechanism of action of a toxin is discovered by careful studies in which the end plate potential, compound nerve action potential, MEPP, and compound muscle action potential are carefully analyzed. Clinical features and the effects of some of these toxins and their mechanisms of action are summarized here.

Toxins and Drugs Affecting Action Potential Generation—Sodium Channels

These toxins inhibit NMT by blocking the Na^+ channels necessary for producing an action potential

in the motor neuron. In the case of tetrodotoxin from the pufferfish, the blocking of NMT is sudden, leading to almost instant death. Toxicity from tetrodotoxin may result from ingesting the toxin from the pufferfish intestine, which is considered a delicacy in Japan (Fugi). If the Fugi is prepared properly, the fish is either harmless or may produce mild toxicity, which Fugi aficionados may find desirable.

Toxin gamma from the Brazilian scorpion[144] and the toxin of the sea anemone also act on Na^+ channels[145] but facilitate NMT. Sea anemone toxin interferes with Na^+ current inactivation and thereby prolongs terminal depolarization. Toxin gamma activates Na^+ channels, increasing MEPP frequency and facilitating transmission. Ciguatoxin, produced by the dinoflagellate (*Gambierdiscus toxicus*) and found in tropical marine life, enhances ACh release by opening the Na^+ channels at the axon terminal.[146] Symptoms following ingestion of toxic fish include paresthesias, dysesthesias, and a paradoxic dysesthesia in which cold objects appear hot. In addition, cardiovascular symptoms, including bradycardia and hypertension; gastrointestinal symptoms, including abdominal pain, nausea, vomiting, and diarrhea; and psychiatric symptoms occur. Treatment is supportive. The venom of the wandering solitary spider, *Phoneutria nigriventer* activates voltage-dependent Na^+ channels prejunctionally and is blocked by tetrodotoxin.[147] This toxin produces repetitive motoneuron terminal action potentials, increasing ACh release. The symptoms of envenomation with this spider are pain, cramps, tremors, convulsions, autonomic instability, and spastic paralysis. Treatment is symptomatic with atropine and sedatives.

Toxins and Drugs Affecting Prejunctional Voltage-Sensitive Potassium Channels

These channels are important in the termination of the motor nerve action potential. K^+ channel blockers prolong the duration of the compound nerve action potential, which ultimately leads to enhancement of transmitter release. One such toxin, dendrotoxin,[148,149] from the mamba snake increases the release of ACh from the nerve terminal. This leads to fasciculation and muscle cramps owing to repetitive activity of the muscle in response to a nerve impulse. This is due to the blockage of K^+ channels presynaptically. Similar actions are seen with scorpion toxin from *Pandinus imperator*.[150] Aminopyridine and 3,4-diaminopyridine, drugs that are useful in treating NMT disorders, also act at this site.[151] The toxin of the Austrian Tiger snake (Notexin)[152] has

TABLE 23.4. Drugs and toxins affecting neuromuscular transmission

Toxin	Effect
Sodium channel	
Tetrodotoxin	Inhibits
Toxin gamma Brazilian Scorpion	Enhances
Sea anemone toxin	Enhances
Phoneutria nigriventer toxin	Enhances
Ciguatoxin	Enhances
Potassium channel	
Dendrotoxin	Enhances
Pandinus imperator	Enhances
Aminopyridine	Enhances
3-4 diaminopyridine	Enhances
Notexin	Inhibits
Calcium channel	
Omega conotoxin	Inhibits
Aminoglycoside	Inhibits
Substance P	Enhances
Angiotensin	Enhances
Calcium channel blockers (verapamil)	Inhibits
Magnesium	Inhibits
Adenosine triphosphate to cyclic adenosine monophosphate	
Trifluoroperazine	Enhances
Forskolin	Enhances
Theophylline	Ehances
Papaverine	Enhances
Imidazole	Inhibits
Sodium fluoride	Enhances
Release of acetylcholine	
Lead	Inhibits
Thallium	Inhibits
Beta bungarotoxin	Inhibits
Alpha latrotoxin	Enhances/inhibits
Crotoxin	Enhances/inhibits
Atraxotoxin	Enhances
Pardaxin	Enhances
Binding of acetylcholine to receptor	
Curare	Inhibits
Pancuronium	Inhibits
Vecuronium	Inhibits
Gallamine	Inhibits
Atracuriam	Inhibits
Nicotine	Enhances/inhibits
Succinylcholine	Enhances/inhibits
Alpha bungarotoxin	Inhibits
Lophotoxin	Inhibits
Cobratoxin	Inhibits
Alpha conotoxin	Inhibits
Acetylcholine receptor channels	
Alpha Conotoxin	Inhibits
Amantidine	Inhibits
Cocaine	Inhibits
Clonidine	Inhibits
Thiamine	Inhibits
Procainamide	Inhibits
Verapamil	Inhibits
Acetylcholinesterase inhibitors	
Fasciculin-2	Enhances
Soman	Enhances

the opposite effect and reduces transmitter release. Notexin also has a direct myotoxic effect.

Toxins and Drugs Affecting Presynaptic Voltage-sensitive Calcium Channels

In response to the depolarization of the axon terminal, Ca^{++} channels open to allow calcium to flow intracellularly. This is associated with transmitter release. Several toxins interfere with the flow of calcium intracellularly. The cone snail toxin, omega conotoxin, inhibits transmitter release by blocking these sites.[153,154] Alpha conotoxin has been used to identify the antibodies found in LEMS that bind to the same voltage-dependent Ca^{++} channels to which omega conotoxin binds.[155] Aminoglycoside antibiotics[156-158] and calcium channel blockers[159] also block this step. These compounds, used in recommended dosages, clinically have no effect on normal patients but interfere with NMT in patients who have underlying NMT disorders. Often unrecognized MG may be *unmasked* by these compounds. Substance P[160] and angiotensin enhance ACh release by increasing calcium channel ion flow.

The calcium channel blockers interfere with the release of ACh prejunctionally.[161] Verapamil and diltiazem, but not nifedipine, block ACh release. Single-fiber EMG studies have shown no effect on NMT in normal subjects,[162] but abnormalities are seen in patients with MG.[159]

Magnesium impairs the release of ACh at the NMJ.[163] Magnesium competitively inhibits the uptake of Ca^{++}. The infusion of magnesium sulfate in preeclamptic women produces areflexia at a level of 9 to 10 mEq/L and weakness at levels above 10 mEq/L. Electrophysiologic studies show a reduction in amplitude of the compound muscle action potential. An incremental response was seen to both 2 c/s and 20 c/s repetitive stimulation.[164] Magnesium sulfate may also unmask a preexisting NMT disorder. In one case, a woman receiving magnesium sulfate developed acute weakness with a level of 3 mEq/L. She had typical electrophysiologic repetitive studies for MG.[165] After the acute effects of the magnesium administration resolved, she was found to have an abnormal single-fiber EMG and an elevated ACh receptor antibody level.

Toxins and Drugs Affecting Adenosine Triphosphate–Cyclic Adenosine Monophosphate Conversion

In this step, the depolarization of the terminal activates adenyl cyclase, which converts ATP to cAMP. This opens the Ca^{++} channel, allowing calcium to enter the motor neuron terminal. The intracellular calcium binds with calmodulin, and intracellular binding protein, leading to transmitter release. Calmodulin is also a potent phosphodiesterase activator in high calcium concentrations and an adenyl cyclase activator in low calcium concentrations. Inhibitors of calmodulin, such as trifluoroperazine, enhance ACh release.[166] Forskolin, an adenyl cyclase activator, enhances NMT.[167] cAMP is broken down by phosphodiesterase. Phosphodiesterase inhibitors, such as theophylline and papaverine, enhance transmission.[167] Imidazole, a phosphodiesterase activator, inhibits transmitter release. Sodium fluoride also enhances transmitter release by acting at this locus. Because of its activity, theophylline is useful as adjuvant therapy in MG.

Toxins and Drugs Affecting the Release of Acetylcholine

These toxins act on the active zones that are believed to be the sites of ACh release. Lead,[169] thallium,[168] beta bungarotoxin, and the toxin from the salivary gland of the Australian tick (*Ixodes holcytes*), which causes tick paralysis, inhibit the release of ACh from the terminal active zones.[1,121] Clinically only the toxin from the tick has any significant effect on NMT. This toxin produces generalized weakness.[170] Treatment is to identify and remove the tick. Electrophysiologic studies reveal reduced conduction velocity of sensory and motor nerves[170,171] and, in one study, a decrement to high-frequency repetitive stimuli.[171] Black widow spider (*Latrodectus mactans*) toxin (alpha latrotoxin) increases the release of ACh and initially causes repetitive firing, which causes muscle cramps.[121] Then transmitter is depleted, and ACh release is reduced. Symptomatically this toxin has other effects that overshadow the NMT effects. Patients experience diffuse stimulation of the nervous system, including vasoconstriction, hypertension, and autonomic instability. Treatment is symptomatic.

Crotoxin from the South American rattlesnake activates nerve terminals, first depressing and then increasing ACh release until all transmitter is released.[172] It is a phospholipase and has myotoxic effects causing irreversible damage to the muscle and mitochondria. Atraxotoxin from the Sidney Funnel spider and pardaxin from the flatfish both enhance transmitter release.[173] Both toxins cause repetitive firing of muscles.[174] Symptoms produced by the toxin of the Sidney Funnel spider are nausea, vomiting, abdominal pain, diarrhea, fasciculation, and hypertension.[175]

Toxins and Drugs Affecting the Acetylcholine Receptor

Curare, a toxin derived from the vine *Strychnos toxifera,* is the prototype of this class of compounds.[2] This toxin was first used by natives for poison arrows because it was noticed that it would cause weakness and respiratory paralysis. Curare was later discovered to bind to muscle ACh receptor, preventing them from being activated by ACh. Many agents used in anesthesia are related to this compound, including pancuronium, vecuronium, gallamine, and atracurium.[2] High-dose curare causes complete blocking of the NMJ, and no compound muscle action potentials are seen with nerve stimulation. With lower dosages, a low-amplitude compound muscle action potential is seen that decrements with low-frequency repetitive stimulation. Nicotine is a depolarizing blocker that binds to and initially activates the receptor and then depolarizes and inactivates it. Its effects are reversed by curare. Succinylcholine acts by a similar mechanism.

Alpha bungarotoxin from the Formosan banded krait irreversibly binds ACh receptor, blocking transmission.[1,172] Radioactively labeled bungarotoxin was used to identify the ACh receptor. Another irreversible blocker of the ACh receptor is lophotoxin from the Pacific sea whip.[176] Cobratoxin from the cobra (*Naja Naja*) is less firmly bound, and neostigmine is useful for the treatment of this type of toxicity.[172,177] Alpha conotoxin from the cone snail (*Conus geographus*) blocks the ACh receptor, reversibly reducing the binding of ACh.[153,178]

Toxins and Drugs Affecting the Acetylcholine Receptor Channels

Certain toxins affect the properties of the ionic channels opened by ACh. Opening these channels longer than normal leads to repetitive firing of the muscle membrane and edrophonium-unresponsive weakness. Alpha conotoxin interferes with NMT by reducing the time course of MEPP decay.[153] This ultimately leads to reduction of MEPP amplitude. Amantidine,[179] cocaine,[180] and clonidine[181] block ionic channels that are open at the muscle end plate, interfering with NMT. Thiamine modifies the time course of the postjunctional channels interfering with NMT.[182] Abnormalities of single-fiber EMG have been seen in subjects taking high-dose thiamine doses greater than 5 g a day.[183] Procainamide, an antiarrhythmic agent that has caused exacerbation of MG, interferes with channel kinetics and interferes with ACh release presynaptically as well.[184] The calcium channel blocker, verapamil, interferes with ACh receptor channels, reducing the time course of channel opening.[185,186]

Toxins and Drugs Acting on Acetylcholinesterase

AChE stops the activity at the NMJ by hydrolyzing ACh into acetic acid and choline.[2] Substances that interfere with AChE at certain concentrations improve NMT but at high concentrations interfere with NMT in the same manner as ACh itself. Fasciculin-2, a toxin from the green mamba snake (*Dendroapis angusticeps*), causes fasciculation and muscle tremor.[187] Neostigmine is not effective in counteracting this toxin. Treatment is aimed at reducing the excessive ACh activity. Organophosphate compounds, such as soman, tightly bind to and deactivate AChE. The resulting increases in ACh produce autonomic hyperactivity and muscle fasciculation.[188] Nerve conduction studies show repetitive firings to single nerve impulses and profound decrements with both high-frequency and low-frequency repetitive stimulation.[189] Treatment is with neuromuscular blocking agents, such as pancuronium, at a dose of 4 mg intravenously followed by 2 mg intravenously every 12 hours, which reduces the cholinergic hyperactivity.[190] Oximes such as N-methyl-2-hydroxy-aminoformyl-pyridinium chlorire (2-PAM) or bis-pyridinium oxime (HI-6) interact with the phosphorylated AChE removing the organophosphate, reactivating AChE.

Unspecified Prejunctional Toxins and Drugs

The compounds tegretol[191] and emetine[192] interfere with the release of transmitter at the NMJ. Corticosteroids have multiple effects on NMT. One steroid, dexamethasone, has been reported to enhance transmitter release.[193]

Unspecified Postjunctional Toxins and Drugs

The following act postjunctionally to interfere with NMT: glucocorticoids, tegretol,[191] chloroquine,[194] oxamniquine,[195] and cleitanthus collinus leaf.[196]

Unknown Toxins

The following substances interfere with NMT, but the site is unknown: halothane,[197] ampicillin, ethanol, and dilantin.

PENICILLAMINE

D-Penicillamine, a drug used to treat rheumatoid arthritis and Wilson's disease, has been associated with the development of MG.[198–200] Patients develop symptoms of MG and have ACh receptor antibodies. The symptoms resolve and antibodies disappear following withdrawal of the drug. Electrophysiologically patients have findings compatible with MG.[201] Penicillamine has been shown to attach to the ACh receptor,[200] but does not interfere with bungarotoxin binding. Penicillamine may produce antigenic modulation of the ACh receptor, inducing the formation of autoantibodies.

REFERENCES

1. Swift TR. Disorders of neuromuscular transmission other than myasthenia gravis. Muscle Nerve 1981; 4:334–353.
2. Jones RM. Neuromuscular transmission and its blockade. Anaesthesia 1985; 40:964–976.
3. Keesey JC. AAEM Minimonograph #33: Electrodiagnostic approach to defects of neuromuscular transmission. Muscle Nerve 1989; 12:613–626.
4. Kuffler SW, Yoshikami D. The number of transmitter molecules in a quantum: An estimate from iontophoretic application of acetylcholine at the neuromuscular synapse. J Physiol (Lond) 1975; 251:465–482.
5. Thesleff S, Molgo J. A new type of transmitter release at the neuromuscular junction. Neuroscience 1983; 9:1–8.
6. Goldberg A, Singer J. Evidence for a role of cyclic AMP in neuromuscular transmission. Proc Nat Acad Sci 1969; 64:134–141.
7. Standaert F, Dretchen K. Cyclic nucleotides and neuromuscular transmission. Fed Proc 1979; 38:2183–2192.
8. Standaert F, Dretchen K, Skirboll LR, Morgenroth V. A role of cyclic nucleotides in neuromuscular transmission. J Pharmacol Exp Therap 1976; 199:553–564.
9. Katz B, Miledi R. The release of acetylcholine from nerve endings by graded electrical pulses. Proc Roy Soc 1967; (Biol)167:23–38.
10. Latorre R, Miller C. Conduction and selectivity in potassium channels. J Membrane Biol 1983; 71:11–30.
11. Rudy B. Diversity and ubiquity of K channels. Neuroscience 1988; 25:729–749.
12. Brigant J, Mullart A. Presynaptic currents in mouse motor endings. J Physiol 1982; 333:619–636.
13. Mallart A. Electric current flow inside perineural sheaths of mouse motor nerves. J Physiol 1985; 368:565–575.
14. Dubois J. Potassium currents in the frog node of Ranvier. Prog Biophys Mol Biol 1983; 42:1–20.
15. Marshall D, Harvey A. Block of potassium channels and facilitation of acetylcholine release at the neuromuscular junction by the venom of the scorpion, *Pandinus Imperator*. Toxicon 1989; 27:493–498.
16. DeLorenzo R. Role of calmodulin in neurotransmitter release and synaptic function. Ann NY Acad Sci 1980; 356:92–109.
17. Potter L. Synthesis, storage and release of ^{14}C acetylcholine in isolated rat diaphragm muscles. J Physiol (Lond) 1970; 206:145–166.
18. Elmqvist D, Quastel D. A quantitative study of endplate potentials in human muscle. J Physiol (Lond) 1965; 178:505–529.
19. Blaber LC. The pre-junctional actions of some nondepolarizing blocking drugs. Br J Pharmacol 1973; 47:109–116.
20. Hubbard JI, Wilson DF. Neuromuscular transmission in a mammalian preparation in the absence of blocking drugs and the effect of d-tubocurarine. J Physiol (Lond) 1973; 228:307–325.
21. Stanec A, Baker T. Pre-junctional and post-junctional effects of tubocurarine and pancuronium in man. Br J Anesthesiol 1984; 56:607–611.
22. Vizi E, Somogyi G, Nagashima H, et al. Tubocurarine and pancuronium inhibit evoked release of acetylcholine from the mouse hemidiaphragm preparation. Br J Anesthesiol 1987; 59:226–231.
23. Foldes F, Chaudhry I, Kinjo M, Nagashima H. Inhibition of mobilization of acetylcholine: The weak link in neuromuscular transmission during partial neuromuscular block with d-tubocurarine. Anesthesiology 1989; 71:218–223.
24. Landau E. Function and structure of the ACH receptor at the muscle endplate. Prog Neurobiol 1978; 10:253–288.
25. Katz B, Miledi R. The binding of acetylcholine to receptors and its removal from the synaptic cleft. J Physiol 1973; 231:549–574.
26. Lindstrom J, Tzartos S, Gullick W. Structure and function of the acetylcholine receptor molecule studied using monoclonal antibodies. Ann NY Acad Sci 1981; 377:1–19.
27. Takeuchi A, Takeuchi N. On the permeability of end-plate membrane during the action of transmitter. J Physiol (Lond) 1960; 154:52–67.
28. Engel A, Lambert E, Mulder O, et al. A newly recognised congenital myasthenic syndrome attributed to a prolonged open time of the acetylcholine induced ion channel. Ann Neurol 1982; 11:553–569.
29. Lambert E, Elmqvist D. Quantal components of endplate potentials in the myasthenic syndrome. Ann NY Acad Sci 183:183–199.
30. Engel A, Lambert E, Gomez M. A new myasthenic syndrome with endplate acetylcholinesterase deficiency, small nerve terminals and reduced acetylcholine release. Ann Neurol 1977; 1:315–330.
31. Elmqvist D. Neuromuscular transmission with special reference to myasthenia gravis. Acta Physiol Scand 1965; 64(suppl 249):1–34.
32. Fatt P, Katz B. Spontaneous sub-threshold activity

at motor nerve endings. J Physiol (Lond) 1952; 117:109–128.

33. Lambert E, Elmqvist D. Quantal components of endplate potentials in the myasthenic syndrome. Ann NY Acad Sci 1971; 183:183–199.

34. Osserman K, Kaplan L. Rapid diagnostic test for myasthenia gravis: Increased muscle strength, without fasciculations, after intravenous administration of edrophonium (tensilon) chloride. JAMA 1952; 150:265–268.

35. Goodman LS, Gilman A. The pharmacological basis of therapeutics, ed 7. New York: Macmillan, 1985:609.

36. Riggs J. Pharmacologic enhancement of neuromuscular transmission in myasthenia gravis. Clin Neuropharmacol 1982; 5:277–292.

37. Rosenbaum R, Bender A, Engel W. Prolonged response to edrophonium in myasthenia gravis. Trans Am Neurol Assoc 1975; 100:233–235.

38. Dirr LY, Donofrio PD, Patton JF, Troost BT. A false-positive edrophonium test in a patient with a brainstem glioma. Neurology 1989; 39(6):865–867.

39. Daroff RB. The office tensilon test for ocular myasthenia gravis. Arch Neurol 1986; 43:843–844.

40. Horowitz S, Krarup C. A new regional curare test of the elbow flexors in myasthenia gravis. Muscle Nerve 1979; 2:478–490.

41. Sethi K, Rivner M, Swift T. Ice pack test for myasthenia gravis. Neurology 1987; 37:1383–1385.

42. Massey J. Electromyography in disorders of neuromuscular transmission. Semin Neurol 1990; 10:6–11.

43. Schumm F, Stohr M. Accessory nerve stimulation in the assessment of myasthenia gravis. Muscle Nerve 1984; 7:147–151.

44. Paton W, Waud D. The margin of safety of neuromuscular transmission. J Physiol (Lond) 1967; 191:59–90.

45. Kelly J, Daube J, Lennon V, et al. The laboratory diagnosis of mild myasthenia gravis. Ann Neurol 1982; 12:238–242.

46. Desmedt J. The neuromuscular disorder in myasthenia gravis: Electrical and mechanical responses to nerve stimulation in hand muscles. In: Desmedt J, ed. New developments in electromyography and clinical neurophysiology. Vol I. Basel: Karger, 1973:241–304.

47. Desmedt J. Nature of the defect of neuromuscular transmission in myasthenia gravis: 'Post-tetanic' exhaustion. Nature 1957; 179:156–157.

48. Henriksson K, Nilsson O, Rosen I, Schiller H. Clinical neurophysiological and morphological findings in Eaton-Lambert syndrome. Acta Neurol Scand 1977; 56:117–140.

49. Gilchrist J, Sanders D. Double step repetitive stimulation in myasthenia gravis. Muscle Nerve 1987; 10:233–237.

50. Stålberg E, Ekstedt J, Broman A. Neuromuscular transmission in myasthenia gravis studied with single fibre electromyography. J Neurol Neurosurg Psychiatry 1974; 37:540–547.

51. Sanders D, Howard J. AAEE Minimonograph #25: Single-fiber electromyography in myasthenia gravis. Muscle Nerve 1986; 9:809–819.

52. Stålberg E, Trontelj J. Single fiber electromyography. Old Woking Surrey, Mirvalle Press, 1979.

53. Jabre J, Chirico-Post J, Weiner M. Stimulation SFEMG in myasthenia gravis. Muscle Nerve 1989; 12:38–42.

54. Trontelj J, Mihelin M, Fernandez J, Stålberg E. Axonal stimulation for end-plate jitter studies. J Neurol Neurosurg Psychiatry 1986; 49:677–685.

55. Trontelj J, Khuraibet A, Mihelin M. The jitter in stimulated orbicularis oculi muscle: Technique and normal values. J Neurol Neurosurg Psychiatry 1988; 51:814–819.

56. Ingram D, Davis G, Schwartz M, Swash M. The effect of continuous voluntary activation on neuromuscular transmission: A SFEMG study of myasthenia gravis and anterior horn cell disorders. Electroencephalogr Clin Neurophysiol 1985; 60:207–213.

57. Yamane M, Nomura Y. Analysis of stapedial reflex in neuromuscular disease. J Otorhinolaryngol 1984; 46:84–96.

58. Kramer L, Ruth R, Johns M, Sanders D. A comparison of stapedial reflex fatigue with repetitive stimulation and single-fiber EMG in myasthenia gravis. Ann Neurol 1981; 9:531–536.

59. DeChicchis AR, Rivner MH, Larson VD. Measurements of acoustic stapedial reflex fatigue in myasthenia gravis. Neurology 1986; 36:161.

60. Simpson J. Myasthenia gravis: A personal view of pathogenesis and mechanism, part I. Muscle Nerve 1978; 1:45–56.

61. Havard C, Scadding G. Myasthenia gravis: Pathogenesis and current concepts in management. Drugs 1983; 26:174–184.

62. Drachman D. Myasthenia gravis (first of two parts). N Engl J Med 1978; 298:136–142.

63. Donaldson D, Ansher M, Horan S, et al. The relationship of age to outcome in myasthenia gravis. Neurology 1990; 40:786–790.

64. Rivner M, Swift T. Thymoma: Diagnosis and management. Semin Neurol 1990; 10:83–88.

65. Behan PO. Immune disease and HLA associations with myasthenia gravis. J Neurol Neurosurg Psychiatry 1980; 43:611–621.

66. Drachman D. Myasthenia gravis (second of two parts). N Engl J Med 1978; 298:186–193.

67. Lindstrom J, Seybold M, Lennon V, et al. Antibody to acetylcholine receptor in myasthenia gravis: Prevalence, clinical correlates and diagnostic value. Neurology 1976; 26:1054–1059.

68. Soliven B, Lange D, Penn A, et al. Seronegative myasthenia gravis. Neurology 1988; 38:514–517.

69. Roses A, Olanow W, McAdams M, Lane R. No direct correlation between serum antiacetylcholine receptor antibody levels and clincal state of individ-

ual patients with myasthenia gravis. Neurology (NY) 1981; 31:220–224.

70. Kornfeld P, Nall J, Smith H, et al. Acetylcholine receptor antibodies in myasthenia gravis. Muscle Nerve 1981; 4:413–419.

71. Tindall R. Humoral immunity in myasthenia gravis: Biochemical characterization of acquired antireceptor antibodies and clinical correlations. Ann Neurol 1981; 10:437–447.

72. Ellis K, Austin J, Jaretzki III A. Radiologic detection of thymoma in patients with myasthenia gravis. Am J Roentgenol 1988; 151:873–881.

73. Aquilonius S, Eckernas S, Hartvig P, et al. Clinical pharmacology of pyridostigmine and neostigmine in patients with myasthenia gravis. J Neurol Neurosurg Psychiatry 1983; 46:929–935.

74. Breyer-Pfuff U, Schmezer A, Maier U, et al. Neuromuscular function and plasma drug levels in pyridostigmine treatment of myasthenia gravis. J Neurol Neurosurg Psychiatry 1990; 53:502–506.

75. Olanow C, Lane R, Roses A. Thymectomy in late-onset myasthenia gravis. Arch Neurol 1982; 39:82–83.

76. Mulder D, Graves M, Herrmann C. Thymectomy for myasthenia gravis: Recent observations and comparisons with past experience. Ann Thorac Surg 1989; 48:551–555.

77. Dau P, Lindström J, Cassel C, et al. Plasmapheresis and immunosuppressive drug therapy in myasthenia gravis. N Engl J Med 1977; 297:1134–1140.

78. Nielsen V, Paulson O, Rosenkvist J, et al. Rapid improvement of myasthenia gravis after plasma exchange. Ann Neurol 1982; 11:160–169.

79. Fateh-Moghadam A, Wick M, Besinger U, Geursen R. High dose intravenous gamma globulin for myasthenia gravis. Lancet 1984; 1:848–849.

80. Gajdos P, Outin H, Elkharrat D, et al. High dose intravenous gamma globulin for myasthenia gravis. Lancet 1984; 1:406–407.

81. Ippoliti G, Cosi V, Piccolo G, et al. High dose intravenous gamma globulin for myasthenia gravis. Lancet 1984; 2:809.

82. Arsura E, Bick A, Brunner N, Grob D. Effects of repeated doses of intravenous immunoglobulin in myasthenia gravis. Am J Med Sci 1988; 295:438–443.

83. Arsura E. Experience with intravenous immunoglobulins in myasthenia gravis. Clin Immunol Immunopathol 1989; 53:S170–S179.

84. Mertens H, Hertel G, Reuther P, Ricker K. Effect of immunosuppressive drugs (azothioprine). Ann NY Acad Sci 1981; 377:691–697.

85. Howard J. Non-steroidal immunosuppressive therapy for myasthenia gravis. Semin Neurol 2:265–269.

86. Tindall RS, Rollins JA, Phillips JT, et al. Preliminary results of a double-blind, randomized, placebo-controlled trial of cyclosporine in myasthenia gravis. N Eng J Med 1987; 316(12):719–724.

87. Pinching A, Peters D. Remission in myasthenia gravis following plasma exchange. Lancet 1976; 2:1373–1376.

88. Vincent A, Lang B, Newsom-Davis J. Autoimmunity to the voltage-gated calcium channel anomalies: The Lambert-Eaton myasthenic syndrome, a paraneoplastic disorder. Trends Neurol 1989; 12:496–502.

89. Newsom-Davis J. Lambert-Eaton myasthenic syndrome: a review. Monographs in Allergy 25:116–124.

90. Fukunaga H, Engel A, Osame M, Lambert E. Paucity and disorganization of pre-synaptic membrane active zones in the Lambert-Eaton myasthenic syndrome. Muscle Nerve 1982; 5:686–697.

91. Eaton L, Lambert E. Electromyography and electrical stimulation of nerves in diseases of motor unit: Observations in myasthenic syndrome associated with malignant tumors. JAMA 1957; 163:1117–1121.

92. O'Neill J, Murray N, Newsom-Davis J. The Lambert-Eaton myasthenic syndrome: A review of 50 cases. Brain 1988; 111:577–596.

93. Rubenstein A, Horowitz S, Bender A. Cholinergic dysautonomia and Eaton-Lambert syndrome. Neurology 1979; 29:720–723.

94. Bromberg MB, Albers JW, McCune WJ. Transient Lambert-Eaton myasthenic syndrome associated with systemic lupus erythematosus. Muscle Nerve 1989; 12:15–19.

95. Hausmanowa-Petrusewicz I, Chorzelski T, Strugalska H. Three-year observation of a myasthenic syndrome concurrent with other autoimmune syndromes in a patient with thymoma. J Neurol Sci 1969; 9:273–284.

96. Ketz E, Fopp M, Weissert M, Bekier A. Polymyositis, myasthenic syndrome and thymoma in a patient with defective cell-mediated immunity. Acta Neurol Belg 1979; 79:469–474.

97. Henriksson K, Nilsson O, Rosén I, Schiller H. Clinical, neurophysiological and morphological findings in Eaton-Lambert syndrome. Acta Neurol Scand 1977; 56:117–140.

98. Jenkyn L, Brooks P, Forcier R, et al. Remission of the Lambert-Eaton syndrome and small cell anaplastic carcinoma of the lung induced by chemotherapy and radiotherapy. Cancer 1980. 46:1123–1127.

99. Berglund S, Eriksson M, von Eyben F, et al. Remission by chemotherapy of the Eaton-Lambert myasthenic syndrome in a patient with small cell bronchogenic carcinoma. Acta Med Scand 1982; 212:429–432.

100. Dau P, Denys E. Plasmapheresis and immunosuppressive drug therapy in the Eaton-Lambert syndrome. Ann Neurol 1982; 11:570–575.

101. Streib E, Rothner AD. Eaton-Lambert myasthenic syndrome: Long-term treatment of three patients with prednisone. Ann Neurol 1981; 10:448–453.

102. Lang B, Newsom-Davis J, Wray D, et al. Autoimmune aetiology for myasthenic (Eaton-Lambert) syndrome. Lancet 1981; 2:224–226.

103. Murray N, Newsom-Davis J. Treatment with oral 4-aminopyridine in disorders of neuromuscular transmission. Neurology (NY) 1981; 31:265–271.

104. Sanders D, Kim Y, Howard J, Goetsch C. Eaton-Lambert syndrome: A clinical and electrophysiological study of a patient treated with 4-aminopyridine. J Neurol Neurosurg Psychiatr 1980; 43:978–985.

105. Lundh H, Nilsson O, Rosen I. Novel drug of choice in Eaton-Lambert syndrome. J Neurol Neurosurg Psychiatry 1983; 40:684–685.

106. Oh S, Kim K. Guanidine hydrochloride in the Eaton-Lambert syndrome: Electrophysiologic improvement. Neurology (Minn) 1983; 23:1084–1090.

107. Seybold M, Lindstrom J. Myasthenia gravis in infancy. Neurology 1981; 31:476–480.

108. Provenzano C, Arancio O, Evoli A, et al. Familial autoimmune myasthenia gravis with different pathogenetic antibodies. J Neurol Neurosurg Psychiatry 1988; 51:1228–1230.

109. Roach E, Buono G, McLean W, Weaver R. Early-onset myasthenia gravis. J Pediatr 1986; 108:193–197.

110. Fenichel G. Clinical syndromes of myasthenia in infancy and childhood. A Review. Arch Neurol 1978; 35:97–103.

111. Ohta M, Matsubara F, Hayashi K, et al. Acetylcholine receptor antibodies in infants and mothers with myasthenia gravis. Neurology (NY) 1981; 31:1019–1022.

112. Engel A. Myasthenia gravis and myasthenic syndromes. Ann Neurol 1984; 10:519–534.

113. Engel A. Congenital myasthenic syndromes. J Child Neurol 1988; 3:233–246.

114. Engel A. Congenital disorders of neuromuscular transmission. Semin Neurol 1990; 10:12–26.

115. Robertson W, Chun R, Kornguth S. Familial infantile myasthenia. Arch Neurol 1980; 37:117–119.

116. Engel A, Lambert E, Gomez M. A new myasthenic syndrome with end-plate acetylcholinesterase deficiency, small nerve terminals and reduced acetylcholine release. Ann Neurol 1977; 1:315–330.

117. Engel A, Lambert E, Mulder D, et al. A newly recognized congenital myasthenic syndrome attributed to a prolonged open time of the acetylcholine-induced ion channel. Ann Neurol 1982; 11:553–569.

118. Vincent A, Cull-Candy S, Newsom-Davis J, et al. Congenital myasthenia: End-plate acetylcholine receptors and electrophysiology in 5 cases. Muscle Nerve 1981; 4:306–318.

119. Smit L, Jennekens F, Veldman A, Barth P. Paucity of secondary synaptic clefts in a case of congenital myasthenia with multiple contractures: Ultrasound morphology of a developmental disorder. J Neurol Neurosurg Psychiatry 1984; 47:1091–1097.

120. Albers J, Faulkner J, Dorovini-Zis K, et al. Abnormal neuromuscular transmission in an infantile myasthenic syndrome. Ann Neurol 1984; 16:28–34.

121. Howard BD, Gunderson Jr CB. Effects and mechanisms of polypeptide neurotoxins that act presynaptically. Ann Rev Pharmacol Toxicol 1980; 20:307–336.

122. Simpson L. Kinetic studies on the interaction between botulinum toxin type A and the cholinergic neuromuscular junction. J Pharmacol Exp Ther 1980; 212:16–21.

123. Cull-Candy S, Lundh H, Thesleff S. Effects of botulinum toxin on neuromuscular transmission in the rat. J Physiol 1976; 260:177–203.

124. Boroff D, Del Castillo J, Evoy W, Steinhardt R. Observations on the action of type A botulinum toxin of frog neuromuscular junctions. J Physiol 1974; 240:227–253.

125. Sellin L. The action of botulinum toxin at the neuromuscular junction. Med Biol 1981; 59:11–20.

126. Swift T, Rivner M. Infectious diseases of nerve. In: Vinken PJ, Bruyn GW, Klawuns HL (eds.). Handbook of clinical neurology. 51 Amsterdam: Elsevier Publishing, 1987:179–194.

127. Sakaguchi G. Clostridium botulinum toxins. Pharmacol Therap 1983; 19:165–194.

128. Barker W Jr, Weissmann J, Dowell V Jr, Kautter et al. Type B botulism outbreak caused by a commercial food product—West Virginia and Pennsylvania. JAMA 1977; 237(5):456–459.

129. Cherington M. Electrophysiologic methods as an aid in diagnosis of botulism: A review. Muscle Nerve 1982; 5(9S):S28–S29.

130. Oh S. Botulism: Electrophysiological studies. Ann Neurol 1977; 1(5):481–485.

131. Gutmann L, Pratt L. Pathophysiologic aspects of human botulism. Arch Neurol 1976; 33(3):175–179.

132. Simpson L. A preclinical evaluation of aminopyridines as putative therapeutic agents in the treatment of botulism. Infec Immun 1986; 52:858–862.

133. Oh S, Halsey J, Briggs D. Guanidine in type B botulism. Arch Intern Med 1975; 135:726–728.

134. Hikes D, Manoli A. Wound botulism. J Trauma 1981; 21:68–71.

135. Rapoport S, Watkins P. Descending paralysis resulting from occult wound botulism. Ann Neurol 1984; 16:359–361.

136. Arnon S. Infant botulism. Ann Radiol Med 1980; 31:541–560.

137. Wilson R, Morris J Jr, Snyder J, Feldman R. Clinical characteristics of infant botulism in the United States: A study of the non-California cases. Pediatr Infect Dis 1982; 4:148–150.

138. Arnon S, Midura T, Damus K, et al. Honey and other environmental risk factors for infant botulism. J Pediatr 1979; 94:331–336.

139. Arnon S, Damus K, Thompson B, et al. Protective role of human milk against sudden death from infant botulism. Pediatrics 1982; 100:568–573.

140. Arnon S, Midura T, Damus K, et al. Intestinal infection and toxin production by *Clostridium botulinum* as one cause of sudden infant death syndrome. Lancet 1978; 1:1273–1277.

141. Cornblath, D, Sladky, J, Sumner A. Clinical electrophysiology of infantile botulism. Muscle Nerve 1983; 6:448–452.

142. Simpson L. Botulinum toxin and tetanus toxin recognized similar membrane determinants. Brain Res 1984; 305:177–180.

143. Fernandez J, Ferrandiz M, Larrea L, Ramio R, Boada M. Cephalic tetanus studied with single fibre EMG. J Neurol Neurosurg Psychiatry 1983; 46:862–866.

144. Oliveira M, Fontana M, Giglio J, Corrado A. Effects of the venom of the Brazilian scorpion, *Titysus serrulatus* and two of its functions on the isolated diaphragm of the rat. Gen Pharmacol 1989; 20:205–210.

145. Erxleben C, Rathmayer W. Effects of the sea anemone, *Anemonia sulcata* toxin II on skeletal muscle and on neuromuscular transmission. Toxicon 1984; 22:387–399.

146. Swift AEB, Swift TR. Ciguatera. J Toxicol Clin Toxicol; in press.

147. Fontana MD, Vital-Brasil O. Mode of action of Phoneutria nigriventer spider venom at the isolated phrenic nerve-diaphragm of the rat. Brazilian J Med Biol Res 1985; 18:557–565.

148. Anderson A, Harvey A. Effects of the potassium channel blocking dendrotoxins on acetylcholine release and motor nerve terminal activity. Br J Pharmacol 1988; 93:215–221.

149. Wu C, Tsai MC, Chen M, et al. Actions of dendrotoxin on K$^+$ channels and neuromuscular transmission in *Drosophilia Melanogaster* and its effects in synergy with K$^+$ channel-specific drugs and mutations. J Exp Biol 1989; 147:21–41.

150. Marshall D, Harvey A. Block of potassium channels and facilitation of acetylcholine release at the neuromuscular junction by the venom of the scorpion, *Pandinus Imperator*. Toxicon 1989; 27:493–498.

151. Gillespie J, Hutter O. The actions of 4-aminopyridine on the delayed potassium current in skeletal muscle fibres. J Physiol (Lond) 1975; 252:70–71P.

152. Mollier P, Chwetzoff S, Bouet F, et al. Tryptophan 110, a residue involved in the toxic activity but not in the enzymatic activity of notexin. Eur J Biochem 1989; 185:263–270.

153. Olivera B, Gray W, Zeikus R, et al. Peptide neurotoxins from fish-hunting cone snails. Science 1985; 230:1338–1343.

154. Sano K, Enomoto K, Maeno T. Effects of synthetic omega conotoxin, a new type Ca^{++} antagonist, on

155. Leys K, Lang B, Johnston I, Newsom-Davis J. Calcium channel autoantibodies in the Lambert-Eaton myasthenic syndrome. Ann Neurol 1991; 29(3):307–314.

156. Fiekers J. Effects of the aminoglycoside antibiotics, streptomycin and neomycin, on neuromuscular transmission I: Pre-synaptic considerations. J Pharmacol Exp Ther 1983; 225:487–495.

157. Atchison W, Adgate L, Beaman C. Effects of antibiotics on uptake of calcium into isolated nerve terminals. J Pharmacol Exp Ther 1988; 245:394–401.

158. Singh Y, Marshall I, Harvey A. The mechanisms of the muscle paralysing actions of antibiotics, and their interaction with neuromuscular blocking agents. Drug Metab Drug Inter 1980; 3:129–153.

159. Lee S, Ho S. Acute effects of verapamil on neuromuscular transmission in patients with myasthenia gravis. Proc Nat Sci Council, Republic of China (B) 1987; 11:307–312.

160. Akasu T. The effects of substance P on neuromuscular transmission in the frog. Neurosci Res 1986; 3:275–284.

161. Chang CC, Lin SO, Hong SJ, Chiou LC. Neuromuscular block by verapamil and diltiazem and inhibition of acetylcholine release. Brain Res 1988; 454:332–339.

162. Adams RJ, Rivner MH, Salazar J, Swift TR. Effects of oral calcium antagonists on neuromuscular transmission. Neurology 1984; 34(1):132.

163. Krendel DA. Hypermagnesemia and neuromuscular transmission. Semin Neurol 1990; 10:42–45.

164. Ramanathan J, Sibai BM, Pillai R, Angel JJ. Neuromuscular transmission studies in pre-eclamptic women receiving magnesium sulfate. Am J Obstet Gynecol 1988; 158:40–46.

165. Bashuk RG, Krendel DA. Myasthenia gravis presenting as weakness after nagnesium administration. Muscle Nerve 1990; 13:708–712.

166. Jinnai K, Takahashi K, Fujita T. Enhancement of spontaneous acetylcholine release from motor nerve terminal by calmodulin inhibitors. Eur J Pharmacol 1986; 130:197–201.

167. Hattori T, Maehashi H. Facilitation of frog neuromuscular transmission by sodium fluoride. Br J Pharmacol 1987; 92:513–519.

168. Wiegand H, Csicsaky M, Krämer U. The action of thallium acetate on neuromuscular transmission in the rat phrenic nerve-diaphragm preparation. Arch Toxicol 1984; 55:55–58.

169. Manalis RS, Cooper GP, Pomeroy SC. Effects of lead on neuromuscular transmission in the frog. Brain Res 1984; 294:95–109.

170. Swift TR, Ignacio OJ. Tick paralysis: Electrophysiologic studies. Neurology (Minn) 1975; 25:1130–1133.

frog and mouse neuromuscular transmission. Eur J Pharmacol 1987; 141:235–241.

171. Morris H. Tick paralysis: Electrophysiologic measurements. Southern Med J 1977; 70:121–122.

172. Mebs D. Snake venoms: Toolbox of the neurobiologist. Endeavour, 1989; 13:157–161.

173. Renner P, Caratsch CG, Waser PG, et al. Presynaptic effects of the pardaxins, polypeptides isolated from the gland secretions of the flatfish, *Pardachirus Marmoratus*. Neuroscience 1987; 23:319–325.

174. Piek T. Arthropod venoms as tools for the study of neuromuscular transmission. Comp Biochem Physiol 68C:75–84.

175. Sutherland SK. The management of Gites by the Sidney Funnel-web spider, *Atrax robustus*. Med J Aust 1978; 1:148–150.

176. Atchison WD, Narahashi T, Vogel SM. End-plate blocking actions of lophotoxin. Br J Pharmacol 1984; 82:667–672.

177. Chang CC, Su MJ, Hong SJ, et al. A comparison of the antagonisms by neostigmine and diaminopyridine against the neuromuscular block caused by cobratoxin and (+) tubocurarine. J Pharmacolog Pharmacol 1978; 38:153–155.

178. McManus OB, Musick JR. Postsynaptic block of frog neuromuscular transmission by conotoxin GI. J Neurosci 1985; 5:110–116.

179. Warnick JE, Malegue MA, Albuquerque EX. Interaction of bicyclo-octane analogs of Amantadine with ionic channels of the nicotinic acetylcholine receptor and electrically excitable membrane. J Pharmacol Exp Therap 1984; 228:73–79.

180. Swanson KL, Albuquerque EX. Nicotinc acetylcholine receptor ion channel by cocaine: The mechanism of synaptic action. J Pharmacol Exp Ther 1987; 243:1202–10.

181. Chiou LC, Chang CC. Effect of clonidine on neuromuscular transmission and the nicotinic acetylcholine receptor. Proc Nat Sci Council, Republic of China (B) 1984; 8:148–154.

182. Enomoto KI, Edwards C. Thiamine blockade of neuromuscular transmission. Brain Res 1985; 358:316–323.

183. Posas HN, Rivner MH, Meador KJ. Stimulated single fiber EMG abnormalities induced by megadose thiamine. Muscle Nerve 1990; 13(9):879.

184. Lee DC, Kim YI, Liu HH, Johns TR. Presynaptic and postsynaptic actions of Procainamide on neuromuscular transmission. Muscle Nerve 1983; 6:442–447.

185. Edeson RO, Madsen BW, Milne RK, Le-Dain AC. Verapamil, neuromuscular transmission and the nicotinic receptor. Eur J Pharmacol 1988; 151:301–306.

186. Edeson R, Madsen B, Milne R. Verapamil alters the amplitude and time course of miniature end plate current. Neuropharmacology 1985; 24:561–565.

187. Anderson AJ, Harvey AL, Mbugua PM. Effects of fasciculin 2, an anticholinesterase polypeptide from green mamba venom, on neuromuscular transmission in mouse diaphragm preparations. Neurosci Lett 1985; 54:123–128.

188. Rousseaux CG, Dua AK. Pharmacology of HI-6, an H-series oxime. Can J Physiol Pharmacol 1989; 67:1183–1189.

189. Besser R, Gutman L, Weilemann LS. Inactivation of end-plate acetylcholinesterase during the course of organophosphate intoxication. Arch Toxicol 1989; 63:412–415.

190. Besser R, Vogt T, Gutmann L. Pancuronium improves the neuromuscular transmission defect of human organophosphate intoxication. Neurology 1990; 40:1275–1277.

191. Tsai MC. A pharmacological study of the effect of carbamazepine on neuromuscular transmission in the rat diaphragm. Neuropharmacology 1985; 24:345–351.

192. Alkadhi KA. Effects of emetine and dehydroemetine at the frog neuromuscular junction. Eur J Pharmacol 1987; 138:257–264.

193. Dalkara T, Onur R. Facilitatory effects of Dexamethasone on neuromuscular transmission. Exp Neurol 1987; 95:116–125.

194. Robberecht W, Bednarik J, Bourgeois P, et al. Myasthenic syndrome caused by direct effect of chloroquine on neuromuscular junction. Arch Neurol 1989; 46:464–468.

195. Adewunmi CO, Ojewole JAO. Effects of Oxamniquine on neuromuscular transmission. Arch Intern Pharmacodyn 1985; 275:231–237.

196. Nandakumar NV, Pagala MKD, Venkatachari SAT, et al. Effect of Cleistanthus Collinus leaf extract on neuromuscular function of the isolated mouse phrenic nerve diaphragm. Toxicology 1989; 27:1219–1228.

197. Nilsson E, Paloheimo M, Müller K, Heinonen J. Halothane-induced variability in the neuromuscular transmission of patients with myasthenia gravis. Acta Anaesthesiol 1989; 33:395–401.

198. Fawcett PRW, McLachlan SM, Nicholson LUB, Argov Z, et al. D-Penicillamine-associated myasthenia gravis: Immunological and electrophysiological studies. Muscle Nerve 1982; 5:328–334.

199. Katz LJ, Lesser RL, Merikangas JR, Silverman JP. Ocular myasthenia gravis after D-Penicillamine administration. Br J Ophthalmol 1989; 73:1015–1018.

200. Bever CT, Chang HW, Penn AS, et al. Penicillamine-induced myasthenia gravis: Effects of penicillamine on acetylcholine receptor. Neurology 1982; 198(32):1077–1082.

201. Albers JW, Beals CA, Levine SP. Neuromuscular transmission in rheumatoid arthritis, with and without penicillamine treatment. Neurology (NY) 1981; 31:1562–1564.

24

Myopathies

Charles K. Jablecki

CONTENTS

ACRONYMS

ADP	adenosine diphosphate
AMP	adenosine monophosphate
ATP	adenosine triphosphate
CK	creatine kinase
CPT	carnitine palmityltransferase deficiency
CRD	complex repetitive myotonia
CSF	cerebrospinal fluid
EDC	extensor digitorum communis
EDX	electrodiagnostic
EMG	electromyography
FSH	facioscapulohumeral
IMP	inosine-5'-monophosphate
MADA	myoadenylate deaminase
MUAP	motor unit action potentials
SP	scapuloperoneal dystrophy

Myopathies are diseases of diverse causes that affect primarily skeletal muscle cells. The term *myopathy* usually brings to mind a typical clinical picture. There is symmetric, proximal limb and girdle muscle weakness and atrophy, and the legs are more affected than the arms. The muscle stretch reflexes and sensation are preserved, and there are no fasciculations. In the typical myopathy, the sensory and motor nerve conduction studies, including repetitive nerve stimulation studies, are normal. Concentric needle electromyography (EMG) usually shows normal spontaneous activity or sparse fibrillation potential activity.[1,2] The motor unit action potentials (MUAPs) are of short duration and low amplitude and are polyphasic or serrated[3,4] (Figure 24.1).

This classic concept of the usual clinical presentation of a myopathy arose from the studies of polymyositis, limb-girdle dystrophy, and endocrine (thyroid, corticosteroid) myopathies. There are many myopathies, however, that do not fit that description, and the aforementioned characterization applies to less than half of the myopathies discussed in this chapter. The diverse presentations of myopathies include the following additional symptoms and signs: (1) asymmetric limb-girdle weakness, (2) primary distal weakness, (3) focal muscle weakness, (4) episodic weakness, (5) episodic muscle pain during or after exercise, (6) muscle cramps, (7) delayed relaxation of contracted muscles (myotonia), and (8) hypotonia or generalized weakness in infants.

The diagnosis of myopathies is not an exact science because in most cases the specific biochemical defects are not known. In the absence of a demonstrable biochemical defect, the diagnosis is based on a combination of findings in four areas: clinical picture, electrophysiology, pathology, and genetics.[5] Nerve conduction studies and EMG are essential parts of the evaluation for several reasons. In most cases, electrodiagnostic studies permit the distinction to be made between disorders of nerve, muscle, or the neuromuscular junction as the cause of muscle weakness. It may not be possible to make this distinction in any other way, including muscle biopsy. Further, EMG permits the sampling of several areas of many muscles in contrast to a single muscle biopsy; a multifocal disorder of muscle such as polymyositis that is apparent on EMG may be missed by a single muscle biopsy.[6] On the other hand, there is generally excellent agreement between electromyographic findings and muscle biopsy histology.

When a patient's clinical history or physical examination suggests a myopathy, the laboratory evaluation logically begins with electrodiagnostic studies,

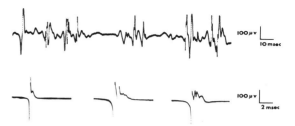

FIGURE 24.1. *Voluntary activity with minimal contraction within the extensor digitorum communis of a 50-year-old woman with myotonic dystrophy recorded in a continuous fashion (upper trace), and isolated, short-duration, low-amplitude motor unit action potentials (lower trace), the center one with a polyphasic configuration and the far right motor unit action potential with a serrated configuration.*

continues with blood studies, and often requires a muscle biopsy. The first objective of the electrodiagnostic studies is to distinguish muscle weakness caused by a myopathy from muscle weakness caused by poor effort, disuse atrophy, a disorder of neuromuscular transmission, motor neuron disease, or a motor neuropathy. When a myopathy is suspected, the second objective of the electrodiagnostic studies is to determine the probable type of myopathy based on the pattern of abnormalities of spontaneous and voluntary activity recorded on needle examination.

With these objectives in mind, the following sequence of electrodiagnostic studies is recommended to evaluate a patient with a suspected myopathy:

1. Sensory nerve conduction study (amplitude, peak latency, conduction velocity) in a clinically affected extremity.
2. Motor nerve conduction study (amplitude, distal latency, conduction velocity, and F wave latency) in a clinically affected extremity, preferably of a nerve to a weak muscle.
3. Repetitive nerve stimulation (train of five stimuli, 2 to 3 per s) of a nerve to a weak muscle before and after 1 minute of sustained, maximal voluntary contraction of the muscle (measurement of decrement, repair of decrement, postactivation exhaustion).
4. Single supramaximal stimulation of a nerve to a weak muscle before and after brief (10 s) maximal contraction (measurement of increment after exercise).
5. Concentric needle EMG of proximal and distal muscles in an upper and lower extremity and

the associated paraspinal muscles in at least one extremity (evaluate insertion, spontaneous, and voluntary activity).

If the patient has symptoms in addition to or other than persistent muscle weakness, additional electrodiagnostic studies are recommended. For example, if the patient complains of episodic muscle weakness, single, supramaximal motor nerve stimulation before and after 5 minutes of exercise monitoring the amplitude (area) of the compound muscle action potential as described by McManus et al.[8] is recommended to evaluate for hypokalemic periodic paralysis. If a patient is seen during an episode of periodic weakness, motor nerve stimulation, direct muscle stimulation, and needle examination are recommended to document a decreased amplitude of the compound muscle action potential and a reduction of voluntary activity consistent with inexcitability of muscle fiber membranes characteristic of periodic paralysis (see section on familial periodic paralysis).

If the patient has frequent muscle cramps, concentric needle EMG of a muscle during the cramp is diagnostically valuable. If electrical activity is noted during the cramp, the problem is probably related to a disorder of the anterior horn cell or motor nerve, although the myopathies of hypothyroidism and some forms of hyperkalemic periodic paralysis are accompanied by cramps with myokymic discharges. On the other hand, an electrically silent muscle cramp strongly suggests a disorder of a muscle glycogen metabolism (see section on disorders of glycogen metabolism).

If the patient complains of muscle stiffness or the clinical examination demonstrates delayed muscle relaxation (clinical myotonia), correlation of the findings on concentric needle EMG with the delayed relaxation of the muscle is extremely helpful in determining whether the disorder is one of muscle metabolism (electrically silent myotonia), electrical instability of the muscle membrane (myotonic discharges, complex repetitive discharges [CRDs]), or electrical instability of the motor neuron (neuromyotonia). This information can be used to narrow the diagnostic possibilities considerably. The results of the electrodiagnostic studies in a patient with a myopathy are as follows:

1. Normal sensory nerve conduction studies unless there is a concomitant neuropathy as described in some *toxic* and mitochondrial myopathies.
2. Normal motor nerve conduction studies except for a low-amplitude compound muscle action potential if there is clinically apparent muscle atrophy.
3. Normal repetitive motor nerve stimulation study before and after exercise unless the electrical excitability of the muscle membrane is altered by muscle activity.
4. A pattern of spontaneous and voluntary activity on needle EMG that helps characterize the specific type of myopathy.

The spontaneous and voluntary activity recorded by needle EMG in myopathies is now discussed in more detail. Spontaneous activity seen in myopathies includes fibrillation potentials, positive sharp waves, CRDs, and myotonic discharges.[2] Fasciculations or myokymic discharges are not seen except rarely in two myopathies: thyrotoxic myopathy and with limb ischemia in hyperkalemic periodic paralyis.[9,10]

Fibrillation potentials and positive sharp waves are commonly seen in inflammatory myopathies, some muscular dystrophies, toxic myopathies, two congenital myopathies (nemaline and myotubular), glycogen storage myopathies, and hyperkalemic periodic paralysis. Experimental animal studies suggest that fibrillation potentials and positive sharp waves occur in some myopathies because focal necrosis of muscle fibers isolates muscle segments from the end plate region; 2 to 3 weeks after isolation, the segments begin to fibrillate.[11]

CRDs are commonly seen in the chronic inflammatory myopathies and in some muscular dystrophies. Single-fiber EMG studies indicate that CRDs arise from ephaptically linked adjacent muscle fibers.[12]

Myotonic discharges occur with delayed muscle relaxation (clinical myotonia) in myotonic dystrophy, myotonia congenita, paramyotonia congenita, myotonia fluctuans, and hyperkalemic periodic paralysis (myotonic form). Myotonic discharges may occur without clinical myotonia in polymyositis, acid maltase deficiency, myotubular myopathy, and chloroquine myopathy. Single-fiber EMG studies indicate that myotonic discharges are generated directly by single muscle fibers.[12] Histologic studies have documented the following changes in the motor unit architecture in muscles of patients with myopathies: loss of muscle fibers, increased variability of muscle fiber diameter, and regeneration of muscle fibers.[13] Interestingly computer simulation of MUAPs based on these histologic changes can reproduce the MUAP configurations recorded in myopathies.[14] It is thought that the architectural changes in the motor

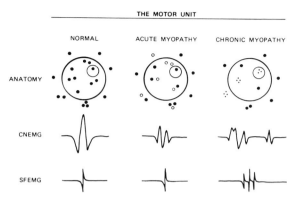

FIGURE 24.2. *Schematic representation of the distribution of muscle fibers in a motor unit in a normal muscle (left), in one with random muscle fiber loss from an acute myopathy (center), and in one with reorganization after muscle fiber splitting and reinnervation from a chronic myopathy (right). The motor unit action potential within the recording area of a concentric needle EMG electrode (large circle) and the synchronized single-fiber potentials within the recording area of a single-fiber EMG electrode (small circle) are illustrated. The various anatomic muscle fiber changes are as follows: solid circles, normal; open circles, denervated; dots, split muscle fibers.*

units are responsible for the abnormal configuration and recruitment pattern of MUAPs recorded by concentric needle EMG in myopathies.[15]

The recruitment pattern of MUAPs in myopathies has been characterized as *rapid* or *increased* to describe the observation that more MUAPs are activated compared with normal muscle for the force of contraction generated.[16–18] This recruitment pattern follows from the effect of the random loss of muscle fibers from the motor units in the muscle. Because the average motor unit contains fewer muscle fibers than normal, more motor units must fire to activate the same total number of muscle fibers. Thus the initial contraction of a muscle weakened by a myopathy is accompanied by the rapid activation of several different MUAPs close to the recording electrode. This pattern of recruitment is quite different from that recorded in a muscle weakened by damage to the motor nerve in which total number of MUAPs is reduced and MUAPs fire rapidly to produce the contracile force.[19] This abnormality of recruitment is as important an electromyographic sign of a myopathy as the changes in configuration of MUAPs usually associated with myopathies.

Low-amplitude, short-duration, polyphasic MUAPs are usually recorded in acute myopathies (Figure 24.2). In chronic myopathies, there may be reorganization of the motor unit with fiber splitting and reinnervation, which produces a decreased number of MUAPs, of which some have high amplitude

and long duration with late components (Figure 24.3).[20,21] Single-fiber EMG studies have confirmed that the electromyographic differences in the configuration of MUAPs between chronic neuropathies and chronic myopathies is one of degree rather than an absolute one. Single-fiber EMG measurements of fiber density and jitter are increased in both disorders, but the increase is greater in chronic neuropathies.[22] Because of this variety of findings, it is best to describe the MUAP characteristics compared with normal findings in each individual case. These characteristics include amplitude, duration, number of phases, and stability of configuration of individual

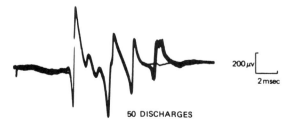

FIGURE 24.3. *Superimposed display of 50 consecutive discharges of a motor unit potential from a weak, atrophic biceps muscle of a 40-year-old man with limb-girdle dystrophy. Note the normal duration and amplitude but polyphasic configuration with one instance of blocking of the last component.*

MUAPs and the pattern of recruitment.[23] Terms such as *myopathic* MUAP and other abbreviations are inaccurate and misleading.

Thus a pattern of findings from the concentric needle EMG examination should emerge on completion of the study. Wilbourn[24] has proposed a simplified but useful organization of myopathies based on the concentric needle EMG findings that forms the basis of the following classification:

1. Normal concentric needle EMG examination (e.g., some congenital, endocrine, and metabolic myopathies—carnitine deficiency, carnitine palmityltransferase (CPT) deficiency, and myoadenylate deaminase (MADA) deficiency; most forms of periodic paralysis between attacks; ocular myopathy).
2. MUAP changes only (increased proportion short-duration, low-amplitude, polyphasic MUAPs) (e.g., oculopharyngeal, facioscapulohumeral (FSH) and scapuloperoneal (SP) muscular dystrophy; most congenital and endocrine myopathies; resolving polymyositis; oculocraniosomatic neuromuscular disease).
3. Fibrillation activity only (e.g., very early polymyositis).
4. Myotonic discharges only: mild/limited (e.g., acid maltase deficiency), prominent (e.g., myotonia congenita).
5. MUAP changes and fibrillation activity (e.g., muscular dystrophy—congenital, Duchenne's, Becker's, limb-girdle, and distal dystrophy; most glycogen storage diseases; nemaline myopathy; myotubular myopathy; active polymyositis, dermatomyositis, and inclusion body myositis; toxic myopathy (alcohol, chloroquine, vincristine, emetine, and colchicine).
6. MUAP changes and myotonic discharges (and fibrillation activity) (e.g., myotonia dystrophy).

It should be emphasized that this classification of the concentric needle EMG findings in myopathies is simplified and that the reader should use it only as a useful guide.

The abnormalities noted here can be documented with monopolar needle electrodes as well as with concentric needle electrodes. EMG with a monopolar needle electrode is generally less painful than EMG with a concentric needle electrode. Most quantitative studies of MUAP parameters, however, have been done with concentric needle electrodes.[25,26] If monopolar needle electrodes are used to evaluate MUAP parameters in a patient suspected of having a myopathy, the findings should be compared with the values reported in the normal population studied

with the same technique. In general, MUAP amplitudes and durations are greater when recorded by monopolar needle electrodes compared with concentric needle electrodes.[27]

The changes in the configuration of MUAPs and their interference pattern are usually assessed *qualitatively* by their appearance on the oscilloscope screen and their sound on a loudspeaker. Methods for the *quantitative* analysis of the configuration of MUAPs have traditionally been complex and time-consuming.[28] With the advancement of computer technology, direct automated analysis of the interference pattern was developed and subsequently has become commercially available. The automated analysis includes measurements of individual MUAP parameters as well as measurement of the relationship between force levels and *turns*, amplitude changes between turns, and other parameters.[29–31] In a limited number of well-established neuromuscular disorders, it has been shown that these techniques demonstrate findings outside the range of normals and that the patterns are consistent with a clinical diagnosis of a *myopathy* or *neuropathy* as the underlying disorder.[31,32] In these studies, the automated *quantitative* analysis of the interference pattern has agreed with the independent *qualitative* assessment by an electromyographer. It has not been clearly shown that these computer-assisted techniques enhance the ability of the clinical electromyographer to detect electromyographic abnormalities in patients with neuromuscular diseases. Thus the *qualitative* analysis of MUAPs and their interference pattern remains the mainstay of clinical EMG. Further, the techniques of automated analysis of electromyographic activity do not compensate for training and experience in the *qualitative* analysis of electromyographic activity.

Although the presentations of myopathies are quite diverse, there are two fairly common presentations, which are discussed in further detail. The first group of patients has selective, relatively symmetric muscle weakness and wasting of long duration. Affected muscles are adjacent to muscle with normal strength. This picture is most commonly caused by hereditary, degenerative diseases of muscle (dystrophies) or of motor neurons (spinal muscle atrophy). The dystrophies are usually distinguished clinically by the absence of spontaneous and contraction fasciculations; electrophysiologically by the presence of a near-normal number of short duration, low-amplitude, and polyphasic MUAPs; and pathologically by muscle biopsies with random muscle cell degeneration. In contrast, the disorders of motor neuron disease may show spontaneous or contraction fasciculations clinically; a reduced number of long-duration, high-amplitude, and polyphasic MUAPs on EMG; and fiber-type grouping on muscle biopsy.[3,7]

The second group of patients with muscle weakness in whom myopathies should be suspected have generalized proximal muscle weakness. The patients may be seen as floppy infants, as children, or as adults. The weakness may have begun abruptly, subacutely, or chronically or have been present since birth. Atrophy may not be prominent. Motor nerve conduction studies, including repetitive nerve stimulations, should be done in these patients in addition to EMG because there are several disorders of the neuromuscular junction with findings on EMG that are similar to those in a myopathy. With repetitive nerve stimulation studies of weak muscles, however, these disorders of neuromuscular transmission (infantile botulism, Lambert-Eaton myasthenic syndrome, myasthenia gravis, and congenital myasthenia) can be identified.[33] Repetitive nerve stimulation studies and tests of motor nerve conduction are usually normal in myopathies, although a decrementing response can be seen in those disorders characterized by myotonia.[34]

Blood studies are conveniently done after the electrodiagnostic study to identify specific causes of myopathies, such as thyroid (serum thyroxine) and adrenal (serum cortisol) dysfunction. Measurements of the serum creatine kinase (CK) level are usually obtained in patients suspected of having a myopathy. A normal serum CK level does not exclude a myopathy: The serum CK level is usually normal in most congenital and endocrine myopathies. Although the serum CK level is usually elevated in inflammatory myopathies, the serum CK level is also elevated in some forms of muscular dystrophy, including limb-girdle muscular dystrophy. Thus the serum CK level cannot be used to make the distinction between an inflammatory and hereditary cause of proximal muscle weakness. Further, elevation of the serum CK level is not specific for myopathy. Serum CK levels are elevated in motor neuron disorders, including spinal muscular atrophy and amyotrophic lateral sclerosis.[35] In normal individuals, aerobic exercise can produce high serum CK levels (greater than 1000 U/L), which take up to a week to return to normal levels.[36]

If the serum CK level is performed after the electromyographic study, it should be done within 2 hours after the test because the EMG procedure itself can produce a slight increase in serum CK levels, which begins 2 hours after the test, peaks in 6 hours, and resolves in 48 hours.[37]

A muscle biopsy is usually performed after completion of the electrodiagnostic and blood studies to make or confirm the diagnosis of a specific myopathy. The preferred site of the muscle biopsy is determined by the clinical features of the disorder with sampling of a moderately, but not severely, affected muscle.[38] Care should be taken to obtain a biopsy specimen of a muscle that has not been examined by needle EMG because inflammatory infiltrates and muscle cell abnormalities that last months can be produced by the slight trauma of the needle electrode.[39]

The needle muscle biopsy technique provides a preferable alternative to the open biopsy technique to obtain muscle tissue for light microscopy, histochemistry, electron microscopy, and biochemical studies, including direct assay for dystrophin.[40] Dystrophin is a large cytoskeletal protein associated with the muscle fiber membrane and is the protein product of the gene related to Duchenne's and Becker's muscular dystrophies.[41]

Because the needle muscle biopsy procedure is rapid and safe, and the scar is less than 1 cm long, the procedure is well accepted by patients, who willingly undergo subsequent biopsies to evaluate the effect of therapies or to provide specimens for additional biochemical studies.[42]

This chapter now turns to a discussion of the clinical and electromyographic findings in the individual myopathies.

MUSCULAR DYSTROPHIES

Muscular dystrophies are genetically determined disorders that cause progressive weakness and atrophy of skeletal muscles.[5,43] The histology of affected muscles shows degeneration of individual muscle cells, internal nuclei, variation of fiber diameter, and infiltration by connective tissue.[44] The pathogenesis of the dystrophies is unknown. Most researchers consider muscular dystrophies to be diseases of muscle; however, in some of the dystrophies, the presence of consistent neural abnormalities has suggested that the disease may be due to disturbances of the trophic function between muscle and nerve and that the more severe manifestations are evident in muscle.[45]

The muscular dystrophies are classified by the following criteria: pattern of inheritance, initial muscle involvement, age of onset, and rate of progression.[45] Most of the diseases are named after the patterns of muscle involvement, although some have eponyms (Table 24.1). Muscle dystrophy should be suspected in any patient with selective muscle weak-

TABLE 24.1. Muscular dystrophies

Congenital (AR)*
Duchenne's (XR)
Becker's (XR)
Oculopharyngeal (AD)
Facioscapulohumeral (AD)
Scapuloperoneal (AD)
Limb-girdle (AR, AD)
Myotonic (AD)

* Inheritance pattern: A, autosomal; D, dominant; R, recessive; X, x-linked.

ness and atrophy. When the disease is advanced, the diagnosis is relatively simple. At onset, however, only a few selected muscles may be involved. The neurologic examination of family members is essential and aids greatly in the diagnosis of a dystrophy. The fact that many of the dystrophies are inherited in an autosomal-dominant fashion makes it possible to establish the presence of similar findings in other less symptomatic individual family members and to confirm the clinical diagnosis. Experience has shown that a simple oral family history is insufficient.

Congenital Muscular Dystrophy

Congenital muscular dystrophy is characterized by generalized hypotonia, muscle atrophy, and contractures at birth; transmission by an autosomal recessive manner; and a muscle biopsy that shows variation of muscle fiber size, central nuclei, and extensive fibrosis and adipose tissue.[46] The serum CK level is usually elevated early in the disease. The sensory and motor nerve conduction studies are normal. EMG shows normal spontaneous activity and short-duration, low-amplitude, polyphasic MUAPs. The course is stable or slowly progressive with development of additional contractures.

Duchenne's Dystrophy

Duchenne's dystrophy is a biochemically, genetically, clinically, and pathologically distinct dystrophy. The disease is inherited in an X-linked recessive pattern; all patients are boys whose mothers are only mildly affected. Pathologically the disease is present at birth, but the clinical symptoms usually become apparent at age 2 to 5 years. Affected young boys have rubbery, hard muscles and mild proximal weakness, which is usually more pronounced in the hips than the shoulders. When the child begins to stand or walk, he has a tendency to fall, and his gait has a slight waddle. As the disease progresses, the patient

has greater difficulty rising from the floor, and he pushes off with his hands (Gower's sign). The patient walks on his toes and develops pseudohypertrophy of the calves. Progressive weakness eventually confines the patient to a wheelchair by age 10 to 12. Death occurs in the second or third decade from respiratory insufficiency, pulmonary infection, or cardiac decompensation in association with marked kyphoscoliosis.[47]

The serum CK level is dramatically elevated (300 to 400 times normal) in the early stages of the disease, but it falls as the disease progresses.[47] Sensory and motor nerve conduction studies are normal. EMG shows fibrillation potentials and short-duration, low-amplitude, polyphasic MUAPs.[3] The nerve conduction studies and electromyographic findings distinguish Duchenne's dystrophy from clinically similar degenerative and inflammatory childhood neuropathies.[3] However, the nerve conduction studies and electromyographic findings do not make the important distinction between potentially treatable polymyositis and Duchenne's dystrophy, with its devastating course and serious genetic implications.[6] A muscle biopsy of the patient is necessary, but routine histology may not be definitive.[48,49] Equally important are the neurologic examinations and laboratory studies of the patient's mother and her siblings to look for evidence of a carrier state. EMG is not as useful as serial determinations of serum CK levels to identify affected female (carrier) family members.[50,51]

The identification of the abnormal gene and its product, dystrophin, now permits direct identification of Duchenne's muscular dystrophy.[41] The muscle biopsy of patients with classic Duchenne's muscular dystrophy contains no dystrophin because the gene with codes for the protein has been deleted. Duchenne's muscular dystrophy may be described as a myopathy owing to dystrophin deficiency.

Becker's Muscular Dystrophy

In 1955, Becker[52,53] described a muscular dystrophy that is very similar to Duchenne's dystrophy. Becker's dystrophy has the same X-linked recessive pattern of inheritance, dramatic elevation of serum CK level and electromyographic findings as are in Duchenne's dystrophy. In contrast to Duchenne's dystrophy, however, Becker's dystrophy has a delayed onset, and patients may survive into adult life. Although there is epidemiologic evidence to suggest this is a separate entity, there are families with Duchenne's dystrophy in which some members follow the less severe course of Becker's dystrophy.[54,55]

An explanation for this clinical heterogeneity lies in the analysis of dystrophin levels in patients with Becker's muscular dystrophy. Becker's muscular dystrophy muscle has reduced but detectable levels of dystrophin, and there is a direct correlation between clinical severity and the degree of dystrophin deficiency. Those individuals with low levels of dystrophin (3% to 10% normal) have a clinical course similar to that of Duchenne's muscular dystrophy, whereas those with higher dystrophin levels (greater than 20% normal) have a less severe course.[56]

Oculopharyngeal Dystrophy

Oculopharyngeal dystrophy is inherited in an autosomal-dominant manner. It has prominent ocular and pharyngeal muscle weakness as well as some weakness of the shoulder and hip girdle musculature.[51] Ptosis is prominent; extraocular muscle weakness is less common.[58] Ptosis usually precedes dysphagia, although the opposite sequence is common in the many cases that can be traced to a single French-Canadian ancestor.[59] The disease usually begins in the fourth to sixth decades and progresses slowly over many years.[60] Histologic studies show variation of muscle fiber size, the presence of small angulated fibers, occasional internal nuclei, and an irregular staining of the intermyofibrillar network with oxidative enzyme reactions giving the appearance of a *rimmed vacuole*.[13] Inflammation may be present in the muscle biopsy, and the serum CK level may be elevated early in the course of the disease.[61] This inflammatory response is seen also in other dystrophies and may be related to a secondary immune reaction triggered by underlying muscle degeneration.[61]

Nerve conduction studies and repetitive nerve stimulation studies of the limb and facial muscles are normal. EMG of proximal muscles usually shows normal spontaneous activity and numerous short-duration, low-amplitude, polyphasic MUAPs with rapid recruitment.[57] As the disease progresses, the interference pattern may be incomplete, presumably owing to further loss of muscle fibers.[62] If the patient is seen early in the course of the disease, examination of other family members may be necessary to make a diagnosis.

Facioscapulohumeral and Scapuloperoneal Dystrophy

The most common FSH syndrome is a familial neuromuscular disease inherited in an autosomal dominant fashion with neurologic abnormalities on muscle biopsy consistent with a dystrophy. FSH dystrophy commonly begins in the first or second decade of life with mild facial weakness, inability to purse the lips owing to weakness of the orbicularis oris, a transverse smile, and incomplete closure of the eyelids. At about the same time or slightly later, the patient develops weakness of the shoulder muscles with selective muscle involvement. Periscapular muscles are involved: the supraspinatus, infraspinatus, rhomboids, serratus anterior, biceps, triceps, and sternal head of the pectoralis major. The deltoids and forearm muscles are relatively spared, resulting in a characteristic appearance comparable to the cartoon character Popeye.[47] Brooke[47] has also described a form of the FSH syndrome that may begin in infancy, progress rapidly, and cause severe crippling weakness.

In the adult form, the serum CK level is elevated in half of the patients; nerve conduction studies are normal.[63] EMG usually shows an increased proportion of low-amplitude, short-duration, polyphasic MUAPs; fibrillation potential activity is rare.[63] Single-fiber jitter measurements in weak facial muscles are normal. Some cases of FSH dystrophy are associated with bilateral weakness of the anterior tibial muscles and footdrop, suggesting that there are forms of FSH dystrophy that clinically resemble SP dystrophy except for the concomitant involvement of facial muscles in FSH dystrophy.[47]

In a group of patients with adult-onset SP muscle weakness and atrophy, it has shown the mild abnormalities of nerve conduction may be present with striking sparing of the extensor digitorum brevis muscle clinically, thus separating the cases from Charcot-Marie-Tooth disease. Careful examination of relatives in suspected cases may provide information to permit identification of the syndrome and its pattern of inheritance.[47]

There are several other diseases that may present with an FSH syndrome. Clinical studies have identified families with electromyographic and histologic patterns compatible with motor neuron disorders, indicating that a form of spinal muscle atrophy may masquerade as FSH dystrophy.[65] Other neuromuscular diseases that can produce weakness in an FSH distribution are congenital myopathies, carnitine deficiency, and inflammatory myopathies.

Limb-Girdle Dystrophy

The diagnosis of limb-girdle dystrophy is a process of elimination. There are numerous diseases that produce the symptoms of progressive weakness and atrophy of the hip and shoulder-girdle muscles. Half of the cases that appear to be limb-girdle dystrophy are in fact due to chronic spinal muscle atrophy.[66] Other disorders that must be considered are late-onset congenital myopathies, mitochondrial myopathies, acid maltase deficiency, carnitine deficiency, polymyositis, and the Lambert-Eaton syndrome.[66] It is possible to separate these disorders from limb-girdle dystrophy and from each other with a combination of family history, examination of family members, serum CK values, muscle biopsies, and electrodiagnostic studies. These other diseases must be carefully excluded before a diagnosis of limb-girdle dystrophy can be made.

The cases that are finally diagnosed as limb-girdle dystrophy remain a heterogeneous group.[47] In some patients, the onset occurs in the second or third decade, primarily in the hip girdle area, with slow progression of over 20 years, with resulting loss in the ability to walk. In other cases, onset is in the fourth decade, and progression is much more rapid, with the inability to walk in a few years. Most forms of limb-girdle dystrophy are autosomal recessive, but some forms are autosomal dominant. Serum CK levels are usually slightly elevated. Muscle biopsies show variation of muscle fiber size, internal nuclei, and fiber splitting. Sensory and motor nerve conduction studies are normal. EMG demonstrates fibrillation potentials and CRDs. This abnormal spontaneous activity, however, is less prominent in limb-girdle dystrophy than in the inflammatory myopathies. Usually there is rapid recruitment of MUAPs that are short duration, low amplitude, and polyphasic. Occasionally in the same patients with the previous findings, there are recording sites where one finds long-duration, high-amplitude, polyphasic MUAPs. This occurrence is probably the result of reinnervation of damaged muscle fibers or regenerating muscle fibers.[62]

Distal Dystrophy

Distal dystrophy is distinguished by the development of weakness and atrophy in the distal limb musculature. The disorder is relatively common in Scandinavia but is rare elsewhere. In 1951, Welander[67] described the clinical findings in 249 cases in 72 pedigrees. The Swedish distal dystrophy is thought to have arisen from a single genetic abnormality and is inherited in an autosomal dominant fashion. The onset usually occurs between the fourth and sixth decades and in the majority of patients becomes symptomatic with clumsiness of the hands with atrophy and weakness. In 10% of the patients, however, the feet are initially involved, with resulting foot-

drop. Men are more commonly affected than women (3:2). The disorder is slowly progressive, but it is clinically limited to the muscles below the elbows and knees. The serum CK level is normal or slightly elevated. The muscle biopsy shows internal nuclei, muscle fiber splitting, and degenerating muscle fibers. Sensory and motor nerve conduction studies in Welander's patients were normal except for low-amplitude motor responses. EMG showed increased insertion activity in affected muscles, although there were no myotonic discharges. This finding was helpful in distinguishing this disorder from myotonic dystrophy, the other common dystrophy with prominent distal muscle wasting. The MUAPs were of short duration and were low amplitude and polyphasic. Even in weak muscles, a full interference pattern could be observed. These observations are quite different from those in patients whose distal muscle weakness is due to spinal muscle atrophy. In 1974, Markesbury et al.[68] described six patients in one kindred with a distal myopathy with early adult onset. They were members of a family in the United States who had physical features similar to those associated with Scandinavian peoples. In 1971, Sumner et al.[69] described five patients in one family with autosomal dominant distal dystrophy with slightly earlier onset (age 15 to 45) and with initial involvement of the hands.

In 1979, Miller et al.[70] described three sporadic cases. These five patients had a disease with an early onset (less than age 35), a rapid course, and the initial involvement of the distal leg musculature. The muscle biopsy confirmed the presence of a myopathy. The sensory and motor nerve conduction studies were normal except for low-amplitude motor responses. EMG in these five patients showed changes in the configuration and recruitment of MUAPs similar to those in Welander's patients. Fibrillation potential activity was much more prominent, however, and probably reflects the rapid progression of the disease rather than the presence of concomitant nerve damage.[69] The primary involvement of distal musculature, normal sedimentation rate, absence of inflammatory changes on muscle biopsy, and lack of response to steroids separate this disorder from polymyositis, which may rarely begin with involvement of distal musculature. Miller et al. suggested that these patients might not have a hereditary origin, although an autosomal recessive inheritance was not excluded.

Autosomal recessive inherited distal dystrophy has been reported in two sisters with early onset of foreleg muscle weakness in their teens.[71] The muscle histology was that of a dystrophy; the electromyographic findings were similar to those in Welander's patients.[71]

Distal dystrophy with autosomal dominant inheritance but with onset in infancy has also been described in several different families.[74-76] Eight additional cases of autosomal recessive–inherited distal dystrophy with onset in the teens and early twenties of weakness in the leg musculature and rapid course, progressing to stepping gait and hand muscle weakness, have been reported.[72,73] Again the electromyographic findings in the weak muscles were similar to those in Welander's patients. Distal dystrophy has several clinically distinct forms distinguished by the pattern of inheritance, age of onset, and site (hand, leg) of onset, which probably represent genetically different family traits.

Myotonic Dystrophy

Myotonic dystrophy, first described by Steinert in 1909, is an autosomal dominant multisystem disease with considerable variability of clinical expression.[77] The onset usually occurs during early adult life. Most patients note the insidious onset of weakness in the forearm extensors, footdrop owing to weakness of the anterior foreleg muscles, or difficulty relaxing muscles after a strong contraction. Dysphagia for cold food such as ice cream and difficulty relaxing forceful eye closure may be described. The evidence of multisystem involvement includes early frontal and temporal balding; less than average intelligence, including an indifference toward the symptoms; posterior subcapsular cataracts; abnormal cardiac conduction; and testicular tubular cell atrophy.

Neurologic examination shows delayed relaxation of muscles (clinical myotonia) that may be observed by percussion of the thenar eminence or tongue and after a strong sustained handshake. Frequently there is wasting of the facial musculature, including the temporalis, masseter, and sternocleidomastoid muscles, which produces a characteristic long face with ptosis, hollow temples, and a hanging jaw. The myotonia is usually enhanced by cold and is reduced with repeated muscle contractions. Less commonly, myotonic muscular dystrophy may present as a floppy infant.[78,79] There is difficulty feeding, swallowing, and sometimes breathing. Clinical myotonia is usually absent in the infant, but in some cases it can be documented by EMG.[80] The infantile form occurs when the affected parent is the mother, suggesting that a maternal factor is essential for its expression.[78] Because of this relationship, neurologic examination of the mother, including electromy-

ographic studies, can provide the diagnosis when similar studies in the infant are normal.

The serum CK levels are normal in early stages of the disease and in infants.[78] The values become moderately elevated as the disease becomes well developed. EMG is extremely helpful in making the diagnosis of myotonic dystrophy.[81] The sensory and motor nerve conduction studies are usually normal. Compound muscle action potentials recording from atrophied distal hand muscles, however, are of low amplitude, and the amplitude declines further with repetitive nerve stimulation of the rested muscle.[82] The decline can be documented in most patients with stimulation rates of 10 to 50 per second and in occasional patients with stimulation at frequencies less than 10 per second, provided that the stimulation train is long enough. The decrement is not present immediately after exercise. This technique is not recommended in the evaluation of patients suspected of myotonic dystrophy because of the discomfort involved. These findings are reviewed to emphasize that the observation of a decrement at stimulation rates of 2 per second and elimination of the decrement immediately after exercise can lead to the erroneous conclusion that there is a defect of neuromuscular transmission in a patient with a myotonic disorder.[83] In contrast to disorders of neuromuscular transmission, however, the amplitude of the compound muscle action potential immediately after exercise is reduced compared with that in the rested muscle (Figure 24.4).[84] Further, reproduction of the decrement with direct muscle stimulation has shown that the decrement occurs independent of neuromuscular transmission in myotonic dystrophy.[82] Because the compound muscle action potentials represent the sum of action potentials recorded from many muscle fibers, the decrement could result from an increasing proportion of muscle fibers becoming excitable or from a progressive decline in the amplitude of the individual action potentials. In goats with a hereditary form of myotonia, intracellular recordings have shown that there is a progressive decline in the amplitude of the compound muscle fiber action potentials with repetitive stimulation. This change in configuration may be related to prolonged afterdepolarization in myotonic fibers.[85] One or both of these mechanisms may be responsible for the decrement seen with repetitive nerve stimulation in human myotonic dystrophy.

Myotonic dystrophy is characterized by the presence of myotonic discharges in affected muscles. The discharges last 2 to 10 seconds and have an initial discharge frequency of approximately 70 per second.[86] Both the amplitude of the potentials and the

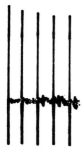 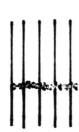

FIGURE 24.4.   *Results of repetitive nerve stimulation at a rate of two per second of the right ulnar nerve in a 50-year-old woman with myotonic dystrophy before (left) and after (right) 30 seconds of sustained contraction. Note the decrementing motor response before exercise and the low amplitude of the initial motor response without a decrementing response after exercise.*

frequency of the discharges wax and wane. The individual potentials in the myotonic discharge have the configuration of positive sharp waves or fibrillation potentials. The sound of the discharges is quite characteristic and aids in their recognition. Myotonic discharges are more prominent in distal muscles than in proximal ones and may be produced by electrode insertion, by percussion of a muscle, and by voluntary muscle contraction. The myotonic discharges may be enhanced by cooling the extremities; sometimes the myotonic discharges are seen only after the extremity has been chilled in ice water for 30 seconds.

Myotonic discharges occur in the infant with myotonic dystrophy, but they have a higher frequency of discharge and are of smaller amplitude, making it possible to mistake the discharges for end plate activity.[79] In some cases of infantile myotonic dystrophy, the discharges were not seen until age 2 or 3.[78] In these cases, it is essential to examine the mother of the infant to make the diagnosis.

The MUAPs in myotonic dystrophy are low amplitude, short duration, and polyphasic. The presence of these abnormal MUAPs serves to differentiate this disease electromyographically from other neuromuscular disorders with myotonic discharges, in particular, myotonia congenita. The distal muscles are more likely to show abnormal MUAPs.[84]

MYOTONIA CONGENITA

Myotonia congenita is characterized by the early onset of painless, delayed skeletal muscle relaxation

accompanied by myotonic discharges on EMG. Because myotonia congenita affects only skeletal muscle, it does not have the systemic involvement seen in myotonic dystrophy. The sensory and motor conduction studies are normal. Repetitive nerve stimulation studies, however, may show a decrementing response, as seen in myotonic dystrophy.[82–84] Also, the different forms of myotonia congenita show a reduction in the amplitude of the compound muscle action potential and the muscle tension immediately after voluntary contractions.[83,84] The electromyographic findings in myotonia congenita are unchanged by cooling the muscle; this observation distinguishes myotonia congenita from paramyotonia congenita, which is dramatically affected by cold.[87]

There are three forms of myotonia congenita. In 1876, Thomsen first described myotonia congenita, a disease from which he suffered, as one with an autosomal dominant inheritance pattern.[47] The onset is frequently in infancy or early childhood and is manifest as muscle stiffness and muscle hypertrophy. Both sexes are affected equally. In Thomsen's disease, the myotonia disappears with exercise. Myotonic discharges in all muscles can be elicited by needle electrode movement, muscle percussion, and voluntary activation. MUAPs are normal in configuration and recruitment. The affected parent has the same electromyographic abnormalities.

The autosomal recessive form of myotonia congenita was described by Becker in 1966.[47] In the autosomal recessive form of the disease, the onset is slightly later but before age 10, muscle stiffness may be more severe, and approximately two-thirds of those affected are males.[88] This disorder resembles myotonic dystrophy because there is a weakness and atrophy of the distal forearm muscles, and pes cavus deformity may be present. As in Thomsen's disease, there are myotonic discharges in all muscles that may be elicited by needle movement, muscle percussion, and voluntary activation. Although the MUAPs are normal in proximal muscles, however, they are small amplitude, short duration, and polyphasic in distal muscles.[89] In contrast to myotonic dystrophy, there is no sign of systemic involvement. The parents of the patients, who are heterozygous for the defect, appear clinically normal. EMG of the parents, however, may show trains of positive waves or myotonic discharges.[90]

In three patients with autosomal recessive myotonia congenita, measurements of the muscle fiber conduction velocity demonstrated a significant decrease with activity and the development of conduction block. This muscle membrane phenomenon can explain the transient paresis with activity after rest and the decrementing response with repetitive nerve (muscle) stimulation described in patients with myotonia congenita.[91] The third form of the disease is a family with autosomal dominant myotonia congenita with painful muscle contractions.[92]

PARAMYOTONIA CONGENITA

In 1866, Eulenberg first described paramyotonia congenita as a rare muscle disease that is transmitted in an autosomal dominant fashion and affects both sexes equally.[47] In his review of 157 patients, Becker stressed that the main characteristics of paramyotonia congenita are myotonia and muscle weakness after exposure to cold.[93] Symptoms are present at birth or in early childhood, and persist throughout life. The muscles of the face, hands, and forearms are the most noticeably affected. The cold-induced myotonia was called *paradoxic* because in contrast to myotonic dystrophy and myotonia congenita, the delayed muscle relaxation is accentuated by repeated muscle contractions.

The patients with paramyotonia congenita complain of muscle weakness and fatigue. Exposure of the muscle to cold precipitates weakness, and flaccid paralysis may develop.[94,95] This weakness often persists for several hours after the muscle has been rewarmed. The paresis is caused by the inexcitability of the muscle cell membrane.[96] These cold-induced episodes of weakness in paramyotonia congenita are similar to those in hyperkalemic periodic paralysis, in which the episodes are induced by elevation of the serum potassium level. Potassium loading producing serum levels above 6 mEq/L, however, does not produce paralysis in paramyotonia congenita.[97] Because the differences between initiating factors have been confirmed at the cellular level, it is apparent that paramyotonia congenita and hyperkalemic periodic paralysis are two different diseases and can be distinguished from each other.[98] It is important to make the distinction between periodic paralysis and paramyotonia congenita because the treatments are different.

In paramyotonia congenita, the clinical myotonia (delayed muscle relaxation) is unique because the mechanical component outlasts the electrical activity by several seconds.[99] The myotonia may be induced by muscle percussion or by voluntary contraction and is much more distinct in cold muscles.[98]

In warm extremities, the sensory and motor nerve conduction studies are normal. When the limbs are cooled, the sensory studies remain normal; however, there is a progressive decline (50%) in the amplitude of compound muscle action potentials, which is accompanied by a corresponding fall in muscle twitch tension.[87,98,99]

EMG in the warm muscle (34°C) may be normal or may show myotonic discharges and fibrillation potential activity, both at rest and following voluntary contractions.[87,98] In the cold muscle (20°C), there is a marked reduction in the spontaneous and voluntary activity. This test is distinctive for paramyotonia congenita and myotonic dystrophy in which the electrical activity is not reduced by cold.[98]

Interestingly continuous electromyographic recordings of paramyotonia congenita muscles cooled from 34° to 20°C showed intense spontaneous fibrillation potential activity before the muscle membrane became inexcitable.[98] This type of spontaneous discharge is identical to that seen in muscles of patients with hyperkalemic periodic paralysis as the muscles become paralyzed in episodes initiated by oral potassium loading.[100] All of these electromyographic findings are consistent with the hypothesis that the basic membrane defect in paramyotonia congenita is a cold-induced depolarization of muscle cell membrane leading to membrane excitability coupled with the presence of an abnormality of mechanical muscle relaxation, which is also aggravated by cold and contributes to the delayed muscle relaxation.[87]

The distinction between paramyotonia congenita and hyperkalemic periodic paralysis has been debated for almost 30 years.[102] There are a sufficient number of distinctions to continue to regard them as distinct entities, although occasional reports indicate that there may be some families with clinical and electromyographic features of both diseases.[102,103]

OTHER MYOTONIC DISORDERS

There are occasional reports of unique familial myopathies in which clinical myotonia is a prominent symptom. Ricker et al.[104] described a family with an autosomal dominant–inherited nondystrophic myopathy with clinical myotonia characterized electromyographically by myotonic discharges but clinically distinct from myotonia congenita, paramyotonia congenita, and hyperkalemic periodic paralysis. In the rested individual, there was percussion myotonia but no grip myotonia and occasional myotonic discharges recorded electromyographically. Muscle stiffness developed 5 to 15 minutes after vigorous exercise. Simultaneous electromyographic recordings and measurements of muscle contraction force demonstrated that the muscle stiffness was caused by myotonic discharges. The clinical myotonia resolved over hours to days. Because of the intermittent nature of the symptoms, the disorder was named *myotonia fluctuans*. Cooling of muscles of affected individuals did not result in muscle stiffness or weakness, in contrast to the effect of cooling of muscles of patients with paramyotonia congenita. Oral potassium loading produced generalized muscle stiffness with myotonic discharges recorded electromyographically, as has been reported in patients with hyperkalemic periodic paralysis, but did not result in muscle weakness, as has been reported in patients with hyperkalemic periodic paralysis. Measurement of muscle membrane chloride conductance in one patient with myotonia fluctuans was normal, in contrast to the abnormal chloride conductance in muscles of patients with myotonia congenita (Thompson's disease). Thus this family appears to have a unique myopathy characterized by exercise-induced myotonia.

FAMILIAL PERIODIC PARALYSIS

The familial forms of periodic paralysis are inherited in an autosomal dominant fashion and are characterized by episodes of flaccid muscle weakness or paralysis. During the attacks, the muscle does not respond to electrical stimulation of the nerve or muscle. The episodes of weakness are usually associated with changes in the serum potassium levels.

Tome,[105] in his review of periodic paralysis, noted that familial cases of periodic paralysis were first described in 1887 by Cousot. In 1934, Biemond and Daniels found decreased serum potassium levels during attacks in one group of patients. In 1956, Gamstorp described another group of patients in whom attacks of periodic paralysis were accompanied by increased serum potassium levels. In 1961, Poskanzer and Kerr reported a family in which potassium levels remained normal throughout attacks. These changes in serum potassium levels with muscle weakness have been used to categorize patients as hypokalemic, hyperkalemic, and normokalemic periodic paralyses. There are some patients, however, in whom this distinction is not clear.[106] In vitro studies of muscle membrane physiology in affected patients have suggested that periodic paralysis is a heterogeneous collection of familial disorders that have similar clinical manifestations.[109]

Hypokalemic Periodic Paralysis

The onset of episodes of hypokalemic periodic paralysis usually begins during the second decade.[110–112] The frequency of the episodes usually declines by the third decade. Although it is clearly inherited in an autosomal dominant manner, the disease is two to three times more common in men than in women. The attacks usually occur at night after a day of heavy exercise. The patient wakes up with weakness or flaccid paralysis of all four limbs. The bulbar musculature is usually spared; however, respiratory insufficiency can develop. Reflexes are reduced or absent, but sensation and consciousness are normal.

Other factors that may precipitate episodes are high carbohydrate intake, sodium, alcohol, stress, cold, and mineralocorticoids.[108] The paralysis may be induced by a subcutaneous injection of insulin with oral glucose. In all cases, there is a time lag between the stimulus and the paralysis. If the stimulus occurs early in the day, the patient will have the attack while awake. The patient senses weakness in the legs, which slowly ascends to involve the arms. If the patient performs mild exercise when the symptoms occur, he or she may delay or abort the attack. Ingestion of potassium chloride in the early phase of the paralysis may also abort the attack.

Between attacks, the neurologic examination and muscle biopsy are usually normal.[108,111] Some patients who have had frequent attacks for 5 to 10 years have mild proximal muscle weakness between episodes.[110] These more severely affected patients have abnormal muscle biopsy specimens with dilated sarcoplasmic reticulum, collections of T system tubules, and vacuoles.[111] The muscle biopsy findings are present both during and between attacks. Lid myotonia and Chvostek's sign have been seen in some families with hypokalemic periodic paralysis.[112]

Electromyographic studies between attacks

Between paralytic episodes, the sensory and motor nerve conduction studies with single supramaximal stimuli are normal. After 5 minutes of maximal voluntary muscle contraction, the muscle twitch tension and corresponding compound muscle action potential amplitudes are reduced.[109] Studies by McManis et al.[113] suggest that this exercise test may be useful to identify patients with periodic paralysis between paralytic attacks. The authors noted a mean reduction of the compound muscle action potential by about 50% during the first 20 to 40 minutes after exercise compared with a decrease in normal control subjects. In one patient, intraarterial infusions of a small quantity (10 μg) of epinephrine produced a 50% to 95% decrease in the twitch tension and compound muscle action potential amplitude; no effect was seen in control subjects. This invasive test, however, is technically difficult and not recommended.

The average muscle fiber conduction velocity can be determined by computer anaysis of muscle activity recorded by surface electrodes. The muscle fiber conduction velocity is reduced in patients with hypokalemic periodic paralysis between attacks. The technique may be of value to confirm the diagnosis and to identify relatives at risk.[114]

Electromyographic studies between paralytic episodes show no abnormal spontaneous activity, including examination of limb muscles in patients with myotonic lid lag.[111,112] Configuration and recruitment of MUAPs are usually normal. However, the more severely affected patients with some weakness between attacks have short-duration, low-amplitude, polyphasic MUAPs in proximal limb muscles.[110]

Electromyographic studies during attacks

During attacks of hypokalemic periodic paralysis, sensory nerve conduction studies remain normal,[115,116] but motor nerve conduction studies become abnormal. The motor conduction velocity remains normal, but the amplitude of the compound muscle action potential falls progressively as the paralysis develops.[117] This decline occurs because the compound muscle action potential does not propagate normally from the end plate region.[111,115,116] The muscle fiber outside the end plate area becomes electrically inexcitable. When the muscle membrane was removed from paralyzed muscle fibers in vitro, the myofibrils contracted normally when stimulated by direct application of calcium.[117] This observation led to the conclusion that the defect in hypokalemic periodic paralysis is the episodic inexcitability of the muscle membrane.

Repetitive nerve stimulation can produce transient improvement of the compound muscle action potential and twitch tension during an attack. With four supramaximal motor nerve stimuli at a rate of 25 c/s, the compound muscle action potential increases up to 50%.[111] Using a proximal nerve block to prevent pain, Campa and Anders[118] performed repetitive nerve stimulation for 1 to 2 minutes at the rate of 10 c/s. They found that the compound muscle action potential of the innervated muscle increased three or four times its initial value and that the amplitude in adjacent, unstimulated muscles remained low. In all the cases, the muscle twitch tension increased as the compound muscle action potential increased. These findings indicate that the clinically beneficial effect of mild exercise during an attack of hypokalemic periodic paralysis is caused by a local muscle membrane phenomenon that results in the transient restoration of impulse propagation in muscle fibers.[118]

As paralysis develops, there is a decrease in insertion activity, and fibrillation potentials are rarely seen.[115,116] The configuration of the MUAP changes as the attack progresses. As the paralysis sets in, there is an increased proportion of short-duration, low-amplitude, polyphasic MUAPs. As the paralysis deepens, there is a reduction in the number of voluntarily activated MUAPs. When the muscle is paralyzed, the MUAPs disappear. As strength returns to the muscle, the events take place in reverse sequence.[116,118]

Hyperkalemic Periodic Paralysis

Hyperkalemic periodic paralysis is inherited in an autosomal dominant pattern and affects both sexes equally.[118–120] Episodes of flaccid paralysis accompanied by a rise in the serum potassium begin in the first decade of life. Gamstorp, in her original description of this disease in 1956, named the entity *adynamia episodica herediteria*.[114]

Attacks are usually precipitated by heavy exercise. The limbs that are more strenuously used are severely affected. The weakness may be focal.[121] For example, after throwing a ball for an hour, the throwing arm alone may become paralyzed after a few hours at rest. When episodes start during sleep after heavy exercise, they are usually generalized. Bulbar and respiratory muscles are usually spared. The attacks may also be precipitated by cold, alcohol, excitement, and ingestion of potassium salts.[121] As in hypokalemic periodic paralysis, attacks can be delayed or aborted by mild exercise at the onset of symptoms. In hyperkalemic periodic paralysis, however, the delay of an attack may lead to a more severe episode.[122]

Muscle biopsy specimens are usually normal or show mild, nonspecific changes. A vacuolar myopathy is seen in patients who have had frequent episodes over several years and who develop mild, persistent shoulder and pelvic girdle weakness and atrophy.[108,119,122,123]

At this time, two distinct familial forms of hyperkalemic periodic paralysis have been identified. Both forms have the paralytic episodes and may develop fixed muscle weakness. The more frequent form has prominent clinical and electromyographic evidence of myotonia—lid lag, delayed relaxation after strong contraction of the eyelids and fists, and delayed relaxation after percussion of the tongue and thenar eminence.[119,122] The other form does not have myotonia.[121,122]

The two forms of hyperkalemic periodic paralysis have been further characterized by the differences in muscle membrane properties. In vitro studies have shown that in both forms, high levels of potassium cause paralysis and depolarization of the membrane.[124–126] In the form without myotonia, paralysis is the result of inexcitability of the membrane. In the form with myotonia, paralysis is due to depolarization block of the membrane; spontaneous activity that was present at rest intensified as depolarization occurred and disappeared when the depolarization block was complete.

Sensory and motor nerve conduction studies including repetitive nerve stimulation at slow rates are normal. EMG shows that between attacks the form of hyperkalemic periodic paralysis without myotonia has normal spontaneous and voluntary activity.[123] During attacks, insertional activity decreases, and the MUAPs decrease in amplitude and duration, the number of MUAPs that can be voluntarily activated decreases, and MUAPs disappear when paralysis is complete.[123]

EMG is distinctive in the form of hyperkalemic periodic paralysis with myotonia. Between attacks, there are fibrillation potentials, trains of positive sharp waves, and myotonic discharges in affected muscle.[101,119,122,125] The myotonic discharges are elicited by needle electrode movement, muscle percussion, and involuntary contraction. As in myotonic dystrophy and myotonia congenita, the myotonic discharges may be enhanced by cooling the muscle.[122] MUAPs are usually normal; they may show a slight increase in the proportion of short-duration, polyphasic MUAPs.[101,122] During attacks, the change in the configuration and recruitment of MUAPs is the same as that seen in the form of hyperkalemic periodic paralysis without myotonia.[101,127]

There is neural hyperexcitability in patients with hyperkalemic periodic paralysis with clinical myotonia. Chvostek's sign and Trousseau's sign may be present.[119] Electromyographic recordings during the development of Trousseau's sign show regular discharges of the MUAPs, which end promptly when the cuff is released.[128]

Normokalemic Periodic Paralysis

In 1961, Poskanzer and Kerr[129] described a family with 21 affected members in whom periodic paralysis occurred without changes in the serum potas-

sium levels. They found that the normokalemic periodic paralysis was an autosomal dominant trait, affected both sexes equally, and became apparent during childhood. Episodes occurred at intervals of 1 to 3 months and lasted up to 3 weeks. The attacks were precipitated by heavy exercise, ingestion of potassium salts or alcohol, cold, and prolonged immobility in one position. The attacks could be prevented or aborted by mild exercise or by ingestion of sodium salts or acetazolamide.

Between episodes, the neurologic examinations were normal with no evidence of myotonia or muscle weakness. Two patients were studied during attacks.[129] The motor nerve conduction velocities were normal. The needle examination showed increased proportions of short-duration, low-amplitude, polyphasic MUAPs in weak muscles. In severely weakened muscles, the number of MUAPs was also reduced. Insertional activity was not increased during the attacks. Muscle biopsy revealed a vacuolar myopathy with tubular aggregates.

There have been other reports of normokalemic periodic paralysis.[130,131] When Brooke[47] restudied some of these patients reported by Tyler, however, Brooke found that they had hyperkalemic periodic paralysis with myotonia. The fact that the serum potassium level is elevated in only about 80% of patients with hyperkalemic periodic paralysis during attacks was probably responsible for this initial confusion.[108] In 1979, Chesson et al.[132] restudied another reported case of normokalemic periodic paralysis and found that some of the patient's attacks were hyperkalemic and some were hypokalemic. Chesson called this form of the disease *biphasic periodic paralysis*. These cases point out the inadequacy of our current classification system based on serum potassium levels. Until the membrane abnormalities are more clearly defined, however, this classification system remains the most useful one.

Acquired Periodic Paralysis

Periodic paralysis may be caused by factors that result in chronic disturbance of the serum potassium levels. Treatment of the causes of the potassium imbalance eliminates the episodes of periodic paralysis. Diuretics, inadequate potassium intake, chronic ingestion of licorice, excessive potassium loss in sweat, and gastrointestinal or renal wasting of potassium can cause hypokalemic periodic paralysis.[105] Renal or adrenal failure, hypoaldosteronism, and metabolic acidosis may cause hyperkalemic periodic paralysis.[105] The important observation is that in these acquired forms of periodic paralysis, the serum potassium is abnormal between attacks. In contrast, the serum potassium level in hereditary periodic paralysis is normal between attacks.

Finally, thyrotoxicosis in people of Asian ancestry can result in hypokalemic periodic paralysis.[133,134] In these patients, serum potassium levels are normal between attacks, but serum thyroxin levels are elevated. During attacks, the serum potassium level falls, and the nerve conduction studies and electromyographic findings are the same as those found during attacks of familial hypokalemic periodic paralysis.[133] These patients, however, do not show the sensitivity to intraarterial injection of epinephrine noted in the familial form of hypokalemic periodic paralysis.[133]

DISORDERS OF GLYCOGEN METABOLISM

Glycogen is the principal storage form of carbohydrate. In normal muscle, glycogen is synthesized to create a store of glucose; subsequent metabolism creates high-energy compounds that are used for muscle contraction and the maintenance of muscle membrane integrity. Glycogen storage diseases are the results of missing or defective enzymes from the glycogen metabolism pathways. To date, 10 glycogen storage diseases have been identified; they have been numbered sequentially as they were discovered.[136] This section reviews the five disorders of glycogen metabolism that have significant muscle involvement (Table 24.2). Often there is an accumulation of glycogen in muscle that can be demonstrated histologically and histochemically. Diagnosis depends on identification of the enzyme deficiency.

The diseases present in two manners.[136] Three of the five (acid maltase deficiency, debrancher deficiency, and brancher deficiency) have slowly progressive muscle weakness that may be generalized or selective. This syndrome is thought to be the consequence of the disruption of the myofibrillar architecture by the accumulation of glycogen in the muscle cells. The other two (myophosphorylase deficiency and phosphofructokinase [PFK] deficiency) show exercise intolerance, with the development of muscle cramps, aches, pains, and myoglobinuria. It has been suggested that this presentation is caused by the muscle's inability to generate adenosine triphosphate (ATP) from glycogen during strenuous exercise. Under stress, the integrity of the muscle membrane is compromised, and rhabdomyolysis leads to myoglobinuria. By far the two most common glycogen

TABLE 24.2. Disorders of glycogen, lipid, and nucleotide metabolism with prominent muscle involvement

Disorders of glycogen metabolism
Acid maltase deficiency
Debrancher enzyme deficiency
Brancher enzyme deficiency
Myophosphorylase deficiency
Phosphofructokinase deficiency
Disorders of lipid metabolism
Systemic carnitine deficiency
Muscle carnitine deficiency
Carnitine palmityltransferase deficiency
Disorder of nucleotide metabolism
Myoadenylate deaminase deficiency

storage disorders that have significant muscle involvement are acid maltase deficiency and myophosphorylase deficiency.

A storage myopathy has been described in which glycogen itself appears to be stored in a nonmetabolizable complex form.[137] The muscle biopsy showed a striking accumulation of polysaccharide material in skeletal muscle with no detectable abnormality of the glycogen pathway. The onset of slowly progressive, primarily proximal limb-girdle muscle weakness was in the thirties. Electromyographic findings were similar to those in glycogen storage disorders, with CRDs and short-duration, low-amplitude polyphasic MUAPs. The weakness was postulated to be due to mechanical effects of accumulated material because no disturbance of energy metabolism has been documented.

Maltase Deficiency (Glycogenosis II)

This disorder is an autosomal recessive disease caused by the deficiency of the lysosomal enzyme acid maltase. The patients appear to be a genetically heterogeneous group with variations of the age of onset from family to family. The age of onset and the severity of the disease are correlated with the degree of reduction of acid maltase activity, which ranges from none to 10% to 20%. Clinically the patients can be divided into three groups.[137]

The most severe (infantile) form (Pompe's disease) has complete acid maltase deficiency and presents as a floppy infant with hepatomegaly and macroglossia; this form progresses to death in less than 2 years. Histologically there are large accumulations of glycogen in all tissues.[137] The second form is first manifest in childhood with delays in reaching motor milestones. There is progressive weakness in limb and trunk muscles; death occurs during the second decade as a result of respiratory insufficiency. The third form presents during the third or fourth decade. Patients have progressive weakness and atrophy of limb and trunk muscles. Fatal respiratory involvement, however, is rare. Because of the distribution of muscle weakness and the course of the disease, this form of acid maltase deficiency may be mistaken for an inflammatory or dystrophic process.

In all forms of acid maltase deficiency, the serum CK level is elevated.[139] Sensory and motor nerve conduction studies are normal.[138,140,141] Electromyographic studies show prominent spontaneous activity; there are fibrillation potentials, trains of positive sharp waves, CRDs, and true myotonic discharges in the absence of clinical myotonia. These findings are widespread in the infantile and childhood forms. In the milder adult form, the spontaneous activity is more apparent in the trunk and paraspinal muscles.[138] Microelectrode studies have demonstrated that the myotonic discharges arise from single muscle fibers.[138] MUAPs are polyphasic and of low amplitude and short duration.[138,140] One adult patient had a reduction in the number of MUAPs with increased duration and amplitude.[141]

The diagnosis is dependent on muscle biopsy and demonstration of acid maltase deficiency by histochemical techniques.[139] In the infantile and childhood forms, there are vacuoles in the muscle fibers that contain periodic acid-Schiff (PAS)–positive material (glycogen). The adult forms may have normal or abnormal muscle histology.[141]

Debrancher Deficiency (Glycogenosis III)

Glycogen is a highly branched molecule. In the normal muscle cell, the configuration permits the rapid use of glycogen during exercise. Two disorders of the branching mechanism have been described.

Debrancher deficiency is a rare autosomal recessive disease in which incomplete mobilization of glycogen takes place. The disease presents in childhood with growth retardation, hepatomegaly, and episodes of hypoglycemia. Hypotonia and weakness develop in adolescence. The weakness is usually proximal, but it may be generalized.[138] Serum CK levels are elevated; nerve conduction studies are normal. EMG usually demonstrates fibrillation potentials and CRDs; MUAPs are of low amplitude and short duration.[139] One patient with prominent distal muscle weakness and atrophy had a decreased number of MUAPs with increased duration and amplitude. Muscle biopsy reveals the accumulation of glycogen

granules in the cytoplasm and PAS-positive material in the vacuoles.[139]

Brancher Deficiency (Glycogenosis IV)

This is another rare autosomal recessive disorder related to the branching of the glycogen molecule.[136] In brancher deficiency, the glycogen structure has a reduced number of branches and is much less soluble. The abnormal glycogen rapidly accumulates in all tissues. The patients are seen as infants who fail to thrive and have hepatosplenomegaly. There may be muscle weakness and atrophy, which is suggestive of Werdnig-Hoffmann disease. The serum CK value is elevated. Nerve conduction studies are normal, and EMG shows an increased number of short-duration, polyphasic MUAPs with scattered fibrillation potential activity. The electromyographic studies serve to distinguish this disorder from Werdnig-Hoffmann disease. Conclusive diagnosis, however, depends on demonstration of the enzyme deficiency in a muscle biopsy.

Myophosphorylase Deficiency (Glycogenosis V)

Myophosphorylase catalyzes the conversion of the skeletal muscle glycogen to glucose during intense exercise under ischemic conditions. In 1953, McArdle described myophosphorylase deficiency, which is usually an autosomal recessive disease.[136] One family was found to have an autosomal dominant inheritance pattern. The male to female ratio of affected individuals is 3:1 in the more common autosomal recessive form.[142]

The biochemical heterogeneity of this disease has been demonstrated. Some families lack the myophosphorylase molecule; other families have a present but defective molecule.[143] Usually the disease becomes symptomatic in childhood; it rarely presents for the first time in adulthood. The symptoms are muscle fatigue and painful contractures after exercise. Following the development of painful contractures, half of the patients note myoglobinuria. Usually the neurologic examination is normal between symptomatic episodes. A few patients have persistent, mild proximal muscle weakness.

Two atypical presentations have been described in two families. A severe form of the disease was seen in a floppy infant; he developed progressive respiratory insufficiency leading to death.[144] A milder form of the disease presented with progressive proximal muscle weakness without the expected painful muscle contractures following strenuous exercise.[145]

The serum CK level is elevated in most patients; nerve conduction studies are normal.[146] Between attacks, EMG is normal in about one-half of the patients; the other patients show scattered fibrillation potentials and short-duration, low-amplitude, polyphasic MUAPs.[147,148]

During muscle contractures induced by vigorous exercise, needle examination shows electrical silence. This important observation distinguishes this metabolic myopathy from other disorders in which during painful muscle cramps, striking, profuse, electrical activity is found.[148] In myophosphorylase deficiency, the muscle contracture may also be initiated by repetitive nerve stimulation at high (50-c/s) rates; this painful procedure is not recommended.[149]

The diagnosis depends on the demonstration of the absence of phosphorylase activity in skeletal muscle by biochemical or histochemical techniques. There may be phosphorylase activity in occasional regenerating muscle fibers; this activity is due to the presence of an active fetal isoenzyme.[150] A PAS-positive material is present in subsarcolemmal vacuoles, and occasional necrotic muscle fibers are present.[44]

Before recent advances in needle biopsy techniques and in muscle histochemistry, the ischemic exercise test was often used.[151] In myophosphorylase deficiency, this test shows a failure of the muscle to produce lactic acid under ischemic conditions. The same results are also seen in muscle glycogenosis VII. The ischemic exercise test is painful and may cause muscle necrosis and myoglobinuria.[47] Therefore this test is no longer recommended for the diagnosis of myophosphorylase deficiency.

Phosphofructokinase Deficiency (Glycogenosis VII)

PFK is an enzyme that catalyzes the phosphorylation of fructose 6-phosphate to fructose 1,6-diphosphate. This reaction is essential for glycolysis and the production of high-energy phosphate compounds. PFK deficiency is a rare, autosomal recessive disease. The clinical findings are similar to those in myophosphorylase deficiency (see under myophosphorylase deficiency).[136] The patients usually present in childhood with easy fatigue and painful contractures of skeletal muscle after strenuous exercise and myoglobinuria. In contrast to patients with myophosphorylase deficiency, however, patients with PFK deficiency frequently have a persistent mild anemia and episodes of nausea and vomiting. The serum CK level is elevated; nerve conduction studies are normal. EMG is frequently normal between attacks. During attacks, there is electrical silence in the painful contracted muscles.[146,150]

The skeletal muscle biopsy confirms the diagnosis. There are subsarcolemmal accumulations of glyco-

gen and no PFK activity. Myophosphorylase activity is normal.

The ischemic exercise test is abnormal; venous lactate levels do not rise during ischemic exercise. This test is now recommended only in cases of suspected disorders of glycolysis in which the biopsies fail to identify myophosphorylase or PFK deficiencies.[47]

DISORDERS OF LIPID METABOLISM

Lipid is an important source of energy in muscle, both at rest and during sustained exercise. There are two well-defined myopathies caused by disorders of lipid metabolism (Table 24.2)[153] Carnitine deficiency and CPT deficiency are rare disorders. Because they are potentially treatable, it is important to distinguish them from other myopathies. These diseases may present with weakness, persistent muscle pain after exertion, or myoglobinuria. In contrast to the glycogen storage disorders, patients with disorders of muscle lipid metabolism do not show contractures during muscle pain, although the muscles may be swollen, tender, and weak. If a patient has these symptoms or signs, a muscle biopsy is necessary to identify a lipid myopathy. In some patients, the muscle histology is normal, and in others, it shows the accumulation of lipid droplets within the muscle cells. The diagnoses of carnitine deficiency and CPT deficiency depend on specialized assays of muscle carnitine concentration and of CPT activity. It must be noted that there are other lipid storage myopathies that have normal levels of carnitine and CPT activity; the defects in these disorders have yet to be identified.[154]

Carnitine Deficiency

Lipid metabolism in muscle involves the oxidation of fatty acids and takes place in the mitochondria. Carnitine acts as the carrier of the fatty acids across the mitochondrial membrane. Carnitine is found in the normal diet (meat especially) and is also synthesized in the liver.

Reduced muscle carnitine levels have been found in both myopathic and systemic forms of carnitine deficiencies. In both conditions, the muscle biopsy specimens usually show a dramatic accumulation of lipid droplets, which are often adjacent to mitochondria and are more frequent in type I muscle fibers.[153] In most patients, the disorders are thought to be inherited in an autosomal recessive fashion.

Systemic carnitine deficiency is characterized by

reduced levels of serum as well as muscle carnitine. DiMauro et al.[153] reviewed this clinical and laboratory feature of eight reported cases. The onset is in early childhood. The disease is progressive and is usually fatal unless it is treated. The symptoms that prompt the patient's parents to seek help are episodes of confusion and vomiting owing to hepatic insufficiency. These episodes occur in the setting of progressive proximal limb and trunk muscle weakness. The serum CK level is increased in most patients; nerve conduction studies are normal. EMG shows short-duration, low-amplitude MUAPs and occasional fibrillation potentials.[155] The diagnosis depends on documentation of reduced serum and muscle carnitine levels. Several specific biochemical abnormalities have been identified that have resulted in systemic carnitine deficiency: defect in carnitine biosynthesis, abnormal renal clearance of carnitine, alterations in cellular carnitine transport or degradation, and defective intestinal absorption of carnitine.[154] In most cases, a good clinical response may be achieved by treatment with oral L-carnitine.[153]

Muscle carnitine deficiency is characterized by decreased concentrations of carnitine in muscle with normal levels in serum.[113] The onset is in adolescence, and there is generalized, slowly progressive, proximal muscle weakness. The serum CK level is usually increased. The nerve conduction studies are usually normal, but abnormalities have been reported in one patient with concomitant clinical evidence of a neuropathy.[156] EMG may be normal or show occasional spontaneous activity (trains of positive sharp waves, fibrillation potentials) and low-amplitude, short-duration MUAPs.[157–159] The diagnosis depends on the finding of normal serum and reduced muscle carnitine levels. One cause of muscle carnitine deficiency is a defect of the transport of carnitine into muscle.[154] Treatment with L-carnitine is effective in some patients.[153] The variability of the responses to treatment suggest that this is a heterogeneous group of diseases.[160]

Carnitine Palmityltransferase Deficiency

CPT catalyzes the combination of fatty acids with carnitine. This linkage is essential for the transportation of fatty acids into muscle mitochondria, where they are metabolized.

CPT deficiencies are characterized by episodic myoglobinuria with muscle pain, swelling, tenderness, and weakness. The episodes are precipitated by fasting and prolonged exercise; the symptoms begin during childhood and adolescence. Between episodes, the patients appear to be normal.[161–163]

The serum CK level is increased during symptomatic periods. An elevated CK level may be induced by fasting; a few patients have elevated CK values when they are otherwise asymptomatic. Nerve conduction studies are normal; EMG is usually normal, but a few patients have shown an increased proportion of low-amplitude, short-duration MUAPs. Abnormal spontaneous activity has not been reported.[161,163,164]

The histology of muscles taken between episodes was normal in two-thirds of the patients; the other third had mildly excessive accumulation of lipid. The diagnosis depends on the demonstration of low levels of CPT activity in muscle. This disease is thought to be transmitted in an autosomal recessive pattern; however, 20 of the 21 reported patients were male. Treatment with a low-fat, high-carbohydrate diet effectively reduces the frequency of attacks.[13,161,164]

DISORDER OF NUCLEOTIDE METABOLISM: MYOADENYLATE DEAMINASE DEFICIENCY

There are several adenylate deaminases in body tissues; MADA is unique to muscle. When adenosine diphosphate (ADP) is converted to ATP, adenosine monophosphate (AMP) is a by-product. If the AMP is not removed, the conversion of ADP to ATP is inhibited. MADA acts as the catalyst in the reaction that converts AMP to inosine-5'monophosphate (IMP) and permits muscle to maintain high levels of ATP during strenuous activity.

MADA activity in muscle biopsy specimens can be assayed histochemically and biochemically.[165] In a variety of neuromuscular diseases that cause muscle destruction, there is decreased MADA activity.[166]

Absence of MADA activity has been reported in two clinical syndromes.[165,167] One group presents as floppy infants with subsequent delayed attainment of motor milestones, persistent hypotonia, and generalized muscle weakness. The serum CK level is normal, and EMG may be normal or show nonspecific abnormalities (they were not described).[165] The other group presents with intolerance to exercise that produces myalgias, muscle stiffness, and soreness. These symptoms begin during adolescence or young adulthood. Between episodes, the neurologic examination is normal; there is no muscle weakness, atrophy, or hypotonia. The serum CK level is normal at rest, but it may be elevated by exercises sufficient to cause myalgias. The nerve conduction studies are normal. EMG is usually normal; the occasional abnormalities are mild and nonspecific with trains of positive sharp waves and abnormal MUAP configurations.[165,167]

In both groups, the diagnosis depends on demonstration of the absence of MADA activity in the muscle biopsy. In the group with early-onset signs, the muscle architecture may be normal or may show variation of muscle fiber diameter, internal muscle nuclei, and fiber-type predominance. In the other group, the muscle histology is usually normal. A biopsy specimen, however, obtained in one patient after onset of symptoms caused by exercise, and the biopsy specimen showed occasional internal nuclei and muscle fiber necrosis. The same patient showed elevation of serum CK levels with exercise.[167] The inheritance pattern of MADA deficiency is uncertain. Case reports have been compatible with autosomal recessive[165] and X-linked patterns.[167] Identification of new patients, analysis of family members, and sequential studies of affected individuals are required to understand whether these two groups of patients have different diseases or reflect different expressions of the same biochemical disorder.

CONGENITAL MYOPATHIES

Congenital myopathies are a diverse group of muscle diseases that have distinctive histologic patterns on muscle biopsy (Table 24.3).[168–180] The diagnosis of a congenital myopathy should be considered in all floppy infants and in cases of relatively stable or slowly progressive muscle weakness in adolescents and young adults. The floppy infants show generalized reduction of body tone, with the limbs externally rotated and abducted when the child is supine. When the child is lifted from the supine position, the head falls back; when the child is supported under the abdomen, the arms, legs, and head all droop, instead of showing the normal extension posture. The differential diagnosis of the floppy infant includes cerebral damage, benign congenital hypotonia, congenital myopathies, and other neuromuscular disorders. Determination of serum CK levels and electrodiagnostic studies are useful in the initial evaluation; however, the diagnosis of a congenital myopathy requires a muscle biopsy. Several congenital myopathies have been discovered by this aggressive approach to the diagnosis of floppy infants and young adults with relatively stable muscle weakness.

The first congenital myopathy to be described was central core disease in 1956.[168] Since then, almost a dozen others have been reported (see Table 24.3). As more congenital myopathies have been described, their clinical profiles have become much more diverse. Even within families, the muscle weakness may become evident at different ages in different family members, and some with biopsy evidence of involvement remain clinically unaffected. Because of this diversity of clinical expression, a congenital myopathy should be considered as a possible diagnosis in a case of slowly progressive, symmetric weakness and atrophy that may or may not have been evident from birth. The three most common congenital myopathies are central core disease, nemaline myopathy, and myotubular myopathy.

Central Core Disease

This disorder was described by Shy and Magee in 1956.[128] The cores appear as well-defined, round, unstained central zones. The cores occupy large areas in type I muscle fibers and are sometimes surrounded

TABLE 24.3. Congenital myopathies

Myopathy	Author
Central core	Shy and Magee, 1956 [168]
Nemaline (rod)	Shy et al, 1963 [169]
	Conen et al, 1963 [170]
Myotubular (centronuclear)	Spiro et al, 1966 [171]
Multicore	Engel et al, 1971 [172]
Fingerprint body	Engel et al, 1972 [173]
Reducing body	Brooke and Neville, 1972 [174]
Fiber type disproportion	Brooke, 1973 [175]
Sarcotubular	Jerusalem et al, 1973 [176]
Cytoplasmic body	Kinoshita et al, 1975 [177]
Zebra body	Lake and Wilson, 1975 [178]
Trilaminar	Ringel et al, 1977 [179]
Spheroid body	Goebel et al, 1978 [180]

by thin, dense rings. Affected patients can develop more core fibers with time. One patient had 3% core fibers at age 4, and all muscle fibers appeared at age 16.[181] There is no clear relationship, however, between the frequency of cores and the clinical severity of the disease.[182] Further, cores characteristic of this disease have been produced experimentally by denervation and tenotomy.[183]

Most patients with central core disease are first seen in early childhood with mild muscle weakness and delayed attainment of motor milestones; a few more severely affected patients present as floppy infants. As adults, the affected individuals show only mild weakness, often primarily of proximal musculature. Some family members with the characteristic histologic findings have only pes cavus or tight heel cords as manifestations of the disorder.[189]

The serum CK level is usually normal. Nerve conduction studies, both sensory and motor, are also normal.[185] EMG in some patients has shown an increased proportion of short-duration, polyphasic, low-amplitude MUAPs.[186] The MUAPs in other patients have been long duration, high amplitude, and polyphasic.[187] Abnormal spontaneous activity has been noted only rarely.[187] The diagnosis depends on muscle biopsy.[168] An autosomal dominant mode of transmission has been documented in most cases.[184,185] Occasional sporadic and autosomal recessive cases have been described.[182,188]

Nemaline (Rod) Myopathy

Nemaline or rod myopathy is a disorder characterized by the presence of rod-shaped bodies within muscle fibers. Two reports published simultaneously in 1963 described this congenital myopathy.[169,170] Conen described the particles as *myogranules*. Shy drew attention to the thread-like (nemaline) undulations produced in the muscle fibers by the accumulation of granules and termed the condition *nemaline* myopathy. Electron microscopic studies demonstrated rod-like structures in the muscle, and the name *rod* myopathy was proposed.[189] Because rod bodies have been documented in diseases quite clinically distinct from nemaline myopathy, it has been suggested that a more significant finding is the predominance of type I fibers with concomitant atrophy.[190,191]

Of the 31 reported patients reviewed by Bender and Wilner,[191] 26 were females. Most presented with the characteristic clinical picture of a floppy infant with both weakness and hypotonia. A high arch palate was frequently present as well as other occasional skeletal deformities in adolescents, including kyphoscoliosis, pes cavus, and an unusually long face.

Generally the serum CK level is normal. Nerve conduction studies are normal.[192,193] Electromyographic studies usually show an increased proportion of short-duration, low-amplitude, polyphasic MUAPs, occasionally with fibrillation potential activity.[169,189] Patients with MUAPs with normal configuration and recruitment have also been seen.[193,194] A longitudinal study of 13 cases of nemaline myopathy reported that the electromyographic findings depend on the duration of the condition: Up to age 3 years, the configurations of the MUAPs were predominantly normal; from age 3 to 10 years, the MUAPs were short duration, low amplitude, and polyphasic; over age 10, most MUAPs were long duration, high amplitude, and polyphasic.[92] The electromyographic findings are nonspecific and indicate the importance of a muscle biopsy to make the diagnosis of nemaline myopathy.

Simple autosomal dominance cannot explain the inheritance pattern of nemaline myopathy, because it is much more common in females than in males. It has been suggested that there is genetic heterogeneity in this disorder.[193] This proposal is supported by the existence of two other clinically distinct profiles of adult-onset myopathies with rod bodies on muscle biopsy: One had SP weakness, and the other had progressive proximal muscle weakness.[195,196]

Myotubular (Centronuclear) Myopathy

In 1966, Spiro et al.[197] described a myopathy with unusual histologic findings. There was a high percentage of centrally located nuclei, with a halo devoid of myofibrils but containing other organelles.[197] Because the fibers resembled fetal myotubules, Spiro called the disorder *myotubular myopathy*. Over 70 cases have been described since Spiro's original report, all identified by the presence of a high frequency of central muscle nuclei.[198] More than half of the cases become manifest during late infancy or adolescence as slowly progressive generalized muscle weakness and atrophy with lordosis and footdrop. One-third of patients have presented with progressive weakness during adult life; rarely the condition presents as a floppy infant with severe weakness and hypotonia. In addition to generalized weakness, some patients have been reported to have ptosis, ophthalmoparesis, and facial weakness.[199,200]

The serum CK level is usually normal. A high percentage of the patients have shown abnormal spontaneous activity on EMG. Fibrillation potentials, CRDs, and true myotonic discharges have been described.[199–202]

Nerve conduction studies have been reported as normal.[200] In some patients, the MUAPs have been noted to be normal.[203] In others, there have been short-duration, low-amplitude, polyphasic MUAPs.[200,204]

Several patterns of inheritance of myotubular myopathy have been noted in different families. Despite the variety of patterns of inheritance, there has been a great deal of similarity in the clinical and pathologic findings.[205] This suggests that different biochemical defects are responsible for the production of each disorder within each family, each with its own inheritance pattern, but that the pathologic and to some degree clinical consequences of the different defects are similar.

INFLAMMATORY MYOPATHIES

Polymyositis

Polymyositis is an acquired inflammatory myopathy of unknown cause. Whitaker[206] indicates in his 1982 review that several pathogenetic mechanisms have been suggested for polymyositis, including a virus, immune complexes, and disorders of cell-mediated immunity. The age distribution curve is bimodal. There are age peaks at 5 to 15 years and 50 to 60 years.[6,206] No single test has been found to be diagnostically definitive. Polymyositis as a disease meets the following criteria:

1. Predominantly proximal, usually symmetric muscle weakness that progresses over weeks or months.
2. Skeletal muscle biopsy shows segmental myonecrosis, regeneration, and a mononuclear cellular infiltrate, with or without perifascicular muscle fiber atrophy.
3. Elevated serum CK levels.
4. Multifocal electromyographic abnormalities (see following).[6,206,207]

Because other inflammatory muscle diseases can produce clinical pictures that meet these criteria, these diseases must be excluded before a diagnosis of polymyositis is made. Diseases to be considered are trichinosis, sarcoid viral myositis, and pyomyositis.[47] Of patients with polymyositis, one-fifth also have an inflammatory collagen vascular disease such as scleroderma, rheumatoid arthritis, lupus erythematosus, or polyarteritis nodosa.[208,209]

Sensory and motor nerve conduction studies are usually normal in polymyositis. In severe cases, there may be low-amplitude motor responses.[210,211] Repetitive nerve stimulation studies should be done. The results are usually normal; however, if significant decrements or increments are recorded, the correct diagnosis may be myasthenia gravis or Lambert-Eaton myasthenic syndrome, which may have clinical presentations similar to polymyositis.[212]

In polymyositis, muscles are affected in a patchy distribution; it is possible to find normal muscle fibers adjacent to affected ones on muscle biopsy.[6] Also, some muscle groups are affected more than others. Therefore different areas within one muscle and many different muscles, including the paraspinal muscles, must be examined electromyographically.[213]

The electromyographic findings vary with the stage of the disease. The findings in the acute phase are spontaneous activity with abundant fibrillation potentials, positive sharp waves, and complex repetitive discharges.[213,215] There is a normal number of MUAPs, and they recruit rapidly with minimal effort. MUAPs are polyphasic and are of short duration and low amplitude.[210,211,213–215] More recent quantitative concentric needle EMG studies have confirmed the increased incidence of short-duration polyphasic MUAPs in acute polymyositis, but the mean amplitude of the MUAPs was normal.[216,217]

The electromyographic findings in the chronic stage demonstrate changes in the MUAP configuration consistent with reinnervation of previously degenerated muscle fibers, probably by collateral sprouts of nerves to muscle fibers isolated by segmental necrosis. Patients examined 2 to 6 years after the initial diagnosis and treatment began showed an increased proportion of long-duration, high-amplitude, polyphasic MUAPs.[5] There was a concomitant increase in the fiber density as determined by single-fiber EMG, and fiber type grouping could be demonstrated on muscle biopsy if the fiber density was greater than 2.6.[210] Thus the electromyographic findings in polymyositis reflect an interaction between random muscle fiber destruction and reinnervation.

There are two atypical forms of presentation of polymyositis. The patients may present with distal or focal muscle weakness.[211,218] There are also several subsets of polymyositis that are characterized by unusual findings on muscle biopsy: eosinophilic polymyositis, localized nodular myositis, and proliferative myositis.[219] The electromyographic findings for all of these disorders are the same as those described earlier.

Dermatomyositis

The diagnosis of dermatomyositis depends on satisfying the four previously described criteria for polymyositis in addition to the concomitant presence of skin abnormalities.[206] In dermatomyositis, there is an erythematous rash over one or more of the following areas: the dorsal surface of the hands, proximal finger joints, elbows, knees, medial maleoli, trunk, neck, and face.[220] The eyelids may have a purple hue. Interestingly there is a higher incidence of cancer in patients with dermatomyositis than in the general population.[221] With the exception of cutaneous involvement and the association with cancer, the clinical features of electromyographic abnormalities are the same as those of polymyositis.

Inclusion Body Myositis

Inclusion body myositis (IBM) is a myopathy that pathologically is characterized by an inflammatory endomysial exudate, rimmed muscle cell vacuoles, and nuclear and cytoplasmic filamentous inclusions (inclusion bodies).[222,223] Clinically IBM resembles polymyositis but responds poorly to steroid therapy.[223,229] Both diseases present as muscle weakness, occasionally with prominent dysphagia.[225] In IBM, however, the clinical course is often relatively benign and protracted; the weakness may be asymmetric; distal as well as proximal muscles are frequently affected; and there may be selective, severe involvement of individual limb muscles.[222,224] In IBM, the serum CK level may be elevated but usually less so than in other inflammatory myopathies.[223]

The amplitude of compound muscle action potentials is low if recorded over atrophic muscles. The motor and sensory nerve conduction velocities and compound sensory nerve action potentials are normal in most patients with IBM. Slight slowing of motor and sensory conduction has been noted in patients in some series, raising the possibility of concomitant nerve damage.[226-228]

Concentric needle EMG studies in IBM demonstrate findings that occur in other inflammatory myopathies: increased insertion activity; fibrillation potentials; and rapid recruitment of short-duration, low-amplitude polyphasic MUAPs. In addition, most patients with IBM also have long-duration, high-amplitude MUAPs in affected muscles. The combination of short-duration and long-duration MUAPs in the same muscle (mixed pattern) is believed by some to be reasonably specific for IBM.[228] Others note that this pattern may be seen in other chronic myopathies and that there is no electromyographic pattern that can reliably distinguish IBM from other inflammatory myopathies; the mixed pattern is believed to reflect chronicity rather than concomitant damage to the motor neurons.[224]

Single-fiber EMG studies of the extensor digitorum communis in seven cases of IBM showed a high fiber density (mean = 6.3) and abnormal jitter (mean = 83 μs).[226] A more recent study of 30 patients showed less striking changes in the fiber density (mean = 2.6) and jitter (mean = 46 μs).[228] The difference in the findings may be related to differences in the degree of distal weakness in the two series of patients; the less abnormal single-fiber EMG findings were seen in a group of patients with primarily proximal weakness and are similar to those found in patients with other chronic myopathies.[228]

Muscle biopsy identification of characteristic vacuoles filled with 15- to 18-nm diameter filaments (inclusion bodies) remains the cornerstone for the diagnosis of IBM.[222,224,229] The finding of identical inclusion bodies in the muscle of a patient diagnosed for 30 years with limb-girdle dystrophy and in the muscle of a patient with new, progressive weakness with previously stable poliomyelitis suggests that IBM should be considered in settings in addition to *steroid-resistant* polymyositis.[230-232]

ENDOCRINE MYOPATHIES

Thyrotoxicosis

Thyrotoxicosis may be caused by a variety of disorders, including thyroid hyperfunction, abnormal thyroid hormone storage, extrathyroid hormone production, and thyroid medication abuse. These disorders produce excessive serum levels of thyroid hormone. Whatever the cause, chronic thyrotoxicosis causes multiple symptoms. The clinical picture includes nervousness, tremor, heat intolerance, palpitations, weight loss, and loss of strength.[233] In thyrotoxicosis caused by Graves's disease, impaired eye movement may be caused by inflammation and fibrosis of the ocular muscles.[234] Some patients with thyrotoxicosis go on to develop either concomitant periodic paralysis with episodic limb weakness or concomitant autoimmune myasthenia gravis with prominent weakness of the bulbar musculature.[133]

Chronic thyrotoxicosis myopathy in the absence of myasthenia gravis is characterized by proximal muscle weakness and atrophy, including the shoulder and hip girdle muscles.[235] The serum CK level and muscle biopsy are usually normal. Motor nerve conduction studies, including repetitive nerve stimulation, are normal.[236] Spontaneous electromyographic activity is usually normal. Rarely there are fasciculation potentials and myokemic discharges.[237] Voluntary MUAPs are short duration and polyphasic.

Treatment of thyrotoxicosis with beta-blocking agents eliminates most of the symptoms; the muscle weakness remains. If the serum thyroid levels are returned to normal for a 4-month period, however, the myopathy resolves, and the MUAPs become normal.

Hypothyroidism

A variety of conditions cause hypothyroidism, which is defined as low serum levels of thyroid hormone. The clinical picture depends on the age at which the chronic deficiency begins. When the deficiency begins at birth, the result is cretinism. When onset is later during childhood, there is growth, maturation, and mental retardation.

Adult-onset hypothyroidism is usually insidious and produces lethargy, cold intolerance, weight gain, and easy fatigue.[238] With exertion, patients may develop muscle pains, cramps, carpal spasms, and pedal spasms; symptoms of carpal tunnel syndrome may develop.[239] The deep tendon reflexes show delayed relaxation.[239] There may be mild proximal muscle weakness, percussion myodema, and development of carpal spasm with limb ischemia (Trousseau's test).[238] Serum CK levels are usually mildly elevated. Muscle biopsy shows type I fiber atrophy and subsarcolemmal granular inclusions.[240]

Electromyographic studies have been reported on patients with adult-onset hypothyroidism. The sensory and motor nerve conduction studies may be normal. (However, see discussion by Bolton, Chapter 21). Spontaneous and voluntary activities are normal.[241] The myoedema produced by percussion is electrically silent.[239] Regular, rhythmic discharges of grouped MUAPs (tetany discharges) are recorded when carpal spasm develops during the Trousseau test (personal observation). With treatment by thyroid hormone replacement, improvement of the adult-onset hypothyroid patient may be dramatic. The neuromuscular signs and symptoms resolve rapidly, and the Trousseau test becomes normal.

Hyperparathyroidism

Hyperparathyroidism is a rare disease that may be caused by a tumor of a single gland or by hyperplasia of all four glands. In these cases, the gland(s) produces excess parathyroid hormone, which causes hypercalcemia and hypophosphatemia. The diagnosis depends on the finding that the serum levels of both calcium and parathyroid hormone are elevated. Because the hypercalcemia may be intermittent, the serum calcium level should be determined several times. It is important to note that hyperparathyroidism may cause a treatable neuromuscular disease that appears similar to amyotrophic lateral sclerosis.[242]

Patients with primary hyperparathyroidism have varying degrees of neurologic involvement. Usually there is symmetric, proximal muscle weakness, which is worse in the legs. The patients note easy fatigue as well as muscle weakness. Dysarthria, dysphagia, atrophy and fasciculations of the tongue, hyperactive muscle stretch reflexes, and Babinski's sign may be present.

The serum CK level is normal. Sensory and motor nerve conduction studies are normal; the reported investigations did not include repetitive nerve stimulation studies.[243,244] EMG shows normal spontaneous activity, but the voluntary activity is abnormal. In some patients, there are short-duration, low-amplitude MUAPs; the other patients show long-duration, high-amplitude MUAPs.

It has been suggested that the short-duration MUAPs reflect damage to the terminal motor axons, not damage to the muscle fibers. This concept is supported by the muscle biopsies, which show only atrophy of type I and type II muscle fibers.[243] The neuromuscular symptoms and signs are reversed by therapy for the hyperparathyroidism.

Hypoparathyroidism

Hypoparathyroidism is usually caused by damage to the parathyroid glands or to their vascular supply during neck surgery. The condition is characterized by hypocalcemia and low serum parathyroid hormone levels. The symptoms may begin several days postoperatively, or they may become apparent months to years after the surgery.

The symptoms of hypoparathyroidism are seizures, carpal spasms, and pedal spasms, all of which reflect increased nerve irritability as a result of the hypocalcemia. Also present are Chvostek's sign and Trousseau's sign. The serum CK level is normal; muscle biopsy shows type II fiber atrophy.[245]

Sensory and motor nerve conduction studies are normal.[246] During spasms, either spontaneous or induced by nerve ischemia (Trousseau's test), there are regular rhythmic discharges of grouped MUAPs (tetany discharges).[247] Random fasciculation may occur between spasms; MUAPs may fire repetitively (doublets, triplets) when activated voluntarily.

Steroid Myopathies

A chronic or acute excess of adrenal corticosteroids produces symmetric, proximal muscle weakness and atrophy; the lower extremities are more affected than the upper extremities. In the severe form, the weakness and wasting are generalized.[248]

An excess of adrenal hormone may be endogenous (Cushing's disease). More commonly, prescription of steroids for the treatment of inflammatory disorders produces excessive levels. Symptoms usually begin 3 to 4 weeks after the patient begins daily steroid doses.[249] Halogenated synthetic corticosteroid compounds are more likely to produce the myopathy.[250] It has also been reported that with high doses of corticosteroids (in grams per day), symptoms may begin 1 to 2 days after initiation of therapy.[251,252]

The laboratory findings are similar in Cushing's disease and chronic iatrogenic steroid myopathy. The serum CK level is normal. A muscle biopsy shows atrophy of type II fibers and the accumulation of lipid droplets in type I fibers.[253,259] Sensory and motor nerve conduction studies are normal. EMG shows normal insertional activity, no spontaneous activity, and a normal number of short-duration and low-amplitude MUAPs in the weak proximal muscles.[255] The patients with Cushing's disease improve after surgery. Patients with iatrogenic steroid myopathies recover with reduction of the steroid dosage or substitution of prednisone for the offending halogenated synthetic steroid compound. Iatrogenic steroid myopathy appears to have been greatly reduced in frequency by the advent of alternate-day steroid therapy.

The laboratory findings in the two reports of acute, severe, generalized muscle weakness during megadose (in grams per day) steroid therapy indicated that the serum CK level was increased to 10 times normal. A muscle biopsy during an acute episode showed vacuolar changes in muscle fibers and regenerating muscle fibers. EMG showed normal spontaneous and voluntary activity. The patients recovered fully a few weeks after reduction of the steroid doses.[251,252]

It is important to note that corticosteroids are commonly used to treat inflammatory myopathies. Sometimes patients on steroid therapy become weaker. It is then necessary to distinguish the reason for the deterioration. The new weakness could be caused by the steroid therapy, in which case the dose should be reduced. On the other hand, the inflammatory myopathy may be progressive, and the patient may require larger doses of corticosteroids.

In this circumstance, an elevated serum CK level or fibrillation potential activity in weak muscles suggests that the inflammatory myopathy is worsening.[249] Ultimately, however, the determination of the cause of increased weakness is made by observing the effect of changes in the steroid therapy.

Acromegaly Myopathy

The neuromuscular complications of acromegaly include the carpal tunnel syndrome and a myopathy. The myopathy is usually mild, but the proximal muscle weakness may be the presenting complaint of the patient. The serum CK level and muscle biopsy are usually normal. EMG shows normal spontaneous activity and short-duration, low-amplitude polyphasic MUAPs in the weak proximal muscles.[256]

TOXIC MYOPATHIES

Many substances have been identified as able to cause toxic myopathies.[257] Five toxins, alcohol, chloroquine, vincristine, emetine, and colchicine, are discussed here. The toxic myopathies are characterized by proximal muscle weakness, atrophy, and muscle cramps. In severe cases, there may be generalized weakness, muscle swelling, muscle tenderness, and myoglobinuria. The severity of the myopathy is related to the dose and duration of exposure to the toxin. Usually the serum CK level is elevated. In mild toxic myopathies, the change in the serum CK may be the only manifestation. In some cases, there is an associated toxic neuropathy. Identification of a toxic myopathy may be difficult when the causative agent is a drug used to treat a disease that can also cause a neuropathy. Because of the regenerative capacity of muscle, elimination of the toxin should result in clinical improvement of the myopathy.[257]

Alcohol

Chronic alcohol abuse causes a myopathy that occurs concomitantly with a cardiomyopathy.[258] Proximal muscle weakness is greater in the legs than in the arms. When a patient who has been a long-time alcoholic has a binge of drinking, an acute myopathy may develop. In the acute form, there is exquisite tenderness, rhabdomyolysis on muscle biopsy, and myoglobinuria, which can lead to renal failure.[259,260]

The nerve conduction studies and electromyographic findings in alcoholic myopathy are variable from patient to patient but are consistent for each patient. Results depend on whether or not the patient also has a peripheral neuropathy and on the severity and duration of the alcoholism. Nerve conduction studies range from normal to slight slowing of conduction. Electromyographic results range from normal spontaneous activity to profuse fibrillation potential activity. The MUAPs may be normal, short duration, low amplitude, and polyphasic or reduced in number with high amplitude and long duration. The electromyographic abnormalities are most evident in weak proximal muscles. These findings are consistent with primary muscle damage with secondary reinnervation or damage to both nerve and muscle.[259,260]

Chloroquine

The antimalarial drug chloroquine is now used to treat connective tissue diseases, in particular, rheumatoid arthritis and systemic lupus erythematosus. Patients who are treated with chloroquine may develop a toxic myopathy for 6 months after initiation of therapy. The painless proximal muscle weakness becomes evident first in the legs. Muscle stretch reflexes may be reduced, but the sensory examination remains normal. The muscle biopsy shows vacuoles and degenerating muscle fibers.

Sensory and motor nerve conduction studies are usually normal, but some patients have slight slowing of motor conduction. There are fibrillation potentials, trains of positive sharp waves, and occasional myotonic discharges in weak proximal muscles, including the paraspinals. In chloroquine myopathy, different areas of the same muscle may show different MUAP abnormalities. Usually the MUAPs are of short duration, of low amplitude, and polyphasic, but some may have increased duration and amplitude.[261,262]

Vincristine

Vincristine is used for cancer chemotherapy. When the drug is given as often as once per week, patients develop myalgias, muscle weakness, and atrophy. They also have paresthesias, which reflect a concomitant neuropathy. Muscle biopsy shows segmental necrosis in proximal muscles and fiber type grouping in distal muscles.

Sensory and motor conduction studies show low-amplitude responses with slight slowing of conduction. EMG of proximal muscles is usually normal; distal muscles show occasional fibrillation potential activity and an increased proportion of polyphasic MUAPs.[263]

Emetine

Emetine is the major constituent of ipecac, a readily available emetic. The drug has been used in alcohol aversion therapy and has been abused by patients with eating disorders. A myopathy has been reported to develop in both situations and has been reproduced in experimental animal studies.[264–268] There is proximal muscle weakness, which may be painful in severe cases. Muscle biopsy shows swollen fibers with abnormal cores and cystoplasmic inclusions. The CPK may be normal or elevated. Sensory and motor nerve conduction studies are normal. EMG usually shows normal spontaneous activity, rarely increased insertion activity, and fibrillation potentials; MUAPs are short duration and low amplitude.[265,266,268]

Colchicine

Colchicine is often used to treat gout. Several patients with gout and renal insufficiency developed symmetric, primarily proximal limb-girdle muscle weakness with customary doses of colchicine.[269] Concentric needle EMG examination of proximal muscles recorded fibrillation potentials, positive sharp waves, and short-duration or low-amplitude MUAPs. The serum CK level was elevated. Muscle biopsy of proximal muscles showed a vacuolar lysosomal myopathy with coexistent mild denervation atrophy.[269,270]

In the same patients, there was also evidence of a mild, concomitant polyneuropathy with mild distal sensory and motor deficits. The distal sensory and motor responses were of low amplitude or absent; the legs were more affected than the arms. If a response was obtained, the latencies, conduction velocities, and F wave studies were essentially normal. Concentric needle EMG examination of distal muscle demonstrated fibrillation potentials, positive sharp waves, and CRDs; MUAPS were long duration and high amplitude. This pattern is consistent with a coexisting axonal sensory motor polyneuropathy.[271]

Three patients were examined after discontinuation of colchicine when symptoms of proximal weakness had improved. The electromyographic abnormalities in the proximal muscles had resolved, but the mild abnormalities in the distal sensory and motor nerve distributions persisted.[271]

Because of the prominent proximal muscle weakness, the elevated CK level, and the concentric needle EMG findings in proximal muscles, an erroneous diagnosis of polymyositis might be made. The mild abnormalities on the sensory conduction studies and the high-amplitude, long-duration MUAPs in distal muscles, however, suggest a toxic cause. The resolution of the proximal muscle weakness and improvement of the concentric needle EMG abnormalities in those muscles within 4 weeks after discontinuation of the colchicine confirm the toxic origin of the myopathy.[271]

OCULAR MYOPATHIES

Several different myopathies cause chronic, slowly progressive external ophthalmoplegia. In 1951, Kiloh and Nevin[272] described them as a single entity. Since then, two distinct groups have been identified as oculopharyngeal dystrophy and oculocraniosomatic neuromuscular disease (OCSND).[273,274] Other patients with extraocular muscle weakness were found to be sensitive to curare and may have had ocular myasthenia gravis.[275,276] Other forms with other associated abnormalities have been described in individual families.[277] Because their symptoms and signs are similar, Kiloh and Nevin[272] saw these diseases as one disorder. Most of the patients have difficulties beginning by age 30, and ptosis usually precedes extraocular muscle weakness. The ptosis may be asymmetric, but it usually becomes bilateral as the disease progresses. Diplopia is unusual because the weakness of the extraocular muscles progresses symmetrically. Rarely there is involvement of facial limb muscles. The serum CK levels are usually normal; nerve conduction studies and EMG are usually unremarkable. Oculopharyngeal dystrophy is discussed more fully elsewhere in this chapter, and OCSND is discussed next.

OCULOCRANIOSOMATIC NEUROMUSCULAR DISEASE

OCSND is a syndrome that was thought to occur sporadically and to be of viral origin.[278] More recently, however, familial forms of OCSND, inherited in an autosomal dominant fashion with variable penetrance, have been described.[279,280] Because of the variable penetrance of signs of the disorder, there are other neuromuscular diseases such as myasthenia gravis and thyrotoxicosis that may present in a similar fashion to OCSND. Therefore the diagnosis of OCSND depends on vigorous efforts to exclude other neuromuscular diseases followed by the satisfaction of most of the following criteria:

1. Progressive external ophthalmoplegia.
2. Heart block.
3. Pigmentary degeneration of the retina.
4. Onset before age 20.
5. Abnormal skeletal muscle biopsy with an excessive amount of clumped, bright red material under the sarcolemma and in the intermyofibrillous space demonstrated by modified Trichrome strain.[281]

Individual cases with some of the findings were originally described by Kearns and Sayre[282] and Shy et al.[283] In their review of 35 cases, Berenberg et al.[281] noted that the cardiomyopathy may be delayed and that the presence of heart block was not essential to make the diagnosis. Further, several other manifestations were common in the literature reports: short stature, sensorineural hearing loss, occasional pyrimidal tract signs, cerebellar incoordination, mild sensorimotor polyneuropathy, and increased cerebrospinal fluid protein.[289]

Olsen et al. described the abnormal muscle fibers seen in biopsy specimens as *ragged red fibers* occurring with a frequency of 1% to 5%. Olsen believed that only patients with OCSND have both ragged red fibers and progressive external ophthalmoplegia. Up to 5% of ragged red fibers, however, are found in muscle biopsy specimens of patients with other neuromuscular diseases in the absence of progressive external ophthalmoplegia.[286,287]

When the syndrome of OCSND is well developed, the progressive external ophthalmoplegia is distinct, and the ragged red fibers are seen in the muscle biopsy specimen, the electrophysiologic studies do not add much to the diagnosis.[47] On the other hand, when ocular and limb muscle weakness occurs in isolation, a careful clinical evaluation, including electrophysiologic studies, is warranted to exclude other neuromuscular diseases.

The nerve conduction studies are generally normal, although slight slowing of motor conduction has occasionally been reported. This along with the demyelinization seen in nerve biopsy specimens may reflect the fact that the disease is a multisystem disorder with variable involvement of peripheral nerves and muscles.[278,281] Repetitive nerve stimulation studies of limb and cranial muscles have not shown a decrementing response except when there was the concomitant occurrence of a disorder of neuromuscular transmission, like myasthenia gravis.[288] Single-fiber EMG studies of either facial or limb muscles of 13 to 16 patients with OCSND have been reported to show increased mean jitter and increased fiber density.[289] Conventional needle EMG has been reported to show an increased proportion of short-duration, polyphasic MUAPs in limb and cranial muscles in over half the patients examined; these findings have been documented with quantitative measurements of MUAP parameters.[278,287]

OTHER MITOCHONDRIAL MYOPATHIES

OCSND is one of several myopathies characterized by subsarcolemmal collections of abnormal mitochondria. There are several other clinical presentations of mitochondrial myopathies, including slowly progressive limb-girdle muscle weakness with normal ocular movements.[290] A significant percentage of mitochondrial myopathies have an associated peripheral neuropathy with reduced or absent deep tendon reflexes and impaired sensation in a distal distribution.[278,281,290,291] The median, ulnar, and sural sensory responses of these patients are absent or of reduced amplitude with slightly prolonged peak latencies.[291] EMG shows short-duration, low-amplitude polyphasic MUAPs in proximal muscles and long-duration, high-amplitude MUAPs in distal muscles.[291] Abnormal mitochondria containing paracrystalline inclusion have been identified in the Schwann cell cytoplasm in sural nerve biopsies as well as in muscle fibers in muscle biopsies of these patients.[291] In some cases, there are neurologic symptoms and signs consistent with concomitant central nervous system involvement.[291]

SUMMARY

Nerve conduction studies and EMG are important tests for the diagnosis of myopathies. When a myopathy is suspected, EMG may confirm that diagnosis or may disclose that a neuropathy or a disorder of the neuromuscular junction is responsible for the clinical picture that resembles a myopathy. EMG may show evidence of a myopathy in patients with nonspecific neuromuscular symptoms. On the other hand, in some myopathies that are documented by muscle biopsy, EMG is normal. Bearing these points in mind, EMG is a useful test for the diagnosis of myopathies, but normal EMG does not exclude a myopathy, particularly a congenital or metabolic myopathy.

REFERENCES

1. Kugelberg E. Electromyograms in muscular disorders. J Neurol Neurosurg Psychiatry 1947; 10:122–133.
2. Buchthal F, Rosenflack P. Spontaneous electrical activity of human muscle. Electroencephalogr Clin Neurophysiol 1966; 20:321–336.
3. Kugelberg E. Electromyography in muscular dystrophies. Differentiation between dystrophies and chronic lower motor neuron lesions. J Neurol Neurosurg Psychiatry 1949; 12:129–136.
4. Buchthal F, Rosenflack P, Ermino F. Motor unit territory and fiber density in myopathies. Neurology 1960; 10:398–408.
5. Bradley WG. The limb girdle syndromes. In: Vinken PJ, Bruyn GW, eds. Handbook of clinical neurology. Diseases of muscle. Amsterdam: North Holland, 1979:433–469.
6. Bohan A, Peter JB. Polymyositis and dermatomyositis. N Engl J Med 1975; 292:344.
7. Black JTR, Bhatt GP, DeJesus PV, et al. Diagnostic accuracy of clinical data, quantitative electromyography and histochemistry in neuromuscular disease. J Neurol Sci 1974; 21:59–70.
8. McManis P, Lambert E, Daube J. The exercise test in periodic paralysis. Muscle Nerve 1986; 9:704–710.
9. Harman JB, Richardson AT. Generalized myokymia in thyrotoxicosis Lancet 1954; 2:473–474.
10. Segura RP, Petajan JH. Neural hyperexcitability in hyperkalemic periodic paralysis. Muscle Nerve 1979; 2:245–249.
11. Desmedt JE, Borenstein S. Relationship of spontaneous fibrillation potentials to muscle fibre segmentation in human muscular dystrophy. Nature 1975; 258:531–534.
12. Stalberg E, Vtrontelj J. Single fiber electromyography. Old Woking, Surrey England: Mirvalle Press Limited, 1979.
13. Dubowitz V, Brooke M. Muscle biopsy: A modern approach. Philadelphia: WB Saunders, 1973.
14. Nandedkar SD, Sander DB. Simulation of myopathic motor unit action potentials. Muscle Nerve 1989; 12:197–202.
15. Buchthal F, Kamieniecka Z. The diagnostic yield of quantified electromyography and quantified muscle biopsy in neuromuscular disorders. Muscle Nerve 1982; 5:265–280.
16. Kugelberg E. Electromyogram in muscular disorders. J Neurol Neurosurg Psychiatry 1947; 10:122–133.
17. Kugelberg E. Electromyography in muscular dystrophies. J Neurol Neurosurg Psychiatry 1949; 12:129–136.
18. Buchthal F, Rosenfalk P. Electrophysiologic aspects of myopathy with particular reference to progressive muscular dystrophy. In: Bourne GW, Golarz MNS, eds. Muscular dystrophy in man and animals. New York: Karger, 1963:193–262.
19. Petajan JH. Clinical electromyographic studies of

diseases of the motor unit. Electroenceph Clin Neurophysiol 1974; 36:395–401.

20. Mechler F. Changing electromyographic findings during the chronic course of polymyositis. J Neurol Sci 1974; 23:237–242.

21. Pickett JB. Late components of motor unit potentials in a patient with myoglobinuria. Ann Neurol 1978; 3:461–464.

22. Shields RW. Single fiber electromyography in the differential diagnosis of myopathic limb girdle syndromes and chronic spinal muscular atrophy. Muscle Nerve 1984; 7:265–272.

23. Daube JR. The description of motor unit potentials in electromyography. Neurology 1978; 28:623–625.

24. Wilbourn AJ. The EMG examination with myopathies. In: Course A: Myopathies floppy infants, and electrodiagnostic studies in children. Rochester, MN: American Academy of Electrodiagnostic Medicine (formerly the AAEE), 1987:18.

25. Buchthal F, Rosenfalk P. Action potential parameters in different human muscles. Acta Psychiatr Scand 1955; 30:125.

26. Sacco G, Buchthal D, Rosenfalk P. Motor unit potentials at different ages. Arch Neurol 1962; 6:366–373.

27. Chu-Andrews J, Johnson RJ. Electrodiagnosis, an anatomical and clinical approach. Philadelphia: JB Lippincott, 1986:230–235.

28. Buchtal F, Kamieniecka Z. The diagnostic yield of quantified electromyography and quantified muscle biopsy in neuromuscular disorders. Muscle Nerve 1982; 5:265–280.

29. Kopec J, Hausmanowa-Petrusewicz I, Rawsky M, Wolynski M. Automatic analysis of the electromyelogram. New Devel Electromyog Clin Neurophysiol 1973; 2:477–481.

30. Stalberg E, Chu J, Brill V, et al. Automatic analysis of the EMG interference pattern. Electroencephalogr Neurophysiol 1983; 56:672–681.

31. Nandedkar SD, Sanders DB, Stalberg EV. Automatic analysis of the electromyographic interference pattern. Part I: Development of quantitative features. Muscle Nerve 1986; 9:431–439.

32. Nandedkar SD, Sanders DB, Stalberg EV. Automatic analysis of the electromyographic interference pattern. Part II: Findings in control subjects and in some neuromuscular diseases. Muscle Nerve 1986; 9:491–500.

33. Stalberg E. Clinical electrophysiology of myasthenia gravis. J Neurol Neurosurg Psychiatry 1980; 43:622–633.

34. Brown JC, Johns RJ. Diagnostic difficulties encountered in the myasthenic syndrome sometimes associated with carcinoma. J Neurol Neurosurg Psychiatry 1974; 37:1214–1224.

35. Sinaki M, Mulder DW. Amyotrophic lateral sclerosis: Relationship between serum creatinine kinase level and patient survival. Arch Phys Med Rehabil 1986; 67:169–171.

36. Nicholson GA, Morgan GJ, Meerkin M, et al. The effect of aerobic exercise on serum creatinine kinase activities. Muscle Nerve 1986; 9:820–824.

36a. Trontelj JV, Zidar J, Denislic M, et al. Facioscapulohumeral dystrophy: Jitter in facial muscles. J Neurol Neurosurg Psychiatry 1988; 51:950–955.

37. Chrissian SA, Stolov WC, Hongladarom T. Needle electromyography: Its effect on serum creatinine phosphokinase activity. Arch Phys Med Rehabil 1976; 57:114.

38. Carpenter S, Karpati G. Pathology of skeletal muscle. New York: Churchill Livingstone 1984:39.

39. Engel WK. Focal myopathic changes produced by electromyographic and hypodermic needles: Needle myopathy. Arch Neurol 1967; 16:509–512.

40. Edwards RHT, Round JM, Jones DA. Needle biopsy of skeletal muscle: A review of 10 years experience. Muscle Nerve 1983; 6:676–683.

41. Wessel HB. Dystrophin: A clinical perspective. Pediatr Neurol 1990; 6:3–12.

42. Edwards RHT. New techniques for studying human muscle function, metabolism, and fatigue. Muscle Nerve 1984; 7:599–609.

43. Walton JN. Muscular dystrophy: Some recent advances in knowledge. Br Med J 1964; 1:1271–1274.

44. Dubowitz V, Brooke MH. Muscle biopsy: A modern approach. Philadelphia: WB Saunders, 1973:169–252.

45. Rowland LP. Muscular dystrophy. Disease-a-Month 1972; 22:1–38.

46. Lazaro RP, Fenichel GM, Kilroy AW. Congenital muscular dystrophy: Case reports and reappraisal. Muscle Nerve 1979; 2:349–355.

47. Brooke MH. A clinician's view of neuromuscular diseases. Baltimore: Williams & Wilkins, 1977:95–124.

48. Dubowitz V. Treatment of dermatomyositis in childhood. Arch Dis Child 1976; 51:494–500.

49. Mastaglia F, Ojeda V. Inflammatory myopathies. Ann Neurol 1985; 17:215.

50. Roses AD, Roses MJ, Metcalf BS, et al. Pedigree testing in Duchenne muscular dystrophy. Ann Neurol 1977; 2:271–278.

51. Gardner-Medwin D, Pennington RJ, Walton JN. The detection of carriers of X-linked muscular dystrophy genes. A review of some methods studied in Newcastle-Upon-Tyne. J Neurol Sci 1971; 13:459–474.

52. Becker PE, Kiefner F. Eine nerve X-chromosomale muskeldystrophie. Arch Physchiatr Nervenkr 1955; 193:427–448.

53. Becker PE. Two new families with benign sex-linked recessive muscular dystrophy. Rev Can Biol 1962; 21:551–566.

54. Furugawa T, Peter JB. X-linked muscular dystrophy. Ann Neurol 1977; 2:414–416.

55. Bradley WG, Jones MZ, Mussini JM, Fawcett PRW. Becker-type muscular dystrophy. Muscle Nerve 1978; 1:111–132.

56. Hoffman EP, Kunkel LM, Angelini C, et al. Im-

proved diagnosis of Becker muscular dystrophy by dystrophin testing. Neurology 1989; 39:1011–1017.

57. Victor M, Hayes R, Adams RD. Oculopharyngeal muscular dystrophy. A familial disease of late life characterized by dysphagia and progressive ptosis of the eyelids. N Engl J Med 1962; 267:1267–1272.

58. Bray GM, Kaarsoo M, Ross RT. Ocular myopathy with dysphagia. Neurology 1965; 15:678–684.

59. Barbeau A. The syndrome of hereditary late onset ptosis and dysphagia in French Canada. In: Kuhn E, ed. Progressive muskeldystrophie, myotonie, myasthenie. Berlin:Springer 1966:102–109.

60. Murphy SF, Drachman DB. The oculopharyngeal syndrome. JAMA 1968; 203:99–104.

61. Bosch EP, Gowans JDC. Munsat T. Inflammatory myopathy in oculopharyngeal dystrophy. Muscle Nerve 1979; 2:73–77.

62. Schmitt HP, Krause K-H. An autopsy study of a familial oculopharyngeal muscular dystrophy (OPMD) with distal spread and neurogenic involvement. Muscle Nerve 1981; 4:296–305.

63. Munsat T, Piper D, Cancilla P, et al. Inflammatory myopathy with facioscapulohumeral dystrophy. Neurology 1972; 22:335–347.

64. Trontelj JV, Zidar J, Denislec M, et al. Facioscapulohumeral dystrophy: Jitter in facial muscles. J Neurol Neurosurg Psychiatry 1988; 51:950–955.

65. Fenichel GM, Emery ES, Hunt P. Neurogenic atrophy simulating facioscapulohumeral dystrophy. A dominant form. Arch Neurol 1967; 17:257–260.

66. Munsat TL. The classification of human myopathies. In: Vinken PJ, Bruyn GW, eds. Handbook of clinical neurology. Diseases of muscle. Amsterdam:North Holland, 1979:275–293.

67. Welander L. Myopathia distalis tarda hereditaria. 249 examined cases in 72 pedigrees. Acta Med Scand 1951; 141(suppl 265):1–124.

68. Markesbery WR, Griggs RC, Leach RP, et al. Late onset hereditary distal myopathy. Neurology 1974; 29:127–134.

69. Sumner D, Crawfurd MO'A, Harrman DGF. Distal muscular dystrophy in an English family. Brain 1971; 94:51–60.

70. Miller RG, Blank NK, Layzer RB. Sporadic distal myopathy with early adult onset. Ann Neurol 1979; 5:220–227.

71. Scoppetta C, Vaccario M, Casali C, et al. Distal muscular dystrophy with autosomal recessive inheritance. Muscle Nerve 1984; 7:478–481.

72. Nonaka I, Sunohara N, Satoyoshi E, et al. Autosomal recessive distal muscular dystrophy: A comparative study with distal myopathy with rimmed vacuole formation. Ann Neurol 1985; 17:51–59.

73. Isaacs H, Badenhorst ME, Whistler T. Autosomal recessive distal myopathy. J Clin Pathol 1988; 41:188–194.

74. Magee KR, Dejong RN. Hereditary distal myopathy with onset in infancy. Arch Neurol 1965; 13:387–390.

75. Van Der Does de Willebois AEM, Bethlem J, Meijer AEFA, et al. Distal myopathy with onset in early infancy. Neurology 1968; 18:383–390.

76. Bautista J, Refel E, Castilla JM, et al. Hereditary distal myopathy with early onset in infancy. Observations of a family. J Neurol Sci 1978; 37:149–158.

77. Harper PS. Myotonic dystrophy. Philadelphia: WB Saunders, 1979.

78. Dodge PR, Gamstorp I, Byers RK, Russell P. Myotonic dystrophy in infancy and childhood. Pediatrics 1965; 35:3–19.

79. Watters G, Williams T. Early onset myotonia dystrophy: Clinical and laboratory findings in five families and a review of the literature. Arch Neurol 1967; 17:137–152.

80. Swift TR, Agnacio OJ, Dyken PR. Neonatal dystrophia myotonia. Electrophysiologic studies. Am J Dis Child 1975; 129:734–737.

81. Polgar JG, Bradley WG, Upton ARM, et al. The early detection of dystrophia myotonica. Brain 1972; 95:761–776.

82. Brown JC. Muscle weakness after rest in myotonic disorders: An electrophysiological study. J Neurol Neurosurg Psychiatry 1974; 37:1336–1342.

83. Aminoff MJ, Layzer RB, Satya-Murti S, et al. The declining electrical response of muscle to repetitive nerve stimulation in myotonia. Neurology 1977; 27:812–816.

84. Streib EW, Sun SF. Distribution of electrical myotonia in myotonic muscular dystrophy. Ann Neurol 1983; 14:80–82.

85. Adrian RH, Bryant SH. On the repetitive discharge on myotonic muscle fibers. J Physiol 1974; 240:505–515.

86. Brumlik J, Drechscler B, Vannin TM. The myotonic discharge in various neurologic syndromes: A neurophysiological analysis. Electromyography 1970; 10:369–383.

87. Subramony SH, Malhorta CP, Mishra SK. Distinguishing paramyotonia congenita and myotonia congenita by electromyography. Muscle Nerve 1983; 6:374–379.

88. Kuhn E, Fiehn W, Seiler D, Schroder JM. The autosomal recessive (Becker) form of myotonia congenita. Muscle Nerve 1979; 2:109–117.

89. Sun SF, Strieb EW. Autosomal recessive generalized myotonia. Muscle Nerve 1983; 6:143–148.

90. Zellweger H, Pavone L, Blondi A, et al. Autosomal recessive generalized myotonia. Muscle Nerve 1980; 3:176–180.

91. Zwarts MJ, Van Weerden TW. Transient paresis in myotonic syndromes, a surface EMG study. Brain 1989; 112:665–680.

92. Sanders DB. Myotonia congenita with painful muscle contractions. Arch Neurol 1976; 33:580–582.

93. Kuhn E, Fiehn W, Seiler D, et al. The autosomal recessive (Becker) form of myotonia congenita. Muscle Nerve 1979; 2:109–117.

94. French EB, Kilpatrick R. A variety of paramyotonia congenita. J Neurol Neurosurg Psychiatry 1957; 20:40–46.

95. Thrush DC, Morris CJ, Salmon MV. Paramyotonia congenita: A clinical histochemical and pathological study. Brain 1972; 95:537–552.

96. Lehmann-Horn F, Rudel R, Dengler R, et al. Membrane defects in paramyotonia congenita with and without myotonia in a warm environment. Muscle Nerve 1981; 4:396–406.

97. Wegmuller E, Ludin HP, Mumenthaler M. Paramyotonia congenita. A clinical, electrophysiological and histological study of 12 patients. J Neurol 1979; 220:251–257.

98. Haass A, Ricker K, Rudel R, et al. Clinical study of paramyotonia congenita with and without myotonia in a warm environment. Muscle Nerve 1981; 4:388–395.

99. Burke D, Skuse NF, Lethlean AK. Contractile properties of the abductor digiti minimi muscle in paramyotonia congenital. J Neurol Neurosurg Psychiatry 1974; 37:894–899.

100. Subramony SH, Wee AS, Mishra SK. Lack of cold sensitivity in hyperkalemic periodic paralysis. Muscle Nerve 1986; 9:700–703.

101. Buchthal F, Engback L, Gamstorp I. Paresis and hyperexcitability in adynamia episodica hereditaria. Neurology 1958; 8:347–351.

102. De Silva S, Kuncl RW, Griffin JW, et al. Paramyotonia congenita or hyperkalemic periodic paralysis? Clinical and electrophysiological features of each entity in one family. Muscle Nerve 1990; 13:21–26.

103. Streib Erich W. Hypokalemic paralysis in two patients with paramyotonia congenita (PC) and known hyperkalemic/exercise-induced weakness. Muscle Nerve 1989; 12:936–937.

104. Ricker K, Lehmann-Horn F, Moxley RT III. Myotonia fluctuans. Arch Neurol 1990; 47:268–272.

105. Tome F. Periodic paralysis and electrolyte disorders. In: Mastaglia FL, Walton J, eds. Skeletal muscle pathology. London:Churchill Livingstone, 1982: 287–308.

106. Chesson AL Jr, Schochet SS Jr, Peters BH. Biphasic periodic paralysis. Arch Neurol 1979; 36:700–704.

107. Rudel R, Lehmann-Horn F, Ricker K, et al. Hypokalemic periodic paralysis: In vitro investigation of muscle fiber membrane parameters. Muscle Nerve 1984; 7:110–120.

108. Pearson C. The periodic paralysis: Differential features and pathological observations in permanent myopathic weakness. Brain 1964; 87:341–354.

109. Engel AG, Lambert EH, Rosevar JW, et al. Clinical and electromyographic studies in a patient with primary hypokalemic periodic paralysis. Am J Med 1965; 38:626–640.

110. Dyken M, Zeman W, Rusche T. Hypokalemic periodic paralysis. Children with permanent myopathic weakness. Neurology 1969; 19:691–699.

111. Engel AG. Evolution and content of vacuoles in pri-

mary hypokalemic periodic paralysis. Mayo Clin Proc 1970; 45:774–814.

112. Resnick JS, Engel WK. Myotonic lid lag in hypokalemic periodic paralysis. J Neurol Neurosurg Psychiatry 1967; 30:47–51.

113. McManis P, Lambert E, Daube J. The exercise test in periodic paralysis. Muscle Nerve 1984; 7:579.

114. Zwarts MJ, Weerden TWV, Links P, et al. The muscle fiber conduction velocity and power spectra in familial hypokalemic periodic paralysis. Muscle Nerve 1988; 11:166–173.

115. Grob D, Johns RJ, Liljestrand A. Potassium movement in patients with familial periodic paralysis. Relationship to the defect in muscle function. Am J Med 1957; 24:356–375.

116. Gordon AM, Green JR, Lagunoff D. Studies on a patient with hypokalemic familial periodic paralysis. Am J Med 1970; 48:185–195.

117. Engel AG, Lambert EH. Calcium activation of electrically inexcitable muscle fibers in primary hypokalemic periodic paralysis. Neurology 1969; 19:851–858.

118. Campa JF, Anders DB. Familial hypokalemic periodic paralysis. Arch Neurol 1974; 31:110–115.

119. McArdle B. Adynamia episodica hereditaria and its treatment. Brain 1962; 85:121–148.

120. Layzer RB. Periodic paralysis and the sodium potassium pump. Ann Neurol 1982; 11:547–552.

121. Bradley WG. Adynamia episodica hereditaria. Clinical, pathological, and electrophysiological studies in an affected family. Brain 1969; 92:345–378.

122. Layzer RB, Lovelace RE, Rowland LP. Hyperkalemic periodic paralysis. Arch Neurol 1967; 16:455–472.

123. Bradley WG, Taylor R, Rice DR, et al. Progressive myopathy in hyperkalemic periodic paralysis. Arch Neurol 1990; 47:1013–1017.

124. Lehmann-Horn F, Rudel R, Ricker K, et al. Two cases of adynamia episodica hereditaria: In vitro investigation of muscle cell membrane and contraction parameters. Muscle Nerve 1983; 6:113–121.

125. Lehmann-Horn F, Kuther G, Ricker K, et al. Adynamia episodica hereditaria with myotonia: A noninactivating sodium current and the effect of extracellular pH. Muscle Nerve 1987; 10:363–374.

126. Ricker K, Camacho L, Grafe P, et al. Adynamia episodica hereditaria: What causes the weakness? Muscle Nerve 1989; 12:883–891.

127. Brooks JE. Hyperkalemic periodic paralysis. Intracellular electromyographic studies. Arch Neurol 1969; 20:13–18.

128. Segura RP, Petajan JH. Neural hyperexcitability in hyperkalemic periodic paralysis. Muscle Nerve 1979; 2:245–249.

129. Poskanzer DC, Kerr DNS. A third type of periodic paralysis with normokalemia and favorable response to sodium chloride. Am J Med 1961; 31: 328–342.

130. Tyler F, Stephens F, Gunn F, et al. Studies in disorders of muscles VII. Clinical manifestations and inheri-

tance of a type of periodic paralysis without hypo-potassemia. J Clin Invest 1951; 30:492–502.

131. Meyers KR, Gilden DH, Rinaldi CF, Hansen JL. Periodic muscle weakness, normokalemia and tubular aggregates. Neurology 1972; 22:269–279.

132. Chesson A, Schochet S, Peters B. Biphasic periodic paralysis. Arch Neurol 1979; 36:700–704.

133. Engel AG. Neuromuscular manifestations of Graves' disease. Mayo Clin Proc 1972; 47:919–925.

134. Kufs WM, McBiles M, Jurney T. Familial thyrotoxic periodic paralysis. West J Med 1989; 150:461–463.

135. Gamstorp I. A study of transient muscular weakness. Clinical, biochemical and electromyographical findings during attacks of periodic paralysis and adynamia episodica hereditaria. Acta Neurol Scand 1962; 38:3–19.

136. Pleasure D, Bonilla E. Skeletal muscle storage disease: Myopathies resulting from errors in carbohydrate and fatty acid metabolism. In: Mastaglia FL, Walton J, eds. Skeletal muscle pathology. New York: Churchill Livingstone, 1982:340–359.

137. Thompson AJ, Swash M, Cox EL, et al. Polysaccharide storage myopathy. Muscle Nerve 1988; 2:349–355.

138. Engel AG, Gomez MR, Seybold ME, et al. The spectrum and diagnosis of acid maltase deficiency. Neurology 1973; 23:95–106.

139. DiMauro S, Hartwig GB. Debrancher deficiency: Neuromuscular disorder in 5 adults. Ann Neurol 1979; 5:422–436.

140. Hogan GR, Gutmann L, Schmidt R, et al. Pompe's disease. Neurology 1969; 19:894–900.

141. Karpati G, Carpenter S, Eisen A, et al. The adult form of acid maltase (a-1, 4-glucosidase) deficiency. Ann Neurol 1977; 1:276–280.

142. Chui L, Munsat T. Dominant inheritance of McArdle's syndrome. Arch Neurol 1976; 33:636–641.

143. Feit H, Brooke M. Myophosphorylase deficiency: Two different molecular etiologies. Neurology 1976; 26:963.

144. DiMauro S, Hartlage PL. Fatal infantile form of muscle phosphorylase deficiency. Neurology 1978; 28:1124–1129.

145. Engel W, Eyerman E, Williams H. Late onset-type of skeletal muscle phosphorylase deficiency. A new family variety with completely and partially affected subjects. N Engl J Med 1963; 268:135–137.

146. DiMauro S. Metabolic myopathies. In: Vinken PJ, Bruyn GW, eds. Handbook of clinical neurology. Amsterdam: North Holland, 1979; 41:175–234.

147. Brandt NJ, Buchtal F, Ebbsen F, et al. Post-tetanic mechanical tension and evoked action potentials in McArdle's disease. J Neurol Neurosurg Psychiatry 1977; 40:920–925.

148. Rowland LP, Lovelace RE, Schotland DL, et al. The clinical diagnosis of McArdle disease. Identification of another family with deficiency of muscle phosphorylase. Neurology 1966; 16:93–100.

149. Dyken ML, Smith DM, Peake RL. An electromy-ographic diagnostic screening test in McArdle's disease and a case report. Neurology 1967; 17:45–50.

150. Roelofs RL, Engel WK, Shauvin PB. Histochemical phosphorylase activity in regenerating muscle fibers from myophosphorylase deficiency patients. Science 1972; 177:795–797.

151. Munsat TL. A standardized forearm ischemic exercise test. Neurology 1970; 20:1171–1178.

152. Tobin WE, Huising F, Porro RS, et al. Muscle phosphofructokinase deficiency. Arch Neurol 1973; 28:128–130.

153. DiMauro S, Trevisan C, Hayes A. Disorders of lipid metabolism in muscle. Muscle Nerve 1980; 3:369–388.

154. Rebouche CJ, Engel AG. Carnitine metabolism and deficiency syndromes. Mayo Clin Proc 1983; 38:533–540.

155. Karpati G, Carpenter S, Engel AG, et al. The syndrome of systemic carnitine deficiency. Neurology 1975; 25:16–24.

156. Markesbery WR, McQuillen MP, Procopis PG, et al. Muscle carnitine deficiency. Associated with lipid myopathy, vacuolar neuropathy, and vacuolated leukocytes. Arch Neurol 1974; 31:320–324.

157. Engel AG, Siekert RG. Lipid storage myopathy responsive to prednisone. Arch Neurol 1972; 27:174–181.

158. Engel AG, Angelini C. Carnitine deficiency of human skeletal muscle with associated lipid storage myopathy: A new syndrome. Science 1973; 179:899–902.

159. Angelini C, Lucke S, Cantarutti F. Carnitine deficiency of skeletal muscle; report of a treated case. Neurology 1976; 26:633–637.

160. Cornelo F, DiDonato S, Peluchetti D, et al. Fatal cases of lipid storage myopathy with carnitine deficiency. J Neurol Neurosurg Psychiatry 1977; 40:170–178.

161. Bank, WJ, DiMauro S, Bonilla E, et al. A disorder of muscle lipid metabolism and myoglobinuria. Absence of carnitine palmityl transferase. N Engl J Med 1975; 292:443–449.

162. Hostetler KY, Hoppel CL, Romine JS, et al. Partial deficiency of muscle carnitine palmityltransferase with normal ketone production. N Engl J Med 1978; 298:553–557.

163. Trevisan CP, Isaya G, Angelini C. Exercise-induced recurrent myoglobinuria: Defective activity of inner carnitine palmitoyltransferase in muscle mitochondria of two patients. Neurology 1987; 37:1184–1188.

164. Engel WK, Vick NA, Glueck CJ, et al. A skeletal muscle disorder associated with intermittent symptoms and a possible defect of lipid metabolism. N Engl J Med 1970; 282:697–704.

165. Fishbein WN, Armbrustmacher VW, Griffin JL. Myoadenylate deaminase deficiency: A new disease of muscle. Science 1978; 200:545–548.

166. Shumate JB, Katnik R, Ruis M, et al. Myoadenylate

deaminase deficiency. Muscle Nerve 1979; 2:213–216.

167. Keleman J, Rice DR, Bradley WG, et al. Familial myoadenylate deaminase and exertional myalgia. Neurology 1982; 32:857–863.

168. Shy GM, Magee KR. A new congenital non-progressive myopathy. Brain 1956; 79:610–621.

169. Shy GM, Engel WK, Somers JE, et al. Nemaline myopathy; a new congenital myopathy. Brain 1963; 86:793–810.

170. Conen M, Murphy EG, Donohue WL. Light and electron microscope studies of "myopathies" in a child with hypotonia and muscle weakness. Can Med Assoc J 1963; 89:983–986.

171. Spiro AJ, Shy GM, Gonatas NK. Myotubular myopathy. Persistence of fetal muscle in an adolescent boy. Arch Neurol 1966; 14:1–14.

172. Engel AG, Gomez MR, Groover RV. Multicore disease. A recently recognized congenital myopathy associated with multifocal degeneration of muscle fiber. Mayo Clin Proc 1971; 46:666–681.

173. Engel AG, Angelini C, Gomez MR. Fingerprint body myopathy. Mayo Clin Proc 1972; 47:377–388.

174. Brooke MH, Neville HE. Reducing body myopathy. Neurology 1972; 22:829–840.

175. Brooke MH. Congenital fiber type disproportion. In: Kakulas BA, ed. Clinical studies in myology. Amsterdam: Excerpta Medica, 1973:147–159.

176. Jerusalem F, Engel AG, Gomez MR. Sarcotubular myopathy. A newly recognized benign, congenital, familial muscle disease. Neurology 1973; 23:897–906.

177. Kinoshita M, Satayoshi E, Suzuki Y. A typical myopathy with myofibrillar aggregates. Arch Neurol 1975; 32:417–420.

178. Lake BD, Wilson J. Zebra body myopathy. Clinical, histochemical and ultrastructural studies. J Neurol Sci 1975; 24:437–446.

179. Ringel SP, Neville HE, Duster MC, et al. A new congenital neuromuscular disease with trilaminar fibers. Neurology 1977; 27:347.

180. Goebel HH, Muller J, Gillen HW, et al. Autosomal dominant "spheroid body myopathy." Muscle Nerve 1978; 1:14–25.

181. Dubowitz V, Roy S. Central core disease of muscle: Clinical, histochemical and electron microscopic studies of an affected mother and child. Brain 1970; 93:133–145.

182. Bethlem J, Van Wisngaarden GK, Meijer AEFH, Fleurs P. Observations on central core disease. J Neurol Sci 1971; 14:293–299.

183. Shafiq SA, Dubowitz V, Peterson HC, et al. Nemaline myopathy: Report of a fatal case, with histochemical and electron microscope studies. Brain 1976; 90:817–828.

184. Telerman-Topper N, Gerard JM, Coers C. Central core disease, a study of clinically unaffected muscle. J Neurol Sci 1973; 19:207–223.

185. Isaacs H, Heffron JJA, Badenhorst M. Central core

186. disease. A correlated genetic, histochemical, ultra-microscopic and biochemical study. J Neurosurg Psychiatry 1975; 38:11277–11286.

186. Mrozek K, Strugalska M, Fidzianska A. A sporadic case of central core disease. J Neurol Sci 1970; 10:339–348.

187. Armstrong RM, Koenigsberger R, Mellinger J, et al. Central core disease with congenital hip displacement: Study of two families. Neurology 1971; 21:369–376.

188. Dubowitz V, Platts M. Central core disease of muscle with focal wasting. J Neurol Neurosurg Psychiatry 1965; 28:432–437.

189. Engel WK, Resnick JS. Late onset rod myopathy: A newly recognized, acquired and progressive disease. Neurology 1966; 16:308–309.

190. Dahl DS, Klutzow FW. Congenital rod disease. Further evidence of innervation abnormalities as the basis for clinicopathological features. J Neurol Sci 1974; 23:371–375.

191. Bender AN, Wilner JP. Nemaline (rod) myopathy: The need for histochemical evaluation of affected families. Ann Neurol 1978; 4:37–42.

192. Karpati G, Carpenter S, Andermann F: A new concept of childhood nemaline myopathy. Arch Neurol 24:291–304.

193. Arts WF, Bethlem J, Dingemans KP, et al. Investigations on the inheritance of nemaline myopathy. Arch Neurol 1978; 35:72–77.

194. Wallgren-Petersson C, Sainio K, Salmi T. Electromyography in congenital nemaline myopathy. Muscle Nerve 1989; 12:587–593.

195. Feigenbaum JA, Munsat TL. A neuromuscular syndrome of scapuloperoneal distribution. Bull Los Angeles Neurol Soc 1970; 35:47–57.

196. Engel WK, Oberc MA. Abundant nuclear rods in adult-onset rod disease. J Neuropathol Exp Neurol 1975; 34:19–32.

197. Spiro AJ, Shy GM, Gonatas, MK. Myotubular myopathy. Arch Neurol 1966; 14:1–14.

198. Serratrice G, Pellissier JF, Faugere MC, et al. Centronuclear myopathy: Possible central nervous system origin. Muscle Nerve 1978; 1:62–69.

199. Radu H, Killyen I, Ionescu V, et al. Myotubular (centronuclear) (neuro-) myopathy. Eur Neurol 1977; 15:285–300.

200. Bergen BJ, Carry MP, Wilson WB, et al. Centronuclear myopathy: Extraocular- and limb-muscle findings in an adult. Muscle Nerve 1980; 3:165–171.

201. Munsat TL, Thompson LR, Coleman RF. Centronuclear ("myotubular") myopathy. Arch Neurol 1969; 20:120–131.

202. Hawkes CH, Absolon MJ. Myotubular myopathy associated with cataract and electrical myotonia. J Neurol Neurosurg Psychiatry 1975; 38:761–764.

203. Sher J, Rimalovski AB, Athanassiades TJ, et al. Familial centronuclear myopathy: A clinical and pathological study. Neurology 1967; 17:727–742.

204. Engel WK, Gold GN, Karpati G. Type 1 fiber hy-

pertrophy and central nuclei: A rare congenital muscle abnormality with a possible experimental model. Arch Neurol 1968; 18L:435–444.

205. Schochet SS, Zellweger H, Ionescu V, McCormick WF. Centronuclear myopathy: Disease entity or syndromes. J Neurol Sci 1972; 27:215–228.

206. Whitaker JN. Inflammatory myopathy: A review of etiologic and pathogenetic factors. Muscle Nerve 1932; 5:573–592.

207. Hudgson P, Peter JB. Classification. Clin Rheum Dis 1984; 10:3–8.

208. Pearson CM, Bohan A. The spectrum of polymyositis and dermatomyositis. Med Clin North Am 1977; 61:439–457.

209. Foote RA, Kimbrough SM, Stevens JC. Lupus myositis. Muscle Nerve 1982; 5:65–68.

210. Henriksson K-G, Stalberg E. The terminal innervation pattern in polymyositis: A histological and SFEMG study. Muscle Nerve 1978; 1:3–13.

211. Lederman RJ, Salanga VD, Wilbourn AJ, et al. Focal inflammatory myopathy. Muscle Nerve 1984; 7:142–146.

212. Jablecki C. Lambert-Eaton myasthenic syndrome. Muscle Nerve 1984; 7:250–257.

213. Streib EW, Wilbourn AJ, Mitsumoto H. Spontaneous electrical muscle fiber activity in polymyositis and dermatomyositis. Muscle Nerve 1979; 2:14–18.

214. Lambert EH, Sayre GP, Eaton LM. Electrical activity of muscle in polymyositis. Trans Am Neurol Assoc 1954; 79:64–69.

215. Buchthal F, Pinelli P. Muscle action potentials in polymyositis. Neurology 1953; 3:424–436.

216. Trojaborg W. Quantitative electromyography in polymyositis: A reappraisal. Muscle Nerve 1990; 13:964–971.

217. Barkhaus PE, Nandedkar SD, Sanders DB. Quantitative EMG in inflammatory myopathy. Muscle Nerve 1990; 13:247–253.

218. Hollinrake K. Polymyositis presenting as distal muscle weakness. A case report. J Neurol Sci 1969; 8:479–484.

219. Bunch TW. Polymyositis: A case history approach to the differential diagnosis and treatment. Mayo Clin Proc 1990; 65:1480–1497.

220. O'Leary PA, Waisman M. Dermatomyositis: A study of forty cases. Arch Dermatol Syphilol 1940; 41:1001–1019.

221. De Vere R, Bradley WG. Polymyositis: Its presentation, morbidity and mortality. Brain 1975; 98:637–666.

222. Carpenter S, Karpati G, Heller I, Eisen A. Inclusion body myositis: A distinct variety of idiopathic inflammatory myopathy. Neurology 1978; 28:8–17.

223. Mikol J. Inclusion body myositis. In: Engel AG, Banker BQ, eds. Myology: Basic and clinical. New York: McGraw-Hill, 1986:1423–1438.

224. Lozt BP, Engel AG, Nishino H, et al. Inclusion body myositis: Observations in 40 patients. Brain 1989; 112:727–747.

225. Wintzen AR, Bots GT, de Bakker HM, et al. Dysphagia in inclusion body myositis. J Neurol Neurosurg Psychiatry 1988; 51:1542–1545.

226. Eisen A, Berry K, Gibson G. Inclusion body myositis (IBM): Myopathy or neuropathy? Neurology 1983; 33:1109–1114.

227. Hartlage P, Rivner M, Henning W, Levy R. Electrophysiologic and prognostic factors in inclusion body myositis. Muscle Nerve 1988; 11:984.

228. Joy JL, Shin J, Baysal AI. Electrophysiological spectrum of inclusion body myositis. Muscle Nerve 1990; 13:949–951.

229. Ringel SP, Kenny CE, Neville HE, et al. Spectrum of inclusion body myositis. Arch Neurol 1987; 11:1154–1157.

230. Calbrese LH, Mitsumoto H, Chou SM. Inclusion body myositis presenting as treatment-resistant polymyositis. J Arch Rheum 1987; 30:397–403.

231. Abarbanel JM, Lichtenfeld Y, Zirkin H, et al. Inclusion body myositis in post-polymyelitis muscular atrophy. J Neurol Scand 1988; 78:81–84.

232. Riggs JE, Schochet SS Jr, Gutmann L, Lerfald SC. Childhood onset inclusion body myositis mimicking limb-girdle muscular dystrophy. J Child Neurol 1989; 4:283–285.

233. Ramsay I. Thyrotoxic muscle disease. Postgrad Med J 1968; 44:931–934.

234. Dresner SC, Kennerdell JS. Dysthyroid orbitopathy. Neurology 1985; 35:1628–1634.

235. Ramsay ID. Muscle dysfunction in hyperthyroidism. Lancet 1966; 14:931–934.

236. Havard CWH, Campbell EDR, Ross HB, et al. Electromyographic and histological findings in the muscles of patients with thyrotoxicosis. J Med 1963; 32:145–163.

237. Harman JB, Richardson AT. Generalized myokymia in thyrotoxicosis. Lancet 1954; 2:473–474.

238. Wilson J, Walton JN. Some muscular manifestations of hypothyroidism. J Neurol Neurosurg Psychiatry 1959; 22:320–324.

239. Lambert EH, Underdahl LO, Beckett S, et al. A study of the ankle jerk in myxedema. J Clin Endocrinol Metab 1951; 11:1186–1205.

240. Spiro AJ, Hiranoi A, Beilin RL, et al. Cretinism with muscular hypertrophy (Kocher-Debre-Semelaigne). Histochemical and ultrastructural study skeletal muscle. Arch Neurol 1970; 23:340–349.

241. Waldstein SS, Bronsky D, Shrifter HB, et al. The electromyogram in myxedema. Arch Intern Med 1958; 101:97–102.

242. Pattern BM, Pages M. Severe neurological disease associated with hyperparathyroidism. Ann Neurol 1984; 15:453–456.

243. Pattern BM, Bilezikian JP, Mallette LE, et al. Neuromuscular disease in primary hyperparathyroidism. Ann Intern Med 1974; 80:182–193.

244. Smith R, Stern G. Myopathy, osteomalacia, hyperparathyroidism. Brain 1967; 90:593–602.

245. Hudgson P, Hall R. Endocrine myopathies. In:

Mastaglia FL, Walton J, eds. Skeletal muscle pathology. New York: Churchill Livingstone, 1982: 403–404.

246. Kugelberg E. Accommodation in human nerves and its significance for the symptoms in circulation disturbances and tetany. Acta Physiol Scand 1944; 8(suppl 24):1–105.

247. Kugelberg E. Activation of human nerves by ischemia. Trousseau's phenomenon in tetany. Arch Neurol Psychiatry 1948; 60:140–152.

248. Golding DN, Murray SM, Pearce GW, et al. Corticosteroid myopathy. Ann Phys Med 1961; 6:171–177.

249. Askari A, Vignos PJ, Moskowitz RW. Steroid myopathy in connective tissue disease. Am J Med 1976; 61:485–491.

250. Perkoff GT, Silver R, Tyler FH, et al. Studies in disorders of muscle. Am J Med 1959; 26:891–898.

251. MacFarlane IA, Rosenthal FD. Severe myopathy after status asthmaticus. Lancet 1977; 2:615.

252. Van Marale W, Woods KL. Acute hydrocortisone myopathy. Br Med J 1980; 281:271–272.

253. Harriman DGF, Reed L. The incidence of lipid droplets in human muscle in neuromuscular disorders. J Pathol 1972; 106:1–24.

254. Pleasure DE, Walsh GO, Engel WK. Atrophy of skeletal muscle in patients with Cushing's syndrome. Arch Neurol 1970; 22:118–125.

255. Muller R, Kugelberg E. Myopathy in Cushing's syndrome. J Neurol Neurosurg Psychiatry 1959; 22:314–319.

256. Pickett JBE III, Layzer RB, Levin SR, et al. Neuromuscular complications of acromegaly. Neurology 1975; 25:638–645.

257. Lane RJM, Mastaglia FL. Drug-induced myopathies in man. Lancet 1978; 2:562–565.

258. Urbano-Marquez A, Estruch R, Navarro-Lopez F, et al. The effects of alcohol on skeletal and cardiac muscle. N Engl J Med 1989; 320:409–415.

259. Perkoff GT, Dioso M, Bleisch V, et al. A spectrum of myopathy associated with alcoholism. Ann Intern Med 1967; 67:481–501.

260. Perkoff GT. Alcoholic myopathy. Ann Rev Med 1971; 22:125–132.

261. Whisnant JP, Espinosa RE, Kierland RR, et al. Chloroquine neuromyopathy. Mayo Clin Proc 1963; 38:501–513.

262. Mastaglia FL, Papadmitriou JM, Dawkins RL, et al. Vacuolar myopathy associated with chloroquine, lupus erythematosus and thyoma. Report of a case with unusual mitochondrial changes and lipid accumulation in muscle. J Neurol Sci 1977; 34:315–328.

263. Bradley WG, Lassman LP, Pearce GW, et al. The neuropathy of vincristine in man: Clinical electrophysiological and pathological studies. J Neurol Sci 1970; 10:107–131.

264. Duane DD, Engel AG. Emetine myopathy. Neurology 1970; 20:733–739.

265. Mateer J, Farrell B, Chou SM, Glutman L. Reversible ipecac myopathy. Neurology 1979; 29:596.

266. Bennett HS, Spiro AJ, Pollack MA, et al. Ipecac-induced myopathy stimulating dermatomyositis. Neurology 1982; 32:91–94.

267. Sugie H, Russin R, Verity MA. Emetine myopathy: Two case reports with pathobiological analysis. Muscle Nerve 1984; 7:54–59.

268. Palmer EP, Guay AT. Reversible myopathy secondary to abuse of ipecac in patients with eating disorders. N Engl J Med 1985; 313:1457–1459.

269. Kuncl RW, Duncan G, Watson D, et al. Colchicine myopathy and neuropathy. N Engl J Med 1987; 316:1562–1568.

270. Riggs JE, Schochet WS, Gutman L, et al. Chronic human colchicine neuropathy and myopathy. Arch Neurol 1986; 43:521–523.

271. Kuncl RW, Cornblath DR, Avila O, Duncan G. Electrodiagnosis of human colchicine myoneuropathy. Muscle Nerve 1989; 12:360–364.

272. Kiloh LG, Nevin S. Progressive dystrophy of the external ocular muscles (ocular myopathy). Brain 1951; 74(9):116–143.

273. Bray GM, Kaarsoo M, Ross RT. Ocular myopathy with dysphagia. Neurology 1965; 15:678–684.

274. Roberts AH, Bamforth J. The pharynx and esophagus in ocular muscular dystrophy. Neurology 1968; 18:645–652.

275. Ross RT. Ocular myopathy sensitive to curare. Brain 1963; 86:67–74.

276. Mathew NT, Jacob JC, Chandy J. Familial ocular myopathy with curare sensitivity. Arch Neurol 1970; 22:68–74.

277. Schotland DL, Rowland LP. Muscular dystrophy. Features of ocular myopathy, distal dystrophy and myotonic dystrophy. Arch Neurol 1964; 10:433–445.

278. Drachman DA. Ophthalmoplegia plus. The neurodegenerative disorders associated with progressive external opthalmoplegia. Arch Neurol 1968; 18:654–674.

279. Kamieniecka Z. Myopathies with abnormal mitochondria. A clinical, histochemical and electrophysiological study. Acta Neurol Scand 1976; 55:57–75.

280. Leshner RT, Spector RH, Seybold M, et al. Progressive external ophthalmoplegia (PEO) with ragged red fibers: An intrafamilial study. Neurology 1978; 28:364–365.

281. Berenberg RA, Pellock JM, DiMauro S, et al. Lumping or splitting? "Ophthalmoplegia-plus" or Kearns-Sayre syndrome. Ann Neurol 1977; 1:37–54.

282. Kearns TP, Sayre GP. Retinitis pigmentosa, external ophthalmoplegia and complete heart block. Arch Ophthalmol 1958; 60:208–289.

283. Shy GM, Silverberg DH, Appel S, et al. A generalized disorder of nervous system, skeletal muscle and heart resembling Refsum's disease and Hurler's syndrome. I. Clinical, pathological, and biochemical characteristics. Am J Med 1967; 42:163–168.

284. Karpati G, Carpenter S, Labrisseau A, et al. The Kearns-Shy syndrome. A multisystem disease with mitochondrial abnormality demonstrated in skeletal muscle and skin. J Neurol Sci 1973; 19:133–151.

285. Olsen W, Engel WK, Walsh GO, et al. Oculocraniosomatic neuromuscular disease with "ragged-red" fibers. Arch Neurol 1972; 26:193–211.

286. Swash M, Schwartz MS, Sargeant MK. The significance of ragged-red fibers in neuromuscular disease. J Neurol Sci 1978; 38:347–355.

287. Kamieniecka Z, Schmalbruch H. Myopathies with abnormal mitochondria: A clinicopathologic classification. Muscle Nerve 1978; 1:413–415.

288. Brust JCM, List TA, Catalano LW, et al. Ocular myasthenia gravis mimicking progressive external ophthamoplegia. Neurology 1974; 24:755–760.

289. Krendel DA, Sanders DB, Massev JM. Single fiber electromyography in chronic progressive external ophthalmoplegia. Muscle Nerve 1985; 8:624.

290. Morgan-Hughes JA. Mitochondrial myopathies. Mastaglia FL, Walton JN eds. Skeletal muscle pathology. Edinburg:Churchill-Livingstone, 1982: 309–339.

291. Yiannikas C, McLeod JG, Pollard JD, Baverstock J. Peripheral neuropathy associated with mitochondrial myopathy. Ann Neurol 1986; 20:249–257.

IV

Electromyographic Studies in Special Settings

25

Pediatric Electromyography   H. Royden Jones, Jr.

CONTENTS

LIST OF ACRONYMS

ABL	Abetalipoproteinemia
AchR	Acetylcholine receptor
AchRAb	Acetylcholine receptor antibodies
AIDP	Acute inflammatory demyelinating polyneuropathy
AIDS	Acquired immune deficiency syndrome
ALD	Adrenoleukodystrophy
ALMN	Adrenoleukomyeloneuropathy
ALS	Amyotrophic lateral sclerosis
AMC	Arthrogryposis multiplex congenita
AraC	Cytosine arabinoside
AST	Aspartate aminotransaminase
AT	Ataxia telangiectasia
BAER	Brain stem auditory evoked response
BMT	Bone marrow transplant
CHN	Congenital hypomyelinating neuropathies
CIC	Circulating immune complex
CIDP	Chronic inflammatory demyelinating polyneuropathy
CK	Creatine kinase
CMAP	Compound muscle action potential
CMG	Congenital myasthenia gravis
CRD	Complex repetitive discharges
CT	Computed tomography
CTS	Carpal tunnel syndrome
CV	Conduction velocity
DNA	Deoxyribonucleic acid
DPT	Diphtheria, pertussis, tetanus
EDMD	Emery-Dreifuss muscular dystrophy
EMG	Electromyography
EP	Evoked potential
ESR	Erythrocyte sedimentation rate
FIMG	Familial infantile myasthenia gravis
GAN	Giant axonal neuropathy
GSD	Glycogen storage disease
HES	Hypereosinophilic syndrome
HIV	Human immunodeficiency virus
HMSN	Hereditary motor sensory neuropathies
HSN	Hereditary sensory neuropathy
IND	Infantile neuroaxonal dystrophy
IP	Incontinentia pigmenti
LEMS	Lambert-Eaton myasthenic syndrome
LLW	Long latency wave
MCV	Motor conduction velocity
MH	Malignant hyperthermia
MNB	Muscle nerve biopsy
MRI	Magnetic resonance imaging
MSS	Marinesco-Sjögren syndrome
MUP	Motor unit potential
NCS	Nerve conduction study
NMG	Neonatal myasthenia gravis
NMTD	Neuromuscular transmission defects

NPD	Niemann-Pick disease
OCRS	Oculocerebral renal syndrome
PTF	Posttetanic facilitation
RMNS	Repetitive motor nerve stimulation
RSS	Rigid spine syndrome
SSER	Somatosensory evoked response
SGOT	Serum glutamic-oxaloacetic transaminase
SLE	Systemic lupus erythematosus
SMA	Spinal muscular atrophy
SNAP	Sensory nerve action potential
SNE	Subacute necrotizing encephalomyelopathy
VER	Visual evoked response
WBC	White blood cells
WHD	Werdnig-Hoffmann disease

Nerve conduction studies (NCS) and electromyographic evaluations are important diagnostic modalities in most forms of pediatric neuromuscular disease.[1-3] Some physicians trained in clinical electromyography (EMG) have relatively minimal experience during their residency training with electromyographic evaluation of children, particularly infants. Most electromyographic laboratories are staffed by neurologists or physiatrists. Even at major academic centers with reputations for expertise in the diagnosis and treatment of childhood neuromuscular diseases, the number of pediatric patients seen compared with adult patients is small. Therefore much experience is required to evaluate the broad spectrum of these illnesses. Although many pediatric neuromuscular diseases are analogous to those seen in the adult, the relative proportion varies greatly in children, as illustrated by the fact that two of the most common clinical indications for adult EMG— carpal tunnel syndrome and nerve root lesions— occur infrequently in childhood. In contrast, more infants have been referred to our laboratory for evaluation of the floppy syndrome than our total experience with mononeuropathies of the extremities.

APPROACH TO THE PEDIATRIC PATIENT

Electromyographers evaluating infants and children need to become familiar with an evolving neurophysiologic database related to maturation of peripheral nerves and muscle. This database provides a reference scale for evaluation of the pediatric patient. Logistic challenges are present, which include the tiny extremities of the newborn that make it technically difficult to perform NCS and EMG. The 1-year-old to 4-year-old child may resist being evaluated and may require sedation. Before deciding about premedication, our physicians review the record and evaluate the child and ideally the parents whenever possible. Infants less than 1 year old do not require sedation. Conversely, most children 1 to 4 years old are premedicated with chloral hydrate, 60 to 70 mg/kg, 30 to 45 minutes before the procedure. This dose usually produces enough sedation to permit accurate attainment of motor and sensory nerve conduction parameters. Another premedication, Demerol compound (Demerol [meperidine, Winthrop Pharmaceuticals, New York, NY], 25 mg; chlorpromazine, 6.25 mg; and promethazine, 6.25 mg, each/mL at a dose of 1 mL-15 kg), tends to oversedate the child, who consequently is unable to recruit motor units during needle EMG. With administration of chloral hydrate, introduction of the needle EMG will waken the child enough to permit adequate motor unit potential (MUP) analysis.

Good rapport with the parents may provide the difference between obtaining an adequate or a poor examination. We try to allay anxieties by discussing the purposes and design of the study. When the parents realize the electromyographer shares their concern for the well-being of their child, they are usually cooperative. Anxieties may be relieved by demonstrating a sensory NCS on a parent. With an infant or young child, the parent usually holds the child on his or her lap. The study is honestly discussed with an older child or an adolescent. The child is encouraged to become a participant in the study by watching the oscilloscope and listening to the loudspeaker.

The evaluation is begun with sensory NCS, which causes the least discomfort. In children, peripheral nerves are close to the surface and require minimal stimulus. During the motor portion of NCS, the child is encouraged to watch the response build on the oscilloscope. When another site on the nerve is tested, we ask them to see whether we can obtain a similar response.

The needle EMG portion of the study is less well tolerated. Never surprise the child with a painful examination. The child should be forewarned, and questions should be answered about pain before the first needle insertion. We never mention the word *needle*, however, but simply state than we are putting tiny wire electrodes into the muscle. We describe the feeling of discomfort like a mosquito bite or a pinch. Avoid the sight of blood whenever possible by being sure hemostasis is achieved before proceeding with the next needle insertion. Try to make the study "fun" by asking the child what the motor units sound like. Commenting on the noise produced, we ask how the child is able to sleep at night with all the noise the muscles are making! This often produces a laugh or at least distracts the child's attention from the electrode. Although physicians may conduct the evaluation alone, it is easier when a resident, technician, or parent assists.

In the intensive care units, adequate motor and sensory NCS and neuromuscular transmission studies can usually be obtained. Electrical interference and artifact, however, often obscure the needle EMG. It is better to perform NCS and EMG in the EMG laboratory, which is isolated from various sources of electrical interference.

The investigation in the child is pursued as it is in the adult. When an isolated problem in one limb in reference to the question of a peripheral nerve or plexus lesion is being studied, several motor and sensory nerves and muscles in that extremity need to be examined. When specific abnormalities are demonstrated, the most affected homologous area in the contralateral extremity is examined for comparison. For more diffuse processes, such as generalized peripheral neuropathies or myopathies, at least two extremities are examined. In processes such as acute inflammatory demyelinating polyneuropathy (AIDP) or spinal muscular atrophies (SMA), in which the possibility of multifocal or diffuse lesions is evaluated, it is also necessary to examine the contralateral extremities or many segments in some extremities to demonstrate multifocal processes.

Maturational Factors

Maturational factors are important in newborns and infants. Peripheral nerve myelination begins at about the fifteenth week of gestation[4] and continues throughout the first 3 to 5 years after birth. A direct relationship exists between diameter of the axon and thickness of the myelin sheath. Conduction velocity (CV) progressively increases in direct proportion to the diameter of the largest axon. The ratio of CV to nerve fiber diameter is about 6:1.[5] In the anterior

cervical nerve roots of newborns and infants, the fiber diameter increased 200% and reached a maximum between ages 2 and 5 years.[6,7] No unusual acceleration of myelination occurs just after birth.[6] The nodes of Ranvier are remodeled, with internodal distances reaching a peak at 5 years.[8]

Evaluation of premature infants indicates that maturation of nerves is primarily related to age from conception rather than age from birth.[6] Changes in CV may permit estimation of fetal development and a distinction between infants with small birth weight or low gestational age.[9] Premature infants of 23 to 27 weeks gestation may have median motor conduction velocity (MCV) as low as 9 to 11 m/second.[10] Infants of different weights but similar age appear to have conduction of equal speeds. Wagner and Buchthal[11] found that the maturation of myelinated nerve fibers appears to be as fast whether in utero or ex utero (Figure 25.1). A scatter of 8 to 15 m/second occurred among the children studied. CVs in the extremities are relatively similar in peripheral nerves of newborns (i.e., 20 to 30 m/s), whereas in older children and adults, the nerves in the arm tend to be 7 to 10 m/second faster than in the legs (Figure 25.2), and all reach adult values at 4 years of age.[11]

Some difference between the maturation of the

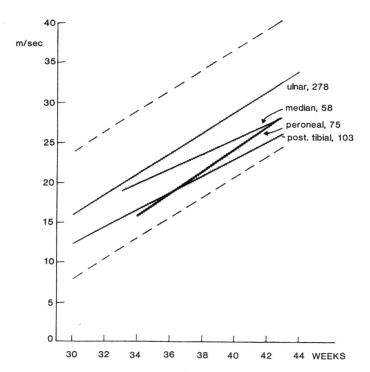

FIGURE 25.1. *Motor conduction velocities related to conceptional age in weeks in healthy newborn. (Reprinted with permission from Wagner AL, Buchthal F. Motor and sensory conduction in infancy and childhood: Reappraisal. Dev Med Child Neurol 1972; 14:197.)*

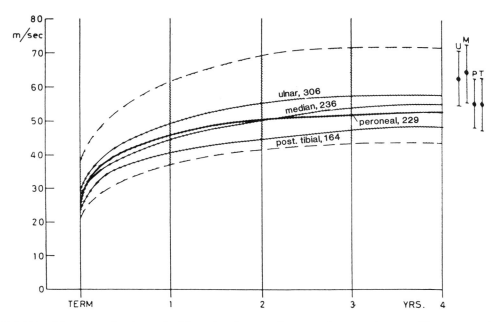

FIGURE 25.2. *Motor conduction velocities related to age from newborn to 4 years old. (Reprinted with permission from Wagner AL, Buchthal F. Motor and sensory conduction in infancy and childhood: Reappraisal. Dev Med Child Neurol 1972; 14:196.)*

median and ulnar motor nerves is noted in the neonatal and early infancy periods.[12] At birth, CV of the median, ulnar, and peroneal nerves approximated half of normal adult values, with the average resting CV of 27 m/second and at 6 months, 36 m/second. At age 5 weeks, the peroneal MCV may be greater than the median and ulnar CV (Table 25.1).[13] Both the ulnar and peroneal nerves gradually increase speed of conduction through infancy, especially during the first 6 months of life. In contrast, the median nerve lags in maturation, and its CV increases significantly between ages 1 and 3 years.[13] At about 3 years of age in children, practically all ulnar MCV values are in the lower adult range.[6] In early childhood, CV of the ulnar and median nerves continues to increase, whereas that of the peroneal nerve does not. The modest difference between ulnar and median MCV gradually disappears by age 4 or 5. The process of peripheral nerve maturation involves not only CV, but also distal latencies and compound muscle action potential (CMAP) amplitudes. Latency determinations for motor fibers have been corrected with a standard distal distance of 2.5 cm (Figure 25.3). The differences for CMAPs are even greater with maturation; they triple in size, in contrast to CVs, which double as the child matures.[6]

Maturational changes of orthodromic sensory conduction corresponded to changes found for motor fibers.[14] In infants, two distinct peaks occurred on the compound sensory nerve action potential (SNAP) on proximal recording of orthodromic conduction that were attributed to differences in maturation of two groups of sensory fibers.[11] An early report[14] noted difficulty in obtaining sensory responses before age 3 months and suggested that absent compound SNAPs are only significant after age 3 months. We routinely obtain sensory conduction in normal newborns, however, and the absence of these responses is of major importance in distinguishing a floppy infant who has SMA (Werdnig-Hoffmann disease [WHD]) from one who has a less common congenital neuropathy. A set of normal values for motor and sensory NCS from normal children 0 to 2 years of age seen at the Mayo Clinic is outlined in Table 25.2.[1]

Fetal nutrition, measured by skinfold thickness, may be an important factor in influencing myelination and consequently affects nerve conduction measurements.[15] A study[16] of 25 infants with *neonatal abstinence syndrome* born to drug-dependent mothers found normal MCV in each neonate with normal results on EMG in 21 of 23, and two neonates had

TABLE 25.1.   Mean motor nerve conduction velocities obtained for children in different age groups

Average Age of Group in Weeks	Velocity in Meters/Second			
	Ulnar	Median	Peroneal	Posterior Tibial
5	34.5 (11)*	33.1 (12)	37.2 (6)	34.3 (11)
18	35.4 (12)	35.8 (11)	39.1 (12)	32.7 (11)
34	46.1 (12)	41.8 (12)	44.1 (12)	38.8 (12)
56	46.7 (10)	40.4 (12)	46.7 (12)	39.8 (12)
88	51.6 (12)	47.5 (12)	49.5 (12)	44.5 (12)
140	52.4 (12)	49.4 (12)	44.2 (11)	43.1 (10)
210	56.1 (12)	54.9 (12)	52.2 (12)	48.4 (12)

* Numbers in parentheses refer to number of children in age group for whom nerve conduction velocity was determined. Reprinted with permission from Baer RD, Johnson EW. Motor nerve conduction velocities in normal children. Arch Phys Med Rehabil 1965; 46:702.

minimal partial denervation. Six infants were less than 10% normal size for gestational age.

In reference to H *reflexes* and F waves, normally an ulnar nerve H *reflex* can be recorded in the infant in contrast to adults. Thomas and Lambert[6] found that the CV of afferent fibers of the H *reflex* between wrist and elbow segments in newborns was approximately 10% faster than the *motor* conduction fibers

of the ulnar nerves. The H *reflex* is carried over group 1 afferent fibers, which are the fastest conducting peripheral fibers. The presence of the H *reflex* in the upper extremities represents lack of central nervous system myelination similar to that which accounts for the presence of the Babinski sign in the newborn and young infant. The H *reflex* was identified on stimulation of the ulnar nerves in 34 of 39

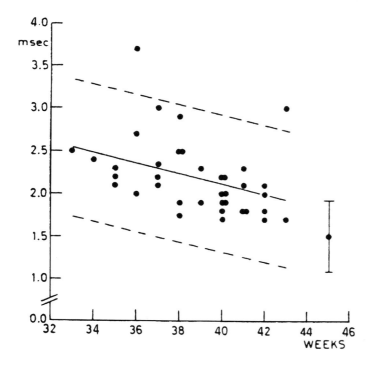

FIGURE 25.3.   *Distal motor latencies of ulnar nerves at 2.5 cm related to conceptional age in healthy newborns. (Reprinted with permission from Wagner AL, Buchthal F. Motor and sensory conduction in infancy and childhood: Reappraisal. Dev Med Child Neurol 1972; 14:197.)*

TABLE 25.2. Motor and sensory nerve conduction studies in infants: Range of normals

	Number	CMAP/SNAP Amplitude (mV/μV)	Conduction Velocity (m/s)	Distal Latency (ms)	Distance (cm)
Neonate					
Motor					
Ulnar	56	1.6–7	20–36.1	1.3–2.9	1–3.4
Median	4	2.6–5.9	22.4–27.1	2–2.9	1.9–3
Peroneal	4	1.8–4	21–26.7	2.1–3.1	1.9–3.8
Sensory					
Median	10	7–15 (A)*	25.1–31.9	2.1–3	3.8–5.4
	1	8–17 (O)	—	—	—
Sural	8		—	3.3	5.5
Medial plantar	3	10–40	—	2.1–3.3	4.4–5.8
1–6 Months					
Motor					
Ulnar	22	2.5–7.4	33.3–50	1.1–3.2	1.7–4.4
Median	6	3.5–6.9	37–47.7	1.6–2.2	2.1–4.1
Peroneal	10	1.6–8	32.4–47.7	1.7–2.4	2.5–4.1
Sensory					
Median	11	13–52 (A) 9–26 (O)	36.3–41.9	1.5–2.3	4.3–6.3
Sural	2	9–10	—	1.7–2.3	5.8
Medial plantar	2	17–26	35.4–35.7	1.5–1.9	4.5–5.5
7–12 Months					
Motor					
Ulnar	28	3.2–10	35–58.2	0.8–2.2	1.9–4.6
Median	13	2.3–8.6	33.3–46.3	1.5–2.8	1.9–4.3
Peroneal	19	2.3–6	38.8–56	1.4–3.2	2.2–5.5
Sensory					
Median	15	14–64 (A) 11–36 (O)	39.1–60	1.6–2.4	5.5–6.8
Sural	5	10–28	40.6	1.7–2.5	5.8–7.6
Medial Plantar	6	15–38	39.4–40.3	1.9–2.7	6.5–7.9
13–24 Months					
Motor					
Ulnar	53	2.6–9.7	41.3–63.5	1.1–2.2	2.4–4.8
Median	16	3.7–11.6	39.2–50.5	1.8–2.8	2.2–4.3
Peroneal	36	1.7–6.5	39.2–54.3	1.6–3.5	2.2–5.8
Sensory					
Median	29	14–82 (A) 7–36 (O)	46.5–57.9	1.7–3	5.7–9.1
Sural	9	8–30	–	1.4–2.8	4.5–8.6
Medial plantar	12	15–60	42.6–57.3	1.8–2.5	6.1–9.3

*(A), antidromic sensory potential; (O), orthodromic sensory potential.

Reprinted with permission from Miller RG, Kuntz NL. Nerve conduction studies in infants and children. J Child Neurol 1986; 1:22.

full-term infants.[6] By age 1 year, however, this response had totally disappeared in the ulnar nerve.

Few studies have defined the normal spectrum of F waves that can be recorded from most limb nerves in newborns and young infants. Shahani and Young[17] studied median nerve F waves in three infants less than 3 months of age and 15 youngsters between 4 months and 2 years of age and found values of 16 ± 1.5 ms for infants less than 3 months of age and 14.4 ± 1.6 ms for the older group. The Mayo Clinic parameters for F wave latencies for infants ages 0 to 2 years are outlined in Table 25.3.[1]

TABLE 25.3.   F wave latencies in infants: Range of normals

Months	Nerve	Number	Latency (ms)	Distance (cm)
1–6	Ulnar	1	17	21
	Peroneal	2	22–25	35–36
7–12	Ulnar	6	13–16	21–30
	Median	3	13–16	23–30
	Peroneal	3	19–23	20–47
	Tibial	2	19–24	43–48
13–24	Ulnar	10	14–17	25–39
	Median	4	14–18	22–27
	Peroneal	10	21–26	30–53
	Tibial	9	25–26	42–52

Reprinted with permission from Miller RG, Kuntz NL. Nerve conduction studies in infants and children. J Child Neurol 1989; 1:24.

Technical Factors with Infantile Nerve Conduction Studies

Because of the inherent small size of infants, when NCS are performed, measurements must be accurate. In the first months of life, the average distance over which CVs are measured is no more than 9 cm. Thus a 1-cm error in measurement accounts for a 12% error in the calculation of CV. Also, the placement of electrodes may be more difficult in the newborn because of the small size of the hand. The G_1 pickup electrode is placed on the thenar or hypothenar eminence. We use a ring electrode as our G_2 reference and place it on the third digit for recording the median CMAP or the fifth finger for recording the ulnar CMAP. Until we adapted this method, the G_2 electrode was sometimes difficult to secure on the unrelaxed often sweaty hand of an infant.

Because the fingers are relatively short and a 2- to 3-cm difference between G_1 and G_2 is needed, the third digit is used to obtain orthodromic median compound SNAP. Antidromic ulnar and musculocutaneous compound SNAPs may be studied with relative ease in the infant. Although forearm sensory CV can be obtained with use of antidromic techniques, the recording of sensory CV is usually not necessary. A normal compound SNAP provides sufficient evidence to exclude any lesion between the dorsal root ganglion and the distal sensory nerve ending. A sural compound SNAP can usually be obtained in children. Sometimes we have difficulty with newborns and young infants because when they lie on their side, they tend to squirm and are unable to support themselves. We have not found many clinical instances in which knowledge of a sural compound SNAP instead of a median compound SNAP has proved to be of considerable help in the differential diagnosis of infants in this age group.

When we test for neuromuscular transmission (NMT) defects in the neonate and child up to age 4 years, it is wise to use sedation. One important difference between children aged 0 to 6 years and the older child is the inability to have the youngest voluntarily exercise to permit examination for presynaptic or postsynaptic defects. Therefore in contrast to older children and adults, in whom it is rarely necessary to use 20- to 50-c/s stimulation, such stimulation may be vitally important with an infant. Although it is well tolerated with adequate sedation, this stimulation sometimes awakens the child, and a technically adequate study may be impossible, necessitating a repeat study later.

When repetitive motor nerve stimulation (RMNS) is performed, it is best to immobilize the infant's arm with a pediatric arm board. Although some laboratories[18] have reported using subcutaneous pin electrodes, surface recording electrodes are adequate, particularly when the child is appropriately sedated. The study should be performed in a warm room with a warm blanket, and the surface temperature should be monitored with a thermister. With cooling, a defect in neuromuscular transmission may be missed.

Because of the relatively short length of the extremities, stimuli may be delivered proximally or distally (the latter is preferred). In general, a distance of at least 4 cm should be maintained between the stimulating and recording electrodes. Rare forms of congenital myasthenia may be recognized by the characteristic evidence of a series of two or more repetitive responses to a single stimulus. This finding is an indication to proceed with repetitive stimulation. In children, supramaximal stimulation may be reached at levels that are considerably lower than those required for adults. Thus evaluation may be completed with less discomfort, and awakening the child may sometimes be avoided. Stimulation begins with 0.5 c/s and is increased to 2 c/s. Brief trains of 1- to 5-second duration with stimulation at rates of 20 to 50 c/s help to look for postexercise facilitation or decrement.

The neuromuscular junction is not fully matured at birth. Unfortunately, only a few control studies of normal infants have been reported. One of the most detailed was the evaluation of 17 newborns, including six premature infants with gestational ages between 34 and 42 weeks, by Koenigsberger et al.[19] Their methods were different from those usually used for adults in that continuous stimulation at rates of 1 to 50 c/s was carried out for 15 seconds, whereas it is difficult to conduct such studies for more than 0.3 to 1.0 seconds in a cooperative adult. In normal newborns, no change in CMAP amplitude was observed at a rate of 1 to 2 c/s. When the stimulus was increased to 5 to 10 c/s, however, five of eight infants showed at least a 10% facilitation. Decremental changes began to occur at rates of 20 c/s and averaged 24% in 12 of 17 normal newborn infants. The degree of decrement was greatest in the most premature infants studied, who were 34 weeks gestation. The neuromuscular junction of the newborn was most sensitive to 50 c/s stimulation; all 17 infants studied demonstrated a decrement averaging 51%. Confirmatory studies have not been carried out because it is difficult to study normal newborns with this uncomfortable procedure. Therefore the rapid and most uncomfortable forms of repetitive stimulation are not as helpful in evaluating postsynaptic infantile NMT defects because of the poor safety factor present in the immature neuromuscular junction. Decremental changes, however, at the rates of 2 to 10 c/s and facilitatory changes at 20 to 50 c/s are significant.

Single-fiber EMG and the assessment of variability in amplitude of repetitively firing MUPs in adults depend on patient cooperation. Thus these techniques cannot be used adequately until children are at least 8 to 12 years of age.

Technical Factors with Infantile Needle Electromyography

As with NCS, any procedure causing discomfort creates increasing anxiety in the child. Careful and accurate examination, however, can be accomplished on most infants. Children younger than 4 years of age cannot be reasoned with, nor does one have the advantage of gaining their participation.

The electromyographer has to tailor the number of muscles examined to the clinical question being considered. The number of muscles examined in children may be limited; however, the electromyographer must not risk an incomplete examination. Because infants do not cooperate, the electromyographer often does not have the chance to observe individual motor units in isolation.

One must be flexible and not always examine insertional activity first, then single motor units, and finally, recruitment. When the child is relaxed and quiet, look at the insertional activity. When the infant is trying to resist, examine the motor units

first. In the newborn, certain muscles are not easily activated, and only abnormalities of insertion can be observed. Other muscles may be activated continuously, thus precluding observation of insertional activity, but they provide an opportunity to evaluate MUPs. This approach is well suited to the generalized diseases present in many newborns and young infants. Less commonly, an infant has a mononeuropathy or plexus lesion that requires study of both insertional activity and MUPs in multiple muscles in the same extremity. This can be accomplished but requires patience and diligence of the electromyographer.

When the floppy infant is examined,[20] flexor muscles such as the tibialis anterior and the iliopsoas are useful in evaluating MUPs. They can be activated by tickling the bottom of the foot, producing a withdrawal response. In the arm, the flexor digitorum sublimis and biceps muscles are frequently reflexly contracted by the newborn or young infant, which permits assessment of MUPs. We do not attempt to use other forms of reflex stimuli, such as the Moro reflex or the various stepping postures. They seem to make the study more cumbersome and more difficult for parents to watch. To evaluate insertional activity extensor muscles, such as the vastus lateralis and gastrocnemius and the first dorsal interosseous and triceps in the arms, are examined that are not reflexly contracted or brought into use by the struggling child.

Normal MUP parameters differ in the infant and young child compared with an adult. The amplitude of the histogram shifts to the left or lower side of adult MUP with normal amplitudes varying between 100 and 700 μV, and MUPs more than 1000 μV in 0- to 3-year-old infants are rare.[21,22] MUPs are biphasic or triphasic. Their recruitment pattern is often disordered but on occasion similar to that of adults. Assessment of MUP characteristics in young children is difficult, and attempts to detect insertional abnormalities may be even more difficult. In infants, MUPs are small, but fibrillation potentials are smaller and may be masked by minimal MUP activation. Vigorous crying may also obscure the characteristic *tick* of subtle fibrillation potentials.

Because of sporadic recruitment of MUPs in infants, a diagnosis is often made based on a gestalt impression. This is easier in infantile SMA, in which definite dropout in the number of MUPs firing occurs, and it is easier to see the rapid recruitment and relatively large size. As in the adult, a diagnosis of a diffuse process affecting motor neurons in the floppy infant is associated with such poor prognostic indication that the presence of fibrillation potentials and concomitant neurogenic MUPs in at least three extremities must be ascertained. At least nine other recognized abnormalities of the motor unit exist in which fibrillation potentials may be associated with the clinical syndrome of the floppy infant, some of which do not merit the poor long-term prognosis of infantile SMA I or WHD.[20] Similarly, caution is necessary when the arthrogrypotic floppy infant is evaluated because findings suggestive of SMA may not carry the same prognosis.[23]

Because the amplitude and duration of normal MUPs in the infant are substantially lower than those in the adult,[21,22] the differentiation between the lower limits of normal and a subtle myopathy is often difficult. In our study of the floppy infant,[24] neurogenic conditions were more easily recognized than myopathic ones. Severe myopathies of infancy, however, may be identified. On occasion, the MUP character is suggestive of, but is not diagnostic of, myopathy or may appear normal. Muscle biopsy is necessary with any possible myopathy.

All needle electrodes used in our laboratory are disposable and are the shortest available, usually 25 mm. Use of the shortest electrodes has considerable psychologic advantages for the child. Concentric electrodes have smaller calibrated recording areas and provide greater sensitivity to changes in amplitude and duration than do monopolar needles. These disposable electrodes are sharp, pierce the skin easily, and produce minimal pain. In contrast to adults, children have minimal subcutaneous tissue, and the underlying muscle is easily accessible.

Rarely with an exceedingly uncooperative infant, the study must sometimes be discontinued. When the infant returns, premedication may be used or the dose increased, or the type of drug may be changed. For the electromyographer who is not accustomed to evaluating children, such results may be an indication to refer the child to a laboratory with greater pediatric experience.

THE FLOPPY INFANT

In the normal newborn, purposeless movements of the extremities are associated with well-defined muscular tone and excellent ability to suck and swallow. Occasionally an infant has minimal or no evidence of significant skeletal muscle activity. When the infant's trunk is supported by an examiner, the head, arms, and legs are limp, with no appreciable tone, and the infant literally forms an inverted U in the examiner's hands (Figure 25.4). Although these in-

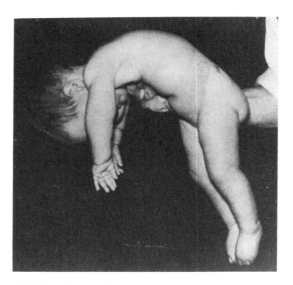

FIGURE 25.4.   *Floppy infant. Classic inverted U position secondary to diffuse hypotonia. (Reprinted with permission from Dubowitz V. The floppy infant, ed 2. Oxford: Butterworth-Heinemann, 1980:21.)*

fants have full eye movements with normal ability to follow and react to a stimulus and the facies appear *bright,* lower bulbar motor function may be lacking. These newborns are often unable to swallow appropriately and eventually may have repetitive episodes of aspiration and recurrent pneumonia. Some infants appear normal at birth, but later, developmental milestones, such as holding up the head, rolling over, or sitting up, are not reached during the first 3 to 6 months, and the infant is obviously floppy. This combination of symptoms eventually leads to referral for neurologic evaluation. Although up to 80% of floppy infants have a primary central nervous system cause, skillful pediatric neurologists are able to select infants most likely to benefit from electrodiagnostic evaluation. Many abnormalities of the motor unit need to be considered in the diagnostic evaluation of the floppy infant (Table 25.4).

Two studies[24,25] have detailed the accuracy and spectrum of electrodiagnostic findings in the evaluation of floppy infants. Packer et al.[25] reported on a retrospective review of EMG on 51 infants less than 1 year old with hypotonia. The final diagnosis, independent of findings on EMG, was based on clinical course, muscle biopsy, or both. The most common mechanism was SMA I or WHD, which accounted for 21 of the 51 patients. Eight patients had a myopathy, and 11 patients had infantile botulism. Re-

TABLE 25.4. Floppy infant: Disorders of motor unit

Anterior horn cell	Postsynaptic
Werdnig-Hoffmann	Neonatal
disease	Myasthenia gravis
Poliomyelitis*	(autoimmune)
(Acid maltase)†	Congenital myasthenia
Neuropathies	Myopathies
Congenital hypomyelinating	Congenital
Congenital axonal	Nemaline rod
Hereditary motor sensory	Central core
Infantile neuronal	Centronuclear
degeneration	Congenital fiber type
Leigh's syndrome	disproportion
Giant axonal	Dystrophies
Guillain-Barré syndrome	Myotonia dystrophica
Dysmaturation	Congenital muscular
neuromyopathy	dystrophy
Leukodystrophies	Inflammatory myopathies
Neuromuscular junction	Enzymatic myopathies
Presynaptic	Acid maltase (type II)
Infantile botulism	Myophosphorylase
Hypermagnesemia—	(type V)
eclampsia	Phosphofructokinase
Aminoglycoside	(type VII)
antibiotics	Cytochrome *c* oxidase
Congenital LEMS	

* Today of historical interest only in Western societies with immunization programs.

† Usually presents as noted with enzymatic myopathies.

HMSN, Hereditary motor sensory neuropathy, LEMS, Lambert-Eaton myasthenic syndrome.

Modified with permission from Jones HR Jr. EMG evaluation of the floppy infant: Differential diagnosis and technical aspects. Muscle Nerve 1990; 13:339.

sults of EMG were normal in 11 patients, five had benign congenital hypotonia, and six had a central nervous system disorder.

We[24] reviewed records of 111 floppy infants studied in our EMG lab and concentrated our study on 41 infants who had combined muscle or nerve biopsy. SMA occurred in 23 of the infants. EMG was most accurate in defining this group. In contrast, EMG was less sensitive in defining the presence of a myopathy, although the correlation was good when EMG showed classic myopathic features. Myopathies were also found in individuals with normal or nonspecific changes on EMG. The importance of evaluating sensory conduction in the floppy infant is illustrated by the fact that we found five patients with hypomyelinating neuropathies, whereas none were identified in the previous study,[25] in which sensory conduction was not reported. The rarity of bot-

ulism in New England as opposed to Philadelphia may explain the single case seen by us[24] and the greater than 20% incidence in the study by Packer et al.[25]

Spinal Muscular Atrophy I—Werdnig-Hoffmann Disease

In 1961, Byers and Banker[26] proposed a classification of the different forms of SMA based on the clinical course. They evaluated 52 patients with SMA confirmed by autopsy in 18 and by biopsy or clinical course or both in 34. They divided the patients into three groups based on onset of illness. In 25 of the 52 infants, SMA I or WHD was present with onset of symptoms in utero (poor fetal movements) or in whom the illness was obvious in the first 2 postnatal months. These infants presented with generalized weakness and they died early. In SMA II, the illness of 19 infants became apparent between the second and twelfth postnatal months, and the weakness initially appeared to be more localized. These infants survived longer, albeit with limited mobility. The eight children with SMA III had findings confined to the proximal musculature. Onset was after age 2 years, although earlier hints of difficulty with some motor delay were found in some infants.

Although these features were proved useful in determining prognosis when dealing with an early onset, occasionally infants may be seen with symptoms at birth who survived more than 4 years.[27] This is particularly true in the group with contractures[28] or arthrogryposis.[23] Genetic studies of this autosomal recessive illness demonstrate that gene locus 5q11.2-13.3[29] appears to be identical for each of the three forms of childhood SMA[30] that are probably caused by different mutations at the same locus[30] or on the basis of allelic heterogeneity, a mechanism similarly noted in Duchenne's muscular dystrophy.[30]

The child with SMA I or WHD assumes a limp *frog leg* posture of the lower extremities and has a prominent abdomen, paradoxic respirations, a bell-shaped trunk, jug handle posture of the upper extremities, and absent deep tendon reflexes (Figure 25.5). Although infants with SMA I are almost totally immobile, the facies are bright and attentive, and they have full extraocular movements. Tongue fasciculations are almost pathognomonic of SMA of any type.[26-28] We have noted on rare occasions, however, that tongue fasciculations may be observed in floppy infants with severe congenital neuropathies. In contrast to adult motor neuron disease, fasciculations in the extremities are not observed in infants with SMA, possibly because they are concealed by subcutaneous fat. On rare occasion, infants with the severe form may be in severe respiratory distress at birth and require intubation. Extubation is never tolerated during their brief life.[31]

Another unusual presentation, possibly a variant of SMA II, was seen in five infants between 3 and 6 months of age with poor head control and with only mild involvement of the extremities.[32] Two infants had tongue fasciculations. Neurogenic changes primarily in the neck and paravertebral muscles were demonstrated on EMG. Results of peroneal MCV were normal. Later respiratory muscle involvement led to death between 2 and 4 years in three children.

Motor NCV and distal latencies are usually normal or near normal for age as expected in primary axonal loss. Slower MCVs, however, have been reported in some children with SMA I. In the study by

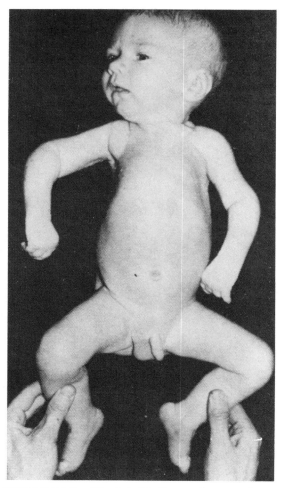

FIGURE 25.5.   *Werdnig-Hoffmann disease. Classic posture with bell-shaped chest and* jug-handle arms. *(Reprinted with permission from Dubowitz V. The floppy infant, ed 2. Oxford: Butterworth-Heinemann, 1980:22.)*

Moosa and Dubowitz,[33] slow ulnar and posterior tibial nerve conduction occurred in 12 of 14 infants with SMA I. They speculated that the fastest conducting fibers, which arise from the largest motor neurons, might be selectively lost. This report made no mention of monitoring temperature; thus cooling of limbs may have been a factor. With temperature controlled at 34°C, Ryniewicz[34] demonstrated maximal MCV slowing in only 27% of ulnar nerves and in 6% of peroneal nerves, which agrees with our[24] experience. In patients with SMA I, CMAP amplitudes may be substantially diminished.[24,35,36] Results of sural and ulnar sensory conductions are normal.[24,34] It may be cumbersome to attempt sural nerve stimulation when the electromyographer has no technical assistant. It is easy, however, to obtain median compound SNAPs in all infants with SMA I.[20,24] When compound SNAPs are unobtainable, the rare infantile neuropathies need to be considered seriously, and sural nerve biopsy should be obtained.

Findings on needle EMG of infants are similar to those of motor neuron disease in adults. At least two muscles innervated by different roots and peripheral nerves in at least three extremities should be examined. The major technical difficulty in the most severely ill patients may be in activating enough MUPs to be certain of their electrical characteristics. Enough MUPS, however, are usually able to be evaluated to note their characteristic appearance, including longer duration (10 to 20 ms) and higher amplitude (0.8 to 6 mV) than normal and firing at an increased rate,[36] at times with spontaneous rhythmic firing.[37] Some MUPs may be more polyphasic and include late components variously labeled as parasites, satellites, or linked potentials.[37] Distribution of these motor units may be bimodal, and concomitantly low-amplitude, short-duration potentials may be found.[37]

Abnormalities on insertion and at rest may be prominent in SMA I.[24,35] Profuse fibrillation potentials may be seen in many infants with SMA I,[35] although they may not be demonstrable initially in less severe disease. Fibrillation potentials may be difficult to detect because of spontaneously firing MUPs.[36] Fasciculation potentials are not reported frequently in SMA I.[35,37]

Great care must be taken in making an unequivocal diagnosis of SMA I because of its important prognostic implications. Most infants with SMA I who are identified in the newborn period die by ages 2 to 4 years[37]; many die before their first birthday.[26] Hausmanowa-Petrusewicz and Karwanska[37] attempted to find an electromyographic marker to differentiate the more malignant form of SMA from the less malignant forms. To date, however, clinical data elaborated by Byers and Banker[26] in combination with standard EMG and muscle biopsy provide practical prognostic criteria except for the benign variety, whose course plateaus.[27,28]

Incontinentia pigmenti with anterior horn degeneration

The Bloch-Sulzberger syndrome or incontinentia pigmenti (IP) is characterized by congenital skin lesions,

skeletal and dental dysplasia, ocular abnormalities, and occasionally generalized hypotonia predominantly affecting girls. Larsen et al.[38] reported a floppy newborn with 3- to 10-mm vesicular bullous lesions on the legs, and soon a progressive generalized erythematous maculopapular rash developed. Skin biopsy demonstrated intradermal eosinophils in vesicles consistent with IP. Proximal limb weakness, areflexia, and recurrent apnea developed at age 2 weeks. Examination demonstrated severe hypotonicity, areflexia, and tongue fasciculations. Peroneal and tibial MCVs were 15 and 11 m/second. No comment was made about compound SNAPs. Needle EMG revealed only rare MUPs and intermittent fibrillations. Postmortem study at 3 months demonstrated anterior horn cells that were greatly decreased in number with varying degeneration. More commonly IP presents with spastic quadriplegia. On literature review, Larsen et al.[38] found only three other infants with IP with flaccid weakness, but none had had neuropathologic spinal cord examination to confirm an association with SMA I.

Peripheral Neuropathies

The peripheral neuropathies that may present as floppy infant syndrome are listed in Table 25.5.

Congenital hypomyelinating neuropathies

Congenital hypomyelinating neuropathies (CHN) represent an uncommon cause for the floppy infant syndrome.[39-44] In 13 years, our laboratory has seen seven patients with infantile neuropathies including four of 111 floppy infants.[24] Each had severe generalized hyptonia; two infants had arthrogryposis.[45]

TABLE 25.5. Floppy infant and infantile neonatal neuropathies

---

Congenital hypomyelinating
Congenital axonal
Hereditary motor sensory
Infantile neuronal degeneration
Leigh's syndrome (subacute necrotizing encephalomyelopathy)
Giant axonal
Acute inflammatory demyelinating polyneuropathy
Chronic inflammatory demyelinating polyneuropathy
Dysmaturation
Leukodystrophies
    Krabbe's disease
    Niemann-Pick disease

Levels of cerebrospinal fluid protein were significantly elevated at birth (199 and 220 mg/dL in two of our five patients who had cerebrospinal fluid examination). The major clue to the diagnosis of CHN in floppy infants is the lack of compound SNAPs. Concomitantly motor involvement is so severe that some had no detectable CMAPs. Needle EMG demonstrated variable fibrillation potentials and on one occasion complex repetitive discharges (CRDs), and dropout in MUPs was severe. In contrast to SMA I, MUP amplitude in patients with CHN tended to be close to normal, although in one patient, a few large units (1 to 6 mV) were noted.[24]

Each infant demonstrated severe hypomyelinating or axonal neuropathy or both on biopsy. At times, electron microscopy was crucial in confirming the evidence or neuropathy in sural nerve biopsies. Gabreëls-Festen et al.[46] reported on six patients with an interesting CHN variant, two of whom were floppy at birth. Each child had an MCV range of 2 to 11 m/second and normal levels of cerebrospinal fluid protein. Sural nerve biopsy revealed tomaculous changes in addition to typical hereditary motor sensory neuropathy (HMSN) III findings.

It is not certain whether CHN is a single disease or whether several mechanisms are involved. Some infants are so severely affected that despite intensive support, their outcome is fatal within a few months of birth. Other authors[39,44] reported survivors, which raises the question of whether some infants with CHN may represent neonatal onset of HMSN III (Dejerine-Sottas disease) or chronic inflammatory demyelinating polyneuropathy.

Hereditary motor sensory neuropathies

Questions have been raised whether HMSN I, which commonly first presents during high school years, may present as a floppy infant syndrome. Ouvrier et al.[47] reported on 10 patients with HMSN I, two of whom appeared as floppy infants in the first 12 months. The precise time of onset of hypotonia, however, was difficult to ascertain (Ouvrier RA. Personal communication, 1988). Similarly, Dubowitz (Dubowitz V. Personal communication, 1988) cannot recall a specific instance of HMSN I presenting as floppy infant syndrome.

Occasionally infants born in families with HMSN I have had neurophysiologic examinations as neonates. In two studies,[48,49] none were truly floppy infants. In the study of Gutmann et al.,[48] although motor NCS were normal in the one affected twin examined at birth, sensory conduction potentials were absent at birth. Of the two patients reported by Vanasse and Dubowitz,[49] one had feeding problems at birth, and the other had congenital scoliosis.

Baker and Upton[50] reported on a hypotonic newborn with a dominantly inherited neuropathy. Motor and sensory NCS first performed on the infant at age 2 years showed demyelination. The infant's mother had similar results. These findings suggested that the infant had HMSN I at birth.[50] This phenotypically unusual infant had associated ptosis, optic atrophy, and chorioretinal dysplasia more compatible with HMSN VI.

Infantile congenital axonal neuropathies also occur.[51,52] Gabreëls-Festen et al.[52] described 18 patients with neuronal HMSN that was different from HMSN II. It is of autosomal recessive inheritance with congenital or early childhood onset and is histologically different on sural nerve biopsy from HMSN II by its lack of regenerative changes. The two infants with onset at birth had limp feet but did not present as diffusely floppy. Motor nerve CVs were variable, absent, decidedly abnormal, or markedly slowed. Sural compound SNAPs were absent.[52]

Hereditary motor neuropathy with neuromyotonia. Hahn et al.[53] described two siblings, one of whom had been clumsy since birth with distal motor neuropathy, cramping, and muscle stiffness with diminished relaxation after exercise, especially in the cold. Motor CMAPs were slightly decreased and distal latencies slightly prolonged, but MCVs and compound SNAPs were normal. EMG demonstrated chronic neurogenic MUPs and at rest frequent neuromyotonia. Neuromyotonia had previously been associated with HMSN II.[54]

Hereditary sensory neuropathies. Three infants having a nonprogressive primary sensory neuropathy with atypical dysautonomia somewhat similar to the Riley-Day syndrome (hereditary sensory neuropathy [HSN] III) have been reported, each of whom was hypotonic at birth with weak or absent reflexes.[55] Motor nerve CVs were normal, and compound SNAPs were absent in each. Sural nerve biopsy results demonstrated that myelinated fibers were completely absent.

Infantile neuronal degeneration

Steiman et al.[56] described two newborns with hypotonia thought to have SMA I and, based on NCS, were thought to have CHN but later proved to have a more diffuse neuronal degeneration. Both died within 5 months. At 5 months, NCS on one newborn showed moderate MCV slowing (14.6 m/s) and no sural compound SNAP. A hypomyelinating neuropathy was confirmed by autopsy. Diffuse central nervous system neuronal loss affected the spinal cord anterior horn cells, brain stem motor nuclei, pons, cerebellum, and thalamus.

Leigh syndrome—subacute necrotizing encephalomyelopathy

Leigh syndrome, an infantile subacute necrotizing encephalomyelopathy (SNE), primarily affects the brain stem. It is a mitochondrial respiratory chain metabolic disorder characterized by metabolic lactic acidosis and ragged red fibers on muscle biopsy. Some patients present as floppy infants. Seitz et al.[57] described a newborn who died with SNE at age 2 months with typical central nervous system findings and prominent demyelination of the sciatic nerve. Goebel et al.[58] undertook a systematic study of peripheral nerve function in four children with SNE, aged 0.5 to 3 years. MCV was 20 to 27 m/second in peroneal nerves and 37 m/second in ulnar nerves. Paranodal demyelination and remyelination were demonstrated by electron microscopy. Jacobs et al.[59] described similar findings, including absent sural compound SNAPs.

Giant axonal neuropathy

One infant[60] with giant axonal neuropathy presented at birth with decreased muscle tone and definite hypotonia by age 2 months. At age 7 months, NCS demonstrated absent compound SNAPs and barely elicitable CMAPs.

Acute Guillain-Barré syndrome and chronic inflammatory demyelinating polyneuropathy

Four reports[61–64] of Guillain-Barré syndrome with onset before age 3 months have been published. One newborn presumed to have infantile Guillain-Barré syndrome presented with diffuse hypotonia, respiratory distress, feeding difficulties, and areflexia.[63] Motor NCS ranged between 7.5 and 15 m/second at age 3 weeks. This infant was normal at 5 months of age. Acute quadriplegia and respiratory arrest developed in a 1-month-old infant.[61] Motor NCS 6 months later were 1.9 to 2.1 m/second. A 4-month-old infant had subacute onset of hypotonia. Motor NCS was 6.5 m/second in the median nerve and unobtainable in the peroneal nerve.[62]

Pasternak et al.[65] reported on acute flaccid paraparesis in a 7-week-old infant 1 week after diphtheria-pertussus-tetanus (DPT) immunization. This infant had a fluctuating course. Despite intermittent improvement with prednisone the child died at age 4 years. Autopsy revealed chronic inflammatory demyelinating polyneuropathy (CIDP). An interesting clinical point was the finding of tongue fasciculations,[65] which we have also seen in two patients with CHN.

Dysmaturation neuromyopathy

Verity and Gao[66] analyzed sural nerves of 10 infants with hypotonia and dysmaturation neuromyopathy and noted abnormalities in large myelinated fiber density in three patients that were different from other patients with CHN.[39–45] Two infants were floppy at birth, and one had arthrogryposis associated with respiratory distress. Five infants had NCS performed; in three patients, NCS were *slowed* or *delayed* and in two infants were normal. EMG showed diffuse fibrillation potentials. At age 2 months, muscle biopsy demonstrated preferential type I fiber hypotrophy.

Leukodystrophies

Consideration is sometimes given in the differential diagnosis of the floppy infant syndrome to two inborn errors of lipid metabolism, Krabbe's disease and metachromatic leukodystrophy.

Krabbe's disease. Clinically Krabbe's disease does not usually present until the infant is 6 to 12 months old. One infant, diagnosed as having Krabbe's disease by amniocentesis at 5 months gestation, was neurologically normal at birth.[67] Sequential NCS were performed beginning at age 5 weeks when the infant appeared well. Peroneal CMAPs were only 0.4 mV, and MCVs could not be calculated. Two weeks later, MCVs were 9.9 and 10.8 m/second. Needle EMG demonstrated decreased numbers of normal-sized MUPs. At 3.5 months, progressive hypotonia ensued. Diffuse fibrillation potentials and positive sharp waves did not appear until the infant was 8 months old. Similar studies on infants with metachromatic leukodystrophy diagnosed prenatally have not been reported to my knowledge.

Niemann-Pick disease. Niemann-Pick disease (NPD) is an inborn error of lipid metabolism subsequent to sphingomyelin accumulation and secondary to sphingomyelinase deficiency. Typically these infants present with intellectual deterioration and hepatomegaly. In a hypotonic areflexic 11-month-old infant with positive Babinski signs (type A NPD), MCVs were slowed (7 to 10 m/s). Needle EMG demonstrated fibrillation potentials with normal MUPs.[68] A 2-year-old child with type C NPD whose neurologic development had plateaued at age 10 months and in whom a spastic paraparesis with dementia developed by age 24 months had electromyographic and NCV results consistent with a moderately severe demyelinating peripheral neuropathy.[69] Nerve biopsy demonstrated massive abnormal lipid inclusions primarily composed of cholesterol.

Neuromuscular Junction—Presynaptic Defects

At the presynaptic or postsynaptic level, NMT defects are rare causes for the floppy infant syndrome.

Infantile botulism

Infantile botulism was originally described by Pickett et al.[70] as a distinct cause for acute onset of severe hypotonia in a previously healthy infant. Each of these infants was normal at birth, and initial development of motor milestones was normal. Suddenly over a few days, difficulty in feeding, inability to suck strongly (whether from bottle or breast), and constipation ensued. The cry was weak, head control was lost, and hypotonia was variable.[70,71] Although some infants may have a relatively mild illness not requiring hospitalization, severe quadriparesis and respiratory failure may develop rapidly in others. One 2-week-old infant had only 5 hours of prodromal symptoms before respiratory arrest developed,[72] and the prolonged subsequent course may have been secondary to use of aminoglycosides.[73]

Characteristic findings on physical examination include diffuse hypotonia; poor sucking with weak cry; decreased gag reflex; dysphagia; ptosis; and, less commonly, enlarged, sluggishly reactive pupils.[74] Reflexes were absent in only one of 12 infants. Ventilatory support was necessary in six of nine hospitalized infants within 2 to 34 days of onset. Thompson et al.[74] warned about the potential for aminoglycoside antibiotics to produce acute respiratory distress in patients with infantile botulism. They noted that three infants later found to have botulism were initially diagnosed as having infantile sepsis and treated with these antibiotics, which led to respiratory arrest in one.[74]

Although infantile botulism primarily occurs between ages 2 and 6 months, three other infants with onset between ages 10 and 17 days have been reported.[75,76] All three had acute hypotonia and respiratory difficulties that led to respiratory arrest in two. In all three electromyographic results were diagnostic and met the criteria of Cornblath et al.[77] An edrophonium (Tensilon, ICN Pharmaceuticals Inc., Costa Mesa, CA) test was positive in one, but such results cannot be used to make a clinical differentiation from some of the congenital myasthenic syndromes.

Test of NMT should be performed on any infant in the first 6 months of life who has been well and in whom diffuse weakness, constipation, and occasionally respiratory distress suddenly develop. An incremental response to repetitive nerve stimulation at rates of 20 to 50 c/s was documented in 23 of 25 (92%) patients with infantile botulism.[77] The mean increment was 73% (range, 23% to 313%). In most instances, 20 c/s stimulation usually demonstrated an increment; however, four patients required 50 c/s stimulation. A distinct feature of adult botulism is prolonged posttetanic facilitation. A 3-month-old infant with infantile botulism[78] had a 21-minute duration posttetanic facilitation after 10 seconds of exercise. In contrast, the response to lower frequency stimulation (2 to 5 c/s) produced variable changes with decrements most prominent in 14 (56%) of 25 infants.[77] Needle EMG demonstrated abnormal spontaneous activity, with fibrillation potentials and positive sharp waves noted in 13 of 24 infants (54%). Short-duration, low-amplitude MUPs were found in 22 of 24 infants (90%).[77]

Magnesium toxicity secondary to eclampsia treatment

Another form of presynaptic infantile NMT defect occurs secondary to magnesium treatment of eclampsia.[79,80] One 1972 report,[80] not using modern NMT defect terminology, demonstrated evidence of *myoneurodepression* with potentiation greater than normal in one child with neonatal hypermagnesemia.

Lambert-Eaton myasthenic syndrome (congenital variant)

Lambert-Eaton myasthenic syndrome (LEMS) has not been demonstrated definitively in newborns or infants. Albers et al.[81] reported on an interesting neonate examined at age 2 weeks with severe hypotonia who had profound decrement at all rates of stimulation between 1 and 50 c/s. At age 2 months, the infant had a 50% to 740% facilitation 15 seconds after a 5-second train of 50-c/s stimulation. Elegant histochemical studies failed to identify the neurophysiologic mechanism. A later report[82] suggested the possibility of a congenital form of LEMS in a child who was initially evaluated at age 1 month for diffuse hypotonia. Repetitive stimulation carried out at age 3 months produced 33% decrement with 1-c/s stimulation, and subsequently 20- to 50-c/s stimulation produced greater than 2000% facilitation.[82]

Neuromuscular Junction—Postsynaptic Defects

Myasthenia gravis

Myasthenia gravis is the most common NMT defect in the newborn.[83,84] Neonatal myasthenia gravis (NMG) is a transitory illness secondary to transfer of maternal acetylcholine receptor antibodies (AChRAb) across the placenta, producing rapidly increasing weakness shortly after birth. The diagnosis is obvious when the mother has myasthenia gravis. In 10% to 15% of mothers with myasthenia gravis, NMG develops in their children, and AChRAbs are present in most of these children. Only two of the 17 infants born to 15 mothers with myasthenia gravis had NMG.[84] All but one had AChRAb present at birth. The mother of that one infant tested negative for AChRAb.

Common symptoms of NMG include hypotonia, poor sucking, feeble crying, bilateral facial paresis, and impaired swallowing. Mechanical ventilation was required in seven of 14 infants.[85] Symptoms improved with administration of anticholinesterase drugs. NMG may be associated with arthrogryposis, severe hypotonia, and polyhydramnios, all indicative of a long-standing prenatal evolution. Although most infants with NMG recover in 1 to 7 weeks, some may not totally improve for 1 year.[85,86] The occurrence of NMG in one infant is a reliable predictor for recurrent NMG in subsequent siblings.[85]

Cardiac arrhythmia and respiratory arrest may occur when edrophonium chloride is administered to infants with NMG.[83] Usually a clinical diagnosis of NMG can be confirmed by intramuscular or subcutaneous injections of neostigmine, 0.04 to 0.1 mg/kg of body weight.[87] Pediatric neurologists in our hospital make a diagnosis of NMG based on the typical maternal history, clinical findings, positive edrophonium response to anticholinesterase medications, and elevated levels of AChRAb in mother and infant. They rarely request EMG for the diagnosis of NMG. The literature is sparse in reference to electromyographic results in infants with NMG. One infant with NMG had 54% decrement at 50 c/s, and the clinically unaffected sibling had none.[87] A control study of three newborns born to mothers without myasthenia gravis demonstrated no NMT defect with 3-c/s stimulation for 10 seconds and at 10 and 50 c/s for 5 seconds.[87] This finding contrasts with another study[19] demonstrating significant decrement in normal infants with 15-second stimulation.

Congenital myasthenia gravis

Newborns with a clinical presentation similar to infantile myasthenia are rarely seen whose mothers do not have myasthenia gravis. Family history may reveal previous siblings with similar difficulty, occasionally with severe respiratory crises leading to death. A review[88] of nine children with congenital myasthenia gravis (CMG) demonstrated that seven of nine were antibody negative, and six of these seven children had symptoms at birth. Elegant physiologic and pathoanatomic studies by Engel[89,90] and others[91,92] have demonstrated various NMT defects in patients with CMG, including defects in the synthesis or mobilization of acetylcholine (ACh), diminished numbers of ACh receptors, a defect in ACh breakdown by acetylcholinesterase (AChE) at the end plate, or physiologic prolongation of the open time for the ACh receptor channel (Table 25.6).

The clinical electromyographer may be able to make some suggestions about the pathophysiology (see Table 25.6). Edrophonium testing is positive in only two of these four syndromes: those in which ACh synthesis or mobilization is defective[89] and those in which the ACh receptors are deficient.[92] The remaining two syndromes, AChE end plate deficiency and the prolonged open channel of the ACh receptor, characteristically demonstrate repetitive CMAPs after single stimulus on motor NCS.[89] Edrophonium testing is unremarkable in these patients. Decremental responses were evidenced on routine 2-c/s stimulation in three of the four syndromes, the exception being syndromes with defective synthesis or mobilization of acetylcholine. These patients, however, had a positive response to 2-c/s stimulation elicited by a few minutes of continuous 10-c/s stimulation.[89]

Familial infantile myasthenia gravis

Familial infantile myasthenia gravis (FIMG) is an autosomal recessive, nonimmunologically mediated illness that usually presents in the newborn or infant and occasionally presents later in childhood.[91,93–96] The recognition of newborn FIMG is of paramount

TABLE 25.6.   Congenital myasthenia (onset at birth with absent acetylcholine receptor antibodies)

	Acetylcholine Synthesis/ Mobilization Defective	*Acetylcholine Receptor Deficiency*	*Acetylcholinesterase End Plate Deficiency*	*Acetylcholine Receptor Prolonged Open Channel*
Genetics	Recessive	Recessive	Recessive	Dominant
Clinical	Ophthalmopa- resis Feeding difficulty Apnea with cry	Ptosis Bulbar	Ptosis Generalized	Ophthalmoparesis Cervical scapular forarm
Diagnostic tests				
Edrophonium (Tensilon)	+	+	−	−
NCS				
Repetitive CMAP*	−	−	+	+
2-c/s decrement	−/+†	+	+	+ (selective)

Adapted with permission from Engel AG. Myasthenia gravis and myasthenic syndrome. Ann Neurol 1984; 16:519–534.

*Repetitive CMAP is linked directly to a single stimulus.

†*Note:* May require a few minutes of continuous 10-c/s stimulation to induce 2-c/s decrement in weak muscle.

NCS, Nerve conduction study; CMAP, compound muscle action potential.

importance because it has the unique potential among the various forms of NMG for anoxic brain damage or death. Typically these infants have a history of feeble cry, intermittent ptosis, poor sucking recurrent dysphagia or dyspnea, and, occasionally, episodic respiratory crisis precipitated by febrile illnesses, vomiting, or excitement sometimes leading to apnea. Episodic drooping of the head may mimic akinetic seizures.[93] The facies may have the tent-like mouth typical of myotonia dystrophica.[93]

Because maternal history does not suggest NMG and the characteristic ptosis or extraocular muscle involvement of CMG is minimal or lacking, clinical suspicion of NMT defect may not be high. A history, however, of siblings dying of undiagnosed episodes of recurrent respiratory depression may be present. Although ACh esterase therapy produces a response[94] and the episodic symptoms occur less frequently as the child matures, classic myasthenia gravis may develop in later childhood or adolescence.[95]

In patients with FIMG, AChRAbs are not present. EMG demonstrates a postsynaptic NMT defect.[90] Ultrastructural studies of the neuromuscular junction have demonstrated abnormally small synaptic vesicles[96] that may have defective metabolism.[90]

Some children with FIMG require emergency treatment with ACh esterase inhibitors. Parents must be instructed to anticipate acute exacerbations, particularly with febrile illnesses, overexertion, or other

excitement and be prepared to inject neostigmine intramuscularly and to use portable ventilatory aids.[90] At times of stress, preemptory hospitalization may be lifesaving, especially with a family history of death from acute respiratory depression.[94]

Neonatal Myopathies

Neonatal myopathies are the second most common motor unit cause for the floppy infant syndrome. In our 11-year review, we[24] found myopathic processes as common as SMA. Some neonatal myopathies are not as easily diagnosed because EMG is not as accurate for neonatal myopathy as it is for neurogenic processes.[24] Neonatal EMG is less sensitive for three reasons. First, in contrast to neurogenic processes that produce striking and widespread changes in motor unit size and firing pattern, myopathic changes are often subtle, especially in infancy when normal motor unit size is considerably smaller than in an older child or adult.[21,22] The appreciation of slight myopathic changes in MUPs from normal infantile motor units is often a challenge. Second, the other sign of a myopathic process, the early recruitment of many MUPs with minimal effort, is appreciated only with the most florid infantile myopathies. The pediatric electromyographer does not often have cooperation of the infant to permit this assessment. Third, infantile needle EMG is prone to time sampling error because newborns do not consistently contract their muscles. Another possible error relates to recent awareness that some infants whom we have identified with a myopathic lesion by biopsy were initially thought, on EMG, to have nonspecific neurogenic changes characterized by occasional positive sharp waves or fibrillation potentials when motor units could not be identified more precisely.[23,24] Although profound fibrillation potentials may be seen in SMA and congenital neuropathies, fibrillation potentials are also seen in at least nine nonneurogenic causes for the floppy infant syndrome, including eight myopathies (Table 25.7) and one NMT defect (i.e., infantile botulism).[20] Therefore when examination of a floppy infant clinically suggests a peripheral motor unit defect, appropriate evaluation must include muscle biopsy even when results of EMG studies are normal or demonstrate mild *neurogenic* changes. When results of EMG are positive, they provide a focus for the best site for biopsy.

The differential diagnosis of electromyographic myopathic findings with the floppy infant is broad (see Table 25.7) and includes congenital myopathies, dystrophies, and rarely polymyositis or enzymatic myopathies. Some common myopathies in the older child, such as those of Duchenne and Becker and less commonly endocrine myopathies and periodic paralyses, are not present in newborns. The common neonatal myopathies of floppy infants are congenital muscular dystrophy, myotonic dystrophy, and congenital myopathies. In our lab we have yet to identify a case of an inflammatory or enzymatic myopathy.

The predominant electromyographic finding with infantile myopathy is increased numbers of short-duration, low-amplitude MUPs usually found in the most proximal muscles. Because of the infant's ten-

TABLE 25.7. Floppy infant and associated neonatal myopathies

Dystrophies
  Congenital muscular
  Myotonic*
Congenital myopathies
  Centronuclear*
  Nemaline rod*
  Fiber type disproportion*
Polymyositis*
Glycogen storage disease
  Type II—Pompe (acid maltase)*
  Type V—McArdle (myophosphorylase)*
  Type VII—Tarui (phosphofructokinase)*
Mitochondrial (cytochrome *c* oxidase) deficiency

  * Myopathies with fibrillation potentials.

dency to contract the iliopsoas muscle spontaneously or on withdrawal to a stimulus to the plantar surface of the foot it is the most useful muscle to identify myopathic motor units. In blatant infantile myopathy, there is rapid recruitment of many myopathic MUPs with minimal effort. This classic finding, however, is not always well appreciated in some infantile myopathies. EMG examination of the mother may provide a diagnosis of previously unrecognized myotonic dystrophy. Repetitive stimulation also needs to be considered in some infants who have myopathic MUPs, particularly infants with symptoms suggestive of infantile botulism or with unexplained ptosis and extraocular muscle weakness.

Dystrophies

Congenital muscular dystrophy. In our[24] laboratory, congenital muscular dystrophy is the most common myopathic cause for a floppy infant, some of whom are arthrogrypotic.[97] Serum creatine kinase (CK) levels may variably be elevated in some infants. MUPs are of short duration and low amplitude, and rarely abnormalities are demonstrated on insertion. Muscle biopsy is necessary to make the diagnosis.

Myotonia dystrophica. Myotonia dystrophica is the other dystrophy that presents as floppy infant syndrome. These infants may have severe hypotonia and a characteristic tenting of the month. The family history may not be recognized; however, careful history and examination of the mother may reveal evidence of myotonia, or she may have had premature cataract surgery.

Newborns with myotonia dystrophica may have two forms of this disorder.[98] The most severe form is transmitted maternally and produces severe generalized hypotonia and weakness that may require respiratory support. Infants who survive this neonatal crisis may present later with an intelligence quotient that is lower than normal. In the other form, Swift et al.[98] indicated that the infant presents with facial diplegia and various arthrogrypotic deformities. Transmission can be by either parent.

Electromyographic examination of newborns may demonstrate myotonic potentials firing at high rates and waxing and waning in frequency and amplitude.[98] Although some have the classic *dive-bomber* sound, often the infantile myotonic potentials are somewhat higher pitched, quieter, and less sustained than those in the adult. Occasionally the myotonic discharges are induced by needle insertion or percussion over the adjacent muscle.[98] Some positively configured myotonic discharges may be confused with end plate noise. In four infants with myotonia, six electromyographic studies demonstrated profuse fibrillation potentials to be the most prominent finding.[99] Myotonic discharges were found in three of the four infants, the earliest noted at 5 days. One infant had no myotonia noted at 3 weeks. In another infant, myotonic discharges increased in degree between the ages of 0 and 17 months, with concomitant diminution of fibrillation potentials. It was difficult to assess MUPs satisfactorily.[99] In addition to myotonia, NCS in some of our infants demonstrated low-amplitude CMAPs.

Electromyographic examinations of the mothers demonstrated myotonia[99] that was previously unsuspected. Sometimes myotonic discharges are not as widespread in newborns as in adults. On occasion, electromyographic examination does not demonstrate myotonia in an infant. A brief needle examination of the mother should be performed because it may prove diagnostic of myotonia dystrophica.

Congenital myopathies

Congenital myopathies include a number of morphologically distinct entities with many clinical similarities, including hypotonia at birth, nonprogressive course, and delayed motor milestones often associated with various skeletal abnormalities.[39] Ptosis and extraocular muscle weakness suggest myotubular myopathy. Some rare congenital NMT defects or myotonia dystrophica, however, have similar findings. In contrast to some other infantile myopathies, congenital myopathies are not associated with elevated levels of CK.

When present, electromyographic abnormalities include short-duration, low-amplitude MUPs that may be recruited rapidly. In most congenital myopathies, abnormalities are not present at rest or on insertion. Abundant fibrillation potentials, however, have been reported in myotubular (centronuclear) myopathy,[100] and they may have concomitant myotonic discharges.[101] Other congenital myopathies that on occasion have fibrillation potentials include nemaline rod myopathy[102] or congenital fiber type disproportion.[103]

Infantile polymyositis

When floppy infants who have elevated CK values are evaluated, three rare conditions, infantile polymyositis, McArdle's disease, and Pompe's disease, must be considered in addition to congenital muscular dystrophy. Infantile polymyositis was described[104,105] in six neonates, five of whom were

floppy at birth. In retrospect, their mothers noticed decreased fetal movements.[104,105] At age 6 months, all but one infant had elevated serum CK levels of 14 to 40 times normal. Five infants had EMG performed, three of the five infants had myopathic MUPs, and one infant had prolonged high-frequency discharges.

Glycogen storage disease

Myophosphorylase deficiency (McArdle's disease—glycogenosis V). An infant with McArdle's disease (myophosphorylase deficiency or glycogen storage disease [GSD] V) presented with progressive weakness beginning at age 4 weeks followed by severe respiratory distress and pronounced weakness of limb and trunk muscles at age 9 weeks that resulted in death.[106] Myopathic MUPs and profuse fibrillation potentials were demonstrated on EMG. Presumably because of the latter, a clinical diagnosis of WHD was made; the infant died 1 week later. Histochemical results revealed complete lack of myophosphorylase. A second infant with myophosphorylase deficiency had some increased polyphasic units but no fibrillation potentials.[107] Levels of CK were twice normal[106] in one infant and low normal[107] in the other infant.

Phosphofructokinase deficiency (Tarui's disease—glycogenosis VII). Fatal phosphofructokinase deficiency (GSD VII) was diagnosed in a newborn with hypotonia and respiratory distress.[108] Abundant fibrillation potentials, positive sharp waves, and full recruitment with slight effort were shown on EMG. The infant died at age 7 months.

Acid maltase deficiency (Pompe's disease—glycogenosis II). Acid maltase deficiency affects skeletal and cardiac muscle as well as motor neurons. Hypotonia developed at birth and at 3 months.[109,110] Values of CK were elevated six to 20 times. Neither child had EMG; however, GSD II may be suspected during EMG by the appearance of many CRDs concomitant with the appearance of myopathic MUPs.[111]

Mitochondrial myopathies

Mitochondrial myopathies occur in the newborn who may have nonspecific myopathic changes and abnormal NCS without signs of clinical neuropathy.[112] Twenty patients with mitochondrial myopathy were studied;[113] 10, including four children, had NCS evidence of peripheral neuropathy. Only five were symptomatic. All 10 had mild peroneal MCV slowing and low-amplitude compound SNAPs. Nine of the 10 with abnormal NCS had a myopathy on EMG. Sural nerve biopsy in four of five patients with clinical peripheral neuropathy demonstrated decreased density of myelinated nerve fibers with axonal degeneration.[113]

Cytochrome c oxidase deficiency. Cytochrome *c* oxidase deficiency has been demonstrated[114] on muscle biopsy in a floppy infant in whom results of EMG were normal, which emphasizes the need for muscle biopsy even when results are normal.

Benign Congenital Hypotonia

Benign congenital hypotonia is a poorly defined syndrome that may present as floppy infant syndrome.[115] Results of muscle enzyme studies, NCS, EMG, and biopsy are normal. When a similar family history is elicited, a benign course can be predicted.

Arthrogryposis Multiplex Congenita

Infants with arthrogryposis multiplex congenita (AMC) are born with multifocal congenital joint contractures that range in degree from equinovarus with bilateral clubfeet to diffuse contractures at all major joints associated with varying degrees of infantile hypotonia[116] (Figure 25.6). Many associated congenital anomalies include low-set ears; flat nose; micrognathia; high arched palate; and maldeveloped heart, lungs, and testes. Drachman and Banker[117] concluded that AMC could be related to neurogenic or myopathic mechanisms. Experimental studies[118] suggested that limited intrauterine fetal movement is responsible for the severe ankylosis. In addition to apparent motor neuron disease,[23] hypotonic AMC has been associated with congenital polyneuropathies[23] and postsynaptic NMT defect.[119,120] In a 25-year prospective study by Banker[121] of 74 infants with AMC, muscle tissue was obtained by autopsy in 53 infants and by biopsy in 21 infants. Neurogenic causes predominated in 69 (93%); dysgenesis of the anterior horn cell was the most common pathologic finding. Based on a progressive clinical course and the finding of tongue fasciculations, however, only two infants had SMA I or WHD.[121] Congenital muscular dystrophy was the most common myopathic cause in two studies.[23,121]

Electromyographic studies of AMC present variable results. Smith et al.[122] studied 17 randomly selected infants and found fibrillation potentials in 14. These fibrillation potentials were scant in some infants. In eight infants, fibrillation potentials were found in the paraspinal musculature. Only four were

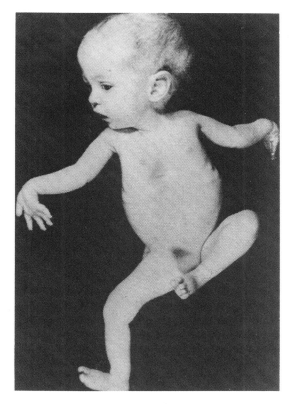

FIGURE 25.6. *Arthrogryposis multiplex congenita. Note severe contractures of hands, left elbow, and right ankle. (Reprinted with permission from Dubowitz V. The floppy infant, ed 2. Oxford: Butterworth-Heinemann, 1980:82.)*

infants less than 1 year old when EMG was performed. Amplitude and duration of MUPs varied; however, none were myopathic. Results of NCS were unremarkable. Three electromyographic studies suggested neurogenic mechanisms for AMC in nine of 10 patients,[123] in 18 of 20 patients,[124] and in seven of 12 patients.[125] Single motor units on full recruitment were found in seven of 12 patients.[125] Although MUPs were of increased duration and polyphasic, most amplitudes were 400 to 1500 μV, and no units were greater than 5000 μV. Fibrillation potentials were noted in only three of seven patients with neurogenic causes. Myopathic changes were present in two children, whereas results in the other three patients were normal.[125] Strehl et al.[126] evaluated 22 infants with AMC, 20 of whom were less than 1 year old when EMG or muscle biopsy or both were performed, including both studies in 14 infants. Ten were thought to be neurogenic and nine were thought to be myopathic, including three with congenital muscular dystrophy, three with myotonic dystrophy, two of unknown cause, and one related to an inheritable connective tissue disorder.

The results of EMG and muscle nerve biopsy were correlated in 35 infants with AMC who were less than 1 year old.[23] Abnormal results on EMG found in 28 infants (80%) were compatible with a diagnosis of SMA I in nine, neuropathy in one, myopathy in six, nonspecific changes in 11, and a mixed pattern in one. Twenty-three infants had muscle nerve biopsy performed; neurogenic changes were noted in four, myopathic in five, indeterminate (probably neurogenic) in one, indeterminate (probably myopathic) in three, dysmature end stage muscle in two, and nonspecific changes in eight. In contrast to a greater than 70% concordance between EMG and muscle biopsy in nonarthrogrypotic floppy infants,[24] the results on infants with AMC were concordant in only 12 of 23 (52%).[23] Autopsy altered the diagnosis in three infants.

Only three of nine infants with AMC designated by EMG to be compatible with SMA had neurogenic muscle nerve biopsy.[23] The remaining six patients included infants with indeterminate, probably myopathic or dysmature, end stage muscle. The latter group of patients had long-term survival in contrast to most floppy infants who had SMA I but not AMC. In our early pediatric experience, we erroneously concluded that floppy infants with AMC with diffuse fibrillation potentials and greatly diminished recruitment with rare long-duration, sometimes high-amplitude, rapidly firing motor units had classic SMA I. Follow-up study, however, of some of these infants has been more benign with a few long-term survivors.

Correlation between biopsy, EMG, and clinical course was much better in infants in whom EMG showed myopathy. Some infants with myopathic biopsy results had normal or nonspecific results on EMG. In conclusion, neither EMG nor muscle nerve biopsy alone is reliably diagnostic, especially EMG suggestive of anterior horn cell disorder. Definitive diagnosis of AMC depends on collation of all data, including careful ongoing follow-up examinations and occasionally complete autopsy.

Overview of Electromyographic Evaluation of the Floppy Infant

The most useful electromyographic parameter in evaluating floppy infants is the assessment of MUPs.[20,24,25] Infants with MUPs of increased dura-

tion and high-amplitude firing at an increased rate usually have SMA. Similar changes have been noted in seven newborns with congenital neuropathy (unpublished data), an illness that can be suspected when no compound SNAPs are present.[24] Most newborns with low-amplitude, short-duration MUPs have a recognizable myopathy.[24,25] Other infantile myopathies may be associated with normal MUPs.

Fibrillation potentials indicate a peripheral motor unit mechanism for the floppy infant; however, their presence is nonspecific being found with disease at any level including the motor neuron, peripheral nerve, NMJ, and some myopathies. In fact, their scattered occurrence, sometimes suggesting nonspecific *neurogenic* changes, was found in some infants whose biopsy revealed myopathy, particularly congenital muscular dystrophy.[24]

Most floppy infants have recognizable signs of hypotonia at birth. A few months of observation by parents and pediatricians, however, may occur before the infants come for EMG. In contrast, a few infants may have a fulminant onset of hypotonia after a totally healthy first weeks or months of life. The differential diagnosis of acute infantile hypotonia (Table 25.8) includes GBS,[61–63] CIDP,[65] infantile botulism,[70–74,77] infantile polymyositis,[104,105] myophosphorylase deficiency,[106,107] and, rarely, infantile acid maltase deficiency.[109–111] Infantile poliomyelitis must be considered in the differential diagnosis in countries where modern immunization techniques are inadequate and very rarely in industrialized countries when the child has not completed a full set of polio immunizations. An electromyographer with knowledge of the various clinical syndromes affecting the motor unit in infancy (Table 25.9) can provide considerable help to the pediatric neurologist in the evaluation of floppy infants. Occasionally examination of a parent may add specific diagnostic definition, especially in diagnosing unsuspected myotonia dystrophica. EMG performed on an infant may define specific illness, such as WHD, congenital neuropathy, infantile botulism, and myotonia dystrophica and may provide the clinician with a useful

TABLE 25.8. Floppy infant with acute onset

Acute inflammatory demyelinating polyneuropathy
Chronic inflammatory demyelinating polyneuropathy
Infantile botulism
Polymyositis
Glycogen storage disease
Poliomyelitis

TABLE 25.9. Nerve conduction study and electromyographic clues to diagnosis of floppy infant

Diagnosis	Motor Conduction	Sensory Conduction	Fibrillation Potentials	Motor Unit Potentials
Werdnig-Hoffmann	↓ CMAP	Normal	+ + +	↓ Numbers, ↑ size
Congenital neuropathy	↓ CMAP	Absent	+ + +	↓ Numbers, some ↑ size
Infantile botulism	Facilitation >20%*	Normal	+ +	↓ Size
Myasthenia gravis	Decrement*	Normal	0	Normal to ↓ size
Congenital myasthenia†	Decrement*	Normal	0	Normal to ↓ size
Myotonia dystrophica	Normal/↓ CMAP	Normal	+ + with myotonia	↑ Numbers, ↓ size
Congenital myopathy	Normal/↓ CMAP	Normal	Normal except + + (A)‡	↑ Numbers, ↓ size
Inflammatory myopathy	Normal/↓ CMAP	Normal	+ + +	↑ Numbers, ↓ size
Glycogen storage enzymatic myopathy	Normal	Normal	+ + + (B)	↑ Numbers, ↓ size

* Repetitive motor nerve stimulation.
† See Table 25.6 for more details.
(A), Myotubular (centronuclear), rarely nemaline rod, and congenital fiber-type disproportion are the three congenital myopathies reported to have spontaneous activity. (B), Types II, V, VII.
CMAP, Compound muscle action potentials. Reprinted with permission from Jones HR Jr. EMG evaluation of the floppy infant: Differential diagnosis and technical aspects. Muscle Nerve 1990; 13:344.

guide in the early management of the floppy infant. Sometimes results of EMG may provide encouragement to parents waiting for results of muscle biopsy because SMA or WHD may be excluded when carefully executed EMG shows normal findings. In contrast, when EMG indicates a diffuse process affecting motor neurons, the responsible clinician can be supportive of the parents, so when the results of muscle biopsy are available, they may be prepared for the seriousness of their child's illness. In the future, computer analysis of MUPs may permit a more accurate definition of subtle myopathies.

SPINAL MUSCULAR ATROPHIES OF CHILDHOOD AND ADOLESCENCE

The SMAs that occur in childhood and adolescence are outlined in Table 25.10.

Childhood Bulbar Paralysis (Fazio-Londe Disease)

Gomez et al.[127] described a young girl with progressive bulbar palsy. Her motor milestones had been normal except for frequent drooling since the age of 1 year. Unilateral ptosis that was unresponsive to anticholinesterase medications, bilateral facial weakness, inspiratory stridor, hoarse voice, and generalized hypotonia with a wide-based gait, subsequent dysphasia, and increased drooling developed in this 3-year-old girl. Results of EMG of the arms and legs

were unremarkable. Extraocular paresis developed, and she died 15 months after onset of the disease. Autopsy demonstrated neuronal atrophy of the motor nuclei of the cranial nerves and the ventral horns in the cervical and thoracic spinal cord. Gomez et al.[127] cited hereditofamilial cases reported in 1892 and 1893 by Fazio and Londe. None had pathologic or electromyographic confirmation. A similar child reported[128] in 1976 had normal MCV and EMG of the extremities; however, EMG of facial muscles showed frequent scattered fibrillation potentials and no voluntary activity.

The childhood bulbar palsies have been reviewed[127] and subcategorized into three groups.[128] They included predominant lower motor neuron disease of the brain stem with less prominent general-

TABLE 25.10. Childhood and adolescent motor neuron disorders

Bulbar paralysis (Fazio-Londe)
Kugelberg-Welander (spinal muscular atrophy III)
Focal monomelic atrophy
Poliomyelitis—mimic with asthma
Juvenile motor neuron disease or amyotrophic lateral
  sclerosis
Paraneoplastic (Hodgkin's disease)
Hexosaminidase A deficiency
Infantile neuroaxonal dystrophy
Primary lateral sclerosis

ized involvement, equal involvement of the spinal and brain stem motor nuclei, and bulbar paresis in association with widespread central nervous system dysfunction, including but not limited to lower motor neurons. In six of the 14 children, the progressive bulbar dysfunction led to death in 6 to 17 months.[127] Childhood bulbar paralysis may be nosologically similar to other childhood SMAs but has a more malignant course secondary to the profound early involvement of brain stem nuclei.[128] We have seen one 7-year-old child who was diagnosed with cerebral palsy at age 9 months because of spastic quadriparesis. Flaccid arms and lower motor bulbar signs developed later. In this child, EMG demonstrated high amplitude (6 to 12 mV) motor units in all extremities with fibrillation potentials in most muscles and with low amplitude CMAPs but otherwise normal motor and sensory NCS. She died of respiratory failure at age 7 years. Autopsy demonstrated focal motor neuron loss in the brain stem and spinal cord with minimal changes in the corticospinal tract. A similar illness reported in two of four siblings suggested an autosomal recessive genetic process.[129]

A juvenile form of progressive bulbar palsy with ptosis, dysphagia, and facial and tongue weakness may mimic myasthenia gravis.[130] The findings of low-amplitude facial CMAPs and neurogenic changes on needle EMG were compatible with a primary motor neuron process.

Kugelberg-Welander Disease—Spinal Muscular Atrophy III

Kugelberg and Welander[131] described a familial juvenile SMA clinically simulating muscular dystrophy. Subsequent investigations attempted to define the nosologic relationship, if any, between infantile SMA I and III. Of 95 patients with SMA III, 35 had onset before age 6 years.[132] Hausmanowa-Petrusewicz et al.[132] studied 12 children having earliest onset of SMA III in whom thorough EMG or muscle nerve biopsy was performed. Only one child had affected siblings. Each had been a product of a normal pregnancy, and the mother had not been aware of a diminution in fetal activity. In retrospect, the initial symptoms were first apparent in 50% at age 2 years when they attempted to walk alone. In other children, first symptoms included a waddling gait and problems running or climbing stairs. Occasionally the symptoms do not become important until early adolescent years. No progression was noted in the 11 children during a 5-year follow-up period.[132]

High-amplitude, long-duration MUPs are demonstrated by EMG in 20% to 40% of the muscles investigated[132] and are often associated with fasciculations and fibrillation potentials, predominantly in the proximal musculature of the lower extremity. This contrasts with more diffuse abnormalities of SMA I. Occasionally myotonic-like discharges were found after 9 to 10 years, and the percentage of large MUPs was increased.[132]

Based on further histochemical and ultrastructural studies, Hausmanowa-Petrusewicz et al.[132] concluded that a fetal defect is responsible for both SMA I and III; however, type III is probably more limited and develops later. This conclusion has been confirmed by the genetic studies of Munsat et al.[30]

Focal Amyotrophies

Hirayama et al.[133] described the insidious onset of a nonprogressive unilateral pure amyotrophy of the upper extremity in Japanese men between the ages of 15 and 22 years. Median, ulnar, and radial innervated muscles were involved in 75%; however, in the rest, a predominant ulnar or radial contribution was noted. Fasciculations were observed in 66%, and a tremor-like involuntary finger movement was observed in 60%. Rapid progression occurred during the first few years, but in most of the patients the illness stabilized within 5 years. Evidence did not suggest poliomyelitis, amyotrophic lateral sclerosis (ALS), or spinal cord diseases. Subsequent investigations suggested the lesion is at the level of the anterior horn cells.[133–136]

In 17 of 20 patients, EMG demonstrated typical chronic neurogenic changes with long-duration, high-amplitude MUPs and occasional fasciculations and fibrillation potentials in the affected extremities.[133] Similar electromyographic changes in the contralateral asymptomatic arm were noted in 25% of patients. No comment was made about NCS. Results of cerebrospinal fluid tests were always normal. Fifteen years later, Sobue et al.[134] reported on 71 patients, one third of whom had bilateral segmental muscular atrophy of the upper extremity. Slight hypoesthesia was observed in the region of the muscular atrophy in 16 patients.

Needle EMG results demonstrated chronic neurogenic changes in 96%; however, fibrillation potentials and positive sharp waves were seen in only 12.5%.[134] Similar changes were observed in the opposite arm in 88%. Monomelic amyotrophy in 23 Indian adolescents or young adults affected the arm

(13 patients) or the leg (10 patients).[135] Additional patients with benign focal amyotrophy of the upper extremities have been reported in non-Asian populations, including 15 patients from North America.[136–138] Bilateral asymmetric neurogenic atrophy and weakness below the elbows insidiously developed in four patients.[137] In contrast to earlier studies, two of the four recovered within 12 to 15 months.[137] These investigators[137] concluded that their patients had a multifocal motor neuropathy with predilection for the ulnar, median, and radial nerves. Certainly multiple or even focal motor neuropathies can have somewhat similar presentations, particularly the tomaculous neuropathies or those with hereditary predisposition to pressure neuropathies.[139] Computed tomography (CT) demonstrated focal cervical cord atrophy in two patients.[138] Evaluation of these patients with magnetic resonance imaging (MRI) will be of future interest.

Poliomyelitis—Mimic with Asthma

Rarely an acute flaccid asymmetric weakness develops in children 4 to 7 days after the occurrence of an acute asthmatic attack that produces a mild cerebrospinal fluid pleocytosis despite earlier poliomyelitis vaccine.[140] NCS or EMG demonstrated normal compound SNAPs and severe signs of primary axonal motor neuropathy.[140,141]

Juvenile Motor Neuron Disease—Amyotrophic Lateral Sclerosis

In juveniles with focal amyotrophy, ALS was excluded; however, the possibility of ALS should be considered even, although it is rare, in this age group. A 12-year-old girl had rapidly progressive paralysis of the arm that led to quadriparesis.[142] Results of EMG demonstrated diffuse fibrillation potentials and fasciculations. She died within a year. Autopsy results demonstrated widespread motor neuronal cytoplasmic inclusions.[142] A 7-year-old child first showed evidence of motor difficulties in keeping up with her peers. Examination when she was 11 years old demonstrated bilateral Babinski signs and pes cavus. Weakness was present by age 12, and she needed a wheelchair when she was in her twenties. Bulbar involvement led to death when she was in her thirties. At autopsy, eosinophilic cytoplasmic inclusions were present in the few remaining anterior horn cells and brain stem motor nuclei.[143] We have seen a 19-year-old woman with progressive arm weakness. Results of EMG demonstrated a severe motor

neurogenic process. She died 18 months after onset of disease. Findings at autopsy revealed typical ALS. In a review of 123 patients with ALS, only one, a 17-year-old girl, had the onset of disease before age 20 years.[144]

Paraneoplastic Motor Neuron Disease

A 14-year-old girl had progressive bilateral weakness, and EMG demonstrated denervation of her arms but normal innervation of her legs. She died within 14 months. At autopsy, cervical, thoracic, and upper lumbar anterior horn cells were almost totally absent, as were neurons in Clark's columns. Both central nervous system and peripheral nervous system demyelination were present. Evidence of Hodgkin's disease was found in the mediastinal lymph nodes.[145]

Hexosaminidase Deficiency and Juvenile Motor Neuron Disease

Progressive proximal weakness developed in a 15-year-old Ashkenazi boy. He had a long history of frequent cramps and a peculiar gait. On EMG, diffuse fibrillation potentials, fasciculations, and large MUPs correlated with the diagnosis of SMA III. Hexosaminidase-A levels were greatly diminished in both serum and leukocytes.[146] A boy who was not of Ashkenazi heritage with partial hexosaminidase deficiency had the onset of symptoms at age 7 years characterized by progressive dysarthria, leg weakness, and muscular twitching. At age 13 years, he had a pseudobulbar dysarthria, mild diffuse weakness of the legs, brisk reflexes, and steppage gait. Diffuse active and chronic neurogenic changes were present on EMG, with the exception that MUP size was normal.[147] A somewhat atypical phenotypic variant with clinical signs of SMA III was reported,[148] and recurrent psychosis with concomitant corticospinal or corticobulbar dysfunction developed. Two of the three patients with hexosaminidase deficiency were Ashkenazi. With two of the children, EMG showed neurogenic changes.

Infantile Neuroaxonal Dystrophy

This rare disorder presents in infants between 18 and 24 months of age, with failure to walk or to develop speech and positive Babinski signs. The original description of infantile neuraxonal dystrophy (IND) was attributed[149] to the 1952 work of Seitelberger.[149] EMG demonstrated a mixture of active and chronic[149,150] denervation potentials. Motor nerve CVs were normal in general; however, case no. 5 at age 7 years had median MCV of 36 m/second.[150] In most instances, normal NCS results help to differentiate the clinical diagnosis of IND from metachromatic leukodystrophy, which has similar clinical manifestations. The characteristic pathologic findings on sural nerve biopsy include the presence of axonal spheroids, similar to those located diffusely in the spinal cord and brain stem gray matter, and variable ovoid fusiform intraaxonal swellings with concomitant patchy areas of axonal degeneration.[150]

Progressive deterioriation in cognitive and motor function developed in an infant with Down's syndrome after 18 months of age.[151] Extensive denervation was found on EMG. Nerve conduction studies demonstrated decreased CMAPs, mild generalized slowing of sensory conduction, and late responses suggesting axonal degeneration.[151] Sural nerve biopsy demonstrated typical findings of IND.

We have seen one child with IND who fit the clinical spectrum perfectly. EMG performed on a 2½-year-old child showed diffuse fibrillation potentials and high-amplitude (8 to 10 mV) large MUPs. Motor CMAPs were borderline in the legs but progressively declined over 2 years, whereas MCVs and compound SNAPs remained normal. Sural nerve biopsy was not diagnostic. Skin biopsy demonstrated many abnormal unmyelinated axons with crystalline inclusions characteristic of IND. Selective cerebellar atrophy was revealed by MRI in infants with IND.[152]

Primary Lateral Sclerosis

A previously healthy 9-month-old infant had progressive weakness in the left arm and leg with signs of corticospinal tract degeneration. Results of EMG and NCS were unremarkable. Swallowing difficulties soon occurred followed by generalized spasticity with fixation of facial expression. Diagnostic possibilities included neuroaxonal dystrophy, neuronal ceroid lipofuscinosis, leukodystrophies, and GSDs. No evidence, however, of mental deterioration, seizures, visual changes or abnormalities on EEG or NCS occurred. This boy died at 4 years of age. Corticospinal tract degeneration was the only finding at autopsy.[153]

NERVE ROOT DISEASE

Cervical or lumbosacral radiculopathies are unusual in children. We have evaluated more than 1600 chil-

dren, aged 0 to 18 years. Only a few had unexplained neck, back, or extremity discomfort and were referred to exclude a radiculopathy. One adolescent (aged 18 years) in whom severe back spasms developed after a sudden turning movement had isolated L-5–S-1 paraspinal denervation. This was the only possible nerve root lesion identified in our pediatric EMG lab in more than 13 years. No specific mechanism was identified. In younger children obtaining relaxation in the lumbosacral paraspinal muscles may be difficult, and consequently occult lesions may be masked.

Lumbosacral Root Disease

Because pediatric lumbosacral disk disease is uncommon, unusual mechanisms need to be considered in children with lumbar nerve root symptoms. A 16-year-old boy, a wrestler, had 1 year of pain in the left buttock, thigh, and calf. EMG was not performed; however, CT demonstrated a mass at L-5–S-1, which at laminectomy proved to be an S-1 schwannoma.[154]

Cervical Root Disease

Although we have not seen classic cervical radiculopathies secondary to discogenic causes in the pediatric population, we evaluated two children with congenital cervical spine lesions. One was a 13-year-old child with a short history of pain in the right shoulder and arm exacerbated by swimming. EMG demonstrated C-7–T-1 denervation. Cervical spine radiography demonstrated anomalous hypoplastic vertebral bodies with incompletely developed interspaces. Another adolescent referred to evaluate a possible brachial plexus lesion with progressive arm weakness and atrophy had C-5–C-8 active denervation in the affected arm with contralateral changes at C-5. Cervical spinal stenosis at C-4–C-7 was demonstrated on myelography.

The latter patient illustrated a problem encountered when cervical paraspinal relaxation is not adequate. Although normal median and ulnar compound SNAPs may support the diagnosis of an intraspinal lesion at C-6–C-8, C-5–C-6 lesions may mimic brachial plexitis. Normal musculocutaneous motor and sensory conduction may be useful in localizing lesions to the C-5–C-6 roots when reliable paraspinal muscle testing is not possible.[155] Radiography of the cervical spine and MRI or myelography or both are of use in defining these congenital spinal lesions.

PLEXUS LESIONS

Brachial Plexopathies

The anatomy of the brachial and lumbar plexus is reviewed in Chapter 8. Most pediatric brachial plexus studies are divided into neonatal and post-neonatal groups. In our laboratory, neonatal lesions are slightly more common.

Neonatal Brachial Plexus Lesions

Eng et al.[156] estimated that the incidence of newborn brachial plexus lesions is approximately 0.4 per 1000 births. In a 1978 study[156] of 135 infants with infantile brachial plexopathies 71 had a complicated birth requiring forceps; 123 presentations were vertex and 11 were breech; only one delivery was by cesarean section. Sever,[157] in 1925, proposed that Erb's palsy is a result of forcible obstetric head traction during cephalic or breech deliveries. Caution is suggested, however, in applying this thesis to all newborns with brachial plexopathies. Two newborns with brachial plexus injury defined by EMG may have had an intrauterine basis.[158] One newborn with Erb's palsy immediately had fibrillations potentials, and a second infant with an Erb-Klumpke lesion had fibrillation potentials in the hand muscles at 4 days old. Three other neonates with Erb's palsies had normal results on EMG soon after birth, which suggested a perinatal injury with potential for electromyographic changes to develop later. Neonatal controls showed no denervation.[158] Based on these data, Koenigsberger[158] suggested that some neonatal plexopathies may be secondary to intrauterine positioning, amniotic bands, or otherwise undefined mechanisms. In general, fibrillation potentials do not occur in the human until 10 days after axonal nerve damage. Animal data[159] suggested that fibrillation potentials may occur in 2 to 4 days with an earlier appearance of fibrillation potentials when the injury was closest to the muscle fibers. It is possible that short distances and immature motor units may permit earlier signs of denervation in the newborn.[160]

The medicolegal implications of Koenigsberger's[158] observation merit further study. To date, however, other studies[156,161,162] of neonatal brachial plexopathies have not included electromyographic evaluation in the immediate neonatal period. One study[162] admonishes pediatricians not to send these newborns for evaluation until age 3 weeks to distinguish neurapraxic lesions from those with axonal damage. Certainly this is of value prognostically. An electromyographic study performed in the immediate neonatal period, however, may provide further pathophysiologic information, especially today with many complicated obstetric situations that require cesarean section.

Classic Erb's lateral plexus palsy was present in 110 of 135 infantile brachial plexopathies. Twenty-one had combined Erb-Klumpke's plexopathy and 4 had isolated posterior brachial plexopathies.[156] All patients had serious abnormalities on EMG, with the exception of eight who had a neurapraxic lesion. Prognosis was best in patients with a lesion in the upper plexus. Overall in 70% of infants, long-term results were good to excellent; in 22%, moderate residual damage was present; and in 8%, a severe incapacity was present.[156] EMG[163] in 24 patients with Erb-Klumpke infantile plexopathies demonstrated proximal recovery in 3 to 4 months, but residual distal weakness remained.

Osteomyelitis-associated brachial neuropathy in young infants

An acute brachial plexus neuropathy associated with osteomyelitis of the proximal humerus was reported in two neonates.[164] In one infant, EMG demonstrated denervation in muscles of the upper trunk. Both infants were febrile, had an erythrocyte sedimentation rate (ESR) greater than 80 mm/hour (Westergren), and blood cultures positive for group B β-hemolytic streptococcus. Osteomyelitis of the proximal humerus was defined by radiography and technetium bone scans. The pathophysiologic mechanism was not defined, although thrombophlebitis and occlusion of the vasa nervorum were possible explanations.[164] We have seen a similar infant with an acute lateral trunk lesion in whom results of initial roentgenography and bone scans were negative but became positive on the fifth day. Group B streptococcus was cultured from blood and spinal fluid. In contrast to Clay's[164] two patients, our patient was normal 3 months later.

Traumatic plexopathies

In our experience, traumatic pediatric plexopathies are related to contact sports, cycling, and, unfortunately, gunshot wounds. In children in whom a definable mechanism is not apparent, the battered child syndrome needs to be considered. We saw one child with an acute brachial plexopathy who had underlying sickle cell trait and plumbism. A precise cause was not initially defined. The child improved but returned 3 months later with a recurrent lesion. Further investigation by the social worker implied that the child was abused by twirling her around by one arm.

Hereditary brachial plexus neuropathy

Dunn et al.[165] described hereditary brachial plexus neuropathy in 12 members of three families with detailed evaluation of three boys, aged 4 to 7 years. These children had repetitive episodes of pain in the shoulder and arm, weakness, and atrophy with gradual recovery. Each child had the interesting physiognomy of a Modigliani facies characterized by hypotelorism. The gene appears to be an autosomal dominant.[165] NCS showed predominant involvement of median and radial sensory fibers with low-amplitude CMAPs, relatively normal motor conduction, and denervation in the affected muscles.

Differential diagnosis includes brachial plexitis;[166–170] however, none of the 82 patients of Parsonage and Turner[166,167] were younger than age 16 years, and only five were between the ages of 16 and 20. Seven of 99 patients seen at the Mayo Clinic were less than 20 years old.[168] In at least three nonfamilial patients, the onset of brachial plexitis was at less than 10 years of age,[169] including one infant at age 11 months.[170] This infant had a more diffuse brachial plexitis with flaccid weakness of the entire arm and subsequent poor recovery.[170]

Four boys with hereditary brachial plexus neuropathy had their first attack between ages 3 and 5 years, and possibly one was at age 6 weeks.[165] Hereditary brachial plexus neuropathy needs to be differentiated from another genetic illness, familial pressure-sensitive neuropathy.[139] The latter patients tend to have lesions affecting nerves known to be sensitive to compression, for example, median, radial, and peroneal; however, some patients present with a painless brachial plexus neuropathy.

Thoracic outlet syndrome

In childhood, thoracic outlet syndrome is an uncommon condition. We have seen only one child in 13 years whose condition fits the strict electrical and clinical definition of neurologic thoracic outlet syndrome described by Gilliatt et al.[171] Ouvrier et al.[172] reported on a 4-year-old child with thenar atrophy and weakness in whom radiography of the cervical spine demonstrated congenital Klippel-Feil anomalies associated with small cervical ribs. Needle EMG demonstrated chronic denervation in thenar muscles

and low-amplitude median compound SNAPs; otherwise results were normal. Surgical exploration revealed an elongated C-7 transverse process that articulated with the first rib, separating the inferior trunk from the middle trunk. Postoperatively improvement occurred during the next 5 years.

Lumbosacral Plexopathies

Neonatal lumbosacral plexus lesions

In contrast to injuries to the brachial plexus, injury to the lumbosacral plexus is rare in newborns. A neonate was born in a precipitous breech delivery and was unable to extend the knee or rotate it internally at birth.[173] Denervation of the quadriceps and adductor magnus muscles was demonstrated on EMG. Excessive traction at birth probably resulted in injury to the L-2–L-4 nerve roots.[173] Four patients have been described, and all had total paralysis of one leg. Recovery was incomplete in three patients[174] and very good in one patient.[175]

Postneonatal lumbosacral plexopathies

Infants are susceptible to stretch injuries to the lumbosacral and brachial plexus. We have seen a 4-month-old infant whose sibling vigorously pulled him by his leg. The next morning, the leg was limp and motionless. A lesion at the lumbosacral plexus was evident on EMG. Other rare causes for lumbosacral plexopathy seen in our pediatric EMG lab include surgical trauma during a lengthening procedure for idiopathic leg length discrepancy and a retroperitoneal mass, such as lymphoma.

Six children, 2 to 16 years of age, had rapid onset of pain, weakness, and atrophy, primarily involving the upper lumbar plexus.[176] A viral illness preceded the onset by 3 to 10 days. The diagnosis of lumbosacral plexopathy was confirmed by EMG. Four children had complete recovery within 3 months, and two had mild residual weakness.[176]

MONONEUROPATHIES

Mononeuropathies in the pediatric population occur infrequently. Between 1979 and 1990, 1369 children, aged 0 to 18 years, were evaluated in our laboratory. Mononeuropathies were documented in 86 of 1369 (6%), which contrasts with 30% in our experience with adult mononeuropathies.[177] Among the children, 46 of 86 involved nerves of the upper extremity: 18 ulnar, 11 radial, 10 median, six long thoracic, and one musculocutaneous.[177] The lesions of the lower extremity included 17 peroneal, 20 sciatic, and three femoral (unpublished data, 1990).

Of 46 upper extremity mononeuropathies, 17 were secondary to fracture, dislocation, lacerations, or puncture wounds.[177] In another pediatric study,[178] 25 of 33 postnatal traumatic neuropathies resulted from fracture in 16 children or laceration in nine children. EMG provided good localization and prognostic data.[178] Although compressive neuropathies are relatively rare in childhood,[179] they are the second most common cause of upper extremity neuropathy.[177] Entrapment is uncommon in our pediatric experience and was identified in only nine of 86 children with mononeuropathies.[177]

Median Nerve

Only 10 patients with median neuropathies have been evaluated in our laboratory. Five were at the wrist, including four from entrapment and one from compression by a cast.[177] Only two children had idiopathic median nerve wrist entrapment commensurate with carpal tunnel syndrome (CTS).[177] One was associated with mucolipidosis III (pseudo-Hurler polydystrophy) and the other idiopathic. Two sisters with mucolipidosis III had bilateral CTS.[180] Starreveld and Ashenhurst noted that CTS may occur in mucopolysaccharidosis II, IV, and VI.[180] A case of asymptomatic CTS with Schwartz-Jampel syndrome was reported.[181] An association between *trigger* finger and bilateral CTS was reported in children.[182] Thenar atrophy was the presenting complaint rather than classic nocturnal paresthesias.[180,182] Typical adult CTS symptoms were found only once in an adolescent less than 15 years old in a 25-year review[183] of 1016 patients. In a father and son, symptoms of CTS began in both at age 2 years and were secondary to congenital thickening of the transverse carpal ligament.[184]

Symptomatic CTS was documented by EMG in four of 16 adults with athetoid dystonic cerebral palsy.[185] Their wrists were kept in continuous hyperflexion.

The finding of thenar hypoplasia may not imply *asymptomatic* CTS. Four children with unilateral or bilateral thenar hypoplasia and normal sensation had roentgenography (Figure 25.7) demonstrating concomitant malformation and hypodevelopment of the thumb phalanges and adjacent carpal bones.[186]

A 6-year-old child had congenital CTS with thenar hypoplasia and melorheostosis with absent

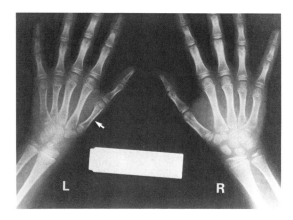

FIGURE 25.7. *Thenar hypoplasia with associated bony abnormalities illustrated by asymptomatic hypodevelopment of left first metacarpal (arrow). (Reprinted with permission from Cavanaugh NCP, Yates DAH, Sutcliffe J. Thenar hypoplasia with associated radiologic abnormalities. Muscle Nerve 1979; 2:432.)*

median CMAP and compound SNAPs.[187] Surgical exploration revealed a large pseudoneuroma. A sural nerve graft restored motor and sensory function 2 years after operation.

The median nerve of a newborn was reported to have been compressed by hematoma[188] at the wrist secondary to radial artery puncture for catheterization and to have been damaged directly in the antecubital fossa by brachial artery catheters.[189]

Of our[177] 10 patients with lesions of the median nerve, four involved the main trunk. Two were secondary to an elbow fracture dislocation or subsequent surgical repair or both, and a third resulted from chronic inflammation of the distal humerus with synovitis and an osteoid osteoma. The fourth lesion was idiopathic. One lesion of the anterior interosseous nerve was sustained after a hockey injury.[177] A posttraumatic median nerve entrapment that occurred within a healed greenstick radius fracture in a 7-year-old child responded well to surgical repair.[190] An 8-year-old child presenting with forearm pain and median nerve distribution weakness had a supracondylar lesion cured by excision of the ligament of Struthers.[191] An aberrant fibromuscular band arising from the supracondylar process and inserting in the deep fascia of the elbow produced median and ulnar nerve compression relieved by surgical excision in a 17-year-old boy.[192]

Ulnar Nerve

Ulnar nerve lesions are the most common upper extremity mononeuropathy in our[177] experience. Eleven of 18 were secondary to trauma, including fracture dislocation (five), laceration (four), and puncture wounds (two). Six of the seven other children had damage to the ulnar nerve secondary to elbow compression or entrapment. The distal ulnar nerve was affected at the wrist in five children; four were secondary to trauma and one to compression, an adolescent who had bicycle-induced compression at the wrist. Ulnar compression occurred at the elbow in three; two were secondary to anesthesia, and the third was related to use of a wheelchair. Entrapment at the elbow was related to an earlier injury in one, to cubital tunnel entrapment in another, and to family history in the last child.[177]

A 13-year-old child had progressive clinical and electromyographic evidence of a deficit localized above the elbow. A 15-cm mass proximal to the elbow was palpated, and biopsy revealed hypertrophic mononeuropathy.[193] Neurofibromas in infants and children may be associated with hypothenar masses and may involve the deep motor branch of the ulnar nerve.[194] After surgical removal, clinical and electromyographic testing may demonstrate some functional return.

Radial Nerve

Eleven (24%) of 46 children with upper extremity mononeuropathies evaluated in our pediatric EMG laboratory[177] involved the radial nerve. Seven were in the upper arm, and four involved the posterior interosseous branch. Three mononeuropathies were secondary to fracture and another three to laceration.

Two newborns presented with isolated unilateral flaccid paralysis of the wrist and finger extensors.[160] Ten other cases have been reported.[195,196] Seven mononeuropathies were associated with prolonged labor lasting longer than 24 hours with need for extraction by forceps or emergency cesarean section. Radial nerve palsy was associated with localized subcutaneous fat necrosis proximal to the radial epicondyle of the ipsilateral humerus in nine of the 10 patients and was evident in both of our patients (Figure 25.8). The prognosis for full recovery within 3 months is good. Pressure directed on the radial nerve during labor may be responsible for the damage.[196]

Other mechanisms for neonatal radial nerve palsy

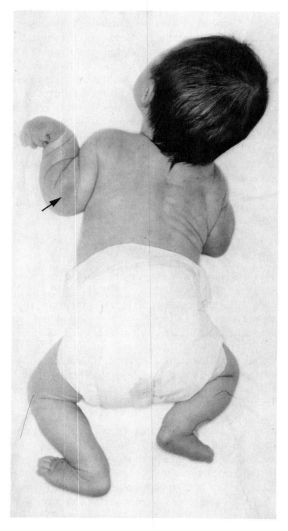

FIGURE 25.8.   *Typical posture of left arm in an infant with radial nerve palsy and associated subcutaneous fat necrosis (arrow). (Reprinted with permission from Ross D, Jones HR Jr, Fisher J, Konkol RJ. Isolated radial nerve lesion in the newborn. Neurology 1983; 33:1355.)*

have included congenital constricting bands of the arm, also involving the median and ulnar nerves.[197] A premature infant (1280 g) sustained radial palsy secondary to repeated blood pressure measurements that used an ultrasonographic Doppler technique with a plastic cuff.[198] This child recovered within 2 months.

Meier and Moll[199] reviewed 261 cases of tomaculous neuropathy published in the literature and noted that 9% involved the radial nerve in the spiral groove of the humerus. Three percent were infants or children less than 10 years old. One of our 11 children with radial nerve palsy had progressive weakness. During operation, the nerve appeared like a string of sausages with multiple areas of tight compression that microscopically consisted of scar tissue.[177] These scars were surgically released. Although postoperative improvement occurred, she eventually required tendon transfers to regain function. Another child with a progressive radial nerve palsy had entrapment by the lateral head of the triceps muscle.[200] This patient also required tendon transfers. These children emphasize the need for early surgical exploration when a progressive course is documented.

Three of four children with posterior interosseous nerve branch involvement had trauma, with two sustaining a laceration and one a fracture. Another child had a posterior interosseous syndrome secondary to an acute compartment syndrome after chemotherapy infiltration.[177] A 16-year-old girl with progressive weakness of the finger and wrist extensors was found at operation to have "compression" i.e., entrapment, of the posterior interosseous nerve between the supinator and aponeurosis of the common extensor.[201]

Long Thoracic Nerve

Isolated involvement of the long thoracic nerve occurred in six of our 46 patients with upper extremity neuropathies. One was a compression neuropathy secondary to a Milwaukee brace[179]; two neuropathies were related to trauma, and three were of unknown cause.[177]

Musculocutaneous Nerve

A body cast was associated with an isolated musculocutaneous compression palsy in one child.[179]

Suprascapular Nerve

This predominantly motor nerve is most likely damaged in the region of the suprascapular or spinoglenoid notch.[172] Mechanisms offered included inflammation, trauma, or compression.[172] It is uncommon for children to have a focal suprascapular nerve lesion, although such a lesion was described[202] in an adolescent who received a shoulder injury in gymnastics class. The role of surgical decompression in this patient was equivocal.

Femoral Nerve

Femoral neuropathies are uncommon; we have seen only three children with femoral lesions in 13 years. Two were postoperative lesions. One was a complication of posterior iliac osteotomy, and the other resulted from an orthopedic lower extremity stretch procedure.

Involvement of the lateral femoral cutaneous nerve branch with resulting numbness in the outer aspect of the thigh was idiopathic in a 12-year-old boy seen in our laboratory. Ouvrier et al.[172] mentioned a 3-year-old child with a similar lesion, possibly caused by an orthopedic harness.

Sciatic Nerve

Sciatic nerve lesions are uncommon; however they are as frequent in children as peroneal lesions. We have seen them in only 20 of 1678 children in 13 years. Previously perinatal lesions from birth trauma,[203] direct intragluteal injection,[204–206] or rarely umbilical vessel injection[207–209] have been recognized as mechanisms for infantile sciatic nerve palsies. We have not seen any of these perinatal sciatic nerve lesions perhaps because of careful obstetric care and not using the gluteal muscles as injection sites. Five children with sciatic nerve damage from intragluteal injection had surgical exploration.[206] A cicatrix was found in each. End-to-end anastomosis resulted in partial improvement in two children and excellent improvement in one child.[206] Of 10 children with sciatic neuropathies,[210] three were caused by compression (two at the sciatic notch). One occurred in a newborn immobilized with pancuronium. An adolescent with congestive heart failure who slept sitting up, with one heel tucked under his buttocks, had an acute sciatic neuropathy. His neuropathy was not unlike that of a healthy child who sat on a concrete step in a similar position.[211] A 2-year-old child had compression damage of the sciatic nerve at the thigh secondary to use of an orthopedic appliance.[210]

In another child, the sciatic neuropathy in some way was related to acute transverse myelitis, conceivably compression.[210] Two children had an acute postoperative sciatic nerve lesion after being placed in the lithotomy position for operation.[210] The precise pathophysiologic mechanism is not well defined for the postlithotomy sciatic nerve injury.[212,213] These injuries still occur despite great diligence in attempting to avoid pressure.[214] Stretch injury may be a mechanism.[215] We have seen one patient with stretch injury associated with closed reduction of a dislocated hip.[210]

Tumors, such as lymphoma,[210] need to be considered in the differential diagnosis of sciatic nerve lesions. MRI was valuable in defining a chloroma (granulocytic sarcoma) that compressed the sciatic nerve in a 10-year-old child's thigh 14 months after the diagnosis of acute leukemia.[216]

In a 60-year review of 35 patients with primary tumors of the sciatic nerve, Thomas et al.[217] reported on a 5-year-old child who presented with a progressive foot deformity. This patient was their youngest and the only one who presented without pain. Results of EMG supported the diagnosis of a sciatic or lower plexus lesion. The value of CT in diagnosing sciatic nerve tumors was emphasized.[217] MRI, however, is now the procedure of choice.

Sciatic entrapment neuropathies are exceedingly rare. Two children, aged 6 weeks and 2 years, were found to have entrapment of the sciatic nerve at the sciatic notch[218] with bony overgrowth of the posterior or the inferior iliac spine as defined by radiography of the hip. Unfortunately, not all childhood sciatic entrapment neuropathies may be defined radiologically, as illustrated by the report[219] of a myofascial band constricting the sciatic nerve. This report illustrates the value of surgical exploration with clinical and EMG evidence of a progressive sciatic neuropathy.

One adolescent presented with an acute sciatic nerve lesion secondary to hypersensitivity vasculitis with hypereosinophilic syndrome.[210] As with other hypereosinophilic syndrome neuropathies, improvement occurred with corticosteroid therapy.[220] Rarely an idiopathic progressive sciatic nerve lesion is found that defies definition despite appropriate radiographic imaging and even surgical exploration.[210]

In our experience with 10 children with sciatic neuropathies, the anatomic level was at the sciatic notch in five, in the thigh in two, and not identified in the remaining three children.[210] The prognosis varied from complete to no recovery; the result had little relationship to the underlying causes.[210]

Peroneal Nerve

Peroneal lesions are one of the two most common lower extremity mononeuropathies. Compression was the cause in 10 of 17 children seen in our EMG

laboratory. Three were related to casts, three to straps at the knee including Buck's traction, a Velcro strap after knee surgery, and to footboard taping necessary for securing neonatal intravenous therapy.[221] Another three were related to anorexia nervosa and one presumably secondary to profound sleep. A review of 70 patients with peroneal nerve palsy included just three children.[222] One was the only child, among 14 compressive peroneal neuropathies, and it was secondary to coma.[222] The other two were in adolescents, one of whom had concomitant ligamentous knee injury and the other an idiopathic progressive peroneal neuropathy.[222]

Three children in our experience had progressive peroneal neuropathies.[221] One was localized to the peroneal head on EMG. Surgical exploration demonstrated a fascial band originating from the peroneus longus tendon that entrapped the peroneal nerve over the fibular head, similar to that of a child reported by Brown et al.[223] Multiple bony exostoses near the fibular head may produce peroneal entrapment.[224] The exostoses may be occult and not demonstrated until CT of the knee is performed.[224] Other causes for progressive peroneal nerve palsy included hemangioma at the main peroneal trunk bifurcation,[225] ganglion cyst,[226,227] intraneural synovial cyst,[228] and sciatic notch tumors.[229] Systemic illnesses rarely associated with childhood peroneal neuropathies include juvenile diabetes mellitus[230] and an acute onset related to anaphylactoid purpura.[231] One child in our experience had primary sensory involvement with calf and toe paresthesias for 1 year. At operation, a schwannoma of the superficial peroneal nerve was found.[221]

Traumatic mechanisms are seen less commonly with peroneal than with sciatic neuropathies. We had three patients whose neuropathy was caused by a traumatic mechanism.[221] One was secondary to an automobile accident, one to a knee laceration, and one to a primary peroneal branch injury that happened in a martial arts class.

Three transient (4 to 9 weeks) peroneal neuropathies were reported[232] in newborns; two were idiopathic. Two patients had EMG, and no peroneal CMAPs could be obtained in either patient. Fibrillation potentials were noted in the peroneal muscles of one infant (aged 4 days) with a purplish excoriation in the lateral popliteal fossa.[232] The possibility of an intrauterine mechanism exists because of the early appearance of the fibrillation potentials.[158,160] Other neonatal causes for peroneal palsy included infiltration of intravenous solutions[233] and a compression presumed secondary to a footboard in two premature infants.[234]

Infantile peroneal neuropathies are of interest in relationship to congenital equinovarus. We have seen a few newborns unable to dorsiflex or evert the foot in whom NCS demonstrated absent or low-amplitude CMAPs recording from the extensor digitorum brevis. Neither had motor units firing within the extensor digitorum brevis, although some had units within the tibialis anterior muscle. No fibrillation potentials were seen.

Conduction block is uncommon in childhood peroneal neuropathy but is found with anorexia nervosa,[221] chronic leg crossing,[229] and some mass lesions, such as bony exostoses[224] or hemangiomas.[225] The lack of conduction blocks, however, does not exclude bony exostoses[224] or entrapment by the peroneus longus tendon.[221] Peroneal nerve ganglions[227] may cause total loss of extensor digitorum brevis response. Surgical exploration may be necessary to exclude these lesions, especially when no systemic process is present, such as with anorexia nervosa,[221] diabetes mellitus,[230] or anaphylactoid purpura.[231]

When no specific conduction block is defined, needle EMG provides localization. Of 17 children seen in our laboratory, ten neuropathies involved the common peroneal nerve, two the deep peroneal nerve, and one the superficial peroneal nerve.[221] Four were not precisely localized but were above the innervation of the tibialis anterior muscle.

Tibial Nerve

Neuropathies of the tibial nerve are rare. A few instances in our pediatric laboratory were concomitant with peroneal nerve injury, usually at the popliteal fossa.

Albrektsson et al.[235] reported on 10 girls, aged 9 to 15 years, with foot pain secondary to tarsal tunnel syndrome with paresthesias of the toes reproduced by tibial nerve percussion near the lateral malleolus. Unfortunately, none had confirmation by NCS or EMG. Nine were free of symptoms after decompression of the distal tibial and medial or lateral plantar nerves.

PEDIATRIC POLYNEUROPATHIES

Although the symmetric polyneuropathies in infants and children often mimic their adult counterparts, the history and examination are more difficult to obtain in children. Valuable additional information is provided by NCS and EMG that may lead to a definitive diagnosis. The pathophysiologic mechanisms are often different in children. Systemic factors, such as diabetes, uremia, and vasculitis, and many drugs or toxins, such as alcohol, are rarely encountered. Evans[236] reviewed 61 patients less than 19 years of age with electromyographic documentation of generalized polyneuropathy and subcategorized these children into six groups. More than 80% fit within three major categories, including acute postinfectious (AIDP) in 17 children, degenerative i.e. hereditary (HMSN, HSN, and spinocerebellar syndromes) in 17 children, and idiopathic in 16 children. Of these 16 children, 11 were associated with an indeterminate encephalopathy, which preceded the neuropathy by a few months to years. Eight of the 11 children had significant nerve CV slowing. The remaining three categories included systemic diseases, such as diabetes, uremia, rheumatoid arthritis, or systemic lupus erythematosus in five children; inborn errors of metabolism, such as metachromatic leukodystrophy in four children; and neuropathies after therapy with vincristine in two children. The incidence of diabetes mellitus was greater in Gamstorp's[237] study. Of the pediatric polyneuropathies in these two studies,[236,237] 30% and 31% were associated with central nervous system disease. The combination of central and peripheral nervous system dysfunction is atypical in adults. The incidence of acute inflammatory demyelinating polyneuropathy (AIDP) varied between 5%[237] and 28%.[236] We have seen 24 children with AIDP in 11 years.

A high incidence of familial neuropathies[236,237] occurred; this finding was supported by a European series of 287 pediatric patients with *pure* chronic, that is, nonpostinfectious, peripheral neuropathies wherein 241 (84%) were genetically determined.[238] Their study emphasizes the need for careful familial evaluation, including NCS or EMG whenever polyneuropathy is diagnosed in a child and when no postinfectious, metabolic, or toxic process is present. Demyelinating neuropathies were most common, including relatively mild autosomal dominant HMSN I (51%).[238] Autosomal recessive HMSN III accounted for 12% of the polyneuropathies and most often occurred in infancy. Consanguinity was more common. It was hoped that cerebrospinal fluid protein analysis might provide a means for differentiating between HMSN I and HMSN III; however, no clear distinction could be made.[238] Hereditary axonal disease, either autosomal dominant (HMSN II) or recessive, accounted for 21% of patients with polyneuropathies.[238]

Ouvrier et al.[172] reviewed 125 children with subacute and chronic polyneuropathies who had sural nerve biopsies performed. Seventy-one percent were specifically hereditary, that is, HMSN I, II, and III; Friedreich's ataxia; and inborn errors of metabolism, such as metachromatic leukodystrophy. Another 18% were hereditary but not identifiable. Only 10% were acquired, including 11 children with CIDP, three with toxic neuropathies, and two with leprosy.

The only reason for not pursuing NCS when evaluating a pediatric peripheral neuropathy is the child whose clinical picture is consistent with HMSN and who has a parent with definite neurophysiologic documentation of a specific form of HMSN.

Hereditary Neuropathies

Hereditary motor sensory neuropathies I through III

The clinical and neurophysiologic findings in HMSN I, II, and, III have been reviewed in another chapter and briefly in this chapter in relation to their unlikely presentation as floppy infant syndrome. In contrast to AIDP and CIDP, these patients have diffuse symmetric slowing without conduction block or temporal dispersion. The differential diagnosis of pediatric demyelinating neuropathies is summarized in Table 25.11.

Leukodystrophies

Krabbe's disease. This autosomal recessive illness secondary to deficiency of galactosylceramide beta-galactosidase presents in infants between ages 2 and 6 months with failure to thrive, irritability, intractable crying, loss of intellectual milestones, variable degrees of hypertonus and spasms, and unexplained febrile episodes. Seven infants with a peripheral neuropathy had levels of cerebrospinal fluid protein elevated between 137 and 360 mg/dL.[239] In four infants, aged 10 to 11 months, NCS or EMG demonstrated median MCV between 12 and 22 m/second and peroneal MCV between 10 and 15 m/second. Distal latencies were mildly prolonged. In three of the four infants, CMAP amplitudes were mildly to moderately diminished, and in one, no CMAP was detected.[239] No report of compound SNAPs was given.[239] Two children with Krabbe's disease seen by us had similar motor NCS and prolonged or absent sensory latencies. Motor units were normal on EMG. Sural nerve biopsies have shown segmental demyelination and Schwann cell cytoplasmic inclusions similar to those found in the brain

TABLE 25.11.   Demyelinating* childhood neuropathies

Acute or Subacute	Chronic
Congenital hypomyelinating	HMSN I, III, IV
AIDP	Krabbe's disease
CIDP	Metachromatic
Glue sniffing	leukodystrophy
Arsenic	Niemann-Pick disease,
Thallium	types A and C
Buckthorn wild cherry	Adrenal
	leukomyeloneuropathy
	Cockayne's syndrome
	Cerebrotendinous xanthomatosis
	Chédiak-Higashi syndrome
	Cherry red spot myoclonus
	syndrome
	Marinesco-Sjögren syndrome
	Giant axonal neuropathy ±†

* As defined by motor nerve conduction velocity less than 80% normal.
† ± = Equivocal.
AIDP, Acute inflammatory demyelinating polyneuropathy; CIDP, chronic inflammatory demyelinating polyneuropathy; HMSN, hereditary motor sensory neuropathy.

of patients with Krabbe's disease; however, the classic globoid cells were not found.[239,240]

Metachromatic leukodystrophy. This autosomal recessive inborn error of metabolism secondary to arylsulfatase-A deficiency occasionally presents as a neuropathy with generalized weakness, hyporeflexia, hypotonia, and unsteady gait after age 1 year.[241] Two 5-year-old children had severe MCV slowing, with median MCV of 16 to 26 m/second and peroneal MCV of 11 to 20 m/second. Distal latency was also prolonged. We have seen six children, aged 1.5 to 6 years, with metachromatic leukodystrophy who presented with gait difficulty and elevated levels of cerebrospinal fluid proteins. MCVs varied between 6 and 31 m/second. Sural compound SNAPs were absent. Median compound SNAPs were absent or of low amplitude and mildly prolonged. Evidence of acute and chronic denervation was found by EMG in only one of the six children with metachromatic leukodystrophy. Sural nerve biopsy showed metachromatic staining of sulfatides deposited within the nerve. Elevated urinary sulfatide excretion and considerable diminution in leukocyte arylsulfatase-A activity were confirmed.[241]

An unusual case of partial arylsulfatase-A deficiency was reported in a previously healthy 8-year-old child in whom proximal greater than distal weakness and hyporeflexia developed within 4 weeks.[242] Nerve CVs were diffusely slowed at 30 m/second, and levels of cerebrospinal fluid protein were 10 times normal. A diagnosis of CIDP was made; however, only partial improvement occurred with prednisone and azathioprine therapy. Further investigation revealed arylsulfatase-A activity about half normal and increased urinary sulfatide excretion. Sural nerve biopsy revealed metachromatic staining. Some improvement had taken place after 8 years; however, nerve CVs were still slow. Both parents had similar low arylsulfatase-A activity. Ouvrier et al.[172] reported on a 10-year-old child with pes cavus, distal weakness, and areflexia with slow nerve CV who was initially diagnosed as having HMSN when her father was found to have high arches. Intellectual decline, however, led to a diagnosis of metachromatic leukodystrophy.

In juvenile metachromatic leukodystrophy, the youngster may be well until midadolescence, when multisystem neurodegeneration evolves manifested by shuffling gait, pseudobulbar dysfunction, and intellectual decline.[243] Diminished nerve CVs help to direct the evaluations to combined central nervous system and peripheral nervous system demyelinating

illness. Bone marrow transplantation (BMT) has been partially beneficial on the rare occasions it has been performed. One child who received BMT at age 11 months began to show steady acquisition of developmental milestones 6 months later.[244] No MCV improvement occurred. Asymptomatic infants, children, and young adolescents with metachromatic leukodystrophy, based on a similar diagnosis in a sibling, should be considered for prompt BMT.[245]

Adrenoleukomyeloneuropathy. Adrenoleukomyeloneuropathy may be a phenotypic variant of adrenoleukodystrophy, both of which are transmitted as sex-linked recessive traits. Although adrenoleukodystrophy presents in childhood, it is not associated with a neuropathy. Patients with adrenoleukomyeloneuropathy may have a polyneuropathy, but the disease presents only in adults. A report[246] of adrenoleukomyeloneuropathy variant with cerebellar signs presenting in early childhood was associated with seizures and impulsive behavior. The child had pes cavus, weakness, broad-based gait, and bilateral Babinski signs. MCVs were slowed, and CMAPs were of low amplitude. Results of needle EMG were unremarkable. An elevated C26/22 ratio was consistent with accumulation of long-chain fatty acids.

Cockayne's syndrome. Cockayne's syndrome is a rare autosomal recessive leukodystrophy with progeria, microcephaly, dwarfism, photosensitivity, mental retardation, nerve deafness, and retinitis pigmentosa. MCVs are consistent with a demyelinating neuropathy.[247,248] Unusual granular lysosomal inclusions have been described in Schwann cells and perineural cells, in contrast to other leukodystrophies.[248]

Cerebrotendinous xanthomatosis. Cerebrotendinous xanthomatosis is an autosomal recessive illness characterized by ataxia, dementia, and corticospinal tract findings. Xanthomatosis tendon infiltration may occasionally be associated with a demyelinating peripheral neuropathy. Three patients with onset in adolescence were the products of first-cousin parents. Two adolescents had brisk reflexes, extensor toe signs, and pes cavus.[249] Motor nerve CV of peroneal and tibial nerves was 12 to 34 m/second and 38 to 40 m/second in median nerves. Compound SNAPs were absent in the legs and were of low amplitude in the arms, and sensory CV was slow in the arms. Results of needle EMG were normal. Sural biopsy demonstrated segmental demyelination and remyelination.

Chédiak-Higashi syndrome.   Chédiak-Higashi syndrome is a rare hereditary disorder characterized by defective pigmentation of the hair and skin, pancytopenia and susceptibility to infection, and lymphoproliferative malignancies. An 11-year-old child with 2 years of progressive distal weakness demonstrated progressive MCV slowing from normal to 30 to 32 m/second with proximal conduction block and normal results on needle EMG.[250] Sural biopsy demonstrated cytoplasmic inclusions similar to those found in leukocytes of patients with Chédiak-Higashi syndrome.

Cherry red spot myoclonus syndrome (sialidosis I).   Debilitating myoclonus occurs in the second or third decade in cherry red spot myoclonus syndrome and is associated with nonpigmentary macular degeneration secondary to lysosomal neuraminidase deficiency. Decreased vision and intermittent tingling developed in an adolescent girl, and by age 21, she had severe action myoclonus.[251] Although peripheral neuropathy was not found on examination, NCS demonstrated MCV to be 25 m/second in peroneal nerves to 41 m/second in median nerves with absent sural compound SNAPs and prolonged H-reflexes; however, results of EMG were normal. Sural biopsy demonstrated segmental demyelination with Schwann cells containing indeterminate abnormal storage material within membrane bound vacuoles.[251]

Spinocerebellar syndromes

Childhood ataxic sensory neuropathies are sometimes associated with inborn errors of metabolism, such as metachromatic leukodystrophy, and present with central nervous system manifestations and demyelinating type MCV. In contrast, patients with idiopathic childhood spinocerebellar syndromes also present with ataxic sensory neuropathy but have normal MCVs despite absent compound SNAPs (Table 25.12).

Friedreich's ataxia.   Friedreich's ataxia is the prototype of the childhood spinocerebellar syndromes. It is an autosomal recessive disorder, with the Friedreich's ataxia gene identified in the pericentromeric region of chromosome 9.[252] Children with Friedreich's ataxia present between 1 and 14 years of age with gait difficulty, generalized clumsiness, dysarthria, clumsy hands, pes cavus, and kyphoscoliosis.[253,254] Examination discloses gait ataxia, pes cavus, and areflexia with diminished vibratory and position sense.[254] Early on, reflexes may be retained.[255] Corticospinal tract dysfunction is present,

TABLE 25.12.   Spinocerebellar syndromes

| | Inheritance | Reflexes | Babinskis Signs | Nerve Conductions | | Evoked Potentials* | | | Magnetic Resonance Imaging |
				Motor	Sensory	VER	BAER	SSER	
Freidreich's ataxia	AR	Ab	↑	N	Ab	↓/D	↓IV/V	D/Ab	Cervical cord atrophy
Cerebellar ataxia with retained reflexes	AR	Pr	↓↑	↓	↓	NA	↓IV/V	D/Ab	Cerebellar atrophy
X-linked	X	Pr	↑	↓	Ab/↓	NA	NA	NA	NA
Ataxia-telangiectasia	AR	↓/Ab	↓	N↓	↓/Ab	↓/D	N	D	NA
Xeroderma pigmentosa	AR	↓/Ab	NA	↓/Ab	Ab	NA	NA	NA	NA
Abetalipoproteinemia	AR	↓	↓↑	N	N/↓	N/D	N	D	NA
Vitamin E deficiency	NG	↓/Ab	↑	N/↓	N/↓	N	N	D/Ab	NA
Marinesco-Sjögren	NA	Ab	NA	↓↓	NA	NA	NA	NA	NA

Ab, Absent; AR, autosomal recessive; D, delayed; NA, not available; NG, not genetic; Pr, present. ↑, extensor; ↓, plantar ↓, slight to mildly abnormal; ↓↓, very abnormal, slow.

* VER, Visual evoked response; BAER, brain stem auditory evoked response; SER, somatosensory evoked response.

but positive Babinski signs may not occur until later ages.

Electrophysiologic studies are important in diagnosis. Reduced or absent compound SNAPs are always noted, and MCV parameters are normal or slightly reduced, compatible with an axonal process.[254–256]

Needle EMG reveals subtle signs of denervation in the lower extremities.[257] Sural biopsies demonstrate considerable reduction in the percentage of large fibers[256] that correlates with the sensory NCS changes and the loss of large neurons in dorsal root ganglia.[257] In a 3- to 7-year follow-up study,[257] no electrophysiologic deterioration occurred whether the patients had a short-term or a long-term history of Friedreich's ataxia. Results of repeated nerve biopsies were unchanged. Caruso et al.[258] examined NCS in 35 relatives of patients with Friedreich's ataxia. Orthodromic distal sensory CV was moderately slowed compared with control subjects. A few compound SNAPs were diminished in amplitude.[258] Results of motor NCS were normal.

The differential diagnosis of children with progressive ataxia and very abnormal sensory NCS with normal to mild motor NCS changes includes many syndromes in addition to Friedreich's ataxia, such as early-onset cerebellar ataxia with preserved reflexes,[259,260] X-linked spinocerebellar degeneration,[261] ataxia-telangiectasia,[262] and xeroderma pigmentosa.[263] It also includes the vitamin E deficiency syndromes, such as abetalipropoteinemia (ABL),[264–267] the spinocerebellar syndrome associated with chronic liver disease,[268–272] intestinal lymphangiectasia,[273] and selective vitamin E malabsorption.[274] Amantidine hydrochloride therapy has shown some symptomatic benefit in ambulatory patients with Friedreich's ataxia.[275]

Cerebellar ataxia with retained reflexes. This autosomal recessive syndrome distinguished from Friedreich's ataxia by Harding[259] is associated with less severe ataxia of the arms, fewer systemic problems, and better prognosis. Electrophysiologic studies are similar[260]; however, MRI findings differ. Cervical cord atrophy occurs in patients with Friedreich's ataxia, and cerebellar atrophy is present in patients with retained reflexes.[260]

Spinocerebellar degeneration of X-linked type. One child between 18 and 24 months of age was seen because of delay in walking. Progressive gait ataxia had occurred when the child was seen between the ages 3 and 16 years.[261] In contrast to Friedreich's ataxia, this syndrome does not affect life expectancy, although older family members may become wheelchair bound by age 30 years. In all patients, MCVs were moderately reduced, compound SNAPs were either absent or of decreased amplitude, and sensory CV was decreased.[261]

Ataxia-telangiectasia. Children with ataxia-telangiectasia have hyporeflexia or areflexia; however, it is uncommon to have extensor plantar responses.[276] Loss of vibratory and position sense is mild and much less profound. These children have recurrent sinopulmonary infections, deficiency of IgA or IgE, and characteristic conjunctival telangiectasia. Striatal dysfunction causes choreoathetosis, masked facies, head tremor, and ocular movement disorders. MCV is slightly diminished, and compound SNAPs are decreased in amplitude or absent.[276] Multimodal evoked potential studies, visual evoked response (VER), brain stem auditory evoked response (BAER), and somatosensory evoked response (SSER) may help differentiate Friedreich's ataxia from ataxia-telangiectasia. Both have similar changes in VERs and SSERs.[262] In some older patients, VERs were of lower amplitude and delayed, and SSERs were abnormal and progressively worsened.[262] In patients with ataxia-telangiectasia, BAERs were normal. In contrast, children with Friedreich's ataxia had progressive loss of waves IV and V.

Xeroderma pigmentosa. Xeroderma pigmentosa is a rare autosomal recessive illness which is common in Japan[263] with clinical signs suggestive of Friedreich's ataxia. These patients also have photosensitivity, telangiectasias, and susceptibility to cutaneous malignancies. Absent compound SNAPs are noted, MCV may be mildly slow, or CMAPs may be absent.[263]

Vitamin E deficiency syndromes—Abetalipoproteinemia. These children have a clinical presentation which mimics Friedreich's ataxia with ataxia, areflexia, scoliosis, and pes cavus and have also had vitamin E deficiency as a consistent abnormality.[264–267] Many patients have malabsorption secondary to steatorrhea or chronic cholestasis. Bassen and Kornzweig[264] noted an association with ABL, prominent acanthocytes, and atypical retinitis pigmentosa. The degree of neurologic involvement is variable and increases with age.[266]

In contrast to Friedreich's ataxia, with its early loss of compound SNAPs, patients with ABL may have preserved or diminished compound SNAPs.[265]

We have seen one child with ABL who had steatorrhea at age 11 years and ataxia at age 12 years. Vitamin E supplementation was started; nevertheless, retinitis pigmentosa developed. NCS and EMG first performed 23 years later demonstrated low-amplitude, normal latency compound SNAPs and absent H wave but normal motor NCS. In five children with ABL, evoked potentials were studied.[267] Vitamin E was less than 3 mg/L (normal, 7 to 12 mg/L). SSERs are the most sensitive, being abnormal in all but one child.[267] Normal VERs are usually found, although one patient had consistent delay, and BAERs are also normal.[267]

Chronic cholestatic liver disease has been associated[268] with vitamin E deficiency in children. Gait ataxia, distal weakness, areflexia, diminished proprioceptive sensation, and gaze paresis have developed in these children.[268] Hyporeflexia was the first sign; reflexes disappeared in children between ages 2 to 10 years. Four children with chronic steatorrhea and cholestasis had a spinocerebellar syndrome with appendicular and gait ataxia, areflexia, extensor toe signs, and ophthalmoplegia.[269] An unusual variant was apparent in a 14-year-old adolescent with 7 years of ataxia in whom severe atrophy of the tongue, sternocleidomastoid, and trapezius muscles and ophthalmoplegia developed.[270] Neurologic function normalized in three children with initiation of vitamin E therapy before age 3 years; limited success occurred in nine children, aged 5 to 17 years.[271] In another study,[272] vitamin E therapy prevented progression, but no improvement occurred. MCVs are normal, and CMAPs and compound SNAPs may be of low amplitude.[271,272] Two patients had a superimposed median neuropathy at the wrist.[272]

Other vitamin E intestinal malabsorption syndromes associated with spinocerebellar syndromes included a report[273] of protein-losing enteropathy secondary to intestinal lymphangiectasia in a 9-month-old infant. Unsteady gait developed at age 13 years, and gait ataxia and areflexia with positive Babinski and Romberg signs followed. A primary axonal motor sensory neuropathy was defined by NCS and EMG. Levels of vitamin E were low; consequently vitamin E therapy was begun. Six months later, her neurologic symptoms had improved; however, NCS were not repeated.

Harding et al.[274] described a 13-year-old patient with a selective vitamin E absorption defect associated with a spinocerebellar syndrome but with no evidence of ABL, steatorrhea, or cholestatic liver disease. Absent tibial and prolonged median SSERs were associated with normal VERS, BAERs, and motor and sensory NCS. Her symptoms improved with vitamin E therapy. The importance of measuring vitamin E levels is emphasized in all patients with spinocerebellar ataxia.

Marinesco-Sjögren syndrome. Patients with Marinesco-Sjögren syndrome, a rare variant of spinocerebellar ataxia, present with ataxia, mental retardation, and congenital cataracts. In contrast to all other spinocerebellar ataxias with predominantly axonal changes, one child demonstrated greatly slowed MCV compatible with demyelination that was confirmed by sural nerve biopsy.[277]

Primary sensory neuropathies

Most childhood primary sensory neuropathies (Table 25.13) are subclassified according to their hereditary characteristics.[278] The clinical features are also distinctive. The neuronal atrophies predominantly affect the peripheral sensory neurons. *Insensitivity* to pain is characterized by a detectable defect in sensory pathways with failure to perceive sensation. In contrast, *indifference* to pain implies normal sensory pathways with lack of concern for a given stimulus.

Hereditary sensory neuropathies I-III. HSN I is an autosomal dominant trait with predominant involvement of the pain and temperature fibers, resulting in dissociated sensory loss and mimicking the changes of syringomyelia. Pathologic lesions are localized to the dorsal root ganglion. These children do not perceive pain. Their feet are subjected to inordinate repetitive trauma with development of painless ulcers under the metatarsal heads during the second decade. When unrecognized, cellulitis and osteomyelitis develop, leading to Charcot joints.

Absent compound SNAPs are noted, and low-amplitude median and tibial SSERs are recorded over the spine, with no responses detected over the scalp.[279] Results of motor NCS and needle EMG are normal. In vitro studies of nerve potentials demonstrated predominant loss of C fibers. A concomitant nerve root or spinal cord abnormality was suggested by the results of SSER.[279]

HSN II is an autosomal recessive congenital sensory neuropathy that begins in infancy. It is characterized by distal self-mutilating acropathy, stress fractures, and digital infections. Pressure and touch sensation is defective and is secondary to predominant involvement of A-alpha fibers.[280] The com-

TABLE 25.13. Sensory neuropathies

	Inheritance	Age at Onset	Fiber Loss	Clinical	Examination	Nerve Conductions	
						Motor	Sensory
HSN* I (Dyck[278])	AD	2nd decade	Unmyelinated	Painless foot ulcer, Charcot joint	↓ Pain and temperature	N	Ab
HSN II (Ohta et al.[280])	AR	Infancy	Small myelinated	Mutilating acropathy	Touch, pressure	N- ± ↓	Ab
HSN III (Aguayo et al.[281])	AR (Ashkenazic)	Infancy		Autonomic lability, absent fungiform papilla on tongue	Postural ↓ BP, ↑ tears, sweating	N- ± ↓	Ab
HSN IV (Landrieu et al.[285])	AD		None	Indifference to pain	Normal	N	N
HSN V (Low et al.[286]) (Dyck et al.[287])	U	2, 6	Small myelinated, unmyelinated	Insensitivity to pain	↓ Pain and temperature	N	N

* HSN, Hereditary sensory neuropathy.
Ab, Absent; AD, autosomal dominant; AR, autosomal recessive; BP, blood pressure; N, normal; U, unknown.
↑ = Increased; ↓ = decreased; ± = equivocal.

pound SNAPs are absent. Sural nerve biopsies confirm a considerable amount of small myelinated fiber loss.[280]

HSN III, the Riley-Day syndrome, has Ashkenazic inheritance and begins in neonates with autonomic dysfunction. These infants tend to feed poorly and have recurrent pulmonary infections, defective lacrimation, excessive perspiration, skin blotching, recurrent unexplained fevers, and labile blood pressure. On examination, they have sensory loss restricted to pain; areflexia, including absent corneal reflexes; and the characteristic loss of fungiform papillae on the tongue. Motor nerve CV is slightly reduced[281] or normal,[282] and compound SNAPs may be absent.

Axelrod and Pearson[283] studied 13 non-Ashkenazic children referred for evaluation of dysautonomia because of failure to thrive, hypotonia, episodic fevers, diminished overflow tears, and decreased pain perception. As in patients with HSN III, all lacked an axon flare after intradermal injection of histamine (1:10,000). No details of sensory NCS were reported.[283] Five children were classified as having HSN II. Three children had congenital autonomic dysfunction with pain loss. Two children were classified as having HSN IV with anhidrosis, two a progressive pan-sensory neuropathy with hypotonia,

and one a congenital sensory neuropathy with skeletal dysplasia.[283] Nordbord et al.[284] described three infants with incomplete sensory defects and dysautonomia. Each had absent compound SNAPs but normal motor NCS. Sural nerve biopsy demonstrated considerable loss of myelinated nerve fibers.

A dominantly inherited variant of congenital indifference to pain is found in patients with HSN IV with normal motor and sensory NCS. Normal morphometric evaluation of sural nerve myelinated and unmyelinated fibers has also been reported.[285]

Other congenital insensitivity neuropathies. A 6-year-old child with recurrent multiple distal ulcerations and Charcot joints had impaired pain and temperature sensation.[286] In contrast to other patients with HSN, motor and sensory NCS were normal. Sural nerve biopsy demonstrated small myelinated fiber loss. A similar child with congenital "indifference to pain," normal compound SNAPs, had decreased A-delta fibers, and moderate loss of C fibers and was classified as having HSN V.[287]

Most children with HSN have primary sensory involvement with cutaneous ulcerations and unrecognized painless fractures, features not seen in most patients with HMSN. Four Navajo children, however, had an autosomal recessive HMSN illness characterized by corneal ulceration, acromutilation, global sensory loss, and elevated levels of cerebrospinal fluid protein.[288] Another Navajo infant with HMSN had an associated leukoencephalomyelopathy, corneal ulceration, and liver disease.[289]

Fabry's disease. Angiokeratoma corporis diffusum is a hereditary X-linked sphingolipidosis secondary to a defect in ceramide hexaminidase. These patients present with lancinating lightning-like pains deep within the limbs that are exacerbated by use or cold weather. Sweating is decreased. Angiokeratomas are present over the abdomen, groin, and genitalia. Results of neurologic examination, motor and sensory NCS, and needle EMG are normal.[290,291] One study[292] found slow motor NCV, at times in only one or two nerves, in eight of 12 male patients with Fabry's disease.

Acquired Demyelinating Polyneuropathies

Acute inflammatory demyelinating polyneuropathy

The incidence of AIDP in children is similar to that of adults (1:100,000).[172] No age predominates in childhood for onset,[293] and AIDP may even occur in infants.[60-63]

Clinical characteristics. Seventy-five percent of children experience an antecedent infection in our experience at a mean of 12 days, with a range of 2 to 28 days.[293] Weakness is the primary complaint with variable distribution, and it may be diffuse—distal greater than proximal or proximal greater than distal.[293-297] Cranial nerve involvement, particularly the third, fourth, sixth, and seventh nerves, is common.[293] Rarely Fisher syndrome[298] occurs in childhood with acute ataxia and ophthalmoparesis.[293] Pain may be so predominant in childhood AIDP as to cause great diagnostic confusion.[293]

The differential diagnosis (Table 25.14) of AIDP includes botulism in infants.[70,71] Transverse myelitis or an intraspinal tumor, especially with muscle pain and stiffness, must be excluded because the reflexes may initially be preserved in AIDP. Myelography or MRI or both may be necessary to exclude a tumor, particularly in the child in whom careful sensory examination is not possible. Acute viral myositis may cause severe calf pain; consequently the child does not walk, which mimics early AIDP. These children, however, do not have symptoms in the upper extremities and the level of CK is usually elevated.

TABLE 25.14. Differential diagnosis of childhood acute inflammatory demyelinating polyneuropathy

Other acute neuropathies*
Tick paralysis
Infantile botulism
Transverse myelitis
Intraspinal tumor
Acute viral myositis
Poliomyelitis
Chinese motor neuronopathy or neuropathy similar to acute inflammatory demyelinating polyneuropathy

* See Table 25.11.

Today poliomyelitis is uncommon; however, with acute muscular pain and weakness, poliomyelitis or other rare neurotropic enteric viruses always need to be considered as the cause. We still see children without proper immunization who immigrated from third world countries and who have acute painful weakness and probably had acute poliomyelitis. In contrast to patients with AIDP, patients with poliomyelitis have asymmetric weakness.

In rural China, epidemics of an illness similar to AIDP occur annually among children, preceded by another illness in 47%.[299] This disease was characterized by a severe ascending weakness involving bulbar muscles (61%) and areflexia, but results of sensory examination were normal, with high levels of cerebrospinal fluid protein. MCVs and compound SNAPs were normal; CMAPs were greatly diminished. Needle EMG demonstrated denervation potentials. Most children had at least some recovery. The authors[299] suggested that the site of the lesion is either at the anterior horn cell or proximal motor nerve, although a lesion at the distal motor nerve terminal cannot be excluded.

At times, pain may be so prominent in childhood AIDP that it precludes reliable neurologic examination. The child may be so irritable that encephalopathy is mimicked. CT or MRI of the head is often necessary, and when results are normal, these studies are followed by a cerebrospinal fluid analysis that may demonstrate albuminocytologic dissociation and lead to evaluation for AIDP. CT is also obtained when a child presents with acute ataxia, necessitating exclusion of a tumor of the posterior fossa, before a diagnosis of AIDP can be made.

When these causes have been eliminated, rare toxic or metabolic processes require consideration. The most important, although rare, is acute tick paralysis.[300-302] Careful search of the child's scalp may disclose a fully engorged pregnant tick. A 3-year-old child seen at The Children's Hospital had clinical features mimicking AIDP. Improvement was dramatic shortly after the tick was removed. A 5-year-old child had NCS or EMG performed before, a few days after, and 6 months after removal of the tick.[303] The reduced CMAP amplitude increased dramatically after removal of the tick. No NMT defect could be detected. These studies and others[304] suggested that the toxin affects large motor or sensory nerves and the motor nerve terminals.

Acute or subacute toxic neuropathies of childhood that may mimic AIDP are described later in this chapter. These toxins include buckthorn wild cherry, insecticides, arsenic, lead, mercury, thallium, glue sniffing, and critical illness polyneuropathy.[305–317] When a history of gastrointestinal distress with polyneuropathy is present, poisoning with arsenic, lead, mercury or porphyria must be considered. AIDP has occurred in one human immunodeficiency virus (HIV)–infected child.[318]

Electrodiagnostic studies. The electrodiagnostic profile in AIDP has been outlined in Chapter 20. In most AIDP studies, children were not separated from adults in the data,[319] or studies were performed several years after the onset.[320] Earlier studies[294–297] were finished before the current clinical and neurophysiologic criteria for AIDP were used. With EMG as prognostic indicator and reports[321,322] suggesting that functional recovery may be better in children, our laboratory[293] studied whether EMG indicators of poor prognosis in adults are equally ominous in children.

We performed NCS or EMG in 23 children with a mean time of 20 days from onset of AIDP and, in most children, near the time of peak neurologic deficit. Using the electrodiagnostic criteria for a diffuse demyelinating neuropathy as defined by Albers and Kelly,[323] we found that 61% of our pediatric patients fulfilled these requirements.[293] The remaining 39% of the children, however, fulfilled criteria for demyelination in at least one nerve. Long latency wave abnormalities with absence or prolongation were noted in 81%; conduction block or temporal dispersion was present in one or more motor nerves in 74%.[293] MCV slowing consistent with demyelination in at least one nerve occurred in 70% and in two or more nerves in 48% of patients. Distal latency prolongation consistent with demyelination was noted in 57% of our pediatric patients with AIDP.[293] The most common motor NCS abnormality was

the CMAP amplitude reduction noted in 83% of children[293]; in 52%, the CMAP amplitude was less than or equal to 20% of the lower limit of normal in at least one nerve. More important, 22% of the children had a mean distal CMAP less than 20%.

Results of sensory NCS were abnormal in 70% of the children. In 52%, one or more compound SNAPs were absent, and an additional 26% had diminished compound SNAP amplitudes or prolonged distal latency.[293]

Fibrillation potentials were present in 27%; however, six of 22 children had EMG within 11 days of onset,[293] which may have skewed the results. Sequential studies that may have shown later evidence of axonal degeneration were not carried out.

The NCS results of younger children with AIDP were compared with those of older children with AIDP, and no difference was found.[293] Electrodiagnostic criteria associated with a poor outcome in adults with AIDP, either low mean CMAP[319] or fibrillation potentials,[324] were found in 39% of our pediatric patients. When follow-up clinical evaluation was obtained on this subgroup with so-called poor prognostic indicators, however, all of the children had recovered without disability.[293] It was our impression that electrodiagnostic indicators of poor prognosis identified in adults with AIDP[319,324] may not apply to children; however, more study is indicated.

Epstein and Sladky[325] retrospectively studied 23 children with AIDP to evaluate the value of plasmapheresis in nine children versus 14 similarly affected historical control subjects. Before treatment, AIDP was similar in both groups. The treated children recovered ambulation in half the time of the control subjects. Randomized multicenter trials are probably necessary with AIDP in childhood to determine whether plasmapheresis[326,327] is effective, particularly comparing it with intravenous serum gamma globulin[328,329] and possibly with a control group.[330]

Acute sensory neuropathy

Nass and Chutorian[331] described three children with a self-limited acute severe hyperpathic symmetric neuropathy somewhat relieved by cold compresses and associated with variable autonomic symptoms. Motor and reflex functions were normal. Results of sensory NCS were abnormal.[331] Severe proprioceptive sensory ataxia and areflexia developed in a 9-year-old child 5 days after being given antibiotics for a febrile illness.[332] The absence of compound SNAPs and H waves and blink reflexes were noted, and MCV and F waves were normal. Sural nerve biopsy demonstrated considerable myelinated fiber loss and moderate unmyelinated fiber loss. Recovery was complete in 3 years.

Chronic inflammatory demyelinating polyneuropathy

Dyck et al.[333] first characterized the clinical spectrum of CIDP. Their work led to the definition of this illness in childhood. Eleven percent of patients with CIDP initially had symptoms during the first decade of life.[333,334] Sladky et al.[335] reviewed six children with CIDP who became symptomatic between 0 and 3 years of age. Two neonates were hypotonic and were referred because they never walked; another child presented with weakness of the hand. Peripheral nerves were enlarged to palpation in four of the six children, and pes cavus was noted in three. The level of cerebrospinal fluid protein was normal[335]; however, in older children the level had elevated.[333,334]

No CMAP was elicited in the legs in four of the six children. MCVs in the arms were less than 10 to 20 m/second in four children and between 35 and 40 m/second in two children.[335] Other abnormalities included focal conduction block, dispersed CMAPs, and variable distal latency prolongation. Sural compound SNAPs were found in only two of the six children; both were prolonged, and the amplitudes were diminished.

Miller et al.[336] differentiated children with CIDP from patients with HMSN I and hereditary leukodystrophies and noted that patients with acquired CIDP demonstrated multifocal slowing, conduction block, and greatly dispersed CMAPs. In contrast, patients with primary hereditary neuropathies of idiopathic or specific metabolic type had uniform slowing, with no temporal dispersion or conduction block.

Two siblings with possible CIDP presenting at age 14 months had awkward gait and typical NCS and cerebrospinal fluid findings. Segmental demyelination with four or five infiltrates of lymphocytes were demonstrated on sural nerve biopsy.[337] The authors[337] suggested that the finding of mononuclear cell infiltrates compatible with CIDP differentiated these children from children with HMSN III. Another criterion for making this distinction might include pharmacologic remission.

A relapsing course was more common with earlier onset. Some children with CIDP are steroid responsive.[338] The time for response to steroids was relatively rapid, ranging between 4 and 14 days. Some children became steroid dependent, requiring plasmapheresis or azathioprine or both to lessen corticosteroid side effects.[335] Evaluations of NCS after treatment have shown an increase in CMAP amplitudes; however, no significant change occurred in MCVs. Previously undetectable compound SNAPs became recordable.[335]

Bird and Sladky[339] reported on three children with corticosteroid-responsive CIDP superimposed on a dominantly inherited familial neuropathy. These children, aged 4 to 14 years, each with pes cavus, had a family history compatible with HMSN I, HMSN II, and possibility Friedreich's ataxia. Each child had proximal weakness. One child, diagnosed with HMSN I 4 years earlier, presented with a history of 4 months of deteriorating gait. In two of the three children, NCS or EMG demonstrated multifocal demyelination compatible with CIDP. The third child with uniform MCV slowing was the only one with even a moderate cerebrospinal fluid protein elevation (82 mg/dL). The authors[339] suggested that some hereditary neuropathies have a genetic susceptibility to CIDP. Although each child's condition responded to administration of corticosteroids, with improved proximal strength, two children showed no distal improvement. Relapses followed the tapering of medication in two children.[339] Therefore clinicians caring for children with HMSN must be alert to the possibility that a superimposed and treatable CIDP may occur.

In children with CIDP whose conditions do not respond to corticosteroids or plasmapheresis, intravenous immunoglobulin may produce dramatic improvement.[340–343] Drugs, such as azathioprine, cyclophosphamide, or possibly even cyclosporine, may be considered.[172] Ouvrier et al.[172] discussed a 4-year-old with a 6-month history of CIDP unresponsive to prednisone therapy. Treatment with cyclophosphamide resulted in total remission and increased MCV.[172]

Glue sniffing is an unusual adolescent addiction that needs to be considered in the diagnosis of CIDP. Ouvrier et al.[172] reported on an adolescent who had sniffed glue and whose biopsy showed paranodal demyelination and large giant axons. The n-hexane component of glue is also in cements used in the shoe industry. Generalized weakness with areflexia, nausea, anorexia, and weight loss rapidly developed in four girls, aged 14 to 16 years.[344] Each worked in a poorly ventilated shoe factory and had direct contact with n-hexane leather cements. Peroneal MCVs were fine except for considerable prolongation of distal latency in one patient. Improvement began 2 months after exposure ceased. Three of the girls had complete recovery; one girl had residual distal weakness.[344]

Recurrent Childhood Neuropathies

The most common childhood recurrent neuropathy is CIDP. Other rare mechanisms need to be considered (Table 25.15).

Porphyria

Porphyria rarely begins in childhood. Ford[345] reported on a child with porphyria whose first episodes of recurrent abdominal pain occurred at age 8 years. Two years later, bilateral wristdrop and footdrop, intense muscle tenderness, and cutaneous hyperesthesia developed. During the next 20 years, she had a few more acute neurologic events, but NCS were not performed. Bolton (personal communication, 1992) performed NCS on a child with porphyria that demonstrated a pure axonal motor neuropathy. The results were similar to the report by Albers et al.[346] of NCS or EMG that showed neuropathy in eight patients with quadriparesis caused by acute porphyria.

Tangier disease

Two sisters, aged 12 and 14, had episodic weakness of the limbs and nonprogressive asymmetric sensory symptoms not anatomically related to the motor abnormalities.[347] The levels of plasma cholesterol were low, with nearly absent alpha-lipoproteins. In the one child studied, results of NCS were normal, and EMG showed denervation. Three of four other patients with Tangier disease had a remitting relapsing multifocal mononeuropathy.[348] Sural nerve biopsy demonstrated prominent demyelination and remyelination.

Refsum's disease

An autosomal recessive progressive hypertrophic demyelinating polyneuropathy, HMSN IV presents with recurrent symmetric episodic weakness associated with retinal pigmentary degeneration, cerebellar ataxia, sensorineural hearing loss, cardiomyopathy, and ichthyosis. Nerve conduction studies may demonstrate considerable slowing of motor and sensory fibers. Elevated levels of serum phytanic acid may distinguish Refsum's disease from CIDP or Friedreich's ataxia. We performed NCS on one 4-year-

TABLE 25.15.   Recurrent childhood neuropathies

Chronic inflammatory demyelinating polyneuropathy
Lead intoxification
Porphyria
Tangier disease
Hereditary motor sensory neuropathy IV—Refsum's disease*
Hereditary motor sensory neuropathy III—Dejerine-Sottas disease*

* Classically they are considered to have remitting relapsing course, but in children not much documentation exists.

old child with Refsum's disease who had no evidence of neuropathy. Results were normal. Similar findings were reported in one child, aged 12 years, with lifelong psychomotor retardation, visual and hearing loss, muscular hypotonia, and slight ataxia. At autopsy, peripheral nerves were normal.[349]

Hereditary motor sensory neuropathy III

Although HMSN III (Dejerine-Sottas disease) is considered to have a relapsing remitting course, a Mayo Clinic review[350] of 11 children failed to demonstrate any child with a remitting relapsing course. Each child became symptomatic within 0 to 2 years of life. Severe slowing of MCVs (less than 6 m/s in all but one child) was demonstrated on NCS. Distal latencies were up to three times longer than normal. The authors[350] emphasized that these slow conduction parameters might be mistaken for absent responses had slower than normal sweep speeds not been used. In contrast to most HMSNs, conduction block with greater than 50% reduction was present. The hypertrophied nerves had a high threshold for stimulation. These findings illustrate the need not to assume a lack of response without first giving maximal stimuli and using prolonged sweep speeds, as emphasized by Bolton et al,[351] when three of five such children had HMSN III, one a metachromatic leukodystrophy variant, and the last CIDP.

Neuropathies in Childhood Systemic Diseases

Diabetes mellitus

Children with diabetes are seldom referred to our EMG laboratory for evaluation of possible neuropathies. The predominant clinical findings in 15 children with diabetic neuropathies were symmetric polyneuropathy in 13 children; the other two children had isolated peroneal neuropathies.[352] Only one child had abnormal MCV. No comment was made about conduction blocks. Interestingly these children were thought to improve with the institution of insulin therapy. MCVs were also studied in 16 consecutive children less than age 16 years with diabetes; four children had slight slowing of peroneal MCV (36.9 to 41.2 m/s). Results of median and ulnar NCS were normal.[352]

Ulnar motor nerve CV changes were normal in 22 children with diabetes.[353] Results of NCS or EMG changes in children with diabetes were abnormal in 5% of 74 electromyographic studies.[354] Gamstorp et al.[355] evaluated 107 children less than age 17 years with insulin-dependent diabetes and demonstrated peripheral neuropathy in 11 children based on clinical and NCS or EMG results. Abnormalities were directly related to duration and control of the diabetes and age.[354,355]

Two adolescents had unusually severe sensory and autonomic diabetic neuropathy that improved with frequent insulin injection or a portable infusion pump.[356] The relationship between glucose control, duration of diabetes, age, and presence of retinopathy versus motor nerve CV was studied in 75 insulin-dependent patients with diabetes, aged 6 to 23 years.[357] A greater than 20% prevalance of delayed NC developed within 5 years after onset of diabetes. Diabetic retinopathy was not present in any patient.

A direct relationship between changes in NCS and autoimmune mechanisms as measured by levels of circulating immune complexes (CIC) in children with type I diabetes was suggested by greater nerve CV slowing in children with CIC.[358] Possibly CIC damaged the myelin sheath, with subsequent segmental demyelination.[358]

Uremia

We have seen only one child in 13 years with chronic renal failure and an axonal polyneuropathy. Evans[236] evaluated 61 children with uremia and found two children with polyneuropathy. Another study[359] included 11 children who required chronic hemodialysis, with normal to mild CV changes. More than half of 47 children in a dialysis transplantation program had NCS changes.[360] The peroneal nerves were most sensitive to modest changes in serum creatinine (1.5 to 2.5 mg/dL). Ulnar MCV did not become significantly decreased until the level of creatinine was greater than 9 mg/dL. After at least eight dialyses were performed, ulnar MCVs considerably increased, whereas peroneal MCVs did not. Transplantation began to affect MCVs 6 months after operation.[360] Ulnar nerve function returned earliest and was normal 3 years later. In contrast, peroneal MCVs continued to be abnormal in half of the children 3 years after transplantation.[360]

Acquired immunodeficiency syndrome or human immunodeficiency virus infection

A review[361] of the literature and a report[362] at a conference on acquired immunodeficiency syndrome (AIDS) on 19 HIV-infected children did not find evidence of neuropathy. Belman,[361] however, reported on two children with AIDS with lymphoid interstitial pneumonitis in whom peripheral neuropathies developed subsequent to the onset of encephalopathy. Some infants with AIDS become greatly distressed when their lower extremities are examined, which suggested the presence of neuropathic painful dysesthesias; however, no patient had NCS performed. A 6-year-old boy with congenital HIV infection was diagnosed with AIDP.[318]

Amyloidosis

Familial amyloid neuropathy may have its onset in patients at age 13 years.[172] Five asymptomatic adolescents with parental amyloid polyneuropathy in whom no EMG was performed had sural nerve biopsies.[363] Minor alterations affected Schwann cells or myelin sheaths in four of the five children. Only one child had severe thickening of the myelin sheath with moderate changes in the axoplasm.

Malignancies—toxic and paraneoplastic neuropathies

The primary association between childhood malignancies and neuropathies relates to toxicity of vincristine. Of 96 survivors of childhood malignancies treated with vincristine, 47 had areflexia and sensory CV prolongation.[364] In contrast, 49 children who did not receive vincristine had normal results on clinical examination and NCS.

We have seen one child who had received vincristine 7 years earlier and who had persistent neuropathy thought to be drug related. NCS, however, defined a demyelinating component compatible with HMSN I. Two adults with Hodgkin's disease and unsuspected HMSN I[365] had acute polyneuropathy after initial therapy with vincristine. A similar adult patient of ours emphasizes the importance of a careful examination for preexisting neuropathy and a family history for HMSN I before initiating vincristine therapy.

Cytosine arabinoside (Ara C) has produced an axonal sensory neuropathy manifested by involuntary movement of the legs and painful toes in an adolescent with leukemia.[366] Administration of carbamazepine produced dramatic improvement.

Paraneoplastic neuropathies are rare in children. An acute axonal polyneuropathy with bulbar involvement developed in 9 months in an adolescent with Hodgkin's disease who did not receive vincristine therapy.[367]

Critical illness polyneuropathy

This axonal neuropathy[368] has been reported in four severely asthmatic children who were taking corticosteroids and were intubated, some of whom were receiving pancuronium.[369] Severe tetraparesis developed in all four children. Low-amplitude CMAPs, normal NCV, and neuropathic needle EMG changes were demonstrated on NCS. Each child recovered within weeks to months. It is postulated that these patients had a pediatric form of critical illness polyneuropathy secondary to axonal transport dysfunction.[369]

Toxic Neuropathies of Childhood

Pancuronium

We have seen an adolescent with asthma who was taking prednisone and who required pancuronium for status asthmaticus. She was quadriplegic on discontinuation of the respirator and pancuronium. When she was examined on EMG, a primary motor neuropathy was found with considerable diminution of CMAPs, some of which were widely dispersed; however, MCVs, distal latencies, F waves, and compound SNAPs were normal. Definite fibrillation potentials were seen distally. Polyphasic MUPs were recorded and were of low amplitude, which suggested nascent reinnervation units. It is not clear whether this was a more generalized motor neuropathy as reported when acutely ill patients with asthma received steroids,[140] direct affects after discontinuation of pancuronium,[370] or another example of critical illness polyneuropathy.[368]

Buckthorn wild cherry

A 5-year-old Mexican girl had difficulty walking that progressed to complete quadriplegia in a few weeks. Ingestion of buckthorn wild cherry had occurred earlier. The level of cerebrospinal fluid protein was normal, and NCS or EMG was not performed. Sural

nerve biopsy demonstrated segmental demyelination.[305] Buckthorn is a poisonous "fruit" found on shrubs in northern Mexico and in southwestern United States.

Insecticides—delayed organophosphate poisoning

A rare polyneuropathy may occur acutely in patients who are exposed to agricultural insecticides. A 13-year-old boy and an adult had a rapidly progressive polyneuropathy mimicking AIDP.[306] The boy had myoclonic jerks at onset. He had a 3-month exposure to cyclodiene insecticides. Both patients had cerebrospinal fluid albuminocytologic dissociation. The boy did not have NCS performed; however, results were normal in the adult farmer.[306]

Arsenic

Arsenic poisoning may mimic AIDP or CIDP.[307] A 17-year-old girl who had depression took arsenious oxide powder, resulting in a progressive motor sensory painful neuropathy.[308] Peroneal MCV was 36 m/second, and sural compound SNAPs were absent.

Lead

Lead neuropathy is rare in childhood, especially in comparison to pica encephalopathy. A 3-year-old with 2 years of pica experienced two episodes of nausea, vomiting, thigh pain, and recurrent subacute motor neuropathy.[309] Although the child was anemic, levels of lead in blood and urine were normal, urinary delta levels of coproporphyrins were positive, and aminolevulinic acid was 9.5 times normal. EMG demonstrated denervation, but NCS were not performed. Treatment with calcium disodium edetate caused a 1000-fold increase in excretion of lead. The child was normal in 6 months. Lead-induced neuropathies in eight other children produced variable acute motor greater than sensory neuropathy and were associated with history of pica, and anemia with usually basophilic stippling of erythrocytes.[309] It was speculated that slow absorption accounted for the child's normal levels of lead in the blood and urine.

Mercury

Mercury rarely causes a peripheral neuropathy in children.[310] Two siblings with exposure to mercury vapor had generalized weakness, ataxic gait, areflexia, and abdominal pain. NCS demonstrated normal to minimally reduced MCV, some reduction in CMAPs, and normal compound SNAPs. Neuropathies (motor greater than sensory) developed in two children treated with ammoniated mercury ointments for dermatologic conditions.[311,312] One child had an elevated level of cerebrospinal fluid protein[312]; however, neither child had NCS or electromyographic studies performed. A 4-year-old child had acrodynia secondary to exposure to fumes in a home recently painted with a latex paint containing an organic mercury preservative.[313]

Thallium

Acute ingestion of thallium may mimic arsenic poisoning, with gastrointestinal distress, neuropathy, and even Mees' lines.[310] It is uncommon in children. An adolescent ingested thallium as a suicidal agent.[314] Motor NCS could not be elicited in the legs or distal arms. The proximal median nerve CV was 20 m/second.

Glue sniffing

Glue sniffing with addiction to n-hexane may occur in adolescents and may result in demyelination[172] with slow nerve CV[315] and neurofilamentous axonal masses on sural nerve biopsy.

Miscellaneous Childhood Neuropathies

Peripheral neuropathy after vaccination

A peripheral neuropathy is an occasional complication of rubella immunization. Distinctive reactions developed in 36 prepubertal children 6 weeks after vaccination that were described as an arm or leg syndrome.[372] In the former, children abruptly awakened with dysesthesias of the hands that lasted 0.5 to 30 minutes and recurred through the night. The leg syndrome was noted first on awakening and was characterized by posterior leg pain resulting in a characteristic gait with the child walking on the toes with the digits flexed. Slow distal sensory conduction was demonstrated on NCS in 11 of the 13 children, with mild median nerve MCV slowing in two children.[371] One year later, these values were normal.[372] Of 39 patients with neurologic complications from smallpox vaccination, five had a symmetric polyneuritis and two a brachial plexitis.[373] Only one of the 39 was a child, aged 2 years, with a foot-slapping gait that stopped within 1 week; NCS or EMG was not performed.[373]

Giant axonal neuropathies

Berg et al.[374] described an unusual chronic polyneuropathy in a 6-year-old child with a history of clumsy gait. She had kinky hair, distal greater than proximal muscle weakness, and areflexia. Sural nerve biopsy demonstrated abnormally large argentophilic masses of tightly woven neurofilaments. A summary[172] of 21 patients noted that motor milestones were delayed, and gait became clumsy consistent with polyneuropathy or spinocerebellar degeneration. Nystagmus and dementia eventually developed. Giant axonal neuropathy may present as the floppy infant syndrome.[60] Findings on NCS[375] in eight children with giant axonal neuropathy included absent compound SNAPs in five, low-amplitude compound SNAPs in two, and varied motor NCS with axonal or demyelinating features or both. Abnormal visual, auditory, and somatosensory potentials are found.[376] Cerebellar and cerebral white matter changes were revealed on MRI.[377] At autopsy, evidence of olivocerebellar, cerebellar peduncle, corticospinal, and posterior column dysfunction is present.[378]

Lowe's oculocerebral renal syndrome

Oculocerebral renal syndrome is an X-linked disorder with hypotonia, mental retardation, cataracts, and renal Fanconi's syndrome. Peripheral nerve studies in 14 boys with oculocerebral renal syndrome revealed decreased CMAP amplitudes in most and decreased compound SNAPs in seven of the 13 boys.[379] MCV and F waves were normal. Only one of nine children had denervation on EMG.

Rett syndrome

Rett syndrome, an unusual but important cause of mental retardation and autism in previously healthy young girls in whom simultaneous regression in language and motor skills develops, is associated with the presence of stereotypic hand movements, bruxism, seizures, and hyperventilation. Hypotonia often appears early. Results of EMG or NCS have not been reported. Nerve biopsies demonstrated mild nonspecific axonal neuropathy in seven of 12 children.[380]

Mitochondrial myopathy with peripheral neuropathy

Peripheral neuropathy is a rare manifestation of mitochondrial myopathy,[112] but an analysis of 20 patients identified 10 with NCS or EMG evidence of peripheral neuropathy.[113] Four were children, and most had a myopathy on EMG. All 10 had mild peroneal MCV slowing and low-amplitude compound SNAPs. Nerve biopsy demonstrated decreased myelinated fiber density with axonal degeneration.

Mitochondria contained paracrystalline inclusions within the Schwann cell cytoplasm in two of four biopsy specimens.

NEUROMUSCULAR TRANSMISSION DISORDERS IN CHILDHOOD

Pediatric neuromuscular junction illnesses are found in a bimodal age distribution. Neonates or infants represent a unique spectrum discussed under Electromyographic Evaluation of the Floppy Infant.

In the older child, the spectrum of neuromuscular junction illness is similar to that of adults. Postsynaptic defects are much more frequent than presynaptic defects. The techniques of NCS and EMG for NMT defect studies are similar to those used on adults. One expection is that single-fiber EMG is technically difficult, especially in younger children. The availability of ACh receptor and the voltage-gated calcium channel binding antibody tests provide further means for diagnosis when a child does not tolerate electrodiagnostic studies or the studies are not diagnostic.

Technical Aspects of Investigation

It is important to gain the child's and parent's confidence before starting repetitive stimulation. Careful interaction is facilitated by having them watch the storage oscilloscope or the recording tapes. Cooperation may provide the crucial difference in achieving technically satisfactory results. Not all children who have NMT defects are sent to the EMG laboratory with that clinical question. Some children may appear to have a primary myopathic appearance clinically. By EMG, they may have normal results on NCS but may need NMT defect testing even when bulbar dysfunction is not present.[381]

Presynaptic Defects

Lambert-Eaton myasthenia gravis

Three children with LEMS presented with proximal myopathic-like weakness.[383,384] A decremental NMT defect with repetitive NCS was present at rest, but after brief exercise or high-frequency repetitive stimulation, each child had classic LEMS facilitation. A 10-year-old child with a 1-month history of progressive weakness, ptosis, extraocular muscle weakness, bone pain, cachexia, and pancytopenia was found to have leukemia.[385] Repetitive NMT defect

testing demonstrated atypical LEMS, with gradual increase in CMAP to 170% of baseline values.

Postsynaptic Defects

Myasthenia gravis

Childhood myasthenia gravis produces predominant ocular and bulbar symptoms[386] that may become more generalized. Results of NCS or NMT defect tests depend on the degree of clinical involvement. The first set of repetitive stimuli is performed on the ulnar or median nerve. When good results are not achieved, a more proximal nerve is used. With a cooperative child, facial nerve stimulation may have the highest yield. High stimulus intensity is usually not required to obtain maximal response. When it is not possible to use the facial nerve, stimulation of the spinal accessory nerve is the best option. Our laboratory uses the same protocol as in adults, but repetitive stimuli are begun at 0.5 to 1 c/s for a few sets to gain the child's confidence, and then the stimulus is set at 2 c/s. Maximal rate (20 to 50 c/s) repetitive stimulation is not necessary except in the youngest child in whom cooperation for 30 seconds of exercise is not possible. Most children older than age 4 years cooperate. If not, as in younger children, premedication may be necessary to permit evaluation for signs of posttetanic potentiation or postexercise exhaustion by using 20 to 50 c/s stimulation. When a postsynaptic defect is defined, intravenously administered edrophonium is indicated to attempt to correct the NMT defect.

Any child who is taking pyridostigmine bromide (Mestinon, ICN Pharmaceuticals, Inc., Costa Mesa, CA) or similar drugs should have these medications discontinued 6 to 12 hours before starting the study. Extremities must be kept warm not only in the winter, but also when air conditioning is operating. Ideally a temperature of 36°C should be achieved to obtain the best chance of defining a defect in NMT.

The presenting complaint of 32 children with myasthenia gravis was bilateral ptosis or ocular muscle weakness or both in 63%[386] Generalized myasthenia developed in less than 1 year in one-third of patients with ocular muscle weakness. The rest (37%) presented with generalized myasthenia. No comments were made about EMG values in initial diagnosis.[386] In 50% of patients with ocular myasthenia and 58% of patients with generalized myasthenia gravis, tests for AChRab were positive. Pyridostigmine was the initial therapy, and depending on its effectiveness, corticosteroids were the next choice.

Lack of response to corticosteroids led to thymectomy. The role of thymectomy may be more important based on a survey[387] of 149 patients with juvenile myasthenia with a median follow-up period of 17 years. A much higher remission rate occurred among children treated with thymectomy. The factors positively correlating with postoperative remission included early operation, the presence of associated autoimmune disorders, onset of symptoms between ages 12 and 16 years, and predominant lower bulbar involvement. This large Mayo Clinic study[387] included 24 of 149 patients treated with prednisone which was initially helpful in six of 20 children who later underwent thymectomy. No child had serious side effects of corticosteroid therapy.[387]

Acute organophosphate poisoning

Acute organophosphate poisoning with inhibition of neuromuscular junction AChE rarely occurs in children. It is characterized by an acute, rapidly progressive muscle weakness with gastrointestinal distress. Ptosis, lid twitches, hypotonia, and areflexia with facilitation also occur.[388] The diagnosis may be unsuspected until NCS provide the important clues of low CMAPs, particularly in the peroneal and tibial nerves,[388] and repetitive CMAPs (Figure 25.9), with a variable decrement to repetitive stimulation, more prominent at rapid rates.[388,389] Administration of edrophonium greatly worsens the decrement.[388] Low serum cholinesterase values confirm the diagnosis.[388,389] Intravenously administered pralidoxine and atropine promote rapid improvement.[388] The finding of repetitive CMAPs after discharges after a single shock to a motor nerve has been reported in some congenital myasthenic syndromes.[89] Auger et al.[390] also noted repetitive CMAP after discharges in three children, aged 4 to 17 years, who had generalized myokymia and muscle stiffness. These CMAPs had a multiple repetitive component (Figure 25.10). The differential diagnosis of repetitive CMAPs also includes trauma to the peripheral nerve, ALS, and hypocalcemic tetany.[390]

MYOPATHIES

In the evaluation of a child with proximal weakness, referring physicians and parents often ask the value of performing NCS and EMG, especially when a biopsy is contemplated, and what the purpose is of subjecting the child to an uncomfortable test that will not necessarily result in a specific definitive diagnosis. Today with newer genetic techniques, these questions have even more relevance. We believe EMG is still an important parameter in making a diagnosis on children presenting with weakness, hypotonia, myalgias, and myotonia[391] (Specht L. personal communication, 1991.). Initially at The Boston Children's Hospital, each child has a clinical examination and test for levels of CK. All children with a

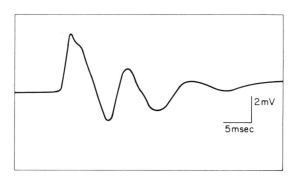

FIGURE 25.9.   *Single repetitive compound muscle action potential in patient with acute organophosphate poisoning. (Reprinted with permission from Maselli R, Jacobsen JH, Spire J-P. Edrophonium: An aid in the diagnosis of acute organophosphate poisoning. Ann Neurol 1986; 19:508.)*

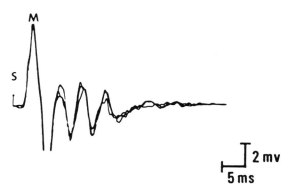

FIGURE 25.10.   *cMAP(M) with multiple repetitive potentials in 14-year-old adolescent with generalized myokymia and muscle stiffness. (Reprinted with permission from Auger RG, Daube JR, Gomez MR, Lambert EH. Hereditary form of sustained muscle activity of peripheral nerve origin causing generalized myokymia and muscle stiffness. Ann Neurol 1984; 15:15.)*

possible myopathy are scheduled for EMG with one exception. Boys with suspected Duchenne's or Becker's dystrophy and greatly elevated CK levels undergo DNA or dystrophin testing or both. When results are positive, no NCS or electromyographic study is indicated. When results are negative, however, NCS and electromyographic evaluation for myopathy is pursued to define the peripheral motor unit site of involvement. Although most children with proximal weakness have myopathies, occasionally motor neuron, peripheral nerve, or neuromuscular junction disorders have similar presentation and need to be excluded by NCS or EMG before muscle biopsy is considered. Demyelinating neuropathies, such as CIDP or unusual NMT defects without bulbar symptoms as may rarely be seen in adolescent LEMS[383-385] or possibly juvenile myasthenia gravis, can be identified on NCS. Needle EMG identifies Kugelberg-Welander disease (SMA III).

Earlier in this chapter, various myopathies that present as floppy infant syndrome have been delineated.

Muscular Dystrophies

Duchenne's and Becker's muscular dystrophies

X-linked dystrophin deficient dystrophies are the most common of the childhood myopathies and are discussed in Chapter 24. A few myopathies are elaborated on here.

Emery-Dreifuss muscular dystrophy

Emery-Dreifuss muscular dystrophy (EDMD), an X-linked syndrome, is a relatively benign myopathy with humeroperoneal distribution associated with contractures of the neck, elbows, and ankles.[392] Rarely EDMD appears in girls of consanguineous parents.[393] Recognition of EDMD is important because of the associated cardiomyopathy and potential conduction block. A summary[393] of 42 patients with X-linked EDMD noted that CK values were elevated three to four times,[394] although rarely they were normal.[393] Myopathic MUPs were demonstrated on EMG.[393,394] Cardiologic assessment is important to exclude atrial ventricular blocks that predispose the patient to sudden death.[394]

Rigid spine syndrome

The rigid spine syndrome (RSS) is a pediatric muscular disorder related to a dystrophy with a benign course. It may be a variant of EDMD because it is characterized by widespread contractures, particularly involving the spine.[395,396] A study[396] of four patients with RSS who were related to 14 other patients suggested that RSS is not a single nosologic entity and is not always X-linked because one child was a girl. Symptoms begin in children between 0.5 and 6 years old, with contractures of spine extensors, scoliosis, and shoulder girdle weakness, with cardiopathy in some children and modest CK elevations. EMG revealed myopathy that was confirmed on muscle biopsy. Although RSS may be relatively benign, progressively severe scoliosis has led to death from right heart failure in patients, aged 13 and 21 years.[396] A 14-year-old boy with RSS died of respiratory arrest. At autopsy, his diaphragm had prominent myopathic changes.[397] A cardiac conduction block may occur.[398]

Another childhood autosomal dominant myopathy associated with lethal cardiac conduction defects is pyloric stenosis.[399] Other pediatric neuromuscular disorders with significant cardiac problems include the Kearn-Sayre syndrome, myotonic dystrophy, Friedreich's ataxia, and multicore myopathy.[400]

Mitochondrial Myopathies

Mitochondrial myopathies encompass a heterogeneous group of inborn errors of mitochondrial metabolism.[112] Some occur in floppy infants, such as the cytochrome oxidase deficiencies.[114] Later these children present with combinations of progressive external ophthalmoplegia; extremity weakness; and sometimes in combination with various central nervous system disorders, including seizures, particularly myoclonic forms; ataxia; movement disorders; deafness; or dementia. Three major subgroups have been defined, including Kearn-Sayre syndrome, the myoclonus epilepsy with ragged red fibers syndrome (MERRF), and the mitochondrial myopathy, encephalopathy, lactic acidosis, and stroke-like episodes syndrome (MELAS).[112,401] A nonspecific but useful biochemical abnormality is systemic lactic acidosis. Occasionally the lactic acid is normal or only slightly increased at rest; however, an exercise stress test may induce a disproportionate increase in venous lactic acid levels. Myopathic MUPs are demonstrated on EMG. Muscle biopsy reveals the characteristic ragged red fibers. No specific treatment exists; however, when severe lactic acidosis is precipitated by various combinations of exercise, infection, or alcohol, the acidosis may be corrected with administration of a sodium bicarbonate solution.[401]

Inflammatory Myopathies

Dermatomyositis or polymyositis

Dermatomyositis or polymyositis occurs in children of all ages. The clinical features and results of EMG are similar to those seen in adults.[402] Gradual onset of proximal weakness was noted in 51 of 60 children; however, an acute onset with myalgia and fever was noted in nine children.[403] Classic dermatologic findings were reported in 73%[403] and 88%[404] of children.

Some interesting variants of inflammatory myopathies include the rare infantile forms. One congenital type with diminished fetal movements may present at birth as a floppy infant.[105] Levels of CK ranged from one to 20 times normal. Myopathic changes were shown on EMG.[405] An acquired infantile variety of inflammatory myopathy has been described.[104] Occasionally the infantile variety has persisted into adolescence. Trials of intravenously administered immune serum globulin have been beneficial.[405]

Other childhood inflammatory myopathies have been associated with Kawasaki disease[406] and acne fulminans.[407] Rarely focal polymyositis has been reported in a child.[408]

In childhood dermatomyositis, laboratory evaluation of CK and serum glutamic-oxaloacetic transaminase (SGOT) (aspartate aminotransaminase levels (AST)) demonstrated increased CK and SGOT in 56%.[403] The value of obtaining both enzymes is illustrated by the finding that at least one enzyme was elevated in 80%[403] to 82%[409] of patients when both enzymes were studied. The ESR is much less helpful in diagnosis, with values greater than 20 mm/hour in only 35% of patients.[403] When levels of CK and SGOT and the ESR are normal or minimally elevated, further diagnostic evaluation, including EMG or muscle biopsy or both, is still warranted in a child with a convincing clinical picture of inflammatory myopathy.

Results of motor NCS are normal except for low-amplitude CMAPs in a few children (four of 22).[409] Results of needle EMG are abnormal in a high percentage of children with inflammatory myopathies.[409] Insertional activity was abnormal in 81% of children, including fibrillation potentials in 76%, positive sharp waves in 50%, and CRDs in 12%. All children had short-duration low-amplitude and rapidly recruited MUPs with an increased percentage in proximal muscles.[409] Changes on EMG may be focal, particularly in childhood inflammatory my-

opathy in which perifascicular atrophy may be the only abnormality. The most peripheral muscle fibers in the distal field of the vascular supply of the muscle fiber may be the only affected area.[410] In subtle instances, the most superficial muscle fibers need careful attention during EMG. Identification of an abnormal area helps to select the best site for biopsy.

Corticosteroid therapy is the treatment of choice.[104,105,402,403] In patients whose condition is refractory to corticosteroids, combined therapy with various immunosuppressive agents, such as methotrexate, intravenously administered immune serum gamma globulin,[407] or cyclophosphamide, may be successful.[411]

A natural history study[404] of 26 children, aged 2 to 11 years, in 1953 demonstrated a 38% mortality rate, with eight deaths occurring 4 to 26 months after onset. A larger series[403] of 60 children in 1982 revealed an 18% mortality rate. Another 25% had an incomplete recovery with serious residual handicaps.[403]

Inclusion body polymyositis

Proximal muscle weakness developed in a 9-year-old child that gradually progressed to severe weakness by age 19 years. Values for CK were greater than 3000 IU.[412] Myopathic changes were demonstrated on EMG. An initial diagnosis of limb-girdle muscular dystrophy was made. His course continually deteriorated, and at age 41 years, he was diagnosed as having inclusion body myositis by electron microscopy. This disease needs to be considered in the differential diagnosis of both limb-girdle dystrophy and steroid-resistant polymyositis.

Benign acute childhood myositis

Children with benign acute childhood myositis have severe transient pain, mainly affecting muscles of the calf that may prevent walking. Calf muscles are tender and mildly swollen. Weakness is mild and confined to the gastrocnemius and soleus muscles. Commonly clinical symptoms occur within 1 or 2 days of an acute upper respiratory infection[413] or acute gastrointestinal illness[414] or in an epidemic form associated with influenza-B infection.[415] The level of CK was elevated in 42 of 50 children[414] (range, 5[413] to greater than 100 times normal[414]). The level of CK returned to normal within 2 weeks, and patchy areas of myopathic units were shown on EMG.[414] Patients improved rapidly within 1 week without definitive therapy.[415]

Primary suppurative myositis (tropical pyomyositis, spontaneous bacterial myositis)

This spontaneous bacterial infection of skeletal muscles is a rare illness in North America but is an endemic problem in tropical South America, Africa, Indochina, and Malaya.[416] Occasionally children with primary suppurative myositis are seen in North America. Some have immigrated from endemic areas,[417] but other children have not been outside the United States.[418] Prolonged morbidity or mortality may result when the correct diagnosis is not made. These illnesses are unrelated to open trauma or to direct extension from infected adjacent areas, such as osteomyelitis. *Staphylococcus aureus* is the causal organism; however, results of blood cultures are positive in less than 5% of patients.[416] Onset is rapid. A painful, palpably large upper thigh or trunk muscle that may initially suggest presence of a hematoma, arthritis, osteomyelitis, or rarely an appendiceal abscess is noted. Six boys, aged 1.5 to 10 years, from Texas were hospitalized because of fever and localized pain.[416] Four boys had previous blunt trauma to the affected area; three injuries involved the psoas muscle. The course was usually benign after antibiotic therapy; however, one child with a 1-week history of fever, low back pain, and paralumbar mass died of an abscess perforation of the psoas muscle into the dural sac, with resultant staphylococcal meningitis. No electromyographic results were reported.[416]

Monomelic Hypertrophy and Myopathy

Two children had congenital unilateral hypertrophy noticeable at birth that led to progressive footdrop in adolescence.[419,420] One child had percussion and electrical myotonia that was lacking in the other child; however, CRDs and fibrillation potentials were identified. Both children had myopathic MUPs.[419,420]

Myoglobinuria or Rhabdomyolysis

Myoglobinuria is an uncommon childhood condition that necessitates electromyographic referral. Various enzymatic and inflammatory myopathies have been identified in adults. Recurrent myoglobinuria was evaluated in 33 children between ages 0.6 and 9 years.[421] Infection was the common precipitating factor. Other factors included fasting, prolonged exercise, exposure to cold, and emotional stress. Clinical findings included weakness (rarely including bulbar signs), hyporeflexia, and muscle tenderness. Levels of CK were strikingly elevated (20,000 to 40,000 IU/L). Results of electromyographic studies performed on six of 33 children were normal in five and suggested a myopathy in one. Results of NCS were normal. In three of 33 children a lipid storage myopathy was documented. In the remaining 30 children no mechanism was identified despite detailed biochemical investigations and muscle biopsy. Renal failure occurred in four children. Ventilatory support was necessary in three children. Six children had cardiac arrhythmias, diminished cardiac output, and cardiac enlargement. Death occurred in 15% of children with a recurrent episode. The remaining patients demonstrated clinical recovery in 1 to 6 weeks.[421]

Neonatal rhabdomyolysis was the presenting feature of X-linked recessive muscular dystrophy.[422] A newborn was found by palpation to have stiff indurated enlarged arm and leg muscles with a CK level of 156,000 IU/L but no myoglobinuria.[423] The induration and elevated CK were felt to be indicative of rhabdomyolysis. Results of EMG were normal when the newborn was 13 days old. Needle muscle biopsy at age 1 year demonstrated nonspecific endomysial and perimysial connective tissue changes. Partial X chromosome deletion compatible with Duchenne's or Becker's dystrophy was demonstrated on DNA analysis.[422]

Lipid storage disease—carnitine palmityl transferase deficiency

Carnitine palmityl transferase deficiency was found in three of 33 children[421] with recurrent myoglobinuria. No other mechanism for myoglobinuria including any glycogen storage disease was found in the other 30 children.

Glycogen storage disease

These metabolic errors are defined in Chapter 24. Neonatal forms of GSD are outlined under Electromyographic Evaluation of the Floppy Infant. A few childhood forms, however, deserve further comment.

McArdle's disease, myophosphorylase deficiency (glycogenosis V). This disease commonly presents in adolescents with exercise-induced muscle soreness and stiffness, cramps, and myoglobinuria. Unusual pediatric variants include the fatal infantile form[106,107] and a 4-year-old child whose condition mimicked a congenital myopathy.[423] This child had difficulty sucking and swallowing at birth, delayed motor milestones, easy fatigability, waddling gait, and proximal weakness. Serum CK level was eight to 14 times normal. Low-amplitude, short-duration MUPs were demonstrated on EMG. Myophosphorylase was absent on biopsy.

Acid maltase deficiency, Pompe's disease (glycogenosis II). This disease is known for its phenotypic heterogeneity, beginning with the fatal floppy infant form.[109,111] Two brothers presented at ages 11 and 12 years with myopathy and waddling gait.[424] Level of CK was moderately elevated, and results of EMG were normal. Acid maltase activity was diminished in both brothers, their mother, and grandparents.

Phosphoglycerate kinase deficiency. Early recognition and treatment of myoglobinuria are important to prevent the potentially devastating consequences of recurrent events. In addition to carnitine palmityl transferase deficiency[421] as a cause of myoglobinuria, a mentally retarded child had recurrent myoglobinuria secondary to phosphoglycerate kinase deficiency.[425]

Malignant hyperthermia

Malignant hyperthermia (MH) occurs precipitously during anesthesia with the common inhalation agents, including halothane and succinylcholine chloride. It may occur in one of 15,000 children.[426] After induction, a rapidly fulminating picture develops with jaw rigidity, arrhythmia, generalized rigidity, shivering, and an extremely high fever. MH may be an isolated autosomal dominant trait or associated with various myopathies, including Duchenne's dystrophy.[427,428] It is important to anticipate MH because when unrecognized, MH is associated with a 70% mortality rate from cardiac arrhythmia or hyperthermia. Immediate treatment with dantrolene sodium is indicated at the earliest suggestion of MH.

In the event that future surgery is needed, pretreatment with dantrolene sodium[429] should be considered, whereas use of volatile agents, such as halothane, and depolarizing relaxants, such as succinylcholine, should be avoided.

A euthermic variety of MH has occurred during muscle biopsy in a boy with clinical features of Duchenne's muscular dystrophy[427] who received anesthesia with halothane. After extubation, tachycardia, ventricular fibrillation, and respiratory arrest associated with a serum potassium level of 7.9 mEq/L developed. Standard resuscitative measures were not successful; however, when dantrolene sodium was given, the arrhythmia and vital signs stabilized. A subsequent study[428] demonstrated that patients with X-linked dystrophies may have positive results on halothane tests and caffeine contracture tests for MH.

Occasionally children with idiopathic elevation of CK levels undergo EMG to look for evidence of occult myopathy. Although we do not often find abnormal results on EMG in these children, the neurologist needs to warn them and their parents that they are potentially at risk for MH. A study[430] of 30 patients with idiopathic persistently elevated CK levels noted a 36% incidence of susceptibility to MH. These children may need to wear a medical alert bracelet.[429]

Toxic Myopathies

Other than corticosteroid-induced myopathy, drug-induced myopathies are uncommon in children. Myopathies developed in two children in renal failure who were taking labetalol. Levels of CK were 10,000 to 27,000 IU/L.[431] EMG showed myopathy in both children, and muscle biopsy demonstrated rhabdomyolysis. Both children had excellent recovery when labetalol was discontinued.[431]

REFERENCES

1. Miller RG, Kuntz NL. Nerve conduction studies in infants and children. J Child Neurol 1986; 1:19–26.
2. Jablecki CK. Electromyography in infants and children. J Child Neurol 1986; 1:297–318.
3. Jones HR Jr, Miller RG, Turk MA, Wilbourn AJ. The pediatric EMG examination: General considerations. AAEE Course A: Panel Discussion 1987:39–46.
4. Gamble HJ, Breathnach AS. An electron-microscope study of human foetal peripheral nerves. J Anat 1965; 99:573–584.
5. Carpenter FG, Bergland RM. Excitation and conduction in immature nerve fibers of the developing chick. Am J Physiol 1957; 190:371–376.
6. Thomas JE, Lambert EH. Ulnar nerve conduction velocity and H-reflex in infants and children. J Appl Physiol 1960; 15:1–9.
7. Cottrell L. Histologic variations with age in apparently normal peripheral nerve trunks. Arch Neurol 1940; 43:1138–1150.
8. Gutrecht JA, Dyck PJ. Quantitative teased-fiber and histologic studies of human sural nerve during postnatal development. J Comp Neurol 1970; 138:117–130.
9. Dubowitz V, Whittaker GF, Brown BH, Robinson A. Nerve conduction velocity: An index of neuro-

logical maturity of the newborn infant. Dev Med Child Neurol 1968; 10:741–749.

10. Cruz Martinez A, Ferrer MT, Martin MJ. Motor conduction velocity and H-reflex in prematures with very short gestational age. Electromyogr Clin Neurophysiol 1983; 23:13–19.

11. Wagner AL, Buchthal F. Motor and sensory conduction in infancy and childhood: Reappraisal. Dev Med Child Neurol 1972; 14:189–216.

12. Gamstorp I. Normal conduction velocity of ulnar, median and peroneal nerves in infancy, childhood and adolescence. Acta Paediatr Scand (Stockh) 1963; 146(suppl):68–76.

13. Baer RD, Johnson EW. Motor nerve conduction velocities in normal children. Arch Phys Med Rehabil 1965; 46:698–704.

14. Gamstorp I, Shelburne SA Jr. Peripheral sensory conduction in ulnar and median nerves of normal infants, children, and adolescents. Acta Paediatr Scand 1965; 54:309–313.

15. Robinson RO, Robertson WC Jr. Fetal nutrition and peripheral nerve conduction velocity. Neurology 1981; 31:327–329.

16. Doberczak TM, Kandall SR, Rongkapan O, et al. Peripheral nerve conduction studies in passively addicted neonates. Arch Phys Med Rehabil 1986; 67:4–6.

17. Shahani BT, Young RR. Clinical significance of late response studies in infants and children (abstr). Neurology 1981; 31:66.

18. Cornblath DR. Disorders of neuromuscular transmission in infants and children. Muscle Nerve 1986; 9:606–611.

19. Koenigsberger MR, Patten B, Lovelace RE. Studies of neuromuscular function in the newborn: 1. A comparison of myoneural function in the full term and the premature infant. Neuropädiatrie 1973; 4:350–361.

20. Jones HR Jr. EMG evaluation of the floppy infant: Differential diagnosis and technical aspects. Muscle Nerve 1990; 13:338–347.

21. Sacco G, Buchthal F, Rosenfalck P. Motor unit potentials at different ages. Arch Neurol 1962; 6:366–373.

22. do Carmo RJ. Motor unit action potential parameters in human newborn infants. Arch Neurol 1960; 3:136–140.

23. David WS, Kupsky WJ, Jones HR Jr. Electromyographic and histologic evaluation of the arthrogrypotic infant (abstr). Muscle Nerve 1991; 14:897.

24. David WS, Jones HR Jr. Electromyographic evaluation of the floppy infant (abstr). Muscle Nerve 1990; 13:857.

25. Packer RJ, Brown MJ, Berman PH. The diagnostic value of electromyography in infantile hypotonia. Am J Dis Child 1982; 136:1057–1059.

26. Byers RK, Banker BQ. Infantile muscular atrophy. Arch Neurol 1961; 5:140–164.

27. Munsat TL, Woods R, Fowler W, Pearson CM. Neurogenic muscular atrophy of infancy with prolonged survival: The variable course of Werdnig-Hoffmann disease. Brain 1969; 92:9–24.

28. Dubowitz V. Infantile muscular atrophy: A prospective study with particular reference to a slowly progressive variety. Brain 1964; 87:707–718.

29. Melki J, Sheth P, Abdelhak S, et al, and the French Spinal Muscular Atrophy Investigators. Mapping of acute (type I) spinal muscular atrophy to chromosome 5q12-q14. Lancet 1990; 2:271–273.

30. Munsat TL, Skerry L, Korf B, et al. Phenotypic heterogeneity of spinal muscular atrophy mapping to chromosome 5q11.2-13.3 (SMA 5q). Neurology 1990; 40:1831–1836.

31. Schapira D, Swash M. Neonatal spinal muscular atrophy presenting as respiratory distress: A clinical variant. Muscle Nerve 1985; 8:661–663.

32. Goutières F, Bogicevic D, Aicardi J. A predominantly cervical form of spinal muscular atrophy. J Neurol Neurosurg Psychiatry 1991; 54:223–225.

33. Moosa A, Dubowitz V. Motor nerve conduction velocity in spinal muscular atrophy of childhood. Arch Dis Child 1976; 51:974–977.

34. Ryniewicz B. Motor and sensory conduction velocity in spinal muscular atrophy: Follow-up study. Electromyogr Clin Neurophysiol 1977; 17:385–391.

35. Kuntz NL, Daube JR. Electrophysiologic profile of childhood spinal muscular atrophy (abstr). Muscle Nerve 1982; 5:S106.

36. Buchthal F, Olsen PZ. Electromyography and muscle biopsy in infantile spinal muscular atrophy. Brain 1970; 93:15–30.

37. Hausmanowa-Petrusewicz I, Karwanska A. Electromyographic findings in different forms of infantile and juvenile proximal spinal muscular atrophy. Muscle Nerve 1986; 9:37–46.

38. Larsen R, Ashwal S. Peckham N. Incontinentia pigmenti: Association with anterior horn cell degeneration. Neurology 1987; 37:446–450.

39. Dubowitz V. The floppy infant. Clinics in developmental medicine, ed 2. London: W Heinemann Medical Books Ltd, 1980:89–94.

40. Anderson RM, Dennett X, Hopkins IJ, Shield LK. Hypertrophic interstitial polyneuropathy in infancy: Clinical and pathologic features in two cases. J Pediatr 1973; 82:619–624.

41. Karch SB, Urich H. Infantile polyneuropathy with defective myelination: An autopsy study. Dev Med Child Neurol 1975; 17:504–511.

42. Kasman M, Bernstein L, Schulman S. Chronic polyradiculoneuropathy of infancy. Neurology 1976; 26:565–573.

43. Kennedy WR, Sung JH, Berry JF. Case of congenital hypomyelination neuropathy. Arch Neurol 1977; 34:337–345.

44. Guzzetta F, Ferrière G, Lyon G. Congenital hypomyelination polyneuropathy: Pathological findings

compared with polyneuropathies starting later in life. Brain 1982; 105:395–416.

45. Seitz RJ, Wechsler W, Mosny DS, Lenard HG. Hypomyelination neuropathy in a female newborn presenting as arthrogryposis multiplex congenita. Neuropediatrics 1986; 17:132–136.

46. Gabreëls-Festen AAWM, Joosten EMG, Gabreëls FJM, et al. Congenital demyelinating motor and sensory neuropathy with focally folded myelin sheaths. Brain 1990; 113:1629–1643.

47. Ouvrier RA, McLeod JG, Conchin TE. The hypertrophic forms of hereditary motor and sensory neuropathy: A study of hypertrophic Charcot-Marie-Tooth disease (HMSN type I) and Dejerine-Sottas disease (HMSN type III) in childhood. Brain 1987; 110:121–148.

48. Gutmann L, Fakadej A, Riggs JE. Evolution of nerve conduction abnormalities in children with dominant hypertrophic neuropathy of the Charcot-Marie-Tooth type. Muscle Nerve 1983; 6:515–519.

49. Vanasse M, Dubowitz V. Dominantly inherited peroneal muscular atrophy (hereditary motor and sensory neuropathy type I) in infancy and childhood. Muscle Nerve 1981; 4:26–30.

50. Baker RS, Upton ARM. Variation of phenotype in Charcot-Marie-Tooth disease. Neuropädiatrie 1979; 10:290–295.

51. Guzzetta F, Ferrière G. Congenital neuropathy with prevailing axonal changes: A clinical and histological report. Acta Neuropathol (Berl) 1985; 68:185–190.

52. Gabreëls-Festen AAWM, Joosten EMG, Gabreëls FJM, et al. Hereditary motor and sensory neuropathy of neuronal type with onset in early childhood. Brain 1991; 114:1855–1870.

53. Hahn AF, Parkes AW, Bolton CF, Stewart SA. Neuromyotonia in hereditary motor neuropathy. J Neurol Neurosurg Psychiatry 1991; 54:230–235.

54. Lance JW, Burke D, Pollard J. Hyperexcitability of motor and sensory neurons in neuromyotonia. Ann Neurol 1979; 5:523–532.

55. Nordborg C, Conradi N, Sourander P, Westerberg B. A new type of non-progressive sensory neuropathy in children with atypical dysautonomia. Acta Neuropathol 1981; 55:135–141.

56. Steiman GS, Rorke LB, Brown MJ. Infantile neuronal degeneration masquerading as Werdnig-Hoffmann disease. Ann Neurol 1980; 8:317–324.

57. Seitz RJ, Langes K, Frenzel H, et al. Congenital Leigh's disease: Panencephalomyelopathy and peripheral neuropathy. Acta Neuropathol (Berl) 1984; 64:167–171.

58. Goebel HH, Bardosi A, Friede RL, et al. Sural nerve biopsy studies in Leigh's subacute necrotizing encephalomyelopathy. Muscle Nerve 1986; 9:165–173.

59. Jacobs JM, Harding BN, Lake BD, et al. Peripheral neuropathy in Leigh's disease. Brain 1990; 113:447–462.

60. Kinney RB, Gottfried MR, Hodson AK, et al. Congenital giant axonal neuropathy. Arch Pathol Lab Med 1985; 109:639–641.

61. Gilmartin RC, Ch'ien LT. Guillain-Barré syndrome with hydrocephalus in early infancy. Arch Neurol 1977; 34:567–569.

62. Carroll JE, Jedziniak M, Guggenheim MA. Guillain-Barré syndrome: Another cause of the "floppy infant." Am J Dis Child 1977; 131:699–700.

63. Al-Qudah AA, Shahar E, Logan WJ, Murphy EG. Neonatal Guillain-Barré syndrome. Pediatr Neurol 1988; 4:255–256.

64. Chambers R, MacDermot V. Polyneuritis as a cause of "amyotonia congenita." Lancet 1957; 1:397–401.

65. Pasternak JF, Fulling K, Nelson J, Prensky AL. An infant with chronic, relapsing polyneuropathy responsive to steroids. Dev Med Child Neurol 1982; 24:504–524.

66. Verity MA, Gao Y-H. Dysmaturation neuromyopathy: Correlation with minimal neuropathy in sural nerve biopsies. J Child Neurol 1988; 3:276–291.

67. Lieberman JS, Oshtory M, Taylor RG, Dreyfus PM. Perinatal neuropathy as an early manifestation of Krabbe's disease. Arch Neurol 1980; 37:446–447.

68. Gumbinas M, Larsen M, Liu HM. Peripheral neuropathy in classic Niemann-Pick disease: Ultrastructure of nerves and skeletal muscles. Neurology 1975; 25:107–113.

69. Marks HG, Spencer D, Sweet BA, Argoff CE. Peripheral nervous system involvement in new variant of Niemann-Pick disease type C (abstr). Ann Neurol 1990; 28:435.

70. Pickett J, Berg B, Chaplin E, Brunstetter-Shafer M-A. Syndrome of botulism in infancy: Clinical and electrophysiologic study. N Engl J Med 1976; 295:770–772.

71. Clay SA, Ramseyer JC, Fishman LS, Sedgwick RP. Acute infantile motor unit disorder: Infantile botulism? Arch Neurol 1977; 34:236–249.

72. Hoffman RE, Pincomb BJ, Skeels MR. Type F infant botulism. Am J Dis Child 1982; 136:270–271.

73. Schwartz RH, Eng G. Infant botulism: Exacerbation by aminoglycosides (letter). Am J Dis Child 1982; 136:952.

74. Thompson JA, Glasgow LA, Warpinski JR, Olson C. Infant botulism: Clinical spectrum and epidemiology. Pediatrics 1980; 66:936–942.

75. Shukla AY, Marsh W, Green JB, Hurst D. Neonatal botulism (abstr). Neurology 1991; 41(suppl 1):202.

76. Donley DK, Knight P, Tenorio G, Oh SJ. A patient with infant botulism, improving with edrophonium (abstr). Muscle Nerve 1991; 41:201.

77. Cornblath DR, Sladky JT, Sumner AJ. Clinical electrophysiology of infantile botulism. Muscle Nerve 1983; 6:448–452.

78. Fakadej AV, Gutmann L. Prolongation of post-tetanic facilitation in infant botulism. Muscle Nerve 1982; 5:727–729.

79. Lipsitz PJ. The clinical and biochemical effects of excess magnesium in the newborn. Pediatrics 1971; 47:501–509.

80. Sokal MM, Koenigsberger MR, Rose JS, et al. Neonatal hypermagnesemia and the meconium-plug syndrome. N Engl J Med 1972; 286:823–825.

81. Albers JW, Faulkner JA, Dorovini-Zis K, et al. Abnormal neuromuscular transmission in an infantile myasthenic syndrome. Ann Neurol 1984; 16:28–34.

82. Bady B, Chauplannaz G, Carrier H. Congenital Lambert-Eaton myasthenic syndrome. J. Neurol Neurosurg Psychiatry 1987; 50:476–478.

83. Fenichel GM. Clinical syndromes of myasthenia in infancy and childhood. Arch Neurol 1978; 35:97–103.

84. Lefvert AK, Osterman PO. Newborn infants to myasthenic mothers: A clinical study and an investigation of acetylcholine receptor antibodies in 17 children. Neurology 1983; 33:133–138.

85. Morel E, Eymard B, Vernet-der Garabedian B, et al. Neonatal myasthenia gravis: A new clinical and immunologic appraisal on 30 cases. Neurology 1988; 38:138–142.

86. Branch CE Jr, Swift TR, Dyken PR. Prolonged neonatal myasthenia gravis: Electrophysiological studies. Ann Neurol 1978; 3:416–418.

87. Wise GA, McQuillen MP. Transient neonatal myasthenia: Clinical and electromyographic studies. Arch Neurol 1970; 22:556–565.

88. Seybold ME, Lindstrom JM. Myasthenia gravis in infancy. Neurology 1981; 31:476–480.

89. Engel AG. Myasthenia gravis and myasthenic syndromes. Ann Neurol 1984; 16:519–534.

90. Engel AG. Congenital myasthenic syndromes. J Child Neurol 1988; 3:233–246.

91. Smit LME, Jennekens FGI, Veldman H, Barth PG. Paucity of secondary synaptic clefts in a case of congenital myasthenia with multiple contractures: Ultrastructural morphology of a developmental disorder. J Neurol Neurosurg Psychiatry 1984; 47:1091–1097.

92. Vincent A, Cull-Candy SG, Newsom-Davis J, et al. Congenital myasthenia: End-plate acetylcholine receptors and electrophysiology in five cases. Muscle Nerve 1981; 4:306–318.

93. Conomy JP, Levinsohn M, Fanaroff A. Familial infantile myasthenia gravis: A cause of sudden death in young children. J Pediatr 1975; 87:428–430.

94. Robertson WC Jr, Chun RWM, Kornguth SE. Familial infantile myasthenia. Arch Neurol 1980; 37:117–119.

95. Gieron MA, Korthals JK. Familial infantile myasthenia gravis: Report of three cases with follow-up until adult life. Arch Neurol 1985; 42:143–144.

96. Mora M, Lambert EH, Engel AG. Synaptic vesicle abnormality in familial infantile myasthenia. Neurology 1987; 37:206–214.

97. Lazaro RP, Fenichel GM, Kilroy AW. Congenital muscular dystrophy: Case reports and reappraisal. Muscle Nerve 1979; 2:349–355.

98. Swift TR, Ignacio OJ, Dyken PR. Neonatal dystrophia myotonica: Electrophysiologic studies. Am J Dis Child 1975; 129:734–737.

99. Kuntz NL, Daube JR. Electrophysiology of congenital myotonic dystrophy. AAEE Course E, 1984:23.

100. Torres CF, Griggs RC, Goetz JP. Severe neonatal centronuclear myopathy with autosomal dominant inheritance. Arch Neurol 1985; 42:1011–1014.

101. Munsat TL, Thompson LR, Coleman RF. Centronuclear ("myotubular") myopathy. Arch Neurol 1969; 20:120–131.

102. Norton P, Ellison P, Sulaiman AR, Harb J. Nemaline myopathy in the neonate. Neurology 1983; 33:351–356.

103. Kimura J. Myopathies. In: Electrodiagnosis in diseases of nerve and muscle: Principles and practice. Philadelphia: FA Davis, 1983:527–548.

104. Thompson CE. Infantile myositis. Dev Med Child Neurol 1982; 24:307–313.

105. Shevell M, Rosenblatt B, Silver K, et al. Congenital inflammatory myopathy. Neurology 1990; 40:1111–1114.

106. DiMauro S, Hartlage PL. Fatal infantile form of muscle phosphorylase deficiency. Neurology 1978; 28:1124–1129.

107. Milstein JM, Herron TM, Hass JE. Fatal infantile muscle phosphorylase deficiency. J Child Neurol 1989; 4:186–188.

108. Servidei S, Bonilla E, Diedrich RG, et al. Fatal infantile form of muscle phosphofructokinase deficiency. Neurology 1986; 36:1465–1470.

109. Finegold DN, Bergman I. High-protein feeding in an infant with Pompe's disease. Neurology 1988; 38:824–825.

110. Verity MA. Infantile Pompe's disease, lipid storage, and partial carnitine deficiency. Muscle Nerve 1991; 14:435–440.

111. Hogan GR, Gutmann L, Schmidt R, Gilbert E. Pompe's disease. Neurology 1969; 19:894–900.

112. DiMauro S, Bonilla E, Zeviani M, et al. Mitochondrial myopathies. Ann Neurol 1985; 17:521–538.

113. Yiannikas C, McLeod JG, Pollard JD, Baverstock J. Peripheral neuropathy associated with mitochondrial myopathy. Ann Neurol 1986; 20:249–257.

114. Heiman-Patterson TD, Bonilla E, DiMauro S, et al. Cytochrome-*c*-oxidase deficiency in a floppy infant. Neurology 1982; 32:898–900.

115. Brooke MH, Carroll JE, Ringel SP. Congenital hypotonia revisited. Muscle Nerve 1979; 2:84–100.

116. Banker BQ. Arthrogryposis multiplex congenita: Spectrum of pathologic changes. Hum Pathol 1986; 17:656–672.

117. Drachman DB, Banker BQ. Arthrogryposis multiplex congenita. Arch Neurol 1961: 5:77–93.

118. Drachman DB, Sokoloff L. The role of movement in

embryonic joint development. Dev Biol 1966; 14:401–420.

119. Holmes LB, Driscoll SG, Bradley WG. Contractures in a newborn infant of a mother with myasthenia gravis. J Pediatr 1980; 96:1067–1069.

120. Smit LME, Barth PG. Arthogryposis multiplex congenita due to congenital myasthenia. Dev Med Child Neurol 1980; 22:371–374.

121. Banker BQ. Neuropathologic aspects of arthogryposis multiplex congenita. Clin Orthop 1985; 194:30–43.

122. Smith EM, Bender LF, Stover CN. Lower motor neuron deficit in arthrogryposis: An EMG study. Arch Neurol 1963; 8:97–100.

123. Amick LD, Johnson WW, Smith HL. Electromyographic and histopathologic correlations in arthrogryposis. Arch Neurol 1967; 16:512–523.

124. Fisher RL, Johnstone WT, Fisher WH Jr, Goldkamp OG. Arthrogryposis multiplex congenita: A clinical investigation. J Pediatr 1970; 76:255–261.

125. Bharucha EP, Pandya SS, Dastur DK. Arthrogryposis muliplex congenita. Part 1: Clinical and electromyographic aspects. J Neurol Neurosurg Psychiatry 1972; 35:425–434.

126. Strehl E, Vanasse M, Brochu P. EMG and needle muscle biopsy studies in arthrogryposis multiplex congenita. Neuropediatrics 1985; 16:225–227.

127. Gomez MR, Clermont V, Bernstein J. Progressive bulbar paralysis in childhood (Fazio-Londe's disease): Report of a case with pathologic evidence of nuclear atrophy. Arch Neurol 1962; 6:317–323.

128. Alexander MP, Emery ES 3d, Koerner FC. Progressive bulbar paresis in childhood. Arch Neurol 1976; 33:66–68.

129. Benjamins D. Progressive bulbar palsy of childhood in siblings. Ann Neurol 1980; 8:203.

130. Albers JW, Zimnowodzki S, Lowrey CM, Miller B. Juvenile progressive bulbar palsy: Clinical and electrodiagnostic findings. Arch Neurol 1983; 40:351–353.

131. Kugelberg E, Welander L. Heredofamilial juvenile muscular atrophy simulating muscular dystrophy. Arch Neurol Psychiatry 1956; 75:500–509.

132. Hausmanowa-Petrusewicz I, Fidzianska A, Niebrój-Dobosz I, Strugalska MH. Is Kugelberg-Welander spinal muscular atrophy a fetal defect? Muscle Nerve 1980; 3:389–402.

133. Hirayama K, Tsubaki T, Toyokura Y, Okinaka S. Juvenile muscular atrophy of unilateral upper extremity. Neurology 1963; 13:373–380.

134. Sobue I, Saito N, Iida M, Ando K. Juvenile type of distal and segmental muscular atrophy of upper extremities. Ann Neurol 1978; 3:429–432.

135. Gouri-Devi M, Suresh TG, Shankar SK. Monomelic amyotrophy. Arch Neurol 1984; 41:388–394.

136. Adornato BT, Engel WK, Kucera J, Bertorini TE. Benign focal amyotrophy (abstr). Neurology 1978; 28:399.

137. Haas DC, Crosley CJ. Juvenile muscular atrophy of the hands and forearms (abstr). Ann Neurol 1982; 12:214.

138. Oryema J, Ashby P, Spiegel S. Monomelic atrophy. Can J Neurol Sci 1990; 17:124–130.

139. Behse F, Buchthal F, Carlsen F, Knappeis GG. Hereditary neuropathy with liability to pressure palsies: Electrophysiological and histopathological aspects. Brain 1972; 95:777–794.

140. Hopkins IJ. A new syndrome: Poliomyelitis-like illness associated with acute asthma in childhood. Aust Paediatr J 1974; 10:273–276.

141. Wheeler SD, Ochoa J. Poliomyelitis-like syndrome associated with asthma: A case report and review of the literature. Arch Neurol 1980; 37:52–53.

142. Nelson JS, Prensky AL. Sporadic juvenile amyotrophic lateral sclerosis: A clinicopathological study of a case with neuronal cytoplasmic inclusions containing RNA. Arch Neurol 1972; 27:300–306.

143. Grunnet ML, Donaldson JO. Juvenile multisystem degeneration with motor neuron involvement and eosinophilic intracytoplasmic inclusions. Arch Neurol 1985; 42:1114–1116.

144. Dantes M, McComas A. The extent and time course of motoneuron involvement in amyotrophic lateral sclerosis. Muscle Nerve 1991; 14:416–421.

145. Rowland LP, Schneck SA. Neuromuscular disorders associated with malignant neoplastic disease. J Chron Dis 1963; 16:777–795.

146. Johnson WG, Wigger HJ, Karp HR, et al. Juvenile spinal muscular atrophy: A new hexosaminidase deficiency phenotype. Ann Neurol 1982; 11:11–16.

147. Cashman NR, Antel JP, Hancock LW, et al. N-acetyl-β-hexosaminidase β locus defect and juvenile motor neuron disease: A case study. Ann Neurol 1986; 19:568–572.

148. Parnes S, Karpati G, Carpenter S, et al. Hexosaminidase-A deficiency presenting as atypical juvenile-onset spinal muscular atrophy. Arch Neurol 1985; 42:1176–1180.

149. Huttenlocher PR, Gilles FH. Infantile neuroaxonal dystrophy: Clinical, pathologic, and histochemical findings in a family with 3 affected siblings. Neurology 1967; 17:1174–1184.

150. Duncan C, Strub R, McGarry P, Duncan D. Peripheral nerve biopsy as an aid to diagnosis in infantile neuroaxonal dystrophy. Neurology 1970; 20:1024–1032.

151. Halperin JL, Landis DMD, Lott IT, Ment L. Neuroaxonal dystrophy and Down's syndrome: Report of a case. Arch Neurol 1982; 39:587–591.

152. Barlow JK, Sims KB, Kolodny EH. Early cerebellar degeneration in twins with infantile neuroaxonal dystrophy. Ann Neurol 1989; 25:413–415.

153. Grunnet ML, Leicher C, Zimmerman A, et al. Primary lateral sclerosis in a child. Neurology 1989; 39:1530–1532.

154. Lahat E, Rothman AS, Aron AM. Schwannoma pre-

senting as lumbar disc disease in an adolescent boy. Ann Neurol 1986; 20:643–644.

155. Flaggman PD, Kelly JJ Jr. Brachial plexus neuropathy: An electrophysiologic evaluation. Arch Neurol 1980; 37:160–164.

156. Eng GD, Koch B, Smokvina MD. Brachial plexus palsy in neonates and children. Arch Phys Med Rehabil 1978; 59:458–464.

157. Sever JW. Obstetric paralysis: Report of eleven hundred cases. JAMA 1925; 85:1862–1865.

158. Koenigsberger MR. Brachial plexus palsy at birth: Intrauterine or due to delivery trauma? (abstr). Ann Neurol 1980; 8:228.

159. Luco JV, Eyzaguirre C. Fibrillation and hypersensitivity to ACh in denervated muscle: Effect of length of degenerating nerve fibers. J Neurophysiol 1955; 18:65–73.

160. Ross D, Jones HR Jr, Fisher J, Konkol RJ. Isolated radial nerve lesion in the newborn. Neurology (NY) 1983; 33:1354–1356.

161. Johnson EW, Alexander MA, Koenig WC. Infantile Erb's palsy (Smellie's palsy). Arch Phys Med Rehabil 1977; 58:175–178.

162. Molnar GE. Brachial plexus injury in the newborn infant. Pediatr Rev 1984; 6:110–115.

163. Kwast O. Electrophysiological assessment of maturation of regenerating motor nerve fibres in infants with brachial plexus palsy. Dev Med Child Neurol 1989; 31:56–65.

164. Clay SA. Osteomyelitis as a cause of brachial plexus neuropathy. Am J Dis Child 1982; 136:1054–1056.

165. Dunn HG, Daube JR, Gomez MR. Heredofamilial brachial plexus neuropathy (hereditary neuralgic amyotrophy with brachial predilection) in childhood. Dev Med Child Neurol 1978; 20:28–46.

166. Parsonage MJ, Turner JWA. Neuralgic amyotrophy: The shoulder-girdle syndrome. Lancet 1948; 1:973–978.

167. Turner JWA, Parsonage MJ. Neuralgic amyotrophy (paralytic brachial neuritis), with special reference to prognosis. Lancet 1957; 2:209–212.

168. Tsairis P, Dyck PJ, Mulder DW. Natural history of brachial plexus neuropathy: Report on 99 patients. Arch Neurol 1972; 27:109–117.

169. Shaywitz BA. Brachial plexus neuropathy in childhood. J Pediatr 1975; 86:913–914.

170. Bale JF Jr, Thompson JA, Petajan JH, Ziter FA. Childhood brachial plexus neuropathy. J Pediatr 1979; 95:741–742.

171. Gilliatt RW, Willison RG, Dietz V, Williams IR. Peripheral nerve conduction in patients with a cervical rib and band. Ann Neurol 1978; 4:124–129.

172. Ouvrier RA, McLeod JG, Pollard JD. Peripheral neuropathy in childhood. New York: Raven Press, 1990.

173. Hope EE, Bodensteiner JB, Thong N. Neonatal lumbar plexus injury. Arch Neurol 1985; 42:94–95.

174. Eng GD. Neuromuscular disease. In: Avery GB, ed.

Neonatology: Pathophysiology and management of the newborn, ed 2. Philadelphia: JB Lippincott, 1981:989–992.

175. Volpe JJ. Injuries of extracranial, cranial, intracranial, spinal cord, and peripheral nervous system structures. In: Neurology of the Newborn, ed 2. Philadelphia: WB Saunders, 1987:631–658.

176. Awerbuch G, Levin JR, Dabrowski E, Nigro MA. Lumbrosacral plexus neuropathy of childhood (abstr). Ann Neurol 1989; 26:452.

177. Jones HR Jr. Mononeuropathies in childhood in the upper extremities: A review of 46 cases (1979–1990) (abstr). J Neurol Sci 1990; 98:S448.

178. Byler DL, Wessel HB. Traumatic peripheral neuropathy in childhood (abstr). Ann Neurol 1988; 24:331–332.

179. Jones HR Jr. Compressive neuropathy in childhood: A report of 14 cases. Muscle Nerve 1986; 9:720–723.

180. Starreveld E, Ashenhurst EM. Bilateral carpal tunnel syndrome in childhood: A report of two sisters with mucolipidosis III (pseudo-Hurler polydystrophy). Neurology 1975; 25:234–238.

181. Cruz Martinez A, Arpa J, Pérez Conde MC, Ferrer MT. Bilateral carpal tunnel in childhood associated with Schwartz-Jampel syndrome. Muscle Nerve 1984; 7:66–72.

182. McArthur RG, Hayles AB, Gomez MR, Bianco AJ Jr. Carpal tunnel syndrome and trigger finger in childhood. Am J Dis Child 1969; 117:463–469.

183. Stevens JC, Sun S, Beard CM, et al. Carpal tunnel syndrome in Rochester, Minnesota, 1961 to 1980. Neurology 1988; 38:134–138.

184. Danta G. Familial carpal tunnel syndrome with onset in childhood. J Neurol Neurosurg Psychiatry 1975; 38:350–355.

185. Alvarez N, Larkin C, Roxborough J. Carpal tunnel syndrome in athetoid-dystonic cerebral palsy. Arch Neurol 1982; 39:311–312.

186. Cavanagh NPC, Yates DAH, Sutcliffe J. Thenar hypoplasia with associated radiologic abnormalities. Muscle Nerve 1979; 2:431–436.

187. Barfred T, Ipsen T. Congenital carpal tunnel syndrome. J Hand Surg 1985; 10A:246–248.

188. Koenigsberger MR, Moessinger AC. Iatrogenic carpal tunnel syndrome in the newborn infant. J Pediatr 1977; 91:443–445.

189. Pape KE, Armstrong DL, Fitzhardinge PM. Peripheral median nerve damage secondary to brachial arterial blood gas sampling. J Pediatr 1978; 93:852–856.

190. Wolfe JS, Eyring EJ. Median-nerve entrapment within a greenstick fracture: A case report. J Bone Joint Surg 1974; 56A:1270–1272.

191. Bilge T, Yalaman O, Bilge S, et al. Entrapment neuropathy of the median nerve at the level of the ligament of Struthers. Neurosurgery 1990; 27:787–789.

192. Mittal RL, Gupta BR. Median and ulnar-nerve palsy: An unusual presentation of the supracondylar process: Report of a case. J Bone Joint Surg 1978; 60A:557–558.

193. Phillips LH 2d, Persing JA, Vandenberg SR. Electrophysiological findings in localized hypertrophic mononeuropathy. Muscle Nerve 1991; 14:335–341.

194. Cavanagh NPC, Pincott JR. Ulnar nerve tumours of the hand in childhood. J Neurol Neurosurg Psychiatry 1977; 40:795–800.

195. Lightwood R. Radial nerve palsy associated with localized subcutaneous fat necrosis in the newborn. Arch Dis Child 1951; 26:436–437.

196. Feldman GV. Radial nerve palsies in the newborn. Arch Dis Child 1957; 32:469–471.

197. Weeks PM. Radial, median, and ulnar nerve dysfunction associated with a congenital constricting band of the arm. Plast Reconstr Surg 1982; 69:333–336.

198. Töllner U, Bechinger D, Pohlandt F. Radial nerve palsy in a premature infant following long-term measurement of blood pressure. J Pediatr 1980; 96:921–922.

199. Meier C, Moll C. Hereditary neuropathy with liability to pressure palsies: Report of two families and review of the literature. J Neurol 1982; 228:73–95.

200. Manske PR. Compression of the radial nerve by the triceps muscle: A case report. J Bone Joint Surg 1977; 59A:835–836.

201. Ford FR. Diseases of the nervous system in infancy, childhood and adolescence, ed 5. Springfield, IL: Charles C Thomas, 1966:1113–1114.

202. Laulund T, Fedders O, Sogaard I, Kornum M. Suprascapular nerve compression syndrome. Surg Neurol 1984; 22:308–312.

203. Sriram K, Sakthivel A. Sciatic nerve palsy in the newborn. Ann Acad Med (Singapore) 1981; 10:472–475.

204. Combes MA, Clark WK, Gregory CF, James JA. Sciatic nerve injury in infants and prevention of impairment resulting from intragluteal injections. JAMA 1960; 173:1336–1339.

205. Curtiss PH Jr, Tucker HJ. Sciatic palsy in premature infants: A report and follow-up study of ten cases. JAMA 1960; 174:1586–1588.

206. Gilles FH, Matson DD. Sciatic nerve injury following misplaced gluteal injection. J Pediatr 1970; 76:247–254.

207. Hudson FP, McCandless A, O'Malley AG. Sciatic paralysis in newborn infants. Br Med J 1950; 1:223–225.

208. San Agustin M, Nitowski HM, Borden JN. Neonatal sciatic palsy after umbilical vessel injection. J Pediatr 1962; 60:408–413.

209. Purohit DM, Levkoff AH, deVito PC. Gluteal necrosis with foot-drop: Complications associated with umbilical artery catheterization. Am J Dis Child 1978; 132:897–899.

210. Jones HR Jr, Gianturco LE, Gross PT, Buchhalter J.

211. Sciatic neuropathies in childhood: A report of ten cases and review of the literature. J Child Neurol 1988; 3:193–199.

211. Deverell WF, Ferguson JH. An unusual case of sciatic nerve paralysis. JAMA 1968; 205:699–700.

212. Loffer FD, Pent D, Goodkin R. Sciatic nerve injury in a patient undergoing laparoscopy. J Reprod Med 1978; 21:371–372.

213. Romfh JH, Currier RD. Sciatic neuropathy induced by the lithotomy position (letter). Arch Neurol 1983; 40:127.

214. Telander RL. Technique and clinical results of ileoanal anastomosis without surgical reservoir: The Mayo Clinic experience. In: Dozois RR, ed. Alternatives to conventional ileostomy. Chicago: Year Book Medical Publishers, 1985:319–332.

215. Burkhart FL, Daly JW. Sciatic and peroneal nerve injury: A complication of vaginal operations. Obstet Gynecol 1966; 28:99–102.

216. Stillman MJ, Christensen W, Payne R, Foley KM. Leukemic relapse presenting as sciatic nerve involvement by chloroma (granulocytic sarcoma). Cancer 1988; 62:2047–2050.

217. Thomas JE, Piepgras DG, Scheithauer B, et al. Neurogenic tumors of the sciatic nerve: A clinicopathologic study of 35 cases. Mayo Clin Proc 1983; 58:640–647.

218. Lester PD, McAlister WH. Congenital iliac anomaly with sciatic palsy. Radiology 1970; 96:397–399.

219. Venna N, Bielawski M, Spatz EM. Sciatic nerve entrapment in a child: Case report. J Neurosurg 1991; 75:652–654.

220. Dorfman LJ, Ransom BR, Forno LS, Kelts A. Neuropathy in hypereosinophilic syndrome. Muscle Nerve 1983; 6:291–298.

221. Jones HR Jr, Felice KJ, Gross PT. Pediatric peroneal mononeuropathy: A clinical and electromyographic study. Muscle Nerve 1993; in press.

222. Berry H, Richardson PM. Common peroneal nerve palsy: A clinical and electrophysiological review. J Neuro Neurosurg Psychiatry 1976; 39:1162–1171.

223. Brown WF, Ferguson GG, Jones MW, Yates SK. The location of conduction abnormalities in human entrapment neuropathies. Can J Neurol Sci 1976; 3:111–122.

224. Levin KH, Wilbourn AJ, Jones HR Jr. Childhood peroneal neuropathy from bone tumors. Pediatr Neurol 1991; 7:308–309.

225. Bilge T, Kaya A, Alatli M, et al. Hemangioma of the peroneal nerve: Case report and review of the literature. Neurosurgery 1989; 25:649–652.

226. Stack RE, Bianco AJ Jr, MacCarty CS. Compression of the common peroneal nerve by ganglion cysts: Report of nine cases. J Bone Joint Surg 1965; 47A:773–778.

227. Cobb CA 3d, Moiel RH. Ganglion of the peroneal nerve: Report of two cases. J Neurosurg 1974; 41:255–259.

228. Nucci F, Artico M, Santoro A, et al. Intraneural

synovial cyst of the peroneal nerve: Report of two cases and review of the literature. Neurosurgery 1990; 26:339–344.

229. Wilbourn AJ, Levin KH, Sweeney PJ. Peroneal neuropathies in children and adolescents (abstr). Can J Neurol Sci 1990; 17:227.

230. Lawrence DG, Locke S. Neuropathy in children with diabetes mellitus. Br Med J 1963; 1:784–785.

231. Ritter FJ, Seay AR, Lahey ME. Peripheral mononeuropathy complicating anaphylactoid purpura. J Pediatr 1983; 103:77–78.

232. Crumrine PK, Koenigsberger MR, Chutorian AM. Footdrop in the neonate with neurologic and electrophysiologic data. J Pediatr 1975; 86:779–780.

233. Kreusser KL, Volpe JJ. Peroneal palsy produced by intravenous fluid infiltration in a newborn. Dev Med Child Neurol 1984; 26:522–523.

234. Fischer AQ, Strasburger J. Footdrop in the neonate secondary to use of footboards. J Pediatr 1982; 101:1003–1004.

235. Albrektsson B, Rydholm A, Rydholm U. The tarsal tunnel syndrome in children. J Bone Joint Surg 1982; 64B:215–217.

236. Evans OB. Pediatrics for the clinician: Polyneuropathy in childhood. Pediatrics 1979; 64:96–105.

237. Gamstorp I. Polyneuropathy in childhood. Acta Paediatr Scand 1968; 57:230–238.

238. Hagberg B, Lyon G. Pooled European series of hereditary peripheral neuropathies in infancy and childhood: A "correspondence work shop" report of the European Federation of Child Neurology Societies (EFCNS). Neuropediatrics 1981; 12:9–17.

239. Dunn HG, Lake BD, Dolman CL, Wilson J. The neuropathy of Krabbe's infantile cerebral sclerosis (globoid cell leucodystrophy). Brain 1969; 92:329–344.

240. Bischoff A, Ulrich J. Peripheral neuropathy in globoid cell leukodystrophy (Krabbe's disease): Ultrastructural and histochemical findings. Brain 1969; 92:861–870.

241. Yudell A, Gomez MR, Lambert EH, Dockerty MB. The neuropathy of sulfatide lipidosis (metachromatic leukodystrophy). Neurology 1967; 17:103–111.

242. Hagberg B. Polyneuropathies in pediatrics. Eur J Pediatr 1990; 149:296–305.

243. Scully RE, Mark EJ, McNeeley BU, eds. Case records of the Massachusetts General Hospital. Weekly clinicopathological exercises: Case 7-1984. N Engl J Med 1984; 310:445–455.

244. Bayever E, Ladisch S, Philippart M, et al. Bone-marrow transplantation for metachromatic leucodystrophy. Lancet 1985; 2:471–473.

245. Krivit W, Shapiro E, Kennedy W, et al. Treatment of late infantile metachromatic leukodystrophy by bone marrow transplantation. N Engl J Med 1990; 322:28–32.

246. Rosen NL, Lechtenberg R, Wisniewski K, et al. Adrenoleukomyeloneuropathy with onset in early childhood. Ann Neurol 1985; 17:311–312.

247. Moosa A, Dubowitz V. Peripheral neuropathy in Cockayne's syndrome. Arch Dis Child 1970; 45:674–677.

248. Grunnet ML, Zimmerman AW, Lewis RA. Ultrastructure and electrodiagnosis of peripheral neuropathy in Cockayne's syndrome. Neurology 1983; 33:1606–1609.

249. Argov Z, Soffer D, Eisenberg S, Zimmerman Y. Chronic demyelinating peripheral neuropathy in cerebrotendinous xanthomatosis. Ann Neurol 1986; 20:89–91.

250. Lockman LA, Kennedy WR, White JG. The Chédiak-Higashi syndrome: Electrophysiological and electron microscopic observations on the peripheral neuropathy. J Pediatr 1967; 70:942–951.

251. Steinman L, Tharp BR, Dorfman LJ, et al. Peripheral neuropathy in the cherry-red spot-myoclonus syndrome (sialidosis type I). Ann Neurol 1980; 7:450–456.

252. Richter A, Melancon SB, Roy M, et al. Further molecular genetic and genealogic studies on the Friedreich's ataxia gene in the Quebec population (abstr). Can J Neurol Sci 1989; 16:266.

253. Ülkü A, Araç A, Özeren A. Friedreich's ataxia: A clinical review of 20 childhood cases. Acta Neurol Scand 1988; 77:493–497.

254. Harding AE. Friedreich's ataxia: A clinical and genetic study of 90 families with an analysis of early diagnostic criteria and intrafamilial clustering of clinical features. Brain 1981; 104:589–620.

255. Salih MA, Ahlsten G, Stålberg E, et al. Friedreich's ataxia in 13 children: Presentation and evolution with electrophysiologic, electrocardiographic, and echocardiographic features. J Child Neurol 1990; 5:321–326.

256. Ouvrier RA, McLeod JG, Conchin TE. Friedreich's ataxia: Early detection and progression of peripheral nerve abnormalities. J Neurol Sci 1982; 55:137–145.

257. Santoro L, Perretti A, Crisci C, et al. Electrophysiological and histological follow-up study in 15 Friedreich's ataxia patients. Muscle Nerve 1990; 13:536–540.

258. Caruso G, Santoro L, Perretti A, et al. Friedreich's ataxia: Electrophysiologic and histologic findings in patients and relatives. Muscle Nerve 1987; 10:503–515.

259. Harding AE. Early onset cerebellar ataxia with retained tendon reflexes: A clinical and genetic study of a disorder distinct from Friedreich's ataxia. J Neurol Neurosurg Psychiatry 1981; 44:503–508.

260. Klockgether T, Petersen D, Grodd W, Dichgans J. Early onset cerebellar ataxia with retained tendon reflexes. Brain 1991; 114:1559–1573.

261. Spira PJ, McLeod JG, Evans WA. A spinocerebellar degeneration with X-linked inheritance. Brain 1979; 102:27–41.

262. Taylor MJ, Logan WJ. Multimodal electrophysiological assessment of ataxia telangiectasia. Can J Neurol Sci 1983; 10:261–265.

263. Kanda T, Oda M, Yonezawa M, et al. Peripheral neuropathy in xeroderma pigmentosum. Brain 1990; 113:1025–1044.

264. Bassen FA, Kornzweig AL. Malformation of the erythrocytes in a case of atypical retinitis pigmentosa. Blood 1950; 5:381–387.

265. Miller RG, Davis CJF, Illingworth DR, Bradley W. The neuropathy of abetalipoproteinemia. Neurology 1980; 30:1286–1291.

266. Wichman A, Buchthal F, Pezeshkpour GH, Gregg RE. Peripheral neuropathy in abetalipoproteinemia. Neurology 1985; 35:1279–1289.

267. Fagan ER, Taylor MJ. Longitudinal multimodal evoked potential studies in abetalipoproteinemia. Can J Neurol Sci 1987; 14:617–621.

268. Rosenblum JL, Keating JP, Prensky AL, Nelson JS. A progressive neurologic syndrome in children with chronic liver disease. N Engl J Med 1981; 304:503–508.

269. Elias E, Muller DPR, Scott J. Association of spinocerebellar disorders with cystic fibrosis or chronic childhood cholestasis and very low serum vitamin E. Lancet 1981; 2:1319–1321.

270. Larsen PD, Mock DM, O'Connor PS. Vitamin E deficiency associated with vision loss and bulbar weakness. Ann Neurol 1985; 18:725–727.

271. Sokol RJ, Guggenheim M, Iannaccone ST, et al. Improved neurologic function after long-term correction of vitamin E deficiency in children with chronic cholestasis. N Engl J Med 1985; 313:1580–1586.

272. Perlmutter DH, Gross P, Jones HR, et al. Intramuscular vitamin E repletion in children with chronic cholestasis. Am J Dis Child 1987; 141:170–174.

273. Gutmann L, Shockcor W, Gutmann L, Kien CL. Vitamin E-deficient spinocerebellar syndrome due to intestinal lymphangiectasia. Neurology 1986; 36:554–556.

274. Harding AE, Matthews S, Jones S, et al. Spinocerebellar degeneration associated with a selective defect of vitamin E absorption. N Engl J Med 1985; 313:32–35.

275. Peterson PL, Saad J, Nigro MA. The treatment of Friedreich's ataxia with amantadine hydrochloride. Neurology 1988; 38:1478–1480.

276. Dunn HG. Nerve conduction studies in children with Friedreich's ataxia and ataxia-telangiectasia. Dev Med Child Neurol 1973; 15:324–337.

277. Alexianu M, Christodorescu D, Vasilescu C, et al. Sensorimotor neuropathy in a patient with Marinesco-Sjögren syndrome. Eur Neurol 1983; 22:222–226.

278. Dyck PJ. Neuronal atrophy and degeneration predominantly affecting peripheral sensory and autonomic neurons. In: Dyck PJ, Thomas PK, Lambert EH, Bunge R, eds. Peripheral neuropathy. Philadelphia: WB Saunders, 1984:1557–1599.

279. Kuntz NL, Daube JR, Dyck PJ. Somatosensory evoked potentials in congenital sensory neuropathy (abstr). Muscle Nerve 1982; 5:560.

280. Ohta M, Ellefson RD, Lambert EH, Dyck PJ. Hereditary sensory neuropathy, type II: Clinical, electrophysiologic, histologic, and biochemical studies of a Quebec kinship. Arch Neurol 1973; 29:23–37.

281. Aguayo AJ, Nair CPV, Bray GM. Peripheral nerve abnormalities in the Riley-Day syndrome. Arch Neurol 1971; 24:106–116.

282. Brown JC, Johns RJ. Nerve conduction in familial dysautonomia (Riley-Day) syndrome. JAMA 1967; 201:200–203.

283. Axelrod FB, Pearson J. Congenital sensory neuropathies: Diagnostic distinction from familial dysautonomia. Am J Dis Child 1984; 138:947–954.

284. Nordbord C, Conradi N, Sourander P, Westerberg B. A new type of non-progressive sensory neuropathy in children with atypical dysautonomia. Acta Neuropathol 1981; 55:135–141.

285. Landrieu P, Said G, Allaire C. Dominantly transmitted congenital indifference to pain. Ann Neurol 1990; 27:574–578.

286. Low PA, Burke WJ, McLeod JG. Congenital sensory neuropathy with selective loss of small myelinated fibers. Ann Neurol 1978; 3:179–182.

287. Dyck PJ, Mellinger JF, Reagan TJ, et al. Not "indifference to pain" but varieties of hereditary sensory and autonomic neuropathy. Brain 1983; 106:373–390.

288. Appenzeller O, Kornfeld M, Snyder R. Acromutilating, paralyzing neuropathy with corneal ulceration in Navajo children. Arch Neurol 1976; 33:733–738.

289. Snyder RD, Singleton R, Helgerson SD, Johnsen SD. Navajo neuropathy with encephalomyelopathy: Clinical features (abstr). Ann Neurol 1989; 26:451.

290. Kocen RS, Thomas PK. Peripheral nerve involvement in Fabry's disease. Arch Neurol 1970; 22:81–88.

291. Ohnishi A, Dyck PJ. Loss of small peripheral sensory neurons in Fabry disease: Histologic and morphometric evaluation of cutaneous nerves, spinal ganglia, and posterior columns. Arch Neurol 1974; 31:120–127.

292. Sheth KJ, Swick HM. Peripheral nerve conduction in Fabry disease. Ann Neurol 1980; 7:319–323.

293. Bradshaw DY, Jones HR Jr. Guillain-Barré syndrome in children: Clinical course, electrodiagnosis, and prognosis. Muscle Nerve 1992; 15:500–506.

294. Banerji NK, Millar JHD. Guillian-Barré syndrome in children, with special reference to serial nerve conduction studies. Dev Med Child Neurol 1972; 14:56–63.

295. Low NL, Schneider J, Carter S. Polyneuritis in children. Pediatrics 1958; 22:972–990.

296. Paulson GW. The Landry-Guillain-Barré-Strohl syndrome in childhood. Dev Med Child Neurol 1970; 12:604–607.

297. Peterman AF, Daly DD, Dion FR, Keith HM. Infec-

tious neuronitis (Guillain-Barré syndrome) in children. Neurology 1959; 9:533–539.

298. Fisher M. Unusual variant of acute idiopathic polyneuritis (syndrome of ophthalmoplegia, ataxia and areflexia). N Engl J Med 1956; 255:57–65.

299. McKhann GM, Cornblath DR, Ho T, et al. Clinical and electrophysiological aspects of acute paralytic disease of children and young adults in northern China. Lancet 1991; 2:593–597.

300. Haller JS, Fabara JA. Tick paralysis: Case report with emphasis on neurological toxicity. Am J Dis Child 1972; 124:915–917.

301. Donat JR, Donat JF. Tick paralysis with persistent weakness and electromyographic abnormalities. Arch Neurol 1981; 38:59–61.

302. Kincaid JC. Tick bite paralysis. Semin Neurol 1990; 10:32–34.

303. Swift TR, Ignacio OJ. Tick paralysis: Electrophysiologic studies. Neurology 1975; 25:1130–1133.

304. Cherington M, Snyder RD. Tick paralysis: Neurophysiologic studies. N Engl J Med 1968; 278:95–97.

305. Calderon-Gonzalez R, Rizzi-Hernandez H. Buckthorn polyneuropathy. N Engl J Med 1967; 277:69–71.

306. Jenkins RB, Toole JF. Polyneuropathy following exposure to insecticides: Two cases of polyneuropathy with albuminocytologic dissociation in the spinal fluid following exposure to DDD and aldrin and DDT and endrin. Arch Intern Med 1964; 113:691–695.

307. Donofrio PD, Wilbourn AJ, Albers JW, et al. Acute arsenic intoxication presenting as Guillain-Barré–like syndrome. Muscle Nerve 1987; 10:114–120.

308. Le Quesne PM, McLeod JG. Peripheral neuropathy following a single exposure to arsenic: Clinical course in four patients with electrophysiological and histological studies. J Neurol Sci 1977; 32:437–451.

309. Seto DSY, Freeman JM. Lead neuropathy in childhood. Am J Dis Child 1964; 107:337–342.

310. Windebank AJ, McCall JT, Dyck PJ. Metal neuropathy. In: Dyck PJ, Thomas PK, Lambert EH, Bunge R, eds. Peripheral neuropathy, vol 2, ed 2. Philadelphia: WB Saunders, 1984:2133–2161.

311. Ross AT. Mercuric polyneuropathy with albuminocytologic dissociation and eosinophilia. JAMA 1964; 188:830–831.

312. Swaiman KF, Flagler DG. Mercury poisoning with central and peripheral nervous system involvement treated with penicillamine. J Pediatr 1971; 48:639–642.

313. Agocs MM, Etzel RA, Parrish RG, et al. Mercury exposure from interior latex paint. N Engl J Med 1990; 323:1096–1101.

314. Davis LE, Standefer JC, Kornfeld M, et al. Acute thallium poisoning: Toxicological and morphological studies of the nervous system. Ann Neurol 1981; 10:38–44.

315. Korobkin R, Asbury AK, Sumner AJ, Nielsen SL. Glue-sniffing neuropathy. Arch Neurol 1975; 32:158–162.

316. Bolton CF, Laverty DA, Brown JD, et al. Critically ill polyneuropathy: Electrophysiological studies and differentiation from Guillain-Barré syndrome. J Neurol Neurosurg Psychiatry 1986; 49:563–573.

317. Goulden KJ, Dooley JM, Peters S, Ronen GM. Critical illness polyneuropathy: A reversible cause of paralysis in asthmatic children (abstr). Ann Neurol 1989; 26:451.

318. Price L, Gominak S, Raphael SA, et al. Acute demyelinating polyneuropathy in childhood human immunodeficiency virus infection (abstr). Ann Neurol 1990; 28:459–460.

319. Cornblath DR, Mellits ED, Griffin JW, et al, and The Guillain-Barré Syndrome Study Group. Motor conduction studies in Guillain-Barré syndrome: Description and prognostic value. Ann Neurol 1988; 23:354–359.

320. Rossi LN, Mumenthaler M, Lütschg J, Ludin HP. Guillain-Barré syndrome in children with special reference to the natural history of 38 personal cases. Neuropädiatrie 1976; 7:45–51.

321. Briscoe DM, McMenamin JB, O'Donohoe NV. Prognosis in Guillain-Barré syndrome. Arch Dis Child 1987; 62:733–735.

322. Cole GF, Matthew DJ. Prognosis in severe Guillain-Barré syndrome. Arch Dis Child 1987; 62:288–291.

323. Albers JW, Kelly JJ Jr. Acquired inflammatory demyelinating polyneuropathies: Clinical and electrodiagnostic features. Muscle Nerve 1989; 12:435–451.

324. Eisen A, Humphreys P. The Guillain-Barré syndrome: A clinical and electrodiagnostic study of 25 cases. Arch Neurol 1974; 30:438–443.

325. Epstein MA, Sladky JT. The role of plasmapheresis in childhood Guillain-Barré syndrome. Ann Neurol 1990; 28:65–69.

326. Jones HR Jr, Bradshaw DY. Guillain-Barré syndrome and plasmapheresis in childhood (letter). Ann Neurol 1991; 29:688–689.

327. Storgion SA, Igarashi M, May WN, Stidham GL. Plasmapheresis for Guillain-Barré syndrome. Pediatr Neurol 1989; 5:389–390.

328. Shahar E, Murphy EG, Roifman CM. Beneficial effect of high-dose intravenous serum gamma globulin in severe Guillain-Barré syndrome (abstr). Ann Neurol 1989; 26:448.

329. Jackson AH, Donnelly JH. The efficacy of high-dose intravenous gammaglobulin in the treatment of Guillain-Barré syndrome in childhood (abstr). Ann Neurol 1990; 28:431.

330. Guillain-Barré Syndrome Study Group. Plasmapheresis and acute Guillain-Barré syndrome. Neurology 1985; 35:1096–1104.

331. Nass R, Chutorian A. Dysaesthesias and dysautonomia: A self-limited syndrome of painful dysaesthesias and autonomic dysfunction in childhood. J Neurol Neurosurg Psychiatry 1982; 45:162–165.

332. Fernandez JM, Davalos A, Ferrer I, et al. Acute sensory neuropathy with remarkable recovery (abstr). J Neurol Sci 1990; 98(suppl):272.

333. Dyck PJ, Lais AC, Ohta M, et al. Chronic inflammatory polyradiculoneuropathy. Mayo Clin Proc 1975; 50:621–637.

334. McCombe PA, Pollard JD, McLeod JG. Chronic inflammatory demyelinating polyradiculoneuropathy: A clinical and electrophysiological study of 92 cases. Brain 1987; 110:1617–1630.

335. Sladky JT, Brown MJ, Berman PH. Chronic inflammatory demyelinating polyneuropathy of infancy: A corticosteroid-responsive disorder. Ann Neurol 1986; 20:76–81.

336. Miller RG, Gutmann L, Lewis RA, Sumner AJ. Acquired versus familial demyelinative neuropathies in children. Muscle Nerve 1985; 8:205–210.

337. Gabreëls-Festen AAWM, Hageman ATM, Gabreëls FJM, et al. Chronic inflammatory demyelinating polyneuropathy in two siblings. J Neurol Neurosurg Psychiatry. 1986; 49:152–156.

338. Colan RV, Snead OC 3d, Oh SJ, Benton JW Jr. Steroid-responsive polyneuropathy with subacute onset in childhood. J Pediatr 1980; 97:374–377.

339. Bird SJ, Sladky JT. Corticosteroid-responsive dominantly inherited neuropathy in childhood. Neurology 1991; 41:437–439.

340. Vermeulen M, van der Meché FGA, Speelman JD, et al. Plasma and gamma-globulin infusion in chronic inflammatory polyneuropathy. J Neurol Sci 1985; 70:317–326.

341. Faed JM, Day B, Pollock M, et al. High-dose intravenous human immunoglobulin in chronic inflammatory demyelinating polyneuropathy. Neurology 1989; 39:422–425.

342. Cornblath DR, Chaudhry V, Griffin JW. Treatment of chronic inflammatory demyelinating polyneuropathy with intravenous immunoglobulin. Ann Neurol 1991; 30:104–106.

343. Vedanarayanan VV, Kandt RS, Lewis DV Jr, DeLong GR. Chronic inflammatory demyelinating polyradiculoneuropathy of childhood: Treatment with high-dose intravenous immunoglobulin. Neurology 1991; 41:828–830.

344. Rizzuto N, Terzian H, Galiazzo-Rizzuto S. Toxic polyneuropathies in Italy due to leather cement poisoning in shoe industries: A light- and electron-microscopic study. J Neurol Sci 1977; 31:343–354.

345. Ford FR. Diseases of the nervous system in infancy, childhood, and adolescence, ed 5. Springfield, IL: Charles C Thomas, 1966:765–767.

346. Albers JW, Robertson WC Jr, Daube JR. Electrodiagnostic findings in acute porphyric neuropathy. Muscle Nerve 1978; 1:292–296.

347. Engel WK, Dorman JD, Levy RI, Frederickson DS. Neuropathy in Tangier disease: α-lipoprotein deficiency manifesting as familial recurrent neuropathy and intestinal lipid storage. Arch Neurol 1967; 17:1–9.

348. Pollock M, Nukada H, Frith RW, et al. Peripheral neuropathy in Tangier disease. Brain 1983; 106:911–928.

349. Torvik A, Torp S, Kase BF, et al. Infantile Refsum's disease: A generalized peroxisomal disorder. Case report with postmortem examination. J Neurol Sci 1988; 85:39–53.

350. Benstead TJ, Kuntz NL, Miller RG, Daube JR. The electrophysiologic profile of Dejerine-Sottas disease (HMSN III). Muscle Nerve 1990; 13:586–592.

351. Bolton CF, Hahn AF, Hinton GG. The syndrome of high stimulation threshold and low conduction velocity (abstr). Ann Neurol 1988; 24:165.

352. Lawrence DG, Locke S. Neuropathy in children with diabetes mellitus. Br Med J 1963; 1:784–785.

353. Hoffman J. Peripheral neuropathy in children with diabetes mellitus. Acta Neurol Scand 1964; 40(suppl 8):1–65.

354. Eeg-Olofsson O, Petersén I. Childhood diabetic neuropathy: A clinical and neurophysiological study. Acta Paediatr Scand 1966; 55:163–176.

355. Gamstorp I, Shelburne SA Jr, Engleson G, et al. Peripheral neuropathy in juvenile diabetes. Diabetes 1966; 15:411–418.

356. White NH, Waltman SR, Krupin T, Santiago JV. Reversal of neuropathic and gastrointestinal complications related to diabetes mellitus in adolescents with improved metabolic control. J Pediatr 1981; 99:41–45.

357. Hoffman WH, Hart ZH, Frank RN. Correlates of delayed motor nerve conduction and retinopathy in juvenile-onset diabetes mellitus. J Pediatr 1983; 102:351–356.

358. Fierro B, Modica A, Cardella F, et al. Nerve conduction velocity and circulating immunocomplexes in Type 1 diabetic children. Acta Neurol Scand 1991; 83:176–178.

359. Chan JC, Eng G. Long-term hemodialysis and nerve conduction in children. Pediatr Res 1979; 13:591–593.

360. Arbus GS, Barnor N-A, Hsu AC, et al. Effect of chronic renal failure, dialysis and transplantation on motor nerve conduction velocity in children. Can Med Assoc J 1975; 113:517–520.

361. Belman AL. AIDS and pediatric neurology. Neurol Clin 1990; 8:571–603.

362. Koch T, Wesley A, Lewis E, et al. AIDS-related peripheral neuropathy in children and young adult hemophiliacs (abstr). Int Conf AIDS 1989; 5:316.

363. Carvalho J, Coimbra A, Andrade C. Peripheral nerve fibre changes in asymptomatic children of patients with familial amyloid polyneuropathy. Brain 1976; 99:1–10.

364. Lowitzsch K, Gutjahr P, Ottes H. Clinical and neurophysiological findings in 47 long-term survivors of childhood malignancies treated with various doses of vincristine. In: Canal N, Pozza G, eds. Peripheral neuropathies. New York: Elsevier/North-Holland Biomedical Press, 1978:459–465.

365. Hogan-Dann CM, Fellmeth WG, McGuire SA, Kiley VA. Polyneuropathy following vincristine therapy in two patients with Charcot-Marie-Tooth syndrome. JAMA 1984; 252:2862–2863.

366. Malapert D, Degos JD. Jambes douloureuses et orteils instables: Neuropathie induite par la cytarabine. Rev Neurol (Paris) 1989; 145:869–871.

367. Kurczynski TW, Choudhury AA, Horwitz SJ, et al. Remote effect of malignancy on the nervous system in children. Dev Med Child Neurol 1980; 22:205–222.

368. Zochodne DW, Bolton CF, Wells GA, et al. Critical illness polyneuropathy: A complication of sepsis and multiple organ failure. Brain 1987; 110:819–842.

369. Goulden KJ, Dooley JM, Peters S, Ronen GM. Critical illness polyneuropathy: A reversible cause of paralysis in asthmatic children (abstr). Ann Neurol 1989; 26:451.

370. Op de Coul AAW, Lambregts PCLA, Koeman J, et al. Neuromuscular complications in patients given Pavulon (pancuronium bromide) during artificial ventilation. Clin Neurol Neurosurg 1985; 87:17–22.

371. Gilmartin RC Jr, Jabbour JT, Duenas DA. Rubella vaccine myeloradiculoneuritis. J Pediatr 1972; 80:406–412.

372. Schaffner W, Fleet WF, Kilroy AW, et al. Polyneuropathy following rubella immunization. Am J Dis Child 1974; 127:684–688.

373. Spillane JD, Wells CEC. The neurology of Jennerian vaccination. Brain 1964; 87:1–44.

374. Berg BO, Rosenberg SH, Asbury AK. Giant axonal neuropathy. Pediatrics 1972; 49:894–899.

375. Tandan R, Little BW, Emery ES, et al. Childhood giant axonal neuropathy: Case report and review of the literature. J Neurol Sci 1987; 82:205–228.

376. Majnemer A, Rosenblatt B, Watters G, Andermann F. Giant axonal neuropathy: Central abnormalities demonstrated by evoked potentials. Ann Neurol 1986; 19:394–396.

377. Donaghy M, Brett EM, Ormerod IEC, et al. Giant axonal neuropathy: Observations on a further patient. J Neurol Neurosurg Psychiatry 1988; 51:991–994.

378. Thomas C, Love S, Powell HC, et al. Giant axonal neuropathy: Correlation of clinical findings with postmortem neuropathology. Ann Neurol 1987; 22:79–84.

379. Chaudhry U, Charnas L. Axonal peripheral neuropathy in Lowe's syndrome (abstr). Muscle Nerve 1989; 12:762.

380. Trevathan E, Naidu S. The clinical recognition and differential diagnosis of Rett syndrome. J Child Neurol 1988; 3(suppl):S6–S16.

381. Cornblath DR. Disorders of neuromusuclar transmission in infants and children. Muscle Nerve 1986; 9:606–611.

382. Dahl DS, Sato S. Unusual myasthenic state in a teenage boy. Neurology 1974; 9:897–901.

383. Chelmicka-Schorr E, Bernstein LP, Zurbrugg EB, Huttenlocher PR. Eaton-Lambert syndrome in a 9-year-old girl. Arch Neurol 1979; 36:572–574.

384. Streib EW, Rothner AD. Eaton-Lambert myasthenic syndrome: Long-term treatment of three patients with prednisone. Ann Neurol 1981; 10:448–453.

385. Shapira Y, Cividalli G, Szabo G, et al. A myasthenic syndrome in childhood leukemia. Dev Med Child Neurol 1974; 16:668–671.

386. Snead OC 3d, Benton JW, Dwyer D, et al. Juvenile myasthenia gravis. Neurology 1980; 30:732–739.

387. Rodriguez M, Gomez MR, Howard FM Jr, Taylor WF. Myasthenia gravis in children: Long-term follow-up. Ann Neurol 1983; 13:504–510.

388. Maselli R, Jacobsen JH, Spire J-P. Edrophonium: An aid in the diagnosis of acute organophosphate poisoning. Ann Neurol 1986; 19:508–510.

389. Wadia RS, Chitra S, Amin RB, et al. Electrophysiological studies in acute organophosphate poisoning. J Neurol Neurosurg Psychiatry 1987; 50:1442–1448.

390. Auger RG, Daube JR, Gomez MR, Lambert EH. Hereditary form of sustained muscle activity of peripheral nerve origin causing generalized myokymia and muscle stiffness. Ann Neurol 1984; 15:13–21.

391. Patterson MC, Gomez MR. Muscle disease in children: A practical approach. Pediatr Rev 1990; 12:73–82.

392. Emery AEH, Dreifuss FE. Unusual type of benign X-linked muscular dystrophy. J Neurol Neurosurg Psychiatry 1966; 29:338–342.

393. Merlini L, Granata C, Dominici P, Bonfiglioli S. Emery-Dreifuss muscular dystrophy: Report of five cases in a family and review of the literature. Muscle Nerve 1986; 9:481–485.

394. Takamoto K, Hirose K, Uono M, Nonaka I. A genetic variant of Emery-Dreifuss disease: Muscular dystrophy with humeropelvic distribution, early joint contracture, and permanent atrial paralysis. Arch Neurol 1984; 41:1292–1293.

395. Banker BQ. Congenital muscular dystrophy. In: Engel AG, Banker BQ, eds. Myology: Basic and clinical. New York: McGraw-Hill, 1986:1367–1384.

396. Poewe W, Willeit H, Sluga E, Mayr U. The rigid spine syndrome—a myopathy of uncertain nosological position. J Neurol Neurosurg Psychiatry 1985; 48:887–893.

397. Harati Y, Zeller RS, Armstrong DL. Emery-Dreifuss muscular dystrophy: An autopsy study (abstr). Neurology 1981; 31:106–107.

398. Vita G, Girlanda P, Santoro M, Messina C. Is rigid spine syndrome a distinct clinical entity? (letter). Muscle Nerve 1983; 6:458–460.

399. Hartlage PL, Soudmand R. An autosomal dominant myopathy with cardiac conduction defects and pyloric stenosis (abstr). Neurology 1981; 31:105–106.

400. Shuaib A, Martin JME, Mitchell LB, Brownell KW. Multicore myopathy: Not always a benign entity. Can J Neurol Sci 1988; 15:10–14.

401. Schapira AH. Mitochondrial myopathies: Mechanisms now better understood (edit). Br Med J 1989; 298:1127–1128.

402. Bunch TW. Polymyositis: A case history approach to the differential diagnosis and treatment. Mayo Clin Proc 1990; 65:1480–1497.

403. Lowry NJ, Murphy EG, Farrell K, Hill A. Polydermatomyositis in children: A review of 60 cases (abstr). Ann Neurol 1982; 12:209.

404. Wedgwood RJP, Cook CD, Cohen J. Dermatomyositis: Report of 26 cases in children with a discussion of endocrine therapy in 13. Pediatrics 1953; 12:447–466.

405. Roifman CM, Schaffer FM, Wachsmuth SE, et al. Reversal of chronic polymyositis following intravenous immune serum globulin therapy. JAMA 1987; 258:513–515.

406. Koutras A. Myositis with Kawasaki's disease. Am J Dis Child 1982; 136:78–79.

407. Noseworthy JH, Heffernan LP, Ross JB, Sangalang VE. Acne fulminans with inflammatory myopathy. Ann Neurol 1980; 8:67–69.

408. Miike T, Ohtani Y, Hattori S, et al. Childhood-type myositis and linear scleroderma. Neurology 1983; 33:928–930.

409. Kuntz NL. Electrophysiology of childhood inflammatory myopathy (abstr). Muscle Nerve 1983; 6:536–537.

410. Carpenter S, Karpati G, Rothman S, Watters G. The childhood type of dermatomyositis. Neurology 1976; 26:952–962.

411. Niakan E, Pitner SE, Whitaker JN, Bertorini TE. Immunosuppressive agents in corticosteroid-refractory childhood dermatomyositis. Neurology 1980; 30:286–291.

412. Riggs JE, Schochet SS Jr, Gutmann L, Lerfald SC. Childhood onset inclusion body myositis mimicking limb-girdle muscular dystrophy. J Child Neurol 1989; 4:283–285.

413. Ruff RL, Secrist D. Viral studies in benign acute childhood myositis. Arch Neurol 1982; 39:261–263.

414. Antony JH, Procopis PG, Ouvrier RA. Benign acute childhood myositis. Neurology 1979; 29:1068–1071.

415. Dietzman DE, Schaller JG, Ray CG, Reed ME. Acute myositis associated with influenza B infection. Pediatrics 1976; 57:255–258.

416. Sirinavin S, McCracken GH Jr. Primary suppurative myositis in children. Am J Dis Child 1979; 133:263–265.

417. Levin MJ, Gardner P, Waldvogel FA. "Tropical" pyomyositis: An unusual infection due to *Staphylococcus aureus*. N Engl J Med 1971; 284:196–198.

418. Altrocchi PH. Spontaneous bacterial myositis. JAMA 1971; 217:819–820.

419. Celesia GG, Andermann F, Wiglesworth FW, Robb JP. Monomelic myopathy: Congenital hypertrophic myotonic myopathy limited to one extremity. Arch Neurol 1967; 17:69–77.

420. Shukla A, Hall CD, Bradley WG, Pendlebury WW. Congenital monomelic hypertrophy with progressive myopathy. Arch Neurol 1991; 48:107–110.

421. Tein I, DiMauro S, Spiro AJ, De Vivo DG. Recurrent myoglobinuria of childhood (abstr). Ann Neurol 1988; 24:310–311.

422. Breningstall GN, Grover WD, Barbera S, Marks HG. Neonatal rhabdomyolysis as a presentation of muscular dystrophy. Neurology 1988; 38:1271–1272.

423. Cornelio F, Bresolin N, DiMauro S, et al. Congenital myopathy due to phosphorylase deficiency. Neurology 1983; 33:1383–1385.

424. Danon MJ, DiMauro S, Shanske S, et al. Juvenile-onset acid maltase deficiency with unusual familial features. Neurology 1986; 36:818–822.

425. Sugie H, Sugie Y, Nishida M, et al. Recurrent myoglobinuria in a child with mental retardation: Phosphoglycerate kinase deficiency. J Child Neurol 1989; 4:95–99.

426. McLeod ME, Creighton RE. Anesthesia for pediatric neurological and neuromuscular diseases. J Child Neurol 1986; 1:189–197.

427. Singer WD, Kelfer HM, Perrin LS, Reynolds RN. A variant of malignant hyperthermia in a child with Duchenne muscular dystrophy (abstr). Ann Neurol 1981; 10:300–301.

428. Heiman-Patterson TD, Natter HM, Rosenberg HR, et al. Malignant hyperthermia susceptibility in X-linked muscle dystrophies. Pediatr Neurol 1986; 2:356–358.

429. Hall SC. Malignant hyperthermia in a child. JAMA 1985; 253:2580.

430. Wedel DJ, Engel AG. Malignant hyperthermia (MH) testing in patients with persistently elevated serum CK (abstr). J Neurol Sci 1990; 98(suppl):453.

431. Willis JK, Tilton AH, Harkin JC, Boineau FG. Reversible myopathy due to labetalol. Pediatr Neurol 1990; 6:275–276.

26

Electromyography in the Critical Care Unit

Charles F. Bolton

CONTENTS

LIST OF ACRONYMS

CT   computed tomography
EEG   electroencephalography

Patients who are acutely and seriously ill are now being managed with increasing frequency in critical care units throughout the world. In the United States, it is estimated that 20% of the inpatient health care budget is devoted to critical care units.[1] The incidence of the various disorders requiring admission to such units depends on the type of unit, whether general medical, general surgical, neurologic, or neurosurgical. In our unit, we estimate at least 50% of patients have significant involvement of the nervous system.

The incidence of neuromuscular problems in such units is much higher than generally recognized. Sepsis and multiple organ failure occur in 40% of patients in a medical critical care unit,[2] and 70% of these patients develop a critical illness polyneuropathy.[3] Because of difficulties in clinically evaluating such patients, identification of neuromuscular problems can be established only through electrophysiologic tests,[4] occasionally supplemented by muscle and nerve biopsy. These tests involve approaches sometimes peculiar to critical care units. For example, assessment of the respiratory neuromuscular system and determining the nature and severity of neuromuscular disorders that may contribute to dependence on the ventilator are especially important. The information gained often helps to establish more effective treatment and provide an accurate prognosis. Considering the high cost of management in critical care units, accurate prognosis is especially important.

CLINICAL ASSESSMENT OF PATIENTS IN THE CRITICAL CARE UNIT

Patients are difficult to assess clinically because a history cannot be obtained because of coma or an endotracheal tube. Relatives are frequently absent, and the charts in critical care units are often voluminous and time-consuming to review. It is often best to obtain the history and other data from both the critical care resident and nurse. Particular attention is paid to evidence of sepsis and multiple organ failure, medications the patient is receiving, injections of neuromuscular blocking agents, and the primary and secondary diagnoses and results of investigations of the nervous system, including computed tomographic (CT) or electromagnetic resonance scans, myelography, electroencephalography (EEG), and examination of the cerebrospinal fluid. Evidence of acquired immunodeficiency syndrome, reaction to hepatitis B antigen, any bleeding tendency, and es-

sential data about current methods of ventilation should all be obtained. Note should be made of procedures, such as insertion of Swan-Ganz catheters; use of vasopressor agents; surgical procedures on the chest and abdomen, particularly those that injure the phrenic nerve or aorta; and insertion of balloon catheters through iliac vessels or the aorta.

Physical examination is impeded by coma, which precludes patient cooperation, and the presence of intravascular lines, catheters, and so forth. The physical examination may therefore be limited to observations of muscular movements induced by reflex activity responses to painful stimulation and abnormalities of deep tendon reflexes and plantar responses. Patients may be weak in a general nonspecific way, with flaccidity, reduced deep tendon reflexes, and absent plantar responses, as a result of conditions varying as widely as acute encephalopathy, acute myelopathy with spinal shock, polyneuropathy, defects in neuromuscular transmission, and myopathy. The only clear-cut sign of myelopathy may be bilateral extensor plantar responses (a sign that may be absent in spinal shock, in total denervation of toe extensors, or in deafferentation of the sole of the foot). Focal wasting of muscle suggests a focal neuropathy. Localized pressure marks on the skin such as redness, swelling, and blistering owing to prolonged recumbency from drug overdose point to sites at which the underlying nerve may have been focally compressed (Figure 26.1).

Rapid, shallow respirations have been traditional signs of neuromuscular respiratory insufficiency. Such signs are often eliminated by the patient being fully ventilated and respirations being triggered at varying rates by the respirator. The pattern of respiration, however, may be observed when the triggering mechanism is removed and the patient allowed to initiate his or her own respirations ventilated with pressure support only. This is best performed later, when doing needle electromyography (EMG) of the diaphragm and chest wall muscles when the clinical and electromyographic responses of the respiratory muscles may be observed at the same time (see later discussion).

ELECTROPHYSIOLOGIC TESTING

A number of technical challenges arise through electromyographic testing in the critical care unit. There may be interference from adjacent machines or poorly grounded plug-ins. The machine must have

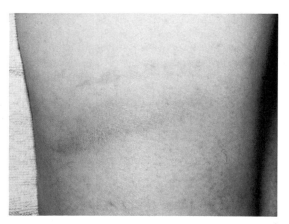

FIGURE 26.1.   *Healing erythematous blistering of the skin of the posterior thigh in a young woman. She was admitted 3 weeks previously after prolonged coma owing to drug overdose. The sciatic nerve, underlying the skin lesion, suffered severe local damage owing to prolonged compression, with distal motor and sensory nerve axonal degeneration. EMG was useful in confirming the site and nature of nerve damage and documenting the partial recovery, which occurred over a matter of months.*

adequately shielded cables. If there is interference from other electrical devices, these should be unplugged, if safe to do so without harming the patient. The skin should be adequately prepared to reduce skin resistance at sites of application of ground and recording electrodes. Even then, 60 cycle artifact may be difficult to eliminate entirely. In this situation, a 60 cycle notch filter on the EMG machine may be useful.

Electrical stimulation of some nerves may not be possible because of intravascular lines, surgical wounds and dressings, casts, or splints. Moreover, because there is a remote chance that a cardiac arrhythmia may be induced by electrical stimuli applied near an intravascular line positioned near the heart, it is wise to choose the opposite limb for nerve stimulation. We, and others, have been concerned for several years that needle EMG of the chest wall or diaphragm might puncture adjacent viscera. By using a technique described later, however, these procedures are now much safer. Finally, while in testing for a defect in neuromuscular transmission, the patient may not be able to contract muscle voluntarily, precluding the possibility of testing for postactiva-

tion facilitation. The technique of stimulated single-fiber EMG is a satisfactory alternative.

A considerable repertoire of electrophysiologic techniques may be applied to the neuromuscular system in the critical care unit, including motor and sensory nerve conduction studies, needle EMG, facial nerve conduction and blink reflexes, somatosensory evoked potential studies, repetitive nerve stimulation studies, stimulated single-fiber EMG,[5–7] and spinal cord stimulation.

DISORDERS THAT MAY BE EXAMINED WITH ELECTROPHYSIOLOGIC TECHNIQUES

Encephalopathy

Encephalopathy may occur as a result of sepsis, metabolic disturbances, and drugs. In acute, diffuse encephalopathies, particularly those caused by drugs or septic encephalopathy,[8,9] the limbs may be flaccid and deep tendon reflexes reduced or absent, making it difficult to determine the presence or absence of an associated neuromuscular problem. EMG tests may provide the only means of detecting a neuromuscular disorder. If motor and sensory nerve conduction, repetitive stimulation, and needle EMG are normal, a peripheral cause for the weakness and flaccidity is unlikely. Then if it is noted on needle EMG that motor unit potentials either fail to recruit or are delayed in recruitment and fire slowly, a central cause for weakness, encephalopathy, is more likely.

Myelopathy

The common myelopathies seen in the unit include traumatic; compression from neoplasm, hemorrhage, or infection in the epidural space; and infarction of the spinal cord secondary to aortic surgery. High cervical lesions may cause respiratory insufficiency, in addition to quadriplegia. Low cervical lesions may produce respiratory insufficiency by interfering with the upper and lower motor neuron supply of the chest wall muscles. Depending on the level of the lesion, there may be very little weakness and sensory loss in the upper limbs. Thoracic cord lesions are usually associated with little impairment of respiration.

Impairment of pain sensation below a definite level on the trunk is important evidence of the level of the spinal cord lesion. This may be tested if the patient is alert enough to grimace to a painful stimulus.

Lesions in the lumbar or sacral regions characteristically produce initial and longstanding flaccid weakness, with reduced deep tendon reflexes, depending on the level of the involvement of the cauda equina. The combination of upper and lower motor neuron signs suggests a lesion at the level of the conus medullaris.

A lesion at any level of the central nervous system may produce urinary retention requiring catheterization. It should be recognized that in acute spinal cord lesions, the limbs may initially be flaccid, with reduced or absent deep tendon reflexes and plantar responses, purely on the basis of spinal shock. This may last days or weeks and simulate a peripheral, rather than a central, cause for the weakness.

The amplitudes of compound muscle action potentials as a result of damage to anterior horn cells may be reduced beginning 5 days since the injury. If sensory conduction is normal and clinical sensory loss is present, the lesion lies proximal to the dorsal root ganglion, usually indicating a myelopathy.

Fibrillation potentials and positive sharp curves appear after 10 to 20 days, depending on the distance between the site of nerve injury and the muscle length of the nerve (i.e., shorter intervals for shorter distances). The pattern of denervation should help to localize the segmental level, whether it is unilateral or bilateral, and roughly the number of segments involved, although because of the considerable overlap in the innervation of most paraspinal muscles, localization may not be precise.

In somatosensory evoked potential (SSEP) studies, scalp recordings would reveal delayed or absent potentials. Normal peripheral nerve and T-12 responses would localize the lesion to above the T-12 level. Absent or delayed T-12 responses suggest the lesion is in the region of the cauda equina or lumbosacral plexus if limb peripheral nerves SSEPs were normal. Unless the spinal cord lesion clearly involves the somasthetic pathways, however, SSEP studies may be normal even in the presence of a spinal cord lesion of considerable size. Further investigations, such as plain films, myelography, magnetic resonance imaging, and examination of the cerebrospinal fluid, may further define the nature and localization of the spinal cord lesion.

Lumbosacral or Brachial Plexopathies

These may be secondary to direct trauma, usually from motor vehicle accidents or surgery. Insertion of catheters into the iliac arteries or aorta may dislodge thrombi, and the resulting embolization impairs vascular supply to nerves producing focal ischemic plex-

opathy.[10] Direct surgical trauma may also induce vascular insufficiency.

In the critical care unit, even fairly severe plexopathies may be overlooked and only a particularly observant nurse or physician may observe the patient's failure to move one limb as well as the others. Abnormalities in motor and sensory nerve conduction and needle EMG may help to localize the lesion to the brachial or lumbosacral plexus. (see Chapter 8.)

Mononeuropathies

These may first become apparent while the patient is in the critical care unit, but because neurologic deficit may be less than a plexopathy, mononeuropathies are often overlooked until the patient has been extubated and discharged from the unit, when the patient complains of weakness and sensory loss within the distribution of the involve nerve. If the patient was admitted postoperatively to the unit, the mononeuropathy may have developed during the operation or post operative period. The radial nerve in the upper arm, ulnar nerve at the elbow, and common peroneal nerve at the fibular head are particularly liable to injury in this way. Phrenic nerves, either bilaterally or unilaterally, may be damaged at the time of surgery by direct trauma or the application of cold, as occurs in the hypothermia associated with cardiac surgery[11] (see discussion later in ths chapter). Motor and sensory nerve conduction and electromyographic studies should properly identify the peripheral nerve and the site of dysfunction as well as its acuteness and whether or not there has been any evidence of regeneration.

As with the brachial and lumbosacral plexopathies, more distal nerves may be damaged as a result of impairment of nutrient blood supply through distal embolization. Thus patients who are being treated in the critical care unit following cardiac or vascular surgery may manifest mononeuropathies, and in our experience, these have usually involved the lower extremity and consist of varying combinations of involvement of femoral or sciatic nerves. Because of difficulties in examining patients in the critical care unit, electromyographic techniques are of great value in properly diagnosing these focal neuropathies. The lesions produce a relatively pure axonal degeneration of motor and sensory fibers.

Patients anticoagulated in the critical care unit run the risk of hemorrhage within confined spaces such as tissue compartments, where sudden rise in tissue pressure may produce severe compression and ischemia of nerves traversing the compartment. The compartments most commonly involved include the iliopsoas and gluteal compartment producing acute femoral or sciatic neuropathies. Other sites may also be involved.[12] If the phenomenon is recognized early, within a few hours, an immediate CT scan should be ordered, to locate the hemorrhage. Surgical decompression may then successfully decompress the nerve. The situation is so acute and emergent that nerve conduction and needle EMG studies are of little value. Fractures and soft tissue trauma may also induce compartment syndromes.

Patients suffering from severe drug overdose may be immobile for many hours. During this time, constant focal pressure on various parts of the body by hard objects may induce local necrosis of skin, subcutaneous tissue, and occasionally the underlying muscle and may also be associated with severe compression of an underlying nerve producing a focal neuropathy. The examiner should look for characteristic erythematous blisters of the skin at the site of compression and suspect injury to an underlying nerve if the latter should lie nearby (see Figure 26.1). Electrophysiologic techniques help to identify these mononeuropathies, which in our experience, have usually been of the axonal type.

Polyneuropathies

Guillain-Barré syndrome developing before admission to the critical care unit and critical illness polyneuropathy developing after admission to the unit are, in our experience, the most common polyneuropathies in this setting. Electrophysiologic studies are of great value in identifying and assessing the nature and severity of the polyneuropathy. Electrophysiologic studies are usually sufficient to distinguish clearly these polyneuropathies from myelopathy, defects in neuromuscular transmission, or primary myopathies, which on a purely clinical basis, may not always be apparent as the cause of the limb weakness or respiratory insufficiency.

Guillain-Barré Syndrome

Patients admitted to a critical care unit because of Guillain-Barré syndrome are usually severely affected enough to require mechanical ventilation.[13] As early as 24 to 48 hours of the onset of Guillain-Barré syndrome, electrophysiologic studies are usually sufficiently characteristic to indicate clearly a demyelinating polyneuropathy.[14,15] The presence of conduction block, predominantly, proximally, or distally[16] (see Chatper 20), and the finding of high motor unit firing frequencies in the presence of reduced recruit-

ment in weak muscles strongly suggests a neuropathy, even though conventional motor and sensory nerve conduction studies may be relatively normal. Phrenic nerve conduction studies and needle EMG of diaphragm are particularly valuable in establishing the type and severity of the involvement of phrenic nerve and diaphragm[17] (see later discussion). Serial studies may provide valuable information about the course and treatments, such as steroids and plasmapheresis.

Acute Axonal Guillain-Barré Syndrome

This uncommon manifestation of Guillain-Barré syndrome[18] presents with a rapidly developing paralysis that reaches complete paralyses often within hours or at the most several days and requires early admission to the critical care unit and full ventilatory assistance. All muscles of the body, including the cranial musculature and even the eye muscles and pupils, may be totally paralyzed. This disorder may simulate brain death clinically, but the electroencephalogram is relatively normal. Peripheral nerves, including the facial nerve, sometimes may be totally unresponsive to supramaxal electrical stimuli of long duration. This neuropathy may represent an unusually severe form of Guillain-Barré syndrome in which initially massive demyelination accounts for the unresponsiveness of the peripheral nerves on stimulation. Axons may become secondarily involved, and fibrillation potentials and positive sharp waves appear in muscles 3 to 4 weeks later. Alternatively, the disorder may be caused by a primary attack on the axon, producing a picture of severe primary axonal degeneration.[18]

Recovery is extremely slow, with patients remaining in the unit for many months. Unfortunately, there may also be severe, persisting disability. The occasional patient however, makes a remarkable recovery, and one of our patients recovered to the point that he was even able to jog. Despite the then poor prognosis and great difficulties in managing these patients, substandard recovery is possible, and patients should be provided with intense long-term support.

Critical Illness Polyneuropathy

This polyneuropathy is a regular complication of the syndrome of sepsis and multiple organ failure.[19–21] It manifests as difficulty in weaning from the ventilator and varying degrees of limb weakness, just as the patient seems to be recovering from the septic syndrome in the critical care unit. It is an important cause of long-term ventilator dependence.[22] Only severe polyneuropathies cause obvious clinical signs, such as severe weakness or paralysis and reduced or absent deep tendon reflexes. Electrophysiologic studies, however, show the presence of an axonal motor and sensory polyneuropathy. Phrenic nerve conduction studies and needle EMG of the diaphragm[23] and chest wall muscles provide additional and more direct evidence of involvement of the neuromuscular respiratory system by this polyneuropathy.[3] Recovery can be expected, provided that the patient survives the septic syndrome and other complications. Recovery occurs within several weeks in milder cases and in months in more severe cases. Serial electrophysiologic studies are often valuable for determining the ultimate prognosis and gauging the recovery.

Critical illness polyneuropathy may readily be distinguished from Guillain-Barré syndrome in most cases,[24] although differentiating between critical illness neuropathy and myopathy may be difficult.[25] Septic myopathy cannot reliably be distinguished from the neuropathy using electromyographic techniques, since both may induce fibrillation potentials and positive sharp waves, and reduced compound muscle action potential amplitudes.

Other Polyneuropathies

Other causes for polyneuropathy in the critical care unit include thiamine deficiency, vitamin E deficiency, pyridoxine abuse, hypophosphatemia, porphyria, and drug induced neuropathies, including antibiotics such as metronidazole, aminoglycoside, and penicillin. These entities are discussed in other chapters.

NEUROMUSCULAR TRANSMISSION DEFECTS

Anesthetic Drugs

These drugs are the most common cause of abnormal neuromuscular transmission in a critical care unit. The frequency of their use varies widely from unit to unit. They are used to reduce metabolic demands, prevent shivering or "fighting" with the ventilator, lower intracranial pressure, and improve chest compliance.[27] In our unit, such drugs are used infrequently, and systematic studies of critically ill patients using repetitive stimulation of nerves have failed to reveal defects in neuromuscular transmission.[24] Weakness in limbs and difficulties in weaning critically ill patients from the ventilator were usually found to be due to critical illness polyneuropathy.[28]

Anesthetic agents, however, have been used more often, particularly the shorter-acting drug, vecuronium. Its effects are said to diminish rapidly within a few hours of cessation. However, we and others[27] (Zuchodne DW, et al. Personal communication) have observed persisting neuromuscular blockade for periods up to 3 weeks following discontinuation of the drug in the presence of renal or liver disease. In patients with sepsis and multiple organ failure, critical illness polyneuropathy is probably present and further contributes to the weakness and difficulties in weaning from the ventilator[27] (Figure 26.2).

Aminoglycoside Toxicity

A defect in neuromuscular transmission has been a recognized complication of this group of antibiotic drugs.[29] So far, however, we have failed to see such a case despite the fact that patients regularly receive this drug to treat prolonged sepsis. These drugs should therefore be considered safe, at least with respect to neuromuscular complications in critically ill patients.

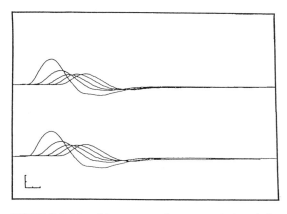

FIGURE 26.2. *Neuromuscular transmission defect caused by the short-acting blocking agent vecuronium. Such a defect, here demonstrated by repetitive nerve stimulation at 3 per second and repeated 10 seconds later without exercise (lower trace), disappeared in 6 hours. (Calibration: 500 microvolts and 2 msec. per division.) It may persist for much longer, however, if there is associated renal or liver failure. Moreover, in this patient, there was an associated critical illness polyneuropathy that further increased muscle weakness; it added to the decrease in compound muscle action potential amplitude and caused fibrillation potentials and positive sharp waves to appear in muscle.*

Myasthenia Gravis

Myasthenia gravis occasionally causes severe and rapidly progressive weakness requiring emergency ventilation and sometimes presents a diagnostic challenge in the critical care unit. Even in established cases, electrophysiologic studies may be required to objectively assess the neuromuscular system following thymectomy or when patients worsen following treatment with steroids or anticholinesterase drugs. Repetitive nerve stimulation usually reveals the typical decrementing response at slow rates of stimulation (see Chapter 23).

Eaton-Lambert Syndrome

Patients with this syndrome may present in the critical care unit with prolonged respiratory paralysis following surgery for an intrathoracic, usually pulmonary, neoplasm. Prolonged neuromuscular blockade may be induced by curare-like drugs because patients with Eaton-Lambert syndrome complicating small cell carcinoma of the lung are especially sensitive to curare, as are patients with myasthenia gravis. As in the latter, repetitive nerve stimulation studies often reveal a decrement at slow rates of stimulation. An important clue to the Eaton-Lambert syndrome, however, is the characteristically reduced amplitudes of the compound muscle action potential in rested muscles in response to single supramaximal stimuli. Reductions in the sizes of compound muscle action potentials in myasthenia gravis in response to single nerve stimuli, are usually more modest or even absent. The typical defect of Eaton-Lambert syndrome is traditionally best shown by repetitive stimulation of a motor nerve immediately following a voluntary muscle contraction or stimulating the nerve at high stimulus frequencies. In both instances, the typical response in the Eaton-Lambert syndrome connects of a twofold or greater rapid increase in the size of the muscle compound action potential. High-frequency stimulation is painful, and patients in critical care units often cannot contract their muscles sufficiently for testing. Stimulated single-fiber EMG gets around the latter difficulties. Demonstration of a small cell carcinoma of the lung points to the Eaton-Lambert syndrome, and a thymoma to myasthenia gravis.

Organophosphate Poisoning

Organophosphate poisoning, usually from exposure to insecticides containing this compound, may prompt admission to a critical care unit. The chemical affects the nervous system at several levels. Involvement of the central nervous system produces increased restlessness then reduced consciousness and occasionally seizures. Stimulation of the sympathetic system may induce hypertension, tachycardia, and dilated pupils. Skeletal neuromuscular junctions may be affected as well, causing weakness, sphincter incontinence, and fasciculations. Muscarinic parasympathetic effects include excessive sweating, salivation, increased pulmonary secretions, bradycardia, hypotension, and constricted pupils. Examination of the neuromuscular system may therefore produce confusing signs. Electrophysiologic studies, however, may clearly establish the diagnosis. Single-pulse or low-frequency stimulation produces a characteristic repetitive discharge (Figure 26.3). Higher frequencies produce a decrementing response of the compound action potential amplitude. In addition to the neuromuscular transmission defect, a primary axonal, predominantly motor, polyneuropathy may develop.[30] Difficulty in weaning from the ventilator may be a complication.[31]

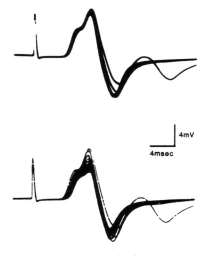

FIGURE 26.3.   *Repetitive discharge in a case of organophosphate poisoning, an important sign of this condition. It appears as a lower amplitude discharge during the late positive phase of the compound action potential. Acetylcholine excess prolongs the end plate potential, causing a repeat firing just as the refractory period ends. Compound action potential decrement occurred with more rapid rates of stimulation. (Ulnar nerve stimulation at wrist, recording hypothenar muscles. Upper trace, 5 stimuli per second; lower traces, 40 stimuli per second.)*

Other neuromuscular transmission defects that may be seen in the critical care unit include hypermagnesemia, wound botulism, and tickbite paralysis. (See Chapter 23 for a detailed discussion of these entities.)

Myopathies

It has been our experience that critical illness polyneuropathy is the most common cause of generalized muscle weakness in the critical care unit even though respiratory muscle fatigue[32] and catabolic myopathy associated with sepsis[33] have been regarded as more traditional causes of weakness. Neither of the latter conditions can be easily defined, either clinically or electrophysiologically. It is our view that sepsis can induce a generalized myopathy as well as a neuropathy. Reduced compound muscle action potential sizes and abnormal spontaneous activity in muscle could result from either the neuropathy or a myopathy. Levels of creatinine phosphokinase have either been normal or mildly elevated, so if muscle is involved, it presumably does not significantly damage muscle membranes. Prolongation of the compound muscle action potential duration occurs early[28] and cannot be explained by a neuropathy because latencies on both proximal and distal stimulation are unaffected. We believe therefore that a primary functional disturbance of the muscle fiber membrane is present. Some support for this has been given by our studies of nuclear magnetic resonance spectroscopy of muscle in patients who had critical illness polyneuropathy. Such patients have a severe reduction in bioenergetic reserves,[26] more than would be expected from an uncomplicated neuropathy.[34] Practically speaking, it may not be possible, even using muscle biopsies, to distinguish a neuropathy clearly from a myopathy because mild, scattered muscle fiber necrosis may at times be difficult to distinguish from early denervation.[20]

A rare severe myopathy that may present for the first time in the critical care unit has been called *panfascicular muscle fiber necrosis,*[35] and may represent an idiosyncratic reaction to infection. It is manifested by acute, severe, generalized weakness of muscle, accompanied at times by swelling and tenderness of the muscles. Creatinine phosphokinase levels are greatly increased, and muscle biopsy shows panfascicular muscle fiber necrosis. Compound muscle action potential amplitudes are reduced, and fibrillation potentials and positive sharp waves may be seen possibly as a result of the acute muscle fiber necrosis. When severe, myoglobinuria may occur,

and if it is also quite severe, acute renal failure may develop. Complete recovery is possible.

Another rare, diffuse myopathy that presents with similar clinical and electrophysiologic features to panfascicular muscle necrosis is pyomyositis.[36,37] This is more likely with suppurative infections in tropical countries and consists of diffuse multiple abscesses throughout skeletal muscles. Muscle biopsy is necessary for accurate diagnosis.

Acid maltase deficiency may present with generalized muscle weakness affecting predominantly the respiratory muscles and requires early intubation and admission to the critical care unit. EMG reveals prominent fibrillation potentials, positive sharp waves, complex repetitive discharges, and myotonic discharges, although clinical myotonia is absent. The diagnosis is established by muscle biopsy and histochemical evidence of acid maltase deficiency.[38] Other causes of primary myopathies in the critical care unit include variety of water and electrolyte disturbances, but these are usually obvious from routine blood tests.

INVESTIGATION OF THE RESPIRATORY NEUROMUSCULAR SYSTEM

The majority of patients in critical care units are ill enough to require assisted ventilation, many requiring intubation and support by a mechanical ventilator. The reasons for this include primary diseases of the lung or mechanical problems with airway or chest wall. In many patients, however, specific dysfunction of the nervous system, either lack of central drive or weakness of the muscles of respiration, is present. The former is usually associated with a wide variety of encephalopathies and the latter by disease of anterior horn cells, peripheral nerves, neuromuscular junction, or muscles of the chest wall or diaphragm and include poliomyelitis, Guillain-Barré syndrome, and myasthenia gravis, but our experience is that the neuromuscular complications of sepsis and traumatic damage to the phrenic nerves are probably the most common causes of these neuromuscular problems.

A lack of central drive in encephalopathies can often be discerned by observing specific patterns of respiration that are of localizing value[39] (Figure 26.4). With assisted ventilation, however, these clinical signs are often interfered with, and in many instances, it is not possible to determine whether there is a lack of central drive or a neuromuscular

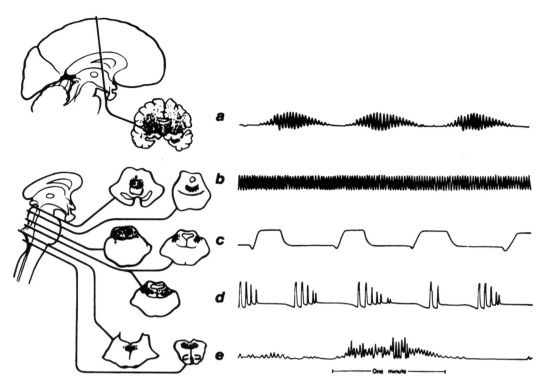

FIGURE 26.4.   *Abnormal respiratory patterns associated with pathologic lesions (shaded areas) at various locations in the brain. (A) Cheyne-Stokes respiration. (B) Central neurogenic hyperventilation. (C) Apneusis. (D) Cluster breathing. (E) Ataxic breathing. Here respiratory movements were recorded with a chest-abdomen pneumograph, but we have found that such patterns can be detected from needle EMG recordings of the diaphragm. (Reprinted with permission from: Plum F, Posner JB. The pathologic physiology of signs and symptoms of coma. In: The Diagnosis of Stupor and Coma, Contemporary Neurology Series; 19, ed. 3, F.A. Davis Company, Philadelphia; 1980, p. 34.*

problem. Neuromuscular dysfunction causes hypoventilation, hypoxia, and potentially apnea. Observation of *respiratory alternans alternation of rib cage* and abdominal movement and *abdominal paradox*—inward movement of the diaphragm during inspiration—suggesting neuromuscular respiratory failure, are often absent in our experience. More sophisticated measurements—vital capacity, high airway occlusion pressure, peak negative pressure on maximal inspiration from full expiration, breathing frequency, and tidal volume[40]—may also provide inconclusive results. Even severe unilateral phrenic nerve palsy due to operative trauma[11] is often unrecognized.

It is not widely appreciated how valuable electromyographic studies may be for more precisely pinpointing the cause of the respiratory insufficiency.

Because clinical examination of cerebral function is difficult in the critical care unit, we have found EEG to be of great value. The nature and degree of abnormality of EEG usually provides indication of the severity of the encephalopathy[8,9] and whether lack of central drive might be a problem. If the patient is on a ventilator, abnormalities of central drive can be assessed by examining the response of the patient to self-triggered ventilation, while ensuring adequate oxygenation with pressure support. The blood pressure, heart rate, and, if possible, venous oxygen tension, should be regularly observed during this period and full ventilation resumed if the patient develops any difficulties. It may be possible to take the patient off the ventilator for a few minutes while observing the pattern of respiration. This procedure may be quite helpful for determining the effectiveness of central drive (see Figure 26.4). Through the use of magnetic stimulation of the brain, it may be possible in the future to test more directly the central drive to anterior horn cells, which subserve the phrenic nerve and nerves supplying chest wall muscles (Brown WF, Personal communication.).

The technique of phrenic nerve conduction, originally described in 1967 by Newsome-Davis,[41] has unfortunately been neglected over the years. One of the reasons may be the fear that it was not as accurate as standard conduction studies of limb nerves. We have used Markand's[17] modification of this technique (Figure 26.5). Studies in our laboratory, however, have shown that the reproducibility of dia-

phragm compound action potential measurements is just as good as thenar compound action potential measurements from median nerve stimulation. Certain technical points must, however, be observed. The most important is the problem of stimulation of the brachial plexus. This results in a compound action potential from chest wall muscles supplied by the brachial plexus, which is volume conducted to the recording electrodes and produces an action potential of reversed polarity and much shorter latency. Repositioning the stimulating electrode so only the phrenic nerve is being stimulated eliminates this problem. The ECG produces a large potential that can interfere with diaphragmatic recordings but is usually and readily avoided by simply repeating the stimulus. The size of the diaphragmatic compound muscle action potential also varies with respiration, being of larger size during inspiration than expiration. However, if supramaximal stimulation of the phrenic nerve is repeated several times during quiet respiration and the two highest amplitude potentials obtained, amplitude measurements are quite reproducible (Figure 26.6). We measure the distance from the point of stimulation on the phrenic nerve to the

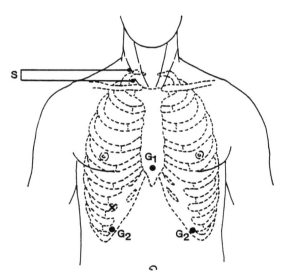

FIGURE 26.5. *The techniques of phrenic nerve conduction and needle EMG of chest wall and diaphragm. The phrenic nerve is stimulated (s) at the posterior border of the sternomastoid muscle. The diaphragm compound action potential is recorded from ipsilateral surface electrodes (G_1 and G_2.) Needle EMG of the chest wall and diaphragm can be recorded with a monopolar electrode inserted at right angles to the chest wall in several interspaces (x) between the anterior axillary and medial clavicular lines. There is at least 1.5 cm between the pleura and the lower costal margin on which the diaphragm inserts. The presence of insertional activity indicates when the needle is in muscle. Bursts of motor unit potentials characteristically occur with each inspiration when the needle is in the diaphragm.*

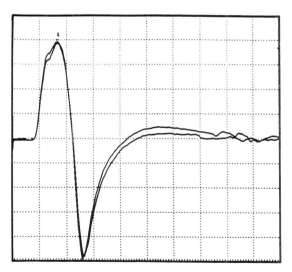

FIGURE 26.6. *Phrenic nerve conduction study in a healthy 50-year-old man. The phrenic nerve was stimulated in the neck, and the compound action potential was recorded with surface electrodes over the ipsilateral diaphragm; G_1, 5 cm above the xyphoid; G_2, 16 cm lateral on the lower costal margin. (200 μV, and 10 ms/div). The latency is 8 ms and negative peak amplitude 800 μV.*

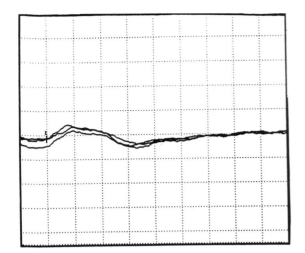

FIGURE 26.7.   *Phrenic nerve conduction study in a 55-year-old woman. She was being ventilated in the critical care unit. She had sepsis, multiple organ failure, and a severe critical illness polyneuropathy. Note low amplitude diaphragm compound action potential at slightly prolonged latency (200 μV and 10 ms/div).*

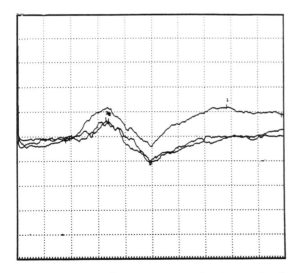

FIGURE 26.8.   *Phrenic nerve conduction study of a 48-year-old man, with very severe Guillain-Barré syndrome, after 1 month in the critical care unit. Note low amplitude diaphragm compound action potential at three times normal latency. (100 μV and 10 ms/division).*

G[1] recording electrode over the xiphoid, although we have found that this measurement varies little in adults. In children, however, this measurement varies considerably.

Markand et al[17] clearly demonstrated the value of phrenic nerve diaphragm studies in both demyelinating and axonal polyneuropathies. We have confirmed this in our own studies over the last 9 years. A purely axonal neuropathy such as critical illness polyneuropathy usually produces only mild increases in latency but considerable reductions in the size of the diaphragmatic compound muscle action potential (Figure 26.7). Demyelinating polyneuropathies such as Guillain-Barré syndrome may produce much greater increases in latency and considerable reductions in the size of compound muscle action potential (Figure 26.8). Studies by Gourie-Devi and Ganapathy[42] have shown there is a reasonably good correlation between phrenic nerve conduction abnormalities and measurements of respiratory function, such as vital capacity. The technique may therefore be used to assess neuromuscular respiratory dysfunction and provide some clue as to the ultimate prognosis.

We originally believed needle EMG of the diaphragm to be too risky for fear of inadvertent puncture of lung, liver, spleen, or colon.[4] We have employed, however, a technique, briefly described many years ago by Koepke,[43,44] which is safe, causes little discomfort, and provides excellent recordings of diaphragm activity.[23] The recording needle is inserted between the ribs between the anterior axillary and medial clavicular lines and just above the costal margin, where there is an approximately 1.5-cm distance between the pleural reflection and the lower costal cartilage on which the diaphragm inserts (see Figure 26.5). The needle does not traverse either the pleural space or the lung. Recordings may be made as the needle passes through external oblique or rectus abdominus muscles, external and intercostal muscles, and finally, the diaphragm. During quiet respiration, the muscles of the chest wall do not fire, but the diaphragm, regularly fires with each inspiration. The firing pattern and other features of motor unit action potentials may be observed (Figure 26.9). Abnormal spontaneous activity may also be detected in the diaphragm (Figure 26.10). In the critical care unit, we now carry out needle EMG from the diaphragm while discontinuing intermittent mandatory ventilation to observe the presence and nature of any spontaneous respiration, the pattern of firing of motor unit potentials with spontaneous respiration, and the appearance of the motor unit action potentials.

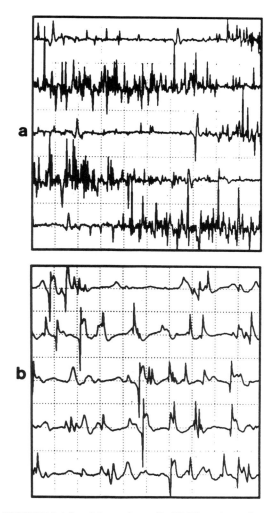

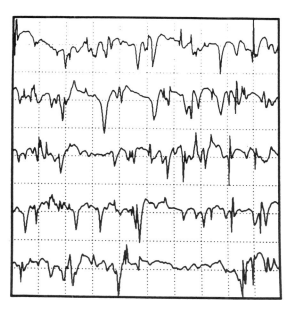

FIGURE 26.10. *Needle EMG of left diaphragm in a patient who had severe denervation as a result of operative trauma to the phrenic nerve. Continuous positive sharp waves and fibrillation potentials are shown. No motor unit potentials fired during inspiration. (100 μV and 10 ms/division, 100 to 10,000 c/s.)*

FIGURE 26.9. *Normal needle EMG activity from the left diaphragm during quiet breathing. (A) At successive slow sweep speeds from top to bottom, bursts of motor unit potentials occur with each inspiration, the bursts and the intervals each lasting 2 seconds. (B) At slower sweep speeds, more detail of motor unit potentials can be seen during a burst. (100 μV and 10 or 200 ms/division, 100 to 10,000 c/s.)*

By applying phrenic nerve–diaphragm studies and needle EMG of the chest wall muscles and diaphragm, it has been possible to determine, in most instances, whether respiratory insufficiency is a result of a disorder of central drive or unilateral or bilateral neuropathy of the phrenic nerves. We have not attempted to detect a defect in neuromuscular transmission from repetitive stimulation of the phrenic nerve because we believe this would be too uncomfortable and accompanied by a greater chance of ECG contamination of the signal by artifact.

Primary myopathies affecting the chest wall muscles or diaphragm may be difficult to detect by these procedures because, similar to neuropathy, they may also reduce the size of the compound muscle action potential amplitude with little change in latency and produce abnormal spontaneous activity in muscle. The only clue that the patient has a primary myopathy may be the finding of motor unit action potentials of the abnormally short duration and often highly polyphasic character commonly seen in myopathies. Motor unit action potentials from the healthy diaphragm, however, are often of short duration and small size, making such interpretation difficult in pathologic conditions. More sophisticated computer techniques may be necessary to identify clearly the presence of a primary myopathy.

REFERENCES

1. Jacobs P, Noseworthy TW. National estimates of intensive care utilization and costs: Canada and the United States. Crit Care Med 1990; 18(11):1282–1286.
2. Tran DD, Groeneveld ABJ, van der Meulen J, et al. Age, chronic disease, sepsis, organ system failure, and mortality in a medical intensive care unit. Crit Care Med 1990; 18:474–479.
3. Witt NJ, Zochodne DW, Bolton CF, et al. Peripheral nerve function in sepsis and multiple organ failure. Chest 1991; 99:176–184.
4. Bolton CF. Electrophysiological studies of critically ill patients. Muscle Nerve 1987; 10:129–135.
5. Trontelj JV, Mihelin M, Fernandez JM, Stalberg E. Axonal stimulation for end-plate jitter studies. J Neurol Neurosurg Psychiatry 1986; 49:677–685.
6. Trontelj JV, Khuraibet A, Mihelin M. The jitter in stimulated orbicularis oculi muscle: Technique and normal values. J Neurol Neurosurg Psychiatry 1988; 51:814–819.
7. Jabre JF, Chirico-Post J, Weiner M. Stimulation SFEMG in myasthenia gravis. Muscle Nerve 1989; 12:38–42.
8. Young GB, Bolton CF, Austin TW, et al. The encephalopathy associated with septic illness. Clin Invest Med 1990; 13:297–304.
9. Bolton CF, Young GB. Neurological complications in critically ill patients. In: Aminoff MJ, ed. Neurology and general medicine. New York: Churchill-Livingstone, 1989:713–729.
10. Wilbourn AJ, Furlan AAJ, Hulley W, Ruschhaupt W. Ischemic monomelic neuropathy. Neurology 1983; 33:447–451.
11. Abd AG, Braun NMT, Baskin MI, et al. Diaphragmatic dysfunction after open heart surgery: Treatment with a rocking bed. Ann Intern Med 1989; 111:881–886.
12. Matsen FA. Compartmental syndromes. New York: Grune & Stratton, 1980.
13. Andersson T, Siden A. A clinical study of the Guillain-Barré syndrome. Acta Neurol Scand 1982; 66:316–327.
14. Albers JW, Donofrio PD, McGonagle TK. Sequential electrodiagnostic abnormalities in acute inflammatory demyelinating polyradiculoneuropathy. Muscle Nerve 1985; 8:528–539.
15. Ropper AAH, Wijdicks EFM, Shahani BT. Electrodiagnostic abnormalities in 113 consecutive patients with Guillain-Barré syndrome. Arch Neurol 1990; 47:881–887.
16. Brown WF, Feasby TE. Conduction block and denervation in Guillain-Barré polyneuropathy. Brain 1984; 107:219–239.
17. Markand ON, Kincaid JC, Pourmand RA, et al. Electrophysiologic evaluation of diaphragm by transcutaneous phrenic nerve stimulation. Neurology 1984; 34:604–614.
18. Feasby TE, Gilbert JJ, Brown WF, et al. Acute axonal form of Guillain-Barré polyneuropathy. Brain 1986; 109:1115–1126.
19. Bolton CF, Gilbert JJ, Hahn AF, Sibbald WJ. Polyneuropathy in critically ill patients. J Neurol Neurosurg Psychiatry 1984; 47:1223–1231.
20. Zochodne DW, Bolton CF, Wells GA, et al. Critical illness polyneuropathy: A complication of sepsis and multiple organ failure. Brain 1987; 110:819–842.
21. Couturier JC, Robert D, Monier P. Polynevrites compliquant des sejours prolonges en reanimation. A propos de 11 cas d'etiologie encore inconnue. Lyon Medical 1984; 252:247–249.
22. Spitzer AR, Maher L, Awerbuch G, Bowles A. Neuromuscular causes of prolonged ventilator dependence. Muscle Nerve 1989; 12:775.
23. Bolton CF, Grand'Maison F, Parkes A, Shkrum M. Needle electromyography of the diaphragm. Muscle Nerve 1992; 15:678–681.
24. Bolton CF, Laverty DA, Brown JD, et al. Critically ill polyneuropathy: Electrophysiological studies and differentiation from Guillain-Barré syndrome. J Neurol Neurosurg Psychiatry 1986; 49:563–573.
25. Bolton CF. Neuropathies in the critical care unit. Brit J Hosp Med 1992; 47:5:358–360.
26. Zochodne DW, Bolton CF, Thompson RT, et al. Myopathy in critical illness. Muscle Nerve 1986; 9:652.
27. Partridge BL, Abrams JH, Bazemore C, Rubin R. Prolonged neuromuscular blockade after long-term infusion of vecuronium bromide in the intensive care unit. Crit Care Med 1990; 18:1177–1179.
28. Zochodne DW, Bolton CF, Laverty D, et al. The effects of sepsis and muscle function: An electrophysiologic and P-31 NMR study. Electroencephalogr Clin Neurophysiol 1987; 66:S115–S116.
29. Phillips I. Aminoglycosides. Lancet 1982; 2:311–314.
30. Jedrzejowska H, Rowinska-Marcinska K, Hoppe B. Neuropathy due to phytosol (Agritox). Acta Neuropathol 1980; 49:163–168.
31. Routier RJ, Lipman J, Brown K. Difficulty in weaning from respiratory support in a patient with the intermediate syndrome of organophosphate poisoning. Crit Care Med 1989; 17:1075–1076.
32. Roussos C, Macklem PT. The respiratory muscles. N Engl J Med 1982; 307:786–797.
33. Clowes GHA, George BC, Villee CA, Saravis CA. Muscle proteolysis induced by a circulating peptide in patients with sepsis or trauma. N Engl J Med 1983; 308:545–552.
34. Zochodne DW, Thompson RT, Driedger AA, et al. Metabolic changes in human muscle denervation: Topical 31P NMR spectroscopy studies. Magn Reson Med 1988; 7:373–383.
35. Penn AS. Myoglobinuria. In: Engel AG, Banker BQ, eds. Myology. Vol 2. New York: McGraw-Hill, 1986:1792–1793.

36. Adamski GB, Garin EH, Ballinger WE, Shulman ST. Generalized non-suppurative myositis with staphylococcal septicemia. J Pediatr 1980; 96:694–697.
37. Armstrong JH. Tropical pyomyositis and myoglobina. Arch Intern Med 1978; 138:1145–1146.
38. Jablecki CK. Myopathies. In: Brown WF, Bolton CF, eds. Clinical electromyography. Boston: Butterworth Publishers, 1987:399–400.
39. Plum F, Posner JB. The diagnosis of stupor and coma, ed 3. Philadelphia: F.A. Davis, 1980:34.
40. Editorial, Lancet, 1987.
41. Newsome-Davis J. Phrenic nerve conduction in man. J Neurol Neurosurg Psychiatry 1967; 30:420–426.
42. Gouri-Devi M, Ganapathy GR. Phrenic nerve conduction time in Guillain-Barré syndrome. J Neurol Neurosurg Psychiatry 1985; 48:245–249.
43. Koepke GH. The electromyographic examination of the diaphragm. Bull Am Assoc Electromyography Electrodiagnosis 1960; 7:8.
44. Koepke GH, Smith EM, Murphy AJ, Dickinson DG. Sequence of action of the diaphragm and intercostal muscles during respiration: I. Inspiration. Arch Phys Med Rehabil 1958; 39:426–430.

Index

The abbreviations f and t stand for figure and table, respectively.